CARDIOVASCULAR INTERVENTION

A Companion to Braunwald's Heart Disease

CARDIOVASCULAR INTERVENTION

A Companion to Braunwald's Heart Disease

Deepak L. Bhatt, MD, MPH, FACC, FAHA, FSCAI, FESC
Executive Director of Interventional Cardiovascular Programs
Brigham and Women's Hospital Heart and Vascular Center
Professor of Medicine
Harvard Medical School
Boston, Massachusetts

ELSEVIER

ELSEVIER

1600 John F. Kennedy Blvd.
Ste 1800
Philadelphia, PA 19103-2899

CARDIOVASCULAR INTERVENTION ISBN: 978-0-323-26219-4

Notices

Knowledge and best practice in this field are constantly changing. As new research and experience broaden our understanding, changes in research methods, professional practices, or medical treatment may become necessary.

Practitioners and researchers must always rely on their own experience and knowledge in evaluating and using any information, methods, compounds, or experiments described herein. In using such information or methods they should be mindful of their own safety and the safety of others, including parties for whom they have a professional responsibility.

With respect to any drug or pharmaceutical products identified, readers are advised to check the most current information provided (i) on procedures featured or (ii) by the manufacturer of each product to be administered, to verify the recommended dose or formula, the method and duration of administration, and contraindications. It is the responsibility of practitioners, relying on their own experience and knowledge of their patients, to make diagnoses, to determine dosages and the best treatment for each individual patient, and to take all appropriate safety precautions.

To the fullest extent of the law, neither the Publisher nor the authors, contributors, or editors, assume any liability for any injury and/or damage to persons or property as a matter of products liability, negligence or otherwise, or from any use or operation of any methods, products, instructions, or ideas contained in the material herein.

Library of Congress Cataloging-in-Publication Data

Cardiovascular intervention : a companion to Braunwald's heart disease / [edited by] Deepak L. Bhatt.
p. ; cm.
Complemented by: Braunwald's heart disease / edited by Douglas L. Mann, Douglas P. Zipes, Peter Libby, Robert O. Bonow, Eugene Braunwald. 10th edition. [2015].
Includes bibliographical references and index.
ISBN 978-0-323-26219-4 (hardcover : alk. paper)
I. Bhatt, Deepak L., editor. II. Braunwald's heart disease. 10th ed. Complemented by (expression):
[DNLM: 1. Cardiovascular Diseases—therapy. 2. Cardiac Surgical Procedures. WG 166]
RC681
616.1′2—dc23

2015004779

Content Strategist: Dolores Meloni
Content Development Specialist: Stacy Eastman
Publishing Services Manager: Catherine Jackson
Senior Project Manager: Carol O'Connell
Design Direction: Xiaopei Chen

Printed in China

Last digit is the print number: 9 8 7 6 5 4 3 2 1

This book is dedicated, with the deepest affection and gratitude …

To my wife, Shanthala, and our sons, Vinayak, Arjun, Ram, and Raj, for their love and for their understanding of the many hours I devote to patients, to procedures, and to academic pursuits

To my parents, for initially setting me on the path of a scholar

To my teachers, for their knowledge, patience, wisdom, and guidance

To my patients, for teaching me what matters most about being a doctor

List of Contributors

Alex Abou-Chebl, MD
Medical Director, Stroke, Baptist Health Louisville, Louisville, Kentucky
Intracranial Intervention and Acute Stroke

Farhad Abtahian, MD, PhD
Cardiology Division, Massachusetts General Hospital, Harvard Medical School, Boston, Massachusetts
Optical Coherence Tomography

Shikhar Agarwal, MD, MPH
Department of Cardiovascular Medicine, Section of Interventional Cardiology, Heart and Vascular Institute, Cleveland Clinic, Cleveland, Ohio
Hypertrophic Cardiomyopathy

Fernando Alfonso, MD
Director, Cardiac Department, Associate Professor of Medicine, Hospital Universitario de La Princesa Madrid, Madrid, Spain
Treatment of In-Stent Restenosis

Amjad T. AlMahameed, MD, MPH
Interventional Cardiologist and Endovascular Specialist, Cape Cod Hospital, Hyannis, Massachusetts
Upper Extremity Intervention

Saif Anwaruddin, MD
Assistant Professor of Medicine, Perelman School of Medicine at the University of Pennsylvania, Co-Director, Transcatheter Valve Program, Hospital of the University of Pennsylvania, Philadelphia, Pennsylvania
Transcatheter Mitral Valve Intervention

Usman Baber, MD
Assistant Professor of Medicine, The Icahn School of Medicine at Mount Sinai, New York, New York
Contrast Selection

Subhash Banerjee, MD
Chief of Cardiology, VA North Texas Healthcare System, Associate Professor, Internal Medicine, University of Texas Southwestern Medical Center, Dallas, Texas
Bypass Graft Interventions

Sripal Bangalore, MD, MHA, FACC, FAHA, FSCAI
Director of Research, Cardiac Catheterization Laboratory, Director, Cardiovascular Outcomes Group; Associate Professor of Medicine, Division of Cardiology, New York University School of Medicine, New York, New York
Vascular Access and Closure

Anthony A. Bavry, MD, MPH
Director, Cardiac Catheterization Laboratories, North Florida/South Georgia Veterans Health System, Associate Professor of Medicine, Division of Cardiovascular Medicine, University of Florida, Gainesville, Florida
Management of Thrombotic Lesions

Stefan C. Bertog, MD
Cardiovascular Center Frankfurt, Frankfurt, Germany
Renal Denervation

Deepak L. Bhatt, MD, MPH, FACC, FAHA, FSCAI, FESC
Executive Director of Interventional Cardiovascular Programs, Brigham and Women's Hospital Heart and Vascular Center, Professor of Medicine, Harvard Medical School, Boston, Massachusetts
Endomyocardial Biopsy

John A. Bittl, MD
Munroe Heart and Vascular Institute, Munroe Regional Medical Center, Ocala, Florida
Hemodialysis Access Intervention

Emmanouil S. Brilakis, MD, PhD
Director, Cardiac Catheterization Laboratories, VA North Texas Healthcare System, Associate Professor, Internal Medicine, University of Texas Southwestern Medical Center, Dallas, Texas
Bypass Graft Interventions

Robert A. Byrne, MB, BCh, PhD
Interventional Cardiologist, Deutsches Herzzentrum München, Technische Universität München, Munich, Germany
Treatment of In-Stent Restenosis

Robert Cecil, PhD
The Imaging Institute and The Heart and Vascular Institute, Department of Radiology, Cleveland Clinic, Cleveland, Ohio
Radiation Safety in the Cardiac Catheterization Laboratory

Georgios Christodoulidis, MD
The Icahn School of Medicine at Mount Sinai, New York, New York
Contrast Selection

Antonio Colombo, MD
Chief Director, Interventional Cardiology Unit, San Raffaele Scientific Institute, Interventional Cardiology Unit, EMO-GVM Centro Cuore Columbus, Milan, Italy
Bifurcations

Darshan Doshi, MD
Herbert and Sandi Feinberg Interventional Cardiology and Heart Valve Center, Columbia University Medical Center/New York-Presbyterian Hospital, and Cardiovascular Research Foundation, New York, New York
Aortic Valvuloplasty and Transcatheter Aortic Valve Replacement

Todd Drexel, MD
University of Minnesota, Minneapolis, Minnesota
Renal Denervation

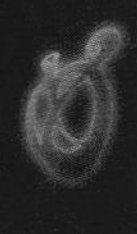

David P. Faxon, MD
Vice Chair of Medicine for Clinical Strategic Planning, Division of Cardiology, Brigham and Women's Hospital; Senior Lecturer, Harvard Medical School, Boston, Massachusetts
Guidelines and Appropriateness Criteria for Interventional Cardiology

Sameer Gafoor, MD
Cardiovascular Center Frankfurt, Frankfurt, Germany
Renal Denervation

Philippe Généreux, MD
Cardiovascular Research Foundation; New York-Presbyterian Hospital/Columbia University Medical Center, New York, New York; Associate Professor, Hôpital du Sacré-Coeur de Montréal, Université de Montréal, Montréal, Canada
Percutaneous Coronary Intervention for Unprotected Left Main Disease

Sachin S. Goel, MD
Interventional Cardiology, Prairie Heart Institute at St John's Hospital, Springfield, Illinois
Patient Foramen Ovale, Atrial Septal Defect, Left Atrial Appendage, and Ventricular Septal Defect Closure

William A. Gray, MD
Associate Professor of Medicine, Columbia University, New York, New York
Carotid and Vertebral Intervention

Howard C. Herrmann, MD
Professor of Medicine, Perelman School of Medicine at the University of Pennsylvania; Director, Interventional Cardiology Program and Cardiac Catheterization Labs, Hospital of the University of Pennsylvania, Philadelphia, Pennsylvania
Transcatheter Mitral Valve Intervention

Frederick A. Heupler, Jr., MD
Director, Diagnostic Catheterization Laboratory, Robert and Suzanne Tomsich Department of Cardiovascular Medicine, Cleveland Clinic, Cleveland, Ohio
Radiation Safety in the Cardiac Catheterization Laboratory

Ilona Hofmann, MD
Cardiovascular Center Frankfurt, Frankfurt, Germany
Renal Denervation

Dani Id, MD
Cardiovascular Center Frankfurt, Frankfurt, Germany
Renal Denervation

Ik-Kyung Jang, MD, PhD
Professor of Medicine, Massachusetts General Hospital, Harvard Medical School, Boston, Massachusetts
Optical Coherence Tomography

Hani Jneid, MD, FACC, FAHA, FSCAI
Assistant Professor of Medicine, Director of Interventional Cardiology Research, Baylor College of Medicine; Director of Interventional Cardiology, The Michael E. DeBakey VA Medical Center, Houston, Texas
Pharmacotherapy in the Modern Interventional Suite

Michael Joner, MD
Deutsches Herzzentrum München, Technische Universität München, Munich, Germany; CEO, Cardiovascular Pathology, CVPath Institute, Gaithesburg, Maryland
Treatment of In-Stent Restenosis

Marwan F. Jumean, MD
Interventional Cardiology and Advanced Heart Failure, The Cardiovascular Center, Tufts Medical Center, Boston, Massachusetts
Interventions for Advanced Heart Failure

David E. Kandzari, MD
Chief Scientific Officer and Director, Interventional Cardiology, Piedmont Heart Institute, Atlanta, Georgia
Chronic Total Coronary Occlusions: Rationale, Technique, and Clinical Outcomes

Samir R. Kapadia, MD
Director, Sones Catheterization Laboratory, Department of Cardiovascular Medicine; Director, Interventional Cardiology Fellowship, The Cleveland Clinic Foundation, Cleveland, Ohio
Radiation Safety in the Cardiac Catheterization Laboratory and Patient Foramen Ovale, Atrial Septal Defect, Left Atrial Appendage, and Ventricular Septal Defect Closure

Navin K. Kapur, MD, FACC, FSCAI
Assistant Professor of Medicine, Director, Acute Circulatory Support Program, Director, Interventional Research Laboratories, Investigator, Molecular Cardiology Research Institute, The Cardiovascular Center, Tufts Medical Center, Boston, Massachusetts
Interventions for Advanced Heart Failure

Adnan Kastrati, MD
Professor of Cardiology, Director, Catheterization Laboratory, Deutsches Herzzentrum München, Technische Universität München, Munich, Germany
Treatment of In-Stent Restenosis

Morton J. Kern, MD, FSCAI, FAHA, FACC
Professor of Medicine, University California Irvine, Orange, California; Chief of Medicine, Veterans Administration Long Beach Heath Care System, Long Beach, California
Fractional Flow Reserve

Scott Kinlay, MBBS, PhD, FAHA, FACC, FSCAI, FSVM, FRACP, FCSANZ
Director, Cardiac Catheterization Laboratory and Vascular Medicine, VA Boston Healthcare System, West Roxbury, Massachusetts; Co-Director, Interventional Cardiology and Vascular Diagnostic & Interventional Clinical and Research Fellowship Program, VA Boston Healthcare System and Brigham and Women's Hospital, Associate Professor in Medicine, Harvard Medical School, Adjunct Associate Professor in Medicine, Boston University Medical School, Boston, Massachusetts
Intervention for Lower Extremity Arterial Disease

Susheel K. Kodali, MD
Herbert and Sandi Feinberg Interventional Cardiology and Heart Valve Center, Columbia University Medical Center/New York-Presbyterian Hospital, and Cardiovascular Research Foundation, New York, New York
Aortic Valvuloplasty and Transcatheter Aortic Valve Replacement

Amar Krishnaswamy, MD, FACC
Associate Director, Interventional Cardiology Fellowship Program; Associate Director, General Cardiology Fellowship Program; Interventional Cardiology, Cleveland Clinic, Cleveland, Ohio
Calcified Lesions

Azeem Latib, MD
Interventional Cardiology Unit, San Raffaele Scientific Institute, Interventional Cardiology Unit, EMO-GVM Centro Cuore Columbus, Milan, Italy
Bifurcations

Martin B. Leon, MD
Professor of Medicine, Herbert and Sandi Feinberg Interventional Cardiology and Heart Valve Center, Columbia University Medical Center/New York-Presbyterian Hospital, and Cardiovascular Research Foundation, New York, New York
Aortic Valvuloplasty and Transcatheter Aortic Valve Replacement

Ronan Margey, MB, FACC, FESC
Consultant Interventional Cardiologist, Special Interest in Vascular and Structural Heart Disease Intervention, Mater Private Hospital Group, Cork and Dublin, Ireland
Pericardiocentesis and Pericardial Intervention

Roxana Mehran, MD
Professor of Medicine (Cardiology) and Health Evidence Policy, Director of Interventional Cardiovascular Research and Clinical Trials, The Zena and Michael A. Wiener Cardiovascular Institute, The Icahn School of Medicine at Mount Sinai, New York, New York
Contrast Selection

Aravinda Nanjundappa, MD, FACC, FSCAI, RVT
Professor of Medicine and Surgery, Director of TAVR program, West Virginia University, Charleston, West Virginia
Endovascular Management of Aortic and Thoracic Aneurysms

Brian P. O'Neill, MD
Division of Cardiology, Temple Heart and Vascular Institute, Temple University, Philadelphia, Pennsylvania
Hemodynamic Support During High-Risk PCI

William W. O'Neill, MD, FACC, FSCAI
Division of Cardiology, Henry Ford Hospital, Detroit, Michigan
Hemodynamic Support During High-Risk PCI

Igor F. Palacios, MD, FACC, FSCAI, FAHA
Director, Structural Heart Disease and Interventional Cardiology, Massachusetts General Hospital, Boston, Massachusetts
Pericardiocentesis and Pericardial Intervention

Lourdes R. Prieto, MD
Director, Pediatric Cardiac Catheterization Laboratory, Department of Pediatric Cardiology, Cleveland Clinic Children's Hospital, Cleveland, Ohio
Patient Foramen Ovale, Atrial Septal Defect, Left Atrial Appendage, and Ventricular Septal Defect Closure

Markus Reinartz, MD
Cardiovascular Center Frankfurt, Frankfurt, Germany
Renal Denervation

John F. Rhodes, Jr., MD
Director of Cardiology, The Heart Program, Miami Children's Hospital, Miami, Florida
Congenital Heart Disease

Nicolas W. Shammas, MD, MS, EJD, FACC, FSCAI
Adjunct Clinical Associate Professor of Medicine University of Iowa Hospitals and Clinics; Founder and Research Director, Midwest Cardiovascular Research Foundation; Section Editor, Advances in Vein Therapies, Journal of Invasive Cardiology; Consultant and Interventional Cardiologist Cardiovascular Medicine, PC, Genesis Heart Institute, Davenport, Iowa
Management of Chronic Venous Insufficiency

Nicholas Shkumat
Department of Radiology, Cleveland Clinic, Cleveland, Ohio
Radiation Safety in the Cardiac Catheterization Laboratory

Horst Sievert, MD, PhD
Cardiovascular Center Frankfurt, Frankfurt, Germany
Renal Denervation

Akhilesh K. Sista, MD
Assistant Professor of Radiology, Weill Cornell Medical College, New York, New York
Interventional Management of Lower Extremity Deep Vein Thrombosis and Pulmonary Embolism

Gregg W. Stone, MD
Professor of Medicine, Columbia University, Director of Cardiovascular Research and Education, Center for Interventional Vascular Therapy, New York Presbyterian Hospital/Columbia University Medical Center; Co-Director of Medical Research and Education, The Cardiovascular Research Foundation, New York, New York
Percutaneous Coronary Intervention for Unprotected Left Main Disease

E. Murat Tuzcu, MD
Professor of Medicine, Vice Chair for Clinical Operations, Department of Cardiovascular Medicine, Section of Interventional Cardiology, Heart and Vascular Institute, Cleveland Clinic, Cleveland, Ohio
Hypertrophic Cardiomyopathy

Laura Vaskelyte, MD
Cardiovascular Center Frankfurt, Frankfurt, Germany
Renal Denervation

Suresh Vedantham, MD
Professor of Radiology and Surgery, Mallinckrodt Institute of Radiology, Washington University School of Medicine, St. Louis, Missouri
Interventional Management of Lower Extremity Deep Vein Thrombosis and Pulmonary Embolism

Christopher J. White, MD
Professor and Chairman of Medicine, Department of Cardiovascular Diseases, Ochsner Clinical School of the University of Queensland, Ochsner Medical Institutions, New Orleans, Louisiana
Renal Artery Intervention: Catheter-Based Therapy for Renal Artery Stenosis and Mesenteric Artery Intervention: Catheter-Based Therapy for Chronic Mesenteric Ischemia

Patrick L. Whitlow, MD, FACC, FAHA
Department of Cardiovascular Medicine, Cleveland Clinic, Cleveland, Ohio
Calcified Lesions

David O. Williams, MD
Professor of Medicine, Harvard Medical School; Senior Physician, Cardiovascular Division, Brigham and Women's Hospital, Boston, Massachusetts
The Birth of Interventional Cardiology

Kevin Wunderle, MS
Department of Radiology, Cleveland Clinic, Cleveland, Ohio
Radiation Safety in the Cardiac Catheterization Laboratory

James B. Young, MD
Professor of Medicine and Executive Dean, Cleveland Clinic Lerner College of Medicine of Case Western Reserve University; George and Linda Kaufman Chair, Kaufman Center for Heart Failure, Heart and Vascular Institute, Cleveland Clinic Foundation, Cleveland, Ohio
Endomyocardial Biopsy

Khaled M. Ziada, MD, FACC, FSCAI
Professor of Medicine, Gill Foundation Professor of Interventional Cardiology, Division of Cardiovascular Medicine, Director, Cardiac Catheterization Laboratories, Director, Cardiovascular Interventional Fellowship Program, Gill Heart Institute–University of Kentucky, Lexington, Kentucky
Intravascular Ultrasound Imaging

Foreword

Cardiac catheterization was developed during the first half of the twentieth century, and together with electrocardiography became one of the two cornerstones of modern cardiology. Appropriately, the credit for applying this technique to patients and to employ it for assessment of cardiac function and to cardiac diagnosis was rewarded by the Nobel Prize in Medicine or Physiology to Forssmann, Cournand, and Richards in 1956. Cardiac catheterization made possible selective angiography, including, of course, coronary arteriography. These invasive techniques allowed measurement of intracardiac pressures and flows and visualization of the cardiac chambers, valves, great vessels, and coronary arteries. Simultaneously, cardiac surgery, especially open heart surgery, made great advances. These two separate approaches to cardiac patients—precise diagnosis in the cardiac catheterization laboratory and successful treatment of cardiovascular and coronary disorders in the operating room—led to a proliferation of both catheterization laboratories and cardiac surgical suites around the world in the 1960s and 1970s.

The 1970s also saw the development of a variety of new imaging techniques, including echocardiography, nuclear imaging, computed tomography, and magnetic resonance imaging, which have allowed noninvasive assessment of cardiac structure and function. This represented an enormous advance and reduced the need for diagnostic cardiac catheterization. Yet, invasive cardiologists did not gradually disappear, and cardiac catheterization laboratories did not close. Instead, after Andreas Gruentzig's gigantic leap forward in 1977, when he demonstrated that atherosclerotic obstructions in coronary arteries could be treated successfully by inflating a balloon near the tip of a cardiac catheter, many invasive cardiologists "morphed" into interventional cardiologists. Soon balloon angioplasty was supplemented by stenting, and this approach was extended to relieving obstructions in the renal, femoral, carotid, and other systemic arteries. Percutaneous treatment of stenotic mitral and aortic valves with balloon valvotomy soon followed. More recently, transcatheter aortic valve replacement has transformed the outlook of patients with aortic stenosis at high risk for surgical valve replacement, and transcatheter mitigation of mitral regurgitation is now under development as well. Catheter-based treatment of many congenital cardiac lesions is being widely practiced. Pumps incorporated into catheters inserted into the left ventricle by interventional cardiologists retrograde through the aortic valve can treat acute heart failure. The proliferation of such interventional procedures and of percutaneous devices is continuing, indeed accelerating.

As a consequence of these important advances, interventional cardiology has become a robust subspecialty, with its own subspecialty board, training programs, journals, and international meetings. It is grounded in conventional cardiology and interfaces with radiology, with both cardiac and vascular surgery, and with pediatrics and neurology as well. There is a growth of so-called "hybrid" interventional suites in which both percutaneous and operative procedures can be performed sequentially in the same patient, in parallel with the development of multidisciplinary "heart teams." As a consequence, the lines that previously separated cardiology from these other disciplines are becoming blurred.

Dr. Deepak L. Bhatt accepted the responsibility of editing *Cardiovascular Intervention*. While this comprehensive text focuses primarily on coronary interventions, it also describes interventions in valvular heart disease, congenital heart disease, advanced heart failure, as well as diseases of various systemic arterial beds and of the aorta. Dr. Bhatt brings a wealth of personal experience to this task. As a practicing interventional cardiologist, he faces the clinical problems that are discussed in this book on a daily basis. He is also an experienced clinical trialist, which provides him with the ability to assess the validity of the myriad studies published in this field as well.

Dr. Bhatt has assembled a group of talented, experienced authors for preparing *Cardiovascular Intervention*. The book is well illustrated and contains 431 figures and 116 tables that summarize an enormous amount of material. It is as up to date as this month's journals and meetings. This text offers great value to trainees and practitioners in this field, as well as to radiologists, cardiovascular surgeons and general cardiologists who interact frequently with interventional cardiologists.

We are proud to welcome *Cardiovascular Intervention* to the growing family of Companions to *Braunwald's Heart Disease.*

Eugene Braunwald
Douglas Zipes
Peter Libby
Robert Bonow
Douglas Mann

Preface

Cardiovascular intervention has saved many lives and improved quality of life. The widespread adoption of cardiovascular intervention worldwide has, in part, led to a decrease in the rate of cardiovascular death for several conditions—though in absolute terms, due to the aging of the population and increasing urbanization, the population at risk is growing and the global cardiovascular epidemic continues.

Few areas in medicine have advanced as meaningfully and rapidly as cardiovascular intervention. The field now encompasses complex coronary intervention, peripheral arterial and venous procedures, cerebrovascular intervention, congenital heart disease, and valvular as well as other structural heart intervention. The care of this panoply of diseases involves multidisciplinary teams increasingly housed in heart and vascular centers, designed around optimizing the patient experience as opposed to the silos of physician and surgeon specialties of the past.

What was previously only treatable with a scalpel can currently be approached with a catheter. This transformation of several open surgical procedures to truly minimally invasive interventional procedures has been of great benefit to patients. Additionally, this evolution potentially allows many more patients to be served even in relatively resource-poor settings and with greater cost effectiveness in all economic environments.

For decades now, innovation and intervention have gone hand in hand. Pioneers in cardiovascular intervention have boldly pushed the boundaries of what is possible. Physicians, scientists, and engineers from industry have served as valuable partners in this exciting journey. The advances in devices, pharmacotherapies, and procedural techniques would not have been possible without this collaboration. As well, the free flow of information across countries and specialties has allowed cardiovascular intervention to mature at an impressive pace for what—viewed within the larger context of medicine—is still a relatively young field.

The resulting explosion of the required knowledge base for practitioners in the field of cardiovascular intervention has created a challenge—how to keep up! In this companion to *Braunwald's Heart Disease,* world-renowned authors provide the latest data to inform decision making in cardiovascular intervention. Furthermore, they provide details on the technical aspects of optimizing procedural care. This focus on both cognitive and procedural elements of cardiovascular intervention provides a needed resource in this dynamic field.

In joining the great lineage of the *Heart Disease* family, *Cardiovascular Intervention: A Companion to Braunwald's Heart Disease* aims to provide the wide variety of health care personnel involved with cardiovascular intervention with evidence-based information critical for successfully ensuring the best possible care. It is meant as an aid to make decisions at the bedside, as a reference text for specific questions, and also as a resource for scientific inquiry and investigation. Cardiovascular intervention is a very visual specialty, and this book has ample figures and abundant videos to provide that necessity. Frequent online supplements will keep the book vibrant in an era of rapid change, with the textbook portion anchoring that knowledge which has stood the test of time. Electronic links with *Braunwald's Heart Disease* and other companion textbooks should make for a comprehensive, current, and visually compelling resource in cardiovascular intervention that is placed within the larger universe of cardiovascular disease care.

My dream is that interventional cardiologists, cardiac and vascular surgeons, interventional radiologists and neurologists, trainees, medical students, nurses and nurse practitioners, physician assistants, industry partners, and others involved with patients undergoing cardiovascular interventions can learn from this book, guiding them in the daily care of their patients. As such, my sincere hope is that these diverse readers find *Cardiovascular Intervention: A Companion to Braunwald's Heart Disease* to be a valuable educational tool that conveys the passion the authors and I feel for the beauty and grandeur of cardiovascular intervention.

Deepak L. Bhatt, MD, MPH, FACC, FAHA, FSCAI, FESC

Acknowledgments

The distinguished authors of this textbook deserve my most heartfelt appreciation. They have produced expert, comprehensive, and timely chapters of which they should be extremely proud. I would like to thank the publishing staff at Elsevier for their assistance in helping make both the content and visuals outstanding. In particular, I would like to thank Dolores Meloni, Executive Content Strategist, and Stacy Eastman, Content Development Specialist, for their exemplary efforts in assembling what I hope will be viewed as the definitive treatise on cardiovascular intervention. I am immensely grateful to Dr. Eugene Braunwald, an inspiring and generous mentor, for having faith in me and for selecting me to serve as editor of this textbook that bears his name—a name synonymous with greatness in medicine.

Contents

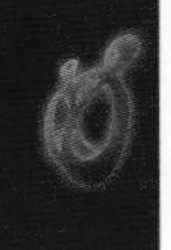

Video Contents

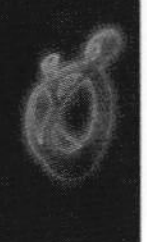

11-5: Example of subclavian steal syndrome. Reversal of flow in the left internal mammary artery graft due to severe proximal left subclavian stenosis.

13 Treatment of In-Stent Restenosis

13-1: Diffuse in-stent restenosis showing features of in-stent neoatherosclerosis by optical coherence tomography (OCT).

13-2: Diffuse in-stent restenosis showing features of in-stent neoatherosclerosis by optical coherence tomography (OCT).

13-2: Diffuse in-stent restenosis showing features of in-stent neoatherosclerosis by optical coherence tomography (OCT).

13-4: Diffuse in-stent restenosis showing features of in-stent neoatherosclerosis by optical coherence tomography (OCT).

13-5: Angiographic classification of restenosis following bare-metal and drug-eluting stenting.

13-6: Angiographic classification of restenosis following bare-metal and drug-eluting stenting.

13-7: Angiographic classification of restenosis following bare-metal and drug-eluting stenting.

13-8: Angiographic classification of restenosis following bare-metal and drug-eluting stenting.

13-9: Angiographic classification of restenosis following bare-metal and drug-eluting stenting.

13-10: Angiographic classification of restenosis following bare-metal and drug-eluting stenting.

13-11: Angiographic classification of restenosis following bare-metal and drug-eluting stenting.

13-12: Angiographic classification of restenosis following bare-metal and drug-eluting stenting.

13-13: Angiographic classification of restenosis following bare-metal and drug-eluting stenting.

13-14: Angiographic classification of restenosis following bare-metal and drug-eluting stenting.

13-15: Angiographic classification of restenosis following bare-metal and drug-eluting stenting.

13-16: Angiographic classification of restenosis following bare-metal and drug-eluting stenting.

13-17: Angiographic classification of restenosis following bare-metal and drug-eluting stenting.

13-18: Angiographic classification of restenosis following bare-metal and drug-eluting stenting.

13-19: Angiographic classification of restenosis following bare-metal and drug-eluting stenting.

13-20: Treatment of drug-eluting stent in-stent restenosis with drug-coated balloon therapy.

13-21: Treatment of drug-eluting stent in-stent restenosis with drug-coated balloon therapy.

13-21: Treatment of drug-eluting stent in-stent restenosis with drug-coated balloon therapy.

13-22: Treatment of drug-eluting stent in-stent restenosis with drug-coated balloon therapy.

14 Management of Thrombotic Lesions

14-1: Saphenous vein graft occlusion. The site of occlusion is proximal to previously placed stent.

14-2: Aspiration thrombectomy.

14-3: Improved, but still poor flow after aspiration thrombectomy.

14-4: Rheolytic thrombectomy.

14-5: Successful reperfusion after rheolytic thrombectomy with the Angiojet Spiroflex device.

15 Fractional Flow Reserve

15-1: Wilson 3VD fractional flow reserve.

15-2: LM FFR (left main fractional flow reserve) Poole.

15-3: Radial percutaneous coronary intervention fractional flow reserve D1.

15-4: Fractional flow reserve with intravascular ultrasound pothena.

16 Intravascular Ultrasound Imaging

16-1: Strut malapposition.

16-2: IVUS imaging to delineate procedural complications.

16-3: Use of IVUS imaging in locating an occluded ostium.

16-4: IVUS-facilitated reentry after subintimal tracking in an occluded femoral artery.

17 Optical Coherence Tomography

17-1: Optical coherence tomography (OCT) pull back across the mid LAD lesion prior to the percutaneous coronary intervention.

17-2: Optical coherence tomography pull back after percutaneous coronary intervention. Images reveal a well-placed drug eluting stent with minimal malapposition.

18 Intervention for Lower Extremity Arterial Disease

18-1: Balloon angioplasty of an occluded anterior tibial artery via the ipsilateral common femoral (antegrade) approach.

18-2: Perforation of the external iliac artery treated with a covered stent.

18-3: Treatment of a chronic total occlusion of the right common iliac artery with an antegrade/retrograde approach.

18-4: Treatment of a thrombosed common femoral to distal superficial femoral artery prosthetic graft and retrograde thrombosis of the iliac artery system.

20 Renal Artery Intervention: Catheter-Based Therapy for Renal Artery Stenosis

20-1: Baseline left renal stenosis.

20-2: Post-stent left renal.

21 Mesenteric Artery Intervention: Catheter-Based Therapy for Chronic Mesenteric Ischemia

21-1: SMA ostial stenosis.

21-2: SMA post-stent.

22 Renal Denervation

22-1: Nonselective abdominal aortography.

22-2: Renal artery engagement.

22-3: Delivery of the denervation catheter into the renal artery.

22-4: Demonstration of the Symplicity catheter.

22-5: Demonstration of the generator.

22-6: Nonselective abdominal aortography.

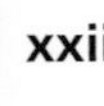

Look for These Other Titles in the Braunwald's Heart Disease Family

BRAUNWALD'S HEART DISEASE COMPANIONS

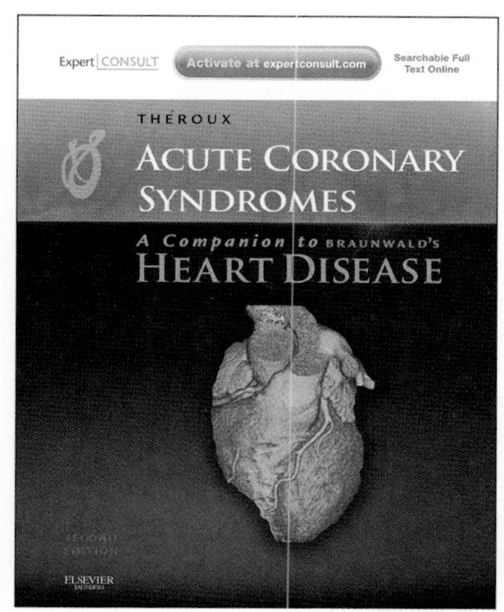

THÉROUX
Acute Coronary Syndromes

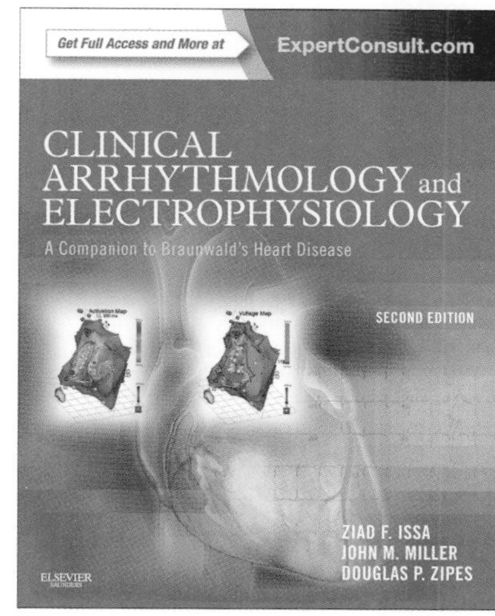

ISSA, MILLER, AND ZIPES
Clinical Arrhythmology and Electrophysiology

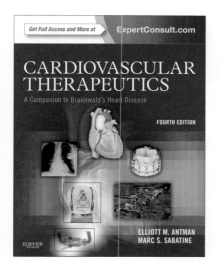

ANTMAN AND SABATINE
Cardiovascular Therapeutics

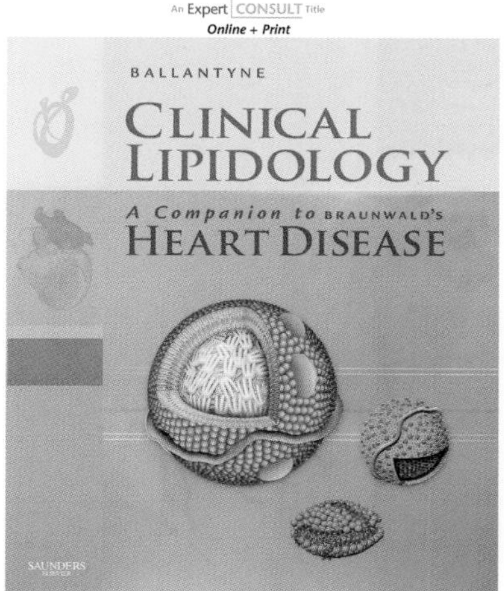

BALLANTYNE
Clinical Lipidology

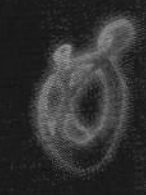

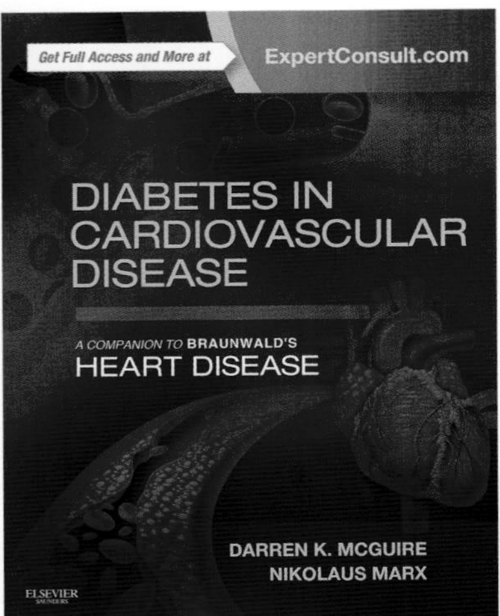

MCGUIRE AND MARX
Diabetes in Cardiovascular Disease

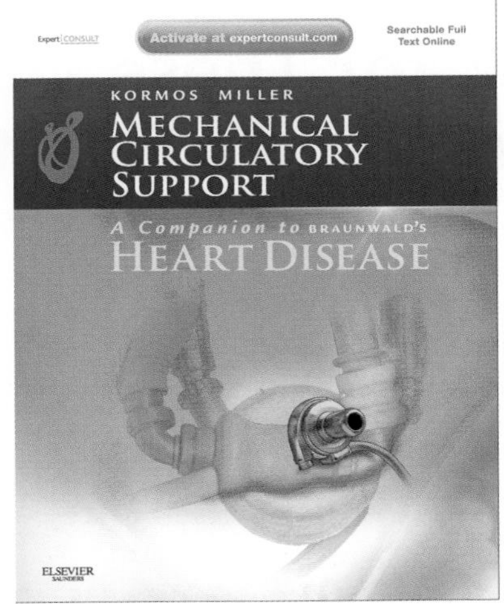

KORMOS AND MILLER
Mechanical Circulatory Support

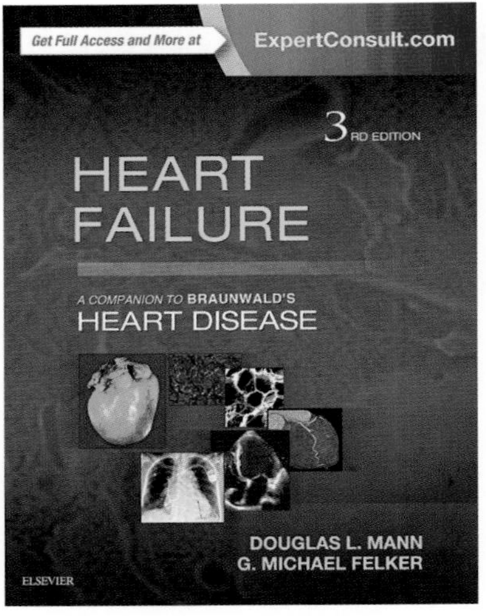

MANN AND FELKER
Heart Failure

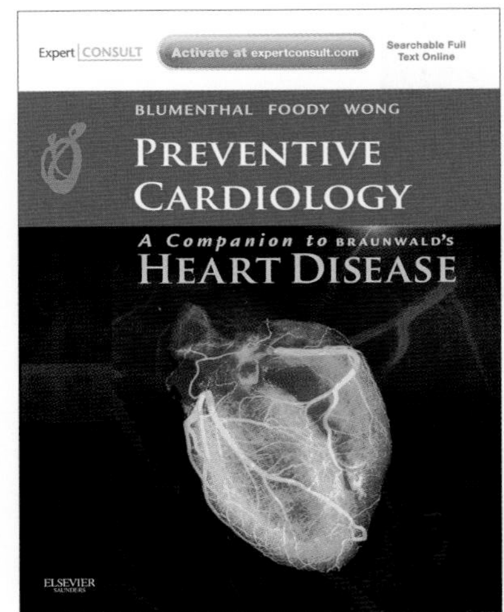

BLUMENTHAL, FOODY, AND WONG
Preventive Cardiology

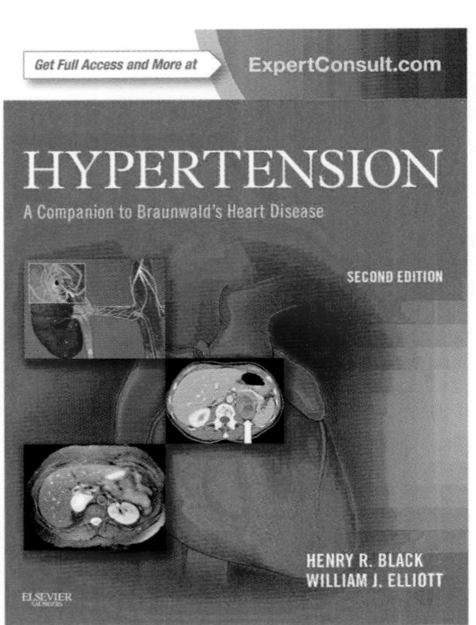

BLACK AND ELLIOTT
Hypertension

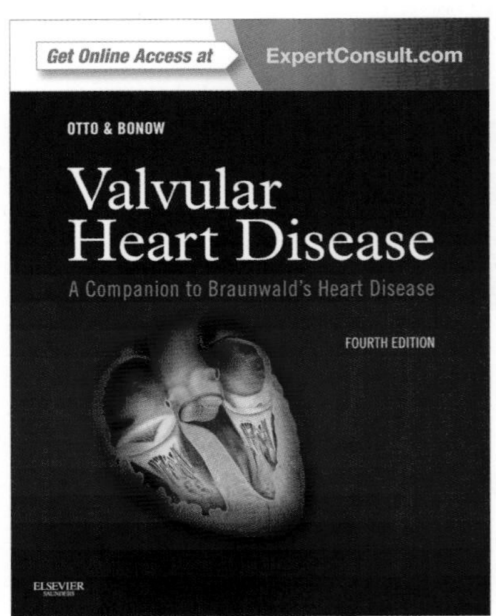

OTTO AND BONOW
Valvular Heart Disease

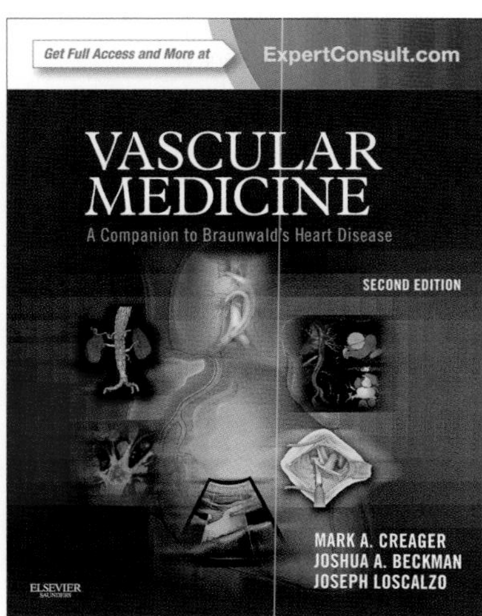

CREAGER, BECKMAN, AND LOSCALZO
Vascular Medicine

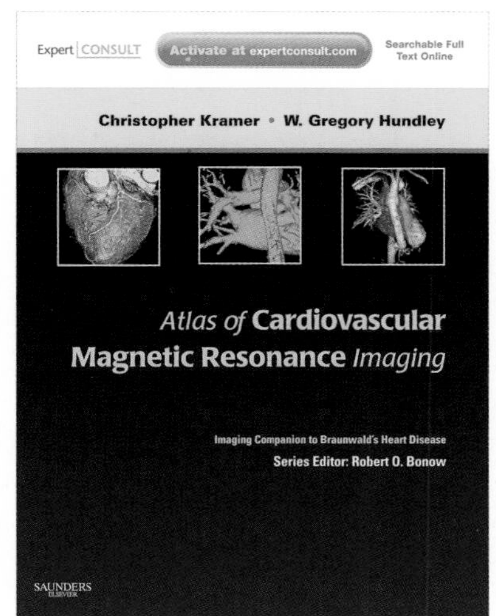

KRAMER AND HUNDLEY
Atlas of Cardiovascular Magnetic Resonance Imaging

BRAUNWALD'S HEART DISEASE REVIEW AND ASSESSMENT

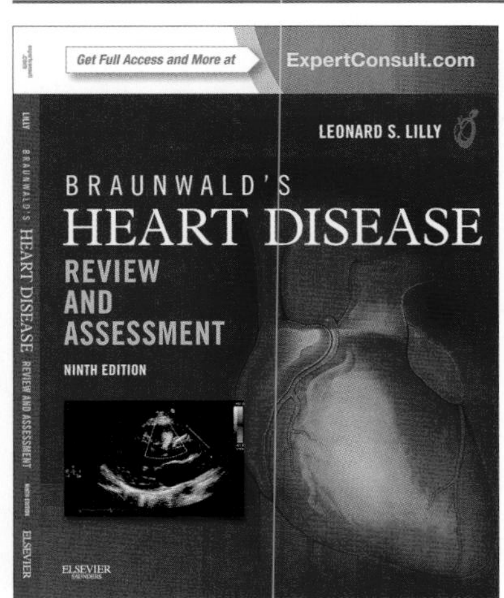

LILLY
Braunwald's Heart Disease Review and Assessment

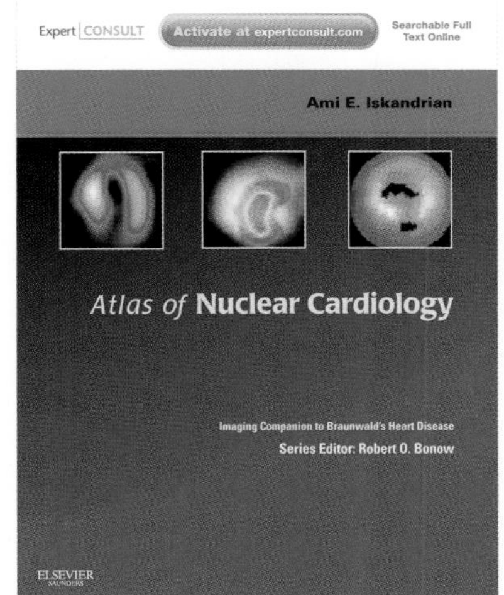

ISKANDRIAN AND GARCIA
Atlas of Nuclear Cardiology

BRAUNWALD'S HEART DISEASE IMAGING COMPANIONS

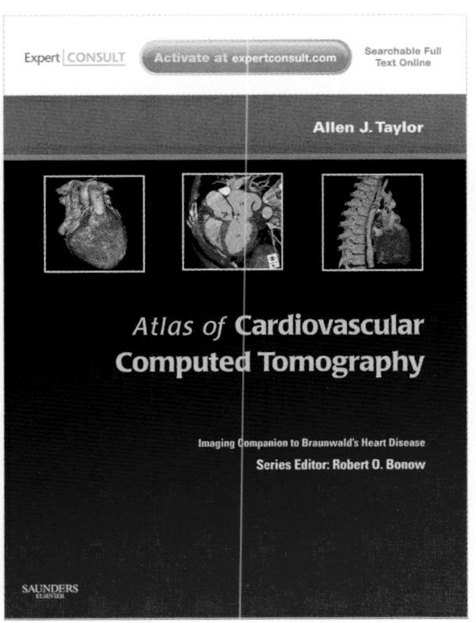

TAYLOR
Atlas of Cardiovascular Computer Tomography

COMING SOON!

BODEN
Chronic Coronary Syndromes

MORROW
Myocardial Infarction

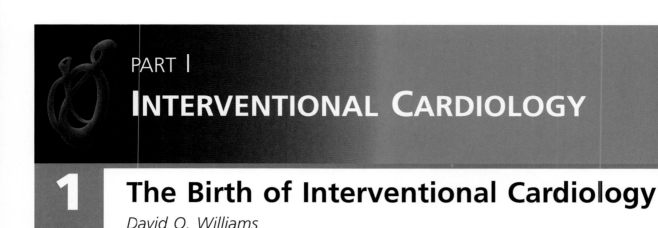

PART I INTERVENTIONAL CARDIOLOGY

1 The Birth of Interventional Cardiology

David O. Williams

THE INNOVATOR OF ANGIOPLASTY

There are few who are acknowledged as true pioneers in medicine, but Andreas Grüntzig was surely one (**Figure 1-1**). He quite simply not only coined the term *interventional cardiology,* he *was* interventional cardiology. For many evenings, he, his wife Michaela, and Walter and Maria Schlumpf sat at the Grüntzig's kitchen table fabricating balloon catheters. These catheters were the prototypes that enabled Grüntzig to eventually effectively treat peripheral and coronary artery disease without surgery. In September 1977, Grüntzig performed the first successful coronary angioplasty on Dolf Bachmann. This event initiated a cascade of innovations that have greatly changed the approaches and techniques for the treatment of patients with coronary disease as well as for others who have required traditional surgical procedures. This chapter will discuss the origin of angioplasty and the story of its inventor.

Andreas Roland Grüntzig was born in Dresden, Germany, June 25, 1939. He was the second child of Charlotta and Wilmar Grüntzig. Andreas was a child of World War II. He had one brother, Johannes, who was older. The boys quickly lost their father, a secondary-school science teacher, who was conscripted as a weatherman for the Luftwaffe.[1]

Based on concerns for her family's safety, Charlotta and her two boys moved from one home to another in Germany, then to South America and then back again. After World War II the fatherless family settled in Leipzig, then a part of East Germany. Day after day, Charlotta and her two boys would go to the local train station, eyeing the German troops returning from the Eastern front. They were waiting for Wilmar, who never arrived.

Although both boys performed well in school, East German rules of the day demanded they become laborers, based on the fact that their father had been educated. This concept did not sit well with either boy. West Germany was potentially accessible to Johannes and Andreas. As teenagers, they would occasionally sneak across the border at night for brief social excursions. Finally to pursue more desirable lives, Andreas, then age 17, and Johannes moved permanently to West Germany. They left their mother behind. How these boys were formally educated in this new country is unclear, but eventually they attended medical school at the University of Heidelberg.

Toward the end of this medical school curriculum, Andreas Grüntzig began a series of clinical rotations. These took him to several European venues. At age 28, he attended the London School of Economics. There he studied epidemiology and statistical methods. This experience was critical and provided the basis for his approach to evaluating the effectiveness and safety of coronary angioplasty.

At age 30, Grüntzig was accepted to the Internal Medicine training program at the University of Zurich (**Figure 1-2**). His educational plans were disrupted when the program director died unexpectedly. Fortunately for Grüntzig, who had just moved to Zurich, Alfred Bollinger offered him a training position in "angiology." Angiology was and remains an established medical discipline of European medicine. Grüntzig accepted. This opportunity exposed him to patients with peripheral artery disease, the substrate for his concept of balloon angioplasty.

While in training, Grüntzig heard a lecture by Eberhard Zeitler of the Aggertal Clinic about the "Dotter procedure" named after U.S. physician Charles Dotter. Dotter lived in Oregon and as a vascular radiologist had developed a technique for dilating atherosclerotic stenoses of peripheral arteries. He called the technique "transluminal dilatation," a

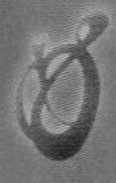

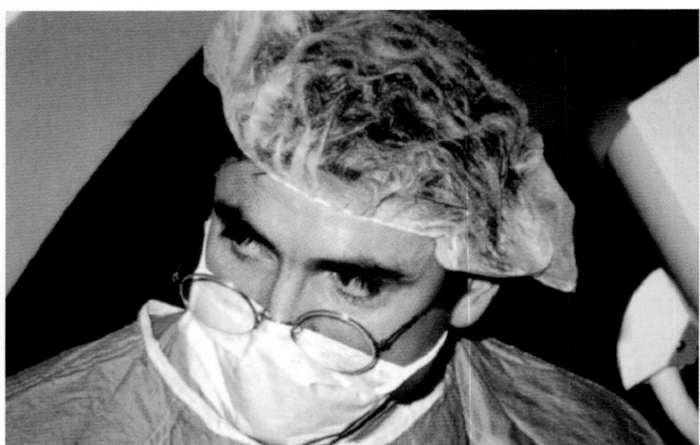

FIGURE 1-1 Andreas Grüntzig during a coronary angioplasty. *(Courtesy Dr. Gary S. Roubin.)*

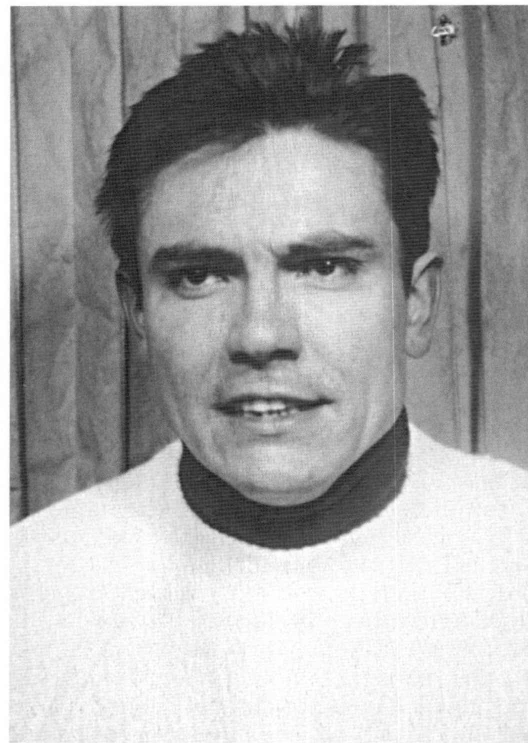

FIGURE 1-2 Photograph Andreas Grüntzig submitted with his application for training in Internal Medicine, University Hospital, Zurich. *(Courtesy Ernst Schneider MD.)*

term Grüntzig would borrow when initially labeling coronary angioplasty.

The Dotter procedure involved crossing a stenotic arterial segment with a guidewire and then sequentially advancing progressively larger, tapered end-hole catheters across the narrowed segment. The actual relief in stenosis severity was quite modest, yet in many instances clinical improvement was substantial. Although this procedure was innovated in the United States, it was not well accepted by American physicians. Zeitler, however, had adopted the technique with enthusiasm. In 1971 he was performing Dotter procedures on a regular basis. Grüntzig met Zeitler, observed him, and eventually assisted him.

After returning to Zurich, Grüntzig began to perform Dotter's procedure with mixed success. Resident vascular surgeons focused on complications of the procedure such as groin hematomas. Moreover improvement of Grüntzig's skill was hampered by limited access to patients. In the back of his mind, however, was the thought of a different approach: namely, a balloon-tipped catheter that could dilate stenotic arteries.

Grüntzig's laboratory for innovation was the kitchen of his and Michaela's two-bedroom flat. The team included Andreas; Michaela; Maria, Andreas' assistant; and her husband, Walter, an engineer by training. Identifying and obtaining materials that could serve appropriately for the catheter shafts and balloons were challenges. Grüntzig eventually selected polyvinyl chloride (PVC) as the balloon material for his catheters. This was a unique substance, particularly strong, and could be easily shaped. In fact, PVC was being used for making disposable bottles of Coca-Cola. Progress was slow but over a period of 2 years, and hours of cutting and gluing, a balloon catheter was fabricated that repeatedly yielded predictable performance.

The initial catheter was a single-lumen system. Once advanced over a guidewire and in proper position, the guidewire was removed and a tip occluding wire was placed in the catheter. Fluid injected into the catheter lumen then filled the balloon by means of side holes or skives in the catheter shaft.

THE FIRST PERIPHERAL ARTERIAL ANGIOPLASTY

It was on February 12, 1974, that Grüntzig used this catheter to dilate the iliac artery of a 67-year-old man in Zurich. The procedure was successful by all parameters: angiographic and hemodynamic assessments and the patient's clinical response.

Although the risks were undoubtedly greater and the technical demands more difficult, coronary disease was always a goal for Grüntzig. Different but significant clinical challenges were unique to the coronary circulation. What would be the consequences of transient coronary occlusion? Would there be irreversible myocardial infarction? Would patients experience ventricular fibrillation? Thoughts such as these stimulated him to develop a two-lumen balloon catheter. One lumen would maintain coronary perfusion; the other lumen would be used for the balloon inflation. Navigation of the catheter would be difficult but aided with a short fixed wire at its tip to assist in entering the correct coronary artery and crossing the stenotic segment.

The logical testing site for the first double-lumen new catheter would be a peripheral artery. In January 1975, Grüntzig used his balloon catheter to dilate an iliac artery stenosis. The procedure was successful! Over the next 2 years, he would perform more than 200 peripheral arterial balloon angioplasties.

THE DEVELOPMENT OF CORONARY ANGIOPLASTY

Creating a "model" to test a coronary angioplasty balloon catheter was the next logical step prior to attempting coronary angioplasty in a patient. To accomplish this, Grüntzig created coronary stenoses in anesthetized open-chest dogs by placing sutures around the coronary arteries. Then with the aid of fluoroscopic guidance, he advanced his balloon-tipped catheters into the constricted coronary and dilated the ligated segment. Grüntzig presented this work at the Miami meeting of the American Heart Association in November 1976. Although his presentation was well attended, the prevailing response was skeptical.

Little is known about the very first attempted coronary angioplasty in man. The patient was a 66-year-old male with cardiogenic shock who had been rejected for cardiac surgery. In an effort to rescue the patient, Andreas attempted coronary angioplasty in Zurich, early 1977. Access was a problem. Following an unsuccessful femoral arterial approach, he eventually obtained access from the left brachial artery. An unwieldy, 9 Fr Teflon guide catheter was inserted. Grüntzig could not engage the catheter into the left coronary ostium and the procedure was aborted.

Grüntzig's next steps were more cautious and modest. With the aid of Richard Myler of San Francisco, Grüntzig pursued a different approach. They evaluated his balloon catheters in the operating room, during coronary bypass operations. Once the coronary arteriotomy was made, catheters were advanced to the lesion and the balloon was inflated. Following a handful of cases, they concluded that Andreas' catheters could dilate coronary lesions.

In September 1977, Andreas met Dolf Bachmann. Like Andreas, Bachmann was 38 years old. Unlike Andreas, he had severe angina, taking up to 15 sublingual nitroglycerine tablets a day. He was adamantly opposed to coronary bypass surgery. Following consultation with Grüntzig, he agreed to be the first patient to have coronary angioplasty. Importantly, he also agreed to coronary bypass surgery should angioplasty fail.

With a surgical operating room on standby, Bachmann's procedure was performed on September 16. Andreas advanced a 3.0-mm short wire-tipped balloon catheter across a left anterior descending lesion and inflated the balloon. A second lumen in the balloon catheter, originally designed to deliver blood flow during balloon inflation, was used to measure coronary arterial pressure proximal and distal to the stenosis. When the balloon catheter crossed the stenosis, the balloon catheter tip pressure fell. Following the initial inflation, the distal pressure rose. According to protocol, the balloon catheter was withdrawn proximal to the lesion, which had improved substantially by angiography. The catheter was then re-advanced across the lesion and a second inflation performed. Angiography following withdrawal of the balloon catheter revealed no significant lesion. The case was a remarkable success. Grüntzig labeled this new procedure percutaneous transluminal coronary angioplasty (PTCA).

The following day Bachmann was completely asymptomatic and so overjoyed that he called a newspaper journalist. Grüntzig, ever a scholar and aware of the adverse potential consequences that might arise from a tabloid report, convinced Bachmann to hold off. The official accounting of this first successful case of PTCA was subsequently published in the February 4, 1978, issue of *Lancet*.

CORONARY ANGIOPLASTY THEN AND NOW

Several aspects of that first case and subsequent ones for the initial years thereafter are noteworthy when compared with coronary intervention performed today. Access to coronary arteries was difficult. Guide catheters were large, 9 Fr, and mostly unresponsive to manipulation and rotation.

There were no over-the-wire balloon catheters. Balloon catheters had only a short fixed wire at the tip and torque was poorly transmitted to the distal end of the catheter. Also balloon catheters were in short supply. It took an entire day to manufacture one balloon catheter and there was only one individual, Hans Gleichner of Schneider Corporation, who could fabricate them. As a consequence, balloon catheters were re-used among patients. Between cases balloon catheters soaked in a bowl containing Cidex, an antiseptic solution. During a case, catheters were removed from the bowl, wiped with a saline sponge and inserted into the patient.

Balloon catheters were routinely withdrawn proximal to the dilated lesion following balloon inflation. There had been fear that leaving catheters distal to lesions would impair coronary perfusion. Techniques were crude and re-crossing initially dilated lesions often resulted in exacerbation of dissection and even abrupt coronary occlusion.

There were no valves on the large 9 Fr sheaths, and serious groin bleeds and the need for blood transfusions were common. Venous sheaths were required as a temporary pacemaker was routinely placed into the right ventricle for every patient. No one had any experience with the incidence of cardiac rhythm disturbance as a consequence of brief coronary occlusion so precautions were initiated.

ACUTE ANGIOPLASTY FAILURE

There was always the concern that angioplasty could fail and the operator would have to deal with the consequences of not only lack of success but the consequence of acute coronary occlusion. With the crude initial tools then available, very early rates of abrupt closure approximated 20% to 30%. A large proportion of patients experienced acute myocardial infarction as a consequence of unsuccessful angioplasty. Consequently, a very close, supportive relationship with cardiac surgery was essential. In the early years, each patient had a formal consultation by a cardiac surgeon prior to PTCA and the procedure was not started unless an operating room was free and an entire surgical team was available.

To minimize abrupt closure, full heparinization was maintained during procedures. If the angioplasty was successful, arterial and venous femoral sheaths were left in place. Patients recovered in the coronary care unit, a site where vigilant observation and nursing care were available. These early cases were difficult for both patients and physicians. Aside from bleeding, procedures took considerable time. With all that was involved and with a lack of training and experience, performing just one case a day could be exhausting.

Several other important lessons became evident early on in the course of angioplasty. One related to the role of PTCA for patients with significant stenosis of their left main coronary artery. Given the difficulties in manipulating angioplasty catheters deep into a coronary artery, left main angioplasty appeared simple. Early in his PTCA experience, Grüntzig was initially successful when he first treated a patient with left main disease. The patient left the hospital in improved condition and follow-up stress testing showed

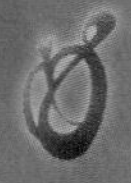

relief of ischemia. But then, Andreas received news that the patient had died suddenly at home. The timing of the death suggested that restenosis rather than acute abrupt closure were the more likely explanation. Realization that restenosis, not uncommon following percutaneous coronary intervention (PCI), located in the left main coronary artery could result in ischemia of sufficient magnitude to cause death, and has limited application of PCI to left main disease even today.

MECHANISM OF BALLOON ANGIOPLASTY

How did balloon angioplasty work? For Grüntzig, the explanation was simple. He likened the explanation to "footprints in the snow." In fact, when he lectured about his procedure, he routinely displayed a slide showing depressions in deep snow from human footprints. Such an explanation made sense and to some degree a component of plaque compression likely did result from balloon inflation. Subsequently pathologic studies indicated that atherosclerotic plaques were actually torn as the diameter of the artery was enlarged circumferentially. Plaque fracturing was accompanied by an increase in the circumference of the external elastic membrane. Pathologic studies from acute and late deaths demonstrated the response to this local injury was neoproliferation of tissue within the dilated arterial wall.[2] Almost in an effort to "repair" damage caused by balloon inflation, media-derived cells proliferated in the crevices of the dilated plaque. Ideally, this proliferation would fill these new crevices and create a smooth and enlarged arterial lumen. However, it became clear that neoproliferation could be more exuberant and extend into the arterial lumen. It could then accumulate to the point where arterial narrowing could develop and the patient become ischemic again. This latter process was termed *restenosis*.

DISSEMINATION OF CORONARY ANGIOPLASTY

Andreas Grüntzig took another bold step in the fall of 1978 at which time he organized a "demonstration course" held at the University Hospital in Zurich to allow others to learn this new form of coronary revascularization. Such an activity was unheard of in cardiology. Certainly demonstrations of surgical procedures had been performed previously but never had anyone publicly demonstrated a procedure performed in a cardiac catheterization laboratory. Furthermore PTCA was in its infancy, and serious consequences such as abrupt coronary occlusion, myocardial infarction, and even death were possible outcomes.

Approximately 35 physicians attended this initial course. We sat in a small, classic amphitheater and observed Andreas perform two PTCA cases a day for 5 days. Each case was televised to the lecture hall from the catheterization laboratory. Of the ten patients treated, approximately half were successful. Of the unsuccessful ones, a substantial proportion had abrupt coronary occlusion and ECG evidence of acute ST-elevation. Each of the unsuccessful treated patients underwent immediate coronary bypass surgery. There were no deaths.

Reactions of attendees were mixed. Some senior cardiologists were appalled and believed this procedure was improper and no match for coronary bypass surgery. Others were impressed by the successfully treated patients and sensed the potential implications of this new procedure.

Notable was the thoroughness, intellectual honesty, and frankness of Grüntzig. He presented the history and clinical presentation of each patient, discussed the potential benefits and risks of both PTCA and coronary artery bypass grafting (CABG), and narrated as he performed each procedure. His demeanor, calmness, and obvious skill were remarkable. Once a case was completed, he returned to the amphitheater and reviewed each step of the prior procedure. The procedures we witnessed were truly astonishing and only exceeded by the skill and daring of the man who performed them.

Following this initial demonstration, angioplasty began to spread. By the end of 1978, Richard Myler, Simon Stertzer, Lamberto Bentivoglio, David Williams, and Peter Block performed PCI in the United States. Other physicians brought patients to U.S. angioplasty sites and observed this new therapeutic approach.

Grüntzig published his initial 50 case experiences in the *New England Journal of Medicine* in July 1979.[3] In that report, coronary lesion dilatation was achieved in 32 (64%) patients and 29 (58%) improved clinically. Of interest, Grüntzig estimated that only 10% to 15% of patients with coronary disease had lesions suitable for PTCA.

Michael Mock, then at the National Heart, Lung, and Blood Institute, initiated a National Institutes of Health (NIH)-funded registry to characterize and describe the patients treated by PTCA and their outcomes. Katherine Detry and Sheryl Kelsey headed the data coordinating center at the University of Pittsburgh. This registry captured consecutive cases performed in Zurich and the United States and became an important mechanism for reporting valuable information about this new procedure.[4]

Grüntzig held additional Zurich demonstration courses in the spring and fall of 1979. There were several differences between these and the first demonstration. First, within a short interval, PTCA had become acknowledged as a legitimate option for coronary revascularization. Grüntzig's openness and objectiveness had added credibility to his achievements and the procedure. Physicians who attend accepted the procedure and thirsted to learn the technique. Second, the news of PTCA had spread such that the number of physicians who attended was now measured in the hundreds. Third, the worldwide experience of PTCA elsewhere was still limited. During this course Grüntzig queried each operator who had performed PTCA and the numbers of cases each had performed. He wrote and totaled their results on the blackboard. This was the worldwide experience. Fourth, there were some physicians who saw PTCA as an opportunity for personal advancement. At times these individuals would jockey for stature and attempt to establish themselves as legitimate authorities. Certainly the tone of this meeting was quite different from that of the first.

ANDREAS GRÜNTZIG, THE MAN

In orchestrating these courses, Grüntzig always included some form of social activity during evenings. These included a boat trip on Lake Zurich, a train to Emmental (the home of Swiss cheese) and a trek to the top of a nearby mountain. Grüntzig was just as comfortable and skillful in these settings as he was in the catheterization lab. Many close personal relationships were formed among attendees that lasted for decades.

As PTCA grew so did the reputation of the man who developed the procedure. Grüntzig became a target for recruitment, particularly for medical institutions in the United States. Eventually Grüntzig joined the faculty of Emory University, which provided the appropriate backdrop to further the growth of PTCA, which he renamed percutaneous coronary intervention (PCI). Andreas' wife, Michaela, joined him there but found the American way of life difficult for her socially and professionally. After a short time, she returned to Zurich and currently resides in the same apartment where she and Andreas developed the very first angioplasty catheters.

With the aid of Spencer King and John Douglas, Grüntzig grew the angioplasty program at Emory. The theme of bi-annual training courses continued with multiple, increasingly complex procedures demonstrated daily. There, Grüntzig met Margret Anne Thornton, an Emory medical student. He was so charmed by this Georgia native that he divorced Michaela and married Margret Anne. Within a short time they purchased an estate in tony Buckhead and a second home in Sea Island, Georgia.

Always a traveler of the fast lane, Grüntzig bought a new car, a Porsche 911. This was followed by a single engine plane, which was perfect for access to their second home in Sea Island, Georgia. Seeking even greater goals, Grüntzig then purchased a twin-engine Beechcraft Baron. This plane, although more challenging to fly, was now affordable for Grüntzig and in fitting with his new stature.

On an overcast Sunday, October 27, 1985, Andreas, Margret Anne, and their two dogs, Gin and Tonic, departed Sea Island for Atlanta. Cloud cover was thick and low. Brief transcripts of recordings from Grüntzig to traffic control state that while in the air, he had difficulty using the autopilot system of the plane. Two hunters in a Georgia forest recall seeing a plane descend from the overcast sky and fly straight into the earth. There was little at the crash site to identify who or what had been in the Grüntzig plane. A funeral service and burial for Andreas and Margret Anne was held in Macon, Georgia, Margret Anne's home. Ironically, three other pioneers of vascular medicine died that year, Melvin Judkins, Mason Sones, and Charles Dotter.

DEVELOPMENT OF INTERVENTIONAL CARDIOLOGY AND MINIMALLY INVASIVE SURGERY

The pioneering work of Grüntzig was followed by a series of innovations that incrementally improved clinical outcomes and advanced the field of interventional cardiology. Many engineers, cardiologists, and entrepreneurs attempted to identify devices that would replace or supplement the balloon catheter. Metallic stents were the first significant advancement.[5-8] Stents addressed two important shortcomings of balloon angioplasty, abrupt closure and late lesion recurrence.

Balloon angioplasty caused localized dissection of the arterial wall. If this dissection was too extensive it caused an intimal flap or created a hematoma within the media, each of which could exacerbate rather than relieve coronary narrowing. Stents provided a rigid scaffold that compressed the arterial wall and minimized the likelihood of abrupt closure. Stents have been so effective that sustained abrupt closure is very rare such that PCI can now be performed safely in the absence of on-site CABG.[9]

A second shortcoming of balloon angioplasty was lesion recurrence. Angiographic assessment of sites of balloon angioplasty indicated a recurrence rate, defined as more than a 50% residual narrowing, of approximately 30% to 40%.[10] Multiple pharmacologic cocktails were proposed and tested to reduce the incidence of restenosis; each failed. New devices for the removal of plaque were intensely investigated.[11,12] None matched the results of coronary stent. While stents prevented the negative remodeling that followed balloon angioplasty, neointimal hyperplasia was more pronounced. Furthermore, if in-stent restenosis did develop, repeat balloon angioplasty was of limited benefit as lesion recurrence was common. Use of local radiation, as a mechanism to prevent neoproliferation, was quite successful in reducing rates of in-stent restenosis.[13,14]

The definitive approach to treat intimal hyperplasia locally was to add potent antiproliferative agents to stents, thus making stents local drug delivery systems.[15] This final combination coupled with improving stent materials and design and adding low profile delivery catheters resulted in very low rates of short-term complications. During later follow-up, however, recurrent symptoms and events can develop and are related to the extent of underlying coronary disease and disease progression.[16]

Coronary balloon angioplasty established the concept of minimally invasive surgery. Angioplasty was the very first procedure to accomplish what could be achieved only by a coronary artery bypass operation. Grüntzig's achievements resulted in efforts to identify alternative less invasive approaches to all types of surgical procedures. Laparoscopic surgery, now the standard of care, is just one example. Transcatheter aortic valve replacement (TAVR) is another example, and one that is revolutionizing the minimally invasive approach to the treatment of valvular heart disease.

Also of interest is that as innovators have attempted to create more advanced therapeutic approaches to coronary disease, balloon angioplasty remains the backbone. Drills, lasers, and suction and cutting devices have been attached to catheters and evaluated as tools to remove atheromatous arterial obstruction and enhance coronary blood flow. Except for unusual circumstances, such as a heavily calcified stenosis, none has proved superior to balloon angioplasty and stenting.[17]

Andreas Grüntzig was an exceptional human being. His courage, innovation, determination, and just plain hard work provided the substance for his enormous contribution. We will never know what other accomplishments he might have achieved had he not died prematurely and so tragically.

ACKNOWLEDGMENT

The author acknowledges the assistance of Carol A. Williams in the preparation of this manuscript.

References

1. Monagan D, Williams DO: *Journey into the Heart*, New York, 2007, Gotham.
2. Ferns GAA, Avades TY: The mechanisms of coronary restenosis: insights from experimental models. *Int J Exp Pathol* 81:63–68, 2000.
3. Grüntzig AR, Senning A, Siegenthaler WE: Nonoperative dilation of coronary-artery stenosis: percutaneous transluminal coronary angioplasty. *N Engl J Med* 301:61–68, 1979.
4. Venkitachalam L, Kip KE, Selzer F, et al: Twenty-year evolution of percutaneous coronary intervention and its impact on clinical outcomes: a report from the NHLBI-sponsored, Multicenter Percutaneous Transluminal Coronary Angioplasty and 1997-2006 Dynamic Registries. *Circ Cardiovasc Interv* 2:6–13, 2009.
5. Schatz RA, Palmaz JC, Tio FO, et al: Balloon-expandable intracoronary stents in the adult dog. *Circulation* 76:450–457, 1987.

6. Sigwart U, Puel J, Mirkovitch V, et al: Intravascular stents to prevent occlusion and restenosis after transluminal angioplasty. *N Engl J Med* 316:701–706, 1987.
7. Roubin GS, Cannon AD, Agrawal SK, et al: Intracoronary stenting for acute and threatened closure complicating percutaneous transluminal coronary angioplasty. *Circulation* 85:916–927, 1992.
8. Fischman DL, Leon MB, Baim DS, et al: A randomized comparison of coronary-stent placement and balloon angioplasty in the treatment of coronary artery disease. *N Engl J Med* 331:496–501, 1994.
9. Aversano T, Lemmon CC, Liu L, et al: Outcomes of PCI at hospitals with and without on-site cardiac surgery. *N Engl J Med* 366:1792–1802, 2012.
10. Holmes DR, Vlietstra RE, Smith HC, et al: Restenosis after percutaneous transluminal coronary angioplasty (PTCA): a report from the National Heart, Lung and Blood Institute. *Am J Cardiol* 53:77C–81C, 1984.
11. Baim DS, Cutlip DE, Sharma SK, et al: Final results of the balloon vs. optimal atherectomy trial (BOAT). *Circulation* 97:322–331, 1998.
12. Reifart N, Vandormeal M, Krajcar M, et al: Randomized comparison of angioplasty of coronary lesions at a single center: eximer laser, rotational atherectomy and balloon angioplasty comparison (ERBAC) study. *Circulation* 96:91–98, 1997.
13. Leon MB, Tierstein PS, Moses JW, et al: Localized intracoronary gamma-radiation to inhibit the recurrence of restenosis after stenting. *N Engl J Med* 344:250–256, 2001.
14. Popma JJ, Suntharalingam M, Lansky A, et al: Randomized trial of 90SR/90Y beta-radiation versus placebo control for treatment of instent restenosis. *Circulation* 106:1090–1096, 2002.
15. Moses JW, Leon MB, Popma JJ, et al: Sirolimus-eluting stents versus standard stents in patients with stenosis in a native coronary artery. *N Engl J Med* 349:1315–1323, 2003.
16. Mohr FW, Morice MC, Kappetein AP, et al: Coronary artery bypass graft surgery versus percutaneous coronary intervention in patients with three-vessel disease and left main disease: 5-year follow-up of the randomized, clinical SYNTAX trial. *Lancet* 381:629–638, 2013.
17. Dill T, Dietz U, Hamm C, et al: A randomized comparison of balloon angioplasty versus rotational atherectomy in complex coronary lesions (COBRA study). *Eur Heart J* 21:1759–1766, 2000.

2 Guidelines and Appropriateness Criteria for Interventional Cardiology

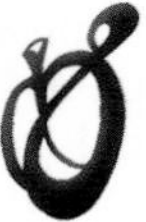

David P. Faxon

INTRODUCTION

Quality of care has been a major focus of medical care since the Institute of Medicine focused attention on the unacceptable degree of variability in care and concern about patient safety and effectiveness. In its classic monograph, *Crossing the Quality Chasm,* the institute identified six aims to improve the quality of health care in the United States.[1] It stressed that health care needs to provide safe, effective, patient-centric, timely, efficient, and equitable care. Efforts to achieve these goals have resulted in the growth and widespread use of a number of tools to improve care, including practice guidelines, appropriateness criteria, performance measures, and methods to put guidelines in practice. Of these tools, practice guidelines have provided the foundation for the other quality efforts. Cardiology has been at the forefront of this process due to a large number of clinical studies and randomized trials upon which to base the guideline recommendations.

Califf et al. has described the "cycle of quality" to emphasize the continuous evolution of quality of care.[2] As shown in **Figure 2-1**, discoveries of new or improved diagnostic tools and optimal treatments are suggested by basic and translational science. Initial observational clinical trials lead to more definitive randomized controlled trials. The evidence derived from these studies forms the basis for consensus-driven guideline recommendations. Guidelines provide the foundation for the patient-specific recommendations of appropriateness criteria where a number of key variables are integrated to best determine optimal use of procedures. Guidelines are also the basis for performance measures where clearly defined and validated variables can be used to monitor the degree of quality and reduce practice variability. New discoveries provide new directions or challenge prior practice and stimulate new clinical trials and the cycle repeats itself.

The explosion of guidelines over the past 20 years has been remarkable. Since 1995, the National Guideline Clearinghouse has identified 2352 practice guidelines, and of these, 491 are in the cardiovascular area (**www.guideline.gov**). The American College of Cardiology Foundation (ACCF) and the American Heart Association (AHA) have published over 100 guidelines since 2005, and the European Society of Cardiology (ESC) has also been active in publishing similar guidelines. The ACCF/AHA have been leaders in publishing appropriateness criteria for cardiovascular tests and procedures. Other organizations, such as the AMA, in collaboration with the ACCF and AHA, have jointly published performance measures. In the cardiovascular field, the ACCF/AHA and ESC guidelines are the most respected and quoted documents.

PRACTICE GUIDELINES

Guideline Development

The ACCF and AHA have adopted a strict and rigorous process for guideline development.[3,4] The joint guideline committee identifies topics of interest and selects a writing committee composed of recognized experts in the field, seasoned clinicians, generalists, and other health care providers from associated disciplines, including nurses and pharmacists. Recent recommendations are to also include a patient advocate. The evidence from clinical registries and trials is collated, rigorously reviewed, and analyzed to assist the committee in formulating its recommendations. These recommendations are categorized into four classes: Class I is defined as procedures or treatment that SHOULD be performed or administered; Class II indications are those where it is REASONABLE to do the procedure/treatment (IIa) or where it MAY BE CONSIDERED (IIb); and Class III is defined as one that is anticipated to have NO BENEFIT or the procedure or treatment would cause HARM. The level of evidence for each recommendation is an important component of the process. Level A is used when the recommendation is supported by either multiple randomized trials or a meta-analysis; Level B is used when the recommendation is supported by either a single randomized trial or nonrandomized studies; and Level C is used when the recommendation is supported by either limited evidence, the consensus opinion of experts, or the standard of care. The final guidelines document is peer reviewed by external experts and revised before the final document is approved by the participating organizations. The process is lengthy, which limits the ability to quickly revise the guidelines as new information from clinical trials alters practice. Efforts to improve the process and increase the speed and rigor of guideline development have been described.[5] While clinical trial data are critical to the formulation of guidelines, the lack of trials in many areas of practice unfortunately has resulted in Level C evidence (expert opinion), responsible for 48% of all guideline recommendations.[6]

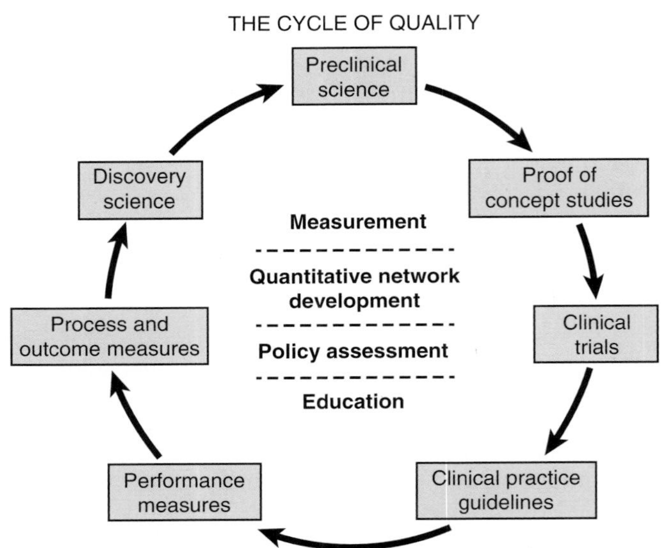

FIGURE 2-1 The cycle of quality. *(Califf RM: The benefits of moving quality to a national level. Am Heart J 156:1019–1022, 2008.)*

For the purposes of this chapter, only current ACCF/AHA guidelines are reviewed and only key recommendations that are directly pertinent to interventional cardiology practice are discussed. Please refer the original documents for a more detailed discussion of the guidelines and the evidence supporting the recommendations.

Guidelines for ST-Elevation Myocardial Infarction

The 2013 STEMI guidelines build upon the recommendations of the prior documents. This and past documents should be referred to for a more in-depth discussion of the recommendations and the evidence supporting them.[7]

The guidelines recommend that the initial management of patients with an acute ST-segment myocardial infarction (STEMI) is the rapid reperfusion of the infarct artery. A reduction in the duration of the coronary occlusion results in a reduction in infarct size and mortality. Of the two reperfusion strategies, fibrinolysis or angioplasty, PCI is the preferred strategy when it can be performed expeditiously. The guidelines recommend that it should be accomplished within a time frame, from the first medical contact (FMC) to the first device, of less than 90 minutes and preferably within 60 minutes in patients who present within 12 hours of the onset of symptoms (Class IA) (**Figure 2-2**). To achieve this goal, it is recommended that all communities create and maintain a regional system of care with integrated emergency medical services (EMS) and hospital systems that meet the guidelines for rapid diagnosis and triage (Class IB). Patients should be transferred by emergency medical systems (EMS) to PCI-capable hospitals for primary PCI.

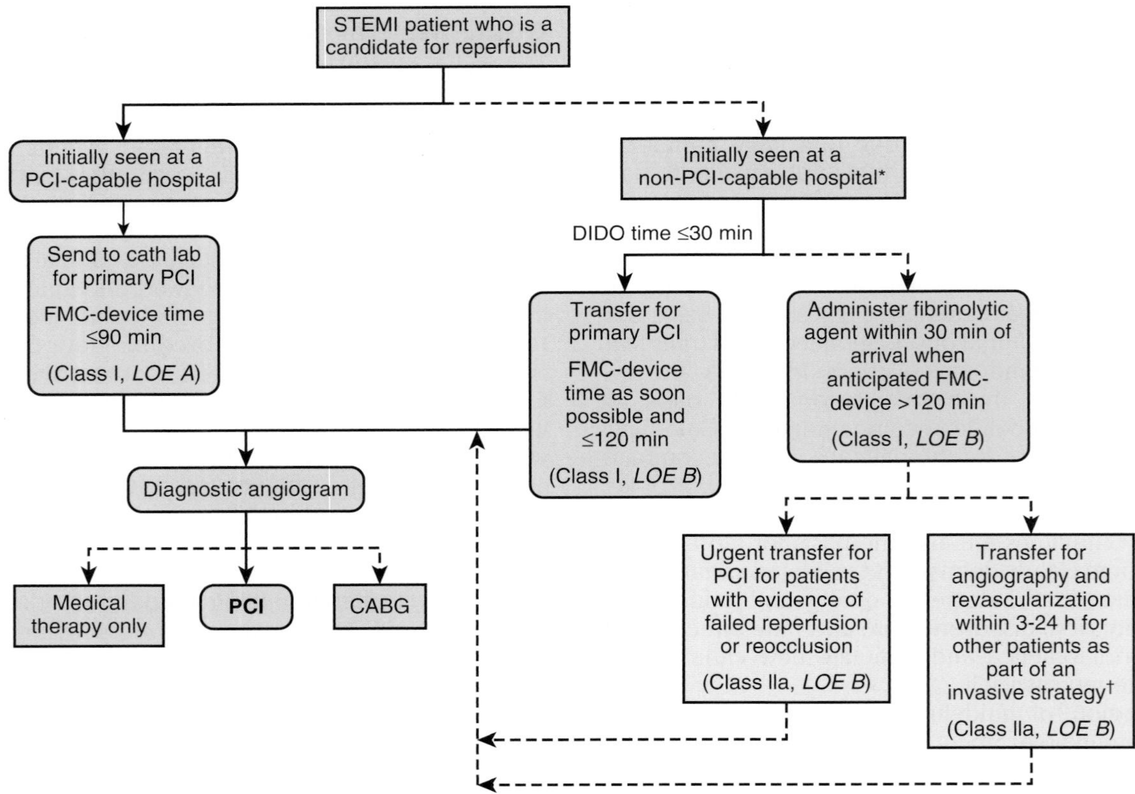

FIGURE 2-2 Acute management for STEMI patients. *(Used with permission from O'Gara PT, Kushner FG, Ascheim DD, et al: 2013 ACCF/AHA guideline for the management of ST-elevation myocardial infarction: a report of the American College of Cardiology Foundation/American Heart Association task force on practice guidelines. Circulation 127:e362–e425, 2013.[7])*

	COR	LOE
Ischemic symptoms <12 h	I	A
Ischemic symptoms <12 h and contraindications to fibrinolytic therapy irrespective of time delay from FMC	I	B
Cardiogenic shock or acute severe HF irrespective of time delay from MI onset	I	B
Evidence of ongoing ischemia 12 to 24 h after symptom onset	IIa	B
PCI of a noninfarct artery at the time of primary PCI in patients without hemodynamic compromise	III: Harm	B

FIGURE 2-3 Indications for primary PCI. *(Used with permission from O'Gara PT, Kushner FG, Ascheim DD, et al: 2013 ACCF/AHA guideline for the management of ST-elevation myocardial infarction: a report of the American College of Cardiology Foundation/American Heart Association task force on practice guidelines. Circulation 127:e362–e425, 2013.[7])*

	COR	LOE
Cardiogenic shock or acute severe HF that develops after initial presentation	I	B
Intermediate- or high-risk findings on predischarge noninvasive ischemia testing	I	B
Spontaneous or easily provoked myocardial ischemia	I	C
Failed reperfusion or reocclusion after fibrinolytic therapy	IIa	B
Stable* patients after successful fibrinolysis, before discharge and ideally between 3 and 24 h	IIa	B

FIGURE 2-4 Indications for coronary angiography when a fibrinolytic agent is given first or the patient does not receive reperfusion therapy. *(Used with permission from O'Gara PT, Kushner FG, Ascheim DD, et al: 2013 ACCF/AHA guideline for the management of ST-elevation myocardial infarction: a report of the American College of Cardiology Foundation/American Heart Association task force on practice guidelines. Circulation 127:e362–e425, 2013.[7])*

When patients present at a non-PCI-capable hospital, immediate transfer to a PCI-capable hospital should be done as rapidly as possible, with a goal of 120 minutes from the FMC to device use (Class Ib) and a door-in to door-out time at the first hospital of 30 minutes or less. When the FMC to device time is anticipated to be more than 120 minutes, a fibrinolytic agent should be given first, unless contraindicated. It is reasonable to then transfer the patient for PCI within 3 to 24 hours (the so-called pharmaco-invasive strategy) (Class IIa-b). When this strategy is chosen, the fibrinolytic agent should be administered within 30 minutes of hospital arrival. The guideline class (COR) and level of evidence (LOE) for these primary PCI strategies are shown in **Figures 2-2, 2-3, 2-4, and 2-5**.

The management of patients with cardiogenic shock or severe heart failure is more aggressive with recommendations for PCI, regardless of the time after the onset of the symptoms or first contact. In this setting urgent transfer to a PCI-capable hospital is critical. Transfer for a failure of fibrinolytic therapy is also a reasonable strategy (so-called rescue angioplasty) (Class IIa-b). The guidelines for coronary angiography and potential PCI when a fibrinolytic agent is given or the patient received no reperfusion is shown in **Figure 2-4**.

The national efforts to improve ischemic time (symptom onset to device/drug) have focused on the FMC to device time and particularly a key component of this time—the door to device time (D2D). Public reporting and efforts such as the AHA Mission Lifeline program and the ACCF D2B

	COR	LOE
Cardiogenic shock or acute severe HF	I	B
Intermediate- or high-risk findings on predischarge noninvasive ischemia testing	I	C
Spontaneous or easily provoked myocardial ischemia	I	C
Patients with evidence of failed reperfusion or reocclusion after fibrinolytic therapy (as soon as possible)	IIa	B
Stable* patients after successful fibrinolysis, ideally between 3 and 24 h	IIa	B
Stable* patients >24 h after successful fibrinolysis	IIb	B
Delayed PCI of a totally occluded infarct artery >24 h after STEMI in stable patients	III: No benefit	B

FIGURE 2-5 Indications for PCI in patients with STEMI who initially received fibrinolytic therapy or who did not receive reperfusion therapy. *(Used with permission from O'Gara PT, Kushner FG, Ascheim DD, et al: 2013 ACCF/AHA guideline for the management of ST-elevation myocardial infarction: a report of the American College of Cardiology Foundation/American Heart Association task force on practice guidelines. Circulation 127:e362–e425, 2013.[7])*

program have been successful in improving D2D times.[8,9] The strategies to achieve this reduction have included prehospital ECG and activation of the cath lab while en route to the hospital, ED activation of the PCI team, a single page for activation of the cath lab, <20 minutes until cath lab staff arrive, and timely feedback to the STEMI care team.[10] While these measures have been effective, the greatest delay in reperfusion is often the delay between the onset of symptoms to the 911 call or the hospital arrival. There are many reasons for this delay, and unfortunately, national efforts to reduce this time have not been successful.[11]

Once the patient arrives at the cath lab, the interventional procedure should be performed expeditiously. Antiplatelet and anticoagulant therapy should be given as soon as possible upon initial medical contact. Dual antiplatelet therapy (aspirin and clopidogrel or prasugrel or ticagrelor) and an anticoagulant (UFH or bivalirudin) should be administered. GP IIb/IIIa agents (abciximab, tirofiban, or eptifibatide) are reasonable in combination with UFH (Class IIa). In current practice, the use of GP IIb/IIa agents has decreased due to concerns about increased bleeding risk, the introduction of the newer more potent P_2Y_{12} antiplatelet agents, and the greater use of bivalirudin.[12] Based on randomized trials, the guideline committee felt it was not unreasonable to perform an aspiration thrombectomy (Class IIa-b). Recent trials have been mixed, and many operators have restricted the use to those situations where there is a large clot burden.[13,14] Drug eluting stents (DES) or bare metal stents (BMS) should be used when possible (Class Ia). Most operators have favored DES, given evidence from large randomized trials of improved long-term outcomes, particularly the reduction in target vessel revascularization without an increased risk of stent thrombosis.[15] BMS should be used when there is an increased risk of bleeding or a concern about compliance with dual antiplatelet therapy for 1 year (Class IC). Initial primary PCI should be restricted to the infarct-related artery, and current guidelines recommend against treatment of other significant stenosis at the same setting. Multivessel PCI is indicated in patients who develop spontaneous symptoms of ischemia (Class Ic) and those patients with an intermediate to high risk of noninvasive testing prior to discharge (Class IIa). These recommendations have been recently challenged following the results of the PRAMI trial that

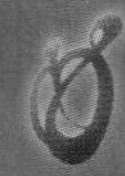

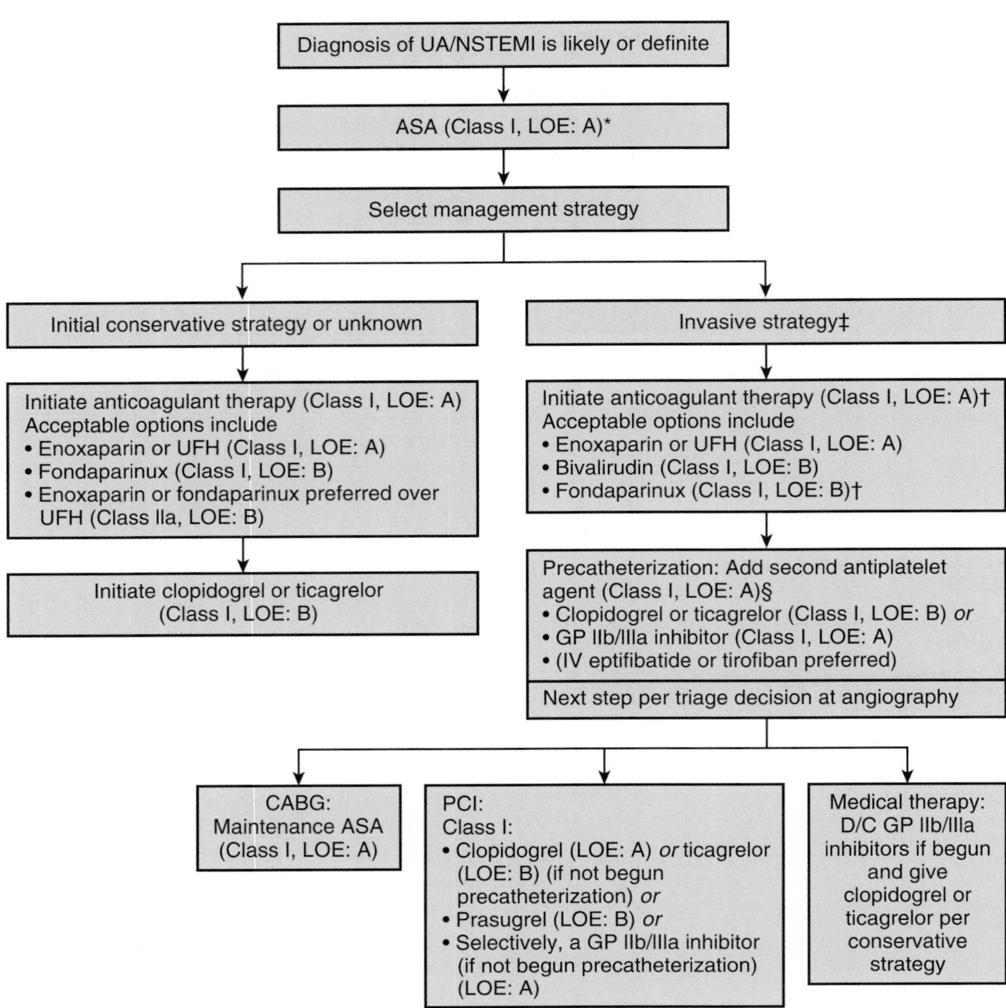

FIGURE 2-6 ACCF/AHA guideline-recommended management of UA/NSTEMI. *(Used with permission from Jneid H, Anderson JL, Wright RS, et al: 2012 ACCF/AHA focused update of the guideline for the management of patients with unstable angina/non-ST-elevation myocardial infarction (updating the 2007 guideline and replacing the 2011 focused update): a report of the American College of Cardiology Foundation/American Heart Association task force on practice guidelines. Circulation 126:875–910, 2012.[19])*

demonstrate improved outcomes with multivessel PCI at the same setting as the primary PCI.[16] A number of large randomized trials are ongoing to help address this issue.

Coronary artery bypass surgery is indicated for patients not amenable to PCI and those who have ongoing or recurrent ischemia, cardiogenic shock, severe heart failure, or other high-risk features (Class Ib). CABG is rarely used as the primary reperfusion strategy, but it is commonly used for other indications during hospitalization, particularly in patients who have extensive coronary disease or have disease that is not amenable to PCI.

The subsequent medical management with dual antiplatelet therapy, oral anticoagulants, beta-blockers, ACE or ARB agents, and statins, in addition to risk factor modification and cardiac rehabilitation, are critically important in improving long-term outcomes and preventing future events. The reader should refer to the STEMI guidelines for specific recommendations.

Guidelines for Unstable Angina/Non–ST-Elevation MI

The ACCF/AHA guidelines for unstable angina and non–ST-elevation MI (UA/NSTEMI) were released in 2007; since then two focused updates have been published, the most recent in 2012.[17-19] This report provides an update on the use of antiplatelet and anticoagulant therapy and management of special groups such as patients with diabetes and chronic kidney disease.

An overview of the guideline recommendations for the management of UA/NSTEMI is shown in **Figure 2-6**. The initial assessment of the patient is to determine the likelihood of acute coronary syndrome based on the history, physical examination, EKG, laboratory tests, cardiac biomarkers, and risk factors. In those in whom the diagnosis is likely or definite, the guidelines recommend that the patient's risk be assessed using one of the available risk scores such as Thrombolysis in Myocardial Infarction (TIMI) or Global Registry of Acute Coronary Events (GRACE) (Class IIa-b). Patients at low risk and/or low likelihood of ACS can be managed in a chest pain unit or in the hospital for 24 hours with serial EKGs and cardiac-specific enzymes. If these tests do not show evidence of ischemia or infarction, the patient should be further risk stratified with a noninvasive test such as a treadmill exercise test (ETT), a nuclear imaging stress test, or a coronary CT angiogram. If these tests are negative or demonstrate a low risk of subsequent events, the patient can be discharged and followed as an outpatient. If the noninvasive test is positive and suggests an

TABLE 2-1 Recommendations for Initial Invasive vs. Initial Conservative Strategies in UA/NSTEMI

GENERALLY PREFERRED STRATEGY	PATIENT CHARACTERISTICS
Invasive	Recurrent angina or ischemia at rest or with low-level activities despite intensive medical therapy Elevated cardiac biomarkers (TnT or TnI) New or presumably new ST-segment depression Signs or symptoms of HF or new or worsening mitral regurgitation High-risk findings from noninvasive testing Hemodynamic Instability Sustained ventricular tachycardia PCI within 6 months Prior CABG High-risk score (e.g., TIMI, GRACE) Mild to moderate renal dysfunction Diabetes mellitus Reduced LV function (LVEF <40%)
Conservative	Low-risk score (e.g., TIMI, GRACE) Patient or physician preference in the absence of high-risk features

Reprinted from Jneid H, Anderson JL, Wright RS, et al: 2012 ACCF/AHA focused update of the guideline for the management of patients with unstable angina/non-ST-elevation myocardial infarction (updating the 2007 guideline and replacing the 2011 focused update): a report of the American College of Cardiology Foundation/ American Heart Association task force on practice guidelines. Circulation 126:875–910, 2012.[19]

CABG, Coronary artery bypass graft; *GRACE,* global registry of acute coronary events; *HF,* heart failure; *LV,* left ventricular; *LVEF,* left ventricular ejection fraction; *PCI,* percutaneous coronary intervention; *TIMI,* Thrombolysis in Myocardial Infarction; *TnI,* troponin I; and *TnT,* troponin T.

increased risk of cardiac events, the patient should be referred for urgent diagnostic cardiac catheterization.

Intermediate- or high-risk patients should be admitted to the hospital for observation, more aggressive medical therapy, and possible cardiac catheterization. It is important to note that cardiac enzyme elevation alone does not automatically imply high risk and can be due to causes other than a myocardial infarction, and likewise, a patient can be high risk without elevation of cardiac enzymes.[20,21]

The decision to proceed with an initial invasive versus conservative strategy is influenced by the risk of the patient, with higher risk patients best treated with an invasive strategy. The guideline recommendations for selecting the appropriate strategy, early invasive versus initial conservative, are shown in **Table 2-1**. The timing of an early invasive strategy has been tested in three trials. The largest, the TIMAC trial, failed to reach its primary endpoint but strongly suggested that an invasive strategy should be performed within 12 to 24 hours, particularly in those patients at highest risk, as determined by the GRACE score (Class IIa-b).[22]

All patients should be given anticoagulant therapy in addition to antiangina medication. The Class I indications for antiplatelet agents are shown in **Figure 2-6 and Table 2-2**. It is recommended that aspirin be given as soon as possible (or clopidogrel if the patient is allergic to aspirin) (Class Ia). Those at moderate to high risk or in whom an initial invasive strategy has been chosen should be given dual antiplatelet therapy on presentation (Class Ia) with a loading and maintenance dose of either clopidogrel or ticagrelor or an IV GP IIb/IIIa inhibitor prior to PCI. If not given before PCI, clopidogrel, ticagrelor, and prasugrel or IC GP IIb/IIIa inhibitors can be given at the time of the PCI procedure. The use of GP IIb/IIIa inhibitors in practice has

TABLE 2-2 Class I Recommendations for Antiplatelet Therapy

2012 FOCUSED UPDATE RECOMMENDATIONS

Class I

1. Aspirin should be administered to UA/NSTEMI patients as soon as possible after hospital presentation and continued indefinitely in patients who tolerate it. ***(Level of Evidence: A)***
2. A loading dose followed by daily maintenance dose of either clopidogrel ***(Level of Evidence: B)***, prasugrel* (in PCI-treated patients) ***(Level of Evidence: C)***, or ticagrelor† ***(Level of Evidence: C)*** should be administered to UA/NSTEMI patients who are unable to take aspirin because of hypersensitivity or major GI intolerance.
3. Patients with definite UA/NSTEMI at medium or high risk and in whom an initial invasive strategy is selected (Appendix 6) should receive dual antiplatelet therapy on presentation. ***(Level of Evidence: A)*** Aspirin should be initiated on presentation. ***(Level of Evidence: A)*** The choice of a second antiplatelet therapy to be added to aspirin on presentation includes one of the following (note that there are no data for therapy with two concurrent $P2Y_{12}$ receptor inhibitors, and this is not recommended in the case of aspirin allergy):
   Before PCI:
   - Clopidogrel ***(Level of Evidence: B)***; or
   - Ticagrelor† ***(Level of Evidence: B)***; or
   - An IV GP IIb/IIIa inhibitor. ***(Level of Evidence: A)*** IV eptifibatide and tirofiban are the preferred GP IIb/IIIa inhibitors. ***(Level of Evidence: B)***

   At the time of PCI:
   - Clopidogrel if not started before PCI ***(Level of Evidence: A)***; or
   - Prasugrel* ***(Level of Evidence: B)***; or
   - Ticagrelor† ***(Level of Evidence: B)***; or
   - An IV GP IIb/IIIa inhibitor. ***(Level of Evidence: A)***
4. For UA/NSTEMI patients in whom an initial conservative (i.e., noninvasive) strategy is selected, clopidogrel or ticagrelor† (loading dose followed by daily maintenance dose) should be added to aspirin and anticoagulant therapy as soon as possible after admission and administered for up to 12 months. ***(Level of Evidence: B)***
5. For UA/NSTEMI patients in whom an initial conservative strategy is selected, if recurrent symptoms/ischemia, heart failure, or serious arrhythmias subsequently appear, diagnostic angiography should be performed. ***(Level of Evidence: A)*** Either an IV GP IIb/IIIa inhibitor (eptifibatide or tirofiban ***[Level of Evidence: A]***), clopidogrel (loading dose followed by daily maintenance dose ***[Level of Evidence: B]***), or ticagrelor† (loading dose followed by daily maintenance dose ***[Level of Evidence: B]***) should be added to aspirin and anticoagulant therapy before diagnostic angiography (upstream). ***(Level of Evidence: C)***
6. A loading dose of $P2Y_{12}$ receptor inhibitor therapy is recommended for UA/NSTEMI patients for whom PCI is planned.‡ One of the following regimens should be used:
   a. Clopidogrel 600 mg should be given as early as possible before or at the time of PCI ***(Level of Evidence: B)***; or
   b. Prasugrel* 60 mg should be given promptly and no later than 1 hour after PCI once coronary anatomy is defined and a decision is made to proceed with PCI[7] ***(Level of Evidence: B)***; or
   c. Ticagrelor† 180 mg should be given as early as possible before or at the time of PCI. ***(Level of Evidence: B)***
7. The duration and maintenance dose of $P2Y_{12}$ receptor inhibitor therapy should be as follows:
   a. In UA/NSTEMI patients undergoing PCI, either clopidogrel 75 mg daily, prasugrel* 10 mg daily, or ticagrelor† 90 mg twice daily should be given for at least 12 months. ***(Level of Evidence: B)***
   b. If the risk of morbidity because of bleeding outweighs the anticipated benefits afforded by $P2Y_{12}$ receptor inhibitor therapy, earlier discontinuation should be considered. ***(Level of Evidence: C)***

Reprinted with permission from Jneid H, Anderson JL, Wright RS, et al: 2012 ACCF/AHA focused update of the guideline for the management of patients with unstable angina/non-ST-elevation myocardial infarction (updating the 2007 guideline and replacing the 2011 focused update): a report of the American College of Cardiology Foundation/American Heart Association task force on practice guidelines. Circulation 126:875–910, 2012.[19] *From ACCF/AHA guidelines.*

*Patients with cardiogenic shock or severe heart failure initially seen at a non–PCI-capable hospital should be transferred for cardiac catheterization and revascularization as soon as possible, irrespective of time delay from MI onset (Class I, LOE: B).

†Angiography and revascularization should not be performed within the first 2 to 3 hours after administration of fibrinolytic therapy.

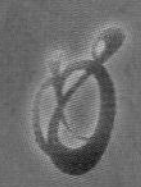

diminished with the availability of potent oral antiplatelet agents and increased bleeding risk of these agents. The guidelines favor their use in those who have recurrent ischemic pain. Studies have shown that upstream use of GP IIb/IIIa inhibitors is not useful. If bivalirudin is used as the anticoagulant, it is reasonable to omit a GP IIb/IIIa inhibitor given the lack of greater efficacy and increased bleeding risk. The recommended anticoagulants (Class I) are unfractionated heparin, enoxaparin, fondaparinux, and bivalirudin. Fondaparinux and enoxaparin are favored for those patients who are managed with a conservative strategy and are not likely to undergo an invasive procedure. If fondaparinux is used, unfractionated heparin should be given in addition if the patient undergoes a PCI due to an increased risk of catheter thrombosis.

Certain subgroups of patients are at higher risk and need special consideration. Patients with diabetes mellitus are well recognized to be at greater risk for short- and long-term adverse events with ACS. The results of randomized trials suggest that the choice of an initial invasive or conservative management strategy in ACS should be similar to patients without diabetes (Class Ia). However, the guidelines recommend CABG rather than PCI for those patients with multivessel disease needing revascularization (Class IIa-b). The results of the FREEDOM trial, which specifically compared DES compared to CABG in diabetic patients, showed superior outcomes with CABG in all subgroups of patients and strongly support the guideline recommendations.[23] There is evidence that patients with Stage 2 or 3 chronic kidney disease are at greater risk for short- and long-term complications as well. The guidelines recommend that an invasive strategy is reasonable in these patients (Class IIa-b). Since contrast nephropathy can increase the risk of patients undergoing invasive procedures, the guidelines recommend that all patients have a calculation of creatinine clearance before PCI and those with CKD have adequate hydration prior to coronary angiography and PCI (Class Ib). The reader should refer to the ACCF/AHA guidelines for UA/NSTEMI for more details concerning the early and late management of these patients.[17]

Guidelines for Stable Ischemic Heart Disease

The 2012 ACCF/AHA guidelines for stable ischemic heart disease (SIHD) built on the prior 2002 guidelines and the 2007 update.[24-26] The earlier documents focused on stable angina, but the most recent guidelines incorporate the full spectrum of SIHD.

The 2012 guidelines recommend that patients with known or suspected SIHD should be initially risk stratified using history, clinical factors, EKG, and an exercise or cardiac imaging study. In addition to determining the likelihood of obstructive coronary disease, exercise testing provides valuable information concerning exercise capacity that can further help in risk stratification and management. The 2012 guidelines provide a detailed discussion of the best noninvasive method to evaluate patients with SIHD, and this document should be referred to for more information on how to choose the proper test. The two exceptions to obtaining a noninvasive test first are those patients with sudden cardiac death or life-threatening ventricular arrhythmias or those with known SIHD who develop signs and symptoms of heart failure, where coronary angiography should be the initial risk-stratifying test (Class IB). In those patients with a prior MI, pathological Q waves, signs or symptoms of heart failure, complex ventricular arrhythmias, or an undiagnosed heart murmur should conduct an assessment of LV systolic and diastolic myocardial function, and an assessment of pericardial and valve structures is recommended (Class Ib). This is most commonly obtained with a 2D echocardiogram.

If the patient does *not* have any high-risk features on noninvasive testing (see **Table 2-3** for criteria), an initial trial of medical therapy should be started before considering coronary angiography. Medical therapy should include

TABLE 2-3 Noninvasive Risk Stratification in SIHD

High Risk (>3% Annual Death or MI)
1. Severe resting LV dysfunction (LVEF <35%) not readily explained by noncoronary causes
2. Resting perfusion abnormalities ≥10% of the myocardium in patients without prior history or evidence of MI
3. Stress ECG findings including ≥2 mm of ST-segment depression at low workload or persisting into recovery, exercise-induced ST-segment elevation, or exercise-induced VT/VF
4. Severe stress-induced LV dysfunction (peak exercise LVEF <45% or drop in LVEF with stress ≥10%)
5. Stress-induced perfusion abnormalities encumbering ≥10% myocardium or stress segmental scores indicating multiple vascular territories with abnormalities
6. Stress-induced LV dilation
7. Inducible wall motion abnormality (involving ≥2 segments or 2 coronary beds)
8. Wall motion abnormality developing at low dose of dobutamine (<10 mg/kg/min) or at a low heart rate (<120 beats/min)
9. CAC score >400 Agatston units
10. Multivessel obstructive CAD (>70% stenosis) or left main stenosis (>50% stenosis) on CCTA
Intermediate Risk (1%-3% Annual Death or MI)
1. Mild/moderate resting LV dysfunction (LVEF 35%-49%) not readily explained by noncoronary causes
2. Resting perfusion abnormalities in 5%-9.9% of the myocardium in patients without a history or prior evidence of MI
3. <1 mm of ST-segment depression occurring with exertional symptoms
4. Stress-induced perfusion abnormalities encumbering 5%-9.9% of the myocardium or stress segmental scores (in multiple segments) indicating one vascular territory with abnormalities but without LV dilation
5. Small wall motion abnormality involving one to two segments and only one coronary bed
6. CAC score 100-399 Agatston units
7. One vessel CAD with ≥70% stenosis or moderate CAD stenosis (50%-69% stenosis) in ≥2 arteries on CCTA
Low Risk (<1% Annual Death or MI)
1. Low-risk treadmill score (score <5) or no new ST-segment changes or exercise-induced chest pain symptoms when achieving maximal levels of exercise
2. Normal or small myocardial perfusion defect at rest or with stress encumbering <5% of the myocardium*
3. Normal stress or no change of limited resting wall motion abnormalities during stress
4. CAC score <100 Agatston units
5. No coronary stenosis >50% on CCTA

Reprinted with permission from Fihn SD, Gardin JM, Abrams J, et al: 2012 ACCF/AHA/ACP/AATS/PCNA/SCAI/STS guideline for the diagnosis and management of patients with stable ischemic heart disease: a report of the American College of Cardiology Foundation/American Heart Association task force on practice guidelines, and the American College of Physicians, American Association for Thoracic Surgery, Preventive Cardiovascular Nurses Association, Society for Cardiovascular Angiography and Interventions, and Society of Thoracic Surgeons. Circulation 126:e354–e471, 2012.[26]

*Although the published data are limited, patients with these findings will probably not be at low risk in the presence of either a high-risk treadmill score or severe resting LV dysfunction (LVEF <35%).

CAC, Coronary artery calcium; *CAD,* coronary artery disease; *CCTA,* coronary computed tomography angiography; *LV,* left ventricular; *LVEF,* left ventricular ejection fraction; *MI,* myocardial infarction.

antiangina medication, lifestyle changes (diet and exercise), and modification of coronary risk factors (hypertension, dyslipidemia, cigarette smoking). In those with high-risk features on noninvasive therapy, further risk stratification should be done with coronary angiography to determine the extent of coronary disease (Class Ib).

Revascularization decisions are based on two primary indications: whether CABG or PCI will improve survival and whether revascularization will improve severe ischemic symptoms not adequately treated with initial medical therapy. It is recommended that a heart team approach be used in making revascularization decisions for patients with left main or complex CAD (Class Ic). Measurement of STS and SYNTAX scores is also recommended to assist in this decision making. The optimal choice in an individual patient requires a careful balance of the risks and benefits of each technique and medical therapy alone.

The specific revascularization recommendations for PCI or CABG are shown in **Figures 2-7 and 2-8**. The guideline recommendations for revascularization to improve survival are unprotected left main, three-vessel disease, or those with two-vessel disease and a proximal LAD lesion. In this setting CABG is favored over PCI (Class Ib). This is in part due to limited studies comparing PCI to medical therapy in multivessel disease and the lower mortality with CABG as compared to PCI in patients with three-vessel disease.

Revascularization to improve symptoms can be accomplished with either CABG or PCI, with CABG favored in those with complex disease (e.g., SYNTAX score >22) and PCI favored in those with prior CABG (Class IIa).

The presence of diabetes is an important consideration in determining the optimal revascularization technique. Randomized trials and a metaanalysis have shown a mortality advantage for CABG over PCI in patients with multivessel disease and diabetes.[27] The FREEDOM trial randomized patients with multivessel disease to PCI with drug-eluting stents or to CABG. The study demonstrated a lower rate of death and MI with CABG. There was not a reduction in cardiovascular death alone.[23] The trial also found no relationship between the SYNTAX score and outcome. Conversely the SYNTAX trial did not find an independent effect of diabetes on outcome but found a strong relationship with the SYNTAX score.[28] The differences in outcomes in these studies may be due to differences in the extent of disease included in each trial.

The management of patients following a successful revascularization procedure is critically important (**Figure 2-9**). Periodic follow-up should be done at least annually, with assessment of symptoms and functional status, adequacy of medical therapy, presence of complications, including heart failure and arrhythmias, and optimal treatment of risk factors and lifestyle changes (Class Ic). Noninvasive testing should be done on those with recurrent symptoms consistent with unstable angina (Class Ib) or those with at least moderate functional limitation or known or likely multivessel disease (Class IIa-b). In general, an exercise test or exercise with a nuclear MPI or echo is preferred.

APPROPRIATENESS CRITERIA

Development Process

The ACCF/AHA guidelines have provided a solid foundation for many areas of clinical practice, but there remain many clinical situations for which there are no guidelines. Even when guidelines are available, they are often based on limited clinical trials or registry data. A study of the ACC/AHA guidelines has shown that Class I recommendations make up only 30% of the guideline recommendations, and of these, only one-third were based on Level A evidence.[6] Almost one half of all recommendations were based on expert opinion (Level C). Another limitation is that they often fail to take into consideration the multiple factors that are weighed in clinical decision making. For instance, age, gender, degree of symptoms, extent of disease, and suitability and risk of PCI or CABG are usually considered when making decisions about revascularization.

Appropriateness criteria have been developed to address these limitations of guidelines and concerns about the documented wide variability in the use of invasive procedures in practice (including both overuse and underuse). Appropriateness criteria are best applied to diagnostic or therapeutic procedures. The development of the criteria used a Modified Delphi process, created by the RAND Corporation. A committee of experts reviews the evidence, including guidelines and observational and randomized trials, and determines the key factors that should be considered in decision making in the use of a test. The committee constructs all of the possible combinations of these factors and ranks the evidence supporting use of the procedure in each clinical situation as "appropriate," "indeterminate," or "inappropriate." More recently these terms have been changed to "appropriate care," "may be appropriate care," and "rarely appropriate care." As with guidelines, the criteria are externally reviewed and approved by the sponsoring organizations.

Summary of Recommendations for Coronary Revascularization

The ACCF/SCAI/STS/AATS/AHA/ASNC appropriateness criteria for coronary revascularization were published in 2009 and updated in 2012.[29,30] In the most recent document, five factors were used to develop >180 separate clinical scenarios. These factors were the clinical presentation (ACS or SIHD), severity of angina (Canadian Cardiovascular Society class), extent of ischemia on noninvasive testing, extent of medical therapy, and extent of anatomic disease (left main, one-, two-, or three-vessel with and without proximal LAD). The committee rated each scenario as appropriate, uncertain, or inappropriate using a score ranging from 1 to 8. The ratings for patients with nonacute indications (SIHD) are shown in **Figure 2-10**. Please refer to the primary document for all the appropriateness criteria. In patients with mild symptoms or no or minimal antiangina therapy, single- or double-vessel disease, and low risk on non-invasive testing, the committee felt it was inappropriate to do PCI. Conversely, it was appropriate in all groups if there was severe angina (CCS Class II-IV), as long as PCI could be done (lack of a CTO) or the stress test was low risk.

Using these criteria, Chan et al. examined the frequency of appropriate indications for PCI from more than 500,000 PCI procedures in the NCDR registry.[31] They found that the majority of patients with acute indications (largely ACS) were appropriate (98.6%), while only 50.4% of nonacute indications (largely SIHD) were appropriate and 11.6% were inappropriate. Others have shown the rate of inappropriate procedures to be as high as 25% in SIHD.[32] The study by Chan also demonstrated great variability in the frequency

Anatomic setting	COR	LOE
UPLM or complex CAD		
CABG and PCI	I—Heart team approach recommended	C
CABG and PCI	IIa—Calculation of STS and SYNTAX scores	B
UPLM*		
CABG	I	B
PCI	IIa—For SIHD when both of the following are present: • Anatomic conditions associated with a low risk of PCI procedural complications and a high likelihood of good long-term outcome (eg, a low SYNTAX score of ≤22, ostial or trunk left main CAD) • Clinical characteristics that predict a significantly increased risk of adverse surgical outcomes (eg, STS-predicted risk of operative mortality ≥5%)	B
	IIa—For UA/NSTEMI if not a CABG candidate	B
	IIa—For STEMI when distal coronary flow is TIMI flow grade <3 and PCI can be performed more rapidly and safely than CABG	C
	IIb—For SIHD when *both* of the following are present: • Anatomic conditions associated with a low to intermediate risk of PCI procedural complications and an intermediate to high likelihood of good long-term outcome (eg, low-intermediate SYNTAX score of <33, bifurcation left main CAD) • Clinical characteristics that predict an increased risk of adverse surgical outcomes (eg, moderate—severe COPD, disability from prior stroke, or prior cardiac surgery; STS-predicted risk of operative mortality >2%)	B
	III: Harm—For SIHD in patients (versus performing CABG) with unfavorable anatomy for PCI and who are good candidates for CABG	B
3-vessel disease with or without proximal LAD artery disease*		
CABG	I	B
	IIa—It is reasonable to choose CABG over PCI in patients with complex 3-vessel CAD (eg, SYNTAX score >22) who are good candidates for CABG	B
PCI	IIb—Of uncertain benefit	B
2-vessel disease with proximal LAD artery disease*		
CABG	I	B
PCI	IIb—Of uncertain benefit	B
2-vessel disease without proximal LAD artery disease*		
CABG	IIa—With extensive ischemia	B
	IIb—Of uncertain benefit without extensive ischemia	C
PCI	IIb—Of uncertain benefit	B
1-vessel proximal LAD artery disease		
CABG	IIa—With LIMA for long-term benefit	B
PCI	IIb—Of uncertain benefit	B
1-vessel disease without proximal LAD artery involvement		
CABG	III: Harm	B
PCI	III: Harm	B
LV dysfunction		
CABG	IIa—EF 35% to 50%	B
CABG	IIb—EF <35% without significant left main CAD	B
PCI	Insufficient data	
Survivors of sudden cardiac death with presumed ischemia-mediated VT		
CABG	I	B
PCI	I	C
No anatomic or physiological criteria for revascularization		
CABG	III: Harm	B
PCI	III: Harm	B

FIGURE 2-7 Revascularization to improve survival compared to medical therapy. *(Used with permission from Fihn SD, Gardin JM, Abrams J, et al: 2012 ACCF/AHA/ACP/AATS/PCNA/SCAI/STS guideline for the diagnosis and management of patients with stable ischemic heart disease: a report of the American College of Cardiology Foundation/American Heart Association task force on practice guidelines, and the American College of Physicians, American Association for Thoracic Surgery, Preventive Cardiovascular Nurses Association, Society for Cardiovascular Angiography and Interventions, and Society of Thoracic Surgeons. Circulation 126:e354–e471, 2012.[26])*

Clinical setting	COR	LOE
≥1 significant stenosis amenable to revascularization and unacceptable angina despite GDMT	I—CABG I—PCI	A
≥1 significant stenosis and unacceptable angina in whom GDMT cannot be implemented because of medication contraindications, adverse effects, or patient preferences	IIa—CABG IIa—PCI	C C
Previous CABG with ≥1 significant stenosis associated with ischemia and unacceptable angina despite GDMT	IIa—PCI IIb—CABG	C C
Complex 3-vessel CAD (eg, SYNTAX score >22) with or without involvement of the proximal LAD artery and a good candidate for CABG	IIa—CABG preferred over PCI	B
Viable ischemic myocardium that is perfused by coronary arteries that are not amenable to grafting	IIb—TMR as an adjunct to CABG	B
No anatomic or physiologic criteria for revascularization	III: Harm—CABG III: Harm—PCI	C C

FIGURE 2-8 Revascularization to improve symptoms. *(Used with permission from Fihn SD, Gardin JM, Abrams J, et al: 2012 ACCF/AHA/ACP/AATS/PCNA/SCAI/STS guideline for the diagnosis and management of patients with stable ischemic heart disease: a report of the American College of Cardiology Foundation/American Heart Association task force on practice guidelines, and the American College of Physicians, American Association for Thoracic Surgery, Preventive Cardiovascular Nurses Association, Society for Cardiovascular Angiography and Interventions, and Society of Thoracic Surgeons. Circulation 126:e354–e471, 2012.[26])*

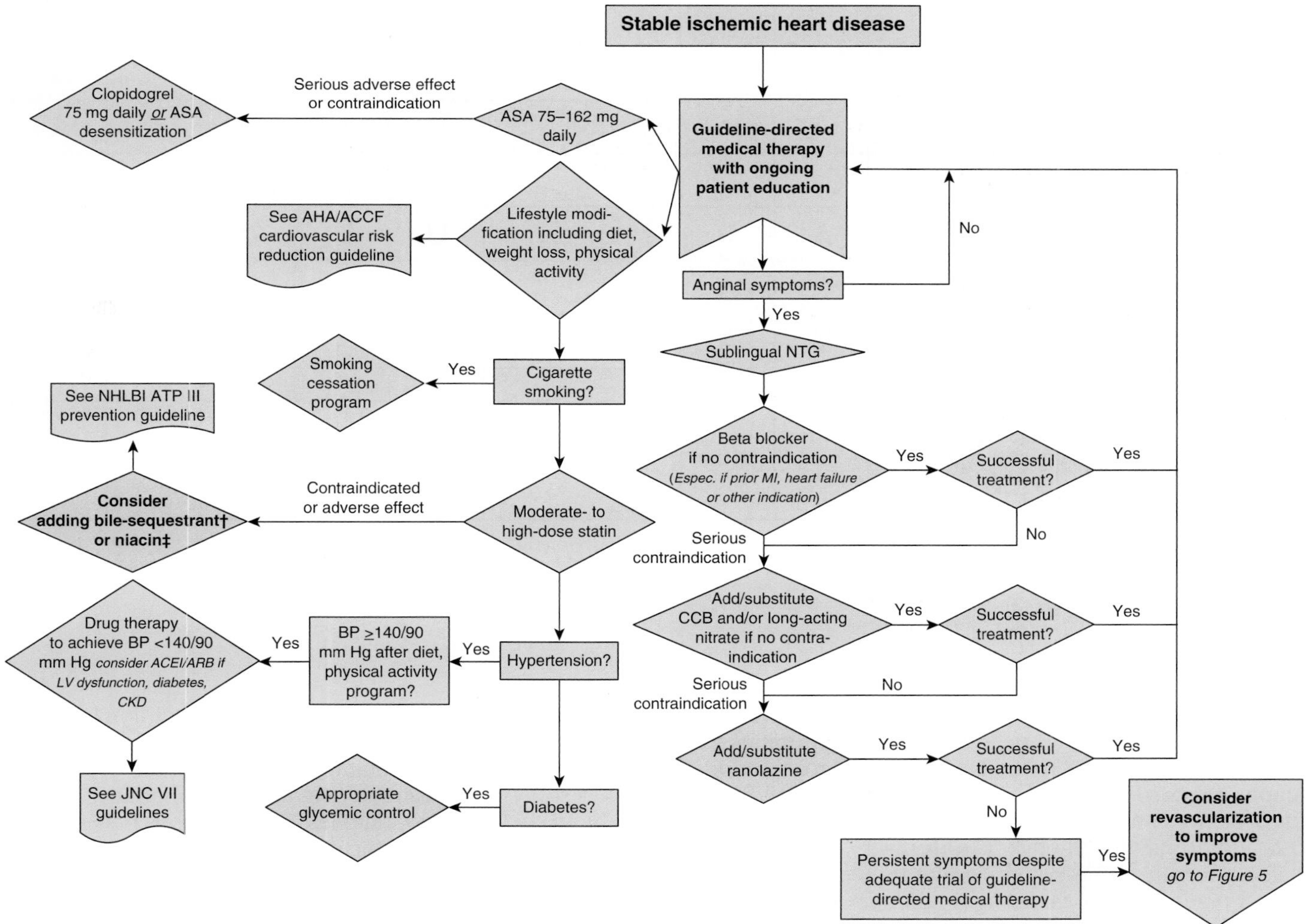

FIGURE 2-9 Treatment of patients with SIHD. *(Used with permission from Fihn SD, Gardin JM, Abrams J, et al: 2012 ACCF/AHA/ACP/AATS/PCNA/SCAI/STS guideline for the diagnosis and management of patients with stable ischemic heart disease: a report of the American College of Cardiology Foundation/American Heart Association task force on practice guidelines, and the American College of Physicians, American Association for Thoracic Surgery, Preventive Cardiovascular Nurses Association, Society for Cardiovascular Angiography and Interventions, and Society of Thoracic Surgeons. Circulation 126:e354–e471, 2012.[26])*

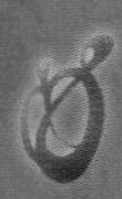

Low risk findings on noninvasive study					
Symptoms Med. Rx					
Class III or IV Max Rx	U	A	A	A	A
Class I or II Max Rx	U	U	A	A	A
Asymptomatic Max Rx	I	I	U	U	U
Class III or IV No/min Rx	I	U	A	A	A
Class I or II No/min Rx	I	I	U	U	U
Asymptomatic No/min Rx	I	I	U	U	U
Coronary anatomy	CTO of 1 vz.; no other disease	1-2 vz. disease; no Prox. LAD	1 vz. disease of Prox. LAD	2 vz. disease with Prox. LAD	3 vz. disease; no Left Main

Asymptomatic					
Stress Test Med. Rx					
High Risk Max Rx	U	A	A	A	A
High Risk No/min Rx	U	U	A	A	A
Int. Risk Max Rx	U	U	U	U	A
Int. Risk No/min Rx	I	I	U	U	A
Low Risk Max Rx	I	I	U	U	U
Low Risk No/min Rx	I	I	U	U	U
Coronary anatomy	CTO of 1 vz.; no other disease	1-2 vz. disease; no Prox. LAD	1 vz. disease of Prox. LAD	2 vz. disease with Prox. LAD	3 vz. disease; no Left Main

Intermediate risk findings on noninvasive study					
Symptoms Med. Rx					
Class III or IV Max Rx	A	A	A	A	A
Class I or II Max Rx	U	A	A	A	A
Asymptomatic Max Rx	U	U	U	U	A
Class III or IV No/min Rx	U	U	A	A	A
Class I or II No/min Rx	U	U	U	A	A
Asymptomatic No/min Rx	I	I	U	U	A
Coronary anatomy	CTO of 1 vz.; no other disease	1-2 vz. disease; no Prox. LAD	1 vz. disease of Prox. LAD	2 vz. disease with Prox. LAD	3 vz. disease; no Left Main

CCS Class I or II Angina					
Stress Test Med. Rx					
High Risk Max Rx	A	A	A	A	A
High Risk No/min Rx	U	A	A	A	A
Int. Risk Max Rx	U	A	A	A	A
Int. Risk No/min Rx	U	U	U	A	A
Low Risk Max Rx	U	U	A	A	A
Low Risk No/min Rx	I	I	U	U	U
Coronary anatomy	CTO of 1 vz.; no other disease	1-2 vz. disease; no Prox. LAD	1 vz. disease of Prox. LAD	2 vz. disease with Prox. LAD	3 vz. disease; no Left Main

FIGURE 2-10 Appropriateness criteria for non-acute indications. *(Used with permission from Patel MR, Dehmer GJ, Hirshfeld JW, et al: ACCF/SCAI/STS/AATS/AHA/ASNC/HFSA/SCCT 2012 appropriate use criteria for coronary revascularization focused update: a report of the American College of Cardiology Foundation appropriate use criteria task force, Society for Cardiovascular Angiography and Interventions, Society of Thoracic Surgeons, American Association for Thoracic Surgery, American Heart Association, American Society of Nuclear Cardiology, and The Society of Cardiovascular Computed Tomography. J Am Coll Cardiol 59:857–881, 2012.[30])*

of inappropriate indications from one hospital to another (range 6% to 16.7% IQR), suggesting that opportunities exist to improve quality. One of the most common reasons for an inappropriate procedure was the presence of mild symptoms or no symptoms, no noninvasive assessment or low risk, and no medical therapy (**Table 2-4**).

The strength of the criteria is that they more accurately reflect practice by considering a number of key factors in the decision for a specific procedure. However, despite consideration of up to five factors, they still do not account for all of the factors that may sway a decision one way or another in a specific patient.[33] In addition, they are derived from an expert panel that relies on expert opinion in a large majority of the criteria.[34] This leads to less confidence that the criteria are representative of practice and reproducible. One study demonstrated significant variability (up to twofold) in the appropriateness classifications between two panels of experts using the same evidence for cardiac catheterization.[35] The criteria have led to a better understanding of the use of procedures in practice and can help to develop better systems to reduce variability. They have also been used during pretest screening to reduce variability. Due to the lower reliability of the criteria, they should not be used as a basis for reimbursement.

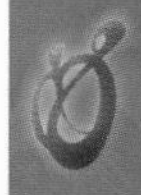

High risk findings on noninvasive study					
Symptoms Med. Rx					
Class III or IV Max Rx	A	A	A	A	A
Class I or II Max Rx	A	A	A	A	A
Asymptomatic Max Rx	U	A	A	A	A
Class III or IV No/min Rx	A	A	A	A	A
Class I or II No/min Rx	U	A	A	A	A
Asymptomatic No/min Rx	U	U	A	A	A
Coronary anatomy	CTO of 1 vz.; no other disease	1-2 vz. disease; no Prox. LAD	1 vz. disease of Prox. LAD	2 vz. disease with Prox. LAD	3 vz. disease; no Left Main

CCS Class III or IV Angina					
Stress Test Med. Rx					
High Risk Max Rx	A	A	A	A	A
High Risk No/min Rx	A	A	A	A	A
Int. Risk Max Rx	A	A	A	A	A
Int. Risk No/min Rx	U	U	A	A	A
Low Risk Max Rx	U	A	A	A	A
Low Risk No/min Rx	I	U	A	A	A
Coronary anatomy	CTO of 1 vz.; no other disease	1-2 vz. disease; no Prox. LAD	1 vz. disease of Prox. LAD	2 vz. disease with Prox. LAD	3 vz. disease; no Left Main

FIGURE 2-10, cont'd

TABLE 2-4 Most Common Reasons to Be Classified as Inappropriate

APPROPRIATE USE CRITERIA SCENARIO NO.*	ANATOMY	PRIOR CABG	SYMPTOMS	CARDIAC RISK (STRESS TEST)	ANTI-ISCHEMIC THERAPY	NO. (%)
Inappropriate PCI 12B	One- or two-vessel CAD, no proximal LAD involvement	No	CCS Class I or II	Low	None/minimal	6662 (39.6)
14A	One- or two-vessel CAD, no proximal LAD involvement	No	Asymptomatic	Intermediate	None/minimal	4127 (24.5)
12A	One- or two-vessel CAD, no proximal LAD involvement	No	Asymptomatic	Low	None/minimal	3083 (18.3)
54B	≥1 Stenoses in non-CABG territory, all bypass grafts patent	Yes	CCS Class I or II	Low	None/minimal	568 (3.4)
56A	≥1 Stenoses in non-CABG territory, all bypass grafts patent	Yes	Asymptomatic	Intermediate	None/minimal	493 (2.9)

Reprinted with permission from Chan PS, Patel MR, Klein LW, et al: Appropriateness of percutaneous coronary intervention. JAMA 306:53–61, 2011.[31]
*Scenario numbers from Patel et al.[30]

OTHER METHODS TO IMPROVE QUALITY

Performance Measures

Performance measures are selected quality metrics that are evidence based, interpretable, definable, actionable, reliable, valid, and feasible to be collected and reported. They are best used to measure quality and compare outcomes among different institutions and they have been used in public reporting.[36] Accordingly they are usually few in number. Recently, the ACCF/AHA/SCAI/AMA-Convened PCIP/NCQA 2013 Performance Measure for Adults Undergoing Percutaneous Coronary Intervention was published.[37] The prior performance measures in cardiology were focused on acute MI and CHF, and the 2013 measures are the first to directly address PCI performance. The committee identified 10 measures that were determined to meet the above criteria and to have a high impact on improving quality (**Table 2-5**). The dimensions of care ranged from diagnostics, patient education, and treatment. Only one, cardiac rehabilitation referral, also involved patient self-management and

TABLE 2-5 The ACC/AHA/SCAI/AMA-Convened PCIP/NCQA 2013 Performance Measure for Adults Undergoing Percutaneous Coronary Intervention

1. Comprehensive documentation of indications for PCI
2. Appropriate indication for elective PCI
3. Assessment of candidacy for dual-antiplatelet therapy
4. Use of embolic protection devices in the treatment of saphenous vein bypass graft disease
5. Documentation of preprocedural glomerular filtration rate and contrast dose used during the procedure
6. Radiation dose documentation
7. Postprocedural optimal medical therapy composite
8. Cardiac rehabilitation patient referral
9. Regional or national PCI registry participation
10. Annual operator and hospital PCI volume

Reprinted with permission from Nallamothu BK, Tommaso CL, Anderson HV, et al: ACC/AHA/SCAI/AMA-Convened PCIP/NCQA 2013 performance measures for adults undergoing percutaneous coronary intervention: a report of the American College of Cardiology/American Heart Association task force on performance measures, the Society for Cardiovascular Angiography and Interventions, the American Medical Association-Convened Physician Consortium for Performance Improvement, and the National Committee for Quality Assurance. Circulation 2013.[37]

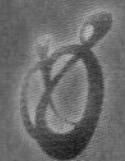

monitoring of disease. A detailed description and rationale for choosing these criteria are available in the references.

While many of the performance measures for PCI are designated for internal quality control, others are intended for monitoring of hospital quality and comparisons among hospitals. If accurate data can be collected on all measures then they will be used to assess hospital quality in the future.

CMS and insurance companies have used the established performance measures for AMI and CHF for pay-for-performance (P4P) financial incentives. Studies to date have failed to show whether P4P actually improves care and quality beyond what is occurring due to other efforts.[38] In addition, it is not clear whether P4P has reduced unnecessary procedures and hospital and health care costs. Future studies are needed to determine whether P4P is an effective method to improve quality.

Public Reporting

Many states publically report risk-adjusted cardiac surgical outcomes by hospital. The goal is to provide information to the public so that individuals can make informed decisions about where to get the best care and to improve quality by incenting hospitals with high mortality rates to improve outcomes. The public reporting of PCI outcomes has only recently been instituted.[39] Whether public reporting can reduce cost and mortality is uncertain. Data from three states with public reporting of PCI (New York, Pennsylvania, and Massachusetts) have shown that the rates of PCI for acute MI were less than in states without public reporting.[40] The differences in the use of PCI were greatest for patients with cardiogenic shock. Interestingly, mortality was not different among the states with and without public reporting. Other studies have suggested a positive impact of public reporting with a reduction in mortality.[41] The decline in mortality in these studies may have been due to improved selection of patients with a decision not to intervene on patients in whom the procedure was futile, but other factors could have contributed as well, including underreporting due to exclusions.[42] Future studies are needed to determine the value of public reporting.

Putting Guidelines into Practice

Guidelines have provided authoritative recommendations for the treatment of cardiovascular disease. The documents are lengthy and difficult to read and integrate into clinical practice. A number of efforts have been introduced to more effectively put guidelines into practice. These have included the AHA Get-with-the-Guidelines. This is a voluntary hospital program to record the following information on a simple web-based form at the time of discharge: patient demographics, hospital course, and the use of secondary prevention guidelines for acute coronary syndromes, stroke, resuscitation, atrial fibrillation, and heart failure. In the participating hospitals, improvement in adherence to performance measures has been shown and better short-term outcomes have been reported in all of the conditions listed above.[43,44] The limitation of this approach is that guidelines, and particularly performance measures, do not deal with areas of the greatest uncertainty, fail to account for variations in local practice, do not account for comorbidities, and do not have a process for continuous quality improvement based on outcomes.

A novel approach to overcome these limitations has been the introduction of the standardized clinical assessment and management plan (SCAMP).[45,46] The goal is to improve quality by narrowing practice variability while providing continuous improvement of the critical pathways. Due to improved use of testing and treatment, SCAMPs also reduce cost as well. The process begins by identifying areas where there is significant practice variability due to uncertainty and lack of adequate data. A group of clinicians formulate a care pathway based on guidelines and expert opinion. Areas of knowledge gaps are clearly identified, and data that need to be collected to understand these gaps and variations in practice patterns are identified. The individual SCAMPs are intended to be brief and focused. The key component is that variations in practice are not prevented or discouraged but rather encouraged. When there is a deviation from the care pathway, the physician is prompted to document the rationale. Data are collected on specialized forms and entered into a database. Following a set time period, which is typically 6 to 12 months, the SCAMP data are analyzed, focusing on the initial areas of uncertainty and practice variations. The committee then revises the SCAMPs based on the outcomes and pays particular attention to the outliers who did not follow the pathway. This results in a continuously updated pathway based on new knowledge and experience that is specific to the institution and practice. Initial experience with 49 SCAMPs in nine states has shown a decrease in practice variation, reduction in the unnecessary use of resources with reduced cost, and improvement in stakeholder's engagement.[45,46]

CONCLUSIONS

The improvement in the quality of care is a fundamental goal for all aspects of medical care. The development of guidelines has been the cornerstone of this effort. Despite their recognized limitations, they provide valuable guidance for clinical practice and are the basis for all of the other methods to improve quality. Appropriateness criteria are most germane to interventional cardiology, since they are best applied to procedures and are likely to help reduce variability and improve quality. Performance measures, P4P, and public reporting may also be helpful, but further study is needed. Iterative clinical pathways such as SCAMPs need further study but provide some advantages over other methods by assessing variability in practice and focusing on areas of greatest uncertainty.

References

1. Geoffrey M: *Crossing the quality chasm*, Washington, DC, 2001, Institute of Medicine.
2. Califf RM: The benefits of moving quality to a national level. *Am Heart J* 156:1019–1022, 2008.
3. Gibbons RJ, Smith S, Antman E: American College of Cardiology/American Heart Association clinical practice guidelines: part i: where do they come from? *Circulation* 107:2979–2986, 2003.
4. Gibbons RJ, Smith SC, Jr, Antman E: American College of Cardiology/American Heart Association clinical practice guidelines: part ii: evolutionary changes in a continuous quality improvement project. *Circulation* 107:3101–3107, 2003.
5. Jacobs AK, Kushner FG, Ettinger SM, et al: ACCF/AHA clinical practice guideline methodology summit report: a report of the American College of Cardiology Foundation/American Heart Association task force on practice guidelines. *Circulation* 127:268–310, 2013.
6. Tricoci P, Allen JM, Kramer JM, et al: Scientific evidence underlying the ACC/AHA clinical practice guidelines. *JAMA* 301:831–841, 2009.
7. O'Gara PT, Kushner FG, Ascheim DD, et al: 2013 ACCF/AHA guideline for the management of ST-elevation myocardial infarction: a report of the American College of Cardiology Foundation/American Heart Association task force on practice guidelines. *Circulation* 127:e362–e425, 2013.
8. Krumholz HM, Herrin J, Miller LE, et al: Improvements in door-to-balloon time in the United States, 2005 to 2010. *Circulation* 124:1038–1045, 2011.
9. Menees DS, Gurm HS: Door-to-balloon time and mortality. *N Engl J Med* 370:181–182, 2014.
10. Bradley EH, Herrin J, Wang Y, et al: Strategies for reducing the door-to-balloon time in acute myocardial infarction. *N Engl J Med* 355:2308–2320, 2006.
11. Denktas AE, Anderson HV, McCarthy J, et al: Total ischemic time: the correct focus of attention for optimal ST-segment elevation myocardial infarction care. *JACC Cardiovasc Interv* 4:599–604, 2011.
12. Stone GW, Witzenbichler B, Guagliumi G, et al: Bivalirudin during primary PCI in acute myocardial infarction. *N Engl J Med* 358:2218–2230, 2008.
13. De Luca G, Navarese EP, Suryapranata H: A meta-analytic overview of thrombectomy during primary angioplasty. *Int J Cardiol* 166:606–612, 2013.

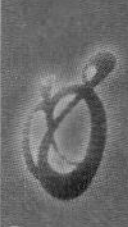

14. Frobert O, Lagerqvist B, Olivecrona GK, et al: Thrombus aspiration during ST-segment elevation myocardial infarction. *N Engl J Med* 369:1587–1597, 2013.
15. Sabate M, Cequier A, Iniguez A, et al: Everolimus-eluting stent versus bare-metal stent in ST-segment elevation myocardial infarction (examination): 1 year results of a randomised controlled trial. *Lancet* 380:1482–1490, 2012.
16. Wald DS, Morris JK, Wald NJ, et al: Randomized trial of preventive angioplasty in myocardial infarction. *N Engl J Med* 369:1115–1123, 2013.
17. Anderson JL, Adams CD, Antman EM, et al: ACC/AHA 2007 guidelines for the management of patients with unstable angina/non ST-elevation myocardial infarction: a report of the American College of Cardiology Foundation/American Heart Association task force on practice guidelines (writing committee to revise the 2002 guidelines for the management of patients with unstable angina/non ST-elevation myocardial infarction): developed in collaboration with the American College of Emergency Physicians, the Society for Cardiovascular Angiography and Interventions, and the Society of Thoracic Surgeons: endorsed by the American Association of Cardiovascular and Pulmonary Rehabilitation and the Society for Academic Emergency Medicine. *Circulation* 116:e148–e304, 2007.
18. Anderson JL, Adams CD, Antman EM, et al: 2011 ACCF/AHA focused update incorporated into the ACC/AHA 2007 guidelines for the management of patients with unstable angina/non-ST-elevation myocardial infarction: a report of the American College of Cardiology Foundation/American Heart Association task force on practice guidelines. *Circulation* 123:e426–e579, 2011.
19. Jneid H, Anderson JL, Wright RS, et al: 2012 ACCF/AHA focused update of the guideline for the management of patients with unstable angina/non-ST-elevation myocardial infarction (updating the 2007 guideline and replacing the 2011 focused update): a report of the American College of Cardiology Foundation/American Heart Association task force on practice guidelines. *Circulation* 126:875–910, 2012.
20. Lindner G, Pfortmueller CA, Braun CT, et al: Non-acute myocardial infarction-related causes of elevated high-sensitive troponin t in the emergency room: a cross-sectional analysis. *Intern Emerg Med* 2013.
21. Sanchis J, Bodi V, Nunez J, et al: New risk score for patients with acute chest pain, non-ST-segment deviation, and normal troponin concentrations: a comparison with the TIMI risk score. *J Am Coll Cardiol* 46:443–449, 2005.
22. Mehta SR, Granger CB, Boden WE, et al: Early versus delayed invasive intervention in acute coronary syndromes. *N Engl J Med* 360:2165–2175, 2009.
23. Farkouh ME, Domanski M, Fuster V: Revascularization strategies in patients with diabetes. *N Engl J Med* 368:1455–1456, 2013.
24. Gibbons RJ, Abrams J, Chatterjee K, et al: ACC/AHA 2002 guideline update for the management of patients with chronic stable angina—summary article: a report of the American College of Cardiology/American Heart Association task force on practice guidelines (committee on the management of patients with chronic stable angina). *Circulation* 107:149–158, 2003.
25. Fraker TD, Jr, Fihn SD, Gibbons RJ, et al: 2007 chronic angina focused update of the ACC/AHA 2002 guidelines for the management of patients with chronic stable angina: a report of the American College of Cardiology/American Heart Association task force on practice guidelines writing group to develop the focused update of the 2002 guidelines for the management of patients with chronic stable angina. *Circulation* 116:2762–2772, 2007.
26. Fihn SD, Gardin JM, Abrams J, et al: 2012 ACCF/AHA/ACP/AATS/PCNA/SCAI/STS guideline for the diagnosis and management of patients with stable ischemic heart disease: a report of the American College of Cardiology Foundation/American Heart Association task force on practice guidelines, and the American College of Physicians, American Association for Thoracic Surgery, Preventive Cardiovascular Nurses Association, Society for Cardiovascular Angiography and Interventions, and Society of Thoracic Surgeons. *Circulation* 126:e354–e471, 2012.
27. Hlatky MA, Boothroyd DB, Baker L, et al: Comparative effectiveness of multivessel coronary bypass surgery and multivessel percutaneous coronary intervention: a cohort study. *Ann Intern Med* 158:727–734, 2013.
28. Kappetein AP, Head SJ, Morice MC, et al: Treatment of complex coronary artery disease in patients with diabetes: 5-year results comparing outcomes of bypass surgery and percutaneous coronary intervention in the syntax trial. *Eur J Cardiothorac Surg* 43:1006–1013, 2013.
29. Patel MR, Dehmer GJ, Hirshfeld JW, et al: ACCF/SCAI/STS/AATS/AHA/ASNC 2009 appropriateness criteria for coronary revascularization: a report of the American College of Cardiology Foundation appropriateness criteria task force, Society for Cardiovascular Angiography and Interventions, Society of Thoracic Surgeons, American Association for Thoracic Surgery, American Heart Association, and the American Society of Nuclear Cardiology: endorsed by the American Society of Echocardiography, the Heart Failure Society of America, and the Society of Cardiovascular Computed Tomography. *Circulation* 119:1330–1352, 2009.
30. Patel MR, Dehmer GJ, Hirshfeld JW, et al: ACCF/SCAI/STS/AATS/AHA/ASNC/HFSA/SCCT 2012 appropriate use criteria for coronary revascularization focused update: a report of the American College of Cardiology Foundation appropriate use criteria task force, Society for Cardiovascular Angiography and Interventions, Society of Thoracic Surgeons, American Association for Thoracic Surgery, American Heart Association, American Society of Nuclear Cardiology, and the Society of Cardiovascular Computed Tomography. *J Am Coll Cardiol* 59:857–881, 2012.
31. Chan PS, Patel MR, Klein LW, et al: Appropriateness of percutaneous coronary intervention. *JAMA* 306:53–61, 2011.
32. Hannan EL, Samadashvili Z, Cozzens K, et al: Appropriateness of diagnostic catheterization for suspected coronary artery disease in New York State. *Circ Cardiovasc Interv* 2014.
33. Marso SP, Teirstein PS, Kereiakes DJ, et al: Percutaneous coronary intervention use in the United States: defining measures of appropriateness. *JACC Cardiovasc Interv* 5:229–235, 2012.
34. Faxon DP: Assessing appropriateness of coronary angiography: another step in improving quality. *Ann Intern Med* 149:276–278, 2008.
35. Hemingway H, Chen R, Junghans C, et al: Appropriateness criteria for coronary angiography in angina: reliability and validity. *Ann Intern Med* 149:221–231, 2008.
36. Bonow RO, Masoudi FA, Rumsfeld JS, et al: ACC/AHA classification of care metrics: performance measures and quality metrics: a report of the American College of Cardiology/American Heart Association task force on performance measures. *Circulation* 118:2662–2666, 2008.
37. Nallamothu BK, Tommaso CL, Anderson HV, et al: ACC/AHA/SCAI/AMA-Convened PCIP/NCQA 2013 performance measures for adults undergoing percutaneous coronary intervention: a report of the American College of Cardiology/American Heart Association task force on performance measures, the Society for Cardiovascular Angiography and Interventions, the American Medical Association-Convened Physician Consortium for Performance Improvement, and the National Committee for Quality Assurance. *Circulation* 2013.
38. Eijkenaar F, Emmert M, Scheppach M, et al: Effects of pay for performance in health care: a systematic review of systematic reviews. *Health Policy (New York)* 110:115–130, 2013.
39. Resnic FS, Welt FG: The public health hazards of risk avoidance associated with public reporting of risk-adjusted outcomes in coronary intervention. *J Am Coll Cardiol* 53:825–830, 2009.
40. Joynt KE, Blumenthal DM, Orav EJ, et al: Association of Public Reporting for Percutaneous Coronary Intervention with utilization and outcomes among Medicare beneficiaries with acute myocardial infarction. *JAMA* 308:1460–1468, 2012.
41. McCrum ML, Joynt KE, Orav EJ, et al: Mortality for publicly reported conditions and overall hospital mortality rates. *JAMA Intern Med* 173:1351–1357, 2013.
42. McCabe JM, Joynt KE, Welt FG, et al: Impact of public reporting and outlier status identification on percutaneous coronary intervention case selection in Massachusetts. *JACC Cardiovasc Interv* 6:625–630, 2013.
43. Tam LM, Fonarow GC, Bhatt DL, et al: Achievement of guideline-concordant care and in-hospital outcomes in patients with coronary artery disease in teaching and nonteaching hospitals: results from the Get with the Guidelines-coronary artery disease program. *Circ Cardiovasc Qual Outcomes* 6:58–65, 2013.
44. Somma KA, Bhatt DL, Fonarow GC, et al: Guideline adherence after ST-segment elevation versus non-ST segment elevation myocardial infarction. *Circ Cardiovasc Qual Outcomes* 5:654–661, 2012.
45. Rathod RH, Farias M, Friedman KG, et al: A novel approach to gathering and acting on relevant clinical information: SCAMPs. *Congenit Heart Dis* 5:343–353, 2010.
46. Farias M, Jenkins K, Lock J, et al: Standardized clinical assessment and management plans (SCAMPs) provide a better alternative to clinical practice guidelines. *Health Aff (Millwood)* 32:911–920, 2013.

3 Vascular Access and Closure

Sripal Bangalore

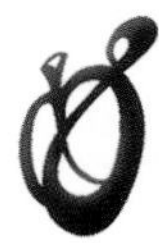

Arterial access for common coronary and vascular procedures can be obtained via the common femoral artery, radial, ulnar, or brachial arteries. More recently, the subclavian artery and direct aortic access are being used for transcatheter aortic valve replacement procedures. Arterial access site complications are common in interventional procedures,[1] and knowledge of the anatomy, optimal access techniques, and optimal techniques to obtain hemostasis postprocedure are critical to minimize such complications.

FEMORAL ARTERIAL ACCESS

Introduction

The common femoral artery (CFA) is the most commonly used site for percutaneous arterial access for coronary diagnostic, interventional, structural heart, and peripheral vascular procedures, although transradial access is on the rise in the United States and worldwide.[2] The femoral artery is often favored for its size, ease of insertion, and ability to provide a relatively less tortuous path to the heart.

Anatomic Considerations

The CFA is a continuation of the external iliac artery and passes through the femoral sheath and branches into the superficial femoral artery (SFA) and the profunda femoris artery (PFA) (**Figure 3-1A**). The femoral sheath has three compartments—from medial to lateral—the femoral canal, which contains the efferent lymphatic vessels and lymph node embedded in areolar tissue; the intermediate compartment, which contains the femoral vein; and the lateral compartment, which contains the femoral artery (**Figure 3-1B**). Lateral to the femoral artery and outside the femoral sheath is the femoral nerve. The relationship is important to avoid accidental puncture of the femoral vein or the femoral nerve. The CFA in the femoral sheath is the ideal site for femoral artery cannulation as the artery is large, less tortuous, less affected by atherosclerosis, and sits against the femoral head, making it easier to palpate and also more compressible to achieve effective hemostasis. In addition, the femoral sheath provides effective scaffolding, thereby limiting the spread of hematoma, acting as a tamponade to the arteriotomy site and preventing pseudoaneurysm formation.[3]

Knowledge of the anatomy of the CFA is essential not only to ensure sheath placement at the ideal site to avoid complications but also to troubleshoot difficulties while cannulating the artery. The access site complications are minimized if access is obtained at the "ideal" femoral puncture, which would avoid either a high puncture or a low puncture and also takes into consideration possible anatomic variations of femoral artery bifurcation. The inguinal ligament is usually 15 mm superior to the midfemoral head, and in the majority of cases (approximately 77%), the bifurcation of the femoral artery is below the level of the femoral head.[4] Hence a "target zone" from the midfemoral head to the lower border of the femoral head is ideal (**Figure 3-2**, Zone B). However, the "ideal" spot (even in the 23% of cases with high femoral artery bifurcation) is ~1 cm lateral to the most medial aspect of the femoral head, midway between its superior and inferior borders (*Rupp's rule*) (**Figures 3-2 and 3-3**).[4]

A "low" cannulation into the superficial femoral artery or the profunda femoris artery increases the risk of ischemic complications because of the smaller size of these branch arteries; increases the risk of bleeding, hematoma, and pseudoaneurysm due to lack of an underlying compressible bony structure or the scaffolding effect of the femoral sheath resulting in ineffective hemostasis; and increases the risk of arteriovenous fistula as the tributaries of the femoral vein overlie the superficial femoral artery, increasing the risk of through and through puncture to access the artery.[3] On the other hand, a "high" cannulation above the inguinal ligament (above the lower border of the inferior epigastric artery on the femoral angiogram) into the external iliac artery makes it harder to compress the artery due to a lack

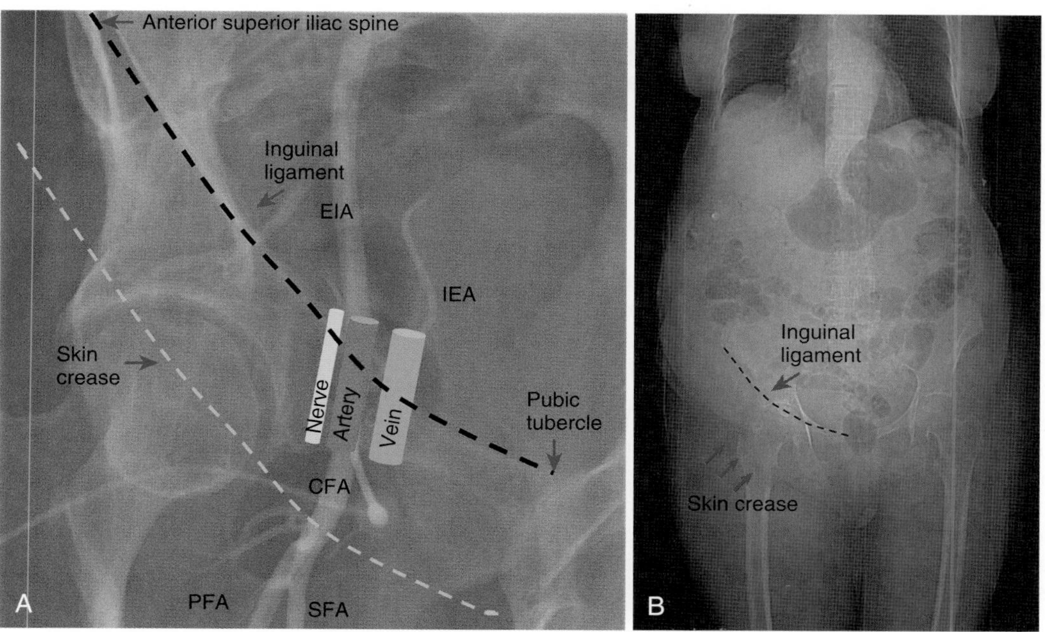

FIGURE 3-1 Femoral artery anatomy. **A,** Relationship of the femoral artery to other neurovascular bundles and the inguinal ligament. **B,** Variability in the relationship between skin crease and the inguinal ligament. *CFA,* Common femoral artery; *EIA,* external iliac artery; *PFA,* profunda femoris artery; *SFA,* superficial femoral artery. *(**A,** Adapted from Bangalore et al: Circulation 124(5):e147–e156, 2011.)*

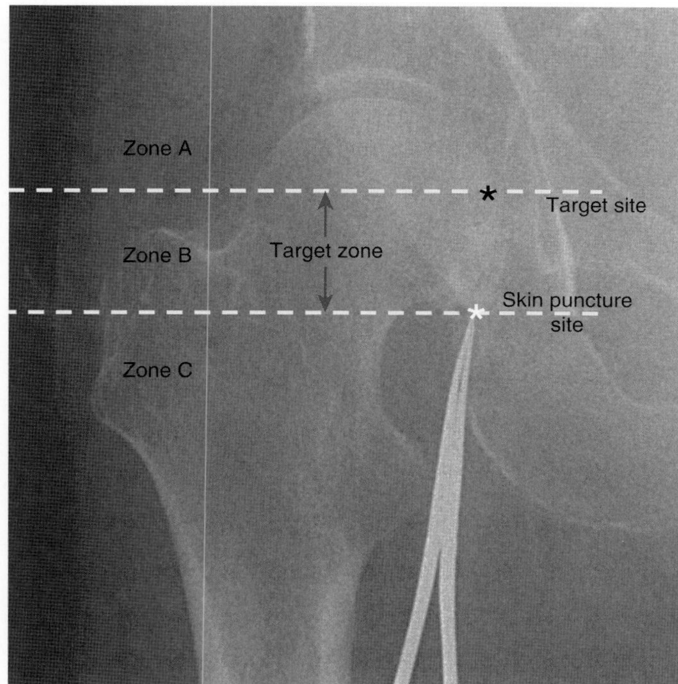

FIGURE 3-2 Target zone for femoral arterial access. The ideal skin puncture site (indicated by the hemostatic clamp and the white star) and the ideal arterial cannulation site (indicated by the black star) are shown.

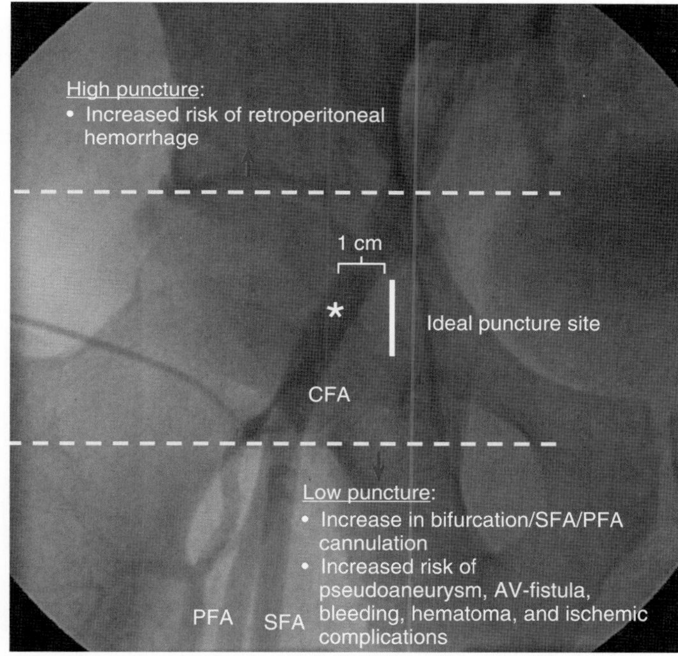

FIGURE 3-3 Rupp's rule: The ideal arterial puncture site is a point 1 cm lateral to the medial-most point of the femoral head in an AP projection on fluoroscopy (indicated by the white star). *CFA,* Common femoral artery; *PFA,* profunda femoris artery; *SFA,* superficial femoral artery.

of underlying bony structure, which increases the risk of retroperitoneal bleeding.[5] In addition, a "high" cannulation of the CFA underneath the inguinal ligament also prevents effective compression by the taut inguinal ligament, thereby increasing bleeding and hematoma.

Preprocedural Considerations

A thorough history and physical examination prior to the procedure may reveal characteristics that indicate the femoral route is not an ideal access site for the patient. Clinically significant history including the indications for the procedure should be obtained and recorded in the patient's chart. Patients with severe peripheral vascular disease, especially with known severe disease of CFA, those with ileofemoral bypass grafts or stents, those with a superficial infection at the groin puncture site or morbid obesity, those with heart failure or low back pain who may not be able to lie supine for prolonged periods of time, those on anticoagulation or thrombolytic therapy, those with recent use of a collagen-plug-based vascular closure device (VCD), and those with recent complications of the femoral artery, such as those with a pseudoaneurysm or AV fistula, may not be ideal candidates for femoral access and should be considered for alternatives, such as radial artery access. However, the above conditions by themselves are not absolute contraindications for femoral access, and in many instances, the procedure can be performed using a small size sheath or in other cases by the use of the contralateral femoral artery. In addition to a routine physical examination, inspection of the groin for any signs of infection, palpation of the femoral and distal pulses (bilateral dorsalis pedis, posterior tibial and popliteal arteries), and auscultation for bruits should be performed and documented in the patient's chart. In addition, a review of prior femoral angiograms, if available, can help plan the optimal location for an ideal femoral arterial puncture. The medications the patient is taking should be reviewed. In addition, laboratory evaluation should include measurement of hemoglobin, hematocrit, platelets, coagulation parameters, creatinine, and electrolytes.

Procedure

One or both the groins should be prepped and draped in a sterile manner. Conscious sedation should be administered using a combination of sedative and analgesic based on local practice and taking into consideration patient age (reduced dose in the elderly) and renal and hepatic functions. Conscious sedation will ensure better patient cooperation during the procedure, although it can be performed using local anesthetic alone. The first step in establishing femoral access is to locate the skin site that corresponds to the "ideal" femoral puncture site. Various external landmarks have been used to access the femoral artery (**Table 3-1**),[6] but the most popular one is by using fluoroscopic landmarks (**Figure 3-2**). In the fluoroscopic technique, the femoral head is visualized under fluoroscopy in posterior-anterior (PA) projection, and a metal clamp is then placed on the skin at the lower border of the femoral head. This corresponds to the skin puncture site, and a puncture at this site at a 30° to 45° angle will cannulate the femoral artery, corresponding to the middle of the femoral head, which is the ideal puncture site. The steps involved in femoral artery cannulation are outlined in **Table 3-2**. After a femoral sheath is inserted, the side port should be connected to the pressure transducer to obtain a femoral artery pressure waveform. Any dampening of the pressure waveform at this stage may indicate atherosclerosis in the CFA or the external iliac or sheath in a dissection plane. It is highly recommended to obtain a femoral angiogram (30°-45° ipsilateral oblique view) prior to coronary angiography (unless the glomerular filtration rate (eGFR) is low) to ensure correct placement of the femoral sheath in the CFA and to detect any complications such as dissection, perforation, or even presence of severe atherosclerotic disease in the CFA. The ipsilateral oblique view should not be used to determine a "high puncture." If a high puncture is suspected based on the ipsilateral oblique view, repeat the femoral angiogram in the P-A or the contralateral oblique view may be helpful to confirm the puncture site. Detection of problems at this stage will help plan subsequent procedures before any anticoagulation is administered (deferral of PCI for high stick or any perforation or dissection) and considerations for access site management at the end of the procedure (manual compression vs. VCD). In addition, flushing the sheath between each catheter exchange can prevent the formation of a clot within the sheath.

Special Considerations

Using a Micropuncture Needle

The standard Seldinger needle used for the femoral artery cannulation is an 18-gauge needle. A micropuncture needle is a 21-gauge needle, which decreases the size of the hole

TABLE 3-1 External Landmarks for Identifying the "Ideal" Femoral Artery Site

Skin/inguinal crease	Skin puncture site 2 cm to 3 cm below the midpoint of the skin crease. Disadvantage: Variability in the relationship between the inguinal ligament and skin crease, especially in the morbidly obese, resulting in a lack of consistency in localization of the ideal puncture site (Figure 3-1A-B).
Bony landmarks	Skin puncture site 2 cm to 3 cm below the midinguinal point (midpoint between the anterior superior iliac spine and pubic tubercle). Disadvantage: Variability in the relationship between the inguinal ligament and the midinguinal point, resulting in a lack of consistency in localization of the ideal puncture site.
Maximal impulse	Skin puncture site at the site of maximal impulse. Disadvantage: Site of maximal pulsation may not correspond to the midfemoral site (ideal puncture site), especially in the obese, resulting in low or high cannulation.
Fluoroscopic landmark	Skin puncture site at a point that corresponds to the lower border of femoral head on fluoroscopy. Provides the most consistent landmark to the midfemoral CFA site.

TABLE 3-2 Steps in Femoral Arterial Cannulation

Step 1: Administer adequate local anesthetic agent (10-20 cc) at the site of the skin entry site over the location of the femoral artery starting with a dermal bleb and working deeper. Anesthetize the area around the artery (above, medial, and lateral).

Step 2*: Palpating the femoral artery with the index and middle finger of one hand, enter the skin at the lower border of head of the femur (identified on fluoroscopy) with an 18-gauge needle at a 30° to 45° angle using the modified Seldinger technique (anterior wall stick). Some operators use fluoroscopy at this stage to ensure that the needle is at the level of the midfemoral head.

Step 3: Once the femoral artery is cannulated with the needle, ensure pulsatile blood flow before advancing a 0.035-inch J-tip guidewire into the femoral, iliac, and onto the descending aorta. If any resistance is encountered, advance the wire under fluoroscopy.

Step 4: A small (2-3 mm) skin nick can be made at this stage (optional) and exchange the cannulation needle to a femoral arterial sheath with the dilator inside it.

Step 5: Remove the J-tip guidewire and the dilator and flush the side port of the sheath using heparinized saline.

Step 6: Perform femoral angiography in the ipsilateral anterior oblique view at a 30° to 45° angulation to visualize the sheath insertion site in relation to the common femoral artery bifurcation. Consider repeat femoral angiography in the PA projection if the cannulation appears too high on the ipsilateral anterior oblique view. Some operators prefer to leave the J-tip guidewire in prior to femoral angiography to avoid injecting into the vessel wall, thereby increasing the risk of dissection.

*Some operators use the nick and tunnel approach at this stage, where a small nick (2-3 mm) is made parallel to the skin crease and an artery forceps is used to create a tunnel. Advantage: Bleeding will manifest as oozing rather than a hematoma. Disadvantage: Need for a separate nick and tunnel if the femoral artery cannulation cannot be obtained at the site of the skin nick.

by 56% and the flow through the hole by nearly sixfold over a standard 18-gauge needle, potentially decreasing complications from errant sticks or inadvertent back wall punctures.[7] However, there are no robust data to support the routine use of micropuncture in all cases to reduce the risk of femoral access site complications. For access using a micropuncture needle, the skin is entered at the site corresponding to the lower border of the femoral head on fluoroscopy using the 21-gauge needle. Some operators use fluoroscopy before entering the vessel to ensure that the tip of the needle is at the desired site and repositioning as needed. After ensuring blood flow from the hub (may not be as pulsatile), a floppy-tipped 0.018-inch guidewire is then advanced into the CFA and the external iliac artery. Advancing the guidewire under fluoroscopy may be preferred as resistance to advancement is better seen than felt with the finer guidewire of the micropuncture set. The needle is now exchanged for a 4 Fr short catheter with a 3 Fr inner dilator. Both the guidewire and the dilator are removed, at which point there should be pulsatile blood flow, followed by introduction of the 0.035/0.038-inch guidewire and exchange of the 4 Fr catheter to the appropriate size femoral sheath. Alternatively, the inner dilator can be used to perform a femoral angiogram. If the cannulation site is too high or low, the dilator is removed and pressure is applied to ensure hemostasis and reaccess are performed at the optimal location.

Using a SmartNeedle Percutaneous Doppler Vascular Access Device

In patients with a difficult to palpate femoral pulse, the SmartNeedle (Vascular Solutions, Inc., Minneapolis, Minn.) may be helpful. The SmartNeedle consists of a detachable Doppler probe inside the lumen of a standard introducer needle. This is connected to a handheld monitor by a cable and the flow is detected by an audio output. Attach the cable of the needle to the connector on the SmartNeedle monitor, turn the monitor on, and adjust the volume as needed. Test the system by dipping the needle in water and moving it back and forth. An audible Doppler signal should be heard. Flush the needle with saline to remove any air. Now insert the needle through the skin with a saline syringe connected, while listening to the Doppler signal. Express a small amount of saline through the tip to clear any air bubbles. Move the needle in a circular motion while listening to the Doppler flow signal. As the needle approaches the artery, the Doppler signal becomes louder and pulsatile, thus assisting femoral arterial cannulation. Arterial flow may be identified as a pulsatile high frequency sound whereas the venous flow is a low frequency sound. Care must be taken not to palpate the artery/vein while advancing the needle, as this can compress the vein and obliterate the venous signal. Once a Doppler signal is detected, the area should be scanned for the loudest signal and then the needle further advanced in the direction. Once the needle enters the artery, there is a pulsatile flow of blood (may not be as brisk as a regular needle due to the probe in place). The Doppler probe is now removed from the needle, a guidewire is inserted, and the other steps are similar to what is described in **Table 3-2**. When compared with a standard needle, the SmartNeedle has been shown to result in a greater proportion of successful femoral arterial cannulations on first attempt and to reduce the risk of hematoma.[8]

Using Ultrasound Guidance

For patients with a difficult to palpate femoral artery pulse, femoral artery cannulation under ultrasound guidance is an option. Arterial cannulation under ultrasound guidance is similar to central venous access using a similar approach. The advantage of this approach is direct visualization of the artery prior to cannulation thereby avoiding cannulation into diseased segments, cannulating branch arteries when there are anatomic variants (high bifurcation), or accidental venous puncture in anatomical variants where the femoral vein (or its tributaries) lies directly above the artery. The disadvantage is the need for a vascular transducer probe and extra time to set up the equipment and for the additional steps involved. The technique involves using a 7-MHz vascular transducer probe draped in a sterile sleeve. The ultrasound is then held at the site of the proposed skin puncture site (determined on fluoroscopy) and moved caudally to visualize the femoral bifurcation and then cranially (**Figure 3-4**). The femoral artery can be differentiated from the femoral vein, as it is less compressible, by the direction of blood flow on color Doppler ultrasonography, and by a triphasic signal (versus a more monophasic signal for the femoral vein) on pulse Doppler ultrasonography (**Figure 3-5**). Once a relatively disease-free segment is identified in the CFA, arterial cannulation can be performed under direct ultrasound guidance holding the ultrasound probe in one hand or by a second operator and the needle in the other hand. Local anesthesia is administered around the artery under direct ultrasound guidance. The Seldinger needle is then used and its position adjusted based on the ultrasound image until the artery is cannulated and confirmed by pulsatile blood. An ultrasound probe with an integral needle guide and built-in needle position sensors are now available (**Figure 3-4**). Together these project on the ultrasound monitor an enhanced virtual image of the needle as it moves through the tissue toward and into the target vessel. Once the path is confirmed on the monitor, the needle is inserted through the needle guide while advancing the needle under direct ultrasound visualization and confirmed by pulsatile blood (**Figure 3-4**). The guidewire is then inserted and the needle exchanged for an appropriate size femoral artery sheath as described previously.

Ultrasound-guided femoral arterial cannulation has been shown to aid vascular access in patients with an absent palpable pulse or after unsuccessful palpation-guided cannulation.[9] However, the data to support ultrasound-guided femoral arterial cannulation in all patients are rather weak. In a randomized trial of ultrasound-guided puncture versus traditional palpation-guided puncture of the femoral artery, ultrasound guidance significantly decreased the number of attempts needed as well as the time for successful arterial puncture only in patients with a weak arterial pulse and in those with a leg circumference of 60 cm or greater.[10] In contrast, time for vessel cannulation was increased in patients with a strong arterial pulse, and there was no difference in femoral arterial complications. In the Femoral Arterial Access With Ultrasound Trial [FAUST], routine real-time U.S. guidance improved CFA cannulation only in patients with high CFA bifurcations but reduced the number of attempts, time to access, risk of venipunctures, and vascular complications in femoral arterial access.[11]

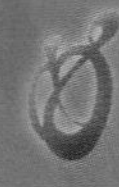

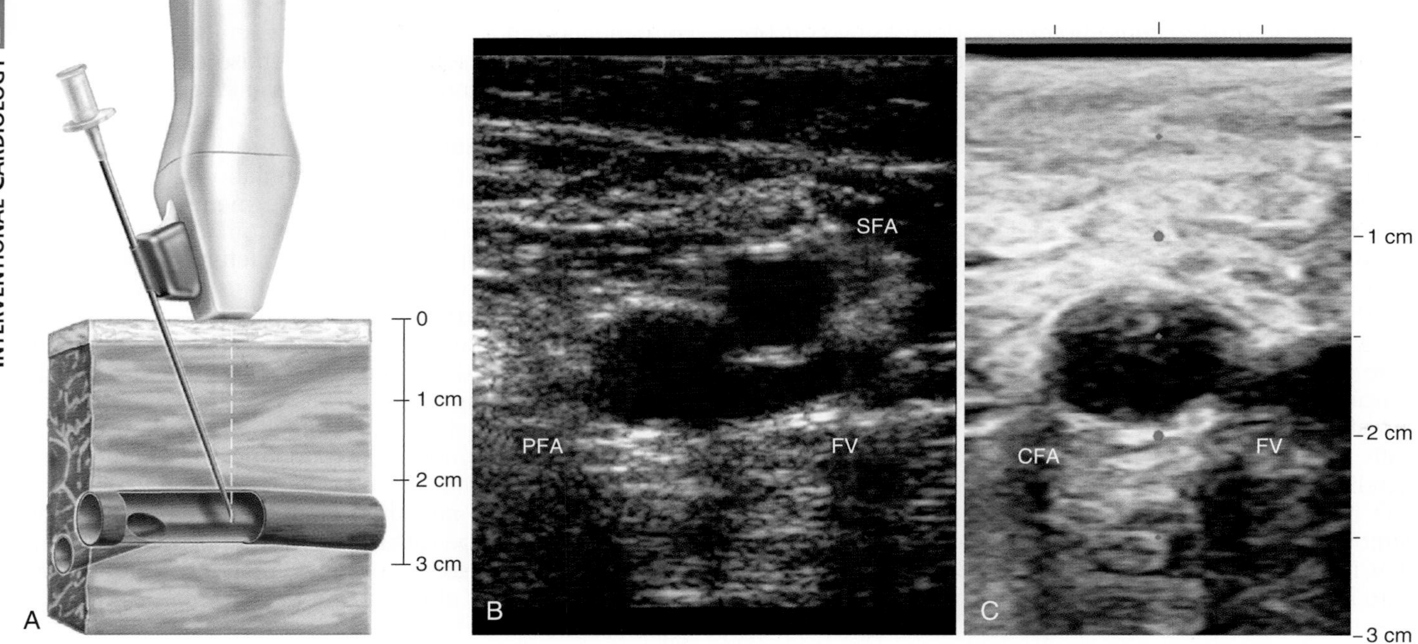

FIGURE 3-4 Ultrasound-guided femoral arterial cannulation. **A,** Ultrasound probe with the needle guide. The attached needle guide fixes the needle's angle of entry to intersect the vessel at the imaging plane 1.5 cm, 2.5 cm, or 3.5 cm below the skin, depending on the needle guide chosen. **B,** Axial view of the femoral artery bifurcation, identifying the separation of the profunda femoral artery (PFA) and superficial femoral artery (SFA). The femoral vein (FV) is differentiated from the arteries using compression. **C,** The probe is moved superiorly until the common femoral artery (CFA) is visualized. During needle advancement, the anterior wall of the vessel is kept under the central target line (green circles), which indicates the path of the needle. *(Reproduced with permission from Seto et al: JACC Cardiovasc Interv 3(7):751–758, 2010.)*

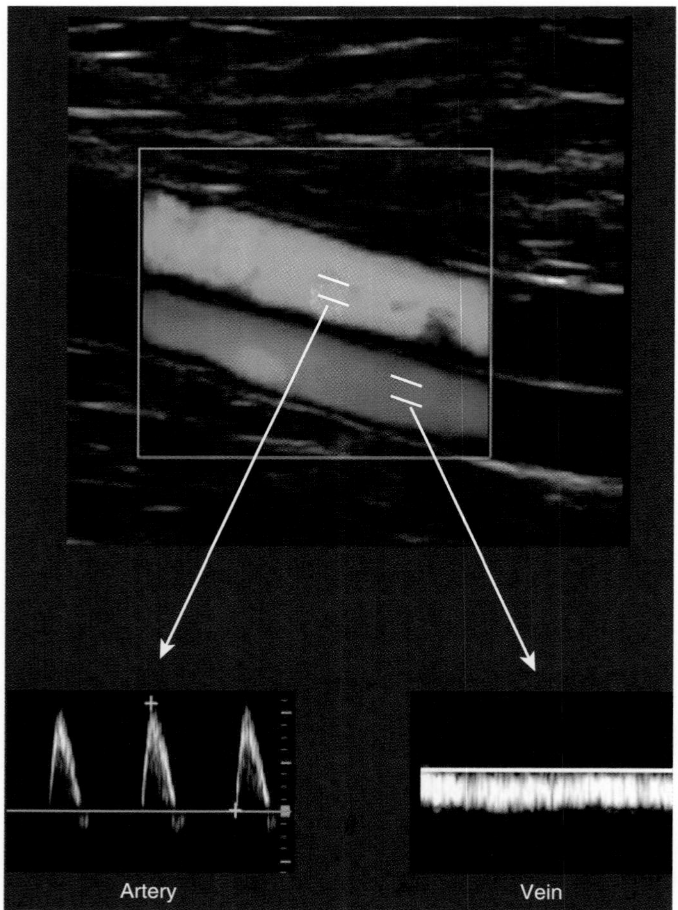

FIGURE 3-5 Color and pulse Doppler ultrasound to differentiate the artery from a vein. *(Adapted from Bangalore et al: Circulation 124(5):e147–e156, 2011.)*

Femoral Arterial Cannulation in a Challenging Patient Subgroup

Morbidly Obese Patients

Femoral arterial cannulation in morbidly obese patients can be a challenge as the artery may be difficult to palpate, the skin at the ideal puncture site may be excoriated, and the folds of adipose tissue may make femoral access a challenge. Considerations should be given for alternatives such as radial access. However, femoral arterial cannulation using a SmartNeedle or under the guidance of ultrasound and using a micropuncture needle can be particularly helpful. Care must be taken to advance the needle at an angle more than the usual 30° to 45° to avoid a high cannulation. In addition, with the needle in the subcutaneous tissue and before puncturing the artery, it may be helpful to use fluoroscopy to ensure proper positioning of the needle. In addition, a long guidewire should preferably be used when exchanging the needle for a femoral artery sheath, and considerations should be given to using a longer femoral artery sheath to ensure that it is well within the artery.

Patients with Ilio-femoral Bypass Grafts

In patients with ilio-femoral bypass grafts, consideration should be given to alternatives such as radial access or use of the nongrafted side (if available). If femoral access is desirable, consideration should be given to micropuncture with the intention of aiming for the hub of the graft. The micropuncture guidewire should be advanced under fluoroscopy and if resistance is encountered, angiography either through the micropuncture needle or after exchanging the needle for a 3 Fr micropuncture dilator should be considered to roadmap the graft. Once a roadmap is established, either the native artery (if patent) or the graft should be wired.

Patients with Calcified Femoral Artery

In some patients the femoral artery calcification is visible on fluoroscopy and can potentially outline the artery and serve as a roadmap of the artery. In such cases femoral artery cannulation can be performed under direct fluoroscopic guidance, aiming the needle (preferably a micropuncture needle) at the CFA at the center of the femoral head. However, consideration should be given to the fact that the artery could have severe atherosclerotic disease, making closure a challenge and increasing the risk of ischemic limb complications. In addition, heavily calcified arteries are less compressible and hence more prone to bleeding. Consideration should therefore be given an alternative route such as radial access.

Postprocedure Care

The risk of complication with femoral arterial access is directly related to the size of the sheath, and consideration should be given to use the smallest size sheath when possible.[12] In addition, the sheath should be left in the artery for the shortest duration required. The sheath should be removed and hemostasis obtained either by manual compression or by using a vascular closure device as described in the next section. Using the sheath for prolonged periods of time for arterial line access should be avoided, especially for sheaths larger than 4 Fr, and considerations should be given to obtain a radial arterial line for longer term use. Patients should be advised of bed rest and closely monitored during the initial postprocedural period. The duration of the bed rest period depends on the site and size of the vascular access, the means by which hemostasis was achieved, puncture-site stability, and the patient's medical conditions. The access site and distal pulsations should be periodically monitored. In addition, urinary output, cardiac symptoms, pain, other indicators of systemic complications, and vital signs should be monitored and recorded in the chart. After the period of bed rest, the initial ambulation of the patient must be supervised and closely monitored for bleeding.

Complications

The femoral access site is a frequent source of complications. The rate of complication varies between <1% and >20%, depending on the patient population studied, type of complication, and the definition used. However, there has been a significant decline in the complication rates in the contemporary era despite performance of PCI in older patients and the use of more potent antiplatelet and antithrombotic agents.[13,14] Femoral access site complications prolong the hospital stay and are associated with a significant increase in cardiovascular events, including death.[15,16] Femoral access site complication is dependent on several patient-specific and procedure-specific factors. Patient-specific risk factors include older age, female gender, lower body mass index, hypertension, peripheral vascular disease, known bleeding diathesis, severe renal impairment, being on anticoagulation preprocedure and postprocedure, peak activated clotting time, and procedure duration.[13,16-19] Procedure-specific risk factors include the use of a larger sheath size (>6 Fr),[13,20] location of the femoral puncture site,[21] and the use of glycoprotein IIb/IIIa inhibitors.[22]

Bleeding/Hematoma

The femoral arterial access site is a frequent source of bleeding and hematoma. The incidence is around 0.8% to 23% and is the most common access-site-related complication.[13,23,24] Patients experiencing major femoral bleeding have a significantly longer postprocedure hospital stay and excess morbidity and mortality in the first 30 days when compared with patients without major femoral bleeding.[13,16,19] Contributing factors include a low or high femoral puncture, ineffective manual compression, a back wall femoral arterial wall puncture, accidental puncture of the vein, and the use of glycoprotein IIb/IIIa inhibitors.[22] A hematoma usually presents as swelling surrounding the puncture site, which is often painful and results in difficulty moving the leg and/or skin discoloration. The presentation depends on the size of the hematoma (small <1 cm, medium 1-5 cm, large >5 cm) and the acuity. A large hematoma can present with signs of hemodynamic instability with tachycardia and/or hypotension. Some patients may present with a vasovagal reaction with bradycardia and hypotension due to severe pain and compression of the underlying artery. Treatment includes manual compression at the site of the hematoma, fluid resuscitation/blood transfusion as needed for hemodynamic instability, prolonged bed rest, and interruption/reversal of anticoagulation/antiplatelet agents if necessary. Close monitoring for recurrence by outlining the hematoma and frequent measurement of the girth of the thigh and serial complete blood cell count are important to detect any further bleeding. Rarely surgical evacuation of the hematoma may be required. Many hematoma resolve within a few weeks; however, care must be taken to prevent infection at the site of the hematoma.

Retroperitoneal Hemorrhage

Retroperitoneal hemorrhage, bleeding that occurs behind the serous membrane lining (peritoneum) the walls of the abdomen/pelvis, is usually due to a high femoral puncture above the inguinal ligament (lower margin of the inferior epigastric artery on fluoroscopy) and/or a posterior wall puncture. The incidence is around 0.1% to 0.4% and can be fatal if not recognized early.[13,14,23,24] Risk factors include female gender, low body surface area, high arterial puncture, glycoprotein IIb/IIIa use, and chronic renal insufficiency.[25,26] Patients usually present with ipsilateral flank or lower back pain, vague abdominal pain, and symptoms and signs of hypotension. Physical examination may show tachycardia and hypotension with Grey Turner's (bruising/blue discoloration of the flanks) or Cullen's (bruising/blue discoloration around the umbilicus) sign (**Figure 3-6**). Often there is no hematoma at the site of the femoral puncture site and the only manifestation may be tachycardia and hypotension, and therefore a high clinical suspicion is required for early diagnosis. Diagnosis can be confirmed by a CT pelvis without contrast (**Figure 3-7**) or on femoral angiography showing frank extravasation of contrast into the pelvis (**Figure 3-8**). Treatment includes fluid resuscitation/blood transfusion as needed for hemodynamic instability, prolonged bed rest, and interruption of anticoagulation if necessary. Serial monitoring of blood pressure and a complete blood count should be performed. Definitive treatment for ongoing hemorrhage includes surgery evacuation of the hematoma with local repair of the artery or contralateral femoral arterial access with balloon tamponade at the site of perforation. In most cases prolonged balloon tamponade will effectively seal the leakage, but in some cases a covered stent may be required.

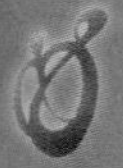

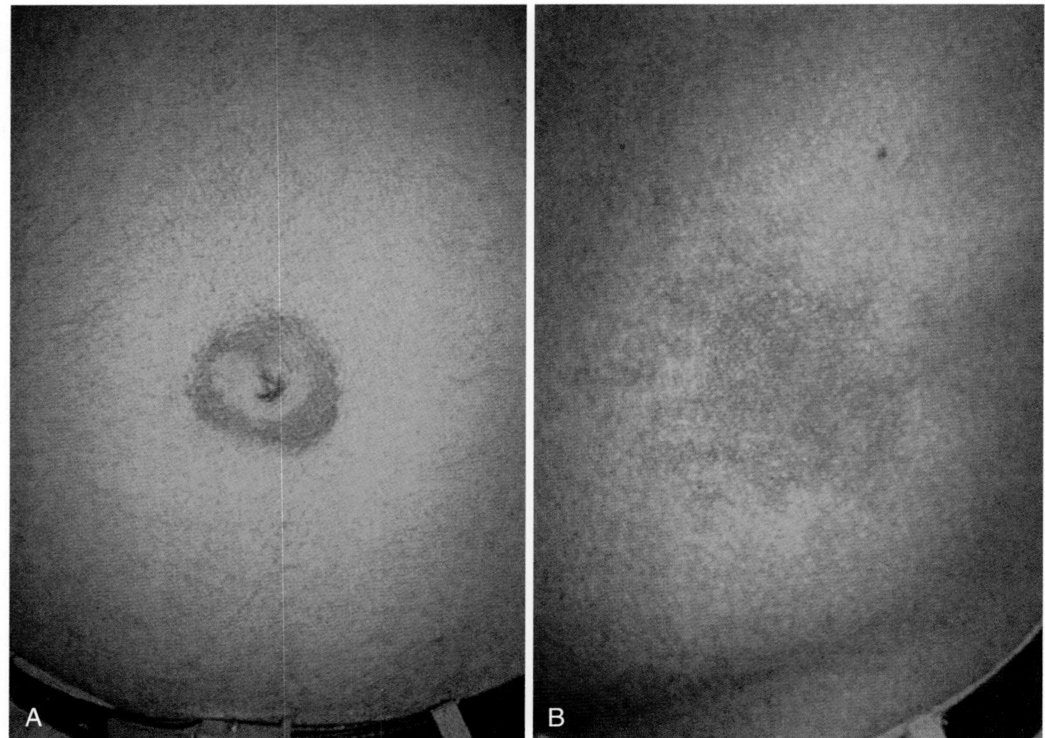

FIGURE 3-6 Cullen's sign **(A)** and Grey Turner's sign **(B)**. *(Reproduced with permission from Chauhan et al: Lancet 372(9632):54, 2008.)*

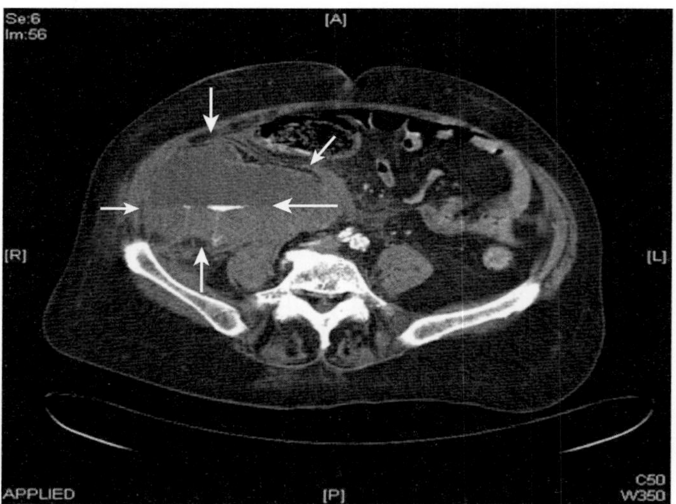

FIGURE 3-7 Abdominal CT with contrast demonstrating a large retroperitoneal hemorrhage (arrows) with fluid level. *(Modified with permission (Open access journal) from Heuer M et al: Int J Case Rep Images 1(3):15–16, 2010.)*

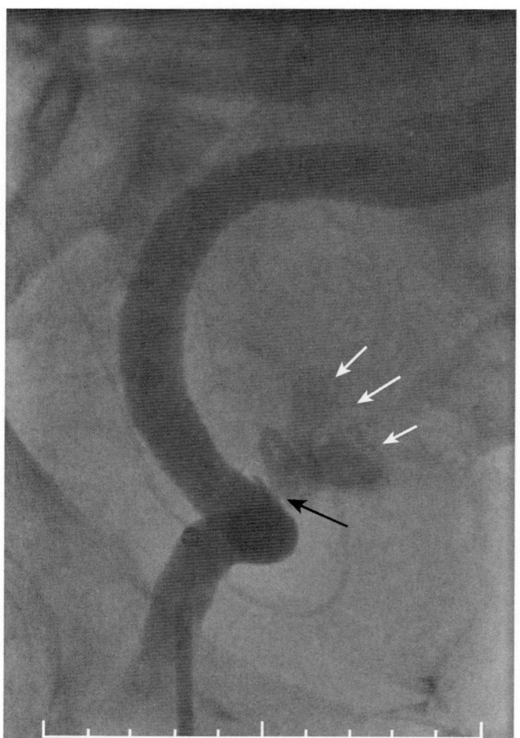

FIGURE 3-8 Retroperitoneal hemorrhage: Femoral angiogram showing a tortuous external iliac artery and contrast extravasation into the pelvis (white arrows). The site of perforation is indicated by the black arrow. Attempt at hemostasis using a covered stent failed and the artery was repaired and hemostasis obtained by surgery. *(Image courtesy Drs. Ivan Pena Singh and Sohah Iqbal, New York University School of Medicine, New York.)*

Arteriovenous Fistula

The incidence of anteriovenous fistula (**Figure 3-9A**) formation after femoral artery cannulation is low (<0.2%).[14,23,24] The risk fctors for AV fistula include a low/high femoral puncture, multiple access attempts, puncture of the overlying femoral vein or its tributaries, and ineffective manual compression. Patients maybe asymptomatic or present with pain and swelling at the groin site. Rarely patients present with symptoms and signs of increased cardiac output or limb ischemia (intermittent claudication, ulcer) or deep venous thrombosis. On physical examination a bruit may be heard on auscultation and a thrill felt on palpation.

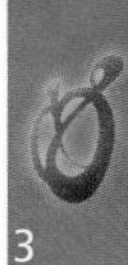

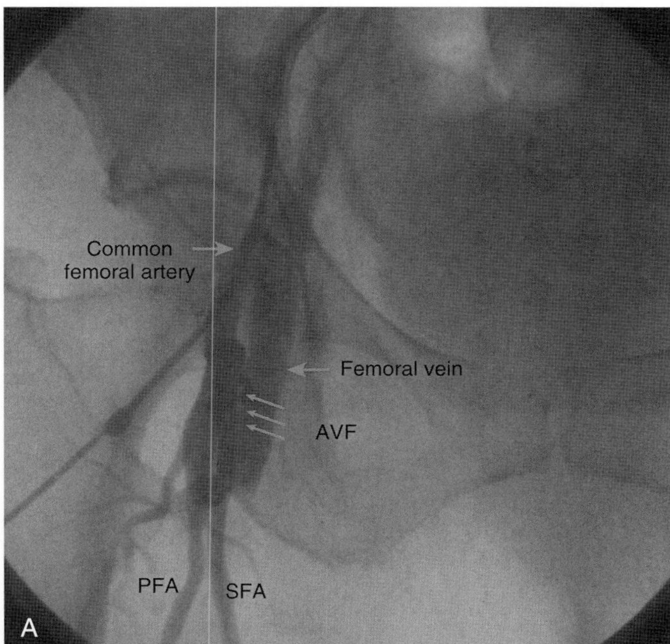

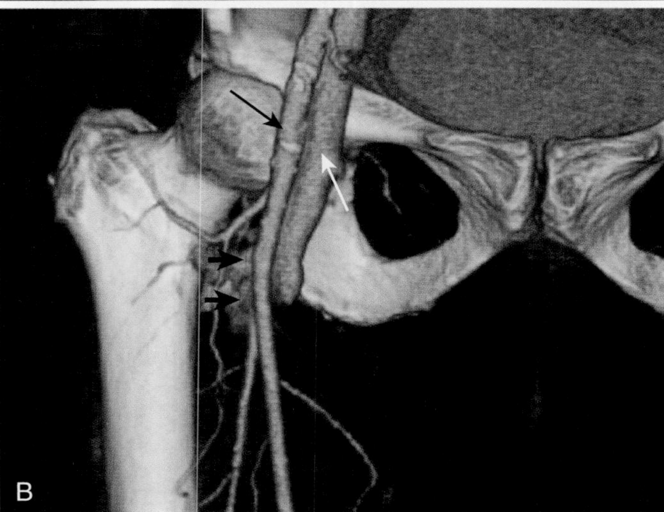

FIGURE 3-9 Arteriovenous fistula. **A,** Femoral angiogram showing communication between the femoral artery and the vein (blue arrows). **B,** 3-D reconstruction of a CT scan showing communication between the common femoral artery (black arrow) and the common femoral vein (white arrow). *(**A,** Adapted from Bangalore et al:* Circulation *124(5):e147–e156, 2011. **B,** Reproduced with permission (Open access journal) from Ozyuksel and Dogan. Case Rep Vasc Med 2013:712089, 2013.)*

Diagnosis is by color Doppler ultrasound and rarely angiography (**Figure 3-9A**) or CT (**Figure 3-9B**) is needed. For small AV fistula and in asymptomatic patients, the treatment is observation and serial ultrasound. Most resolve with time. For large AV fistula, ultrasound-guided compression is the treatment of choice. Other options include use of a balloon tamponade, covered stent, endovascular coils, and if all else fails, surgical repair.

Pseudoaneurysm

A pseudoaneurysm (PSA) is defined as an arterial rupture of one or more layers of its walls, contained by overlying fibromuscular tissue, which communicates with an artery by a neck or sinus tract. The incidence of pseudoaneurysm is 0.3% to 9.0%.[14,23,24] Risk factors for pseudoaneurysm include a low femoral puncture site and ineffective manual compression after sheath removal. The patient usually presents with swelling/pain or a large hematoma at the site. A large pseudoaneurysm can present with symptoms of nerve compression (limb weakness and paresthesia). A pseudoaneurysm can rupture causing abrupt swelling and severe pain. A physical examination may reveal a pulsatile mass with a bruit and/or thrill. Diagnosis is made on color Doppler ultrasonography (**Figure 3-10A**). It can also be diagnosed by angiography or CT (**Figure 3-11**). Treatment depends on the size of the pseudoaneurysm. A small pseudoaneurysm (≤2 cm) usually resolves spontaneously and requires manual/mechanical compression, prolonged bed rest, and cessation of anticoagulation, followed by observation and serial ultrasonography. A large pseudoaneurysm can be treated by ultrasound-guided manual/mechanical compression or ultrasound-guided thrombin injection (**Figure 3-10B**) into the pseudoaneurysm sac. Rarely surgical repair may be required.

Artery Occlusion

Limb ischemia after femoral arterial cannulation is rare with an incidence of <0.8%.[14,23,24] It is usually due to occlusion of the artery by thromboembolism. Common risk factors include small caliber artery, peripheral vascular disease, the use of larger size sheaths, low cannulation into the superficial femoral or profunda femoris artery, the use of a vascular closure device with intraarterial components (such as Angio-Seal), or a sheath that is left behind for a prolonged period of time. In addition, digital ischemia may be due to cholesterol emboli (**Figure 3-12**). Classic signs and symptoms include the five P's: pain, pallor, paresthesia, pulselessness, and paralysis. Diagnosis is by Doppler ultrasonography studies. Angiography is needed to localize the site of occlusion. Treatment includes anticoagulation, contralateral access, and angiography, with thrombectomy and possible angioplasty or stenting, or intraarterial fibrinolytic administration. In some cases surgical thrombectomy with vascular bypass grafting may be required. In rare cases ischemic complication can be due to the use of a vascular closure device such as Perclose or the Angio-Seal (**Figure 3-13A-C**). In addition to dislodgment of plaque by the footplate of these devices, intraarterial deposition of collagen (with Angio-Seal) or subintimal dissection of the common femoral artery (with Perclose) has been described as the etiology of ischemic complications.[27]

Dissection

Femoral artery dissection is a rare (0.2%-0.4%) complication of femoral artery cannulation.[24] Risk factors include presence of atherosclerosis in the CFA or the external iliac artery, vessel tortuosity, and dissection during advancement of the guidewire or during femoral angiography. Diagnosis is made during femoral angiography and most patients are asymptomatic. In rare cases the patient presents with symptoms and signs of ischemic limb after the sheath is removed. Treatment includes observation as most dissections are retrograde and spontaneously heal. In rare cases if ischemic complications arise, contralateral access and angiography and possible angioplasty or stenting or surgical repair should be considered.

Femoral Neuropathy

Femoral neuropathy is due to injury to the femoral nerve during access and/or compression of the femoral nerve by

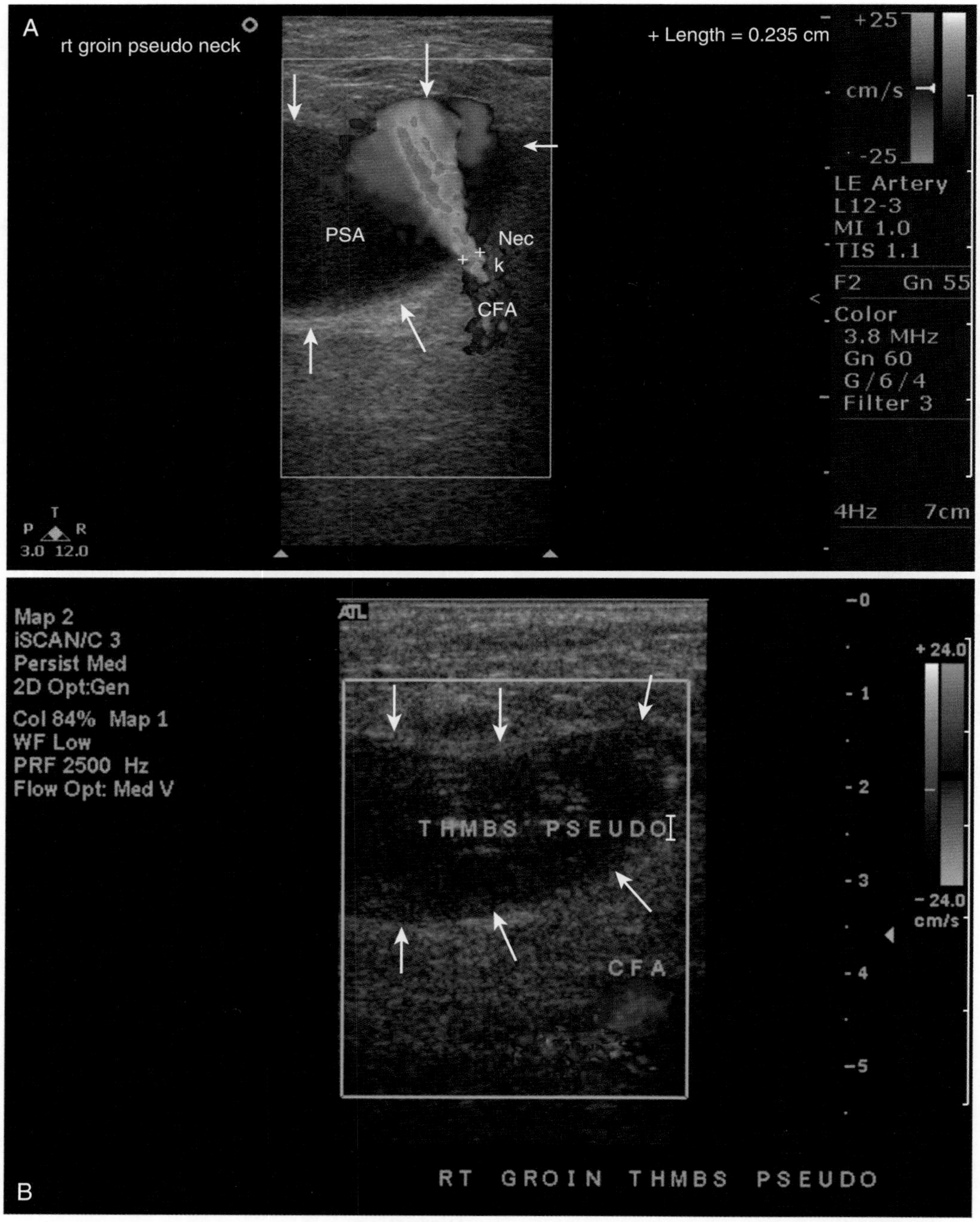

FIGURE 3-10 Pseudoaneurysm. **A,** Color Doppler ultrasound showing a pseudoaneurysm (PSA) communicating with the common femoral artery (CFA) via a short neck. **B,** Color Doppler ultrasound of a patient post ultrasound-guided thrombin injection showing a thrombosed pseudoaneurysm with no communication with the common femoral artery (CFA).

a hematoma or pseudoaneurysm. The incidence is around 0.2%.[23] Patients present with pain/paresthesia at the femoral access site with radiation down the limb or with leg weakness. Physical examination may reveal focal neurological signs including decreased sensory perception, decreased motor strength, or decreased patellar tendon reflexes. Treatment should be aimed at the underlying cause (hematoma/pseudoaneurysm), treatment of symptoms, and physical therapy.

Groin Site Infection

Access site infection is rare (<0.1%)[23] but can be potentially serious resulting in sepsis. Risk factors include obesity with folds of adipose tissue at the access site, presence of superficial infection at the site of entry, diabetes mellitus, compromised sterile technique during access or closure, prolonged indwelling sheath time, and use of a vascular closure device. Patients present with pain, swelling, discharge at the access site, fever, and/or an increase in the white blood cell count. Treatment includes administration of antibiotics and symptomatic treatment for pain relief. In rare case and especially when a vascular closure device is used, surgical debridement with removal of any indwelling component of the closure device may be necessary. Infection associated with the vascular closure device is an extremely serious complication that requires aggressive medical and surgical

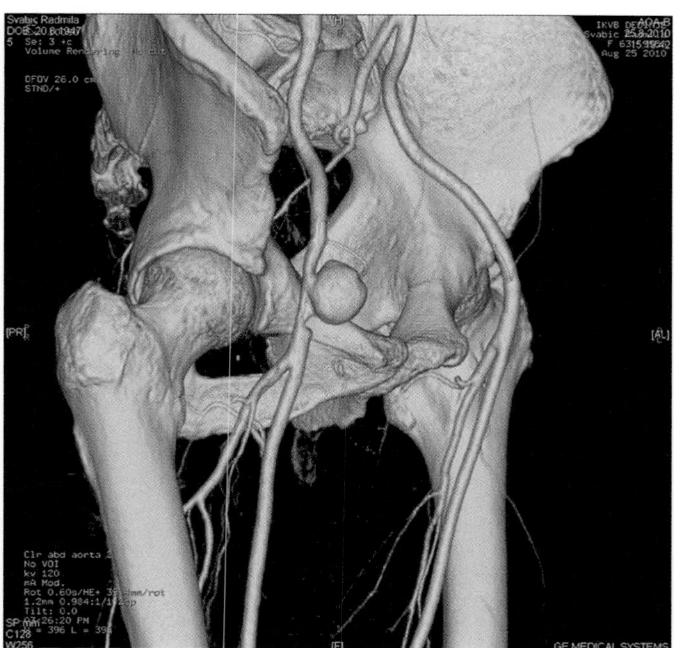

FIGURE 3-11 Pseudoaneurysm: 3-D CT reconstruction of a patient with femoral pseudoaneurysm (black arrow). *(Reproduced with permission (Open access journal) from Predrag Matic et al: Case Rep Vasc Med 2012, Article ID 292945, 4 pages, 2012. doi:10.1155/2012/292945.)*

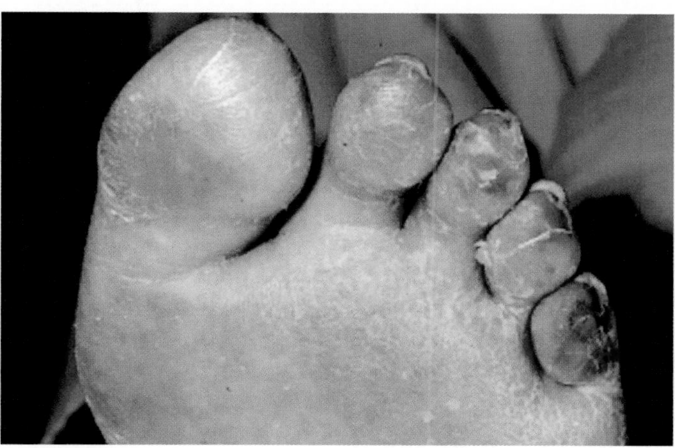

FIGURE 3-12 Cholesterol emboli: Peripheral embolic lesions in toes. *(Reproduced with permission from Dupont et al: BMJ 321:1065, 2000.)*

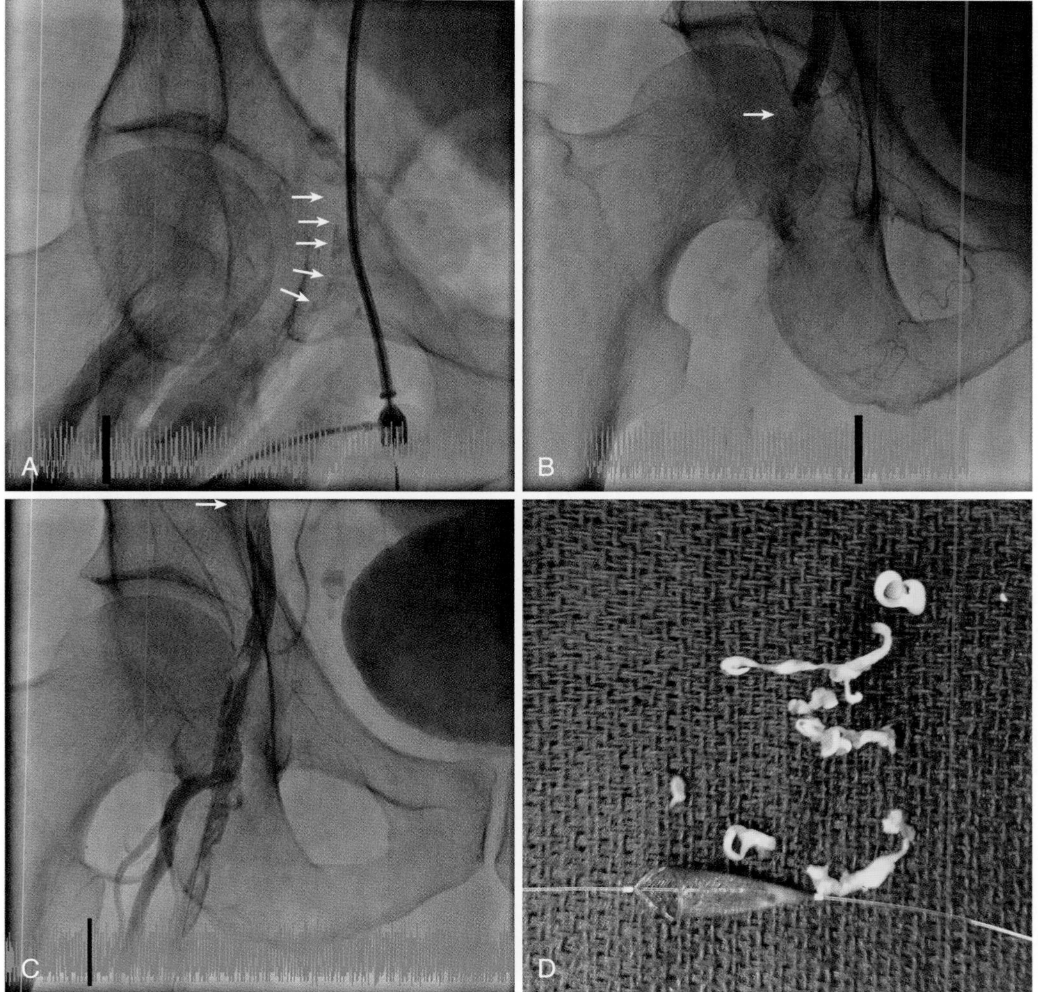

FIGURE 3-13 Femoral artery occlusion. **A,** Heavily calcified common femoral artery (white arrows). **B,** No flow at the site of calcification after deployment of the Angio-Seal device. **C,** Reestablishment of flow after wiring and thrombectomy showing thrombus at the site of calcification (white arrow). **D,** Collagen plug retrieved after atherectomy using the SilverHawk Plaque Excision system. *(**A-C,** Image courtesy Dr. Sohah Iqbal, New York University School of Medicine, New York. **D,** Image courtesy Drs. Pawan Hari and Anvar Babaev, New York University School of Medicine, New York.)*

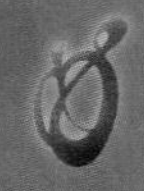

intervention and carries high rates of morbidity and mortality.[28] The majority of patients with infection present 7 to 10 days after deployment of the device and need prolonged antibiotic therapy (up to 28 days) and arterial debridement and reconstruction.

FEMORAL ARTERIAL ACCESS SITE CLOSURE

Introduction

Securing hemostasis after performing a procedure via the femoral arterial access is an important part of the procedure, and complications can be serious. The risk of complications (both ischemic as well as bleeding) is directly related to the duration the sheath is left in place. It is therefore recommended that the femoral arterial sheath be left in for the least amount of time possible and removed immediately after diagnostic procedures if no anticoagulation was used. There are four ways of obtaining hemostasis post procedure: (1) manual compression, (2) mechanical compression, (3) assisted compression devices/topical hemostasis accelerators, and (4) VCDs.

Manual Compression

Manual compression is considered the gold standard for obtaining hemostasis after femoral arteriotomy and is the most commonly used hemostasis technique worldwide. Correct technique is essential to ensure adequate hemostasis but also to minimize complications such as bleeding/hematoma and pseudoaneurysm formation. The femoral sheath should be removed immediately following diagnostic procedures if no anticoagulation is used or when the activated clotting time (ACT) is <150 s to 160 s or PTT <45 s when heparin is used, 6 to 8 hours after last enoxaparin dose, 2 hours after stopping bivalirudin or when the fibrinogen level is >150 mg/dL when fibrinolytics are used. VCD should be considered if the sheath is to be removed on a fully anticoagulated patient. The general principles of manual compression include application of pressure at the correct site and for adequate periods of time. It is important to note that the artery puncture site is 2 cm superior and medial to the skin entry site and as such, manual compression should be applied over the arteriotomy site and not directly over the skin puncture site. The duration of compression varies with the size of the catheter and on other factors such as patient's blood pressure and anticoagulation status. A rough rule is to apply manual compression for 5 minutes for each 1 Fr, although effective hemostasis can be obtained for an arterial sheath of 4 Fr or 5 Fr in under 10 to 15 minutes and for venous sheath of 8 Fr or 9 Fr in under 5 to 10 minutes. Adjunctive use of a mechanical compression device should be considered for compressing the access site for an extended period of time. The steps in manual compression are outlined in **Table 3-3**. The advantage of manual compression is that it is associated with the lowest complication rate and there is no foreign body left behind either intraarterial or extraarterial.[29-31] The disadvantage includes the need to wait for prolonged periods of time for anticoagulation to wear off prior to sheath removal, discomfort (both to the operator and the patient) during the sheath removal, prolonged period of bed rest post manual compression with longer time to ambulation, complications due to ineffective compression (bleeding, hematoma, pseudoaneurysm, or AV fistula formation), and a potential increase in time to hospital discharge. More recently, ambulation as early as 1 hour after removing a 5 Fr[12,32] or 1.5 hours after removing a 6 Fr sheath[33,34] has been shown to be safe, thereby decreasing the time to hospital discharge.

TABLE 3-3 Steps in Manual Compression for Femoral Artery Hemostasis

Preprocedure:

- Check to ensure that adequate time has passed since the last anticoagulation (as described in the text).
- Ensure that the patient's blood pressure is not high and treat as needed.
- Connect the patient to the monitor to assess heart rate continuously and blood pressure every 1 to 2 minutes.
- Lower the bed level to the comfort of the operator (prevents operator from straining his/her back).
- Move the patient close to the side edge of the bed next to the operator removing the sheath (prevents operator from straining his/her back).
- Notify the nurse of the procedure to be ready with medications in case of vasovagal reaction.
- Inspect the access site for any signs of existing hematoma.
- Assess the distal pulses (dorsalis pedis and posterior tibial).

Procedure:

- Clean the sheath and surrounding area with antiseptic solution.
- Remove the sutures holding the sheath in place.
- Bleed back the sheath to expel any thrombus.
- Palpate the artery cranially (1-2 cm cranially) from the skin exit site of the sheath using three fingers.
- Apply gentle pressure over the arteriotomy site (not the skin exit site) with the three fingers, remove the sheath, allow for back bleed from the arteriotomy site to flush any remaining thrombus. Too much pressure at this stage can compress or crush the sheath and strip clots that may have formed.
- Continue compression along the length of the artery using the three-finger approach. Alternately, place a rolled gauze along the length of the artery and apply pressure using the palm of the hand.
- Lock the elbows of both arms and lean forward using the upper body weight to apply pressure.
- Duration of compression varies with the size of the catheter (rough rule is to hold for 5 minutes for every 1 Fr). However, for arterial sheaths of 4 Fr or 5 Fr, hemostasis may be achieved in under 10 to 15 minutes and for venous sheaths smaller than 8 Fr or 9 Fr in under 5 to 10 minutes.
- Remove the venous sheath (if any) 5 minutes after removing the arterial sheath (prevents arteriovenous fistula formation).
- During the last 5 minutes of compression, let the pressure down to 25% of initial pressure.
- For any symptoms and signs of vasovagal reaction (nausea, vomiting, diaphoresis, bradycardia, or hypotension), decrease pressure on the artery (while ensuring hemostasis) and administer atropine/intravenous fluids if needed.
- Assess and record the distal pulses (dorsalis pedis and posterior tibial).

Postprocedure:

- Clean the area with an antiseptic solution.
- Cover with a small transparent dressing (opaque dressing can obscure bleeding/hematoma and should be avoided).
- Monitor for any signs of bleeding (access site inspection, heart rate, and blood pressure monitoring).
- Instruct patient bed rest with the corresponding leg straight. A rough rule for the duration is 1 hour for each French size of the sheath (e.g., 6 Fr = 6 hr).
- Instruct the patient not to lift his/her head up or strain during coughing as any increase in intraabdominal pressure can cause the arteriotomy site to open up, resulting in bleeding.

Mechanical Compression

Mechanical compression involves the use of a mechanical device for external compression to obtain hemostasis. This can be used as a stand-alone device (no manual compression) or as an adjunct to manual compression for an extended period of compression. There are two main types of mechanical compression: The C-clamp [CompressAR

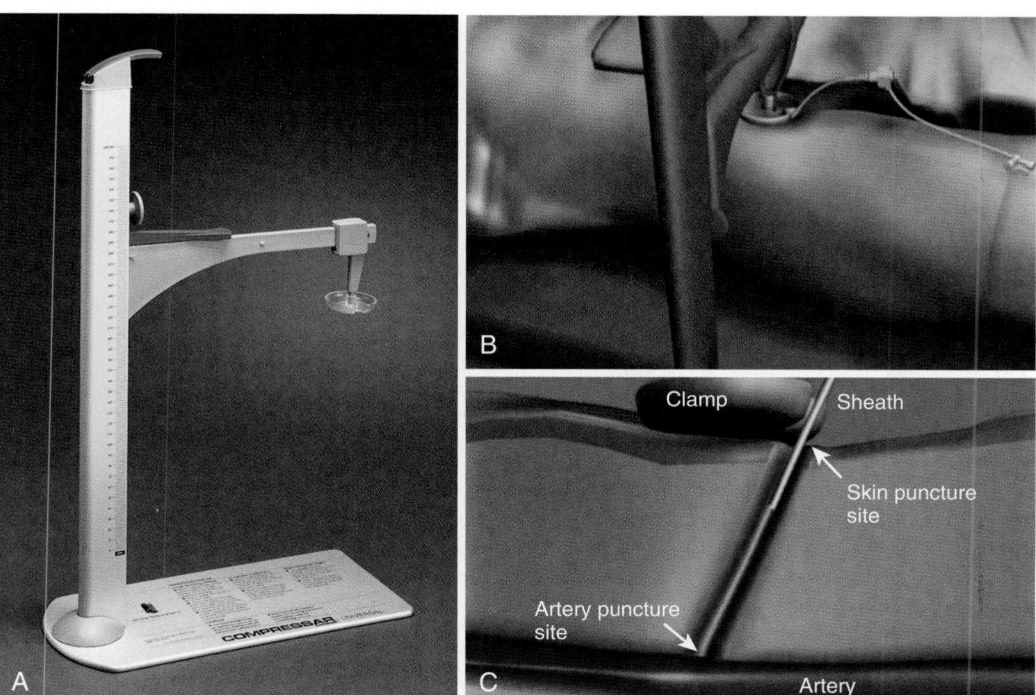

FIGURE 3-14 **A,** C-clamp [CompressAR (Advanced Vascular Dynamics)] showing a flat metal base, pivoting metal shaft, adjustable arm level, and a translucent pad attached to the tip of the C-clamp arm. **B,** C-clamp use technique: The C-clamp arm is lowered into position ensuring that the sheath is positioned center to the disc at the V-notch just outside the perimeter of the disc. **C,** C-clamp use technique: The C-clamp is positioned such that the clamp is above the artery puncture site (arrow) and not the skin puncture site (arrow). *(Reprinted with permission from Advanced Vascular Dynamics™, © 2014. All rights reserved.)*

(Advanced Vascular Dynamics); Clamp Ease (Pressure Products, Inc.)] and pneumatic (FemoStop, Radi Medical Systems AB, St. Jude Medical, Inc.). The C-clamp consists of a flat metal base, a pivoting metal shaft attached to the base, an adjustable arm lever with arm slide, and an upper and lower arm lock mechanism to hold the desired level of pressure (**Figure 3-14A**). The preprocedural considerations are similar to those outlined in **Table 3-3**. Raise the arm to the top of the stand and rotate the shaft so that the arm is pointed away from the patient. Position the base of the C-clamp beneath the bed mattress and directly below the patient's hip on the site of the femoral sheath. Rotate the C-clamp arm into the desired position. Attach a disposable translucent pad to the tip of the C-clamp arm. Palpate the access site 1 cm to 2 cm proximal to the skin entry site and gently lower the C-clamp arm into position, ensuring that the sheath is center to the disc at the V-notch just outside the perimeter of the disc (**Figure 3-14B**). Do not place anything between the pad and the skin including gauze pads. Lock the top lever. With one hand on the arm lever preparing to push down, use the other hand to remove the sheath and immediately apply enough pressure from the arm lever to obtain adequate hemostasis after ensuring adequate bleed back to flush remaining thrombus. Tighten the lever with adequate pressure so as to ensure hemostasis but at the same time ensuring that the peripheral pulse is not fully obliterated (**Figure 3-14C**). If bleeding is noticed, increase pressure as needed. If pulse is obliterated, ensure that this does not last beyond 2 to 3 minutes. When it is time to release compression, gradually raise and lower the arm lever to release pressure at small increments and check the site for any bleeding. If bleeding is noticed, press down on the arm lever until hemostasis is obtained. Repeat the procedure until the C-clamp can be fully removed without any bleeding. Postprocedure care is similar to that outlined in **Table 3-3**.

Pneumatic compression devices such as the FemoStop use a small transparent inflatable dome, an adjustable belt placed underneath the patient's hips, and a pump with a manometer to adjust pressure to an optimal level (**Figure 3-15A**). The preprocedural considerations are similar to those outlined in **Table 3-3**. Position the belt underneath the patient's hips in line with the puncture site, ensuring that the length of the belt is equal on either side of the hip (**Figure 3-15B**). Check pedal pulses and record this in the patient's chart. Position the dome over the arteriotomy site (1-2 cm cranial and medial to the skin puncture site) and attach the belt to either end, making sure that the arch is level and square across the groin area (**Figure 3-15C**). Retract the sheath far enough to allow the hub to be free from underneath the dome. Pull the belt straps on either end to ensure that the arch is perpendicular to the femoral arteriotomy site. If a venous sheath is used, inflate the dome 20 mm to 30 mm Hg and remove the venous sheath prior to removal of the arterial sheath. Inflate the dome 60 mm to 80 mm Hg, remove the arterial sheath, and quickly increase pressure in the dome 10 mm to 20 mm Hg greater than the patient's systolic blood pressure or until hemostasis is achieved. After a maximum of 3 minutes of suprasystolic pressure, lower pressure to maintain a palpable pedal pulse while ensuring hemostasis. Postprocedure monitoring is as outlined in **Table 3-3**. After an appropriate duration of compression, deflate pressure 10 mm to 20 mm Hg every 2 to 3 minutes until zero. If bleeding ensues, inflate 10 mm to 20 mm Hg or until hemostasis is obtained and wait for 10 minutes before starting to wean off the pressure. Once

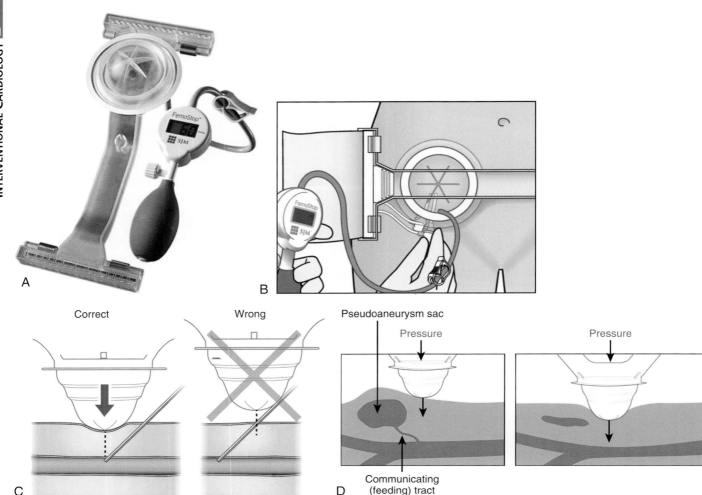

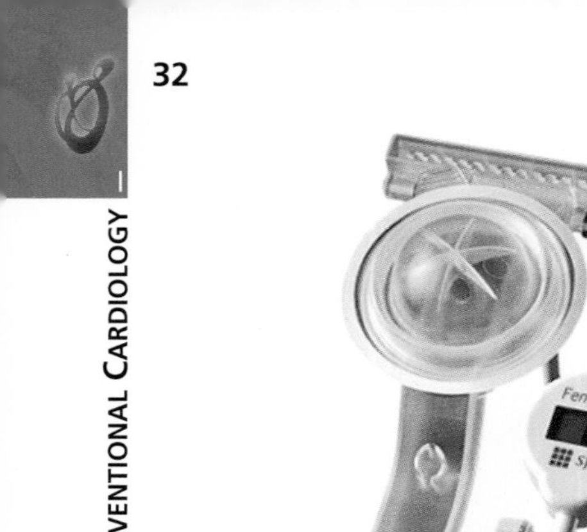

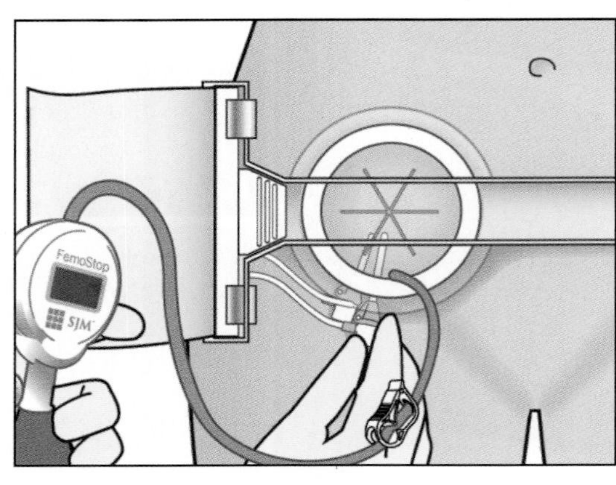

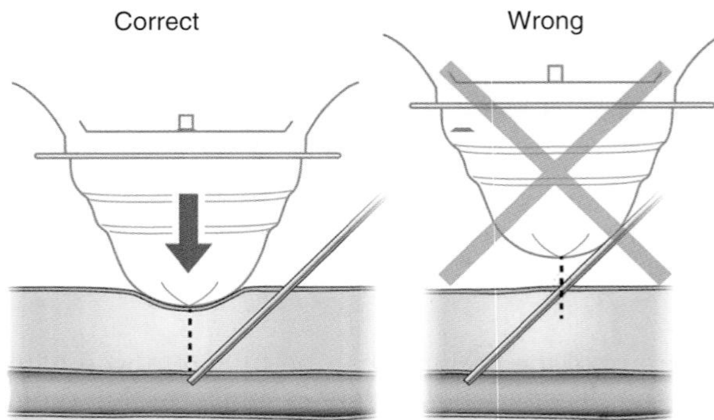

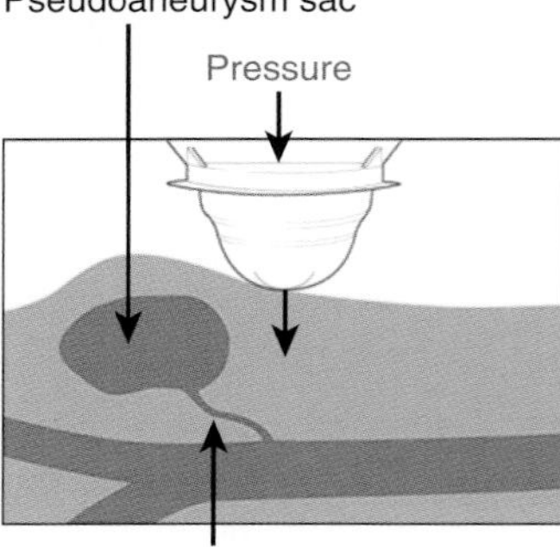

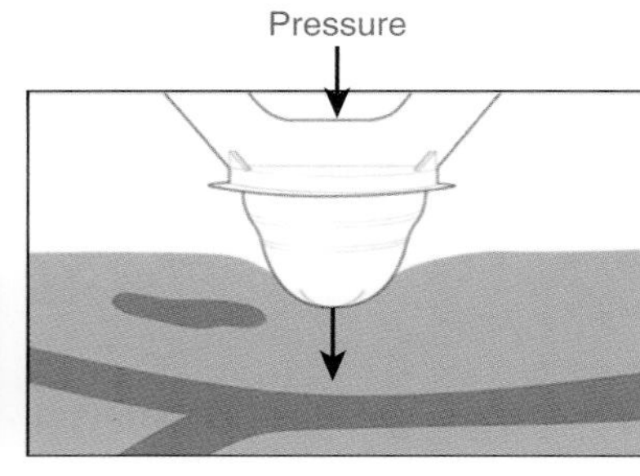

FIGURE 3-15 **A,** FemoStop [St. Jude Medical] device. **B,** FemoStop [St. Jude Medical] device use technique: Withdraw the femoral sheaths partially out and position the belt underneath the patient's hips in line with the puncture site, ensure that the length of the belt is equal on either side of the hip, and connect it to the FemoStop device such that the hubs of the sheath are outside the bulb of the device. **C,** FemoStop [St. Jude Medical] device use technique: The bulb is placed over the arterial puncture site and not the skin puncture site. **D,** FemoStop [St. Jude Medical] device use for treatment of pseudoaneurysm: The bulb is placed over the site of the communicating tract under ultrasound guidance and pressure is applied for a prolonged period of time. *(Reprinted with permission from St. Jude Medical™, © 2014. All rights reserved.)*

hemostasis is obtained, dress the site with a transparent sterile dressing as outlined in **Table 3-3**. The FemoStop is generally more comfortable for the patient compared with either manual compression or the C-clamp, direct contact with the blood is less, and the manometer allows for accurate control of pressure, potentially permitting patent hemostasis. In addition, it is also approved for ultrasound-guided compression of pseudoaneurysm (**Figure 3-15D**).

Assisted Compression Devices/Topical Hemostasis Accelerators

These consist of topical agents that hasten local clotting at the puncture site and are used along with manual/mechanical compression. The preprocedural considerations are similar to those outlined in **Table 3-3**. After cleaning the area around the sheath with antiseptic solution, palpate the artery 1 cm to 2 cm superior and medial to the skin puncture site. Apply firm pressure at the arteriotomy site (not the skin puncture site) and place the hemostasis patch over the puncture site. Ask the patient to take a deep breath in and then exhale while simultaneously removing the sheath, allowing for back bleeding from the tissue tract to help expel any remaining thrombus. The bleeding also helps activate the hemostatic agent on the patch (**Figure 3-16**). After 3 minutes of occlusive pressure over the arteriotomy site, slowly release pressure while maintaining firm pressure directly over the puncture site and hemostasis pad. Apply sterile gauze and transparent dressing over the pad after hemostasis is obtained. These devices can potentially reduce the duration of manual compression. The commonly available topical hemostasis accelerators are listed in **Table 3-4**. The efficacy of topical hemostasis accelerators has been compared with manual compression alone in small randomized trials with variable results, and there are no robust data to suggest that they shorten the time to ambulation.[35-37]

Vascular Closure Device

VCDs, first introduced in the 1980s, are an effective alternative to both manual and mechanical compression after angiography. They function by mechanical closure of the arteriotomy site and are usually deployed in the catheterization laboratory even in a fully anticoagulated patient. Data from over 1.8 million PCI procedures in the United States indicate that VCD is used in >60% of patients and is therefore the predominant modality to obtain hemostasis in the

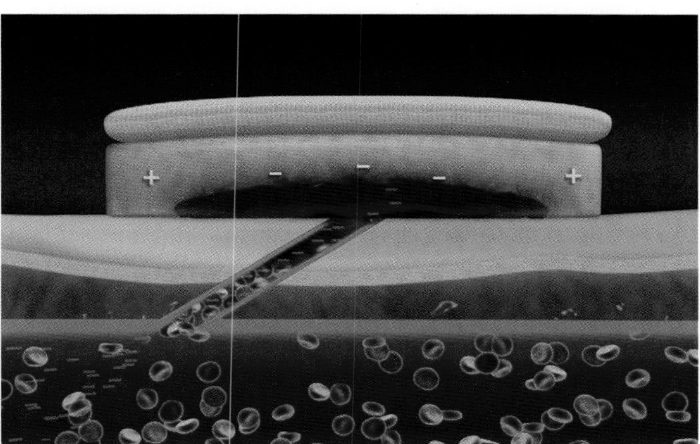

FIGURE 3-16 Topical hemostatic agent (Clo-Sur P.A.D.). The pad is positively charged, which reacts with negatively charged red blood cells to accelerate clotting in the tissue tract. *(Reprinted with permission from Merit Medical System™, © 2014. All rights reserved)*

TABLE 3-4 Topical Hemostasis Accelerator

PRODUCT NAME	ACTIVE AGENT	MECHANISM OF ACTION
CELOX Vascular (Advanced Vascular Dynamics)	Chitosan	A natural polysaccharide that works independent of the body's normal clotting mechanisms.
D-Stat Dry (Vascular Solutions)	Thrombin based	Thrombin-based agent that accelerates clotting. Other versions have silver chloride for an antimicrobial barrier.
HemCon Patch PRO (Hemcon)	Chitosan derivative with antibacterial barrier	Positive ionic charge of the polymer attracts and binds red blood cells, promoting hemostasis. Also provides antibacterial barrier. Does not contain procoagulants and is effective on anticoagulated patients.
Neptune Pad (Biotronik)	Calcium alginate	Facilitates clotting cascade while providing an antimicrobial barrier.
QuikClot (Z-medica)	Kaolin	Kaolin activates the clotting cascade and platelet adhesion.
Scion Clo-Sur Plus PAD (Merit Medical Systems, Inc.)	Polyprolate acetate (form of chitosan)	Positive ionic charge of the polymer attracts and binds red blood cells, promoting hemostasis.
StatSeal ADVANCED (Medline)	Topical hemostatic powder	Stimulates the body's natural clotting cascade.
Syvek Patch, PS, NT (Marine Polymer Technologies)	Poly-*N*-acetyl-gluocosamine	Accelerates clot formation through red blood cell and platelet aggregation. Localized vasoconstrictive effect.
V + Pad (Angiotech)	D-glucosamine	Stimulates the body's natural clotting cascade.

United States.[24] Early studies showed an increased risk of vascular complications with VCDs when compared with manual compression.[28-30,38-41] However, other studies have either shown equivalent efficacy[31,42] or superiority of these devices in reducing the risk of complications when compared with manual compression.[43-46] In the largest series so far, data from over 1.8 million PCI procedures demonstrated a significantly lower bleeding or vascular complication rate with Angio-Seal, Perclose, StarClose, Boomerang Closure Wire, and hemostasis patches when compared with manual compression alone.[24] Of note, all types of hemostasis strategies including manual compression showed reduced complication rates over time, perhaps an attestation to either improvement in technology or awareness or both. The advantages of these devices are reduction in the time to hemostasis, early patient mobilization, decrease in the hospital length of stay, facilitation of outpatient PCI, same-day discharge, and improvement in patient satisfaction.[45,47-52] The disadvantages of these devices are the costs associated with them and various complications as discussed below. In an analysis of 23,813 patients undergoing coronary interventional procedure, the risk of VCD failure (defined as unsuccessful deployment or failure to achieve immediate access site hemostasis) was highest with the StarClose device (9.5%), followed by the Perclose device (6.1%), with the lowest rate being that for the Angio-Seal device (2.1%).[53] In addition, patients with VCD failure had a significant increase in the risk of subsequent vascular complications, major (any retroperitoneal hemorrhage, limb ischemia, or any surgical repair) and minor (any groin bleeding, hematoma (≥5 cm), pseudoaneurysm, or arteriovenous fistula), compared with patients with successful deployment of a closure device.[54] This is likely because most VCDs are deployed in fully anticoagulated patients and failure can result in serious complications. In addition, VCDs can serve as a nidus for infection (please see the section on groin infection).

The commonly available VCDs are listed in **Table 3-5**. There are many classification systems for VCDs based on the mode of action, whether a foreign body is left behind, and whether this foreign body is extraluminal or intraluminal or temporary vs. permanent.[7]

TABLE 3-5 Vascular Closure Device Used in Clinical Practice

ACTIVE APPROXIMATORS	PASSIVE APPROXIMATORS
Angio-Seal (St. Jude Medical, Inc., St. Paul, Minn.)	Boomerang (Cardiva Medical, Mountain View, Calif.)
AngioLink (Medtronic CardioVascular, Santa Rosa, Calif.)	Duett (Vascular Solutions, Inc., Minneapolis, Minn.)
FISH (Morris Innovative Research, Bloomington, Ind.)	Mynx (AccessClosure, Mountain View, Calif.)
Perclose (Abbott Vascular, Santa Clara, Calif.)	VasoSeal (Datascope Corp., Montvale, N.J.)
StarClose (Abbott Vascular, Santa Clara, Calif.)	ExoSeal (Cordis Corporation, Miami Lakes, Fla.)
SuperStitch (Sutura, Inc., Fountain Valley, Calif.)	
Catalyst (Cardiva Medical, Inc., Sunnyvale, Calif.)	

Only FDA-approved devices are listed.
Adapted from Bangalore S, Bhatt DL: Femoral arterial access and closure. Circulation 124(5):E147–E156, 2011.

1. *Active approximators vs. passive approximators:* Active approximators actively approximate the arteriotomy site with the use of an anchor and collagen plug (Angio-Seal), suture (Perclose), or nitinol clip (StarClose). On the other hand, passive approximators passively seal the arteriotomy site using either a sealant or gel foam (Mynx, FISH, Exoseal) or thrombin, which facilitates clot formation.
2. *Foreign body vs. no foreign body:* VCDs such as the Angio-Seal, Perclose, StarClose, Mynx, etc., all leave behind a foreign body (anchor, plug, suture, clip, sealant), which can potentially be a source for infection. Novel devices such as the AXERA Access Device (Arstasis) provide self-sealing access that creates shallow-angle, longer arterial access and are designed to obtain hemostasis without the implantation of a foreign body (**Figure 3-17A-B**).[56] Similarly, the Cardiva Catalyst (Cardiva Medical, Inc.) consists of a biconvex, low profile Catalyst Disc that is deployed over a wire inside the artery blocking the arteriotomy site. A biocompatible coating aids the natural hemostatic process in the tissue tract. Once hemostasis is obtained, the disc is collapsed and removed from the body, leaving no part of the device behind (**Figure 3-18**).
3. *Extraluminal vs. intraluminal:* VCDs such as StarClose and Mynx leave an extraluminal foreign body, whereas Angio-Seal and Perclose leave behind an intraluminal foreign body.
4. *Temporary vs. permanent:* VCDs such as Angio-Seal and Mynx leave behind foreign body, which gets reabsorbed over a period of time. However, devices such as the Perclose and the StarClose leave behind a permanent foreign body.

We will discuss the four commonly used VCDs—the collagen-plug-based (Angio-Seal), the suture-based (Perclose), the nitinol-clip-based (StarClose), and the sealant-based (Mynx) devices.

Collagen-Plug-Based Devices—Angio-Seal

The Angio-Seal device (St. Jude Medical, St. Paul, Minn.) is the most commonly used VCD in the United States, likely due to the short learning curve and high success rate (>97%).[57] It contains a small (2 × 10 mm), flat, absorbable rectangular anchor, an absorbable collagen plug, and an absorbable suture. It works on the principle of active approximation where the intravascular anchor at the site of arteriotomy approximates the collagen plug (in the tissue tract) held together by a suture. The intravascular anchor, collagen plug, and the suture resorb in 3 months.

The device consists of (a) an insertion sheath with an arteriotomy locator, (b) a delivery device that contains the anchor and the collagen plug held together by the suture, and (c) a 0.035-inch or 0.038-inch 70-cm J-tip guidewire. The insertion technique is outlined in **Table 3-6** (**Figure 3-19A-C**). The anchor, collagen plug, and suture all get reabsorbed over the next 90 days, leaving nothing permanently in the artery. Reaccess is therefore recommended >90 days, but if earlier reaccess is necessary, it is recommended to access 1 cm proximal to the prior cannulation site. Of note, the Angio-Seal device is available only in 6 Fr or 8 Fr size. However, Angio-Seal has been used successfully to close 10 Fr arteriotomy using a "double wire" technique.[58] In this technique two Angio-Seal J-tip guidewires are inserted into the 10 Fr sheath and the sheath is removed. The Angio-Seal

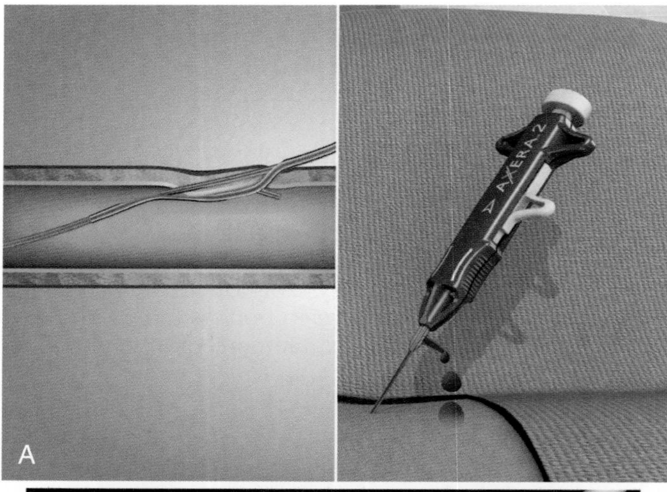

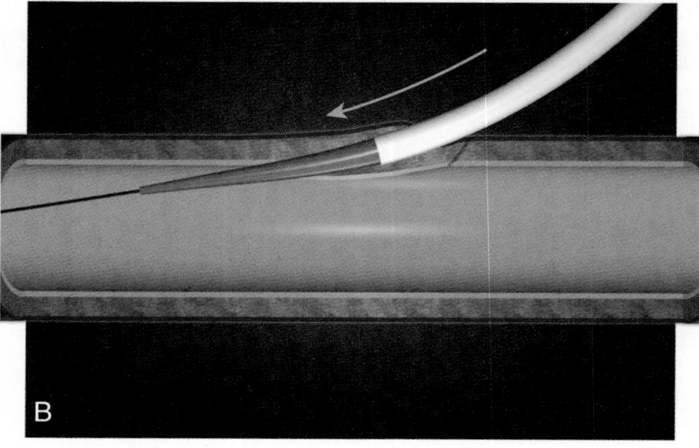

FIGURE 3-17 AXERA Access Device (Arstasis). **A,** The device creates a shallow-angle, longer arterial access, and is designed to obtain hemostasis without the implantation of a foreign body. The image shows a needle passing through the wall of the artery at a shallow angle, creating a longer arterial access. **B,** Sheath entry into the artery at a shallow angle, resulting in a longer arterial access. *(Reprinted with permission from Arstasis™, © 2014. All rights reserved.)*

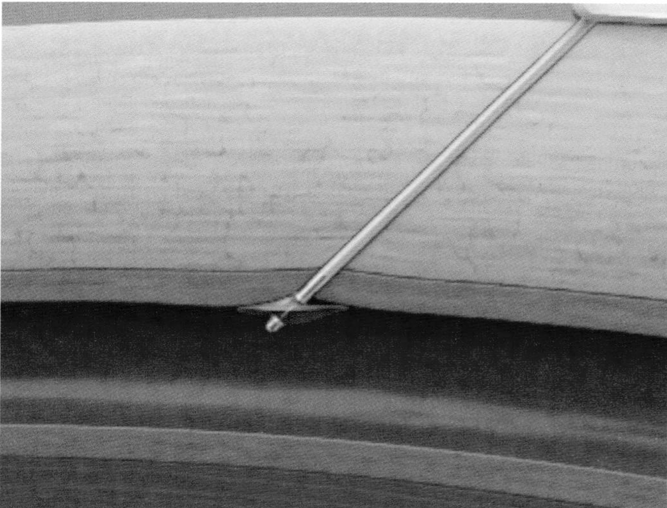

FIGURE 3-18 Cardiva catalyst device (Cardiva Medical Inc.). A biconvex, low profile Catalyst Disc is deployed over a wire inside the artery blocking the arteriotomy site. A biocompatible coating aids the natural hemostatic process in the tissue tract. A newer version of the device called the VASCADE vascular closer system is now available. VASCADE VCS is an extravascular, bioabsorbable femoral access closure system that leaves no permanent components behind, and has demonstrated significant reduction in minor complications as compared with manual compression (1% vs. 7%) in a multicenter, prospective randomized trial of 420 patients. Data from the Rapid Extravascular Sealing Via PercutanEous Collagen ImplanT (RESPECT) trial. *(Journal of Invasive Cardiology, 2015 [in press]). (Reprinted with permission from Cardiva Medical Inc.™, © 2014. All rights reserved.)*

TABLE 3-6 Steps in Insertion of Angio-Seal Device

Preprocedure:

- Obtain ipsilateral femoral angiogram (30°-45°) to verify the position of the femoral arterial cannulation and to ensure no complications (dissection, perforation).
- Factors unfavorable for the use of the Angio-Seal device include a small caliber of the artery (<4 mm), low cannulation (bifurcation, superficial femoral artery, profunda femoris artery), high cannulation (above the level of inferior epigastric artery), moderate to severe peripheral artery disease at the sheath insertion site, and an allergy to beef products, polyglycolic/polylactic acid polymers, or collagen products.
- Clean the femoral artery cannulation site with an antiseptic solution.
- Bleed back on the sheath to flush out any thrombus and flush the sheath with saline.

Procedure:

- Choose a 6 Fr or 8 Fr Angio-Seal device based on the femoral artery sheath size.
- Insert the J-tip guidewire into the sheath and remove the sheath over the wire.
- Insert the arteriotomy locator into the insertion sheath until a click is heard. Insert this over the J-tip guidewire and advance until a pulsatile flow is observed from the arteriotomy locator.
- Withdraw the insertion sheath and the arteriotomy locator until the pulsatile flow ceases and advance just enough when the pulsatile flow starts again (optional). The insertion sheath is now distal to the arteriotomy site and within the artery lumen.
- Hold the insertion sheath steady with one hand and remove the arteriotomy locator and guidewire by flexing upward.
- Insert the delivery device through the insertion sheath and advance until it snaps fit. This deploys the anchor.
- Hold the insertion sheath steady and pull the device cap back until it assumes a fully rear locked position. This sets the anchor.
- Slowly withdraw the assembly until resistance is felt. The anchor is now up against the arterial wall. This also exposes the collagen plug.
- Hold the assembly back and push the tamper tube down to push the collagen plug closer to the anchor.
- A clear stop is exposed on the suture. Cut the suture below the clear stop and remove the tamper tube.
- Cut the suture below the skin level, leaving behind as little of the suture as possible.
- The Angio-Seal device is now deployed.

Postprocedure:

- Check the femoral and distal pulse and document this in the chart.
- Apply a small transparent dressing over the arteriotomy site.
- The anchor, collagen plug, and suture will all get reabsorbed (over 90 days).
- Reaccess at the site can be performed 90 days after the procedure. If reaccess is needed prior to that, consider reaccess 1 cm cranial or caudal to the puncture site.

For more details, please see product information for use.

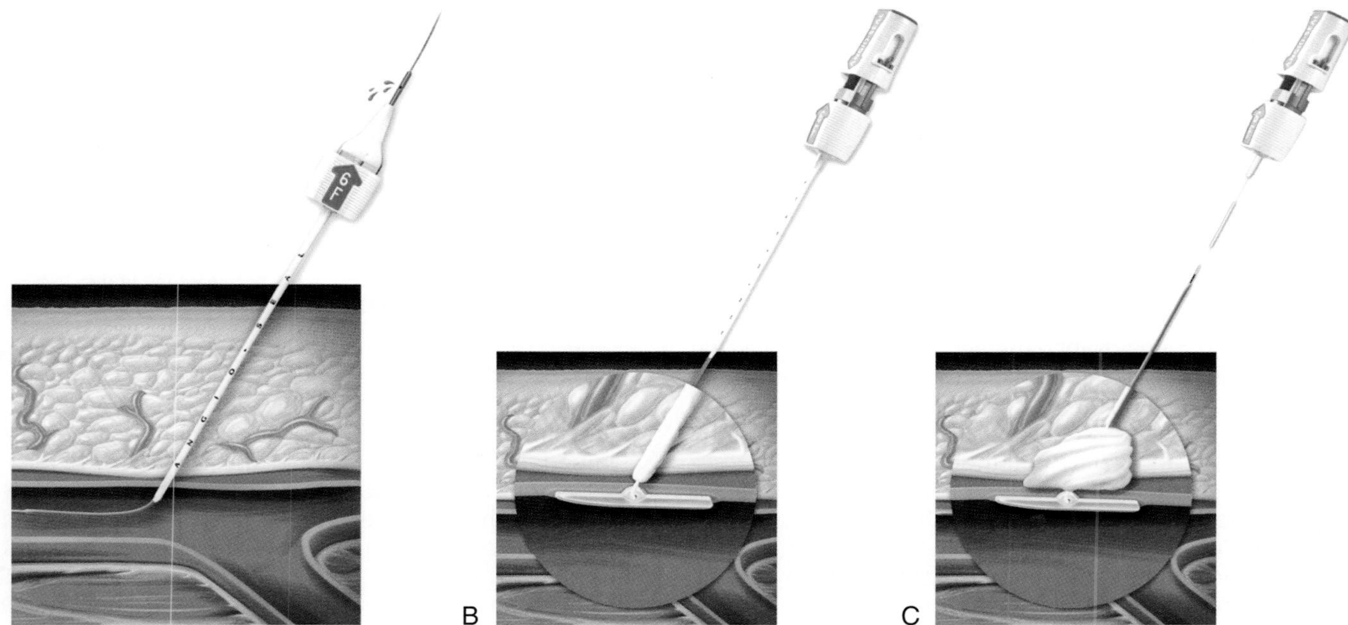

FIGURE 3-19 Angio-Seal device (St. Jude Medical) deployment technique. **A,** The Angio-Seal insertion sheath with an arteriotomy locator is exchanged for the femoral artery sheath over a guidewire and advanced till a pulsatile flow is noted from the arteriotomy locator. **B,** Deployment of the anchor. The collagen plug is also visible. **C,** The collagen plug is pushed closer to the anchor by a tamper tube. *(Reprinted with permission from St. Jude Medical™, © 2014. All rights reserved.)*

device is deployed over one guidewire. If hemostasis is obtained after deployment of one Angio-Seal, the second wire is carefully removed while maintaining back pressure on the collagen plug. If hemostasis is not obtained after the first Angio-Seal device, a second device is then deployed over the second guidewire.[58]

Collagen-Plug-Based Devices—Mynx

The Mynx VCD (AccessClosure, Mountain View, Calif.) is an extravascular closure device that utilizes a synthetic hydrogel (polyethylene glycol sealant) that is deployed outside the artery while a balloon occludes the arteriotomy site from within the artery. The hydrogel absorbs blood and other subcutaneous fluids and expands and adheres to the surface of the artery to achieve hemostasis, and the balloon is deflated and removed through the tract, leaving behind only the sealant. As such, no foreign body is left within the artery and the sealant reabsorbs in 30 days. The device works on the principle of passive approximation.

The device consists of (a) a MynxGrip device including balloon catheter and the sealant and (b) a 10-mL syringe for balloon inflation. It is indicated for vascular closure of sheaths sizes 5 Fr to 7 Fr. The insertion technique is outlined in **Table 3-7** (**Figure 3-20A-C**). The device success rate is 91% to 93%, and the device leads to rapid hemostasis (mean time 1.3 minutes) and ambulation (mean time 2.6 hours).[59,60]

Suture-Mediated Closure Devices

The Perclose ProGlide (Abbott Vascular, Santa Clara, Calif.) is a suture-mediated device that works on the principle of active approximation, leaving behind a monofilament nonabsorbable polypropylene suture. The 6 Fr ProGlide is designed for closure of 5 Fr to 21 Fr sheaths, while the Prostar XL, uses two braided polyester sutures, is for closure of 8.5 Fr to 24 Fr sheaths (CE Mark). For sheath sizes >8 Fr, preclose technique with at least two ProGlide devices can be employed. Perclose ProGlide and Prostar XL work on the principle of mechanical closure and is therefore not clot dependent.

The Perclose ProGlide device consists of (a) delivery device with a plunger, handle, guide, and sheath, containing the pre-tied suture knot; (b) a snared knot pusher; and (c) a suture trimmer. The insertion technique is outlined in **Table 3-8** (**Figure 3-21A-C**). When compared with the Angio-Seal device, the Perclose device has a higher learning curve, a higher failure rate,[57,61] and a longer time to hemostasis.[61] However, the reported infection rate (approximately 0.3%) is comparable to that with the Angio-Seal device.[62]

For sheath sizes greater than 8 Fr, a preclose technique may be employed using two or more ProGlide devices. After cannulating the femoral artery, insert a 6 Fr sheath and obtain a femoral angiogram to ensure that the anatomy is suitable for the use of a ProGlide device. Exchange the sheath over a wire and insert the first of the two ProGlide devices over the guidewire until the guidewire exit port of the device sheath is just about at the skin line. Remove the guidewire and then advance the device until brisk pulsatile blood flow is seen at the marker lumen. Rotate the device to approximately 30 degrees toward the patient's right side (approximately the 10 o'clock position), deploy the foot by lifting the lever, and gently pull the device back until resistance is felt and there is no more pulsatile flow at the marker lumen. While retracting the device gently, deploy the needles by pushing on the plunger assembly. Remove the plunger assembly and cut the suture limb using QuickCut or a sterile scissor/scalpel. Relax the device and return the foot to the closed position by pushing the lever down to the body of the device. Retract the device to release the pre-tied suture knot and continue to withdraw until the guidewire exit port is visible above the skin line. Gently pull both the suture limbs out from the distal end of the guide. Use a hemostat or clamp to hold the two suture limbs together and place it to a side. Reinsert the guidewire through the guidewire exit port. Remove the device while holding compression above the puncture site to maintain hemostasis. Insert the second ProGlide device over the guidewire and repeat the above steps, now deploying the needle about 60 degrees to the first device (approximately the 2 o'clock position). The two suture limbs from the second device should be similarly clamped and placed on the opposite side to that of the first one without locking the suture knot. Insert the guidewire again through the guidewire exit port, remove the device, and exchange it for an appropriate size femoral artery sheath. The procedure is then carried out through this sheath. At the end of the procedure, insert a J-tipped guidewire through the sheath. Insert the blue suture limb (rail limb) onto the snared knot pusher, wrap it around the left index finger, and advance the knot pusher with the thumb of the left hand onto the sheath. With pressure on the knot pusher onto the sheath from the left hand, remove the sheath with the right hand while pushing the knot pusher onto the guidewire. Do not lock or excessively tighten the knot while the guidewire is still in the vessel. Now free the second suture, insert the rail limb of the suture through a snared knot pusher, wrap it around the index finger of the left hand, and push the knot pusher down to the guidewire. Do not lock or excessively tighten

TABLE 3-7 Steps in Insertion of MynxGrip Vascular Closure Device

Preprocedure:
• Obtain ipsilateral femoral angiogram (30°-45°) to verify the position of the femoral arterial cannulation and to ensure no complications (dissection, perforation). • Factors unfavorable for the use of the Mynx device include a small caliber of the artery (<5 mm), severe peripheral artery disease at the sheath insertion site, prior surgical procedure, stent placement or vascular graft in the common femoral artery, patients with bleeding disorders or uncontrolled hypertension, and those with morbid obesity. • Clean the femoral artery cannulation site with an antiseptic solution. • Bleed back on the sheath to flush out any thrombus and flush the sheath with saline.
Procedure:
• Use the appropriate MynxGrip device—5 Fr or 6/7 Fr based on the femoral artery sheath size. • Fill the locking syringe with 2 mL to 3 mL of saline, attach it to the stopcock, draw the vacuum, and then inflate the balloon until the black marker on the inflation indicator is fully visible. Check for any leaks in the balloon. Deflate the balloon and leave the syringe at neutral. • Insert the MynxGrip into the femoral artery sheath up to the white shaft marker. The balloon is now just distal to the femoral artery sheath. • Inflate the balloon using the locking syringe until the black marker on the inflation indicator is fully visible and close the stopcock. • Grasp the handle and withdraw the catheter until there are two points of tactile resistance. The first point is when the balloon abuts the distal end of the sheath and the second point is when the balloon abuts the arteriotomy site. • Open the stopcock on the procedure sheath. There should be no blood coming out, confirming hemostasis by the inflated balloon. • With slight back tension on the device, advance the shuttle until a definitive stop is felt. This advances the sealant into position. • Withdraw the femoral artery sheath until the shuttle locks in place while still holding back tension on the device. • Grasp the white tube at the skin level and advance until the green marker is fully exposed. This advances the sealant on to the arteriotomy surface. • Hold in place for up to 30 seconds. Then lay the device down for up to 90 seconds. • Lock the syringe to a full negative. Hold gentle pressure on the groin and open the stopcock to deflate the balloon. • Keep the advancer tube in place and remove the device. Remove the advancer tube and hold pressure for up to 60 seconds. • Assess for hemostasis and apply pressure if needed.
Postprocedure:
• Check the femoral and distal pulse and document this in the chart. • Apply a small transparent dressing over the arteriotomy site. • The sealant dissolves in 30 days.

For more details, please see product information for use.

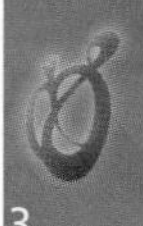

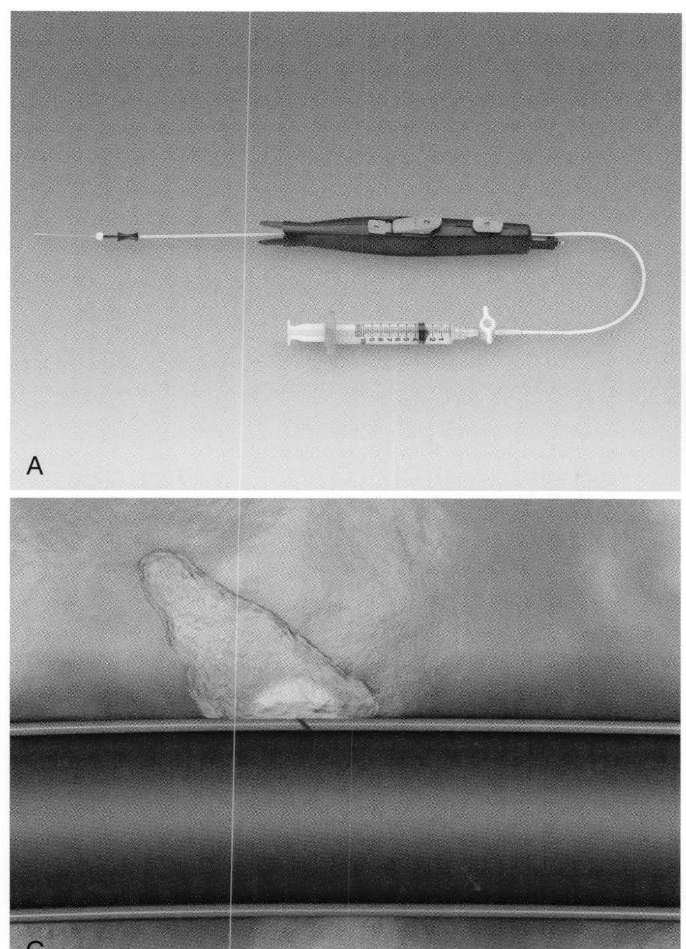

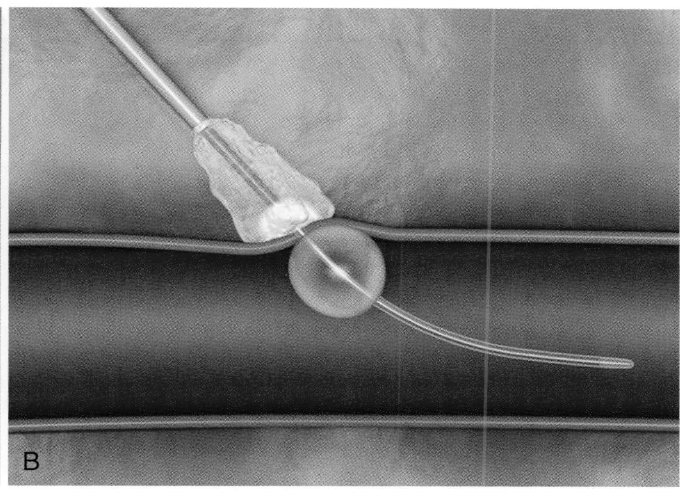

FIGURE 3-20 Mynx device (AccessClosure, Inc.) deployment technique. **A,** Mynx-Grip device including balloon catheter and the syringe. **B,** Inflated balloon at the arteriotomy site. Sealant with the white tube is also shown. **C,** Retraction of the device leaving behind the sealant, which promotes hemostasis. *(Reprinted with permission from AccessClosure, Inc.™, © 2014. All rights reserved.)*

the knot while the guidewire is still in the vessel. Assess for hemostasis. If hemostasis is not obtained, one more Pro-Glide device can be deployed, with this one facing the 12 o'clock position and repeating the above steps. If hemostasis is achieved, push down on the knot pusher on one or both of the rail sutures and ask an assistant to remove the guidewire while advancing both the pushers. Assess for hemostasis and tighten the knot by holding the rail suture limb steady, pulling the nonrail suture limb on both the wires, and trimming the suture limbs using a suture trimmer. Using the pre-close technique, successful hemostasis was achieved in 94% of patients undergoing percutaneous endovascular aortic valve repair in a metaanalysis of 36 studies and 2257 patients with 3606 arterial accesses. The complication rate was low (3.6%) and complications requiring open surgery were only 1.6%.[63] In addition, the technical success rate for sheath sizes 12 Fr to 16 Fr has been shown to be around 99% and that for sheath size 18 Fr to 24 Fr around 91%.[64] When compared with the Angio-Seal device, the risk of device failure was higher with the Perclose device.[54]

Clip-Based Device—StarClose

The StarClose device (Abbott Vascular, Redwood City, Calif.) uses a 4-mm nitinol clip that is deployed outside the arterial wall. The clip grasps the edges of the arteriotomy, drawing them together for closure. It thus works on the principle of active approximation, using a mechanical approximation without leaving behind any intravascular components. However, the clip is permanently left behind on the surface of the artery. The device is approved for closure of 5 Fr to 6 Fr arteriotomies but has also been used with larger sheath sizes (7-8 Fr). The device success was 91% for 7 Fr and 90% for 8 Fr sheaths with a major vascular complication rate of 4.1% and 2.5%, respectively.[65] Although not recommended for closure of cannulation at or near the femoral artery bifurcation, the device appears to be safe with a low rate of vascular complications (0.9%).[66]

The device consists of the StarClose clip applier and a 6 Fr exchange system. The clip applier contains the nitinol clip, which is delivered through the exchange sheath. The insertion technique is outlined in **Table 3-9** (**Figure 3-22A-D**). There are no reaccess restrictions for the StarClose device, although this has not been well studied. In porcine models, reaccess even through the center of the clip was feasible and reclosure using a second StarClose device was successful with achievement of a secure closure.

RADIAL ARTERIAL ACCESS AND CLOSURE

Introduction

The radial artery is a common site for arterial access for continuous blood pressure monitoring and for arterial blood gas measurement. Transradial access for coronary diagnostic procedures was introduced by Campeau[67] and

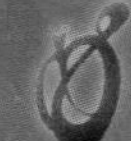

TABLE 3-8 Steps in Insertion of Perclose Vascular Closure Device

Preprocedure:

- Obtain the ipsilateral femoral angiogram (30°-45°) to verify the position of the femoral arterial cannulation and to ensure no complications (dissection, perforation).
- Factors unfavorable for the use of the Perclose device include those with small femoral arteries (<5 mm), severe peripheral artery disease at the sheath insertion site, severe calcification at the insertion site, prior surgical procedure, stent placement or vascular graft in the common femoral artery, low cannulation (bifurcation, superficial femoral artery, profunda femoris artery), high cannulation (above the level of inferior epigastric artery), or cannulation at the femoral artery bifurcation.
- Clean the femoral artery cannulation site with an antiseptic solution.
- Bleed back on the sheath to flush out any thrombus and flush the sheath with saline.

Procedure:

- Use the appropriate size Perclose ProGlide for 5 Fr to 21 Fr or ProStar for 8.5 Fr to 10 Fr.
- Insert a 0.035-inch or 0.038-inch J-tipped guidewire through the femoral artery sheath and remove the sheath.
- Advance the Perclose device over the guidewire until the guidewire exit port is just about at the skin line.
- Remove the guidewire and continue to advance the device until pulsatile blood flow is seen at the marker lumen.
- Deploy the foot by lifting the lever on the body of the device.
- Pull the device back until the foot is against the arterial wall (resistance is felt at this stage and blood flow at the marker lumen ceases).
- Stabilize the device by maintaining gentle traction and deploy needles by pushing on the plunger.
- Pull the plunger assembly back to completely remove the plunger and needle from the body of the device and use the quickcut suture trimming mechanism or a sterile scalpel/scissors to cut the suture from the anterior needle.
- Relax the back tension of the device and bring the foot to its original closed position by pushing the lever down.
- Retract the device to release the suture knot. Continue to retract until the two suture limbs are seen in the distal guide. Free the suture limb from the device. The blue suture limb is the rail suture whereas the white suture limb is the lock suture
- Load the rail limb of the suture onto a snared knot pusher.
- Wrap the rail suture limb around your left forefinger and bring down the knot pusher to the level of the Perclose device.
- Remover the device completely with your right hand while pulling on the rail suture limb and advancing the knot pusher with the thumb of the left hand.
- With the knot pusher held in position and keeping the rail suture limb taut, tighten the knot by pulling on the nonrail suture limb while being coaxial to the tissue tract.
- Relax the pressure on the knot pusher and observe for hemostasis. If hemostasis is not achieved, advance the knot pusher and hold it down until hemostasis is achieved. Tighten the knot by pulling on the nonrail (white) suture limb.
- Remove the knot pusher and use the knot trimmer to cut the excess length of the suture limbs.

Postprocedure:

- Check the femoral and distal pulse and document this in the chart.
- Apply a small transparent dressing over the arteriotomy site.
- There is no reaccess restriction for the Perclose device.

For more details, please see product information for use.

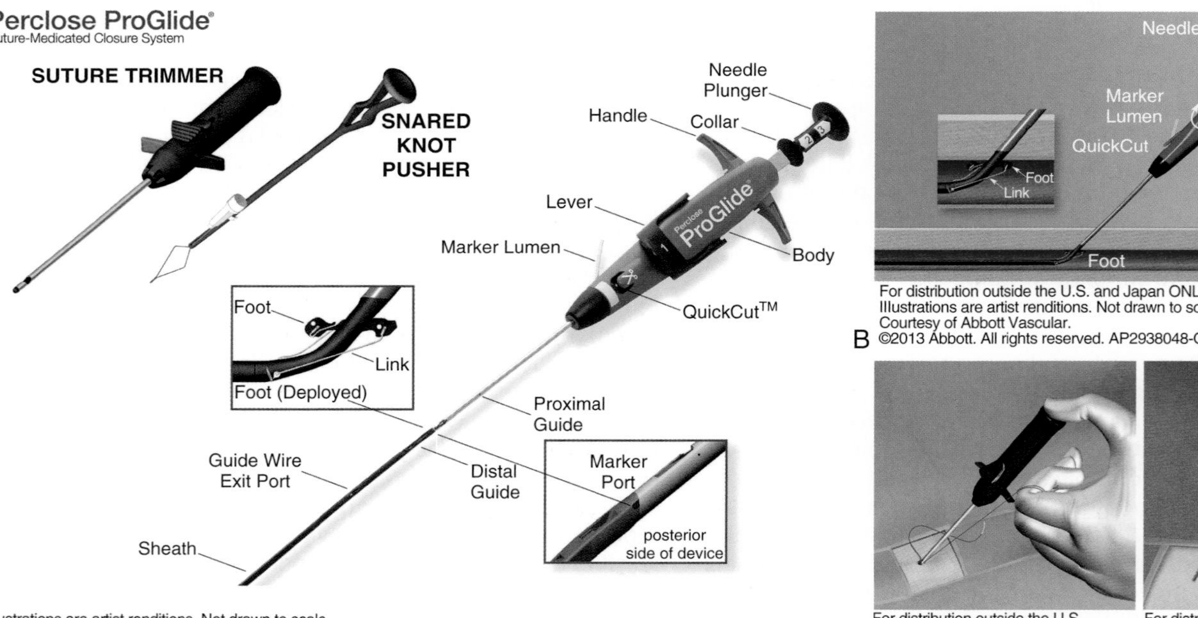

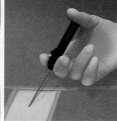

FIGURE 3-21 Perclose ProGlide device (Abbott Vascular) deployment technique. **A,** Component of the Perclose ProGlide device. **B,** Device advanced into the artery with pulsatile blood flow from the maker lumen. **C,** Using the snared knot pusher on the blue rail to push the knot down to the arteriotomy site. Right panel shows the suture trimmer that is placed on the suture limb, and the suture is trimmed as close to the arteriotomy site as possible. *(Courtesy Abbott Vascular, © 2012-2013. All rights reserved.)*

TABLE 3-9 Steps in Insertion of the StarClose Vascular Closure Device

Preprocedure:

- Obtain the ipsilateral femoral angiogram (30°-45°) to verify the position of the femoral arterial cannulation and to ensure no complications (dissection, perforation).
- Factors unfavorable for the use of the StarClose device include those with small femoral arteries (<5 mm), sheath size >6 Fr, severe peripheral artery disease at the sheath insertion site, severe calcification at the insertion site, prior surgical procedure, stent placement or vascular graft in the common femoral artery, low cannulation (bifurcation, superficial femoral artery, profunda femoris artery), high cannulation (above the level of inferior epigastric artery), cannulation at the femoral artery bifurcation, or hypersensitivity to nickel titanium.
- Clean the femoral artery cannulation site with an antiseptic solution.
- Bleed back on the sheath to flush out any thrombus and flush the sheath with saline.
- Create a 5-mm to 7-mm skin nick at the sheath site, and perform blunt dissection of the tissue tract using a hemostat clamp to accommodate insertion of the clip delivery tube into the tissue tract.

Procedure:

- Exchange the femoral artery sheath over a J-tipped guidewire to the StarClose exchange sheath.
- Remove the guidewire.
- Insert the clip applier into the hub of the exchange sheath and advance until the clip applier locks into the sheath hub (click is heard).
- Retract the assembly by 3 cm to 4 cm and deploy the locator wings by pressing down on the plunger.
- Initiate splitting of the sheath by pressing down on the thumb advancer and advance the assembly down to ensure that it can be delivered through the tissue tract.
- Stabilize the device with the left hand at a 45° angle and retract until resistance is felt. The locator wings are now up against the arterial wall.
- With continued stabilization with the left hand, press down on the thumb advancer to fully split the sheath all the way down until a click is heard.
- Raise the clip applier to a 60° to 75° angle and press the assembly down gently. Femoral artery pulsation can usually be felt at this stage.
- With gentle downward pressure, deploy the clip by pressing on the deployment button.
- Hold downward pressure for 2 to 3 seconds.
- Apply counterpressure with the left hand with the index and middle fingers at the sheath exit site and slowly remove the assembly device.
- Inspect for hemostasis and apply manual pressure as needed.

Postprocedure:

- Check the femoral and distal pulse and document this in the chart.
- Apply a small transparent dressing over the arteriotomy site.
- There is no reaccess restriction for the StarClose device, although this is not well-studied.

For more details, please see product information for use.

for coronary interventional procedures by Kiemeneij and Laarman.[68] Initially used as a "backup" access, transradial angiography and intervention are now the preferred alternatives to the traditional femoral approach worldwide, with rapid adoption in the United States.[2] In an analysis of over 2.8 million coronary procedures performed in the United States, 16.1% of procedures, accounting for one in six procedures in 2012, were performed via the transradial route.[2] This is the predominant and preferred approach in many countries in Europe and Asia.[69] In addition to use for diagnostic and interventional coronary procedures, transradial access has been used to treat peripheral artery disease, renal artery disease, and for carotid intervention.[70,71] The advantages of radial access for coronary procedures include reduced bleeding even with aggressive use of anticoagulation and antiplatelet therapies, reduced vascular complication rates, reduced cost, rapid ambulation, reduced length of stay, and increased patient satisfaction when compared with the femoral access.[2,72,73] In the RIVAL trial, 90% of patients randomized to undergo the transradial approach reported preference for the same approach if a repeat procedure was needed, as opposed to 49% in the transfemoral arm.[74] As discussed previously, bleeding and vascular complications are a major source of morbidity and mortality.[75] However, a reduction in mortality with radial access when compared with femoral has only been shown in high-risk subgroups such as those with ST-segment elevation myocardial infarction,[74,76-78] without increase in door to balloon times. Disadvantages of radial access include longer fluoroscopy time and radiation exposure,[79,80] steeper learning curve,[81] limitation of guide catheter size, access failure/crossover, and complications related to the access site such as radial artery occlusion. In addition, in patients with a left internal mammary artery graft, the procedure can be challenging, especially if the right radial artery is used. However, the procedure can be safely performed using the left radial access.[82] Studies have shown that the gap between radial and femoral approaches for access-site crossover, procedure time, and radiation exposure decreases with increasing operator volume and experience.[72,83,84] **Table 3-10** compares radial and femoral arterial access for coronary angiography and intervention.

Anatomic Considerations

Knowledge of the anatomy of the radial artery and the circulation of the hand is important for proper radial artery cannulation and to troubleshoot complications. The radial artery originates from the brachial artery below the elbow and runs on the lateral aspect of the forearm underneath the supinator longus muscle to the wrist, where it lies on top of the styloid process of the radius bone and the scaphoid bone. The artery then passes across the base of the fifth metacarpal bone and joins the deep communicating branch of the ulnar artery to form the deep palmar arch. The superficialis branch of the radial artery joins the palmar part of the ulnar artery to complete the superficial palmar arch. At the region of the styloid process, the radial artery is superficial, has a diameter of 2 mm to 3 mm, and is not adjacent to other neurovascular structures, making it an ideal site for radial artery cannulation.

Preprocedural Considerations

While radial access can be performed safely in the majority of patients, it should be avoided in patients with Raynaud's syndrome, thromboangiitis obliterans (Buerger's disease) (increased risk of radial artery occlusion), those with full-thickness burn over the insertion site, known carpal tunnel syndrome, skin infection at the insertion site, or ipsilateral hemodialysis fistulae. Prior to radial artery cannulation, palpating the radial artery and testing for collateral circulation/patency of the palmar arch of the hand is recommended. This can be performed by either the Allen test or the Barbeau test. In addition, a thorough history and physical examination, a review of laboratory and medication data, and a review of prior angiograms should be performed when available, as outlined in the section on femoral artery access.

Modified Allen Test

Originally described by Dr. Edgar Van Nuys Allen in 1929, the Allen test is a simple bedside visual test to assess for collateral circulation/dual circulation via the palmar arch of

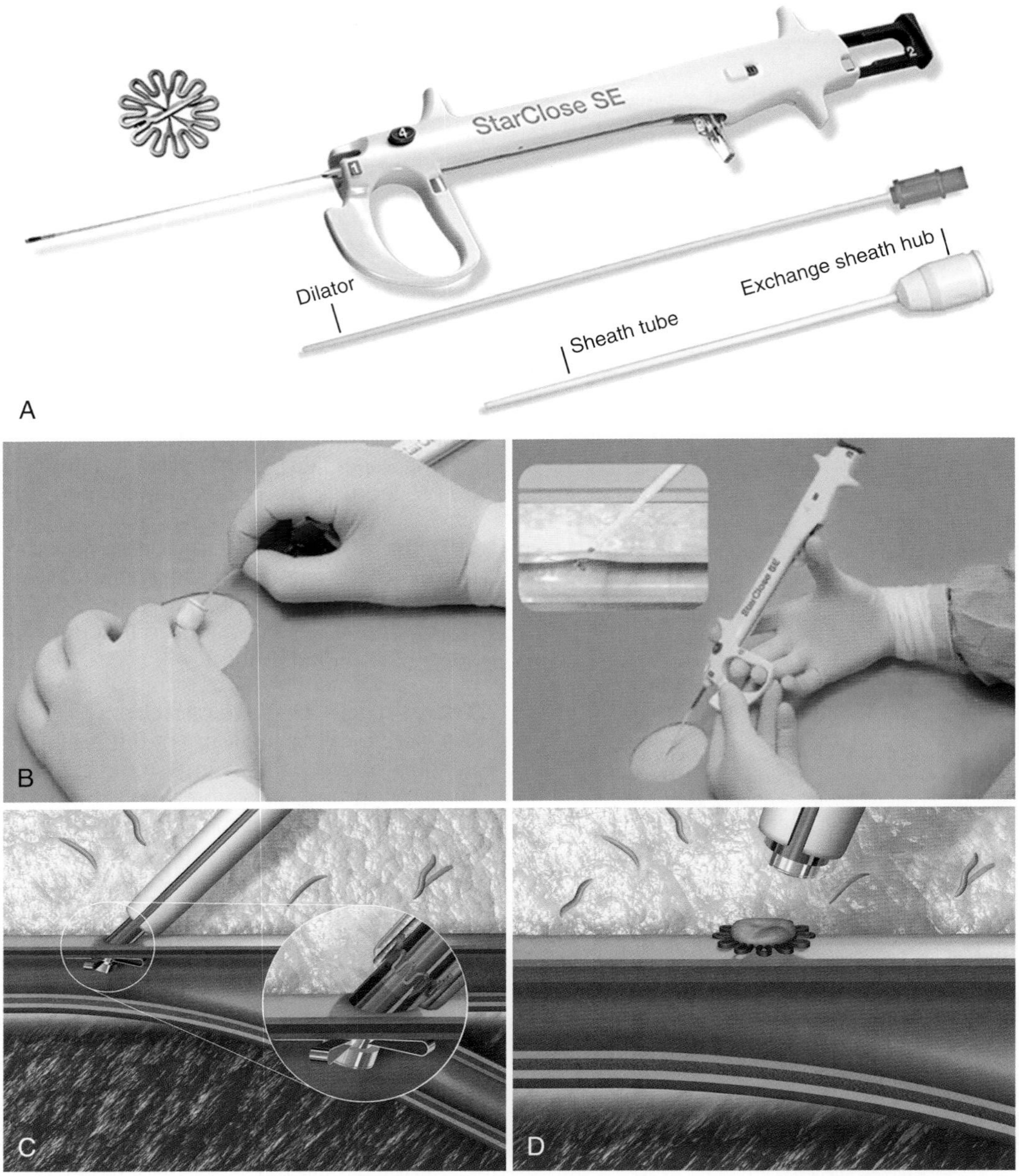

FIGURE 3-22 StarClose device (St. Jude Medical) deployment technique. **A,** Component of the StarClose device showing the nitinol clip, clip applier, dilator, and sheath. **B,** Insertion of the clip applier into the hub of the sheath. Right panel shows the technique for partial splitting of the sheath. **C,** The foot plate deployed at the arteriotomy site. The nitinol clip is shown inside the clip applier. **D,** Deployment of the nitinol clip. *(Reprinted with permission from St. Jude Medical™, © 2014. All rights reserved.)*

the hand (**Figure 3-23A**). Occlude both the radial and the ulnar artery at the wrist. Ask the patient to forcefully clench the hand several times to expel blood from the hand. Ask the patient to then open the hand avoiding wrist and finger hyperextension or wide separation of digits (can result in a false positive or a falsely abnormal test). The hand should appear blanched (**Figure 3-23B**). Release pressure over the ulnar artery and record the time it takes for maximal blush in the palm (**Figure 3-23C**). If the color returns within 5 to 9 seconds, the modified Allen test is considered negative (normal) and the radial artery cannulation can be performed safely. If not, the test is considered positive (abnormal). To date, there is no consensus regarding the optimum cutoff time for a positive modified Allen test. It is preferable to use the term normal/abnormal as the negative/positive connotation may create confusion. The results of the Allen test should be recorded in the patient's chart. The disadvantage of the Allen test is that it is more subjective and several conditions can result in false positive or negative studies.

Barbeau Test

Originally described by Gerald Barbeau in 2004,[86] the Barbeau test is an objective way of assessing for the ulnopalmar arterial arch with the use of pulse oximetry and plethysmography using a pulse oximeter. Place the plethysmography sensor on the index finger or the thumb of the upper extremity to be tested and observe the oximetry waveforms. Compress both the radial and ulnar arteries at the wrist for 2 minutes. The response to the ulnar artery release can be graded as the following: Type A: no damping of pulse tracing immediately after radial artery compression; Type B: damping of pulse tracing; Type C: loss of pulse

TABLE 3-10 Comparison of Radial and Femoral Arterial Access for Coronary Angiography and Intervention

VARIABLES	RADIAL ACCESS	FEMORAL ACCESS
Anatomical Features		
Vessel caliber	2 mm to 3 mm	6 mm to 10 mm
Vascular course	Variable	Constant
Vessel location in relation to skin	Constant, superficial	Variable, related to body habitus
Nearby neurovascular structures	No	Yes
Procedural Features		
Procedural success	Marginally lower than for femoral access	Marginally higher than for radial access
Procedural time	Comparable	Comparable
Contrast load	Comparable	Comparable
Fluoroscopy time	Marginally longer than for femoral access	Marginally shorter than for radial access
Choice of sheath sizes	Restricted	Unrestricted
Learning curve	Longer than for femoral access	Shorter than for radial access
Crossover to alternative arterial access	Higher than for femoral access	Lower than for radial access
IMA graft cannulation	Variable	Simple
Complications		
Access-site bleeding	Lower than for femoral access	Higher than for radial access
Access-vessel occlusion	Up to 30%	Up to 5%
Access-site pseudoaneurysm	0.05%	Up to 5%
PCI Outcomes		
Rate of MACE	Comparable	Comparable
Mortality	Reduced in STEMI more than for femoral access	Increased in STEMI than radial access
Patient Care		
Patient preference	Higher than for femoral access	Lower than for radial access
Time to ambulation	Immediate	2 to 6 hours
Length of hospital stay	Shorter than for femoral access	Longer than for radial access

Data from Byrne RA, Cassese S, Linhardt M, et al: Vascular access and closure in coronary angiography and percutaneous intervention. Nat Rev Cardiol 10(1):27–40, 2013.

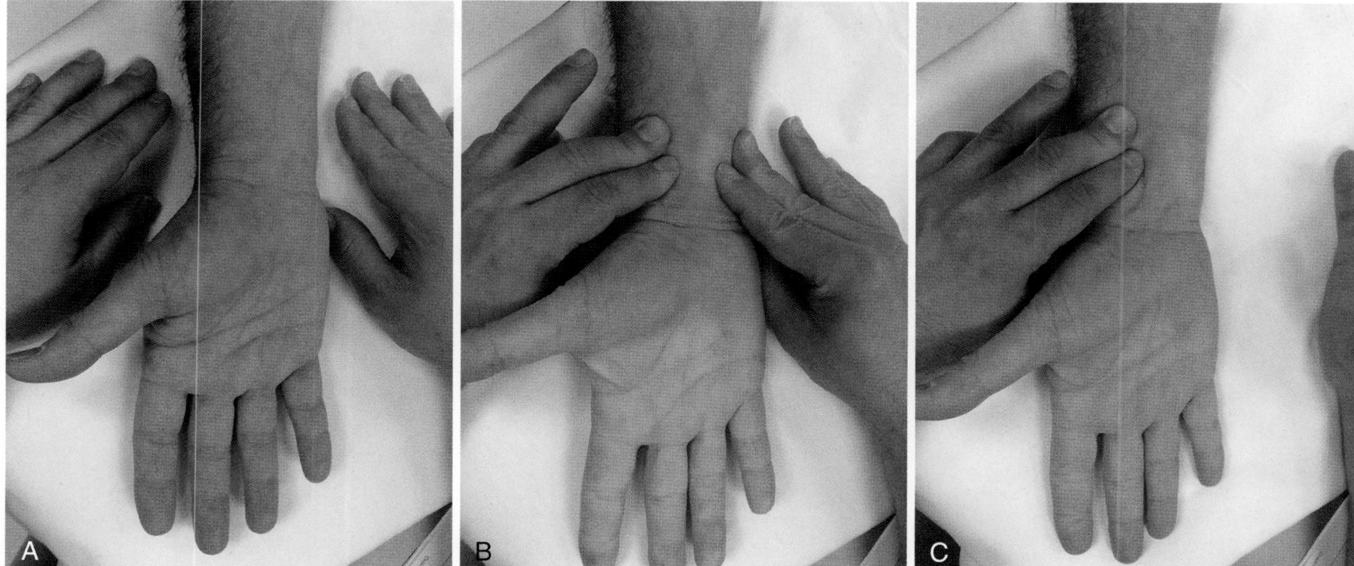

FIGURE 3-23 Modified Allen test to assess dual circulation of the hand. **A,** At baseline prior to compression of the radial and the ulnar arteries. **B,** Blanching of the hand after compression of radial and ulnar artery and after opening and closing the hand to expel blood. **C,** Release of the ulnar artery and blushing of the palm within 5 to 9 seconds indicating a normal modified Allen test. *(Picture courtesy Dr. John Coppola, New York University School of Medicine, New York.)*

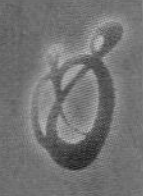

tracing followed by recovery of pulse tracing within 2 minutes; Type D: loss of pulse tracing without recovery within 2 minutes (**Figure 3-24**). The Barbeau test is found to be more sensitive than the Allen test.[86] In the modified Barbeau test, both the radial and ulnar arteries are compressed, resulting in a flat line on the plethysmography. The ulnar artery pressure is now realized and return of the plethysmography waveform is indicative of good ulnar circulation (**Figure 3-25A-C**).

The role of the Allen and Barbeau tests to predict the risk of ischemic complications following radial artery cannulation is controversial, and some experts believe postprocedural "patent hemostasis" is more important. An abnormal Allen/Barbeau test may not necessarily indicate poor distal blood flow as shown by photoplethysmography,[87] fluorescein dye injection,[88] or thumb capillary lactate levels (as noted in the RADAR trial).[89] Moreover, the test assesses for collateral circulation via the palmar arch but other routes of collateral circulation also exist (via the interosseous artery). In addition, in patients with an abnormal test who had a radial artery harvested for a bypass graft, no postoperative hand ischemia has been reported.[90] On the other hand, reports of ischemic injury have been reported even after a normal Allen test.[91] Ischemic injury after radial cannulation can also be due to distal embolization or nerve compression.

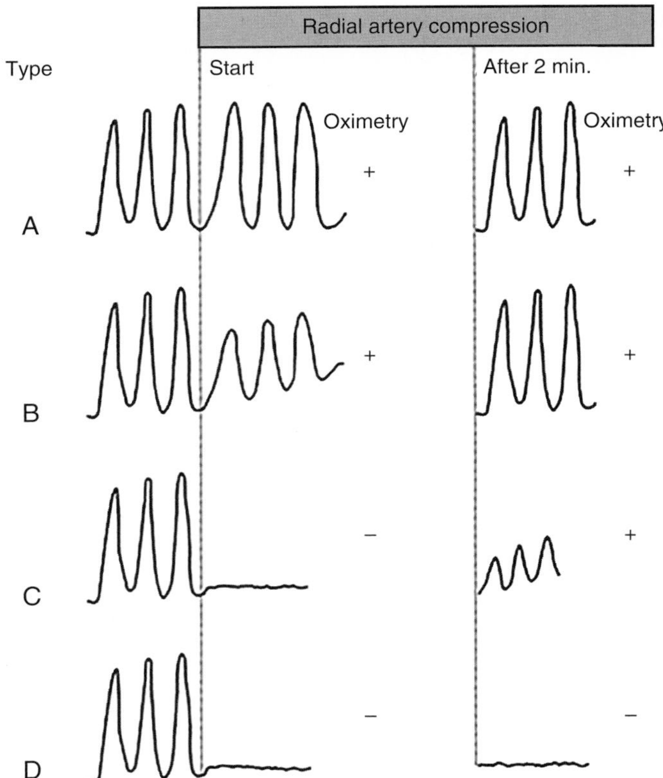

FIGURE 3-24 Barbeau test to assess dual circulation of the hand. Type **A** to **D** based on the original description by Barbeau. *(Reproduced with permission from Barbeau et al: Am Heart J 147(3):489-493, 2004.)*

Procedural Considerations

Prior to the commencement of the procedure, a "time-out" should be performed to verify the patient's identity, review the patient's medical history and indications for the

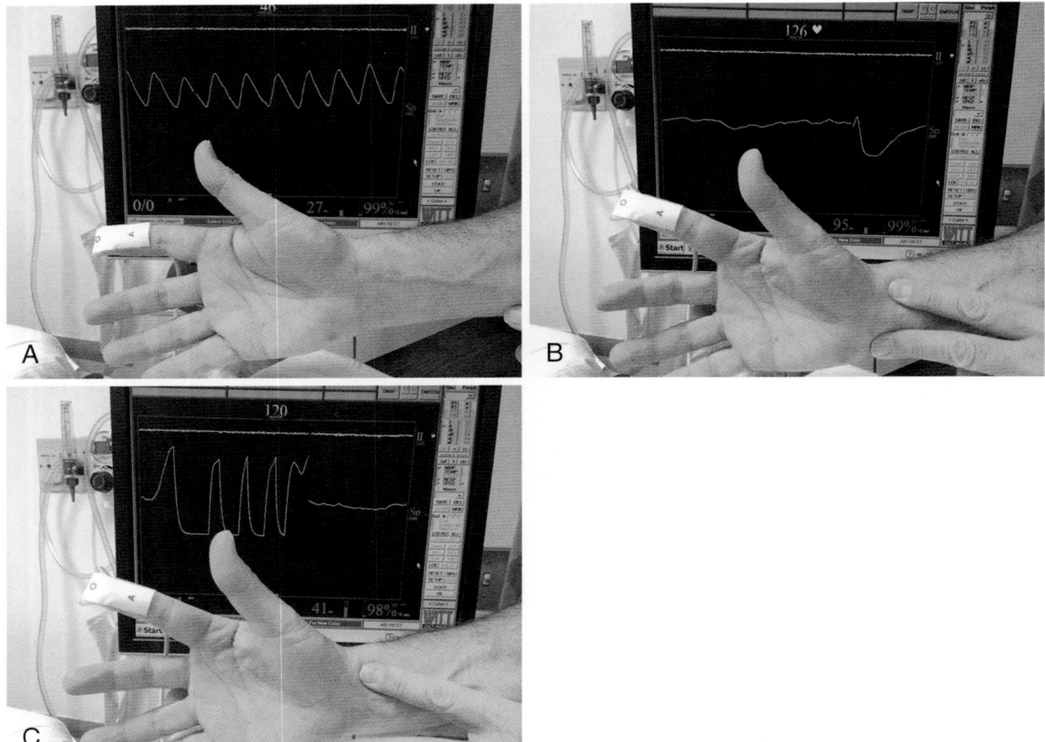

FIGURE 3-25 Modified Barbeau test to assess dual circulation of the hand. **A,** Baseline. Sensor on the index finger with normal plethysmography waveforms and oxygen saturation. **B,** Occlusion of both the radial and ulnar artery with flat lining of the plethysmography waveforms. **C,** Release of the ulnar artery and return of the plethysmography waveforms to baseline. *(Picture courtesy Dr. John Coppola, New York University School of Medicine, New York.)*

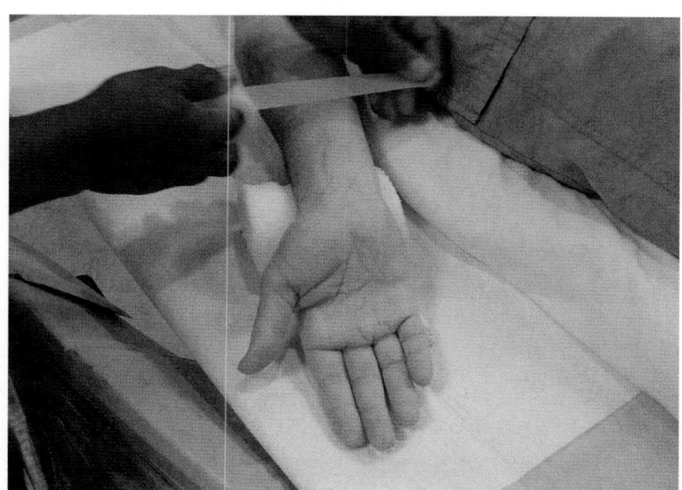

FIGURE 3-26 Positioning of the right hand for transradial access. A rolled gauze or towel is placed underneath the patient's wrist so as to hyperextend it. *(Picture courtesy Dr. John Coppola, New York University School of Medicine, New York.)*

procedures, review the laboratory data, and confirm that the patient has provided written informed consent. The patient is then prepared and draped under sterile conditions.

Positioning

A number of arm boards/radial boards have been devised to assist in proper positioning of the patient's arms for adequate radial access and to ensure comfort to the patient during the procedure. With the patient in a supine position, the arm should be maintained in a neutral position with the palm up and the wrist exposed. The access site should be clipped of hair if present. The wrist should be hyperextended to 30° using a roll of gauze or towel and the hand and forearm secured to the board using tape (**Figure 3-26**). The arm should then be prepared and draped under sterile conditions. Some operators prepare the femoral site for "backup," although this is rarely needed with more experienced operators.

Conscious Sedation and Local Anesthesia

Conscious sedation is administered with the use of a sedative (e.g., versed) and an analgesic (e.g., fentanyl). Local anesthesia (e.g., lidocaine) is administered at the site of the radial artery using a 25-gauge needle or an insulin syringe to first create a dermal bleb. The amount of local anesthesia to be administered must be sufficient to provide comfort for the patient while not obliterating the radial artery pulsation. Care must be taken not to inject lidocaine into the artery as it can cause serious arrhythmias.

Technique

The radial artery can be cannulated using a 20- to 21-gauge needle. Specialized access kits are now available. Some of the access kits have a 21-gauge needle and others have a microcatheter over a metal needle. The ideal puncture site for the radial artery is 2 cm to 3 cm proximal to the flexor crease of the wrist. If the pulse is not easily palpable, distal compression of the radial artery close to the palmar crease can increase the pulse amplitude at the more proximal site of puncture. Access can be obtained either with a through and through puncture (often preferred) (Video 3-1) or an anterior wall puncture (Video 3-2). With the through and through puncture technique, the needle with the microcatheter is advanced into the artery at a 30° to 45° angle until a flash of blood is seen (**Figure 3-27A-B**). The needle is then advanced through the posterior wall of the artery until the flash stops (**Figure 3-27B**). The needle is now removed from the microcatheter and the microcatheter is slowly withdrawn until pulsatile blood flow is seen (**Figure 3-27C**). The 0.018 or 0.021 inch guidewire is then inserted and the microcatheter exchanged for the appropriate size sheath with the dilator (**Figure 3-27D**). It may sometimes be necessary to perform a skin nick prior to advancement of the sheath, especially for sheath size >5 Fr. Care should be taken to ensure that the bevel of the scalpel is facing up and away from the artery to prevent accidental transection of the radial artery. The dilator and the guidewire are then removed, the sheath flushed with saline, and an intraarterial vasodilator cocktail (verapamil/diltiazem or nitroglycerin) administered.[92] Hydrophilic sheaths are generally used to minimize trauma and vasospasm. In addition, an anticoagulant such as unfractionated heparin or bivalirudin should be administered to prevent radial artery thrombosis.[93] The recommended regimen is intraarterial or intravenous unfractionated heparin at a dose of at least 50 U/kg up to a maximum of 5000 units.[94] In patients with heparin-induced thrombocytopenia, bivalirudin should be used.[94]

Closure and Postprocedural Care

Closure

Similar to that of the femoral artery, the radial artery sheath should be left in place for the shortest duration required to minimize complications. Prior to removal of the sheath, the sheath should be back bled to flush out thrombus and flushed with saline. Closure can be obtained by manual compression or by using specialized devices that maintain pressure on the wrist. The TR band is one such device, which consists of a transparent band with a dual compression balloon. Prior to application of this device, the introducer sheath should be withdrawn by 2 cm to 3 cm (Video 3-3). The green marker on the TR band is aligned 2 mm to 3 mm proximal to the puncture site and the strap is tightened with the adjustable fastener (**Figure 3-28A, B**). The syringe should be filled with 18 mL of air (maximal volume allowed) and attached to the TR band. Inject half the volume into the TR band balloon and remove the sheath with one hand while injecting the rest of the air with the other. Now slowly withdraw air 1 cc at a time until a flash of blood is seen at the puncture site. Now inject 1 cc to 2 cc of air to obtain hemostasis. Excess blood can be wiped away from underneath the band with sterile gauze. The TR band assures adequate hemostasis without compromising blood flow of the radial artery. Keep the syringe with the patient for later use during deflation. Assess for radial artery patency using the reverse Barbeau test. Place the pulse oximeter on the first or second finger of the affected arm. Occlude the ulnar artery to assess patency of the radial artery. Observe for waveforms on plethysmography. If no waveforms are seen on plethysmography when occluding the ulnar artery, the TR band should be slowly deflated while holding pressure on the ulnar artery, until the waveform returns (so-called patent hemostasis). Now the radial artery is patent. Maintain the wrist in a neutral position or with a small pillow underneath to ensure patient comfort. Perform periodic physical examinations while waiting to remove the TR band. This should

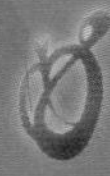

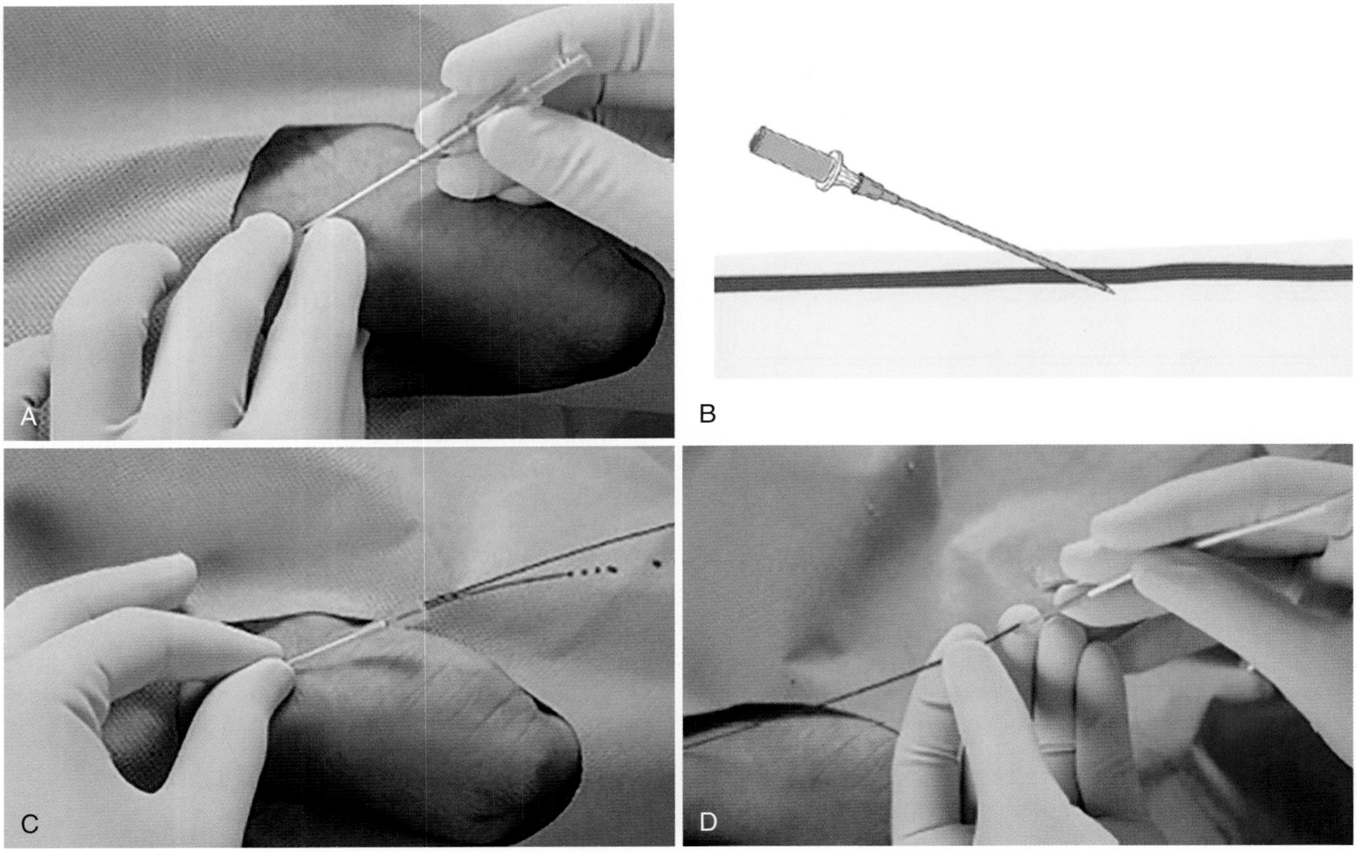

FIGURE 3-27 Transradial access. **A,** Ideal puncture site is 2 cm to 3 cm proximal to the crease of the wrist. The artery should be entered at a 30° to 45° angle. **B,** Through and through puncture technique. Once a flash is seen upon entry of the artery, the needle is advanced, puncturing the posterior wall until no blood flow is seen at the needle hub. **C,** The needle is removed and the microcatheter slowly advanced back until pulsatile blood flow is seen. A guidewire is inserted. **D,** The microcatheter is exchanged for an appropriate size sheath over the guidewire. *(Reproduced with permission from Patel's Atlas of Transradial Intervention. HMP Communications LLC [HMP].)*

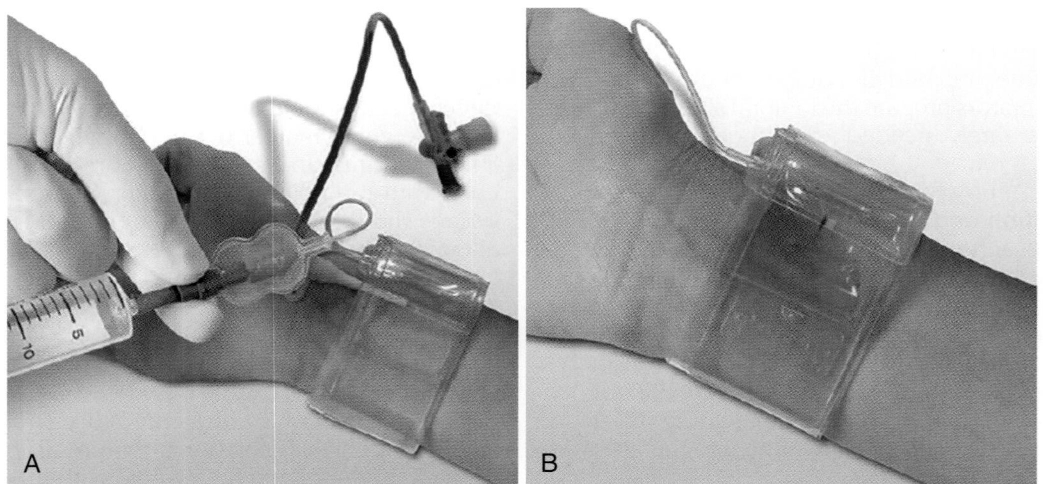

FIGURE 3-28 Transradial access site closure using a TR band (Terumo). **A,** The radial sheath is pulled back by 2 cm to 3 cm and the TR band applied such that the green marker is over the arteriotomy site (not the skin puncture site). The balloon is injected into the port (maximum of 18 cc). **B,** The sheath is removed and air is removed from the balloon until a flash of blood is seen, at which point 1 cc to 2 cc of air is reinjected until hemostasis is obtained. *(Reprinted with permission from Terumo™, © 2014. All rights reserved [permission pending].)*

include inspection for any signs of bleeding, edema, color of extremity, temperature, capillary refill, pain, and power. Prevent use of the affected extremity and maintain a neutral position.

When it is time to remove the TR band (30 minutes after diagnostic catheterization or 2 hours after the end of PCI or cessation of bivalirudin infusion), remove 1 cc to 2 cc of air and watch for any bleeding. If any signs of bleeding are observed, insert air until hemostasis is obtained and retry removing air in 5 to 10 minutes. If no bleeding is observed, 1 cc to 2 cc of air must be removed every 2 to 3 minutes until all the air is removed and hemostasis obtained. The TR band can now be removed, the site dressed with a sterile transparent dressing, and the site observed for any bleeding.

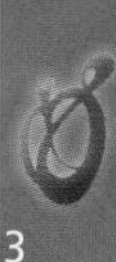

Postprocedure Care

Patients should have radial artery patency assessed before discharge and also at the first postprocedure visit. Patients should be instructed not to manipulate the wrist for 24 hours post procedure and to not lift any objects over 3 to 5 pounds for the next 2 days. The following discharge instructions may be appropriate, although this is not driven by evidence and variations based on local practice are common:

- Protect your wrist from bending for 48 hours. Deep bending of your wrist could cause bleeding.
- Do not lift, push, or pull anything over 5 pounds for 48 hours and over 10 pounds for a week.
- Do not write or type for 48 hours.
- Do not use your hand/arm to support your weight when rising from a chair or bed for 48 hours.
- Do not drive a car for 48 hours unless instructed by your doctor. Someone else should drive you home.
- Do not operate a lawnmower, motorcycle, chainsaw, or all-terrain vehicle for 48 hours.
- No soaking the arm or swimming for one week. Showering is fine.
- All activities are permitted after a week if no problems occur.
- Call your doctor for any bleeding, swelling, or pain at the site.

Complications and Challenges

Radial Artery Occlusion

A relatively common complication of radial access is early and late radial artery occlusion, virtually all of which are asymptomatic and the majority will spontaneously recanalize within a month. The incidence is variable from 1.1% to 20% and depends on the patient population and diagnostic test adopted. Risk factors for radial artery occlusion include large sheath size (sheath-to-artery ratio), occlusive hemostasis, and lack of anticoagulation use. Other risk factors for radial artery occlusion such as longer sheath and nonhydrophilic coating are controversial.[95] Asymptomatic radial artery occlusion can be detected by plethysmography or by color Doppler ultrasound. Symptomatic patients present with signs and symptoms of arterial insufficiency—the five P's: pain, paresthesia, paralysis, pallor, and pulselessness—which is extremely rare given dual blood supply to the hand.[96] Radial artery occlusion, even if asymptomatic, can limit future radial access and limit the use of the radial artery for dialysis fistula as a conduit for bypass grafts or invasive arterial pressure monitoring and hence should be prevented when possible. The incidence of radial artery occlusion can be minimized by using smaller sheath sizes less than the radial artery diameter, using anticoagulation, avoiding repeated access of the radial artery, and utilizing patent hemostasis after sheath removal.[94,97] Other measures that may potentially reduce the risk of radial artery occlusion include use of hydrophilic sheaths, use of drugs to reduce radial artery spasm, and limiting the duration of radial artery compression.[94] Using the above measures, the rate of radial artery occlusion is around 1.1% to 1.8%.[97] Treatment for asymptomatic patients is observation alone. If radial artery occlusion is noted early after the procedure (3-4 hours after removal of the TR band), ipsilateral ulnar artery compression for 1 hour to promote radial artery reopening has been shown to be successful.[98] In addition, treatment with anticoagulation (enoxaparin or fondaparinux) for 4 weeks increases the rate of recanalization.[99] Patients who are extremely symptomatic will need revascularization either by percutaneous technique or by surgery, though this appears to be very rare.

Access Failure

Many studies have evaluated the predictors of radial access failure. Access failure for the transradial procedure can be a failure to cannulate the artery, failure to advance the catheter to the ascending aorta due to spasm, loops or tortuosity, or failure to obtain adequate guide support, all of which necessitate conversion to alternate access routes (femoral, ulnar, or contralateral radial artery). There are a few patient-related factors such as advanced age, female, and short stature that are associated with increased failure.[100]

- ***Radial Artery Spasm (Figure 3-29A, B):*** Radial artery spasm can be prevented by adequate sedation before the procedure (even prior to the administration of a local anesthetic). This will minimize the circulating catecholamine-induced vasospasm. In addition, administering an intraarterial vasodilator cocktail after access is obtained can minimize spasm. Intraarterial verapamil/diltiazem with or without nitroglycerin is routinely used, although the cocktail has been variable. In addition, using smaller size sheaths with a hydrophilic coating and smaller size catheters can minimize spasm.
- ***Radial Loops (Figure 3-30):*** These are a common arterial anomaly that can be an obstacle for advancement of wires and catheters and increase the risk of radial artery spasm and perforation. Most radial loops can be traversed with a guidewire (preferably a hydrophilic wire) or by using a 0.014 inch coronary wire. Balloon-assisted tracking involves use of a coronary balloon that is nominally inflated to assist passage of a guide catheter over a 0.014 inch wire by creating a smoother transition from catheter tip to wire. Once the catheter is passed beyond the loop, the loops usually straighten. In rare cases, switching over to a different access may be required.
- ***Subclavian/Brachiocephalic Artery Tortuosity (Figure 3-31):*** Increased subclavian/brachiocephalic artery tortuosity due to unwinding of the aorta is commonly seen in the elderly and in those with hypertension. Common maneuvers to help navigate this include asking patients to take a deep breath to straighten the segment and or to use an angled hydrophilic guidewire. Switching to a left radial approach can be considered.
- ***Lack of Guide Support (Figure 3-32):*** Switching the guide based on the need and considering specific transradial guide catheters can help as they have secondary curves that use the contralateral aortic wall for support. In addition, sheathless guide catheters that allow a larger inner diameter catheter without increasing the outer diameter have been developed to provide more support.[101] Not fully inserting the introducer sheath (which has a larger outer diameter than the guide catheter) into the radial artery may also allow use of larger size guides without causing radial artery spasm. Switching to the left radial approach can also be considered.

Perforation

Perforation of the radial artery is usually caused by forceful manipulation of the hydrophilic wire, sheath, or catheter. The incidence is around 1%. The site of perforation can be along the course of the artery. However, common sites are the

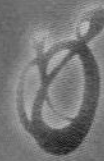

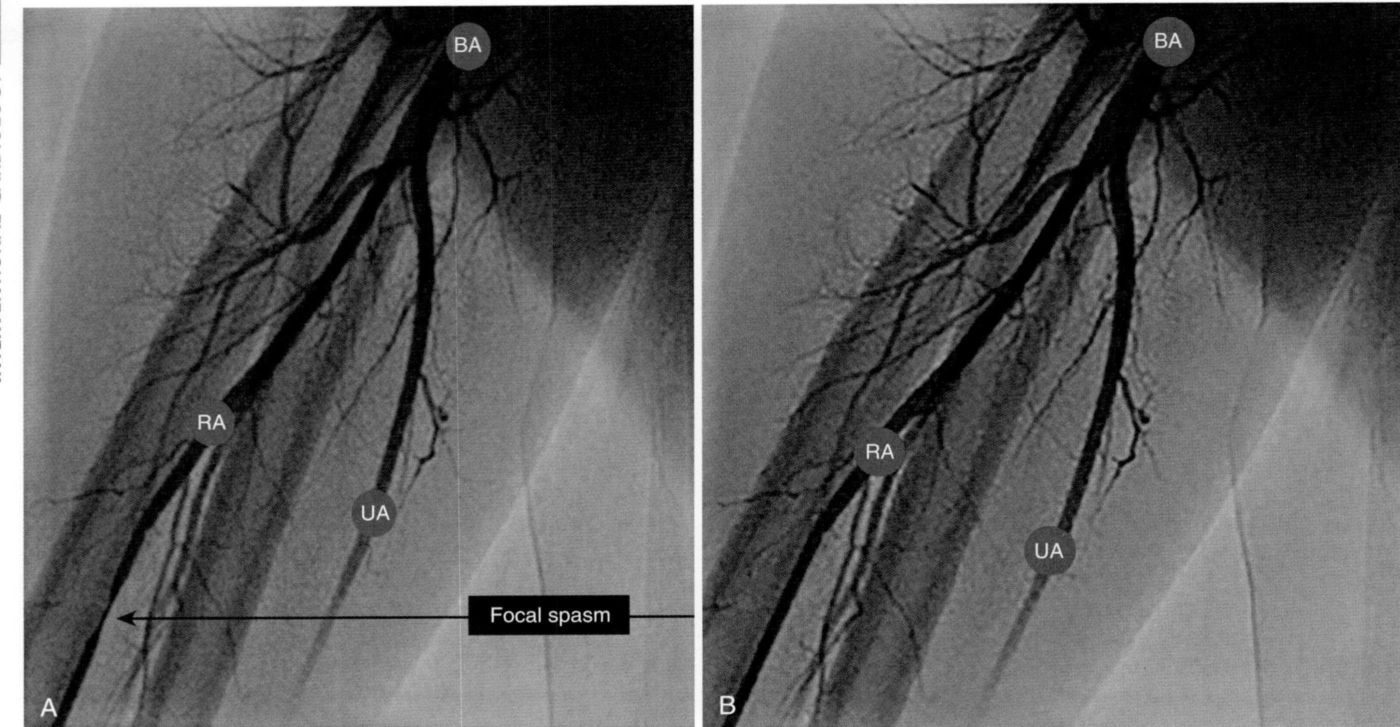

FIGURE 3-29 Radial artery spasm. **A,** Focal spasm seen just distal to the radial artery sheath (black arrow). **B,** Spasm relieved after administration of an intraarterial vasodilator cocktail. *BA,* Brachial artery; *RA,* radial artery; *UA,* ulnar artery. *(Reproduced with permission from Patel's Atlas of Transradial Intervention. HMP Communications LLC [HMP].)*

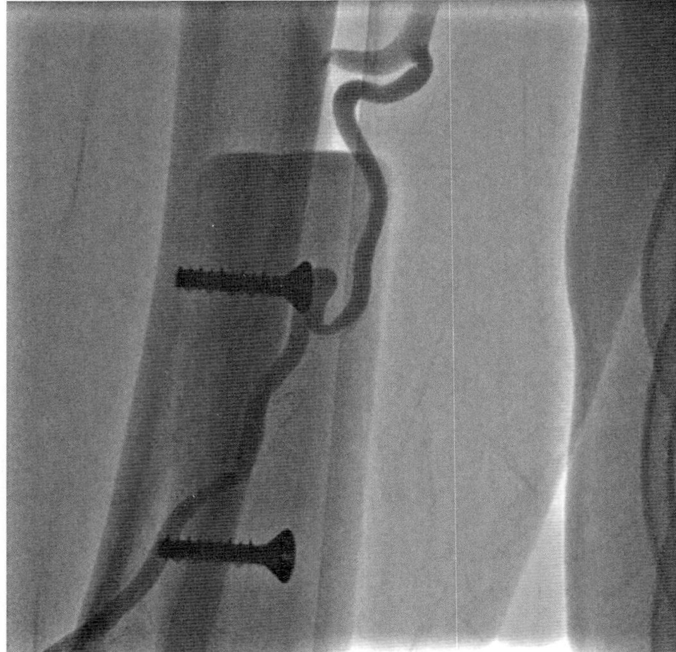

FIGURE 3-30 Radial artery loop and tortuosity. *(Image courtesy Dr. Sudhanva Hegde, Kings County Medical Center, New York.)*

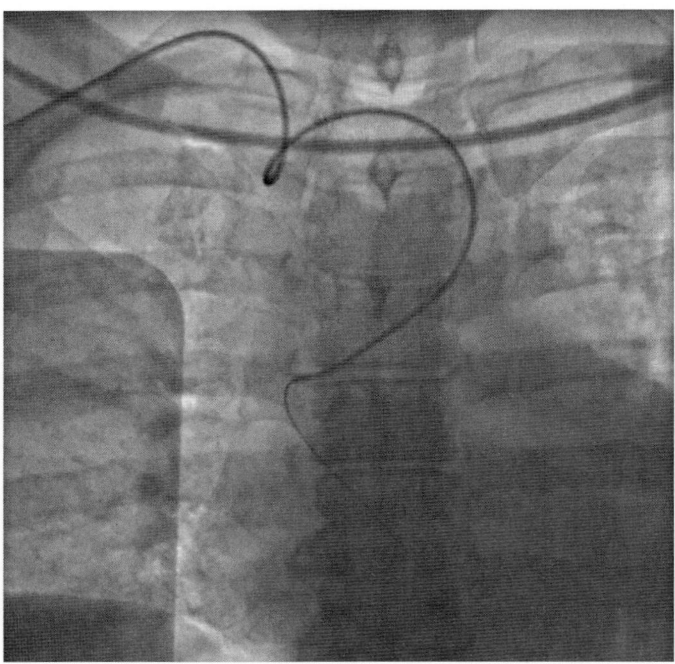

FIGURE 3-31 Subclavian/Brachiocephalic artery tortuosity. *(Image courtesy Dr. Sudhanva Hegde, Kings County Medical Center, New York.)*

forearm and the arm. Risk factors include radial loops and tortuosities. Diagnosis is on angiography demonstrating contrast extravasation. Failure to achieve hemostasis can lead to hematoma formation and/or compartment syndrome in the forearm. If perforation is detected at the time of guide catheter advancement, the catheter should be advanced across the site of the perforation and the coronary procedure carried out. The guide serves as an internal hemostasis to prevent contrast extravasations even in fully anticoagulated patients. At the end of the coronary procedure, the guide should be withdrawn over a wire just distal to the site of perforation and repeat angiography performed to evaluate for the perforation (**Figure 3-33A, B**). Most perforations can be sealed with the above technique.

Application of the blood pressure cuff to the forearm for external compression with inflation to 30 mm to 50 mm Hg may also be helpful. Treatment of hematoma and compartment syndrome is described below.

Hematoma

The incidence of hematoma is 14.4%.[102] Hematoma may occur at the site of the sheath insertion or along the course of the artery—forearm, arm, and even infraclavicular. Hematoma at the sheath insertion site is usually due to ineffective compression. Forearm hematoma is due to radial artery perforation during the introduction of the wire, sheath, or catheter. Most small hematomas are asymptomatic. Larger hematoma can cause symptoms of hand ischemia, especially when collateral circulation of the hand is poor. Treatment is by manual compression and reversal of anticoagulation if required. Effective compression of the forearm can be achieved by using a blood pressure cuff, though such nonspecific compression may sometimes facilitate development of compartment syndrome. Treatment of compartment syndrome is described below.

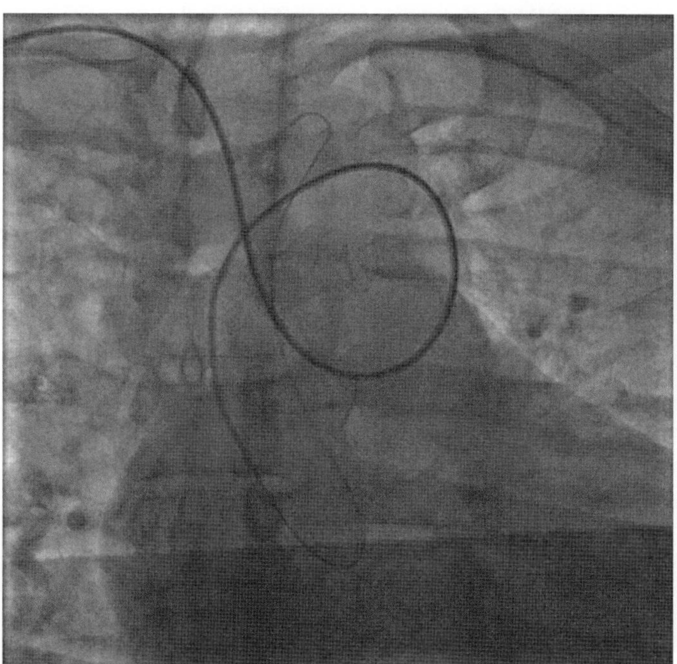

FIGURE 3-32 Low insertion of the brachiocephalic artery into the descending aorta. *(Image courtesy Dr. Sudhanva Hegde, Kings County Medical Center, New York.)*

Compartment Syndrome

This is a very rare complication with a reported incidence of 0.1% to 0.4%.[103] This is caused by radial artery perforation in the forearm. The forearm has the anterior compartment, which contains muscles and neurovascular bundles covered by the antebrachial fascia (deep fascia of the forearm). As such, any bleeding contained within the fascia can cause high fluid pressure (which prevents venous and lymphatic drainage with edema), nerve damage, and eventually muscle damage collectively called compartment syndrome. Patients present with symptoms and signs of ischemia with the five P's—pain, paresthesia, paralysis, pallor, and pulselessness. Pain is usually out of proportion to the injury, especially with passive extension of the fingers (pathognomonic sign). Radial and ulnar pulses are usually intact. Treatment is by urgent surgery (extensive fasciotomy). Late consequences include limb ischemia, hand paralysis, septicemia, and death.

Radial Artery Pseudoaneurysm (Figure 3-34)

Similar to femoral artery pseudoaneurysm, radial artery pseudoaneurysm is due to ineffective hemostasis resulting in a aneurysmal dilatation lined by fibrous tissue and

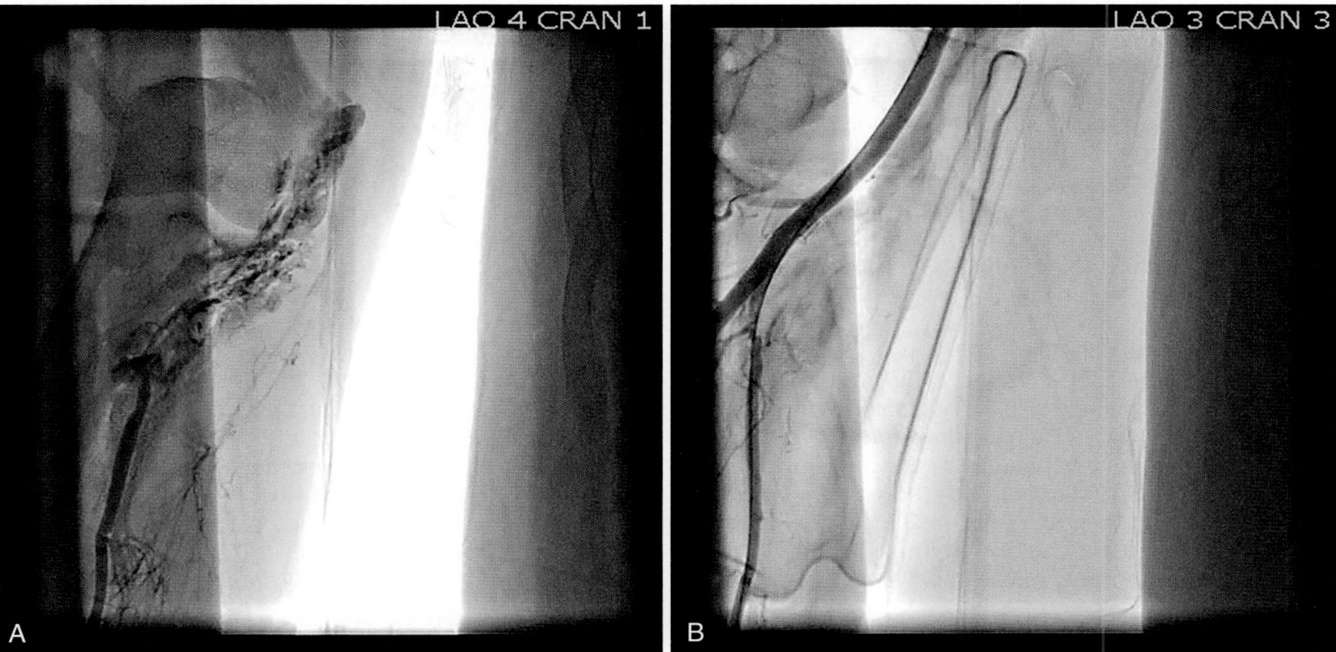

FIGURE 3-33 Radial artery perforation. **A,** Guidewire-induced radial artery perforation at the beginning of the procedure in a patient presenting with ST segment elevation myocardial infarction. The true lumen was wired, a guide catheter was passed over it, and percutaneous coronary intervention was performed on the culprit artery. **B,** Perforation site at the end of the procedure showing no active extravasation of contrast.

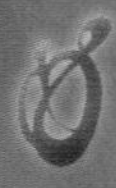

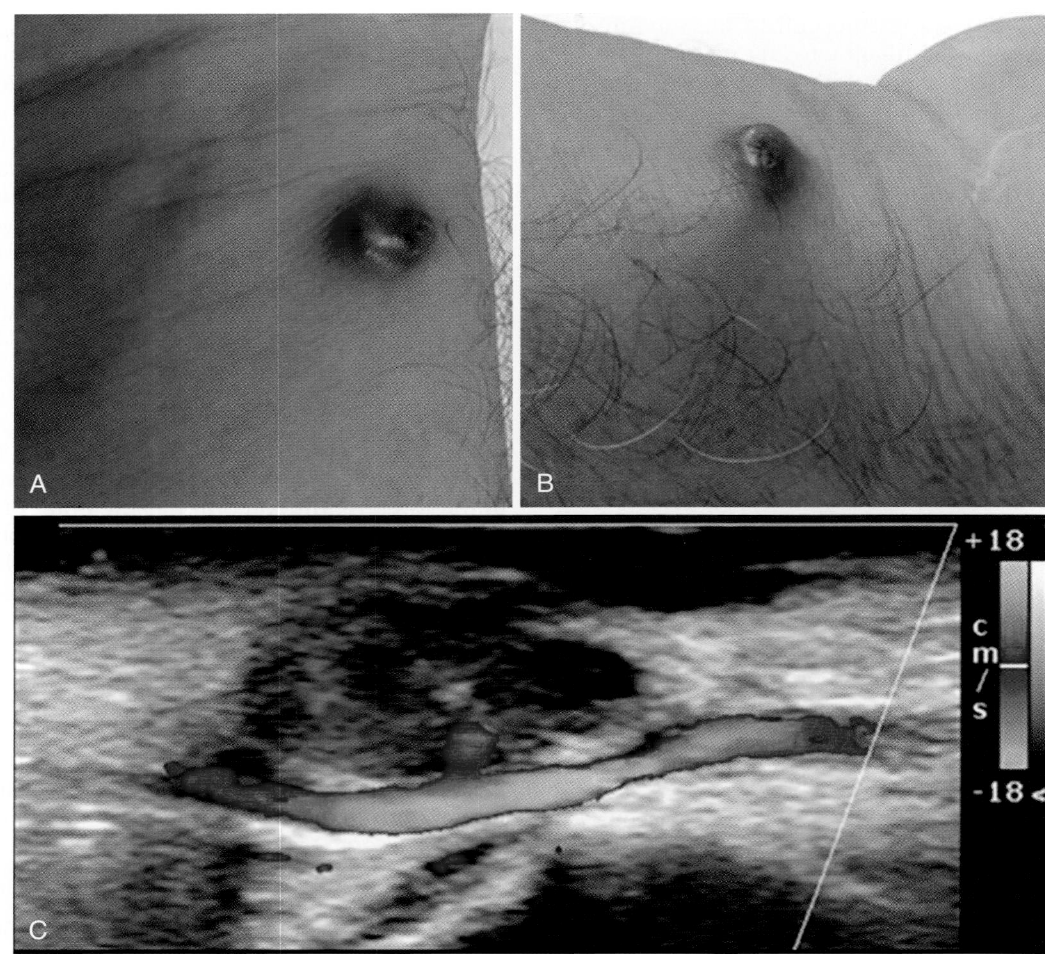

FIGURE 3-34 Late development of radial artery pseudoaneurysm. **A** and **B** show swelling at the radial artery puncture site 5 months after transradial procedure. **C,** Duplex ultrasound of the radial artery showing a large, patent vessel with a short neck of blood flow into a partially thrombosed pseudoaneurysmal sac. *(Image courtesy Drs. Ravikiran Korabathina, Bayfront Health, St. Petersburg, Fla.; and John T. Coppola, New York University School of Medicine, New York.)*

thrombus with communication with the artery via a tract. The incidence is about 0.1%.[103] Risk factors for pseudoaneurysm include multiple puncture attempts, aggressive anticoagulation therapy, use of large sheaths, and ineffective manual compression.[103] Patients present with pain and/or swelling at the arterial puncture site. Diagnosis is by color Doppler ultrasound. Treatment involves prolonged manual compression, cessation/reversal of anticoagulation as needed, ultrasound-guided compression/thrombin injection, and, in rare cases, surgery.

Radial Arteriovenous Fistula

Arteriovenous fistula between the radial artery and the veins is a rare complication (0.3%) occurring during cannulation of the artery.[104] Patients may present with pain and swelling and rarely with signs and symptoms of high output cardiac failure. Examination reveals a palpable thrill and/or a bruit. Diagnosis is confirmed by color Doppler ultrasonography. Treatment is by prolonged manual compression. If this fails, surgery or use of covered stents may be considered.

Sterile Granuloma

Sterile granuloma at the entry site is due to chronic inflammation at the arterial entry site due to hydrophilic coated sheaths (incidence up to 2% with certain older brands of sheath).[105] Patients present 2 to 3 weeks after the procedure with swelling. There are usually no systemic signs of fever or increased white blood cell count. Differential diagnosis includes infection or pseudoaneurysm. Ultrasonography should be performed to rule out pseudoaneurysm. Diagnosis is by biopsy that shows sterile granulomas with chronic inflammation and giant cell reaction. Treatment involves surgical drainage.

Radial Artery Avulsion

This is a rare complication due to excessive radial artery spasm during sheath removal.[106] In cases of excessive spasm, treatment should include intraarterial vasodilators, use of sedation, and slow retraction of the sheath over extended periods of time. In some cases, the sheath should be left in place and an attempt at removal should be performed several hours later. In very rare cases, general anesthesia may be necessary to completely resolve the spasm.

ULNAR ARTERIAL ACCESS AND CLOSURE

The ulnar artery can be used as an alternative to the radial artery for percutaneous coronary and peripheral vascular procedures. The artery is usually smaller than the radial artery (although this is variable), has a deeper course in the forearm and wrist making it difficult to palpate, and lies in close proximity to the neurovascular bundle at the wrist. Preprocedural considerations, access technique, and post-procedure care including closure are similar to those described under radial access. Transulnar access has been found to have a higher crossover rate due to access failure when compared with transradial access. However, in a few patient subsets, the ulnar artery pulse may be stronger than the radial and can serve as an access site for failed transradial access.

BRACHIAL ARTERIAL ACCESS AND CLOSURE

Introduction and Anatomy

With the increase in transradial procedures, brachial artery access is less preferred as it has a higher complication profile. The advantage of brachial access over radial access is the larger size of the artery, which can accommodate larger sheath sizes. However, brachial access carries with it the risk of distal ischemia and embolization. The brachial artery is a continuation of the axillary artery below the lower border of the teres major muscle, runs down the ventral surface of the arm into the cubital fossa on the medial aspects of the biceps brachialis, and divides into the radial and ulnar arteries. The artery is in close proximity with the median nerve, which is medial to the artery at the level of the cubital fossa. In addition, a fascia covers the brachial artery and hence a hematoma can risk compartment syndrome.

Procedure

The arm is abducted on an arm board and the brachial artery site in and around the antecubital fossa is prepped and draped. Preprocedural considerations are similar to those described under the radial access section. The artery is palpated just proximal to the antecubital fossa where the biceps tendon can be felt. A 21-gauge micropuncture kit is preferred to minimize complications. The artery is entered with the modified Seldinger technique and exchanged for a suitable size sheath. Anterior wall puncture is preferable to a through and through puncture to reduce the risk of hematoma. Brachial artery access can also be performed under ultrasound guidance. After access is obtained, intraarterial administration of a vasodilator cocktail will help minimize spasm. Anticoagulation with heparin (or bivalirudin for patients with heparin-induced thrombocytopenia) also can potentially reduce the risk of ischemic complications.

Closure and Complications

After the procedure the sheath should be left in for a short period of time and removed immediately after diagnostic catheterization or after the effect of anticoagulants has worn off after interventional procedures (as described under the femoral arterial access section). The most commonly employed technique is manual compression. The reported rates of complication are high and many patients with access complication require surgical correction (for brachial artery thrombosis or pseudoaneurysm).[107] Topical hemostatic agents may be used as an adjunct to manual compression. In addition, various vascular closure devices such as the Angio-Seal have been used for brachial artery hemostasis with a high success rate.[108] However, complications such as brachial artery occlusion and pseudoaneurysm can occur.[108]

VENOUS ACCESS AND CLOSURE

Right Heart Catheterization via the Basilic Vein

Anatomy

The basilic vein arises from the dorsum of the hand, traverses through the medial part of the forearm and arm, continues as the axillary vein and the subclavian vein, which joins with the internal jugular vein to form the brachiocephalic vein, which drains into the superior vena cava and then into the right atrium. The basilic vein at the elbow is being increasingly used for right heart catheterization.

Procedure

Have the nurse insert an intravenous heplock in the basilic vein in the prep area. Usually an 18-gauge or a 20-gauge line should be placed. Exchange the line for a 5 Fr sheath in the cardiac catheterization laboratory after prepping and draping the area. A 5 Fr Swan-Ganz catheter is now advanced while injecting saline through it into the axillary and subclavian vein into the brachiocephalic vein, SVC, and the right atrium. In some patients, the subclavian vein joins the internal jugular vein into the brachiocephalic vein at an angle that may make the passage of the Swan-Ganz catheter difficult. In such cases a 0.021- or 0.025-inch Swan wire or a 0.014- or 0.018-inch coronary guidewire can be used and the catheter advanced over this wire.

Complication

In rare cases, perforation of the vein, especially at the point of insertion into the internal subclavian vein, can result in infraclavicular hematoma.

Other Venous Access—Femoral/ Internal Jugular

Procedure

Central venous access via either the femoral vein or the internal jugular vein using ultrasound guidance is gaining popularity. Under sterile conditions, the area is prepped and draped. Ultrasound is then performed to locate the vein. The vein is distinguished from the artery as it is more compressible than the artery and with the triphasic Doppler signal from the artery. Once the ideal site is obtained, local anesthesia should be administered starting with the skin and working deeper (can be done under ultrasound guidance). An 18-gauge or a 20-gauge needle is then used to enter the vein under direct ultrasound guidance and using the modified Seldinger technique.

Closure

Manual compression is the most commonly used modality to obtain hemostasis after cannulation of the veins. However, VCDs such as the Perclose can be used to close larger veins such as the femoral vein (not an FDA-approved indication). Care must be taken not to pull back on the device too much as the thin-walled veins can tear. This is ideal for fully anticoagulated patients and those who receive thrombolytic agents. In addition, in patients undergoing structural heart procedure with the insertion of a sheath >10 Fr size, preclosure of the vein using the technique described under the

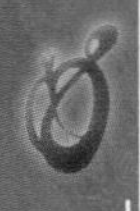

Perclose section has been found to be successful with a very low complication rate.[109]

Complications

Common complications include bleeding or hematoma at the site. Other complications include AV fistula formation.

CONCLUSIONS

Vascular access remains the key initial step of most procedures in the interventional suite. Careful planning is necessary to choose the optimal access site, though for arterial access, the radial artery is gaining popularity. Nevertheless, femoral arterial access will remain important for procedures that need larger diameter access sites, such as for percutaneous valves or hemodynamic support devices. Hemostasis is also a critical part of the procedure, and this stage is crucial to minimize what has become the most common source of complications in patients undergoing interventional procedures—vascular complications.

References

1. Babu SC, Piccorelli GO, Shah PM, et al: Incidence and results of arterial complications among 16,350 patients undergoing cardiac catheterization. *J Vasc Surg* 10(2):113–116, 1989.
2. Feldman DN, Swaminathan RV, Kaltenbach LA, et al: Adoption of radial access and comparison of outcomes to femoral access in percutaneous coronary intervention: an updated report from the national cardiovascular data registry (2007-2012). *Circulation* 127(23):2295–2306, 2013.
3. Rapoport S, Sniderman K, Morse S, et al: Pseudoaneurysm: a complication of faulty technique in femoral arterial puncture. *Radiology* 154(2):529–530, 1985.
4. Rupp SB, Vogelzang RL, Nemcek AA, Jr, et al: Relationship of the inguinal ligament to pelvic radiographic landmarks: anatomic correlation and its role in femoral arteriography. *J Vasc Interv Radiol* 4(3):409–413, 1993.
5. Ellis SG, Bhatt D, Kapadia S, et al: Correlates and outcomes of retroperitoneal hemorrhage complicating percutaneous coronary intervention. *Catheter Cardiovasc Interv* 67(4):541–545, 2006.
6. Grier D, Hartnell G: Percutaneous femoral artery puncture: practice and anatomy. *Br J Radiol* 63(752):602–604, 1990.
7. Turi ZG: Overview of vascular closure. *Endovascular Today* Wayne, PA: Bryn Mawr Communications. 24–32, 2009.
8. Blank R, Rupprecht HJ, Schorrlepp M, et al: [Clinical value of Doppler ultrasound controlled puncture of the inguinal vessels with the "Smart Needle" within the scope of heart catheter examination]. *Z Kardiol* 86(8):608–614, 1997.
9. Wacker F, Wolf KJ, Fobbe F: Percutaneous vascular access guided by color duplex sonography. *Eur Radiol* 7(9):1501–1504, 1997.
10. Dudeck O, Teichgraeber U, Podrabsky P, et al: A randomized trial assessing the value of ultrasound-guided puncture of the femoral artery for interventional investigations. *Int J Cardiovasc Imaging* 20(5):363–368, 2004.
11. Seto AH, Abu-Fadel MS, Sparling JM, et al: Real-time ultrasound guidance facilitates femoral arterial access and reduces vascular complications: FAUST (Femoral Arterial Access With Ultrasound Trial). *JACC Cardiovasc Interv* 3(7):751–758, 2010.
12. Chhatriwalla AK, Bhatt DL: Walk this way: early ambulation after cardiac catheterization–good for the patient and the health care system. *Mayo Clin Proc* 81(12):1535–1536, 2006.
13. Doyle BJ, Ting HH, Bell MR, et al: Major femoral bleeding complications after percutaneous coronary intervention: incidence, predictors, and impact on long-term survival among 17,901 patients treated at the Mayo Clinic from 1994 to 2005. *JACC Cardiovasc Interv* 1(2):202–209, 2008.
14. Applegate RJ, Sacrinty MT, Kutcher MA, et al: Trends in vascular complications after diagnostic cardiac catheterization and percutaneous coronary intervention via the femoral artery, 1998 to 2007. *JACC Cardiovasc Interv* 1(3):317–326, 2008.
15. Yatskar L, Selzer F, Feit F, et al: Access site hematoma requiring blood transfusion predicts mortality in patients undergoing percutaneous coronary intervention: data from the National Heart, Lung, and Blood Institute Dynamic Registry. *Catheter Cardiovasc Interv* 69(7):961–966, 2007.
16. Manoukian SV, Feit F, Mehran R, et al: Impact of major bleeding on 30-day mortality and clinical outcomes in patients with acute coronary syndromes: an analysis from the ACUITY Trial. *J Am Coll Cardiol* 49(12):1362–1368, 2007.
17. Akhter N, Milford-Beland S, Roe MT, et al: Gender differences among patients with acute coronary syndromes undergoing percutaneous coronary intervention in the American College of Cardiology-National Cardiovascular Data Registry (ACC-NCDR). *Am Heart J* 157(1):141–148, 2009.
18. Kinnaird TD, Stabile E, Mintz GS, et al: Incidence, predictors, and prognostic implications of bleeding and blood transfusion following percutaneous coronary interventions. *Am J Cardiol* 92(8):930–935, 2003.
19. Moscucci M, Fox KA, Cannon CP, et al: Predictors of major bleeding in acute coronary syndromes: the Global Registry of Acute Coronary Events (GRACE). *Eur Heart J* 24(20):1815–1823, 2003.
20. Grossman PM, Gurm HS, McNamara R, et al: Percutaneous coronary intervention complications and guide catheter size: bigger is not better. *JACC Cardiovasc Interv* 2(7):636–644, 2009.
21. Turi ZG: An evidence-based approach to femoral arterial access and closure. *Rev Cardiovasc Med* 9(1):7–18, 2008. Winter.
22. Exaire JE, Tcheng JE, Kereiakes DJ, et al: Closure devices and vascular complications among percutaneous coronary intervention patients receiving enoxaparin, glycoprotein IIb/IIIa inhibitors, and clopidogrel. *Catheter Cardiovasc Interv* 64(3):369–372, 2005.
23. Nasser TK, Mohler ER, 3rd, Wilensky RL, et al: Peripheral vascular complications following coronary interventional procedures. *Clin Cardiol* 18(11):609–614, 1995.
24. Tavris DR, Wang Y, Jacobs S, et al: Bleeding and vascular complications at the femoral access site following percutaneous coronary intervention (PCI): an evaluation of hemostasis strategies. *J Invasive Cardiol* 24(7):328–334, 2012.
25. Tiroch KA, Arora N, Matheny ME, et al: Risk predictors of retroperitoneal hemorrhage following percutaneous coronary intervention. *Am J Cardiol* 102(11):1473–1476, 2008.
26. Farouque HM, Tremmel JA, Raissi Shabari F, et al: Risk factors for the development of retroperitoneal hematoma after percutaneous coronary intervention in the era of glycoprotein IIb/IIIa inhibitors and vascular closure devices. *J Am Coll Cardiol* 45(3):363–368, 2005.
27. Derham C, Davies JF, Shahbazi R, et al: Iatrogenic limb ischemia caused by angiography closure devices. *Vasc Endovascular Surg* 40(6):492–494, 2006–2007.
28. Sohail MR, Khan AH, Holmes DR, Jr, et al: Infectious complications of percutaneous vascular closure devices. *Mayo Clin Proc* 80(8):1011–1015, 2005.
29. Dangas G, Mehran R, Kokolis S, et al: Vascular complications after percutaneous coronary interventions following hemostasis with manual compression versus arteriotomy closure devices. *J Am Coll Cardiol* 38(3):638–641, 2001.
30. Koreny M, Riedmuller E, Nikfardjam M, et al: Arterial puncture closing devices compared with standard manual compression after cardiac catheterization: systematic review and meta-analysis. *JAMA* 291(3):350–357, 2004.
31. Nikolsky E, Mehran R, Halkin A, et al: Vascular complications associated with arteriotomy closure devices in patients undergoing percutaneous coronary procedures: a meta-analysis. *J Am Coll Cardiol* 44(6):1200–1209, 2004.
32. Doyle BJ, Konz BA, Lennon RJ, et al: Ambulation 1 hour after diagnostic cardiac catheterization: a prospective study of 1009 procedures. *Mayo Clin Proc* 81(12):1537–1540, 2006.
33. Gall S, Tarique A, Natarajan A, et al: Rapid ambulation after coronary angiography via femoral artery access: a prospective study of 1,000 patients. *J Invasive Cardiol* 18(3):106–108, 2006.
34. Chhatriwalla AK, Bhatt DL: You can't keep a good man (or woman) down. *J Invasive Cardiol* 18(3):109–110, 2006.
35. Nguyen N, Hasan S, Caufield L, et al: Randomized controlled trial of topical hemostasis pad use for achieving vascular hemostasis following percutaneous coronary intervention. *Catheter Cardiovasc Interv* 69(6):801–807, 2007.
36. Mlekusch W, Dick P, Haumer M, et al: Arterial puncture site management after percutaneous transluminal procedures using a hemostatic wound dressing (Clo-Sur P.A.D.) versus conventional manual compression: a randomized controlled trial. *J Endovasc Ther* 13(1):23–31, 2006.
37. Balzer JO, Schwarz W, Thalhammer A, et al: Postinterventional percutaneous closure of femoral artery access sites using the Clo-Sur PAD device: initial findings. *Eur Radiol* 17(3):693–700, 2007.
38. Brown DB: Current status of suture-mediated closure: what is the cost of comfort? *J Vasc Interv Radiol* 14(6):677–681, 2003.
39. Cura FA, Kapadia SR, L'Allier PL, et al: Safety of femoral closure devices after percutaneous coronary interventions in the era of glycoprotein IIb/IIIa platelet blockade. *Am J Cardiol* 86(7):780–782, A789, 2000.
40. Kahn ZM, Kumar M, Hollander G, et al: Safety and efficacy of the Perclose suture-mediated closure device after diagnostic and interventional catheterizations in a large consecutive population. *Catheter Cardiovasc Interv* 55(1):8–13, 2002.
41. Wagner SC, Gonsalves CF, Eschelman DJ, et al: Complications of a percutaneous suture-mediated closure device versus manual compression for arteriotomy closure: a case-controlled study. *J Vasc Interv Radiol* 14(6):735–741, 2003.
42. Applegate RJ, Sacrinty MT, Kutcher MA, et al: Propensity score analysis of vascular complications after diagnostic cardiac catheterization and percutaneous coronary intervention 1998-2003. *Catheter Cardiovasc Interv* 67(4):556–562, 2006.
43. Arora N, Matheny ME, Sepke C, et al: A propensity analysis of the risk of vascular complications after cardiac catheterization procedures with the use of vascular closure devices. *Am Heart J* 153(4):606–611, 2007.
44. Tavris DR, Gallauresi BA, Lin B, et al: Risk of local adverse events following cardiac catheterization by hemostasis device use and gender. *J Invasive Cardiol* 16(9):459–464, 2004.
45. Chevalier B, Lancelin B, Koning R, et al: Effect of a closure device on complication rates in high-local-risk patients: results of a randomized multicenter trial. *Catheter Cardiovasc Interv* 58(3):285–291, 2003.
46. Vaitkus PT: A meta-analysis of percutaneous vascular closure devices after diagnostic catheterization and percutaneous coronary intervention. *J Invasive Cardiol* 16(5):243–246, 2004.
47. Gerckens U, Cattelaens N, Lampe EG, et al: Management of arterial puncture site after catheterization procedures: evaluating a suture-mediated closure device. *Am J Cardiol* 83(12):1658–1663, 1999.
48. Kussmaul WG, 3rd, Buchbinder M, Whitlow PL, et al: Rapid arterial hemostasis and decreased access site complications after cardiac catheterization and angioplasty: results of a randomized trial of a novel hemostatic device. *J Am Coll Cardiol* 25(7):1685–1692, 1995.
49. Nasu K, Tsuchikane E, Sumitsuji S: Clinical effectiveness of the Prostar XL suture-mediated percutaneous vascular closure device following PCI: results of the Perclose AcceleRated Ambulation and DISchargE (PARADISE) Trial. *J Invasive Cardiol* 15(5):251–256, 2003.
50. Slaughter PM, Chetty R, Flintoft VF, et al: A single center randomized trial assessing use of a vascular hemostasis device vs. conventional manual compression following PTCA: what are the potential resource savings? *Cathet Cardiovasc Diagn* 34(3):210–214, 1995.
51. Ward SR, Casale P, Raymond R, et al: Efficacy and safety of a hemostatic puncture closure device with early ambulation after coronary angiography. Angio-Seal Investigators. *Am J Cardiol* 81(5):569–572, 1998.
52. Baim DS, Knopf WD, Hinohara T, et al: Suture-mediated closure of the femoral access site after cardiac catheterization: results of the suture to ambulate aNd discharge (STAND I and STAND II) trials. *Am J Cardiol* 85(7):864–869, 2000.
53. Vidi VD, Matheny ME, Govindarajulu US, et al: Vascular closure device failure in contemporary practice. *JACC Cardiovasc Interv* 5(8):837–844, 2012.
54. Bangalore S, Arora N, Resnic FS: Vascular closure device failure: frequency and implications: a propensity-matched analysis. *Circ Cardiovasc Interv* 2(6):549–556, 2009.
55. Bangalore S, Bhatt DL: Femoral arterial access and closure. *Circulation* 124(5):E147–E156, 2011.
56. Turi ZG, Wortham DC, Sampognaro GC, et al: Use of a novel access technology for femoral artery catheterization: results of the RECITAL trial. *J Invasive Cardiol* 25(1):13–18, 2013.
57. Applegate RJ, Grabarczyk MA, Little WC, et al: Vascular closure devices in patients treated with anticoagulation and IIb/IIIa receptor inhibitors during percutaneous revascularization. *J Am Coll Cardiol* 40(1):78–83, 2002.
58. Bui QT, Kolansky DM, Bannan A, et al: "Double wire" Angio Seal closure technique after balloon aortic valvuloplasty. *Catheter Cardiovasc Interv* 75(4):488–492, 2010.
59. Scheinert D, Sievert H, Turco MA, et al: The safety and efficacy of an extravascular, water-soluble sealant for vascular closure: initial clinical results for Mynx. *Catheter Cardiovasc Interv* 70(5):627–633, 2007.
60. Azmoon S, Pucillo AL, Aronow WS, et al: Vascular complications after percutaneous coronary intervention following hemostasis with the Mynx vascular closure device versus the Angio-Seal vascular closure device. *J Invasive Cardiol* 22(4):175–178, 2010.
61. Martin JL, Pratsos A, Magargee E, et al: A randomized trial comparing compression, Perclose Proglide and Angio-Seal VIP for arterial closure following percutaneous coronary intervention: the CAP trial. *Catheter Cardiovasc Interv* 71(1):1–5, 2008.
62. Cherr GS, Travis JA, Ligush J, Jr, et al: Infection is an unusual but serious complication of a femoral artery catheterization site closure device. *Ann Vasc Surg* 15(5):567–570, 2001.
63. Jaffan AA, Prince EA, Hampson CO, et al: The preclose technique in percutaneous endovascular aortic repair: a systematic literature review and meta-analysis. *Cardiovasc Intervent Radiol* 36(3):567–577, 2013.

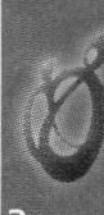

64. Lee WA, Brown MP, Nelson PR, et al: Total percutaneous access for endovascular aortic aneurysm repair ("Preclose" technique). *J Vasc Surg* 45(6):1095–1101, 2007.
65. Branzan D, Sixt S, Rastan A, et al: Safety and efficacy of the StarClose vascular closure system using 7- Fr and 8- Fr sheath sizes: a consecutive single-center analysis. *J Endovasc Ther* 16(4):475–482, 2009.
66. Bangalore S, Vidi VD, Liu CB, et al: Efficacy and safety of the nitinol clip-based vascular closure device (Starclose) for closure of common femoral arterial cannulation at or near the bifurcation: a propensity score-adjusted analysis. *J Invasive Cardiol* 23(5):194–199, 2011.
67. Campeau L: Percutaneous radial artery approach for coronary angiography. *Cathet Cardiovasc Diagn* 16(1):3–7, 1989.
68. Kiemeneij F, Laarman GJ, Odekerken D, et al: A randomized comparison of percutaneous transluminal coronary angioplasty by the radial, brachial and femoral approaches: the access study. *J Am Coll Cardiol* 29(6):1269–1275, 1997.
69. Bertrand OF, Rao SV, Pancholy S, et al: Transradial approach for coronary angiography and interventions: results of the first international transradial practice survey. *JACC Cardiovasc Interv* 3(10):1022–1031, 2010.
70. Sanghvi K, Kurian D, Coppola J: Transradial intervention of iliac and superficial femoral artery disease is feasible. *J Interv Cardiol* 21(5):385–387, 2008.
71. Patel T, Shah S, Ranjan A, et al: Contralateral transradial approach for carotid artery stenting: a feasibility study. *Catheter Cardiovasc Interv* 75(2):268–275, 2010.
72. Jolly SS, Amlani S, Hamon M, et al: Radial versus femoral access for coronary angiography or intervention and the impact on major bleeding and ischemic events: a systematic review and meta-analysis of randomized trials. *Am Heart J* 157(1):132–140, 2009.
73. Cooper CJ, El-Shiekh RA, Cohen DJ, et al: Effect of transradial access on quality of life and cost of cardiac catheterization: a randomized comparison. *Am Heart J* 138(3 Pt 1):430–436, 1999.
74. Jolly SS, Yusuf S, Cairns J, et al: Radial versus femoral access for coronary angiography and intervention in patients with acute coronary syndromes (RIVAL): a randomised, parallel group, multicentre trial. *Lancet* 377(9775):1409–1420, 2011.
75. Chhatriwalla AK, Amin AP, Kennedy KF, et al: Association between bleeding events and in-hospital mortality after percutaneous coronary intervention. *JAMA* 309(10):1022–1029, 2013.
76. Mehta SR, Jolly SS, Cairns J, et al: Effects of radial versus femoral artery access in patients with acute coronary syndromes with or without ST-segment elevation. *J Am Coll Cardiol* 60(24):2490–2499, 2012.
77. Romagnoli E, Biondi-Zoccai G, Sciahbasi A, et al: Radial versus femoral randomized investigation in ST-segment elevation acute coronary syndrome: the RIFLE-STEACS (Radial Versus Femoral Randomized Investigation in ST-Elevation Acute Coronary Syndrome) study. *J Am Coll Cardiol* 60(24):2481–2489, 2012.
78. Mamas MA, Ratib K, Routledge H, et al: Influence of access site selection on PCI-related adverse events in patients with STEMI: meta-analysis of randomised controlled trials. *Heart* 98(4):303–311, 2012.
79. Shah B, Bangalore S, Feit F, et al: Radiation exposure during coronary angiography via transradial or transfemoral approaches when performed by experienced operators. *Am Heart J* 165(3):286–292, 2013.
80. Lange HW, von Boetticher H: Randomized comparison of operator radiation exposure during coronary angiography and intervention by radial or femoral approach. *Catheter Cardiovasc Interv* 67(1):12–16, 2006.
81. Looi JL, Cave A, El-Jack S: Learning curve in transradial coronary angiography. *Am J Cardiol* 108(8):1092–1095, 2011.
82. Sanmartin M, Cuevas D, Moxica J, et al: Transradial cardiac catheterization in patients with coronary bypass grafts: feasibility analysis and comparison with transfemoral approach. *Catheter Cardiovasc Interv* 67(4):580–584, 2006.
83. Jolly SS, Niemela K, Xavier D, et al: Design and rationale of the radial versus femoral access for coronary intervention (RIVAL) trial: a randomized comparison of radial versus femoral access for coronary angiography or intervention in patients with acute coronary syndromes. *Am Heart J* 161(2):254–260, e251–254, 2011.
84. Jolly SS, Cairns J, Niemela K, et al: Effect of radial versus femoral access on radiation dose and the importance of procedural volume: a substudy of the multicenter randomized RIVAL trial. *JACC Cardiovasc Interv* 6(3):258–266, 2013.
85. Byrne RA, Cassese S, Linhardt M, et al: Vascular access and closure in coronary angiography and percutaneous intervention. *Nat Rev Cardiol* 10(1):27–40, 2013.
86. Barbeau GR, Arsenault F, Dugas L, et al: Evaluation of the ulnopalmar arterial arches with pulse oximetry and plethysmography: comparison with the Allen's test in 1010 patients. *Am Heart J* 147(3):489–493, 2004.
87. Stead SW, Stirt JA: Assessment of digital blood flow and palmar collateral circulation. Allen's test vs. photoplethysmography. *Int J Clin Monit Comput* 2(1):29–34, 1985.
88. McGregor AD: The Allen test–an investigation of its accuracy by fluorescein angiography. *J Hand Surg* 12(1):82–85, 1987.
89. Valgimigli M, Campo G, Penzo C, et al: Trans-radial coronary catheterization and intervention across the whole spectrum of Allen's test results. *J Am Coll Cardiol*. In press.
90. Hata M, Sezai A, Niino T, et al: Radial artery harvest using the sharp scissors method for patients with pathological findings on Allen's test. *Surg Today* 36(9):790–792, 2006.
91. Mangano DT, Hickey RF: Ischemic injury following uncomplicated radial artery catheterization. *Anesth Analg* 58(1):55–57, 1979.
92. Coppola J, Patel T, Kwan T, et al: Nitroglycerin, nitroprusside, or both, in preventing radial artery spasm during transradial artery catheterization. *J Invasive Cardiol* 18(4):155–158, 2006.
93. Plante S, Cantor WJ, Goldman L, et al: Comparison of bivalirudin versus heparin on radial artery occlusion after transradial catheterization. *Catheter Cardiovasc Interv* 76(5):654–658, 2010.
94. Rao SV, Tremmel JA, Gilchrist IC, et al: Best practices for transradial angiography and intervention: a consensus statement from the Society for Cardiovascular Angiography and Intervention's transradial working group. *Catheter Cardiovasc Interv* 2013.
95. Rathore S, Stables RH, Pauriah M, et al: Impact of length and hydrophilic coating of the introducer sheath on radial artery spasm during transradial coronary intervention: a randomized study. *JACC Cardiovasc Interv* 3(5):475–483, 2010.
96. Rhyne D, Mann T: Hand ischemia resulting from a transradial intervention: successful management with radial artery angioplasty. *Catheter Cardiovasc Interv* 76(3):383–386, 2010.
97. Pancholy S, Coppola J, Patel T, et al: Prevention of radial artery occlusion-patent hemostasis evaluation trial (PROPHET study): a randomized comparison of traditional versus patency documented hemostasis after transradial catheterization. *Catheter Cardiovasc Interv* 72(3):335–340, 2008.
98. Bernat I, Bertrand OF, Rokyta R, et al: Efficacy and safety of transient ulnar artery compression to recanalize acute radial artery occlusion after transradial catheterization. *Am J Cardiol* 107(11):1698–1701, 2011.
99. Zankl AR, Andrassy M, Volz C, et al: Radial artery thrombosis following transradial coronary angiography: incidence and rationale for treatment of symptomatic patients with low-molecular-weight heparins. *Clin Res Cardiol* 99(12):841–847, 2010.
100. Dehghani P, Mohammad A, Bajaj R, et al: Mechanism and predictors of failed transradial approach for percutaneous coronary interventions. *JACC Cardiovasc Interv* 2(11):1057–1064, 2009.
101. Sciahbasi A, Mancone M, Cortese B, et al: Transradial percutaneous coronary interventions using sheathless guiding catheters: a multicenter registry. *J Interv Cardiol* 24(5):407–412, 2011.
102. Scheer B, Perel A, Pfeiffer UJ: Clinical review: complications and risk factors of peripheral arterial catheters used for haemodynamic monitoring in anaesthesia and intensive care medicine. *Crit Care* 6(3):199–204, 2002.
103. Tizon-Marcos H, Barbeau GR: Incidence of compartment syndrome of the arm in a large series of transradial approach for coronary procedures. *J Interv Cardiol* 21(5):380–384, 2008.
104. Kwac MS, Yoon SJ, Oh SJ, et al: A rare case of radial arteriovenous fistula after coronary angiography. *Korean Circ J* 40(12):677–679, 2010.
105. Kozak M, Adams DR, Ioffreda MD, et al: Sterile inflammation associated with transradial catheterization and hydrophilic sheaths. *Catheter Cardiovasc Interv* 59(2):207–213, 2003.
106. Abu-Ful A, Benharroch D, Henkin Y: Extraction of the radial artery during transradial coronary angiography: an unusual complication. *J Invasive Cardiol* 15(6):351–352, 2003.
107. Alvarez-Tostado JA, Moise MA, Bena JF, et al: The brachial artery: a critical access for endovascular procedures. *J Vasc Surg* 49(2):378–385, discussion 385, 2009.
108. Lupattelli T, Clerissi J, Clerici G, et al: The efficacy and safety of closure of brachial access using the Angio-Seal closure device: experience with 161 interventions in diabetic patients with critical limb ischemia. *J Vasc Surg* 47(4):782–788, 2008.
109. Mahadevan VS, Jimeno S, Benson LN, et al: Pre-closure of femoral venous access sites used for large-sized sheath insertion with the Perclose device in adults undergoing cardiac intervention. *Heart* 94(5):571–572, 2008.

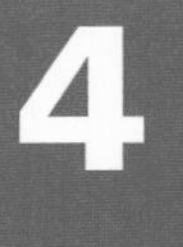

Pharmacotherapy in the Modern Interventional Suite

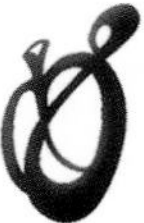

Hani Jneid

The major aims of pharmacotherapy during percutaneous coronary intervention (PCI) and invasive cardiac procedures are to avoid the adverse consequences related to iatrogenic plaque rupture during balloon angioplasty and stent deployment, to reduce the hazards of thrombus formation on the intracoronary PCI equipment, and to mitigate myocardial ischemia and all periprocedural complications. The informed, effective, and judicious use of drugs in the modern interventional suite allows invasive cardiovascular procedures to be performed safely while maintaining hemodynamic and electrical stability of patients and minimizing complications.

PATHOPHYSIOLOGY OF ARTERIAL THROMBOSIS

Thrombosis is fundamental to the process of arterial injury associated with both acute coronary syndromes (ACSs) and PCIs. The pathogenesis of coronary arterial thrombosis is characterized by atherosclerotic plaque disruption (usually rupture or erosion), followed by platelet activation and aggregation and resultant thrombus formation. Irrespective of whether plaque disruption occurs spontaneously or as a result of mechanical disruption during balloon angioplasty, platelets first adhere to the injured endothelium by binding to Class I glycoproteins (GP)[1] (**Figure 4-1**). Thrombin and other agonists, such as adenosine diphosphate (ADP) and epinephrine, activate the platelets and precipitates conformational changes in the GP IIb/IIIa receptor and platelet degranulation.[1] This results in the release of more vasoactive substances such as serotonin, thromboxane A2 (TXA2), and more ADP, which are important mediators of thrombosis that stimulate further platelet activation and recruitment. Activation of the ADP-specific purinergic P2Y$_{12}$ receptor results in activation of the GP IIb/IIIa receptor, granule release, amplification of platelet aggregation, and stabilization of the platelet aggregate.[2] TXA2 is another key platelet agonist which is derived from arachidonic acid through conversion by cyclooxygenase-1 and thromboxane synthase.[3] The binding of these agonists to their platelet receptors ultimately activates the GP IIb/IIIa receptor, which promotes the interaction of adjacent platelets through fibrinogen, forming cross-bridges between activated platelets and leading to platelet aggregation (**Figure 4-2**).

The platelet-clot is stabilized by fibrin derived from the coagulation cascade[4] (**Figure 4-3**). Initiation of blood coagulation occurs mainly through tissue factor (TF), a membrane GP that becomes exposed to blood after plaque disruption. Thrombin is another potent platelet agonist that activates platelet by binding protease-activated receptor

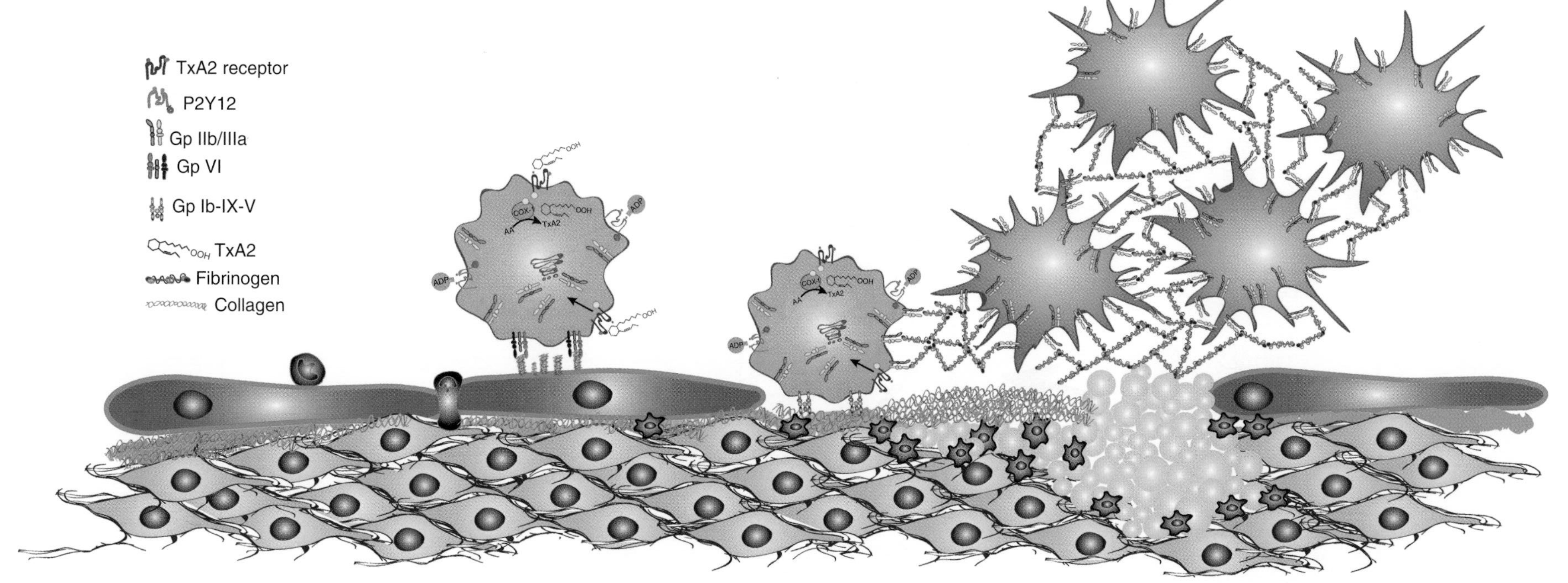

FIGURE 4-1 Following vascular injury, platelet adhesion is generally the first step during which single platelets bind through specific membrane receptors (e.g., glycoprotein [GP] Ib/IX/V, GP VI) to the extracellular matrix constituents of the vessel wall (e.g., collagen, von Willebrand factor, fibronectin). Platelets then become activated and release multiple mediators including thromboxane A2 (TXA2) and adenosine diphosphate (ADP) that bind to TXA2 and $P2Y_{12}$ receptors, respectively. Activation of the GP IIb/IIIa receptor, release of more vasoactive substances from the platelets, and platelet aggregation finally ensue.

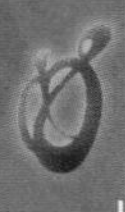

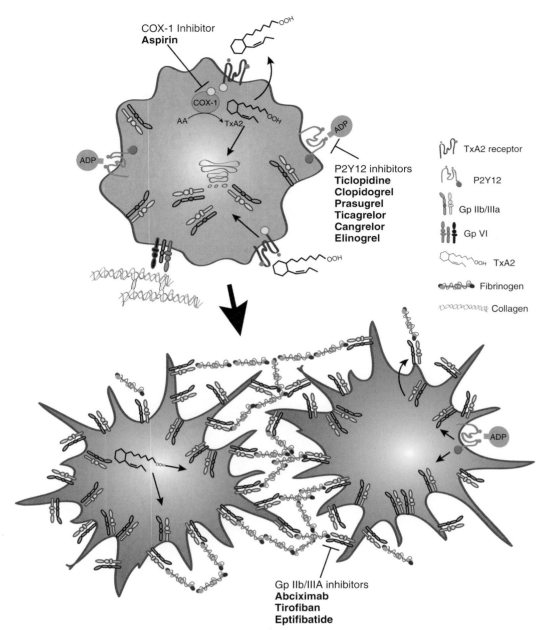

FIGURE 4-2 Thrombin and other agonists, such as adenosine diphosphate (ADP) and epinephrine, activate platelets and precipitate conformational changes in the glycoprotein (GP) IIb/IIIa receptor and platelet degranulation. This results in the release of more vasoactive substances such as serotonin, thromboxane A2 (TXA2), and more ADP, which bind to their receptors and cause activation of the GP IIb/IIIa receptor, further granule release, and ultimately promotes the common final pathway of platelet aggregation through the cross-linking of GP IIb/IIIa receptors on adjacent platelets by fibrinogen.

(PAR-1) on the platelet surface.[5] Thrombin-mediated cleavage of fibrinogen into fibrin is even more important for hemostasis than thrombin-mediated platelet activation.[5]

ASPIRIN

When aspirin was marketed in 1899 for its efficacy in relieving rheumatological conditions, its manufacturer issued a reassurance for the public that it had no harmful effects on the heart. More than a century later, aspirin is one the most commonly used medications worldwide. It is an inexpensive, safe, and effective antiplatelet drug that irreversibly inhibits cyclooxygenase, an enzyme responsible for the formation of eicosanoids (such as PGI_2 and TXA2).[6] Because TXA2 promotes platelet aggregation, the acetylation of cyclooxygenase by aspirin decreases its generation in platelets and therefore platelet aggregability throughout the platelet's 7- to 10-day lifetime.[7] Aspirin reaches appreciable plasma levels by 20 minutes and exerts its platelet-inhibitory effect within 60 minutes (**Table 4-1**). The use of enteric-coated and buffered formulations does not reduce the gastrointestinal bleeding (GIB) complications, as these are largely related to aspirin's systemic effects.[8]

Aspirin Dosage

In a collaborative meta-analysis performed by the Antithrombotic Trialists' collaboration, low-dose aspirin (75-150 mg daily) was shown effective for long-term use.[9] A substudy from the PCI-CURE trial demonstrated that low-dose aspirin (≤100 mg) is effective in preventing ischemic

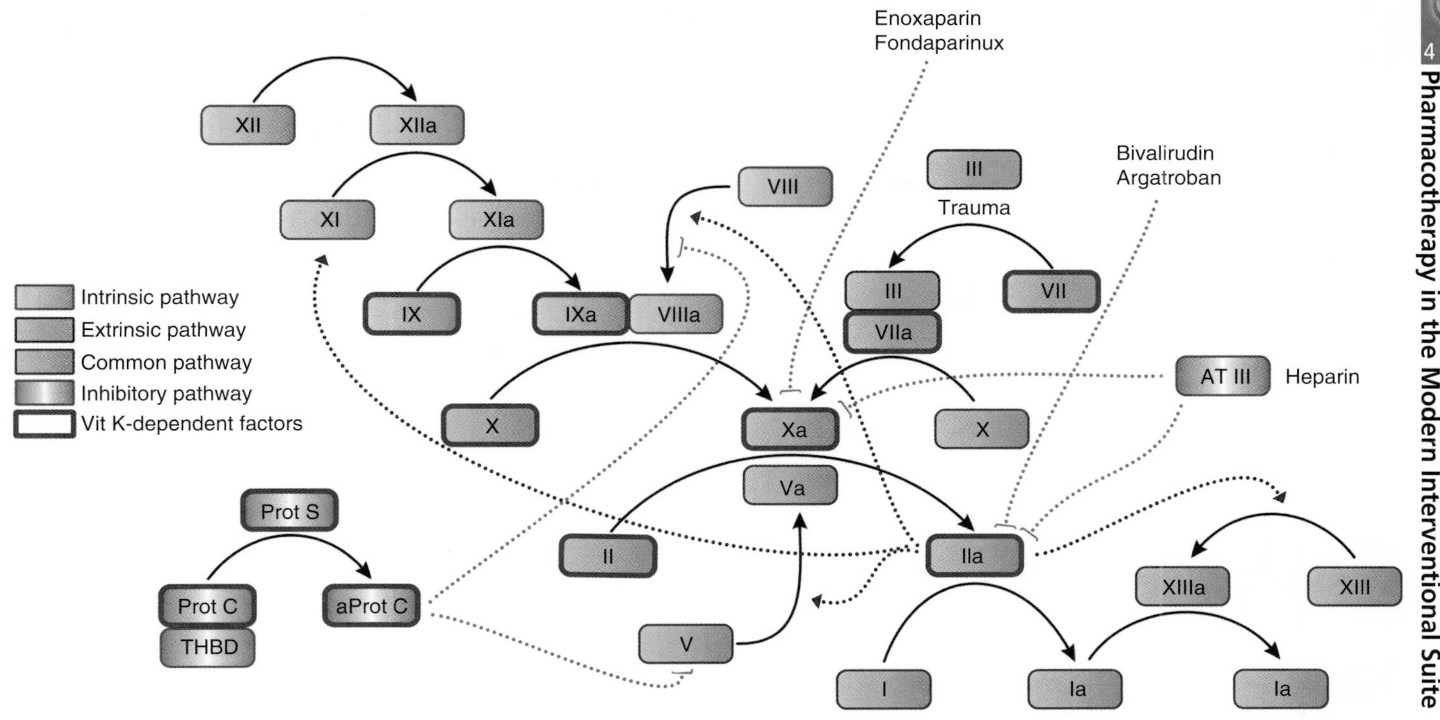

FIGURE 4-3 Coagulation proteins usually circulate in an inactive form in the blood. The coagulation cascade, triggered by vascular injury and exposure of tissue factor (TF) in the plaque to blood, consists of the intrinsic and extrinsic pathways. These two initially separate pathways ultimately converge on the common pathway and activate prothrombin to the active enzyme thrombin which is important to catalyze the production of fibrin. Targets of the various anticoagulants used during PCI are shown.

events and causes lesser bleeding risk compared with higher doses.[10] The 2011 ACC/AHA PCI guideline recommended treating patients with 81-325 mg before PCI when already receiving chronic aspirin therapy.[11] However, if they are aspirin naive, they should receive at least one non-enteric aspirin 325-mg dose before PCI (given at least 2 hours and preferably 24 hours before the procedure).[11] The 2011 PCI guideline also reiterated that it is reasonable to use a daily 81-mg aspirin dose in preference to higher maintenance doses. The use of low-dose aspirin (81 mg in the United States, 75 mg or 100 mg elsewhere) is supported by the saturability of its antiplatelet effect at low doses, the lack of dose-response relationship in studies evaluating its clinical anti-ischemic effects, and the dose-dependent response associated with its bleeding side effects.

ORAL $P2Y_{12}$ RECEPTOR INHIBITORS

For over a decade, dual antiplatelet therapy (DAPT) with aspirin and clopidogrel has been the mainstay of antiplatelet management after PCI.[12] Atherothrombotic events, however, continue to occur in a relevant proportion of subjects despite the benefit of this combination, which has led to the clinical development of newer and more potent antiplatelet drugs. Two of these, prasugrel and ticagrelor, have been approved for clinical use by the FDA in 2009 and 2011, respectively (**Table 4-1** and Video 4-1).

Ticlopidine

Ticlopidine was the first clinically used $P2Y_{12}$ receptor inhibitor and demonstrated superiority (as part of a DAPT regimen with aspirin) in reducing stent thrombosis and ischemic complications during coronary stenting.[13,14] In a meta-analysis of studies comparing ticlopidine with clopidogrel in patients receiving coronary stents, clopidogrel had more tolerability and fewer side effects and was at least as effective as ticlopidine in reducing major adverse cardiovascular events (MACEs).[15] Ticlopidine is a thienopyridine administered orally twice daily (250 mg bid). Its use was eclipsed by the use of safer and more potent $P2Y_{12}$ receptor inhibitors, especially given its significant hematologic toxicity (e.g., neutropenia, agranulocytosis).

Clopidogrel

Mechanism of Action

Clopidogrel is a thienopyridine analog that binds irreversibly to the platelet ADP $P2Y_{12}$ receptor, and inhibits the binding of ADP to its receptor. It has a quicker onset of action and appears to be safer than ticlopidine. It is a prodrug that requires a two-step hepatic bioconversion to its active metabolite.

Evidence

Clopidogrel has a similar clinical efficacy as ticlopidine in preventing stent thrombosis.[16,17] Because of its better safety profile, it has replaced ticlopidine as the favored thienopyridine following stent implantation. The Clopidogrel for the Reduction of Events During Observation (CREDO) trial showed that long-term therapy (1 year) with clopidogrel following elective PCI significantly reduces the risk of MACEs.[18] A pre-treatment strategy with clopidogrel at least 6 hours before PCI resulted in lower incidence of the composite MACE in patients undergoing elective PCI compared with no reduction with treatment administered <6 h before PCI.[18] The PCI-CURE trial demonstrated that among patients with non-ST-elevation acute coronary syndrome (NSTE-ACS) undergoing PCI, pretreatment with clopidogrel followed by long-term therapy (for a mean of 8 months—on

TABLE 4-1 Oral Antiplatelet Drugs in Patients Undergoing PCI

DRUG	ROUTE	REVERSIBILITY	DOSE	HALF-LIFE	TIME TO PLATELET INHIBITION	INDICATIONS	CONTRAINDICATIONS	TRANSITION TO CABG SURGERY	COMMENTS
Aspirin	Oral	Irreversible	81-325 mg daily	Dose dependent: 15-20 min for parent compound; 2-3 hours after a single dose, and up to 2-19 hours for higher doses	Varies according to formulation: within 30-60 min for immediate-release tablets; up to 45 min for coated tablets	All patients with CAD and/or clinical atherosclerotic CV disease	Hypersensitivity (i.e., anaphylaxis, urticaria, or bronchospasm) to aspirin, gastrointestinal or active bleeding, severe thrombocytopenia	Recommended to be continued unless contraindications present—to be re-instituted within 6 h after CABG surgery	Available as a variety of formulations including a rectal suppository; higher doses associated with GI toxicity; desensitization studies are considered in cases of allergy where long-term use needed
Clopidogrel	Oral	Irreversible	Loading dose: 300-600 mg (a 600-mg loading dose is recommended at the time of PCI) Maintenance dose: 75 mg daily Following a loading dose of 600 mg, a 150 mg daily dose may be considered for the first 6 days and then 75 mg daily (as part of a double-dose clopidogrel regimen among ACS patients undergoing PCI).	6 h	2 h	All patients with CAD and/or clinical atherosclerotic CV disease	Patients with active pathological bleeding (peptic ulcer, ICH); patients with hypersensitivity to clopidogrel; severe thrombocytopenia	5 days	Manufacturer warning of diminished effectiveness in poor metabolizers; labeling: avoid concomitant use with omeprazole or esomeprazole; CYP2C19 genotyping available although unproven; desensitization studied and considered for specific allergies where long-term use needed
Prasugrel	Oral	Irreversible	Loading dose: 60 mg daily Maintenance dose: 10 mg daily (5 mg daily in patients with age ≥75 or weight <60 kg)	2-15 h	1-2 h	Patients with ACS who are managed with PCI (after angiography to delineating the coronary anatomy)	Patients with active pathological bleeding (peptic ulcer, ICH); patients with hypersensitivity to prasugrel; severe thrombocytopenia Patients with previous TIA/stroke SHOULD NOT receive prasugrel (black box warning by FDA)	7 days	Much less variability in response; no benefit in medically managed patients or those ≥75 yo unless prior MI or DM. A 5 mg dose is used in the elderly (≥75 yo), but remains unproven for CV outcomes
Ticagrelor	Oral	Reversible	Loading dose: 180 mg daily Maintenance dose: 90 mg twice daily	6-13 h	2 h (maximum platelet inhibition)	Patients with ACS including patients who are managed with PCI or conservatively)	Active bleeding, previous ICH, severe thrombocytopenia, severe bradycardia	5 d	Aspirin maintenance dose should not exceed 100 mg daily. CYP3A4/5 substrate, so it is predisposed to numerous interactions: phenobarbital, carbamazepine, dexamethasone, rifampin, phenytoin may all decrease effectiveness Proven efficacy and safety in ACS patients with CKD (compared with clopidogrel)

ACS, Acute coronary syndrome; *CABG,* coronary artery bypass graft; *CAD,* coronary artery disease; *CKD,* chronic kidney disease; *CV,* cardiovascular; *h,* hour; *ICH,* intracranial hemorrhage; *min,* minute; *PCI,* percutaneous coronary intervention; *TIA,* transient ischemic attack.

the background of aspirin therapy) was associated with a lower MACEs rate and no increase in major bleeding.[12] The PCI-Clopidogrel as Adjunctive Reperfusion Therapy (CLARITY) trial extended the efficacy of clopidogrel to patients receiving fibrinolytics for ST-elevation myocardial infarction (STEMI).[19]

Indications

Clopidogrel is indicated for both ACS and non-ACS patients undergoing PCI on top of aspirin.

Dosage

A loading dose of 600 mg of clopidogrel should be given to both ACS and non-ACS patients before PCI (Videos 4-2AB). However, the loading dose of clopidogrel for patients undergoing PCI after fibrinolytic therapy should be 300 mg within 24 hours and 600 mg >24 hours after receiving fibrinolytic therapy. A 75-mg daily maintenance dose of clopidogrel is recommended thereafter.[11,19]

Variability in Responsiveness to Clopidogrel

Limitations of clopidogrel include a broad variability in platelet inhibition, with a percentage of low responders ranging from 5% to 40%, mostly attributable to genetic, cellular, and clinical mechanisms including non-compliance.[20,21] Poor responsiveness to clopidogrel is related to increased adverse ischemic outcomes.[21]

The Clopidogrel and Aspirin Optimal Dose Usage to Reduce Recurrent Events—Seventh Organization to Assess Strategies in Ischemic Syndromes (CURRENT-OASIS 7) trial investigators demonstrated that in patients undergoing PCI for ACS, a 7-day double-dose clopidogrel regimen was associated with a reduction in MACE and stent thrombosis compared with the standard dose.[22] This was proposed as a possible strategy to reduce the variability in response to clopidogrel.[23] However, the aforementioned findings were from a subgroup analysis from a trial that did not meet its prespecified primary outcome in the overall population studied.[24] Recent prospective randomized trials of platelet function testing (PFT) did not demonstrate clinical benefit. It is unclear whether treatment modification based on current PFT platforms can actually impact clinical outcomes.[25] Updated American and European practice guidelines have issued a Class IIb recommendation for PFT to facilitate the choice of $P2Y_{12}$ receptor inhibitor in selective high-risk patients treated with PCI, although routine testing is not recommended (Class III). Importantly, recent data suggest that low on-treatment platelet reactivity to ADP may still be associated with a higher risk of bleeding, lending credence to the concept of a therapeutic window for $P2Y_{12}$ inhibitor therapy.[21]

Interaction with Proton Pump Inhibitors

The use of some proton pump inhibitors (PPIs) in conjunction with clopidogrel was shown to interfere with clopidogrel metabolism and to be associated with worse clinical outcomes in experimental and observational studies, respectively. The Clopidogrel and the Optimization of Gastrointestinal Events (COGENT) trial demonstrated no increase in cardiovascular ischemic events and a lower GI bleeding rate with the combination of clopidogrel and 20 mg omeprazole (in a single pill).[26] Thus, most patients can be safely treated with a PPI and clopidogrel, although there should be a clear indication for PPI therapy.

The Role of Genotyping

Clopidogrel is a pro-drug that requires conversion to its active metabolite, through a 2-step process in the liver that involves several *CYP450* isoenzymes, of which the *CYP2C19* isoenzyme is the most important.[27] At least 3 genetic polymorphisms of the *CYP2C19* isoenzyme are associated with loss of function. Genotyping for a *CYP2C19* loss of function variant in patients treated with clopidogrel may be considered if results of testing may alter management.[23,27] Genotyping should be made on individual basis, as no definitive outcome data support its utility and cost effectiveness in the general population.

Prasugrel

Mechanism of Action

Prasugrel is a thienopyridine pro-drug that requires conversion to an active metabolite before binding to the platelet $P2Y_{12}$ receptor to confer antiplatelet effects.[28] Prasugrel inhibits ADP-induced platelet aggregation faster, more consistently, and to a greater extent than clopidogrel.

Evidence

The Trial to Assess Improvement in Therapeutic Outcomes by Optimizing Platelet Inhibition with Prasugrel–Thrombolysis in Myocardial Infarction 38 (TRITON–TIMI 38) compared prasugrel head-to-head with clopidogrel among ACS (STEMI and NSTEMI) patients undergoing PCI.[29] During a 15-month median follow-up, prasugrel was superior to clopidogrel in reducing the relative risk of the composite endpoint of cardiovascular death, myocardial infarction (MI), or stroke by 19% (2.2% absolute risk reduction), which was driven predominantly by a significant reduction in nonfatal MI.[29] Stent thrombosis and urgent target vessel revascularization were also reduced by prasugrel. However, prasugrel was associated with higher rate of the key safety endpoint (major bleeding) and more life-threatening and fatal bleeding events.[29]

Indications

Prasugrel is indicated for the treatment of ACS (STEMI and NSTEMI) patients undergoing PCI on top of aspirin (ASA). The utility of prasugrel in non-ACS patients undergoing PCI is not well studied and is off-label. Its risk-benefit ratio in medically treated ACS patients is similar to clopidogrel, but given that it is more expensive than clopidogrel, prasugrel in general should not be used in the medical management of ACS.[30]

Dosage

A 60-mg loading dose of prasugrel should be administered as soon as possible for STEMI patients and once the coronary anatomy is delineated and before PCI among NSTEMI patients.[29] A 10-mg daily maintenance dose of prasugrel should be continued thereafter.

Additional Considerations

Post hoc analyses demonstrated that underweight patients (<60 kg) and the elderly (≥75 years old) had no net clinical benefit, while patients with prior stroke or transient ischemic attack (TIA) experienced net clinical harm with prasugrel.[29] Prasugrel should not be given to ACS patients with a prior history of stroke or TIA ("black box warning" by the FDA).[11] Despite greater and more consistent inhibition of ADP-dependent platelet function and MACE

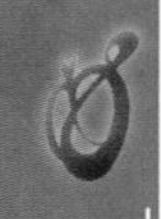

reduction, there is still inter-patient variability in on-treatment platelet reactivity with prasugrel, albeit less than with clopidogrel.[31-33]

Ticagrelor

Mechanism of Action

Unlike the thienopyridines clopidogrel and prasugrel, ticagrelor is a reversible and direct-acting oral antagonist of the ADP receptor $P2Y_{12}$.[34] It provides faster, greater, and more consistent $P2Y_{12}$ inhibition than clopidogrel.[34]

Evidence

The Study of Platelet Inhibition and Patient Outcomes (PLATO) trial was a randomized controlled trial comparing ticagrelor versus clopidogrel for the prevention of vascular events among 18,624 ACS patients (STEMI and NSTEMI).[35] Compared with clopidogrel, ticagrelor reduced the composite endpoint of vascular death, MI, or stroke by 16% (absolute risk reduction of 1.9%), which was driven by reduction in both MI and vascular death events. Notably, ticagrelor treatment resulted in absolute risk reduction in overall mortality of 1.4% compared with clopidogrel at 12-month follow-up.[35] Although ticagrelor was not associated with an increased rate of trial-defined major bleeding, it had a higher rate of major non-CABG-related bleeding and more fatal intracranial bleeding.[35]

Indications

Ticagrelor is indicated in ACS patients (STEMI and NSTEMI) undergoing PCI, as well as in medically treated ACS, on top of low-dose aspirin (75 mg, 81 mg, or 100 mg).[35,36]

Dosage

An oral loading dose of 180 mg of ticagrelor should be administered as early as possible or at time of PCI, followed by a maintenance dose of 90 mg twice daily.

Additional Considerations

Because of its reversible inhibition of the $P2Y_{12}$ receptor, ticagrelor is associated with quicker functional recovery of circulating platelets and a faster offset of effect than clopidogrel. This may theoretically pose a problem for noncompliant patients, especially given its twice-daily dosing regimen.[23] The FDA issued a *Boxed Warning* indicating that aspirin daily maintenance doses of >100 mg decrease the effectiveness of ticagrelor and cautioned against its use in patients with active bleeding or a history of intracranial hemorrhage. Among clopidogrel non-responders, the direct-acting ticagrelor therapy inhibited platelet reactivity below the cut points associated with ischemic risk.[32] Ticagrelor also demonstrated superior efficacy and comparable safety to clopidogrel among patients with chronic kidney disease (CKD) (eGFR <60 mL/min).[37] Thus, ticagrelor is a useful $P2Y_{12}$ receptor inhibitor in CKD patients.[38]

Duration of Therapy with Oral $P2Y_{12}$ Receptor Inhibitors

Irrespective of the stent type, patients undergoing PCI for ACS should receive an oral $P2Y_{12}$ receptor inhibitor for at least 12 months,[12,29,35] on the background of aspirin therapy. Among non-ACS patients undergoing PCI with a drug-eluting stent (DES), an oral $P2Y_{12}$ receptor inhibitor should be administered for at least 12 months.[39] On the other hand, non-ACS patients undergoing PCI with a bare-metal stent (BMS) should receive an oral $P2Y_{12}$ receptor inhibitor for a minimum of 1 month and ideally up to 12 months (although a shorter 2-week course may be acceptable if the patient is at very high bleeding risk).[11,18]

Recently, the Optimized Duration of Clopidogrel Therapy Following Treatment With the Zotarolimus-Eluting Stent in Real-World Clinical Practice (OPTIMIZE) trial compared 3-month versus 12-month DAPT durations in low-risk patients (stable CAD or low-risk ACS) who underwent PCI using zotarolimus-eluting stents.[40] A 3-month DAPT duration was proven non-inferior to a 12-month regimen with respect to the composite endpoint (all-cause death, MI, stroke, or major bleeding) and did not increase the risk of stent thrombosis.[40]

If the risk of bleeding outweighs the anticipated anti-ischemic benefits, earlier discontinuation (≤12 months) of the $P2Y_{12}$ receptor inhibitor is reasonable. On the other hand, maintenance therapy >12 months may also be reasonable in certain patients at higher risk of ischemic events (e.g., long stenting with overlapping DESs, increased thrombosis risk).[11] According to the 2014 American College of Cardiology (ACC) and American Heart Association (AHA) perioperative guideline,[41] elective non-cardiac surgery after PCI DES may be considered after 180 days if the risk of further delay is greater than the expected risks of ischemia and stent thrombosis.

Choice of Oral $P2Y_{12}$ Receptor Inhibitor Therapy

Prasugrel and ticagrelor each showed superiority to clopidogrel in a randomized controlled trial,[29,35] with ticagrelor in particular demonstrating a respectable mortality benefit. Nevertheless, the 2011 American College of Cardiology Foundation (ACCF), AHA, and the Society of Cardiovascular Angiography and Interventions (SCAI) PCI and the 2012 ACCF/AHA ACS guidelines provided equal footing for the use of any of the oral $P2Y_{12}$ receptor inhibitors (clopidogrel, prasugrel, ticagrelor) within the realm of their FDA-approved labels, though the European guidelines gave clear preference to ticagrelor and prasugrel over clopidogrel in the absence of contraindications.[11,23] This was driven then by multiple factors, including the lack of data on cost-effectiveness, real-world outcomes, and bleeding rates as well as the uncertainty about the value of these novel therapies compared with the generic clopidogrel. The 2014 AHA/ACC NSTE-ACS (non-ST-elevation acute coronary syndrome) guideline stated that it is reasonable to choose ticagrelor or prasugrel over clopidogrel for $P2Y_{12}$ inhibition in appropriate clinical settings (in ACS patients and for prasugrel in PCI-treated ACS patients only).[42]

Use of Oral $P2Y_{12}$ Receptor Inhibitors with Fibrinolytic Therapy

Timely fibrinolytic therapy should be administered to achieve prompt reperfusion among acute STEMI patients presenting to a non-PCI-capable hospital and who cannot be transferred to a PCI-capable hospital for primary PCI within 120 minutes.[43] In these patients, the use of a 75-mg daily dose of clopidogrel (on top of aspirin) has been shown to reduce short-term mortality and major cardiovascular (CV) events without increasing major bleeding hazards.[44] There is a paucity of data demonstrating the clinical utility and safety of the newer oral $P2Y_{12}$ receptor inhibitors in patients receiving fibrinolytic therapy.

Timing of Discontinuation of Oral $P2Y_{12}$ Receptor Inhibitor Therapy

Among patients undergoing planned coronary artery bypass graft (CABG), clopidogrel and ticagrelor should be discontinued for at least 5 days and prasugrel for at least 7 days before elective surgery in order to reduce the need for blood transfusion.[11,23,43,45] Among patients undergoing urgent CABG, these agents should be discontinued for at least 24 hours to reduce major bleeding complications.[45]

Oral Glycoprotein IIb/IIIa Receptor Inhibitors

Four oral GP IIb/IIIa inhibitors were examined in randomized clinical trials and demonstrated increased mortality risk and significantly higher bleeding rates.[46] The development and use of oral GP IIb/IIIa inhibitors were therefore halted.

INTRAVENOUS ANTIPLATELET DRUGS

Intravenous Glycoprotein IIb/IIIa Receptor Inhibitors

There are three clinically used intravenous GP IIb/IIIa inhibitors: abciximab, tirofiban, and eptifibatide (**Table 4-2**). Although these agents have a role in selective clinical settings, their use has diminished with the advent and widespread use of $P2Y_{12}$ receptor inhibitors and newer anticoagulants.

Mechanism of Action

The GP IIb/IIIa receptor is the most abundant receptor on the platelet surface and is responsible for the last common pathway of platelet aggregation, and GP IIb/IIIa receptor inhibitors interfere with platelet cross-linking and thrombus formation by competing with fibrinogen and von Willebrand factor for the GP IIb/IIIa binding.

Evidence

Evidence supporting the use of IV GP IIb/IIIa receptor inhibitors predates the era of widespread DAPT and the advent of bivalirudin. Earlier studies showed the efficacy of IV GP IIb/IIIa receptor inhibitors in reducing periprocedural ischemic complications—mostly periprocedural MI—during PCI among patients treated with aspirin and heparin.[47-51]

In the contemporary era, the strongest evidence supporting the use of GP IIb/IIIa inhibitors came from the *ISAR-REACT-2* randomized controlled study of 2022 NSTE-ACS patients undergoing PCI who were adequately pretreated with DAPT (with all patients receiving 600 mg of clopidogrel at least 2 hours before the procedure).[52] In this study, abciximab conferred a significant 3% absolute risk reduction and a 25% relative risk reduction at 30 days in the composite ischemic endpoint of death, MI, or urgent target vessel revascularization.[52] The benefits of abciximab were confined to patients presenting with elevated troponin. In the era of adequately treated patients with DAPT, the benefits of GP IIb/IIIa inhibitors are inconsistent and less conclusive among STEMI patients,[53,54] and the benefits appear to be among patients with the highest risk profile.[55] Similarly, contemporary trials of patients pretreated with aspirin and clopidogrel have not demonstrated any benefit with GP IIb/IIIa inhibitor therapy in patients with stable symptoms undergoing elective PCI.[56]

Therefore, these agents should not be used routinely but rather selectively, such as in patients with large thrombus burden and those who are not adequately pre-loaded with a $P2Y_{12}$ receptor inhibitor.

Indications

In patients undergoing primary PCI and who are treated with unfractionated heparin (UFH), it is reasonable to administer a GP IIb/IIIa inhibitor whether or not patients were pretreated with an oral $P2Y_{12}$ receptor inhibitor. These agents are also useful in NSTE-ACS patients with high-risk features (e.g., elevated troponin) who are treated with UFH and not adequately pretreated with clopidogrel. However, their use during PCI is still reasonable among high-risk NSTE-ACS patients, even when adequately treated with DAPT.[11] Similarly, GP IIb/IIIa inhibitors are reasonable to use among high-risk stable CAD patients undergoing PCI, especially when not pre-treated with DAPT.[11]

In clinical scenarios where pre-loading with $P2Y_{12}$ inhibitors is not routinely performed, IV GP IIb/IIIa inhibitors should be strongly considered. IV GP IIb/IIIa inhibitors are advocated in patients with refractory ischemia, those undergoing high-risk PCI, or as bailout therapy for thrombotic complications occurring during PCI (e.g., distal embolization, jailed side branch, wire on thrombus, side-branch closure, obstructive dissection, intracoronary thrombus, persistent residual stenosis, prolonged ischemia). IV GP IIb/IIIa inhibitors should not be routinely used during PCI for vein graft diseases as they have not shown to be beneficial in this setting.[57] The use of GP IIb/IIIa inhibitors is likely to further decline with the use of the newer and more potent $P2Y_{12}$ receptor inhibitors.

Dosage

Double-bolus eptifibatide (180-mcg/kg bolus followed 10 minutes later by a second 180-mcg/kg bolus) and high-bolus dose tirofiban (25 mcg/kg) have been adopted to achieve a high degree of platelet inhibition, similar to abciximab.[58,59] IV abciximab is usually administered as a 0.25-mg/kg bolus followed by a maintenance dose of 0.125 μg/kg/min for up to 12 hours (**Table 4-2**).

Duration of Therapy

Abciximab is usually given intra-procedurally and for up to 12 hours post-PCI, while eptifibatide and tirofiban are administered for 18-24 hours. Longer infusions are associated with increased bleeding hazards and thrombocytopenia and should be avoided unless absolutely necessary. Shorter durations of infusions (<18 hours) may be safe even in high-risk NSTE-ACS,[60] and in certain clinical scenarios can be even abbreviated to <2 hours.[61]

Additional Considerations

In a meta-analysis examining the benefits of abciximab among STEMI patients, adjunctive abciximab is associated with a significant reduction in short- and long-term mortality in patients treated with primary angioplasty, but not in those receiving fibrinolysis.[62] The 30-day reinfarction rate is significantly reduced in patients treated with either reperfusion strategy, although increased major bleeding was observed with abciximab in association with fibrinolysis.[62] Routine use of GP IIb/IIIa receptor inhibitors is not recommended in patients receiving bivalirudin as the primary

TABLE 4-2 Intravenous Antiplatelet Drugs in Patients Undergoing PCI*

DRUG	ROUTE	DOSE	DOSE ADJUSTMENT	ROUTE OF ELIMINATION	HALF-LIFE	INDICATIONS	CONTRAINDICATIONS
Abciximab	Intravenous	250-µg/kg IV bolus followed by a maintenance dose of 0.125 µg/kg/min for up to 12 hours (maximum 10 µg/min)	None	Proteolytic cleavage	30 minutes	In patients undergoing elective PCI with stenting and receiving UFH, it is reasonable to use a GP IIb/IIIa inhibitor when patients are not adequately pretreated with clopidogrel. Even among stable CAD patients who are adequately pretreated with clopidogrel, it may be reasonable to administer a GP IIb/IIIa inhibitor. Among NSTE-ACS patients with high-risk features who are not adequately pretreated with clopidogrel and who are receiving UFH, it is useful at the time of PCI to administer a GP IIb/IIIa inhibitor. Even among NSTE-ACS patients adequately pre-treated with clopidogrel, it is reasonable at the time of PCI to administer a GP IIb/IIIa inhibitor. In patients undergoing primary PCI for STEMI treated with UFH, it is reasonable to administer a GP IIb/IIIa inhibitor, whether or not patients were pretreated with clopidogrel.	Hypersensitivity; active bleeding; recent GI/GU bleed; recent surgery; recent CVA; bleeding diathesis; thrombocytopenia; severe hypertension Should not be used as an upstream strategy for ACS patients
Eptifibatide	Intravenous	Double-bolus is advocated: IV 180-µg/kg bolus followed 10 min later by a second IV 180-µg/kg bolus Maintenance dose: 2 µg/kg/min (up to 15 mg/h) for up to 72 h	Cr Cl <50 mL/min/1.73 m^2: 180-µg/kg/min IV bolus, followed by 1 µg/kg/min for up to 72 h Contraindicated in patients on hemodialysis	Primarily renal	2.5 h	In patients undergoing elective PCI with stenting and receiving UFH, it is reasonable to use a GP IIb/IIIa inhibitor when patients are not adequately pretreated with clopidogrel. Even among stable CAD patients adequately pretreated with clopidogrel, it may be reasonable to administer a GP IIb/IIIa inhibitor. Among NSTE-ACS patients with high-risk features who are not adequately pretreated with clopidogrel and who are receiving UFH, it is useful at the time of PCI to administer a GP IIb/IIIa inhibitor. Even among NSTE-ACS patients adequately pretreated with clopidogrel, it is reasonable at the time of PCI to administer a GP IIb/IIIa inhibitor. In patients undergoing primary PCI for STEMI treated with UFH, it is reasonable to administer a GP IIb/IIIa inhibitor, whether or not patients were pretreated with clopidogrel.	Hypersensitivity; active bleeding; recent GI/GU bleed; recent surgery; recent CVA; bleeding diathesis; thrombocytopenia; severe hypertension Should not be used routinely as an upstream strategy for ACS patients undergoing PCI
Tirofiban	Intravenous	High-bolus dose is advocated: 25 µg/kg over 3 min, followed by a maintenance dose of 0.15 µg/kg/min for up to 18 h	Cr Cl <30 mL/min/1.73 m^2 → reduce maintenance dose by 50%	Primarily renal	2 h	In patients undergoing elective PCI with stenting and receiving UFH, it is reasonable to use a GP IIb/IIIa inhibitor when patients are not adequately pretreated with clopidogrel. Even among stable CAD patients adequately pretreated with clopidogrel, it may be reasonable to administer a GP IIb/IIIa inhibitor. Among NSTE-ACS patients with high-risk features who are not adequately pretreated with clopidogrel and who are receiving UFH, it is useful at the time of PCI to administer a GP IIb/IIIa inhibitor. Even among NSTE-ACS patients adequately pretreated with clopidogrel, it is reasonable at the time of PCI to administer a GP IIb/IIIa inhibitor. In patients undergoing primary PCI for STEMI treated with UFH, it is reasonable to administer a GP IIb/IIIa inhibitor, whether or not patients were pretreated with clopidogrel.	Hypersensitivity; active bleeding; recent GI/GU bleed; recent surgery; recent CVA; bleeding diathesis; thrombocytopenia; severe hypertension Should not be used routinely as an upstream strategy for ACS patients undergoing PCI

*Cangrelor is an adenosine triphosphate analog that reversibly binds to and inhibits the $P2Y_{12}$ ADP receptor. It is an intravenous reversible drug with a half-life of 3-6 min. When given as a bolus plus infusion, it quickly and consistently inhibits platelets to a high degree, with normalization of platelet function within 60 min after discontinuation. It is not yet approved by the FDA as of this writing.

ACS, Acute coronary syndrome; *CAD,* coronary artery disease; *CVA,* cardiovascular accident; *GI,* gastrointestinal; *GP,* glycoproteins; *GU,* genitourinary; *NSTE-ACS,* non-ST-elevation acute coronary syndrome; *PCI,* percutaneous coronary intervention; *UFH,* unfractionated heparin.

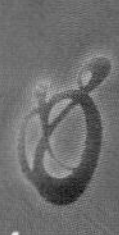

anticoagulant but may be considered as a bailout strategy in selective cases.[11]

The benefits of intracoronary (IC) GP IIb/IIIa inhibitors are inconsistent.[11,63,64] IC abciximab (0.25-mg/kg bolus) may be reasonable to use instead of the IV route among high-risk STEMI patients,[11,65,66] especially as it was shown to be at least as safe as IV abciximab.[67] In the large Intracoronary Abciximab and Aspiration Thrombectomy in Patients with Large Anterior Myocardial Infarction (INFUSE-AMI) trial, patients with large anterior STEMI undergoing primary PCI with bivalirudin anticoagulation, infarct size was significantly reduced by an IC abciximab bolus delivered to the infarct lesion site but not by manual aspiration thrombectomy.[68]

Timing of Administration of Glycoprotein IIb/IIIa Receptor Inhibitor

Upstream pre-catheterization use of GP IIb/IIIa inhibitors among STEMI patients undergoing PCI is not recommended given the lack of efficacy,[54,69] and the increased risk of bleeding (irrespective of the reperfusion strategy). Among patients with NSTE-ACS pre-treated with DAPT, routine upstream administration of eptifibatide (≥12 hours before angiography), was not superior to its provisional use during PCI and was actually associated with increased risk of bleeding and transfusions.[70]

Choice of Intravenous Glycoprotein IIb/IIIa Receptor Inhibitor

In a meta-analysis of five RCTs comparing abciximab with the small-molecule GP IIb/IIIa inhibitors among patients undergoing primary PCI, no outcome differences (short-term mortality, re-infarction, bleeding) were seen between the STEMI groups.[71] Another meta-analysis among STEMI patients undergoing primary PCI confirmed similar results between abciximab and the small molecules in terms of angiographic, electrocardiographic, and clinical outcomes.[72] Thus, all GP IIb/IIIa inhibitors seem to perform equally, even in the highest thrombotic risk subset of patients, and the benefits of GP IIb/IIIa receptor inhibitors do not appear to be drug-specific but rather a class effect.

Timing of Discontinuation of Glycoprotein IIb/IIIa Receptor Inhibitors

Eptifibatide and tirofiban should be discontinued ≥2-4 hours before urgent CABG, while the longer-acting abciximab should be discontinued ≥12 hours. Platelet transfusions are indicated in patients receiving glycoprotein IIb/IIIa receptor inhibitors who have active life-threatening bleeding, especially among patients treated with abciximab (though repeat transfusions may be necessary). They are, however, not directly effective in reversing the effects of the small molecules, eptifibatide or tirofiban, though they are still useful to reverse any aspirin or clopidogrel effect. Fresh frozen plasma or cryoprecipitate alone or in combination with platelet transfusions can help reverse the antiplatelet effects in patients treated with eptifibatide and tirofiban. In addition, tirofiban is dialyzable and immediate hemodialysis can be done when needed.

Cangrelor

Cangrelor, a non-thienopyridine adenosine triphosphate (ATP) analog, is a direct-acting, selective, and specific inhibitor of the $P2Y_{12}$ receptor with a very short half-life (3-6 minutes). Platelet function normalizes within 30-60 minutes after its discontinuation. Thus, cangrelor is likely to play a role in patients who require rapid, predictable, and profound but reversible platelet inhibition. The CHAMPION PCI[73] and CHAMPION PLATFORM[74] RCTs examined cangrelor administered during PCI and showed no benefit of cangrelor compared with clopidogrel or placebo with respect to ischemic outcomes. On the other hand, the CHAMPION PHOENIX trial included 11,145 patients who were undergoing urgent or elective PCI and were receiving guideline-recommended therapies to receive a bolus/infusion of cangrelor or 300- to 600-mg loading dose of clopidogrel.[75] Cangrelor significantly reduced the rate of ischemic events including stent thrombosis during PCI, without increasing severe bleeding events.[75] Pooled patient-level data from all three aforementioned trials comparing cangrelor with control (clopidogrel or placebo) for prevention of PCI-related thrombotic complications demonstrated that cangrelor reduced PCI thrombotic complications, albeit at the expense of increased bleeding.[76]

INTRAVENOUS ANTICOAGULANT DRUGS

An anticoagulant (**Table 4-3**) should be administered to all patients undergoing PCI, in addition to at least two antiplatelet drugs, in order to prevent intracoronary thrombus formation at the site of arterial injury or on the interventional equipment (e.g., guidewire, catheter). Before the procedure, all patients should be evaluated for bleeding risk which also predicts post-PCI mortality. Strategies to reduce bleeding risk should be implemented, such as the use of lower bleeding-risk agents (e.g., bivalirudin), weight-adjusted dosing of heparin, ACT and activated partial thromboplastin time (aPTT) monitoring, dose adjustment in CKD patients, and use of radial artery access.[77]

Unfractionated Heparin

Unfractionated heparin (UFH) is the oldest and most commonly used anticoagulant during PCI. It is easy to administer, fast-acting, easily monitored, and can be reversed with protamine. The ability to reverse it makes it the preferred anticoagulant for use during PCI of chronic total occlusion (CTO) lesions.

Mechanism of Action

UFH is an indirect anti-thrombin drug made of a mixture of glycosaminoglycans of varying lengths with a high affinity for the anti-thrombin enzyme.

Evidence

Although it is widely used, there are no prospective RCTs demonstrating its efficacy (vs. placebo) during PCI.

Indications

In the absence of other anticoagulants and despite the paucity of high-level evidence, IV UFH is indicated during PCI.[11] Anticoagulation with UFH monotherapy, on the background of aspirin alone, is insufficient during PCI to protect against thrombotic complications[11] and, in this instance, at least a second antiplatelet agent (an oral $P2Y_{12}$ agent or an IV GP IIb/IIIa inhibitor) should be added.

Dosage

Dosing differs depending on whether an IV GP IIb/IIIa inhibitor is used or not. In the absence of GP IIb/IIIa inhibitor

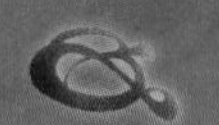

TABLE 4-3 Commonly Used Parenteral Anticoagulant Drugs during PCI

PARENTERAL ANTICOAGULANT MEDICATIONS	ROUTE	DOSE	DOSE ADJUSTMENT	ROUTE OF ELIMINATION	HALF-LIFE	CONTRAINDICATIONS
Unfractionated heparin	Intravenous	70-100 U/kg without GP IIb/IIIa or 50-70 U/kg with GP IIb/IIIa to re-bolus (e.g., 1000-5000 U) according to ACT levels	Without GP IIb/IIIa: adjust to achieve a target ACT of 250-300 s (HemoTec assay) or 300-350 s (Hemochron assay) with GP IIb/IIIa: adjust to achieve an ACT of 200-250 s	Liver and reticulo-endothelial system	1.5 h (range 1-6 h) [follows zero-order kinetics]	Active bleeding, HIT/HITT
Enoxaparin	Subcutaneous	1 mg/kg SC every 12 h for medically treated ACS IV 0.3 mg/kg enoxaparin should be administered at the time of PCI to patients who received <2 therapeutic subcutaneous doses or received the last subcutaneous dose 8-12 h before PCI. If undergoing PCI >12 h after the last subcutaneous enoxaparin dose, patients should receive full-dose de novo anticoagulation regimen. If undergoing PCI ≤8 h of the last subcutaneous dose (and already received multiple subcutaneous doses), no more enoxaparin is needed. If no prior anticoagulation is given, an IV bolus of 0.5-0.75 mg enoxaparin should be administered during PCI.	Decrease to 1 mg/kg SC daily in patients whose Cr Cl <30 mL/min	Liver, renal clearance if 10% of active dose	4.5 hours (range 3-6 hours)	Active bleeding, HIT/HITT
Fondaparinux	Subcutaneous	2.5 mg SC daily	Avoid if Cr Cl <30 mL/min/1.73 m^2	Primarily renal	17-21 hours	Severe renal impairment, hypersensitivity, active bleeding, weight <50 kg, thrombocytopenia
Bivalirudin	Intravenous	0.75-mg/kg IV bolus followed by 1.75 mg/kg/h during PCI (and up to 4 hours post procedure, if needed) If continued anticoagulation is needed after the initial 4-h post PCI, the infusion may be continued for up to an additional 20-h period at 0.2 mg/kg/h.	Cr Cl = 10-30 mL/min/1.73 m^2: reduce infusion to 1 mg/kg/h	Renal (20%), proteolytic cleavage (80%)	25 min (normal renal function)	Hypersensitivity, active bleeding

ACT, Activated clotting time; *Cr Cl*, creatinine clearance; *HIT*, heparin-induced thrombocytopenia; *HITT*, heparin-induced thrombotic thrombocytopenia; *IV*, intravenous; *GP IIb/IIIa*, glycoprotein IIb/IIIa; *PCI*, percutaneous coronary intervention; *SC*, subcutaneous.

therapy, a 70- to 100-U/kg bolus of UFH should be administered during PCI (and before wiring the coronary artery) to achieve a target ACT of 250-300 seconds (when using the HemoTec assay) or 300-350 seconds (when using the Hemochron assay). In the presence of an IV GP IIb/IIIa inhibitor, a 50- to 70-U/kg bolus of UFH should be used to achieve an ACT of 200-250 seconds. Additional boluses should be administered as needed (usually in 2000- to 5000-U increments) to maintain the aforementioned ACT goals during PCI. Although still widely used, both the Hemochron and HemoTec assays for measuring ACT are imprecise.[78] Moreover, the relationship between ACT levels and outcomes and thus the utility of measuring ACT during PCI are really uncertain.[79] Similar dosing regimen and ACT goals apply to PCIs performed using the radial approach.

Additional Considerations

UFH has many limitations including platelet activation, inability to bind clot-bound thrombin, narrow therapeutic window, and an unpredictable anticoagulant effect. It can also cause heparin-induced thrombocytopenia (HIT) or even the rare heparin-induced thrombotic thrombocytopenia (HITT) syndrome.[80] Following PCI, a femoral sheath is usually removed when the ACT <150-180 seconds (or when the aPTT becomes <50 seconds). UFH should not be administered to patients who already received recent subcutaneous enoxaparin because of difficulty in dosing and increased bleeding rate.[81]

Enoxaparin

Mechanism of Action

Enoxaparin is a low-molecular-weight heparin (3-5 kDa) with greater activity against factor Xa than thrombin. It has more predictable and consistent anticoagulation effects,[82] and carries lower risk of HIT and HITT than UFH.

Evidence

Comparative studies showed inconsistent benefits of enoxaparin over UFH during PCI.[81,83-86] A large meta-analysis of randomized trials (n = 13 studies; 7318 patients) comparing low-molecular-weight (mostly enoxaparin) versus UFH as anticoagulants during PCI demonstrated a significant reduction in the risk of major bleeding with low-molecular-weight heparins (OR 0.57; 95% CI = 0.40 to 0.82) but without differences in ischemic outcomes.[87]

Indications

IV enoxaparin may be reasonable during PCI for patients who have not received prior anticoagulant therapy or who have received upstream subcutaneous enoxaparin for NSTE-ACS (Class IIb).[11]

Dosage

Enoxaparin can be administered subcutaneously (usually as upfront therapy in ACS patients) or IV (usually during PCI). ACS patients who are initially treated medically usually receive 1 mg/kg subcutaneous enoxaparin twice daily. An additional dose of 0.3 mg/kg IV enoxaparin should be administered at the time of PCI to patients who have received less than two therapeutic subcutaneous doses or received the last subcutaneous dose 8-12 hours before PCI.[88] Patients undergoing PCI >12 hours after the last subcutaneous enoxaparin dose should receive a full-dose de novo anticoagulation regimen, while those who undergo PCI ≤8 hours of the last subcutaneous dose (and already received multiple subcutaneous doses) are usually adequately anticoagulated and do not require additional treatment (Videos 4-3AD). For those who have not received prior anticoagulant therapy, an IV bolus of 0.5-0.75 mg/kg enoxaparin was established to be safe and efficacious compared with UFH in the Safety and Efficacy of Enoxaparin in PCI Patients, an International Randomized Evaluation (STEEPLE) trial.[89] Anti-Xa levels are not routinely measured during PCI.

Additional Considerations

Despite a better safety profile and more evidence, enoxaparin carries a weaker class of recommendation compared with UFH according to the 2011 ACCF/AHA/SCAI PCI guideline (Class IIb vs. Class I).[11] Enoxaparin is generally less popular because of many shortcomings, including but not limited to longer half-life, inability to reverse completely with protamine, complexity of dosing, and the need for dose adjustment among patients with CKD.

Bivalirudin

Mechanism of Action

Bivalirudin is a synthetic polypeptide that acts as a direct thrombin inhibitor. Unlike heparins, bivalirudin binds to thrombin in both its clot-bound and fluid phases and inactivates thrombin directly. Additional advantages of bivalirudin include its short-half-life (25 minutes), lack of need for anticoagulation monitoring, and lack of platelet activation. In addition, it does not cause HIT or HITT and is the agent of choice (along with argatroban) in these patients.

Evidence

Bivalirudin has been studied in multiple PCI settings: elective PCI,[90-92] NSTE-ACS,[92,93] and STEMI.[94] Overall, bivalirudin is associated with reduced bleeding and is, for the most part, non-inferior in terms of ischemic outcomes to the combination of UFH and IV GP IIb/IIIa inhibitor. Importantly, bivalirudin reduced cardiac mortality in patients with STEMI undergoing primary PCI (an effect that can be only partially attributable to differences in bleeding).[95] This mortality benefit is controversial and was not observed in the more contemporary European Ambulance Acute Coronary Syndrome Angiography (EUROMAX) trial.[96] EUROMAX, which used upstream bivalirudin and had increased radial access and novel $P2Y_{12}$ inhibitor use, reconfirmed, however, the risk of early stent thrombosis with bivalirudin in primary PCI.[96] Adequate clopidogrel pre-treatment (with 600-mg dose) is likely to mitigate any potential hazards of early thrombosis that may arise with bivalirudin.[97] Recently, the How Effective Are Antithrombotic Therapies in Primary PCI (HEAT-PPCI) trial compared anticoagulation with bivalirudin versus UFH during primary PCI for STEMI, on the background of similar GP IIb/IIIa inhibitor use (14%).[98] In this single center study, UFH reduced the incidence of MACE compared with bivalirudin and did not increase bleeding risk.[98] These provocative findings were attributed by some to methodological shortcomings (e.g., open-label design, single center, adjudication of events).[99]

Indications

Bivalirudin is useful as an anticoagulant with or without prior UFH treatment across the full spectrum of CAD patients undergoing PCI (Class I recommendation, similar to UFH).[11]

Bivalirudin should replace UFH as the anticoagulant of choice among patients with HIT.

Dosage

Bivalirudin is administered as a 0.75-mg/kg IV bolus followed by 1.75-mg/kg/h IV infusion for the duration of the PCI procedure (and up to 4 hours after the procedure if needed) **(Table 4-3)**.

Additional Considerations

The lower bleeding rate imparted by bivalirudin is eliminated when used concomitantly with an IV GP IIb/IIIa inhibitor. Notably, the bailout rates with GP IIb/IIIa inhibitors in the major bivalirudin trials were consistently around 7%.[90,93,94] Some shortcomings of bivalirudin are (1) it has no antidote and cannot be reversed (Videos 4-4AB), thus, it should generally be avoided during CTO PCI; (2) when used alone (and without adequate DAPT pretreatment), ACS patients may sustain slightly excess thrombotic risk (especially acute stent thrombosis risk); (3) it is more expensive than unfractionated heparin.

Fondaparinux

Mechanism of Action

Fondaparinux is a synthetic pentasaccharide that indirectly inhibits factor Xa but has no effect on thrombin.

Evidence

The Fifth Organization to Assess Strategies in Acute Ischemic Syndromes (OASIS-5) trial assessed fondaparinux use in ACS patients undergoing PCI and demonstrated similar rates of ischemic event at 9 days, but substantially improved bleeding and long-term mortality rates compared with enoxaparin.[100]

Indications

Fondaparinux is indicated for NSTE-ACS patients and should be continued for the duration of hospitalization or until PCI is performed.[42] Concerns about catheter-associated thrombosis were evident in clinical trials,[100,101] and fondaparinux should therefore never be used alone during PCI. An anticoagulant with anti-IIa activity (either UFH or bivalirudin) should be administered with fondaparinux to mitigate this risk.[11]

Dosage

ACS patients are usually treated with a once-daily subcutaneous injection of 2.5 mg of fondaparinux for the duration of hospitalization or until PCI.

Additional Considerations

Fondaparinux is limited by its long half-life (17-20 hours) and is contraindicated in patients with severe CKD (because of its predominant renal excretion). Monitoring of anti-Xa activity is not needed, and fondaparinux does not affect aPTT or ACT levels.

Other Parenteral Anticoagulants

Argatroban is another IV direct thrombin inhibitor that was approved in 2002 by the FDA for patients undergoing PCI who have HIT or are at risk of developing it.[102] Unlike bivalirudin, it can be used in patients with chronic kidney disease (CKD). However, it is excreted by the liver and should be avoided in patients with significant hepatic dysfunction.

Duration of Anticoagulation Therapy after Percutaneous Coronary Intervention

Prolonged anticoagulation after PCI results in excessive bleeding and prolonged length of stay with no reduction in ischemic outcomes. Unlike oral DAPT, anticoagulants should not be routinely continued after PCI,[13] unless a compelling reason exists for the use of triple agents (e.g., atrial fibrillation, prosthetic valve).

VASODILATORS AND ANTIHYPERTENSIVE DRUGS

Hypertension Urgency/Emergency

A large proportion of patients referred for cardiac catheterization have baseline hypertension (HTN), predominantly essential HTN. Often these patients experience HTN exacerbation in the cardiac catheterization laboratory. Anxiety, missing antihypertensive medication doses prior to the procedure, and volume overload during PCI can all be predisposing factors. Poorly controlled HTN during coronary angiography and/or PCI may predispose patients to myocardial ischemia and create myocardial oxygen demand-supply mismatch. It is therefore important to become familiar with the treatment of acute HTN crises in the cardiac catheterization with the goal to alleviate myocardial ischemia but without compromising coronary perfusion or depressing the heart contractile function. Vasodilators such as nitroglycerin are especially attractive as they mitigate the effects of HTN, reduce wall stress, alleviate ischemia, and promote coronary vasodilation. Hypertensive emergencies are usually characterized by ongoing end-organ damage and warrant the use of parenteral agents of rapid onset and offset action. However, sudden rapid declines in blood pressure (BP) may be hazardous and should be avoided.

The No-Reflow Phenomenon

No-reflow occurs usually as a result of distal embolization, vasospasm, and/or endothelial injury, and often complicates PCI of degenerated vein grafts, ectatic coronary arteries, and heavily thrombotic lesions. It is more common after STEMI and is reported to occur in approximately 30% of patients undergoing primary PCI.[103] In one study of 489 patients with STEMI treated at four primary PCI centers, no-reflow was the only independent predictor of MACE at one-year follow-up.[104] No-reflow may be associated with more cases of congestive heart failure, cardiogenic shock, and death. Therefore, prompt treatment is essential. IC vasodilators (e.g., adenosine, nitroprusside) are reasonable for the treatment of PCI-associated no-reflow (Class IIb according to the 2011 ACCF/AHA/SCAI PCI guideline[11]). In the case of no-reflow, it is best to administer the vasodilator drug in the distal portion of the vessel via a micro-catheter (or through the lumen of a distally advanced balloon catheter) rather than at the tip of the guide catheter, to ensure delivery to the microvascular bed.

Selective Vasodilators and Antihypertensive Medications (Table 4-4)

Nitroglycerin

Nitroglycerin (NTG) is a vasoactive nitric oxide (NO) donor that reduces ischemia through its predominant venodilatory effect which reduces preload, left ventricular wall stress, and myocardial oxygen demand. NO helps inhibit platelet

TABLE 4-4 Overview of Commonly Used Parenteral Anti-Hypertensive Drugs in Cardiac Catheterization

ANTI-HYPERTENSIVE MEDICATIONS	*Dose*		*Drug Kinetics and Metabolism*		*Systemic Effects*			ADVERSE EFFECTS
	INITIAL	MAXIMUM			CO	HR	SVR	
Nitroglycerin	Initial: 5 mcg/min increased by 5 mcg/min every 3-5 min up to 20 mcg/min; then increase by 10-20 mcg/min every 3-5 min	200 mcg/min	$t_{1/2}$: 1-4 min	Hepatic, plasma	↔/↓	↔/↑	↓	Hypotension, headache, rash, tachyphylaxis, methemoglobinemia
Nitroprusside	Initial: 0.25-0.3 mcg/kg/min increased by 0.5 mcg/kg/min to 3 mcg/kg/min	10 mcg/kg/min	$t_{1/2}$: 2 min	Plasma	↑	↔/↑	↓↓	Cyanide poisoning, cardiac dysrhythmia, hypotension, hemorrhage, bowel obstruction, metabolic acidosis, methemoglobinemia
Esmolol	50 mcg/kg/min (titrate by 50 mcg/kg/min every 5 min)	300 mcg/kg/min	$t_{1/2}$: 9 min Onset: immediate	Esterases, renal	↓	↓↓	↓	Bradycardia, dizziness, drowsiness, hypotension, heart block
Labetalol	IV: bolus 10-20 mg over 2 min; then 0.5-2 mg/min (titrate by 0.5 mg/min every hour)	8 mg/min not to exceed 300 mg/day	$t_{1/2}$: 2.5-8 h (normal renal function)	Hepatic (glucuronidation), biliary, renal (minimal ~5%)	↓	↓↓	↓	Bradycardia, dizziness, drowsiness, hypotension, heart block, orthostatic hypotension, syncope
Nicardipine	Initial: 5 mg/hr increased by 2.5 mg/hr every 5-15 min Maintenance: 3 mg/hr	15 mg/hr	$t_{1/2}$: 2-4 h	Hepatic, plasma	↓	↔/↑	↓	Acute hepatitis, myocardial ischemia, headache, hypotension

CO, Cardiac output; *h,* hour; *HR,* heart rate; *min,* minute; *SVR,* systemic vascular resistance; $t_{1/2}$, half-life.

adhesion and also has also anti-inflammatory activity. It is commonly administered via the IV or sublingual routes in the cardiac catheterization laboratory. Given its short duration of action, an IV infusion of NTG (5-10 mcg/min; up to 200 mcg/min) is relatively selective for the venous capacitance vessels and is especially useful in patients with PCI-complicated ischemia and/or heart failure. At higher doses (>200 mcg/min), IV NTG can vasodilate large conductance vessels and is effective in treating HTN urgency. NTG also dilates the epicardial coronary arteries and large arterioles (>100 μm), so they can improve coronary perfusion and mitigate vasospasm (e.g., catheter-induced spasms) when used intracoronary (IC) (usually 100- to 400-mcg IC boluses) (Videos 4-5AB). NTG has no effect on the microcirculation, does not induce hyperemia, and has limited use in the treatment of no-reflow phenomenon.

Adenosine

IC adenosine (40- to 100-mcg boluses) is often used during PCI to vasodilate the microcirculation to prevent or treat the no-reflow phenomenon.[105,106] In a meta-analysis of 10 RCTs comparing adenosine versus placebo among patients with ACS, adenosine was associated with a 75% reduction in post-PCI no reflow.[107] However, no benefits on mortality or clinical outcomes were observed with the adjunctive use of adenosine therapy.[107]

Both IC boluses and IV infusion of adenosine are utilized to induce maximal hyperemia during invasive physiological assessment of intermediate coronary lesions, such as fractional flow reserve (FFR). While IC adenosine (40- to 100-mcg boluses or higher) is easier to use, more cost effective, and has fewer systemic side effects, IV adenosine (usually at 140 mcg/kg/min, sometimes at 180 mcg/kg/min) achieves more consistent and prolonged hyperemia and is particularly useful to evaluate ostial lesions and when slow pull-back across a diffusely diseased vessel is needed.[108] A small study (n = 45) recently demonstrated that high incremental doses of IC adenosine (up to 600 mcg) allows obtaining FFR values similar to IV adenosine and was not associated with increased side effects.[109]

Adenosine is also valuable in diagnosing and treating supraventricular tachycardias that occur during PCI. Adenosine can induce AV block and bradycardia, necessitating the use of a temporary transvenous pacemaker in some instances, and should be cautiously used in patients with conduction abnormalities and in patients with advanced bronchospastic airway disease. Fortunately, it has a short half-life and its effect is usually quickly dissipated (5-10 seconds) through metabolism by the red blood cells.

Nitroprusside

Sodium nitroprusside is a direct NO donor and potent vasodilator that rapidly reduces ventricular filling pressure and systemic vascular resistance. It has a very rapid onset of action (2-5 minutes) and its effect quickly dissipates after discontinuing the infusion. IV nitroprusside is therefore

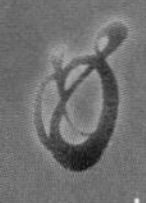

ideal for treatment of heart failure (HF) and among patients with post-MI mechanical complications. Prolonged infusions, particularly in the setting of renal or hepatic disease, may result in the uncommon but serious side effect of cyanide or thiocyanate toxicity. IC nitroprusside (100- to 200-mcg boluses) is also effective in treating slow flow/no reflow[110-112] and may be beneficial in its prevention.[113]

Ca^{2+} Channel Antagonists

Ca^{2+} channel antagonists reduce BP and improve coronary flow through peripheral and coronary arterial vasodilation, suppress myocardial contractility, and also reduce HR (through suppression of SA node automaticity and AV conduction). They are therefore very good anti-ischemic and anti-HTN agents, but can also precipitate HF in predisposed patients (especially the cardio-selective agents). Verapamil, diltiazem, and the dihydropyridines have fundamental differences with respect to pharmacological characteristics and effects. The cardio-selective verapamil and diltiazem have potent anti-HTN effects but also exert negative chronotropic and inotropic effects on the heart, while dihydropyridines exert predominantly vascular effects (with minimal effects on cardiac contractility) and are also very effective HTN drugs. Dihydropyridines, such as nicardipine, are more potent vasodilators than verapamil, which is more potent than diltiazem. IV nicardipine (5-15 mg/h) can be used during HTN urgencies, although it can exacerbate myocardial ischemia and cause hypotension.

IC nicardipine is a safe and highly effective pharmacological agent to reverse no reflow during PCI (mean dose in a study was 460 mcg).[114] Early administration of IC verapamil during direct PCI also improves post-procedural myocardial perfusion, as evaluated by TIMI myocardial perfusion grade.[115] IC diltiazem (50-200 mcg) or verapamil (50-200 mcg) can reverse no reflow more effectively than nitroglycerin during primary PCI for acute MI.[116] The efficacy of diltiazem and verapamil is similar, although diltiazem seems safer.[116] In one study of 347 identified STEMI subjects treated with PCI, nicardipine, nitroprusside, and verapamil were equally effective in improving flow.[103] Overall, pharmacologic treatment normalized coronary flow in 40% of patients assessed by myocardial blush grade and in 79% of patients assessed using the TIMI score.[103]

β Adrenergic Receptor Antagonists

β adrenergic receptor antagonists are effective in treating HTN crises and reducing myocardial O_2 consumption through negative chronotropic and inotropic effects and by decreasing arterial BP. In patients with limited cardiac reserve who are critically dependent on adrenergic stimulation, β receptor blockers may cause profound reduction in left ventricular function and cause or exacerbate HF and cardiogenic shock. For the latter reasons, β blockers are not advocated any more as an upfront clinical performance measure to be implemented within 24 hours of presentation after acute myocardial infarction (AMI),[117] and their parenteral use should be particularly avoided given the increased hazards of cardiogenic shock.[118]

IV labetalol (10- to 20-mg bolus, followed by 0.5- to 2-mg/min infusion up to 300-mg total cumulative dose) may be useful during adrenergic crises in the catheterization laboratory, as in patients presenting with cocaine-associated ACS and HTN crisis.[119] Given its short half-life, IV esmolol (50-300 mcg/kg/min) may be particularly useful in patients with acute aortic syndromes presenting for preoperative angiography (often in conjunction with IV nitroprusside) to rapidly reduce BP and the shear stress on the aortic wall (though most of these patients should go directly to surgery without angiography).

VASOPRESSORS AND INOTROPIC DRUGS

Hypotension

There are a myriad of reasons for hypotension occurring during coronary interventions. Appropriate treatment depends on prompt and accurate diagnosis of the precipitating etiology. A sudden drop in BP within minutes of radiocontrast material is usually attributable to an anaphylactic reaction with vasodepressor response (confirmed by low left-ventricular end diastolic pressure, LVEDP, on left heart catheterization). Treatment in this case should be immediate volume resuscitation and epinephrine. Following complicated femoral arterial access, vascular hemorrhage is usually suspected. Wire exit and coronary perforation are in the differential diagnosis, and pericardiocentesis and discontinuation/reversal of anticoagulants should be instituted in such cases. Arrhythmias and valvular lesions (e.g., critical aortic stenosis, acute ischemic mitral regurgitation) have differing therapies (e.g., anti-arrhythmics, cardioversion, balloon valvuloplasty, revascularization). Cardiogenic shock is usually diagnosed by right heart catheterization and arterial hemodynamic monitoring (combination of elevated intracardiac pressures, depressed cardiac index, and low systemic arterial pressure) and should be treated with a combination of vasopressors/inotropes, percutaneous ventricular assist devices (pVADs), and revascularization in most instances. In all the aforementioned scenarios, vasopressors are the initial treatment strategy (with or without volume repletion) irrespective of the inciting etiology and on top of the definitive treatment (such as revascularization, blood transfusions, vascular repair).

Acute Heart Failure/Cardiogenic Shock

Acute HF may develop in the cardiac catheterization laboratory as a result of multiple inter-related etiologies: volume overload from increased contrast use, pulmonary vascular redistribution during prolonged cases, iatrogenic from inappropriate and overzealous β blockers or Ca^{2+} channel blockers, arrhythmias, myocardial ischemia during PCI (in cases of acute closure, distal embolization, myocardial stunning), and a myriad of other causes. Initial therapy requires airway protection with intubation and mechanical ventilation, in addition to inotropic support, aggressive diuresis and possibly pVADs. Also, around 6% to 8% of patients with AMI develop cardiogenic shock, of which up to 60% to 75% may develop during hospitalization. Many of those occurred in the cardiac catheterization laboratory and require adding vasopressors to inotropic support.[120]

Selective Vasopressors and Inotropes (Table 4-5)

Phenylephrine

It is a synthetic α-agonist catecholamine that causes predominantly peripheral vasoconstriction. It is used to treat acute hypotension resulting from myocardial ischemia, stunning or no-reflow during PCI, or complicating dynamic left ventricular outflow obstruction. It is usually given IV in 50- to 100-mcg incremental boluses.

TABLE 4-5 Overview of Commonly used Parenteral Vasopressors and Inotropes in the Cardiac Catheterization Laboratory

				Systemic Effects				
VASOPRESSORS	DOSE	*Drug Kinetics and Metabolism*		CO	HR	SVR	ADVERSE EFFECTS	ROUTE OF ADMINISTRATION
Dopamine	Initial: 5-10 mcg/kg/min Maximum: 50 mcg/kg/min (adults)	$t_{1/2}$: 2-5 min	Renal, hepatic, plasma	5-10 mcg/kg/min: ↑ >10 mcg/kg/min: ↑	5-10 mcg/kg/min: ↑ >10 mcg/kg/min: ↑↑	5-10 mcg/kg/min: ↔/↑ >10 mcg/kg/min: ↑↑	Angina, ectopic beats, dyspnea nausea/ vomiting, headache, tachycardia	Continuous intravenous infusion
Norepinephrine	Initial: 8-12 mcg/min, titrate to desired response Maintenance: 2-4 mcg/min Maximum: 30 mcg/min Post cardiac arrest: 0.1-0.5 mcg/kg/min	$t_{1/2}$: 1 min	Renal, hepatic, plasma	↔/↓	↑	↑↑	Arrhythmia, reflex bradycardia, headache, extravasation, dyspnea	Continuous intravenous infusion
Phenylephrine	Initial: 20-180 mcg/min or 0.5 mcg/kg/min; titrate to desired response Maintenance: 40-60 mcg/ min (given also as 100-mcg IV boluses for transient hypotension episodes in the catheterization lab)	$t_{1/2}$: 5 min	Hepatic	↔	↔/↓	↑	Arrhythmia, extravasation, pulmonary edema, myocardial infarction	Continuous intravenous infusion
Epinephrine	Hypotension/shock: Initial: 0.1-0.5 mcg/kg/min to be titrated to the desired response Anaphylaxis: IM/SC: 0.2-0.5 mg (1 : 1000) every 5-15 min IV: 0.1 mg (1 : 1000) over 5 min; or may infuse at 1-4 mcg/min Asystole/pulseless VT or VF: Usually: 1 mg IV every 3-5 min until restoration of spontaneous circulation	$t_{1/2}$: 2 min	Uptake and metabolism in the adrenergic neurons (by monoamine oxidase, etc.) Hepatic metabolism for circulating drug	↑	↑	↔/↓ at low doses ↑ at high doses	Arrhythmias, splanchnic vasoconstriction and mesenteric ischemia, hypertension, pallor, anxiety, pulmonary edema	Continuous intravenous infusion Intravenous, intramuscular and subcutaneous routes are used during anaphylaxis Intravenous, intra-osseous, and endotracheal routes are acceptable for asystole and pulseless VF/VT
Vasopressin	Cardiac arrest: 40 units given once as an alternative to the first or second dose of epinephrine Maintenance: 0.02-0.04 units/min	$t_{1/2}$: 10-20 min; ~18 min	Hepatic, renal	↔	↔	↑	Arrhythmia, extravasation, dyspnea, water intoxication syndrome, anaphylaxis	Intravenous/ intraosseous/ endotracheal, continuous intravenous infusion
Inotrope								
Dobutamine	Initial: Acute cardiac decompensation: –1-20 mcg/kg/min Maximum: 40 mcg/kg/min	$t_{1/2}$: 2 min	Hepatic	↑	↑	↔/↓	Arrhythmia, angina, nausea, dyspnea, tachycardia	Continuous intravenous infusion
Milrinone	Initial loading dose (optional): 50 mcg/kg over 10 min Maintenance: 0.125-0.750 mcg/kg/min	$t_{1/2}$: 2.5 h	Hepatic (12%)	↑	↑	↓	Arrhythmias, hypotension, chest pain/angina, headache	Continuous intravenous infusion

CO, Cardiac output; *h*, hour; *HR*, heart rate; *min*, minute; *SVR*, systemic vascular resistance; $t_{1/2}$, half-life.

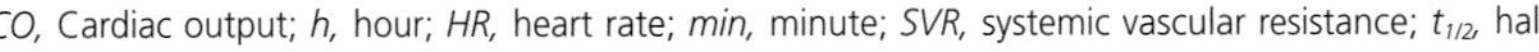

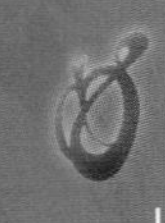

Dopamine

It is an endogenous parenteral catecholamine-like agent that is useful in the treatment of hypotension, HF, and cardiogenic shock. Its pharmacodynamic effects differ with escalating doses, with low doses (2 mcg/kg/min) usually causing splanchnic vasodilation and enhanced natriuresis, moderate doses (2-8 mcg/kg/min) inducing β-1 adrenergic receptor activation in the heart, and high doses (>8 mcg/kg/min) stimulating peripheral vasoconstriction and predominant vasopressor effects by acting as an α-1 sympathomimetic. A maximal inotropic effect is likely seen at a 5-mcg/kg/min dose. Dopamine is useful to treat hypotension and shock in the cardiac catheterization laboratory by imparting a vasopressor effect and increasing cardiac output. However, it can cause tachycardia and exacerbate arrhythmias and myocardial ischemia, which may limit its use.

Norepinephrine

It is an endogenous catecholamine with selective β-1 (but no β-2) sympathomimetic activity and strong α-1 and -2 sympathomimetic effects. IV norepinephrine (2-4 mcg/min up to 30 mcg/min) is a potent vasoconstrictor with fewer inotropic and chronotropic effects than epinephrine and dopamine and causes less arrhythmia than either agent. In a multicenter randomized controlled trial (RCT) of 1679 shock patients, dopamine was compared head-to-head against norepinephrine as first-line vasopressor therapy to restore and maintain blood pressure.[121] While no significant inter-group differences in 28-day mortality were observed, there were more arrhythmias among dopamine-treated patients.[121] In the subgroup of 280 patients with cardiogenic shock, norepinephrine was associated with lower mortality.[121] Norepinephrine may produce mesenteric vasoconstriction and cause splanchnic ischemia and resultant septicemia.

Dobutamine

It is a parenteral sympathomimetic that activates both β-1 and β-2 but has few effects on α-adrenergic receptors. It is the preferred inotrope following an AMI when a pure inotropic response is desired, but not a vasopressor effect that may exacerbate ischemia. Dobutamine does not increase the infarct size or cause significant arrhythmias, and is also preferred to dopamine in HF patients because of its vasodilatory actions (through β-2 receptor activation). An IV infusion of 2-20 mcg/kg/min is typically used. Hypotension may ensue sometimes with its use, and thus low-dose dopamine may be co-administered with it. Infrequently, low to moderate-dose dobutamine infusion may be used in the cardiac catheterization laboratory to induce pharmacologic stress and examine contractile reserve and valvular stenosis severity (e.g., in low-output aortic stenosis).

Epinephrine

Epinephrine is a sympathomimetic drug that activates α, β-1, and β-2 adrenergic receptors. At low doses, it increases the cardiac output through its β-1 adrenergic effects (as the α receptor–induced vasoconstriction is offset by the β-2 receptor–induced vasodilation). At higher doses, the α adrenergic receptor vasoconstrictor effect predominates, causing an increase in cardiac output and systemic vascular resistance. In the cardiac catheterization laboratory, it is used for the treatment of asystole and pulseless ventricular tachycardia/ventricular arrhythmias (VT/VF) (usually 1 mg IV every 3-5 minutes until return of spontaneous circulation) and for the treatment of anaphylaxis (0.2- to 0.5-mg IM/subcutaneous injections to be repeated every 5-15 minutes as needed; 0.1-mg IV bolus over 5 minutes; or 1- to 4-mcg/min IV infusion for refractory patients). It can be used for treatment of bradycardia and severe hypotension as well.

Additional Agents

Vasopressin is an anti-diuretic hormone analog that has important vasopressor actions, especially in patients with extreme shock. It can be administered IV as 0.01-0.04 U/min. During cardiac arrest, a 40-U bolus may be administered IV (or endotracheal). IV milrinone (0.125-0.750 mcg/kg/min) is an inotropic agent that inhibits phosphodiesterase III and increases cardiac contractility and is independent of the action of the β adrenergic receptors. It is useful in patients with HF, but can induce peripheral arterial and venous dilation and consequent hypotension, as well as exacerbate arrhythmias.

PROCEDURAL SEDATION: ANXIOLYTICS AND ANALGESICS

Most PCIs are performed under minimal sedation (anxiolysis) or moderate sedation (depressed consciousness with the ability to respond to verbal commands) (**Table 4-6**).[122] Deep sedation is infrequently used in the catheterization laboratory and usually requires the presence of an anesthesiologist for airway protection.

Benzodiazepines (e.g., midazolam, lorazepam, diazepam) are sedating agents used to provide anxiolysis and anterograde amnesia. Midazolam is very commonly used because of its short half-life and is usually given as 0.5- to 1-mg IV boluses to be repeated every 5 minutes for up to a maximum of 0.1-0.2 mg/kg. Benzodiazepines should, however, be complemented by an opioid (e.g., fentanyl, morphine sulfate), which can provide an analgesic effect (**Table 4-7**). Fentanyl (25- to 100-mcg IV boluses) is fast acting, has rapid offset of action after small bolus doses, does not release histamine, and imparts minimal cardiovascular depression. Fentanyl is therefore the preferred analgesic in patients undergoing PCI, especially those with poor cardiac function. IV propofol is a very fast acting sedative (<1 min) with short duration of action that can be used for monitored anesthesia care sedation (0.5 mg/kg slow injection over 3-5 min followed by 25-75 mcg/kg/min infusion); however, it can cause profound hypotension and cardiorespiratory depression. Thus, its use in non-intubated patients by the non-anesthesiologists is not routinely recommended.

MISCELLANEOUS DRUGS

Anti-arrhythmic Medications

Arrhythmias may occur in patients undergoing invasive cardiac procedures. They can be caused by myocardial ischemia, increased sympathoadrenal tone from pain or anxiety, catheter manipulation of cardiac structures (e.g., during right heart catheterization), or occur as a result of poor left ventricular contractile function. IV lidocaine is a class IB drug that is particularly useful in the treatment of ventricular arrhythmias occurring in the setting of myocardial ischemia. Lidocaine-associated pro-arrhythmias are uncommon; however, central nervous system side effects may occur,

TABLE 4-6 Overview of Commonly Used Parenteral Sedatives in Cardiac Catheterization

	Dose		Drug Kinetics and Metabolism					
ANXIOLYTICS	INITIAL	MAXIMUM				PREFERRED ROUTE OF ADMINISTRATION	REVERSAL AGENT	ADVERSE EFFECTS
Benzodiazepines								
Midazolam	0.02-0.04 mg/kg IV; usual dose is 1-2 mg IV bolus (consider lower initial doses in the elderly or when given concomitantly with analgesics); 0.07-0.08 mg/kg or 5 mg IM 30-60 min prior	Until desired clinical response or 0.1-0.2 mg/kg; usually no more than 5 mg IV needed for induction unless prior history of heavy alcohol use	Onset: 2-5 min Duration: less than 2 h (single dose)	$t_{1/2}$: 2-6 h (prolonged in renal failure, elderly, cirrhosis, and HF)	Hepatic	Intravenous injection (may give intramuscular)	Flumazenil (0.2 mg every min up to 1 mg)	Amnesia, respiratory depression, hypotension, headache, drowsiness/over-sedation, nausea/vomiting, pain and injection site reactions
Lorazepam	0.044 mg/kg IV; usual dose is 2 mg; 0.05 mg/kg or 2 mg IM 2 h prior	4 mg IV/IM	Onset: 2-3 min Duration: Up to 8 h	$t_{1/2}$: ≈12-14 h	Hepatic	Intravenous injection (may give intramuscular)		Amnesia, respiratory depression, hypotension, drowsiness/over-sedation, dizziness, headache, propylene glycol toxicity (lactic acidosis, hyper-osmolality, hypotension) with IV use in renal failure, pain and injection site reactions
Non-benzodiazepine								
Propofol	50-150 mcg/kg/min (3-9 mg/kg/h)	Until desired clinical response or 200 mcg/kg/min (12 mg/kg/h)	Onset: 30 seconds Duration: 3-10 min	$t_{1/2}$ (Biphasic): initially ≈40 min; terminal 4-7 h but up to 1-3 d if prolonged infusion (≈10 d)	Hepatic	Intravenous injection/infusion	None	Respiratory depression, hypotension, pruritus, involuntary movement, pain or injection site reactions, apnea, hypertriglyceridemia, zinc deficiency
Etomidate	0.2-0.4 mg/kg IV for induction, 5-15 mcg/kg/min for maintenance	0.6 mg/kg IV for induction, 20 mcg/kg/min for maintenance	Onset: 30-60 seconds Duration: 3-5 min	$t_{1/2}$: ≈1.25-2.6 h	Hepatic	Intravenous injection/infusion		Respiratory depression, pain and injection site reaction, involuntary movements, nausea/vomiting, apnea, adrenal suppression, propylene glycol toxicity (renal failure)

d, Day; *HF,* heart failure; *h,* hour; *IM,* intramuscular; *IV,* intravenous; *min,* minute; $t_{1/2}$, half-life.

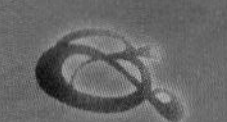

TABLE 4-7 Overview of Commonly Used Parenteral Analgesics in Cardiac Catheterization

	Dose		*Drug Kinetics and Metabolism*					
ANALGESICS	**INITIAL**	**MAXIMUM**				**PREFERRED ROUTE OF ADMINISTRATION**	**REVERSAL AGENT**	**ADVERSE EFFECTS**
Fentanyl	25-100 mcg IV/IM up to every 3 min	Doses greater than 200 mcg rarely needed unless chronic opioid user	Onset: (IV) immediate to within a minutes (IM) ≈7-8 min Duration: (IV): dose dependent ≈0.5-1 hour after single dose but increases with repeated doses (IM) 1-2 hours (respiratory effects may persist longer than analgesia)	$t_{1/2}$: 2-4 h (increases with repeated doses)	Hepatic/ Intestinal	Intravenous injection (may give subcutaneous or via continuous IV infusion)	Naloxone (0.2-2 mg IV; may repeat in 2-3 minutes not to exceed 10 mg)	Respiratory depression, apnea, hypotension, over-sedation, nausea/vomiting, constipation, cardiac dysrhythmia, headache, pruritus
Morphine	1-4 mg IV/IM up to every 5 min	Doses greater than 6 mg rarely needed unless chronic opioid user	Onset: 5-10 min Duration: 4 h	$t_{1/2}$: 2-4 h	Hepatic	Intravenous injection (may give intramuscular/ subcutaneous or via continuous IV infusion)		Respiratory depression, anaphylaxis, hypotension, agitation, over-sedation, nausea/vomiting, urinary retention, constipation, xerostomia, pruritus, blurry vision

d, Day; *HF,* heart failure; *h,* hour; *IM,* intramuscular; *IV,* intravenous; *min,* minute; $t_{1/2}$, half-life.

TABLE 4-8 Overview of Commonly Used Parenteral Anti-arrhythmic Medications in Cardiac Catheterization

ANTI-ARRHYTHMIC MEDICATIONS	*Dose* INITIAL	MAXIMUM	*Drug Kinetics and Metabolism*		ADVERSE EFFECTS	ROUTES OF ADMINISTRATION
Amiodarone	Pulseless VT or VF: 300-mg IV bolus; if refractory, administer additional 150-mg bolus Stable VT or AF: 150 mg IV piggyback; then start maintenance infusion Maintenance: 1 mg/min for 6 h followed by 0.5 mg/min for 18 h; then transition to PO regimen	2.2 g over 24 h	$t_{1/2}$: 40-55 d (range 26-107 d)	Hepatic, biliary (minor)	Acute side effects: hypotension, bradycardia, congestive heart failure, cardiac dysrhythmia, acute respiratory distress syndrome, anaphylaxis, ataxia, nausea/vomiting Chronic side effects: pulmonary fibrosis, hepatitis/hepatotoxicity, thyroid dysfunction, phototoxicity, corneal deposits, neurologic toxicity	Intravenous
Lidocaine	Pulseless VT or VF if amiodarone is not available: 1-1.5 mg/kg; if refractory, repeat 0.5-0.75 mg/kg every 5-10 min Maintenance: 1-4 mg/min; if hepatic dysfunction, heart failure, or low muscle mass then 1-2 mg/min	3 mg/kg	$t_{1/2}$: initially 7-30 min in distribution phase then 1.5-2 h Onset rapid if given IV with duration of 10-20 min	Hepatic, plasma	CNS side effects (nystagmus, seizure, tremor, etc.), cardiac dysrhythmia, articular chondrolysis, loss of consciousness, methemoglobinemia	Intravenous/intra-osseous/endotracheal

AF, Atrial fibrillation; *d,* day; *h,* hour; *IM,* intramuscular; *IV,* intravenous; *min,* minute; $t_{1/2}$, half-life; *VF,* ventricular fibrillation; *VT,* ventricular tachycardia.

with nystagmus being an early sign of lidocaine toxicity (**Table 4-8**). IV amiodarone is effective in acutely terminating ventricular tachycardia[123] and is supplanting lidocaine as first-line therapy in these patients (**Table 4-8**).[124] It is often used in the treatment of atrial fibrillation with rapid ventricular response. Prompt electrical cardioversion and defibrillation remain the cornerstone therapies for unstable arrhythmias and ventricular fibrillation. Adenosine is an anti-arrhythmic agent that slows AV nodal conduction and interrupts re-entry pathways through the AV node. It has a very rapid onset and a brief duration of action (<10 seconds half-life) and is typically used for the treatment of paroxysmal supraventricular tachycardia (6- to 12-mg IV boluses) in the cardiac catheterization laboratory. Atropine is an anticholinergic agent with a rapid onset of action and short half-life (2-3 hours) that is often used in the cardiac catheterization laboratory to treat bradycardia (0.5 mg IV every 3-5 minutes, not to exceed 3 mg).

Diuretics

Loop diuretics are the most powerful diuretic agents and act to reduce sodium chloride reabsorption in the kidney. They are the agents of choice in patients who develop acute pulmonary edema and volume overload in the cardiac catheterization laboratory. In the presence of normal renal function, a 40-mg furosemide IV bolus (equivalent to 1 mg bumetanide or 20 mg torsemide) can achieve a maximal diuretic effect with a 15-minute onset of action. However, in the presence of CHF or renal insufficiency, a twofold to fivefold increase in dose may be needed. Loop diuretics may cause hypovolemia, hypotension, and electrolyte abnormalities.

CONCLUSIONS

There is a large armamentarium of pharmacotherapies that invasive cardiologists can choose from. As new evidence, indications, and medications are forthcoming, it is important that invasive cardiologists are continuously updated and constantly familiar with the evolving trends. It is also preferable that operators and all staff in the cardiac catheterization laboratory focus on the use of a few medications from each class, develop deep knowledge about them, and consistently utilize them. Physicians and staff should know the intricacies related to the drugs they use, including the evidence, indications, dosage, onset, and duration of action, reversal, drug-drug interactions, excretion/metabolism, need for dose adjustment among patients with renal or hepatic failure, and side effects (including rare ones). Protocols for commonly used therapies should be written and consistently implemented. Finally, it is important that physicians are mindful of the cost of therapies and their overall value to patients' care and the catheterization laboratory in the contemporary environment of constrained resources.

References

1. Capodanno D, Ferreiro JL, Angiolillo DJ: Antiplatelet therapy: new pharmacological agents and changing paradigms. *J Thromb Haemost* 11(Suppl 1):316–329, 2013.
2. Dorsam RT, Kunapuli SP: Central role of the P2Y12 receptor in platelet activation. *J Clin Invest* 113(3):340–345, 2004.
3. Jneid H, Bhatt DL, Corti R, et al: Aspirin and clopidogrel in acute coronary syndromes: therapeutic insights from the CURE study. *Arch Intern Med* 163(10):1145–1153, 2003.

4. Angiolillo DJ, Ferreiro JL: Antiplatelet and anticoagulant therapy for atherothrombotic disease: the role of current and emerging agents. *Am J Cardiovasc Drugs* 13(4):233–250, 2013.
5. Leger AJ, Covic L, Kuliopulos A: Protease-activated receptors in cardiovascular diseases. *Circulation* 114(10):1070–1077, 2006.
6. Jneid H, Bhatt DL: Advances in antiplatelet therapy. *Expert Opin Emerg Drugs* 8(2):349–363, 2003.
7. Patrignani P, Filabozzi P, Patrono C: Selective cumulative inhibition of platelet thromboxane production by low-dose aspirin in healthy subjects. *J Clin Invest* 69(6):1366–1372, 1982.
8. Kelly JP, Kaufman DW, Jurgelon JM, et al: Risk of aspirin-associated major upper-gastrointestinal bleeding with enteric-coated or buffered product. *Lancet* 348(9039):1413–1416, 1996.
9. Antithrombotic Trialists C: Collaborative meta-analysis of randomised trials of antiplatelet therapy for prevention of death, myocardial infarction, and stroke in high risk patients. *BMJ* 324(7329):71–86, 2002.
10. Jolly SS, Pogue J, Haladyn K, et al: Effects of aspirin dose on ischaemic events and bleeding after percutaneous coronary intervention: insights from the PCI-CURE study. *Eur Heart J* 30(8):900–907, 2009.
11. Levine GN, Bates ER, Blankenship JC, et al: 2011 ACCF/AHA/SCAI guideline for percutaneous coronary intervention. A report of the American College of Cardiology Foundation/American Heart Association Task Force on Practice Guidelines and the Society for Cardiovascular Angiography and Interventions. *J Am Coll Cardiol* 58(24):e44–e122, 2011.
12. Mehta SR, Yusuf S, Peters RJ, et al: Effects of pretreatment with clopidogrel and aspirin followed by long-term therapy in patients undergoing percutaneous coronary intervention: the PCI-CURE study. *Lancet* 358(9281):527–533, 2001.
13. Schomig A, Neumann FJ, Kastrati A, et al: A randomized comparison of antiplatelet and anticoagulant therapy after the placement of coronary-artery stents. *N Engl J Med* 334(17):1084–1089, 1996.
14. Leon MB, Baim DS, Popma JJ, et al: A clinical trial comparing three antithrombotic-drug regimens after coronary-artery stenting. Stent Anticoagulation Restenosis Study Investigators. *N Engl J Med* 339(23):1665–1671, 1998.
15. Bhatt DL, Bertrand ME, Berger PB, et al: Meta-analysis of randomized and registry comparisons of ticlopidine with clopidogrel after stenting. *J Am Coll Cardiol* 39(1):9–14, 2002.
16. Moussa I, Oetgen M, Roubin G, et al: Effectiveness of clopidogrel and aspirin versus ticlopidine and aspirin in preventing stent thrombosis after coronary stent implantation. *Circulation* 99(18):2364–2366, 1999.
17. Taniuchi M, Kurz HI, Lasala JM: Randomized comparison of ticlopidine and clopidogrel after intracoronary stent implantation in a broad patient population. *Circulation* 104(5):539–543, 2001.
18. Steinhubl SR, Berger PB, Mann JT, 3rd, et al: Early and sustained dual oral antiplatelet therapy following percutaneous coronary intervention: a randomized controlled trial. *JAMA* 288(19):2411–2420, 2002.
19. Sabatine MS, Cannon CP, Gibson CM, et al: Effect of clopidogrel pretreatment before percutaneous coronary intervention in patients with ST-elevation myocardial infarction treated with fibrinolytics: the PCI-CLARITY study. *JAMA* 294(10):1224–1232, 2005.
20. Depta JP, Bhatt DL: Aspirin and platelet adenosine diphosphate receptor antagonists in acute coronary syndromes and percutaneous coronary intervention: role in therapy and strategies to overcome resistance. *Am J Cardiovasc Drugs* 8(2):91–112, 2008.
21. Tantry US, Bonello L, Aradi D, et al: Consensus and update on the definition of on-treatment platelet reactivity to adenosine diphosphate associated with ischemia and bleeding. *J Am Coll Cardiol* 62(24):2261–2273, 2013.
22. Mehta SR, Tanguay JF, Eikelboom JW, et al: Double-dose versus standard-dose clopidogrel and high-dose versus low-dose aspirin in individuals undergoing percutaneous coronary intervention for acute coronary syndromes (CURRENT-OASIS 7): a randomised factorial trial. *Lancet* 376(9748):1233–1243, 2010.
23. Jneid H, Anderson JL, Wright RS, et al: 2012 ACCF/AHA focused update of the guideline for the management of patients with unstable angina/non-ST-elevation myocardial infarction (updating the 2007 guideline and replacing the 2011 focused update): a report of the American College of Cardiology Foundation/American Heart Association Task Force on Practice Guidelines. *J Am Coll Cardiol* 60(7):645–681, 2012.
24. Investigators C-O, Mehta SR, Bassand JP, et al: Dose comparisons of clopidogrel and aspirin in acute coronary syndromes. *N Engl J Med* 363(10):930–942, 2010.
25. Price MJ, Berger PB, Teirstein PS, et al: Standard- vs high-dose clopidogrel based on platelet function testing after percutaneous coronary intervention: the GRAVITAS randomized trial. *JAMA* 305(11):1097–1105, 2011.
26. Bhatt DL, Cryer BL, Contant CF, et al: Clopidogrel with or without omeprazole in coronary artery disease. *N Engl J Med* 363(20):1909–1917, 2010.
27. Mega JL, Close SL, Wiviott SD, et al: Cytochrome p-450 polymorphisms and response to clopidogrel. *N Engl J Med* 360(4):354–362, 2009.
28. Niitsu Y, Jakubowski JA, Sugidachi A, et al: Pharmacology of CS-747 (prasugrel, LY640315), a novel, potent antiplatelet agent with in vivo P2Y12 receptor antagonist activity. *Semin Thromb Hemost* 31(2):184–194, 2005.
29. Wiviott SD, Braunwald E, McCabe CH, et al: Prasugrel versus clopidogrel in patients with acute coronary syndromes. *N Engl J Med* 357(20):2001–2015, 2007.
30. Roe MT, Armstrong PW, Fox KA, et al: Prasugrel versus clopidogrel for acute coronary syndromes without revascularization. *N Engl J Med* 367(14):1297–1309, 2012.
31. Michelson AD, Frelinger AL, 3rd, Braunwald E, et al: Pharmacodynamic assessment of platelet inhibition by prasugrel vs. clopidogrel in the TRITON-TIMI 38 trial. *Eur Heart J* 30(14):1753–1763, 2009.
32. Gurbel PA, Bliden KP, Butler K, et al: Response to ticagrelor in clopidogrel nonresponders and responders and effect of switching therapies: the RESPOND study. *Circulation* 121(10):1188–1199, 2010.
33. Fuster V, Bhatt DL, Califf RM, et al: Guided antithrombotic therapy: current status and future research direction: report on a National Heart, Lung and Blood Institute working group. *Circulation* 126(13):1645–1662, 2012.
34. Storey RF, Husted S, Harrington RA, et al: Inhibition of platelet aggregation by AZD6140, a reversible oral P2Y12 receptor antagonist, compared with clopidogrel in patients with acute coronary syndromes. *J Am Coll Cardiol* 50(19):1852–1856, 2007.
35. Wallentin L, Becker RC, Budaj A, et al: Ticagrelor versus clopidogrel in patients with acute coronary syndromes. *N Engl J Med* 361(11):1045–1057, 2009.
36. Mahaffey KW, Wojdyla DM, Carroll K, et al: Ticagrelor compared with clopidogrel by geographic region in the Platelet Inhibition and Patient Outcomes (PLATO) trial. *Circulation* 124(5):544–554, 2011.
37. James S, Budaj A, Aylward P, et al: Ticagrelor versus clopidogrel in acute coronary syndromes in relation to renal function: results from the Platelet Inhibition and Patient Outcomes (PLATO) trial. *Circulation* 122(11):1056–1067, 2010.
38. Basra SS, Tsai P, Lakkis NM: Safety and efficacy of antiplatelet and antithrombotic therapy in acute coronary syndrome patients with chronic kidney disease. *J Am Coll Cardiol* 58(22):2263–2269, 2011.
39. Grines CL, Bonow RO, Casey DE, Jr, et al: Prevention of premature discontinuation of dual antiplatelet therapy in patients with coronary artery stents: a science advisory from the American Heart Association, American College of Cardiology, Society for Cardiovascular Angiography and Interventions, American College of Surgeons, and American Dental Association, with representation from the American College of Physicians. *Circulation* 115(6):813–818, 2007.
40. Feres F, Costa RA, Abizaid A, et al: Three vs twelve months of dual antiplatelet therapy after zotarolimus-eluting stents: the OPTIMIZE randomized trial. *JAMA* 310(23):2510–2522, 2013.
41. Fleisher LA, Fleischmann KE, Auerbach AD, et al: 2014 ACC/AHA Guideline on Perioperative Cardiovascular Evaluation and Management of Patients Undergoing Noncardiac Surgery: Executive Summary: a report of the American College of Cardiology/American Heart Association Task Force on Practice Guidelines. *J Am Coll Cardiol* 2014.
42. Amsterdam EA, Wenger NK, Brindis RG, et al: 2014 AHA/ACC Guideline for the Management of Patients With Non-ST-Elevation Acute Coronary Syndromes: a report of the American College of Cardiology/American Heart Association Task Force on Practice Guidelines. *J Am Coll Cardiol* 2014.
43. O'Gara PT, Kushner FG, Ascheim DD, et al: 2013 ACCF/AHA guideline for the management of ST-elevation myocardial infarction: a report of the American College of Cardiology Foundation/ American Heart Association Task Force on Practice Guidelines. *Circulation* 127(4):e362–e425, 2013.
44. Chen ZM, Jiang LX, Chen YP, et al: Addition of clopidogrel to aspirin in 45,852 patients with acute myocardial infarction: randomised placebo-controlled trial. *Lancet* 366(9497):1607–1621, 2005.
45. Hillis LD, Smith PK, Anderson JL, et al: 2011 ACCF/AHA guideline for coronary artery bypass graft surgery. A report of the American College of Cardiology Foundation/American Heart Association Task Force on Practice Guidelines. Developed in collaboration with the American Association for Thoracic Surgery, Society of Cardiovascular Anesthesiologists, and Society of Thoracic Surgeons. *J Am Coll Cardiol* 58(24):e123–e210, 2011.
46. Yousuf O, Bhatt DL: The evolution of antiplatelet therapy in cardiovascular disease. *Nat Rev Cardiol* 8(10):547–559, 2011.
47. Topol EJ, Califf RM, Weisman HF, et al: Randomised trial of coronary intervention with antibody against platelet IIb/IIIa integrin for reduction of clinical restenosis: results at six months. The EPIC Investigators. *Lancet* 343(8902):881–886, 1994.
48. Investigators E: Platelet glycoprotein IIb/IIIa receptor blockade and low-dose heparin during percutaneous coronary revascularization. *N Engl J Med* 336(24):1689–1696, 1997.
49. Investigators E: Randomised placebo-controlled and balloon-angioplasty-controlled trial to assess safety of coronary stenting with use of platelet glycoprotein-IIb/IIIa blockade. *Lancet* 352(9122):87–92, 1998.
50. Hamm CW, Heeschen C, Goldmann B, et al: Benefit of abciximab in patients with refractory unstable angina in relation to serum troponin T levels. c7E3 Fab Antiplatelet Therapy in Unstable Refractory Angina (CAPTURE) Study Investigators. *N Engl J Med* 340(21):1623–1629, 1999.
51. Therapy EIESotPIIRwI: Novel dosing regimen of eptifibatide in planned coronary stent implantation (ESPRIT): a randomised, placebo-controlled trial. *Lancet* 356(9247):2037–2044, 2000.
52. Kastrati A, Mehilli J, Neumann FJ, et al: Abciximab in patients with acute coronary syndromes undergoing percutaneous coronary intervention after clopidogrel pretreatment: the ISAR-REACT 2 randomized trial. *JAMA* 295(13):1531–1538, 2006.
53. Ellis SG, Tendera M, de Belder MA, et al: Facilitated PCI in patients with ST-elevation myocardial infarction. *N Engl J Med* 358(21):2205–2217, 2008.
54. Mehilli J, Kastrati A, Schulz S, et al: Abciximab in patients with acute ST-segment-elevation myocardial infarction undergoing primary percutaneous coronary intervention after clopidogrel loading: a randomized double-blind trial. *Circulation* 119(14):1933–1940, 2009.
55. De Luca G, Navarese E, Marino P: Risk profile and benefits from Gp IIb-IIIa inhibitors among patients with ST-segment elevation myocardial infarction treated with primary angioplasty: a meta-regression analysis of randomized trials. *Eur Heart J* 30(22):2705–2713, 2009.
56. Kastrati A, Mehilli J, Schuhlen H, et al: A clinical trial of abciximab in elective percutaneous coronary intervention after pretreatment with clopidogrel. *N Engl J Med* 350(3):232–238, 2004.
57. Roffi M, Mukherjee D, Chew DP, et al: Lack of benefit from intravenous platelet glycoprotein IIb/IIIa receptor inhibition as adjunctive treatment for percutaneous interventions of aortocoronary bypass grafts: a pooled analysis of five randomized clinical trials. *Circulation* 106(24):3063–3067, 2002.
58. Gilchrist IC, O'Shea JC, Kosoglou T, et al: Pharmacodynamics and pharmacokinetics of higher-dose, double-bolus eptifibatide in percutaneous coronary intervention. *Circulation* 104(4):406–411, 2001.
59. Danzi GB, Capuano C, Sesana M, et al: Variability in extent of platelet function inhibition after administration of optimal dose of glycoprotein IIb/IIIa receptor blockers in patients undergoing a high-risk percutaneous coronary intervention. *Am J Cardiol* 97(4):489–493, 2006.
60. Hess CN, Schulte PJ, Newby LK, et al: Duration of eptifibatide infusion after percutaneous coronary intervention and outcomes among high-risk patients with non-ST-segment elevation acute coronary syndrome: insights from EARLY ACS. *Eur Heart J Acute Cardiovasc Care* 2(3):246–255, 2013.
61. Fung AY, Saw J, Starovoytov A, et al: Abbreviated infusion of eptifibatide after successful coronary intervention The BRIEF-PCI (Brief Infusion of Eptifibatide Following Percutaneous Coronary Intervention) randomized trial. *J Am Coll Cardiol* 53(10):837–845, 2009.
62. De Luca G, Suryapranata H, Stone GW, et al: Abciximab as adjunctive therapy to reperfusion in acute ST-segment elevation myocardial infarction: a meta-analysis of randomized trials. *JAMA* 293(14):1759–1765, 2005.
63. Deibele AJ, Jennings LK, Tcheng JE, et al: Intracoronary eptifibatide bolus administration during percutaneous coronary revascularization for acute coronary syndromes with evaluation of platelet glycoprotein IIb/IIIa receptor occupancy and platelet function: the Intracoronary Eptifibatide (ICE) Trial. *Circulation* 121(6):784–791, 2010.
64. Bertrand OF, Rodes-Cabau J, Larose E, et al: Intracoronary compared to intravenous abciximab and high-dose bolus compared to standard dose in patients with ST-segment elevation myocardial infarction undergoing transradial primary percutaneous coronary intervention: a two-by-two factorial placebo-controlled randomized study. *Am J Cardiol* 105(11):1520–1527, 2010.
65. Shimada YJ, Nakra NC, Fox JT, et al: Meta-analysis of prospective randomized controlled trials comparing intracoronary versus intravenous abciximab in patients with ST-elevation myocardial infarction undergoing primary percutaneous coronary intervention. *Am J Cardiol* 109(5):624–628, 2012.
66. De Luca G, Verdoia M, Suryapranata H: Benefits from intracoronary as compared to intravenous abciximab administration for STEMI patients undergoing primary angioplasty: a meta-analysis of 8 randomized trials. *Atherosclerosis* 222(2):426–433, 2012.
67. Thiele H, Wohrle J, Hambrecht R, et al: Intracoronary versus intravenous bolus abciximab during primary percutaneous coronary intervention in patients with acute ST-elevation myocardial infarction: a randomised trial. *Lancet* 379(9819):923–931, 2012.
68. Stone GW, Maehara A, Witzenbichler B, et al: Intracoronary abciximab and aspiration thrombectomy in patients with large anterior myocardial infarction: the INFUSE-AMI randomized trial. *JAMA* 307(17):1817–1826, 2012.
69. Ellis SG, Tendera M, de Belder MA, et al: 1-year survival in a randomized trial of facilitated reperfusion: results from the FINESSE (Facilitated Intervention with Enhanced Reperfusion Speed to Stop Events) trial. *JACC Cardiovasc Interv* 2(10):909–916, 2009.
70. Giugliano RP, White JA, Bode C, et al: Early versus delayed, provisional eptifibatide in acute coronary syndromes. *N Engl J Med* 360(21):2176–2190, 2009.

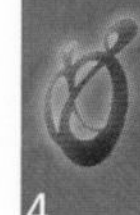

71. Gurm HS, Tamhane U, Meier P, et al: A comparison of abciximab and small-molecule glycoprotein IIb/IIIa inhibitors in patients undergoing primary percutaneous coronary intervention: a meta-analysis of contemporary randomized controlled trials. *Circ Cardiovasc interv* 2(3):230–236, 2009.
72. De Luca G, Ucci G, Cassetti E, et al: Benefits from small molecule administration as compared with abciximab among patients with ST-segment elevation myocardial infarction treated with primary angioplasty: a meta-analysis. *J Am Coll Cardiol* 53(18):1668–1673, 2009.
73. Harrington RA, Stone GW, McNulty S, et al: Platelet inhibition with cangrelor in patients undergoing PCI. *N Engl J Med* 361(24):2318–2329, 2009.
74. Bhatt DL, Lincoff AM, Gibson CM, et al: Intravenous platelet blockade with cangrelor during PCI. *N Engl J Med* 361(24):2330–2341, 2009.
75. Bhatt DL, Stone GW, Mahaffey KW, et al: Effect of platelet inhibition with cangrelor during PCI on ischemic events. *N Engl J Med* 368(14):1303–1313, 2013.
76. Steg PG, Bhatt DL, Hamm CW, et al: Effect of cangrelor on periprocedural outcomes in percutaneous coronary interventions: a pooled analysis of patient-level data. *Lancet* 382(9909):1981–1992, 2013.
77. Jolly SS, Yusuf S, Cairns J, et al: Radial versus femoral access for coronary angiography and intervention in patients with acute coronary syndromes (RIVAL): a randomised, parallel group, multicentre trial. *Lancet* 377(9775):1409–1420, 2011.
78. Doherty TM, Shavelle RM, French WJ: Reproducibility and variability of activated clotting time measurements in the cardiac catheterization laboratory. *Catheter Cardiovasc Interv* 65(3):330–337, 2005.
79. Chew DP, Bhatt DL, Lincoff AM, et al: Defining the optimal activated clotting time during percutaneous coronary intervention: aggregate results from 6 randomized, controlled trials. *Circulation* 103(7):961–966, 2001.
80. Warkentin TE: Drug-induced immune-mediated thrombocytopenia–from purpura to thrombosis. *N Engl J Med* 356(9):891–893, 2007.
81. Ferguson JJ, Califf RM, Antman EM, et al: Enoxaparin vs unfractionated heparin in high-risk patients with non-ST-segment elevation acute coronary syndromes managed with an intended early invasive strategy: primary results of the SYNERGY randomized trial. *JAMA* 292(1):45–54, 2004.
82. Martin JL, Fry ET, Sanderink GJ, et al: Reliable anticoagulation with enoxaparin in patients undergoing percutaneous coronary intervention: the pharmacokinetics of enoxaparin in PCI (PEPCI) study. *Catheter Cardiovasc Interv* 61(2):163–170, 2004.
83. Gibson CM, Murphy SA, Montalescot G, et al: Percutaneous coronary intervention in patients receiving enoxaparin or unfractionated heparin after fibrinolytic therapy for ST-segment elevation myocardial infarction in the ExTRACT-TIMI 25 trial. *J Am Coll Cardiol* 49(23):2238–2246, 2007.
84. Montalescot G, Gallo R, White HD, et al: Enoxaparin versus unfractionated heparin in elective percutaneous coronary intervention 1-year results from the STEEPLE (SafeTy and efficacy of enoxaparin in percutaneous coronary intervention patients, an international randomized evaluation) trial. *JACC Cardiovasc Interv* 2(11):1083–1091, 2009.
85. Montalescot G, Ellis SG, de Belder MA, et al: Enoxaparin in primary and facilitated percutaneous coronary intervention: a formal prospective nonrandomized substudy of the FINESSE trial (Facilitated INtervention with Enhanced Reperfusion Speed to Stop Events). *JACC Cardiovasc Interv* 3(2):203–212, 2010.
86. Brieger D, Collet JP, Silvain J, et al: Heparin or enoxaparin anticoagulation for primary percutaneous coronary intervention. *Catheter Cardiovasc Interv* 77(2):182–190, 2011.
87. Dumaine R, Borentain M, Bertel O, et al: Intravenous low-molecular-weight heparins compared with unfractionated heparin in percutaneous coronary intervention: quantitative review of randomized trials. *Arch Intern Med* 167(22):2423–2430, 2007.
88. Cohen M, Levine GN, Pieper KS, et al: Enoxaparin 0.3 mg/kg IV supplement for patients transitioning to PCI after subcutaneous enoxaparin therapy for NSTE ACS: a subgroup analysis from the SYNERGY trial. *Catheter Cardiovasc Interv* 75(6):928–935, 2010.
89. Montalescot G, White HD, Gallo R, et al: Enoxaparin versus unfractionated heparin in elective percutaneous coronary intervention. *N Engl J Med* 355(10):1006–1017, 2006.
90. Lincoff AM, Bittl JA, Harrington RA, et al: Bivalirudin and provisional glycoprotein IIb/IIIa blockade compared with heparin and planned glycoprotein IIb/IIIa blockade during percutaneous coronary intervention: REPLACE-2 randomized trial. *JAMA* 289(7):853–863, 2003.
91. Lincoff AM, Kleiman NS, Kereiakes DJ, et al: Long-term efficacy of bivalirudin and provisional glycoprotein IIb/IIIa blockade vs heparin and planned glycoprotein IIb/IIIa blockade during percutaneous coronary revascularization: REPLACE-2 randomized trial. *JAMA* 292(6):696–703, 2004.
92. Schulz S, Mehilli J, Ndrepepa G, et al: Bivalirudin vs. unfractionated heparin during percutaneous coronary interventions in patients with stable and unstable angina pectoris: 1-year results of the ISAR-REACT 3 trial. *Eur Heart J* 31(5):582–587, 2010.
93. Stone GW, McLaurin BT, Cox DA, et al: Bivalirudin for patients with acute coronary syndromes. *N Engl J Med* 355(21):2203–2216, 2006.
94. Stone GW, Witzenbichler B, Guagliumi G, et al: Bivalirudin during primary PCI in acute myocardial infarction. *N Engl J Med* 358(21):2218–2230, 2008.
95. Stone GW, Clayton T, Deliargyris EN, et al: Reduction in cardiac mortality with bivalirudin in patients with and without major bleeding: the HORIZONS-AMI trial (Harmonizing Outcomes with Revascularization and Stents in Acute Myocardial Infarction). *J Am Coll Cardiol* 63(1):15–20, 2014.
96. Steg PG, van 't Hof A, Hamm CW, et al: Bivalirudin started during emergency transport for primary PCI. *N Engl J Med* 369(23):2207–2217, 2013.
97. Dangas G, Mehran R, Guagliumi G, et al: Role of clopidogrel loading dose in patients with ST-segment elevation myocardial infarction undergoing primary angioplasty: results from the HORIZONS-AMI (harmonizing outcomes with revascularization and stents in acute myocardial infarction) trial. *J Am Coll Cardiol* 54(15):1438–1446, 2009.
98. Shahzad A, Kemp I, Mars C, et al: Unfractionated heparin versus bivalirudin in primary percutaneous coronary intervention (HEAT-PPCI): an open-label, single centre, randomised controlled trial. *Lancet* 2014.
99. Berger PB, Blankenship JC: Is the heat on HEAT-PPCI appropriate? *Lancet* 2014.
100. Fifth Organization to Assess Strategies in Acute Ischemic, Syndromes I, Yusuf S, Mehta SR, et al: Comparison of fondaparinux and enoxaparin in acute coronary syndromes. *N Engl J Med* 354(14):1464–1476, 2006.
101. Yusuf S, Mehta SR, Chrolavicius S, et al: Effects of fondaparinux on mortality and reinfarction in patients with acute ST-segment elevation myocardial infarction: the OASIS-6 randomized trial. *JAMA* 295(13):1519–1530, 2006.
102. Dhillon S: Argatroban: a review of its use in the management of heparin-induced thrombocytopenia. *Am J Cardiovasc Drugs* 9(4):261–282, 2009.
103. Rezkalla SH, Dharmashankar KC, Abdalrahman IB, et al: No-reflow phenomenon following percutaneous coronary intervention for acute myocardial infarction: incidence, outcome, and effect of pharmacologic therapy. *J Interv Cardiol* 23(5):429–436, 2010.
104. Bruder O, Breuckmann F, Jensen C, et al: Prognostic impact of contrast-enhanced CMR early after acute ST segment elevation myocardial infarction (STEMI) in a regional STEMI network: results of the "Herzinfarktverbund Essen." *Herz* 33(2):136–142, 2008.
105. Fischell TA, Carter AJ, Foster MT, et al: Reversal of "no reflow" during vein graft stenting using high velocity boluses of intracoronary adenosine. *Cathet Cardiovasc Diagn* 45(4):360–365, 1998.
106. Stoel MG, Marques KM, de Cock CC, et al: High dose adenosine for suboptimal myocardial reperfusion after primary PCI: a randomized placebo-controlled pilot study. *Catheter Cardiovasc Interv* 71(3):283–289, 2008.
107. Navarese EP, Buffon A, Andreotti F, et al: Adenosine improves post-procedural coronary flow but not clinical outcomes in patients with acute coronary syndrome: a meta-analysis of randomized trials. *Atherosclerosis* 222(1):1–7, 2012.
108. Jeremias A, Whitbourn RJ, Filardo SD, et al: Adequacy of intracoronary versus intravenous adenosine-induced maximal coronary hyperemia for fractional flow reserve measurements. *Am Heart J* 140(4):651–657, 2000.
109. Leone AM, Porto I, De Caterina AR, et al: Maximal hyperemia in the assessment of fractional flow reserve: intracoronary adenosine versus intracoronary sodium nitroprusside versus intravenous adenosine: the NASCI (Nitroprussiato versus Adenosina nelle Stenosi Coronariche Intermedie) study. *JACC Cardiovasc Interv* 5(4):402–408, 2012.
110. Hillegass WB, Dean NA, Liao L, et al: Treatment of no-reflow and impaired flow with the nitric oxide donor nitroprusside following percutaneous coronary interventions: initial human clinical experience. *J Am Coll Cardiol* 37(5):1335–1343, 2001.
111. Wang HJ, Lo PH, Lin JJ, et al: Treatment of slow/no-reflow phenomenon with intracoronary nitroprusside injection in primary coronary intervention for acute myocardial infarction. *Catheter Cardiovasc Interv* 63(2):171–176, 2004.
112. Jaffe R, Dick A, Strauss BH: Prevention and treatment of microvascular obstruction-related myocardial injury and coronary no-reflow following percutaneous coronary intervention: a systematic approach. *JACC Cardiovasc Interv* 3(7):695–704, 2010.
113. Su Q, Li L, Naing KA, et al: Safety and effectiveness of nitroprusside in preventing no-reflow during percutaneous coronary intervention: a systematic review. *Cell Biochem Biophys* 68(1):201–206, 2014.
114. Huang RI, Patel P, Walinsky P, et al: Efficacy of intracoronary nicardipine in the treatment of no-reflow during percutaneous coronary intervention. *Catheter Cardiovasc Interv* 68(5):671–676, 2006.
115. Hang CL, Wang CP, Yip HK, et al: Early administration of intracoronary verapamil improves myocardial perfusion during percutaneous coronary interventions for acute myocardial infarction. *Chest* 128(4):2593–2598, 2005.
116. Huang D, Qian J, Ge L, et al: REstoration of COronary flow in patients with no-reflow after primary coronary interVEntion of acute myocaRdial infarction (RECOVER). *Am Heart J* 164(3):394–401, 2012.
117. Krumholz HM, Anderson JL, Bachelder BL, et al: ACC/AHA 2008 performance measures for adults with ST-elevation and non-ST-elevation myocardial infarction: a report of the American College of Cardiology/American Heart Association Task Force on Performance Measures (Writing Committee to develop performance measures for ST-elevation and non-ST-elevation myocardial infarction): developed in collaboration with the American Academy of Family Physicians and the American College of Emergency Physicians: endorsed by the American Association of Cardiovascular and Pulmonary Rehabilitation, Society for Cardiovascular Angiography and Interventions, and Society of Hospital Medicine. *Circulation* 118(24):2596–2648, 2008.
118. Chen ZM, Pan HC, Chen YP, et al: Early intravenous then oral metoprolol in 45,852 patients with acute myocardial infarction: randomised placebo-controlled trial. *Lancet* 366(9497):1622–1632, 2005.
119. McCord J, Jneid H, Hollander JE, et al: Management of cocaine-associated chest pain and myocardial infarction: a scientific statement from the American Heart Association Acute Cardiac Care Committee of the Council on Clinical Cardiology. *Circulation* 117(14):1897–1907, 2008.
120. Francis GS, Bartos JA, Adatya S: Inotropes. *J Am Coll Cardiol* 63(20):2069–2078, 2014.
121. De Backer D, Biston P, Devriendt J, et al: Comparison of dopamine and norepinephrine in the treatment of shock. *N Engl J Med* 362(9):779–789, 2010.
122. American Society of Anesthesiologists Task Force on S, Analgesia by N-A: Practice guidelines for sedation and analgesia by non-anesthesiologists. *Anesthesiology* 96(4):1004–1017, 2002.
123. Levine JH, Massumi A, Scheinman MM, et al: Intravenous amiodarone for recurrent sustained hypotensive ventricular tachyarrhythmias. Intravenous Amiodarone Multicenter Trial Group. *J Am Coll Cardiol* 27(1):67–75, 1996.
124. Dorian P, Cass D, Schwartz B, et al: Amiodarone as compared with lidocaine for shock-resistant ventricular fibrillation. *N Engl J Med* 346(12):884–890, 2002.

5 Hemodynamic Support During High-Risk PCI

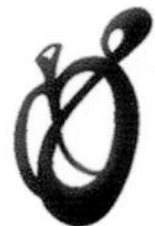

William W. O'Neill and Brian P. O'Neill

INTRODUCTION

Coronary balloon angioplasty (PTCA), introduced in 1977,[1] was initially limited to treatment of focal, noncalcified, proximal, concentric coronary lesions. Initially case selection was confined to patients with normal left ventricular function and single vessel coronary artery disease.[2] Complex lesions (eccentric, bifurcation, chronic total occlusion) and patients with multivessel coronary disease simply could not be technically approached. Dramatic advances in guidewire technology, advances in balloon technology, new atherectomy devices, and the introduction of flexible, easily deployable stents have dramatically expanded the complexity of the lesions that can be treated successfully. As the age of the population and the life expectancy of patients with overt coronary artery disease (CAD) increase, clinicians are increasingly faced with elderly, highly symptomatic patients with multiple comorbidities that make PCI and CABG prohibitively risky. In this setting, the coronary interventionalist is asked to perform a PCI. To safely undertake these high-risk procedures, hemodynamic support may be required. Who requires hemodynamic support and what method of support is safest and most effective are the subjects of this chapter.

RATIONALE FOR DEFINITION OF HIGH RISK

Through the 1990s and up to 2005, scores of studies were published regarding "high-risk" percutaneous coronary intervention (HRPCI).[3] Studies were mainly single center registries or a few prospective multicenter registries.[4-6] Wide variations in outcomes were reported. The consistent characteristic that appeared to enhance risk was severely impaired ventricular function.

Keelan[7] has demonstrated a thirtyfold increase in risk of death for patients with ejection fractions less than 40% compared to patients with normal ejection fraction. There are multiple reasons why underlying impaired left ventricular (LV) function increases risk. First, in order to have ejection fractions less than 40%, patients have survived an extensive acute myocardial infarction (MI). This often results in the presence of a chronic total occlusion. As survivors of acute MI, these patients present later with recurrent symptoms related to worsening of another coronary artery. Thus patients are later into the natural history of their disease and usually have multiple vessel disease. As CAD patients age, other comorbidities such as diabetes, chronic kidney disease (CKD), and chronic obstructive lung disease (COPD) increase procedural risk. During the interventional procedure, patients with severely depressed LV function pose a special challenge. Typically the operator is treating a stenosis that subtends a large segment of the normally contracting left ventricle and that often subtends a distant myocardial segment that has blood flow through the collaterals. Repeated interruptions of blood flow that occur with contrast injections, balloon inflation, and stent manipulation can lead to ischemia of normally contracting myocardial segments. This results in marked elevation of LV filling pressure and can quickly lead to sustained hypotension or cardiovascular collapse. For this reason the two main prospective randomized trials, hemodynamic support with Impella 2.5 versus the intra-aortic balloon pump[8] and the balloon pump-assisted Coronary Intervention Study,[9] have both used severely impaired LV function as the primary risk segregator. In addition, the BCIS investigators chose an advanced jeopardy score ≥8/12 and the Protect II investigators added the presence of a last patent coronary vessel as inclusion criteria (**Table 5-1**). These simple, concise criteria have in fact defined a patient population with a thirtyfold increase in mortality risk during hospitalization compared to routine elective multiple vessel angioplasty (**Table 5-2**). Future clinical trials and prospective quality assurance endeavors

TABLE 5-1 Definition of High-Risk PCI

	BCIS	PROTECT II
Inclusion	PCI native vessel or SVBG	PCI native vessel or SVBG
	LVEF ≤30% on Echo	PCI last patent vessel
	Jeopardy score ≥8/12	LVEF ≤30% with 3 VD
		LVEF ≤35% with UPLM
Exclusion	Acute MI or shock	Acute MI or shock
	Acute VSD or MR	Acute VSD or MR
	More than mild AR on echo	LV thrombus on echo
	Planned staged procedure	Creatinine ≥3
		AS with AVA ≤1.5 cm^2

AR, Aortic regurgitation; *AS,* aortic stenosis; *AVA,* aortic valve area; *LVEF,* left ventricular ejection fraction; *MI,* myocardial infarction; *MR,* mitral regurgitation; *PCI,* Percutaneous coronary intervention; *SVBG,* saphenous vein bypass graft; *UPLM,* unprotected left main; *VSD,* ventricular septal defect.

Jeopardy score (Modified Duke Jeopardy score, which allows subclavian and left main lesions).

In comparison to Syntax, BCIS, and Protect II, trials treated older patients with impaired LV function who have more after a history of CABG or prior MI. MACE events continued to increase between 30 and 90 days.

*In protect II, 66% of patients were formally turned down for surgery by site surgeons. It is not known if the remaining 32% were ever evaluated for CABG.[8]

TABLE 5-2 Baseline Characteristics and Outcome

BCIS, PROTECT II, and SYNTAX TRIALS			
	SYNTAX	**BCIS**	**PROTECT II**
Age (years)	65 ± 10	71 ± 10	68 ± 10
History CHF (%)	NR	6	87
History CABG (%)	0	15	33
Prior MI (%)	32	73	68
Syntax score (mean)	28	32	30
LVEF ≤35%	2.3%	100%	95%
LMCA PCI (%)	39	27	22
Surgery candidate	100%	NR	<32%*
30-day death (%)	2	2	7.6
90-day death (%)	3	5	10
30-day MACE (%)	6	15	10
90-day MACE (%)	15	NR	22

From Syntax, BCIS, and Protect II: Outcomes of trials. Serruys PW, Morice MC, Kappetein AP, et al: Percutaneous coronary intervention versus coronary-artery bypass grafting for severe coronary artery disease, N Engl J Med 360:961–972.

CABG, Coronary artery bypass; *CHF,* congestive heart failure; *LMCA,* left main coronary artery; *LVEP,* ejection fraction; *MACE,* major adverse cardiac events; *MI,* myocardial infarction.

*68% of patients in Protect II had formal denial of surgical candidacy by site surgeon.

should use these benchmark inclusion criteria and outcome data for comparative safety analysis.

CLINICAL PRESENTATION

This chapter initially discusses management of elective or urgent patients who are treated outside the setting of acute MI or cardiogenic shock. These patients present late in the natural history of coronary atherosclerosis. Average age is >70 years. A large proportion of the population has diabetes mellitus, renal function is impaired, and they are highly symptomatic. NYHA symptoms III or IV were present in 60% of the patients in BCIS and 65% of Protect II. Symptoms could be worsening heart failure or angina. In fact, since

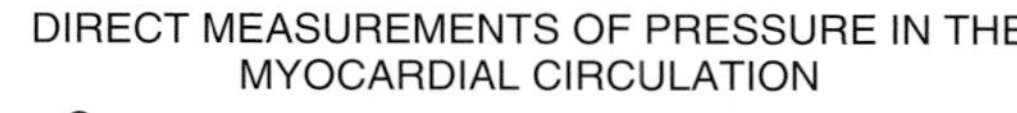

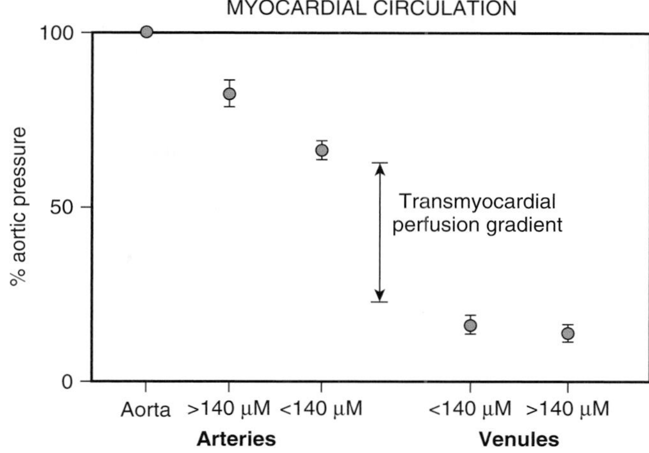

FIGURE 5-1 Myocardial perfusion. Using a micropuncture technique demonstrated the contribution of arterial and venous vessels to vascular pressure in the left ventricle. The vast majority of pressure drops occur between small caliber arteries and vessels. Coronary sinus (or right atrial pressure) contributes little to the perfusion gradient. Assuming an LVED of 10 mm Hg, a minimum aortic diastolic pressure of 40 mm Hg is needed to ensure antegrade transmural blood flow. *(Adapted with permission from Marcus ML: The coronary circulation in health and disease, New York, 1983, McGraw-Hill.)*

a large segment of these patients have diabetes, it is often difficult to differentiate worsening heart failure from worsening ischemia. In the Protect II study, 26% of the patients had peripheral vascular disease and 64% were evaluated and turned down for CABG by the site surgeons. Thus these elderly, highly symptomatic patients have limited therapeutic options apart from high-risk PCI. Age, poor ventricular function, diabetes, CKD, and peripheral vascular disease all increase procedural risk. In addition, coronary angiography, IVUS interrogation, coronary balloon inflation, rotational atherectomy, or complex stent procedures (kiss, crush, coulotte) may compromise coronary blood flow to the vital myocardial segments. Without hemodynamic support, these coronary manipulations can result in cardiovascular collapse. To avoid cardiac collapse, clinicians may choose to perform unassisted procedures with minimal coronary angiography, lack of IVUS interrogation, brief balloon, stent inflation, and incomplete revascularization. Even with these precautions, in the BCIS study, 10% of the control, unsupported patients suffered from severe hypotension, and 12% of the patients required rescue intraaortic balloon pump (IABP). To optimize patient safety and long-term clinical effectiveness, a controlled, well-planned, supported PCI procedure must be considered.

CORONARY BLOOD FLOW AND MYOCARDIAL ENERGETICS DURING HIGH-RISK PCI

Coronary blood flow physiology is well defined in mammalian models (**Figure 5-1**).[10] It is known that under conditions of maximal stress, a fourfold increase in resting blood flow can occur. Coronary occlusions begin to impact vasodilator reserve at 50% area occlusion and eliminate vasodilator capacity at 80% occlusion. After this, resting coronary blood flow dramatically decreases with small increases in occlusion severity. It is also well understood that in mammals, a perfusion gradient of 30 mm Hg to 50 mm Hg is required to drive blood through the myocardium (**Figure 5-2**).[11] In systole, when aortic and ventricular pressures are the same and when ventricular compression occurs, little forward blood flow occurs. Thus mammalian coronary blood flow is largely diastolic. As coronary occlusion worsens, the phasic nature diminishes and blood flow is largely driven by the mean arterial pressure with requirement for a 30 mm Hg to 50 mm Hg gradient for perfusion. How do these principles translate to this high-risk population? First, generally all three major coronary territories are affected with severe atherosclerosis. One or more coronaries may be chronically totally occluded from previous infarctions. Patients are presenting with worsening of non–infarct-related vessels with lesions severe enough to diminish vasodilatory reserve or decrease resting coronary blood flow. The remaining patent vessels provide collateral flow to the occluded territories and likely have severe lesions. The demand for increased coronary blood flow to supply collateral flow and the usual hyperkinesis of the noninfarct zones cause the patent coronaries to be at a maximal state of coronary vasodilation. In this setting, blood flow is entirely driven by perfusion gradient (**Figure 5-3**).[10] No incremental vasodilation is possible, since the patent vessels have severe underlying lesions. Thus the coronary tree has no capacity for augmentation of blood flow (**Figure 5-4**). Coronary blood flow is driven entirely by the transmyocardial perfusion gradient and diastolic interval. When patients become distressed, tachycardia, elevated LVEDP, and systolic hypotension occur. These factors dramatically increase myocardial oxygen demand (MVO_2) (**Figure 5-5**)[12] or decrease supply. At the same time, decreased perfusion gradients and coronary blood flow can lead to a rapid cycle of worsening ischemia and lowering of blood pressure, which leads to less coronary blood flow, worsening myocardial contracture, and irreversible shock. To prevent this catastrophe, measures to maximize the myocardial perfusion gradient, minimize MVO_2, and maintain adequate cardiac output for vital organ perfusion are required.

In addition to coronary blood flow physiology, an understanding of myocardial energetics is required to determine optimal support strategies for these patients. Myocardial energetics can be studied using pressure volume relationships. Suga[13] and Burkhoff[14] demonstrated that pressure volume loops are an ideal way to define cardiac performance throughout the cardiac cycle (**Figure 5-6**). Ideally, interventions that decrease the end diastolic pressure-volume relationship improve myocardial energetics by

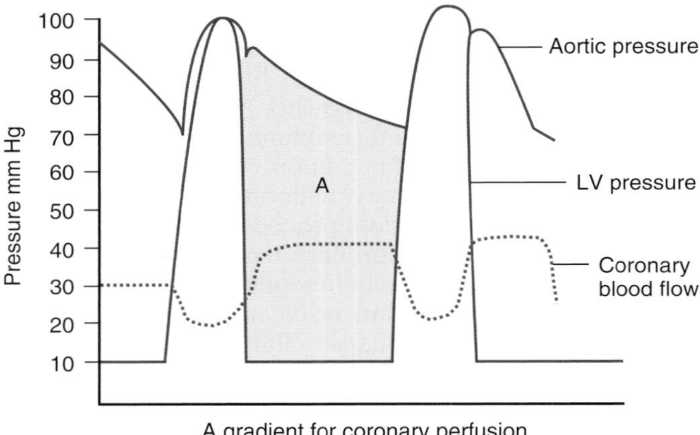

FIGURE 5-2 Coronary blood flow + LV + aortic pressure. In the absence of severe coronary lesions, coronary blood flow is largely diastolic (dotted line). CBF is regulated by coronary arteries that dilate in response to physiologic stimuli. Any factors that decrease the diastolic interval or decrease the diastolic perfusion gradient will diminish CBF. Hypotension lowers diastolic pressures; ischemia raises LVEDP. These two events occur frequently during HRPCI and can decrease coronary blood flow to the point of cardiovascular collapse. *(Courtesy Dr. William W. O'Neill.)*

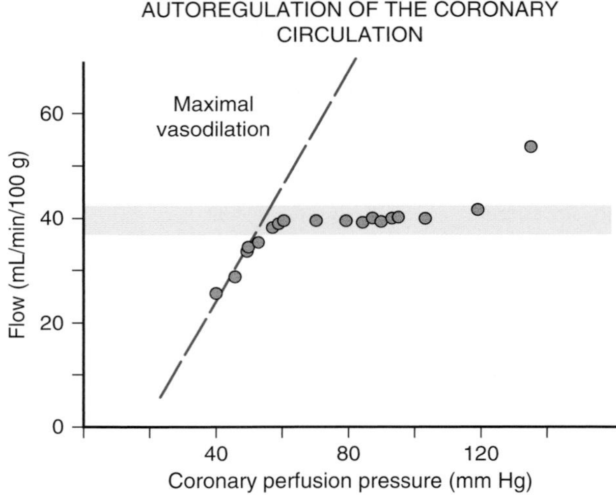

FIGURE 5-3 Maximal flow during vasodilatation. The normal maximal circulation can autoregulate over a wide range of pressures during conditions of maximal dilation. Once coronary perfusion pressure drops below 50 mm Hg, a rapid decline in CBF will occur. Coronary blood flow will cease once perfusion gradients less than 20 mm Hg occur. *(Adapted with permission from Marcus ML: The coronary circulation in health and disease, New York, 1983, McGraw-Hill.)*

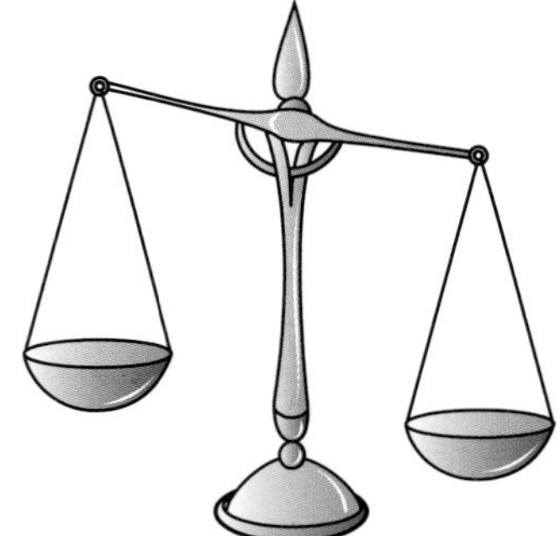
Increase CBF
• Coronary vasodilation
• Increase aortic pressure
• Decrease LVEDP
Decrease CBF
• Increase LVEDP
• Decrease perfusion pressure
• Severe coronary stenosis
• Tachycardia
• Repeat contrast injections
• Coronary manipulation
• Balloon inflation
• No reflow

FIGURE 5-4 Factors impacting coronary blood flow during high-risk PCI. Clinicians face an uphill battle during high-risk PCI. They have limited means to maintain or improve CBF while faced with numerous factors that tend to decrease or abolish CBF during intervention. *CBF*, Coronary blood flow.

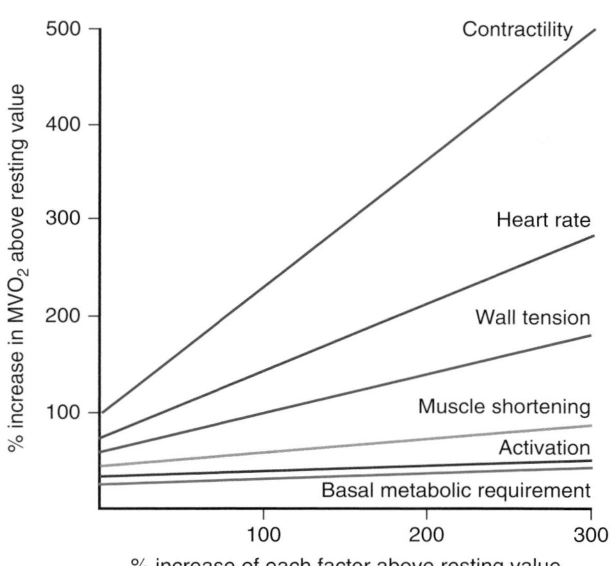

FIGURE 5-5 Factors increasing MVO_2. An ideal support strategy for HRPCI should rest the left ventricle so that contractility, wall tension, and perhaps heart rate could be decreased, thereby decreasing myocardial oxygen demand (MVO_2). Conversely, during HRPCI, the use of inotropes may increase systolic pressure but at the expense of an increase in MVO_2. This sets up a supply-demand mismatch. *(Adapted with permission from Marcus ML: The coronary circulation in health and disease, New York, 1983, McGraw-Hill.)*

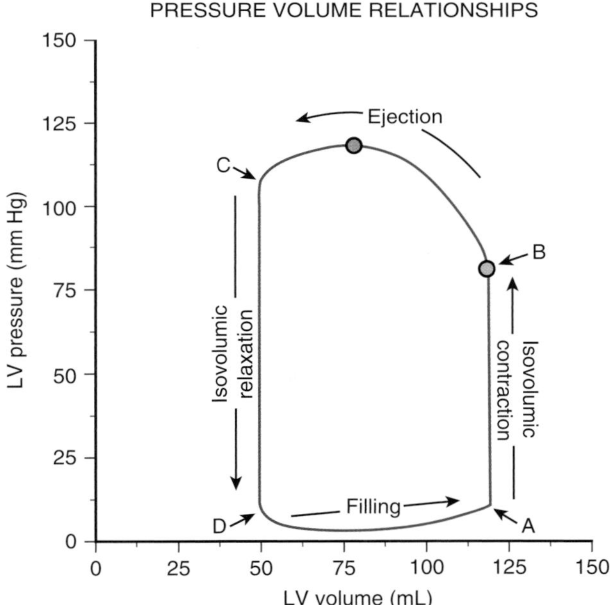

FIGURE 5-6 Pressure valve relationships. The science of hemodynamic support and cath cardio intervention.[14] Diastolic and systolic compliance is best considered at end diastole and systolic contractility at end systole. To optimize cardiac performance, LVEDP decrease and LVESP increase are required. *(Reproduced with permission from Burkhoff D, Naidu SS: The science behind percutaneous hemodynamic support: a review and comparison of support strategies. Catheter Cardiovasc Interv 80(5):816–829, 2012.)*

decreasing ventricular wall tension and thus decreasing MVO_2. At the same time, interventions that increase the end systolic pressure-volume relationship increase the transmyocardial perfusion gradient and improve coronary blood flow. When the transmyocardial pressure gradient drops below 30 mm Hg due to a decrease in mean arterial pressure or an elevation of LVEDP, dangerous reductions in coronary blood flow will occur and cardiac collapse will soon follow. Thus the goal of hemodynamic support is threefold. First, maintaining a mean arterial pressure ≥60 mm Hg is required to maintain coronary flow. Second, maintaining a cardiac power ≥0.6 watts will prevent systemic hypoperfusion.[15] Finally, decreasing ventricular diastolic pressure will enhance the coronary perfusion gradient and decrease LV wall tension. Burkhoff and Naidu summarized the impact of hemodynamic support strategies on these three variables using a circulation simulator.[16]

Each hemodynamic support maneuver has been modeled (**Figure 5-7**). First, inotropic agents appear to augment MAP and cardiac output but do so at the expense of increasing diastolic filling pressure (PCWP) and thus increasing MVO_2. Inotropes increase MVO_2 by increasing contractility, heart rate, and wall tension. If LVEDP is increased proportionally more than MAP, myocardial perfusion pressure is lowered and coronary blood flow will drop. At high levels of alpha adrenergic tone, coronary vasoconstriction will occur and coronary blood flow will drop further. Thus isotropes alone are a poor strategy that provides only modest support of MAP at the expense of increased MVO_2 and potentially less coronary blood flow.

The addition of an intraaortic balloon pump to an inotropic support provides more support of mean arterial pressure and cardiac output but does so at the expense of elevations of wall tension and MVO_2. It is likely that the increased MVO_2 demand will not be matched by increased coronary blood flow and this will set up a substrate for myocardial ischemia. The impact of IABP on coronary blood flow has been of interest for three decades. Soon after its introduction, it became apparent that IABP could stabilize patients with recurrent, medically refractory unstable angina. Williams et al. measured LAD blood flow by placing thermodilution catheters into the great cardiac vein in six patients with refractory angina who had severe proximal LAD lesions.[17] They found that the greater cardiac vein flow decreased from 78 ± 11 to 69 ± 8 mL/min, $p = 0.048$, when IABP support was initiated. In addition, systolic pressure was significantly reduced and augmented diastolic pressure was increased. They concluded that the mechanism of the relief of angina related to the decreased afterload and decreased MVO_2 rather than increased coronary blood flow. Yoshanti measured coronary pressures using the Radi Wire (Radi Medical Systems, Uppsala, Sweden) in 16 patients with unstable angina.[18] Pressures were measured distal to 16 culprit lesions and 5 normal vessels. The distal diastolic pressures were unchanged after initiation of IABP distal to the severe stenotic segments (42.8 ± 17 to 44 ± 21, p = NS). In the normal vessels, pressures increased with initiation of IABP (78 ± 9 to 97 ± 8 mm Hg, $p < 0.05$). Kern et al. measured coronary flow velocity with a Doppler tipped catheter (Millar Instruments).[19,20] They found that the coronary flow velocity was unchanged distal to severe lesions after IABP was turned on. After PTCA of the lesion, coronary flow velocity significantly increased with IABP support. Thus IABP support may be of benefit when severe hypotension occurs and one or more coronary arteries are free of disease. In this circumstance, augmentation of diastolic pressure will enhance coronary blood flow. Since most patients undergoing HRPCI have multivessel disease, IABP support will be of little value in maintaining or supporting coronary blood flow.

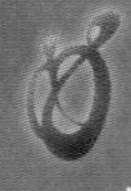

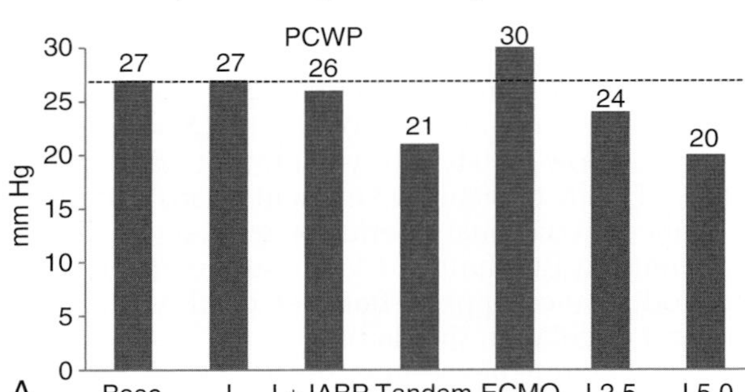

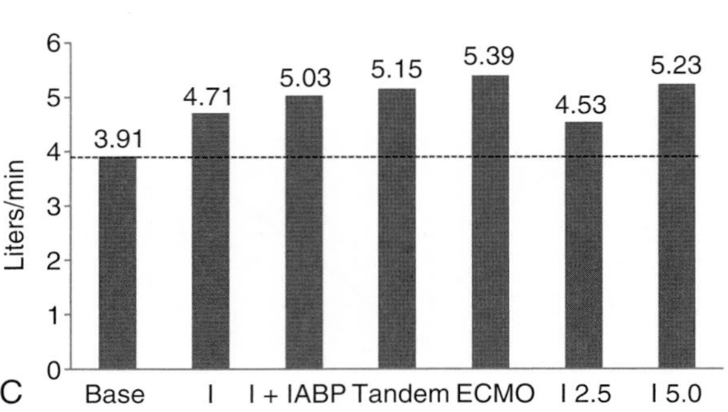

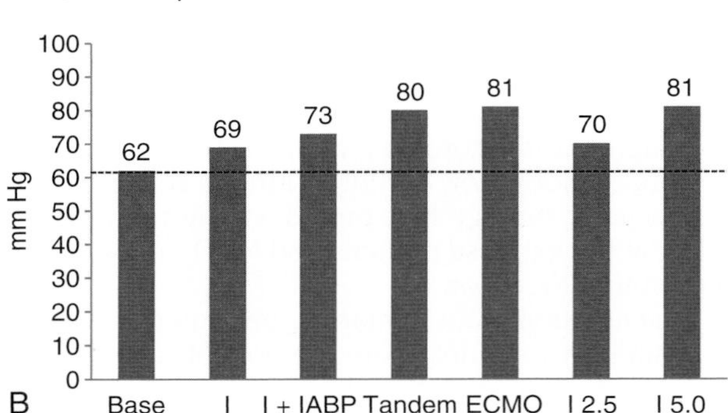

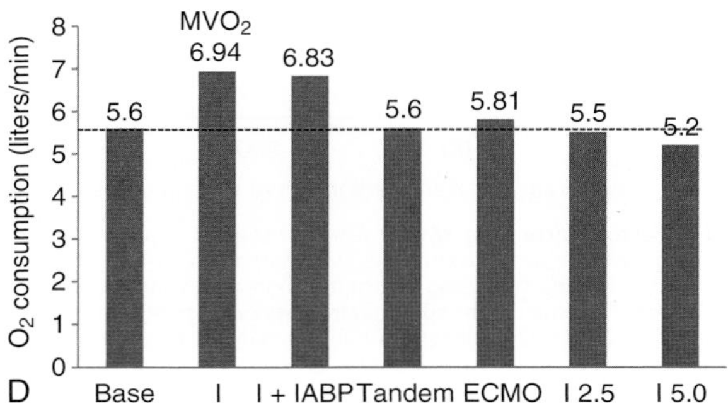

FIGURE 5-7 Modeling. Burkhoff modeled changes in hemodynamics that occur with various support strategies. Wedge pressure (PCWP) **(A)**, cardiac output **(C)**, mean aortic pressure **(B)**, and myocardial oxygen consumption changes **(D)** are calculated. The dotted line is a baseline value, and support strategies can be seen to raise or drop each parameter. *(Reproduced with permission from Burkhoff D: Pressure-volume loops in clinical research: a contemporary view. J Am Coll Cardiol 62(13):1173–1176, 2013.)*

The TandemHeart Pump (Cardiac Assist Inc., Pittsburgh, Pennsylvania) substantially decreases filling pressure and augments mean arterial pressure as well as cardiac output.[21] Since wall tension is reduced and mean arterial pressure is elevated, MVO_2 is reduced and coronary blood flow should be increased. Of the hemodynamic support devices, Impella is the only one that directly drains the left ventricle and augments forward cardiac flow. As cardiac output is increased from 2.5 to 5 L, filling pressures are reduced, mean arterial pressure is elevated, and myocardial perfusion gradient is elevated. This device has the ideal properties of maintaining mean arterial pressure and forward cardiac output while decreasing MVO_2. The device seems well suited for short- and long-term hemodynamic support. Finally, Extracorporeal Membrane Oxygenator (ECMO), also known as Peripheral Cardiopulmonary Bypass (CPS), is unequivocally useful when both right and left heart failure occurs. It provides excellent support for cardiac output and MAP. Unfortunately, it does so at the expense of elevated filling pressure and elevated MVO_2. For patients with severe multivessel CAD, it is likely that a longer duration of the use of this device sets up a substrate for myocardial ischemia. In the short term, the device provides superb support of the cardiac output and mean aortic pressure. To summarize, the previous discussion of modeling provides the clinician with the theoretic basis to choose from a variety of support strategies. In addition to these factors, patient body surface area, status of peripheral circulation, urgency of the need for hemodynamic support, and operator training and experience using the individual devices play a major role in defining an optimal support strategy for individual patients. Ideally these complex interventions should be performed in referral centers with expertise and access to many types of support and with open communication either in-house or rapidly available LVAD and transplant referral support.

HISTORY OF DEVELOPMENT OF LV SUPPORT DEVICES FOR HRPCI

The 1985 to 1986 National Heart Lung and Blood Institute (NHLBI) registry of coronary angioplasty documented outcomes for PCI in the pre-stent era.[22] The presence of depressed LV function identified a group of patients who often had multivessel CAD. When the LV ejection fraction was less than or equal to 35%, there was a 3% mortality rate compared to a 0.1% mortality rate for patients with LV EF greater than 45%. Left ventricular support with IABP was first developed to improve outcomes. The IABP had been in use since 1968[23] and was widely used to support patients in cardiogenic shock. Voudris reported the first European experience[24] and Kahn reported the U.S. experience with IABP to support HR PTCA.[25] Both groups used depressed LV function and/or unprotected left main angioplasty as entry criteria.

HISTORY OF USE OF IABP DURING HRPCI

The Mid America Heart group led by Dr. Goeffrey Hartzler pioneered the use of balloon angioplasty in patients with multivessel coronary artery disease.[26] Similarly, this group first reported on adjunctive use of IABP in high-risk cases.

Kahn et al. reported on 28 patients with a mean ejection fraction of 24%, three vessel diseases in 93%, and LMCA in 255 patients who had balloon angioplasty performed with IABP support.[25] They found that augmented diastolic pressure greater than 90 mm Hg occurred in all cases. During hospitalization, no deaths were reported. Soon after, Voudris reported the initial European experience with supported HRPCI. In a 1-year period, 27/1385 patients in Toulouse, France, had supported HRPCI.[24] Ejection fraction less than 40% was present in 24/27 cases. No deaths or MI occurred during initial hospitalization. The impact of poor ventricular function on outcomes was brought into clear focus by the NHLBI report in 1993. Holmes et al. reported on 244/1802 patients treated in the 1985 to1986 NLHBI PTCA registry who had EF ≤ 45% 9.[27] Angioplasty was less successful (76% vs. 84%, $p < 0.01$) and 4-year survival was lower than patients with normal LV function. With the advent of coronary stent implantation, PCI of unprotected left main intervention began in the early 1990s. Briguori et al. reported the Milan, Italy, experience with stent implantation in 219 consecutive patients.[28] Of these patients, 69 had prophylactic IABP support and 150 had conventional unsupported procedures. Severe hemodynamic instability occurred in 8% of the unsupported group and none of the IABP group. Major adverse events were higher in the unsupported group (9.5% vs. 1.5%, $p = 0.032$). Thus both depressed LV function and unprotected left main stent therapy started to be considered "high-risk PCI." More registry data continued to be reported concerning the value of IABP support. Mishra et al. summarized the Washington Heart Center experience with prophylactic versus rescue IABP support.[29] During a period from January 2000 to December 2004, outcomes of 68 patients with prophylactic IABP support were compared to 46 patients with IABP support started as a rescue for hemodynamic compromise. At 6 months' follow-up, mortality was lower (8% vs. 29%, $p < 0.01$) and MACE events were lower (12% vs. 32%, $p = 0.02$) for patients with elective IABP support. While these single center reports suggested a safety advantage for elective IABP support, Curtis et al. found a more mixed picture in the National Cardiovascular Registry.[30] They reported outcomes from January 2005 to December 2007 in 181,599 high-risk PCI procedures; 1170 had cardiogenic shock, 80% had ST-elevation acute MI, 2% underwent unprotected LMCA PCI, and 20% had EF less than 30%. An IABP was used in 44% of cardiogenic shock patients, 28% of patients with UPLM, and 14% of patients with EF less than 30%; overall IABP support was used in 10.5% of HRPCI cases and varied widely from hospital to hospital. The hospitals were divided into quartiles of IABP use (6.5%, 6.6% to 9.2%, 9% to 14%, >14%). No convincing evidence was found that IABP use improved outcomes. The wide variation in IABP use rates across U.S. hospitals suggested enormous operator preference and a lack of strong evidence for the elective use of prophylactic balloon pump therapy.

The IABP is constructed of a polyethylene balloon that is mounted onto a catheter that can be delivered through a sheath or sheathless to provide hemodynamic support in patients undergoing high-risk PCI. Although it may be inserted in the femoral artery without fluoroscopic guidance in an emergent situation, fluoroscopy is preferable when available to help with positioning. Prior to insertion of the balloon pump, a one-way valve is attached to the over the wire lumen and a large syringe may be used to apply negative pressure to downsize the balloon to facilitate passage through the sheath. Using the standard technique, a Cook needle is used to access the femoral artery. A small incision may be made with a scalpel in the subcutaneous tissue, and a sheath may then be delivered over a 0.035-inch wire. After the sheath is inserted, most kits contain a 0.018-inch wire that is inserted through the sheath into the ascending aorta. The balloon is advanced over this wire and delivered 2 cm distal to the left subclavian artery. After position is verified, the inflation-deflation of the balloon pump is normally timed with ECG monitoring of the console. The balloon can be filled with up to 50 cc of helium, which allows rapid inflation and deflation to provide both augmentation in coronary perfusion and unloading of the left ventricle during systole. In addition to placement through the femoral artery, the balloon pump may also be inserted into the axillary artery for those patients with severe peripheral arterial disease. In the future, balloon pump shafts small enough for 6-F access, in which case it is conceivable that radial access for balloon pump support may be feasible, at least for short-term use. Most balloon pump consoles may provide augmentation to heart rates up to 150 beats per minute and may operate on battery power for limited time periods (Maquet Quick Reference Guide IABP insertion/CS300 Operation, 2014 Maquet). When heart rates greater than 130 beats per minute occur, a 2:1 ratio of pumping allows optimal balloon pump inflation-deflation. Daily x-rays should be performed to assure that catheter migration does not occur. In addition, knee splints are useful to place on the leg with the balloon pump inserted so as to immobilize the leg and prevent catheter dislodgment. If incremental support is required, balloon pumps may be exchanged for larger sheath sizes.

To do this, a stiff 260-cm 0.018-inch guidewire is advanced through the lumen of the balloon pump shaft and the balloon pump is withdrawn. Negative pressure should be maintained with a large bore syringe while the balloon pump is removed. Once the balloon pump is removed, firm pressure is maintained at the puncture site while a 6F or 7F sheath dilator is advanced. The dilator remains in place, the 0.018 wire is removed, and a 0.035 guidewire can then be advanced for upsizing of the sheaths. If concern exists at the time of the initial balloon pump insertion, a regular 8F sheath can be used, the balloon pump can simply be removed, and a 0.035 guidewire can be advanced. The balloon pump may be inserted into the femoral or axillary artery to provide hemodynamic support.

BCIS INVESTIGATION

The equipoise that existed around routine IABP support for HRPCI allowed United Kingdom investigators to conduct the Balloon-Pump Assisted Coronary Intervention Study (BCIS).[9] This prospective randomized trial tested the strategy of routine, elective balloon pump support versus a provisional or standby strategy. Between December 2005 and January 2009, 301 patients with severe LV dysfunction or high jeopardy score were randomized to IABP support or conventional care. It is not known how many patients were treated outside of this study in these centers. Physicians had to be unsure of whether the support was necessary in order to randomize patients. The primary endpoint of MACCE (death, acute MI, cerebrovascular event, or further revascularization) occurred in 23/151 of elective IABP patients

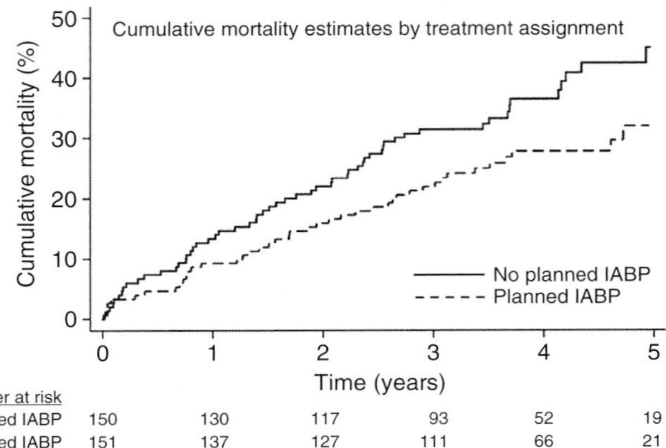

FIGURE 5-8 **BCIS survival.** Five-year survival rate for IABP or control patients is depicted. A steady increase in mortality over time is seen for control-treated patients. *(Reproduced with permission from Perera D, Stables R, Clayton T, et al: Long-term mortality data from the balloon pump-assisted coronary intervention study (BCIS-1): a randomized, controlled trial of elective balloon counterpulsation during high-risk percutaneous coronary intervention. Circulation 127(2):207–212, 2013.)*

versus 24/150 control patients (p = NS). The 6-month mortality rate was 4.6% versus 7.4% (p = 0.32) for IABP versus the control group. During the procedure major complications were less frequent in the IABP group (1.3% vs. 10.7%, p < 0.001). Rescue IABP for profound procedural hypotension occurred in 18 (12%) of the control patients. The authors concluded that no evidence existed for a safety advantage to routine IABP use, although a trend to lower mortality at 6 months was encouraging.

The BCIS investigators followed all patients for 5 years.[31] The original trend toward improved survival was enhanced after 5-year follow-up (**Figure 5-8**). At a mean follow-up of 51 months, 42/301 patients in the IABP group had expired versus 58/300 patients in the control group (p = 0.039), thus a 33% risk reduction had occurred. The mechanism for enhanced survival is unclear, yet similar trends are seen in the other revascularization trials, including Shock[32] and Protect II.[8] In aggregate these trials suggest longer follow-up is required to fully assess the impact of hemodynamic support in these high-risk patients.

With the recognition that more robust hemodynamic support might be required, Shawl[33] and Vogel[5] reported experience with femoral-femoral cardiopulmonary bypass (CPS) during elective angioplasty. Schreiber[34] compared CPS to IABP in the William Beaumont Hospital experience. In this nonrandomized consecutive series, CPS use resulted in the greater angioplasty success (97% vs. 87%, p = 0.005), but vascular complications requiring surgical repair were higher in the CPS groups, and the transfusions were higher in the CPS group (60% vs. 27%, p = 0.0001). No formal randomized trials of CPS compared to unsupported care or other support devices have been conducted. IABP was well known and easy to use but might result in less complete revascularization and could not provide extreme support when intrinsic myocardial function was absent. While CPS provided excellent systemic support, the large arterial cannulas and blood interface with the membrane oxygenator caused excessive bleeding and vascular complications. More worrisome, Stack et al. showed that initiation of CPS caused frank myocardial ischemia as demonstrated by myocardial lactate production in this high-risk PTCA population.[35] In addition, Pavlides[36] demonstrated that regional wall motion of myocardial segments supplied by vessels with greater than 50% stenosis worsened with initiation of CPS. For these reasons, alternative hemodynamic support methods that provided both systemic and myocardial support were sought.

HISTORY OF TANDEMHEART DEVELOPMENT

As elevated left-sided filling pressures are a hallmark of those patients with severe LV dysfunction, support devices that unload the LV during PCI are important to decrease wall tension and MVO_2. One of these devices is the TandemHeart (Cardiac Assist Inc., Pittsburgh, Pennsylvania, USA) percutaneous ventricular assist device (pVAD) (**Figure 5-9**). The TandemHeart is a centrifugal continuous flow pump.[37] A 21-Fr venous inflow cannula is placed through the femoral vein up and across the interatrial septum via a transseptal puncture into the left atrium. A second 14 Fr to 19 Fr cannula is then placed into the femoral artery. Oxygenated blood is removed from the left atrium and delivered to the descending aorta, effectively unloading the left ventricle in both systole and diastole. At a maximum speed of 7500 rotations per minute (RPM), the TandemHeart can deliver up to 4 L of flow per minute.

The TandemHeart has proven to be a very effective device in providing improvements in hemodynamics in cardiogenic shock as a bridge to cardiac transplant[39,40] and as a bridge to recovery in myocarditis.[41] It has also shown a potential role as a right ventricular (RV) support device in a case of acute RV infarction in an inferior ST-segment elevation MI.[42]

Several studies have compared the TandemHeart to IABP counterpulsation in cardiogenic shock. In a 12-center study of 42 patients, Burkhoff et al. demonstrated superior improvement in cardiac index and mean arterial blood pressure of the TandemHeart over IABP.[21] Sixty percent of these patients underwent revascularization either prior to or concomitantly with initiation of support, and many of the patients who were randomized to the TandemHeart group had a balloon pump placed before TandemHeart insertion. The overall 30-day mortality and rate of severe adverse events were similar between the two.[15] Thiele et al. randomized 41 patients to Tandem Heart versus IABP, presenting with acute MI and cardiogenic shock.[43] Thirty-day mortality was similar between the two groups; however, there was a higher rate of severe bleeding and limb ischemia in the TandemHeart group.[43] Finally, in one of the largest series from Kar et al.,[44] 117 patients in cardiogenic shock underwent implantation of the TandemHeart. Eighty-two percent of these patients received IABP counterpulsation prior to placement of a TandemHeart. The experience of the operators with the device was demonstrated by a 48% rate of placement of TandemHeart during CPR. Those patients who were bridged to transplant after TandemHeart had improved survival versus those who underwent bridge to LVAD or bridge to recovery. Rates of groin hematoma and limb ischemia were low, respectively.[44]

The experience with TandemHeart in high-risk PCI is restricted primarily to single center registry studies. Two small studies with fewer than 10 patients each demonstrated 100% procedural success with TandemHeart-assisted PCI in high-risk patients with severe LV dysfunction[45] and in unprotected left main disease in patients who were deemed

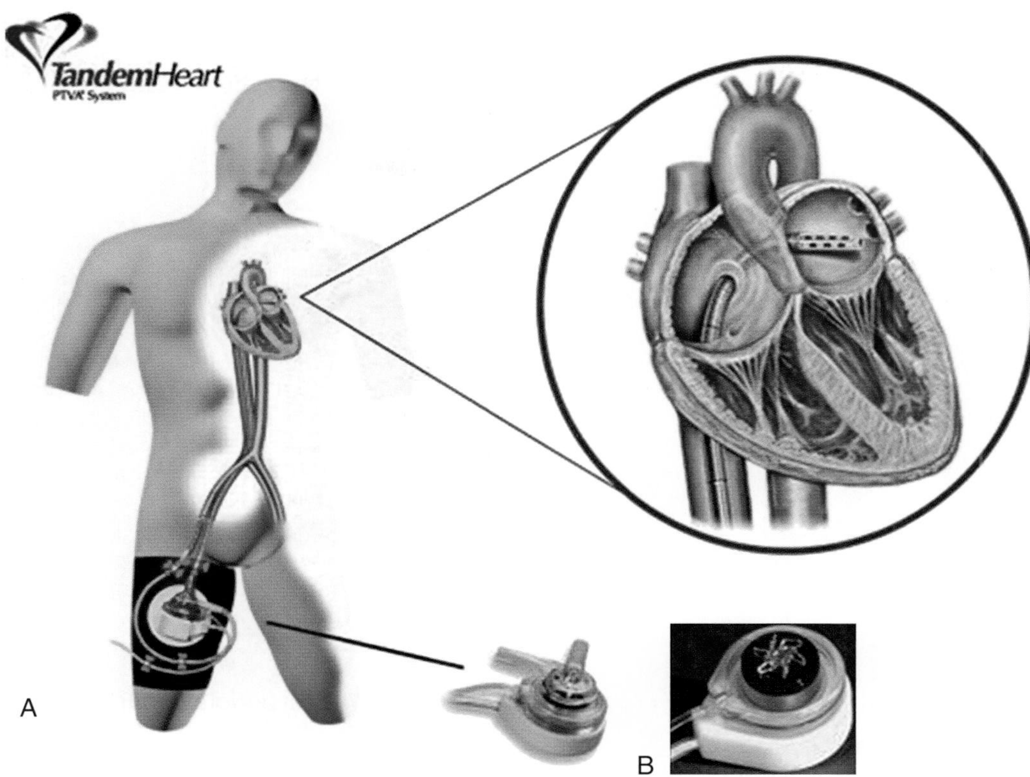

FIGURE 5-9 Cardiac assist device (A, B). TandemHeart placement occurs through the femoral artery and vein. A large venous catheter is placed through the intraatrial septum to sump oxygenated blood from the left atrium, and this blood is sent through the centrifugal pump back into the femoral artery. *(Reproduced with permission from Vranckx P, Otten A, Schultz C, et al: Assisted circulation using the Tandemhear, percutaneous transseptal left ventricular assist device, during percutaneous aortic valve implantation: the Rotterdam experience. EuroIntervention 5(4):465–469, 2009.)*

unsuitable for CABG.[38] Schwartz et al. showed, in a cohort of 32 TandemHeart patients, a 100% success rate with device initiation and a 97% angiographic success rate.[46] One patient suffered an embolic stroke, which was presumed to be from aortic atheroma, and there were two cases of limb ischemia, which resolved with device removal or repositioning. Finally, Kovacic et al. compared the use of TandemHeart versus Impella 2.5 in a group of patients who were deemed at high risk. PCI success rate was 99% in both groups.[46] The 30-day rate of death, death or MI, and death, MI, or target lesion revascularization was similar between the two groups. There was a single case of left atrial perforation with initiation of the TandemHeart.[46] These studies in aggregate demonstrate the high technical success rate for revascularization in those patients who are supported with the TandemHeart during high-risk PCI.

TRANSVALVULAR AXIAL FLOW PUMPS

The first transvalvular axial pump was developed by Wampler's group.[47] The Hemopump was an intraarterial LVAD that was initially tested in a surgical environment. The device was a 7-mm transvalvular axial flow blood pump. It was powered by an external console with power delivered to the pump by a flexible drive cable. Frazier et al.[48] described its use in 12 patients, 8 of whom had postcardiotomy shock, 2 with acute allograft reaction, and 1 with MI shock. Support ranged from 26 to 139 hours and 10/12 patients were successfully weaned off support. The large catheter size (21F) mandated surgical access and repair.

For this device to be applicable to the cath lab setting, a smaller shaft size was required. For this reason, a 14F catheter was developed. Panos et al.[49] described the use of this device in 13 patients who were treated in Geneva between 1993 and 1996. The device had a 14F outer diameter and could provide flow rates of 1.5 to 2.2 L/min (**Figure 5-10**). A modest increase in cardiac index (2.0 (+/–) 0.3 to 2.2 ± 0.5, p = 0.04) and modest decrease in PCWP (17 ± 8 to 14 ± 8, p = 0.004) occurred. No in-hospital mortality occurred. Dubois-Rande demonstrated that PWCP decreased but no changes in coronary blood flow occurred when 13 patients undergoing HRPCI were treated.[50] While this initial experience was encouraging, during subsequent testing an unacceptably high rate of cable fractures was reported and the device was abandoned. At least the concept of a transvalvular axial flow device was established.

HISTORY OF IMPELLA DEVELOPMENT

After the Hemopump demonstrated proof of the concept of a transvalvular axial flow hemodynamic support, Cardiosystems Gmbh from Aachen, Germany, developed a series of LVAD and RVAD devices. The LV system was a mircroaxial flow pump 6.4 mm in diameter. The pump was placed at the tip of the catheter and this was designed to be inserted through a graft placed on the aorta and advanced retrograde across the aortic valve. Initially rotor speeds of up to 32,000 RPM could supply up to 5.2 L of flow. The electrical power was provided through the shaft of the catheter and the Impella housing was flushed continuously with

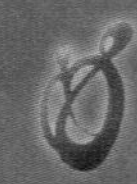

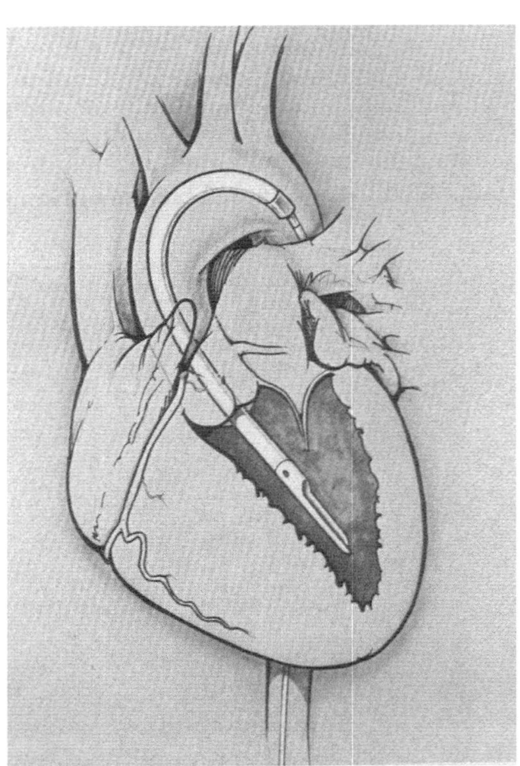

FIGURE 5-10 Transfemoral Hemopump placement. The Hemopump was placed from the femoral or iliac arteries. A long flexible drive shaft was connected to the catheter tip. The drive shaft was attached to an external motor. The length and high speeds required made frequent drive shaft fracture a major obstacle to chronic support. *(Reused with permission from Frazier OH, Wampler RK, Duncan JM, et al: First human use of the Hemopump, a catheter-mounted ventricular assist device. Ann Thorac Surg 49(2):299–304, 1990.)*

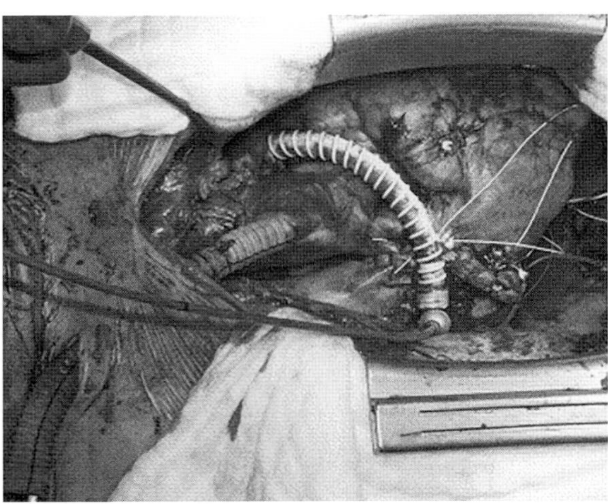

FIGURE 5-11 RV support. Open thorectomy. The patient's head is to the left. An aortic graft allows access to the aortic valve for the left heart support and a graft is sewn from the right atrium to the pulmonary artery for the right heart support. *(Reused with permission from Jurmann MJ, Siniawski H, Erb M, et al: Initial experience with miniature axial flow ventricular assist devices for postcardiotomy heart failure. Ann Thorac Surg 77(5):1642–1647, 2004.)*

hyperosmolar, heparinized solution to prevent clotting in the pump. A right ventricular device (RVAD) was also designed. It too was meant to be inserted during cardiac surgery.

These implants were developed as adjuncts to beating heart surgery.[51] At this time, beating heart surgery was gaining traction as a potentially safer way of performing CABG without use of the pump oxygenator. Surgeons had difficulty in performing anastomosis in the back and inferior border of the left ventricle during off-pump surgery. When the heart was lifted to explore these areas, profound hypotension occurred. The Impella catheters were designed to be placed by puncture of the aorta for the LV support and by puncture or grafting onto the pulmonary artery for RV support (**Figure 5-11**). Meyns et al. published a small randomized trial of support with Impella versus normothermic cardiac bypass.[52] Although support of the heart during off-pump surgery was the initial reason for development, other uses soon became evident. From January 2001 to September 2002, 16 patients in cardiogenic shock refractory to inotropic support were treated by Meyns et al.[52] Excellent hemodynamic support was achieved with cardiac output increased (4.1 to 5.5 L/min, $p = 0.01$), mean PCWP decreased (29 ± 10 to 18 ± 7, $p = 0.04$), and mean arterial pressure increased (74.9 ± 13 to 80.6 ± 17 mm Hg, $p = 0.003$). The increased cardiac flow caused a reduction in serum lactate levels at 6 hours of support. In spite of these beneficial hemodynamic and biochemical findings, only a 37% survival rate occurred. A common theme with ECMO and the TandemHeart began to emerge. All three devices provided excellent short-term support that were life saving in the short term. Without a more definitive end strategy (LVAD or transplant), less than 50% of these extreme shock patients survive. From May 2002 to November 2002, Jurmann et al. treated six patients with postcardiomyotomy heart failure; three patients were in cardiogenic shock and one patient had posttransplant graft failure.[53] This group described the intraoperative use of the LVAD, which is inserted through a graft sewn on the ascending aorta. The LV Impella device was inserted through the graft and placed across the aortic valve. The right ventricular support device (RVAD) was externalized through the right jugular vein. The inlet portion was advanced to the right atrium and the outlet portion was grafted using a prosthesis. This was sewn onto the pulmonary artery. Thus biventricular support with flows up to 5 L/min could be provided. Similarly, Garatti et al.[54] treated five patients from September 2002 to April 2003; two patients had fulminant myocarditis, two were bridged to transplant, and one had postcardiomyotomy failure. The device was maintained for 3 to 18 days. Two patients were weaned at 15 and 18 days; one patient was transplanted successfully at day 10. Superb hemodynamic support was achieved.

After this initial experience, a second generation Impella microaxial pump was developed. The Impella Recover LP 2.5 device decreased shaft size to allow passage of the device through a 13F sheath. Dens et al. first reported outcomes in 13 patients in the shock and 27 patients undergoing HRPCI.[55] The initial device caused hemolysis in nine patients and the device malfunctioned in three. The device was modified and no further failures occurred. The device improved cardiac output (4.4 to 4.81 L/min, $p = 0.018$) and decreased wedge pressure (22 ± 7.5 to 16 ± 6 mm Hg, $p = 0.0008$) after 6 hours. While the Impella devices were originally designed as surgically implanted micro-VADS, downsizing of the catheter and shaft as well as placement of the pigtail on the tip allowed the potential for transfemoral access (**Figure 5-12**). The initial use of the Impella Recover 2.5 device in HRPCI is described by Valgimigli et al.[56] A 56-year-old patient with four previous myocardial infarcts and chronic EF of 27% was admitted with unstable angina.

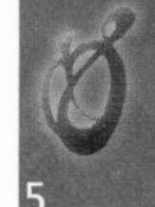

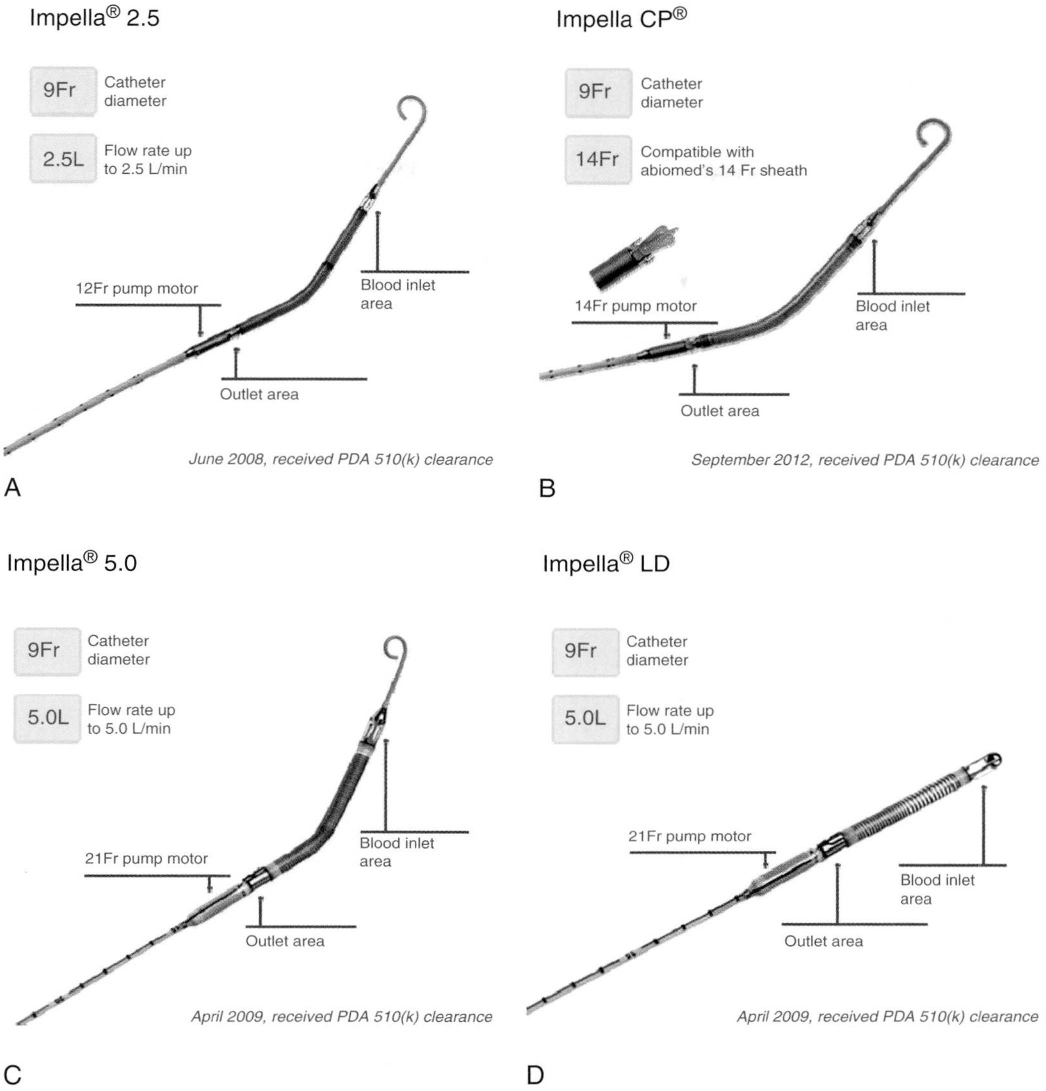

FIGURE 5-12 Current commercially available Impella catheters. The Impella 2.5 **(A)** requires a 13F sheath and will generate up to 2.5 L/min of forward cardiac flow. The Impella CP **(B)** requires a 14F sheath and will generate up to 4 L/min flow. The Impella 5.0 **(C)** requires a 22F sheath and is placed surgically or by transcaval access. The Impella LD **(D)** is meant to be placed during heart surgery through an aortic cannula. All devices have a 9F shaft. *(Reproduced with permission from Abiomed, Danvers, MA.)*

There was a severe, ulcerated culprit lesion of a large dominant left circumflex vessel. Before PCI was performed, hemodynamic changes and pressure volume loops were obtained (**Figure 5-13**). During high flows (RPM = 50,000) left ventricular volumes were reduced, systolic pressure was elevated, and LV filling pressures were reduced. These changes would all be expected to decrease MVO_2 while maintaining or increasing coronary blood flow. Remmelink et al. confirmed the beneficial effects of Impella support on coronary hemodynamics.[57] This group studied 11 patients undergoing HRPCI and assessed coronary pressures and flow velocity nondisease coronaries or after stent implantation of a last patent vessel. They found that coronary pressures were elevated by Impella support. Coronary flow velocity was increased and coronary microvascular resistance was reduced with increasing levels of support. Unfortunately no data were collected on pressure and flow distal to stenotic segments. At the same time, Remmelink et al. further elaborated the hemodynamic benefit of the Impella catheter.[58] This group further analyzed wall stress and LV volume. During high-level support, systolic pressure was maintained while LVEDP was dramatically reduced and wall stress was reduced (**Figure 5-14**). The beneficial effects on coronary flow and microvasuclar resistance along with decreases in LV wall stress appeared to be ideal for hemodynamic support during HRPCI.

CLINICAL TRIALS OF IMPELLA IN HRPCI

Henriques et al. reported a series of 19 HRPCI patients with the Impella LP 2.5 supported system.[59] This report summarized the Academic Medical Center Experience from October 2004 to August 2005. In this study, echocardiograms were reported and no increase in aortic regurgitation was found. They first described the preclosure techniques of placing double Perclose (Abbott Laboratory, Abbott Park, Illinois) devices for vascular closure in 15/19 patients (**Figure 5-15**). This series included all patients with EF ≤ 40% and 12/19 patients with EF ≤ 25%. Ten patients had PCI of the left main or last patent vessel. Successful Impella

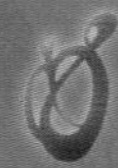

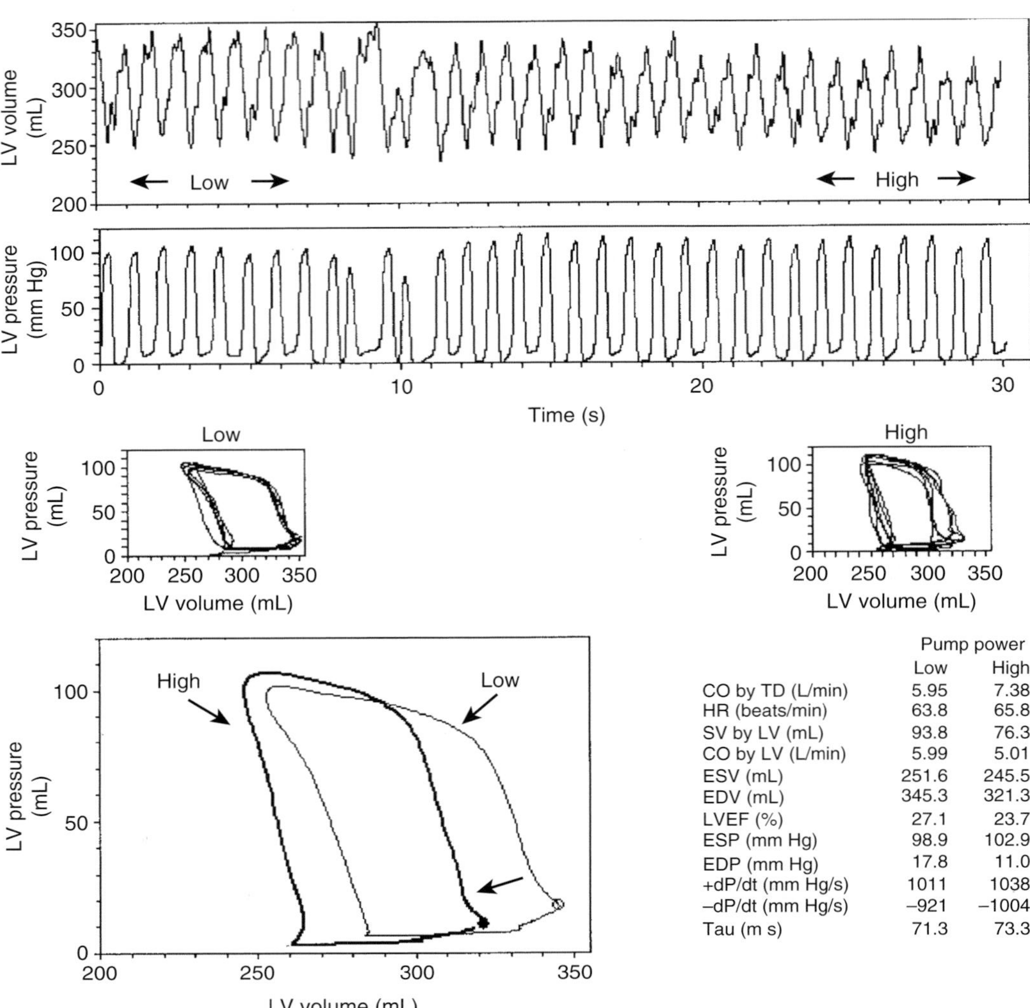

	Low	High
CO by TD (L/min)	5.95	7.38
HR (beats/min)	63.8	65.8
SV by LV (mL)	93.8	76.3
CO by LV (L/min)	5.99	5.01
ESV (mL)	251.6	245.5
EDV (mL)	345.3	321.3
LVEF (%)	27.1	23.7
ESP (mm Hg)	98.9	102.9
EDP (mm Hg)	17.8	11.0
+dP/dt (mm Hg/s)	1011	1038
–dP/dt (mm Hg/s)	–921	–1004
Tau (m s)	71.3	73.3

FIGURE 5-13 Pressure volume loops during Impella support. During high flows, left ventricular (LV) volumes diminish (upper panel) while LV pressures remain constant (second row). Average of P-V loops are present in the lower row. During high-flow LV end diastolic pressures are decreased while systolic pressures are maintained or augmented. *(Reproduced with permission from Valgimigli M, Steendijk P, Sianos G, et al: Left ventricular unloading and concomitant total cardiac output increase by the use of percutaneous Impella Recover LP 2.5 assist device during high-risk coronary intervention. Catheter Cardiovasc Interv 65(2):263–267, 2005.)*

placement occurred in all patients. One of the patients was excluded due to the presence of intraventricular thrombus. The Impella was successfully removed in the elective cases and no vascular complications occurred. Thus elective HRPCI appeared feasible but needed to be prospectively tested.

The device received a Conformite Europeenne (CE) mark in 2004. Sjauw published the initial European (Europella) registry.[61] This report summarized the clinical outcome in 144 consecutive patients who underwent HRPCI. PCI was considered high risk due to left main disease, last patent coronary vessel, or multivessel disease with low EF. A 30-day mortality rate of 5.5% occurred. In addition, 5.5% of the patients required blood transfusions and one stroke was reported. These results were at least comparable to previous registry reports of HRPCI.

In July 2006, the U.S. safety and feasibility trial was initiated. Dixon et al. reported outcomes on 20 patients undergoing HRPCI.[62] The study was performed to provide U.S. operators with experience and to determine MACE endpoints for sample size calculation for the pivotal randomized trial. To be included, patients were required to have EF ≤ 35% and were about to undergo PCI of LMCA or last patent vessel. Patients with MI within the previous 24 hours, with documented LV thrombus, with presence of mechanical aortic prosthetic valve, or aortic stenosis with the valve area ≤1.5 cm^2 were excluded. Of the 20 patients enrolled, 14 underwent of the LMCA PCI and 6 had the last patent vessel treated. The mean duration of support was 1.7 ± 0.6 hours. Mean pump flow was 2.2 L/min. All devices were successfully removed and no reports of device malfunction occurred. At 30 days, an adverse safety endpoint had occurred in 20% of patients. Echocardiograms performed at baseline and 30 days found no damage to the aortic valve and an improved ejection fraction (25 ± 10 to 33 ± 10, p < 001). Two patients had lab evidence of mild hemolysis. There were two deaths at 12 and 14 days after PCI. During the procedure, all patients had freedom from hemodynamic compromise, although one patient had moderate aortic regurgitation during Impella support, which resolved with a device explant. The results of this trial were encouraging and allowed planning for the definitive randomized trial of Impella during HRPCI.

The Impella 2.5 device received FDA approval in June of 2008. Two series were reported on the use of Impella in elective PCI. A single center report from the Detroit Medical

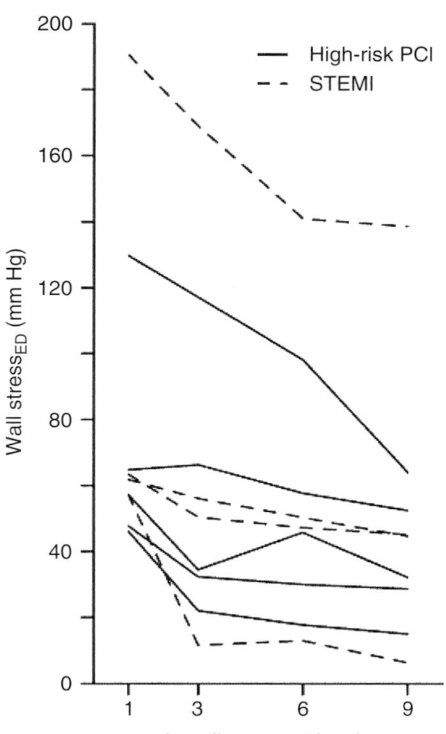

FIGURE 5-14 Pressure volume loops during Impella support. Increasing support decreases LV wall stress in both HRPCI as well as STEMI patients being treated with PCI therapy. *(Reproduced with permission from Remmelink M, Sjauw KD, Henriques JP, et al: Effects of left ventricular unloading by Impella Recover LP2.5 on coronary hemodynamics. Catheter Cardiovasc Interv 70(4):532–537, 2007.)*

Center experience from August 2008 to April 2010 found a 5% mortality rate. A complex patient population was treated. LVEF was 23 ± 15%, Syntax score was 30 ± 9, and left main intervention occurred in 55% of patients.[63]

Maini et al. reported on a larger multicenter registry.[64] The USpella registry reported on 175 patients treated at U.S. sites after FDA approval. A 99% angiographic success occurred. The Syntax score was reduced from 36 ± 15 to 18 ± 15 ($p < 0.01$), and LVEF improved from 31 ± 15 to 36 ± 14, $p < 0.0001$. At 30 days, MACE was 8% and survival was 96%. Both U.S. registries suggested the use of Impella 2.5 in HRPCI resulted in high angiographic success and low rate complications. It remained, however, for a prospective, multicenter randomized trial to define the proper role for this device during HRPCI.

PROTECT II

After completion of the Protect I, Abiomed (Danvers, Massachusetts) petitioned the FDA to conduct a pivotal randomized trial.[8] At the same time, it applied for 510(k) clearance based on data obtained in Europe and the Protect I trial. In negotiations with the FDA and using the Protect I data, a 30% MAE (Major Adverse Events) was assumed for control-treated patients and a reduction to 20% MAE by Impella was hypothesized. A sample size of 654 patients was required to achieve an 80% power and two-sided alpha error of 5%. A 30-day endpoint was a standard FDA-required time frame. In addition, since these high-risk patients may not stabilize at 30 days, a 90-day endpoint was prospectively

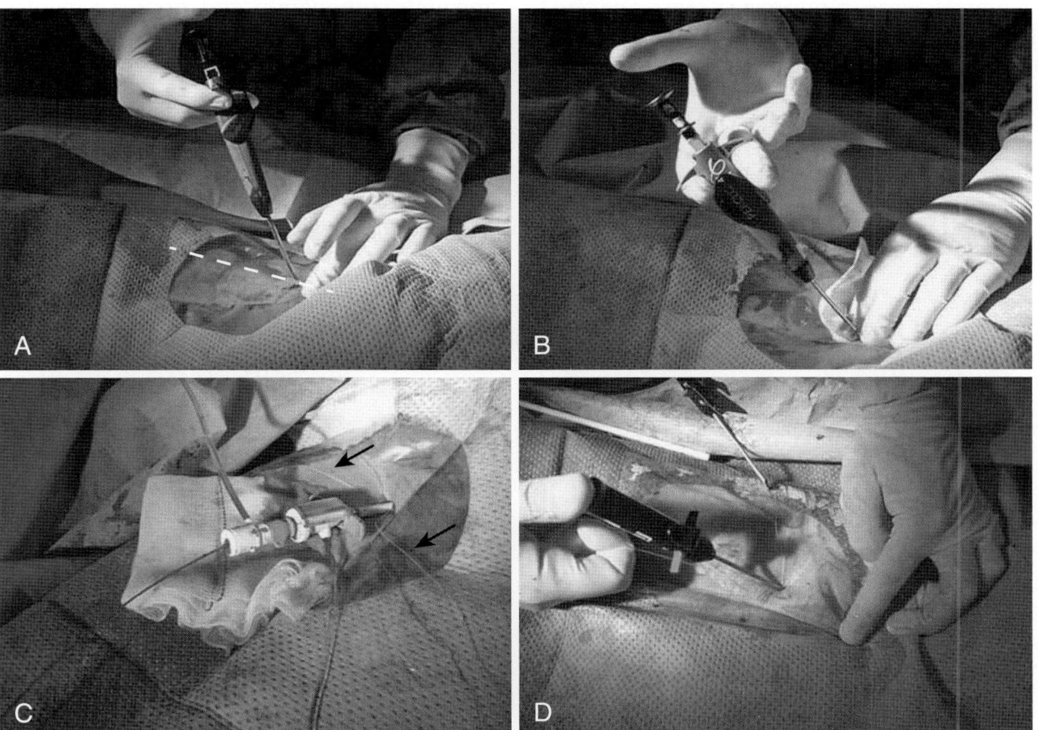

FIGURE 5-15 Preclose technique for large vessel hemostasis. Prior to placing Perclose (Abbott Labs, Chicago, IL, ICC) sutures, femoral angiography is performed to assure access is in the common femoral artery. Two Perclose devices are placed at 90-degree angles **(A** and **B)**. The large sheath is then inserted **(C)**. At the end of the procedure, both sutures are tied sequentially **(D)**. If bleeding persists, manual pressure can be applied. This technique should not be used when sheaths remain in place for chronic support. *(Reproduced with permission from Dangas GD, Kini AS, Sharma SK, et al: Impact of hemodynamic support with Impella 2.5 versus intra-aortic balloon pump on prognostically important clinical outcomes in patients undergoing high-risk percutaneous coronary intervention (from the PROTECT II randomized trial). Am J Cardiol 113(2):222–228, 2014.)*

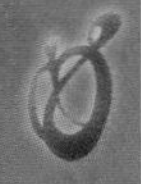

mandated. Both intention to treat and per protocol analysis were reported to test the treatment and device strategies.

Prospective subgroup analysis was predetermined. First, there was a concern that, since the device was new, a learning curve might exist. Since the company could not afford the cost of supporting a learning curve at each site, a learning curve analysis whereby each center's first patient was excluded was performed. Second, there was a concern that the use of rotational atherectomy might cause excessive cardiac enzyme elevations; for this reason, an analysis of patients treated with and without rotational atherectomy was conducted. Finally, STS level and treatment of LMCA versus three-vessel disease was also evaluated prospectively.

The Protect II study commenced enrollment in November 2007. In July 2008, FDA 510(k) clearance for the device occurred. This commercial approval led to a slowdown in recruitment, as some high volume centers chose to stop enrollment in the trial and only treat HRPCI patients with commercially available Impella support. An independent Data Safety Monitoring Board (DSMB) was charged with a review of safety and provided an unblinded analysis at 25% and 50% recruitment levels. At the 50% enrollment level, the DSMB recommended cessation of the enrollment since 30-day efficacy endpoints were similar, and the board concluded that a significant difference would be unlikely. By the time this recommendation was received, 70% of the enrollment target had been achieved. The entire trial experience was analyzed and reported. In retrospect, it is unfortunate that the DSMB did not take the 90-day endpoint into the efficacy analysis and could not have known the strong influence of a learning curve that existed for the device (**Figure 5-16**).

In total, 448 patients were randomized and analyzed according to Intention to Treat (ITT) principles; 427 patients were adjudicated to meet entry criteria and were analyzed by per protocol (PP) principles. Thus both the strategy (ITT) and the device (PP) were tested. During the PCI procedure, the Impella provides unequivocally better hemodynamic support. There were fewer hypotensive events (0.45 ± 1.37 vs. 0.96 ± 2.05 event/patient, p = 0.001) with Impella versus IABP support. Cardiac power was better preserved with less of a drop in cardiac power (–0.04 ± 0.24 vs. –0.14 ± 0.27 watts, p = 0.001) for Impella support. In other words, fewer hypotensive events and better cardiac power protection occurred with Impella therapy. The primary endpoints are demonstrated in (**Figure 5-17**). A review of the Kaplan-Meier event-free survival curves demonstrates that little difference existed between the two groups out to 30 days. At 90 days, however, there was a difference in outcomes, with Impella-treated patients having a higher rate of event-free survival. The events after the 30-day endpoint occurred in an outpatient population. These events were overt and included death, reinfarction, stroke, repeat hospitalization, and repeat coronary intervention. In addition to the overall results, two prospectively designed subgroup analyses have been reported.

First, Cohen et al. demonstrated that Impella-assigned patients had rotational atherectomy used at a higher frequency (8 vs. 14%, p = 0.08).[65] In addition, Impella-treated patients had more aggressive atherectomy with longer duration of passes and more frequent passes for left main obstructions. This resulted in a higher rate of cardiac enzyme elevation, which resulted in a higher rate of periprocedural MI. For 88% of patients treated without atherectomy, a major benefit existed at both 30- and 90-day endpoints (**Figure 5-18**).

A second substudy publication describes the learning curves that existed. Henriques et al.[66] analyzed outcomes for the entire population, and the first patient who enrolled was removed from the trial. Since many of the centers used Impella for the first time in this trial, the learning curve was

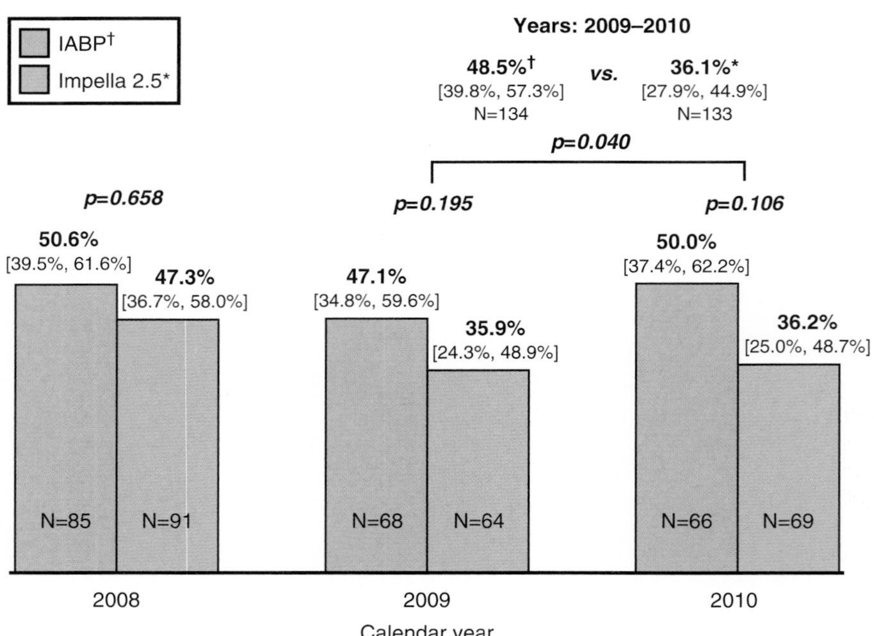

FIGURE 5-16 Learning curve for Impella therapy in Protect II. Major adverse outcomes are presented based on the year patients were treated. Since IABP is a well-established therapy, event rates were similar in all three years; conversely event rates significantly dropped in years 2009 and 2010 for Impella-treated patients. *(Reproduced with permission from Henriques JP, Remmelink M, Baan J, Jr, et al: Safety and feasibility of elective high-risk percutaneous coronary intervention procedures with left ventricular support of the Impella Recover LP 2.5. Am J Cardiol 97(7):990–992, 2006.)*

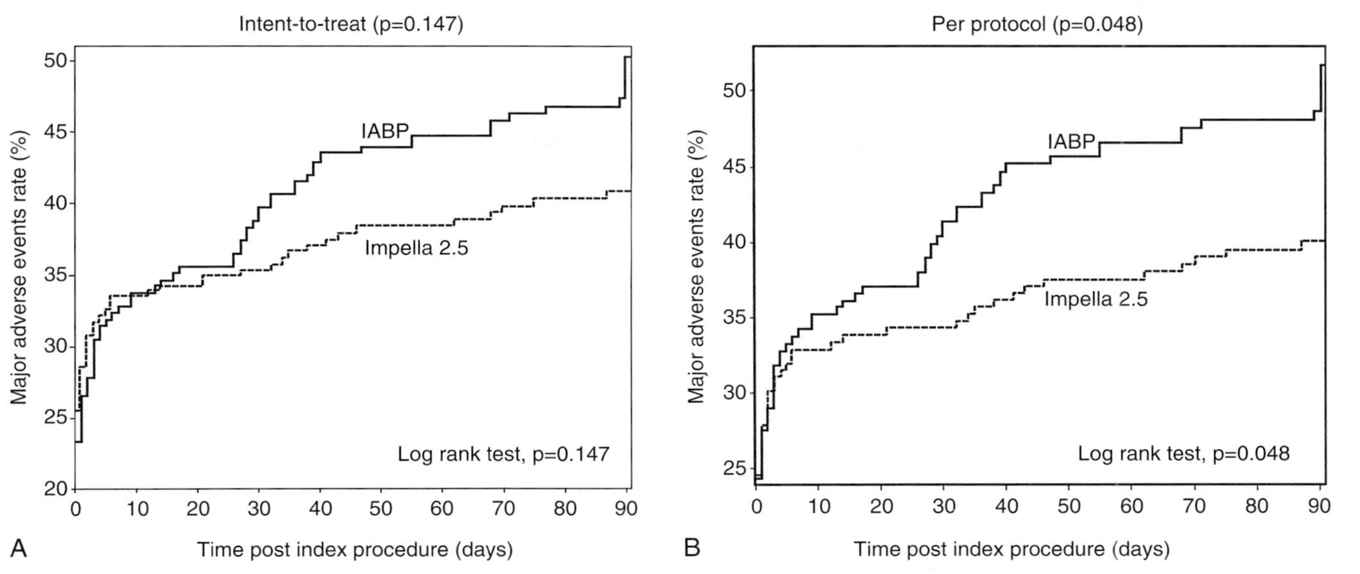

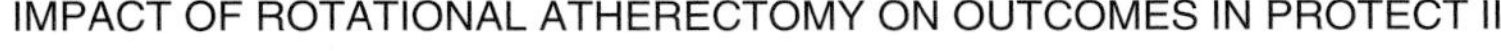

FIGURE 5-17 P II overall results (A, B). Event curves demonstrate that after 30 days, many overt clinical events occur, particularly in IABP-treated patients. *(Reproduced with permission from O'Neill WW, Kleiman NS, Moses J, et al: A prospective, randomized clinical trial of hemodynamic support with Impella 2.5 versus intra-aortic balloon pump in patients undergoing high-risk percutaneous coronary intervention: the PROTECT II study. Circulation 126(14):1717–1727, 2012.)*

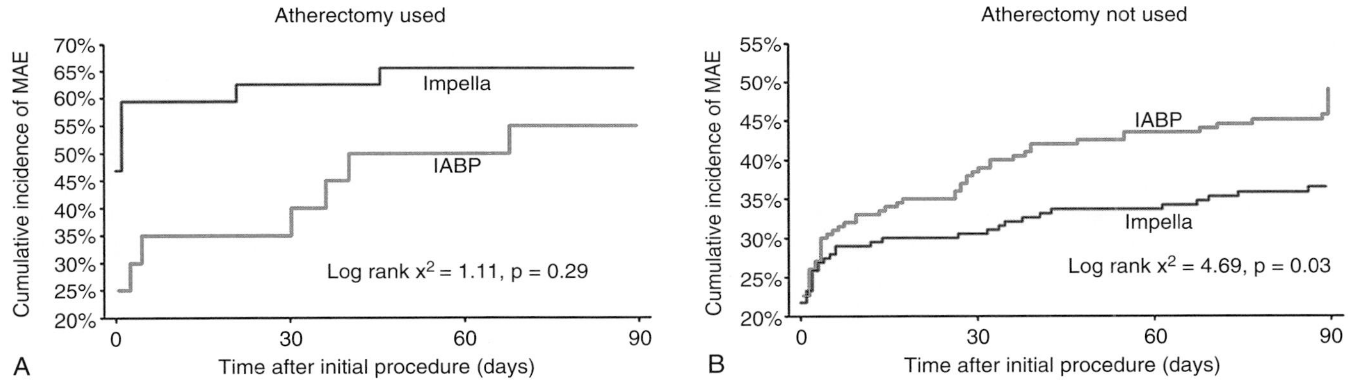

FIGURE 5-18 Cohen MRA. Event curves for patients treated with atherectomy are depicted in the left panel **(A)** and patients with stent therapy alone in the right panel **(B)**. For 885 patients treated without atherectomy, a significant reduction in MAE occurred at both 30 days and 90 days. *(Reproduced with permission from Cohen MG, Ghatak A, Kleiman NS, et al: Optimizing rotational atherectomy in high-risk percutaneous coronary interventions: insights from the PROTECT Iotalota study. Catheter Cardiovasc Interv 2013.)*

embedded in the overall results. Once operators became proficient, a significant improvement in outcome occurred for Impella-treated patients. In addition to these two prospective subgroups' publications, two other important post hoc analyses have been published. Dangas et al. reported on the major impact that the definition of periprocedual MI has on the outcomes in Protect II.[60] Before the Protect II trial was conducted, the FDA recommended a historic definition of periprocedural MI, which was an elevation of cardiac enzymes 3 times the upper limit of normal for each institution. This definition has been called into question since Stone et al. published a metaanalysis of 8000 patients treated in modern device trials.[67] Stone demonstrated that prognostically important cardiac enzyme elevation was 8 times the upper limit. When an 8× level was analyzed by Dargas in the Protect II population, a significant improvement in event-free survival occurred for Impella-treated patients both at 30- and 90-day time points (**Figure 5-19**). Overall, no difference in the incidence of negligible MI or large prognostically significant MI occurred. A doubling incidence of small MI (>3 to <8× elevation of cardiac enzymes) (9/124 vs. 18/225, p = 0.078) occurred for Impella-treated patients. A multivariable analysis demonstrated that Impella use resulted in a 25% risk reduction (odds ratio, 0.76, CI 0.61 to 0.96, p = 0.02) at 90 days.

Kovacic et al. presented an initial analysis of outcomes for patients based on the number of lesions treated.[68] When one vessel is intervened, little difference occurs between Impella and IABP. Conversely, when two or more vessels are treated, a marked reduction in cardiac power occurs in the IABP-treated patients compared to Impella. The 90-day outcomes were significantly improved for Impella-treated patients when two or more vessels were treated.

When the overall trial results and subgroup reports are considered together, a clear picture for the value of Impella in HRPCI emerges. First, when a new device is tested, a

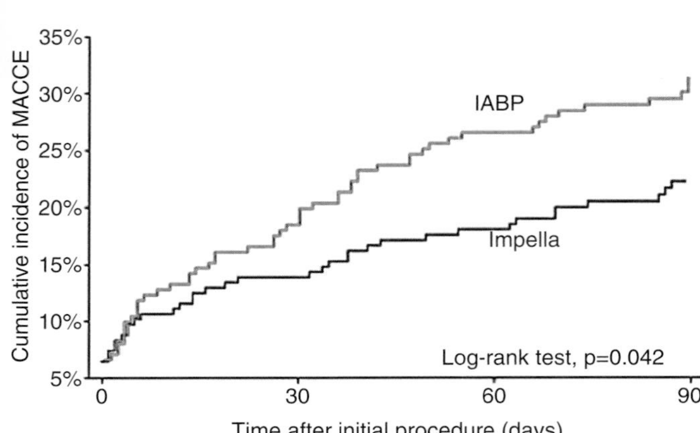

FIGURE 5-19 **MACCE.** Major adverse cardiac and cerebrovascular events with a >8× increase in CK MB were compared for Impella and balloon pump patients. A significantly lower risk for MACCE occurred over the 90-day follow-up for the Impella group. *(Reproduced with permission from Dangas GD, Kini AS, Sharma SK, et al: Impact of hemodynamic support with Impella 2.5 versus intra-aortic balloon pump on prognostically important clinical outcomes in patients undergoing high-risk percutaneous coronary intervention (from the PROTECT II randomized trial). Am J Cardiol 113(2):222–228, 2014.)*

learning curve exists and procedural outcomes are expected to improve over time. In the Protect II study, outcomes were far better after the learning curve was overcome. Next and perhaps most important, trials of HRPCI must report long-term outcomes in analysis of efficacy. The traditional 30-day surgical endpoint is insufficient. Both the Shock[69] and BCIS[31] trials were neutral at 30 days and showed superiority for balloon pump therapy at 1 year or 5 years. Outpatient events continue to occur over the first 90 days, so it is insufficient to use in-hospital or 30-day outcomes to assess efficiency of a support strategy. Furthermore, the definition of periprocedural MI that uses prognostically relevant (>8×) enzyme elevations shows that Impella support decreases adverse events compared to IABP. The patients most likely to benefit are treated with stent implantation unassisted by rotational atherectomy. When atherectomy is used, fewer, shorter passes are recommended. Finally, the advantage of Impella over IABP is most pronounced when multiple vessels are intervened. In these patients, Impella provides far superior hemodynamic support and results in improved event-free survival at 90 days.

OPTIMAL USE OF IMPELLA FOR HEMODYNAMIC SUPPORT

To provide maximum safety and efficiency of support, an organized preprocedure plan is required. Since a 13F to 14F arterial sheath is required, knowledge of iliofemoral vessel dimension is necessary. A preprocedure contrast CT of the abdominal aorta and iliofemoral vessels is useful in this regard. If this is not available, a 5F or 6F pigtail catheter can be introduced and a lower abdominal angiogram is done to allow choice of the best femoral vessel. Vessels with excessive tortuosity or heavy calcium deposits at the iliofemoral junction should be avoided. Once the target femoral vessel is chosen, a preclose technique can be used for post-procedure femoral vessel closure. If this is not an option, manual pressure after ACT normalizes is an alternate hemostasis strategy. Ideally, target vessel puncture should be guided by ultrasound or contrast injections from the contralateral vessel. This will assure that the femoral puncture is in the common femoral artery and below the inguinal ligament. We favor the ultrasound-guided approach, since this reliably allows access to the common femoral artery and avoids excessive calcium in the anterior wall that might make suture-mediated closure unsuccessful.

Once the femoral vessel is adequately prepared, a pigtail catheter is advanced into the left ventricle. A 0.18-inch platinum plus wire is advanced through the pigtail and used as the rail for advancement of the Impella. The 0.18-inch wire provides sufficient body to deliver the device into the left ventricle. Importantly, if resistance is encountered when advancing through the iliofemoral vessel, forceful advancement will lead to damage to the vessel or the device. The catheter should be withdrawn and a large sheath (14F) should be advanced into the abdominal aorta. This technique may be necessary when vessels are tortuous or heavily calcified.

Once the Impella is advanced into the ventricle, the device is turned on full flow (P9 level). If pressure alarms go off or if optimal flow does not occur, the device needs to be repositioned. Typically, the energy of forcing blood through the device forces the device further into the ventricle, so the device needs to be withdrawn. Not infrequently during the procedure, the device needs to be repositioned. Usually after one or two moves, a stable position can be achieved. If the device is to remain in place after the procedure, a knee immobilizer of the instrumented leg is required so that the knee is not flexed. Knee flexing poses a risk of device migration. Once a stable position has been achieved, coronary intervention can commence. At the end of the PCI procedure, the Impella is turned down to a P2 level, and if the patient is stable, the device is removed from the ventricle and turned off for removal from the body. Hemostasis is then achieved by closure of the instrumented vessel. If manual presence is required, the sheath should be left in the proper place until the ACT normalizes. Manual presence for 45 minutes with further mechanical pressure for 4 to 6 hours assures adequate hemostasis.

ALTERNATIVE ACCESS SITES

All transarterial hemodynamic support devices require femoral vessel dimensions that range from 8F with IABP to 17F with TandemHeart or ECMO. If femoral access is not possible, alternate conduits can be used (**Figure 5-20**). Traditionally the iliac artery can be accessed through a lateral flank retroperitoneal approach.[70] A vascular graft can be sewn on the iliac artery and the graft can be tunneled to exit through the femoral area. This technique has the advantage of stable access with closure by suture occlusion of the distal graft segment without need for retroperitoneal reexploration. This technique has been used for the Impella 5.0, which requires a 22F sheath. Similarly, an access graft can be sewn on the right subclavian artery and the graft can be tunneled for exit in the pectoral area. This technique is used for placement of the Impella 5.0, when a longer duration of the support is needed. Patients can sit in a semirecumbent position and can bathe and eat. The device can be removed and the distal graft segment sewn shut. Direct puncture and suture-mediated hemostasis of the left axillary artery has been performed.[71] Recently, Greenbaum et al.[72] demonstrated that large bore arterial sheaths can be placed through a transcaval approach, with arterial closure achieved by using a VSD or PDA occluder (St. Jude's Medical, Memphis,

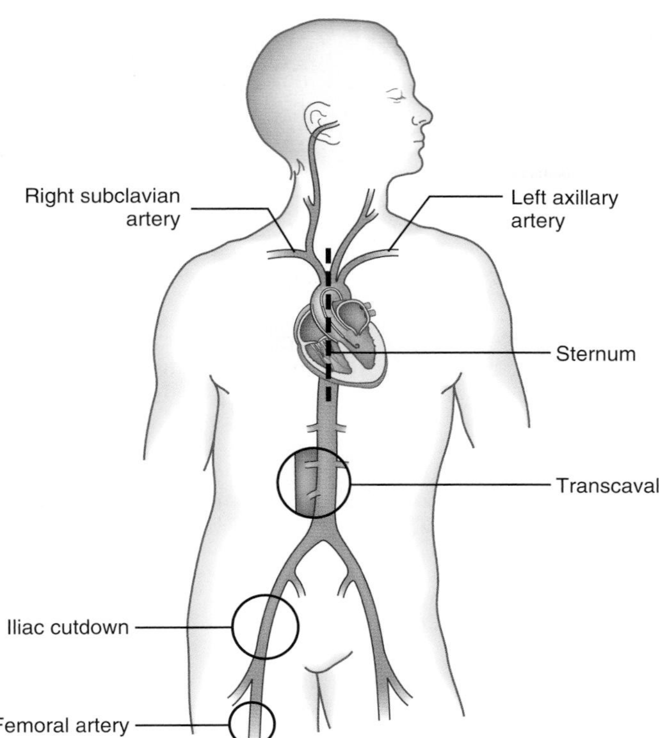

FIGURE 5-20 Access for large bore hemodynamic support devices. Arterial access is a major challenge for the safety of large bore LV support devices. Typically, percutaneous puncture of the common femoral artery is the first choice. When the femoral cannulation is not possible, surgical cutdown of the iliac artery through a lateral peritoneal approach and cutdown of either the right or left axillary artery can occur. For longer support, a chimney graft can be inserted into the right subclavian artery. A direct puncture of the aorta with a ministernotomy is feasible in the surgical population. *(Courtesy Dr. William W. O'Neill.)*

Tennessee). This approach will allow transfemoral access of even the Impella 5.0 without concern for limb ischemia.

CASE EXAMPLE

The use of Impella 2.5 support was demonstrated in a patient treated at the Henry Ford Cath Lab in August 2013. This was an 85-year-old Jehovah's Witness who was catheterized at a referral institution 2 weeks prior to admission. She presented with an NSTEMI and underwent cath. She was found to have impaired LV function, total occlusion of the proximal right coronary artery, and a complex calcified bifurcation left main lesion with calcified lesions of the proximal LAD and obtuse marginal as well. After catheterization, she developed radiocontrast nephropathy and was deemed not a surgical candidate. The patient was referred for HRPCI. Over a 2-week period, renal function returned to baseline.

Initially, an abdominal angiogram (Video 5-1) was performed and both iliac arteries were suitable for access. The Impella 2.5 device was delivered through a sheath in the left femoral artery and a preclose technique was used. Once the Impella was in place, p-8 flow rates were obtained and an output of 2.4 L/min was attained (Video 5-2). A complex intervention was initiated, with atherectomy performed in LMCA (Videos 5-3, 5-4, 5-5) as well as LAD and OM branches (**Figure 5-21**). Subsequently, simultaneous balloon inflations were performed in LAD and circumflex. During this time, no coronary blood flow was possible (Video 5-6). During balloon inflation, pulsatile flow ceased, yet pulmonary artery pressures were maintained and MAP remained at 100 mm Hg. Immediately after balloon deflation, systemic pressure returned to baseline (**Figure 5-22**). Finally, stent deployment occurred in the LAD, OM, and bifurcation left main vessels. The final angiogram demonstrates wide angiographic patency of the three treated vessels (Video 5-7). Impella was removed immediately after intervention (Video 5-8) and hemostasis was achieved with suture closure.

This case exemplifies the principles of hemodynamic support for HRPCI. First, this elderly, highly symptomatic female was deemed ineligible for CABG. Thus either an HRPCI or hospice care was available. Once a decision for intervention was reached, hemodynamic support was indicated due to the complex anatomy and poor LV function. In addition, the heavily calcified vessels mandated use of rotational atherectomy. Technical aspects of the case were complex; initially, even wire manipulation could cause cardiac collapse without support. Next, the use of atherectomy could cause coronary no reflow, which could be catastrophic. Extensive stenting of multiple vessels was required and meticulous complex stenting guided by IVUS was also required to complete this procedure. Even when coronary blood flow was abolished during simultaneous balloon inflation, the patient remained alert, communicative, and with a stable cardiac rhythm. In this fashion, a careful, complete, and methodical coronary intervention could be performed.

COMPLICATIONS OF IMPELLA

Like all invasive devices, complications with use of the Impella have been reported. The most worrisome complications arise from femoral access. The 13F to 14F sheath is inserted in the femoral artery and can cause injury, requiring surgical repair. Proper preprocedure angiography and guided arterial puncture of the common femoral artery should minimize this risk. In the Protect II study,[8] vascular surgery was required in 1.4% of IABG- and 0.9% of Impella-treated patients (p = NS). This complication thus should be quite uncommon.

If the device is left in place, a peel-away sheath is removed and an occluder device is advanced so that only the 9F shaft of the Impella remains in the femoral artery. It is essential to immobilize the instrumented leg so that catheter dislodgment will not occur.

The most common complication with prolonged support is catheter migration. Pressure alarms should detect this. Catheter repositioning using echo or fluoroscopic guidance may be required. If the inlet part is entrapped in a papillary muscle, high shear rates can occur and hemolysis may develop. Hemolysis is rare during short-term support. Hemolysis occurred in 21% of the patients treated with Impella in Protect II. Tanawuttiwat et al. reported a case of fiber wrapped around the inlet part of an Impella device, which led to severe hemolysis.[73] Elhussein et al. reported placement of an Impella 5.0 for support, which led to flail mitral leaflet and severe mitral regurgitation.[74] Conversely, Toggweiler[75] reported a case where the Impella catheter migrated and the shaft was lying on the anterior leaflet of the mitral valve. Functional mitral stenosis occurred as a result.

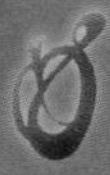

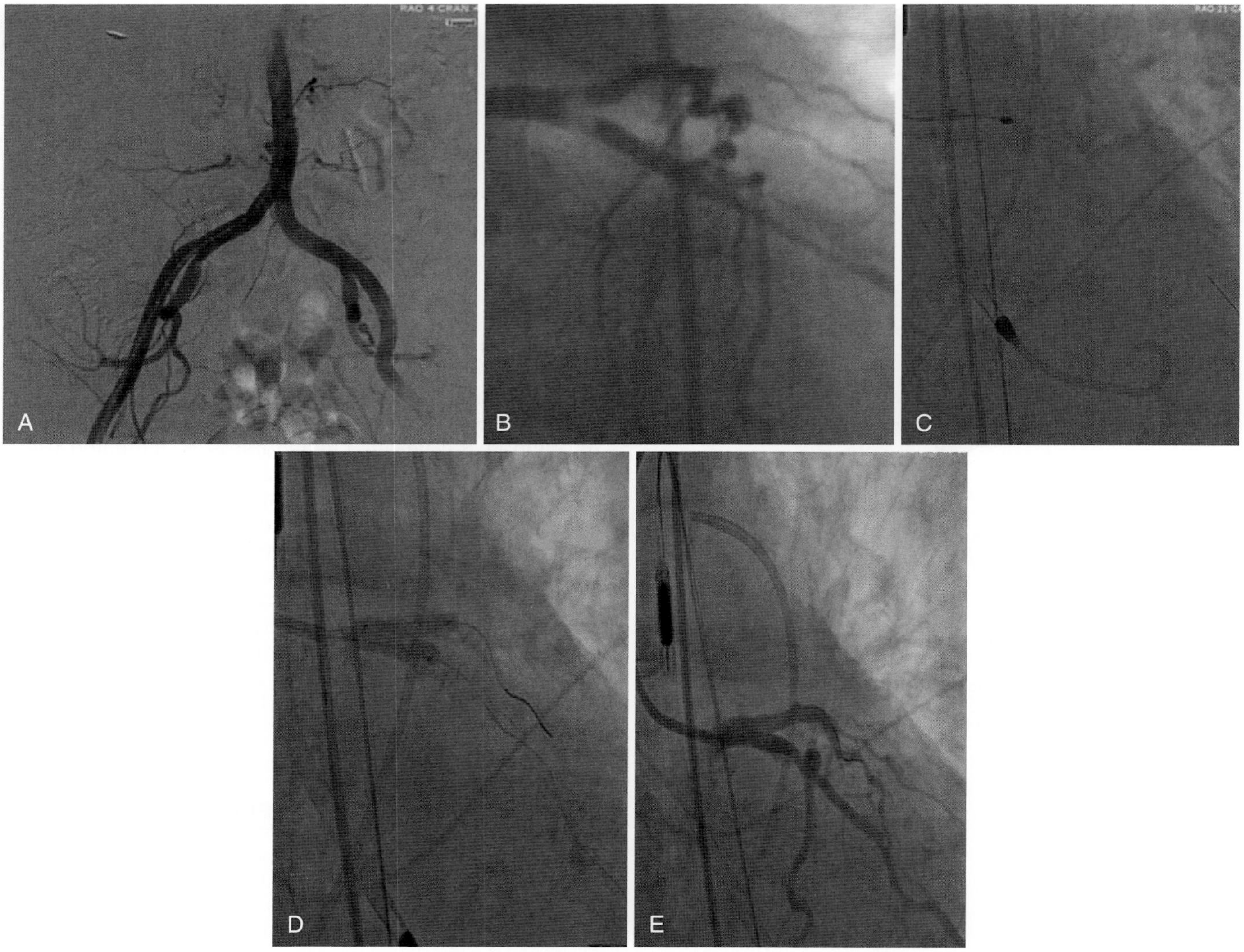

FIGURE 5-21 High-risk PCI procedure. A, Abdominal angiogram demonstrates that both femoral vessels are of adequate caliber for intervention. **B,** *PRE,* Preprocedure angiogram shows a highly calcified bifurcation distal LMCA lesions. **C,** *MRA,* use of rotational atherectomy in LMCA, LAD, and circumflex vessels. **D,** *Balloon,* simultaneous balloon inflation in the LAD and LCX. **E,** *Post,* final angiogram after stent implantations in LAD, LCX, and LMCA. *(Courtesy Dr. William W. O'Neill.)*

Ranc et al.[76] reported acute thrombosis of the inlet part of an Impella 5.0 that was inserted to manage a patient in cardiogenic shock. They theorized that the acute thrombosis that occurred 27 hours after implantation was related to subtherapeutic anticoagulation or entrapment of an intraventricular thrombus. These reports highlight the vigilance that is required for optimal safety of use. Patients must be therapeutically anticoagulated to avoid thrombotic complications and thrombosis of the inlet shaft. Careful echocardiographic screening should occur to avoid use of the device when LV thrombus is present. Careful positioning of the catheter in the ventricle with intermittent checks to assure optimal position should occur after placement. Often slight withdrawal is needed soon after device activation.

When the device is left in place, daily chest x-rays and daily echocardiograms should be obtained. Interference of mitral valve function should be considered if hemodynamic instability occurs. Repositioning of the device is ideally performed with fluoroscopy. With these precautions, excellent durable support of cardiac output can be safely achieved.

NOVEL USES OF IMPELLA

The availability of a transvalvular hemodynamic support device has allowed clinicians to support patients for indications apart from HRPCI or cardiogenic shock. Garatti et al. first reported use of the Impella 100 (1R 100) for patients bridged to transplant or in the case of fulminant myocarditis bridged to recovery.[77]

One of the main limitations of ECMO support is that the left ventricle is not decompressed. A series of reports[78-81] demonstrated the reliability of the combination of Impella and ECMO support. Pozzi reported an innovative use of the Impella 5.0 through a right axillary artery approach.[82] Typically, Impella is first placed through transfemoral access, but severe ventricular failure or pulmonary failure necessitates the initiation of ECMO support. This combination allows for support of the right ventricle and optimal oxygenation, decreases LV wall stress, and allows for adequate systemic output. In addition, the presence of Impella allows earlier weaning off of the ECMO once recovery occurs. This combination appears to have excellent efficacy for patients with fulminant myocarditis. Patane[83] and La Torre[84]

FEMORAL ARTERY AND PULMONARY ARTERY PRESSURES DURING LMCA BALLOON INFLATION

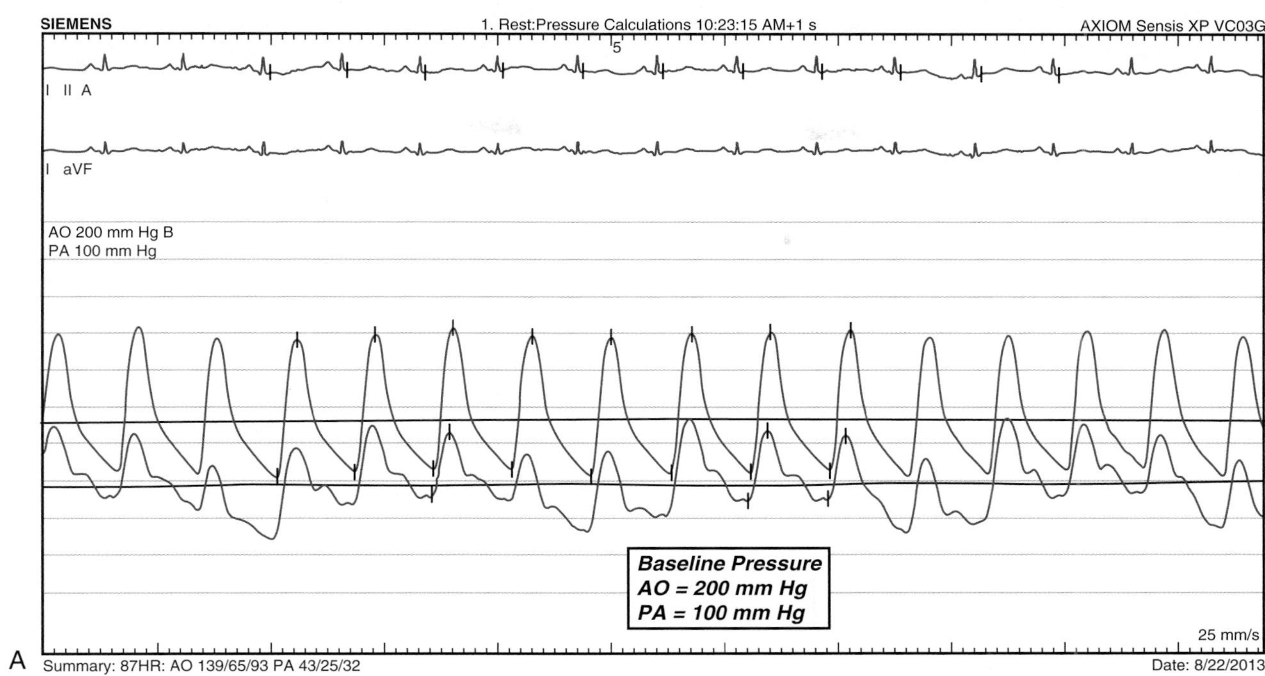

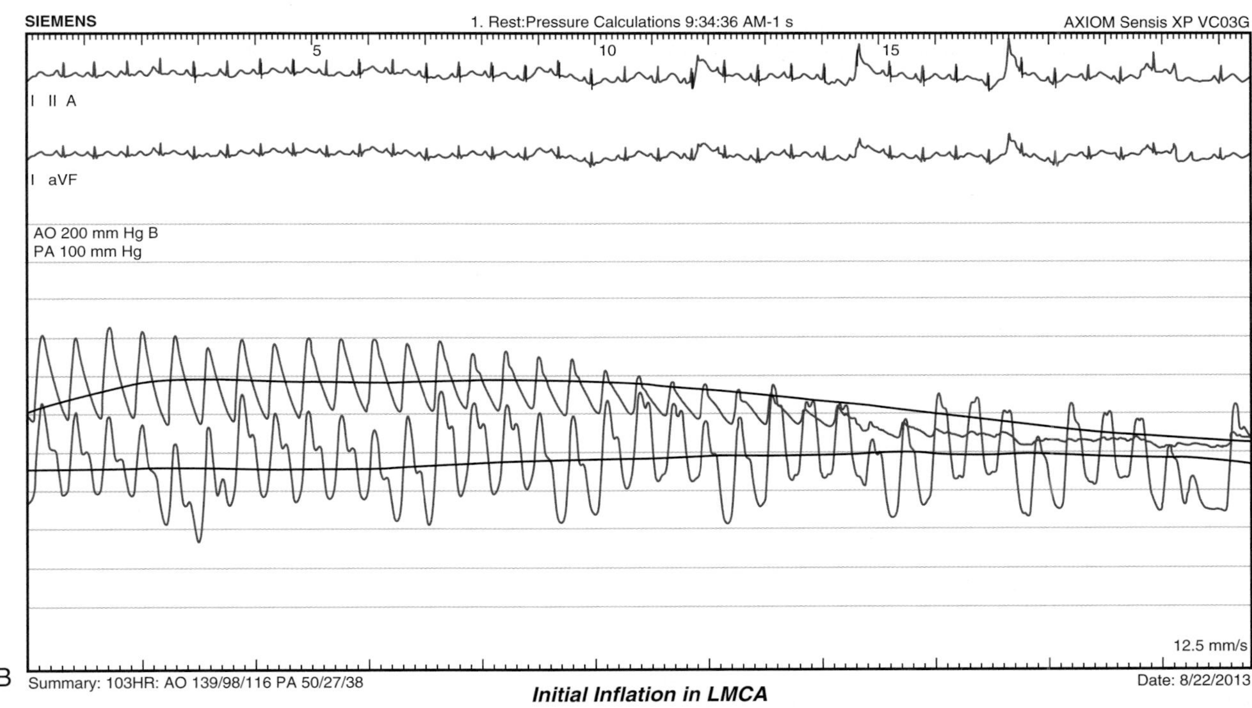

FIGURE 5-22 Femoral artery and pulmonary artery pressures during LMCA balloon inflations. Baseline aortic (AO) and pulmonary artery (PA) pressures are recorded **(A).** As balloons are inflated in both LAD and LCX **(B)**, aortic pulse pressure diminishes yet mean aortic pressure is maintained at 100 mm Hg. NOTE: There is very little difference in pulmonary artery pressure or contour. Immediately after balloon deflation (lower panel), the aortic and pulmonary artery pressures normalize**.** *(Courtesy Dr. William W. O'Neill.)*

described use of the Impella 5.0 to stabilize patients with acute ventricular septal defect after acute MI. It is known that immediate operation is fraught with risk because infarction zones are not well demarcated and suture tears with failure of the patch can be lethal. La Torre described placement of a support device. Left to right shunting and pulmonary artery pressure decreased and liver and renal function stabilized. They reported a 60% survival rate with this approach.

Londono and Martinez[85,86] reported the use of Impella in combination with balloon valvuloplasty for patients with critical aortic stenosis and impaired LV function. These patients are at extreme risk for cardiac collapse when rapid RV pacing is performed for the BAV. The insertion of an

Impella device allows BAV to occur without collapse and with improvement in the valve area from 0.6 to 1.0 cm ($p < 0.001$).

Another innovative use of Impella involves support of cardiac output during ventricular tachycardia EP mapping. Miller described the initial Mount Sinai experience in 20 patients who underwent scar VT mapping and ablation.[87] Full support allowed adequate cerebral saturation to be maintained in 95% of patients. Only 1/20 patients developed cognitive dysfunction. Thus hemodynamic support appeared sufficient to allow time for mapping and ablation in these patients. It is expected that enhanced cardiac output with the newest Impella CP device might prove even more effective. Lu et al.[88] also reported on the use of Impella or peripheral CPB to support patients for VT ablation. These initial reports suggest an important role for Impella support during this procedure.

FUTURE ADVANCES

Transfemoral support with Impella has largely been studied with the Impella 2.5 device. Recently, the Impella CP device has become available. This device requires a 14F sheath for access. It can deliver up to 4 L of forward flow. The device appears ideal for patients of a large body size (>80 kg) or when minimal intrinsic cardiac output exists. It is currently being evaluated in the USPella registry and within 1 to 2 years its utility in support of patients treated in cardiogenic shock will be established. A large, National Danish "Dan Shock" randomized trial is currently enrolling patients. This trial is testing the use of Impella CP versus conventional therapy as adjunctive treatment for PCI in cardiogenic shock. The device is being placed prior to PCI. Outcomes are expected in 2016.

A major advance in hemodynamic support will occur with testing of the Impella RP device. This device has been designed to provide percutaneous support of the right ventricle. The device has a shape to allow the inlet to sit at the right atrial-vena cava junction and the outlet to sit in the main pulmonary artery. A 22F sheath is inserted in the right femoral vein. The device is advanced over guidewire and can provide up to 4 L of forward flow. Initial use to manage RV shock after acute MI has been reported.[89] Currently the Recover Right clinical trial is testing the device in 30 patients in a single arm Humanitarian Device Exemption (HDE) trial. Enrollment is expected to be complete in 2014 and the device should be clinically available in 2015.

CONCLUSIONS

As the population in the Western world ages, clinicians will be increasingly faced with highly symptomatic, elderly patients with advanced coronary disease. Technical advances have made percutaneous revascularization a therapeutic option for cases not approachable 10 to 15 years ago. Many of these patients will present with extremely depressed ventricular function. In these patients, support of the ventricular function and maintenance of coronary blood flow are essential for an uncomplicated procedure. The BCIS and the Protect II have demonstrated that intraprocedural course and intermediate to long-term event-free survival are improved with hemodynamic support. In spite of this support, in-hospital mortality and long-term survival are markedly worse than patients with normal LV function. This group of patients needs to be reported independently, since operator and hospital experience vary widely and therefore outcomes will vary widely. Ideally, centers with special expertise should organize and report outcomes to assure optimal results for these patients.

References

1. Gruntzig AR, Senning A, Siegenthaler WE: Nonoperative dilatation of coronary-artery stenosis: percutaneous transluminal coronary angioplasty. *N Engl J Med* 301(2):61–68, 1979. doi:10.1056/NEJM197907123010201.
2. Mullin SM, Passamani ER, Mock MB: Historical background of the National Heart, Lung, and Blood Institute Registry for Percutaneous Transluminal Coronary Angioplasty. *Am J Cardiol* 53(12):3C–6C, 1984.
3. Morrison DA, Sethi G, Sacks J, et al: A multicenter, randomized trial of percutaneous coronary intervention versus bypass surgery in high-risk unstable angina patients. The AWESOME (Veterans Affairs Cooperative Study #385, angina with extremely serious operative mortality evaluation) investigators from the Cooperative Studies Program of the Department of Veterans Affairs. *Control Clin Trials* 20(6):601–619, 1999.
4. Sharma S, Lumley M, Perera D: Intraaortic balloon pump use in high-risk percutaneous coronary intervention. *Curr Opin Cardiol* 28(6):671–675, 2013. doi:10.1097/HCO.0b013e3283652dcc.
5. Vogel RA, Shawl F, Tommaso C, et al: Initial report of the National Registry of Elective Cardiopulmonary Bypass Supported Coronary Angioplasty. *J Am Coll Cardiol* 15(1):23–29, 1990.
6. Teirstein PS, Vogel RA, Dorros G, et al: Prophylactic versus standby cardiopulmonary support for high risk percutaneous transluminal coronary angioplasty. *J Am Coll Cardiol* 21(3):590–596, 1993.
7. Keelan PC, Johnston JM, Koru-Sengul T, et al: Comparison of in-hospital and one-year outcomes in patients with left ventricular ejection fractions < or =40%, 41% to 49%, and > or =50% having percutaneous coronary revascularization. *Am J Cardiol* 91(10):1168–1172, 2003.
8. O'Neill WW, Kleiman NS, Moses J, et al: A prospective, randomized clinical trial of hemodynamic support with Impella 2.5 versus intra-aortic balloon pump in patients undergoing high-risk percutaneous coronary intervention: the PROTECT II study. *Circulation* 126(14):1717–1727, 2012. doi:10.1161/CIRCULATIONAHA.112.098194.
9. Perera D, Stables R, Thomas M, et al: Elective intra-aortic balloon counterpulsation during high-risk percutaneous coronary intervention: a randomized controlled trial. *JAMA* 304(8):867–874, 2010. doi:10.1001/jama.2010.119.
10. Rouleau J, Boerboom LE, Surjadhana A, et al: The role of autoregulation and tissue diastolic pressures in the transmural distribution of left ventricular blood flow in anesthetized dogs. *Circ Res* 45(6):804–815, 1979.
11. Nellis SH, Liedtke AJ, Whitesell L: Small coronary vessel pressure and diameter in an intact beating rabbit heart using fixed-position and free-motion techniques. *Circ Res* 49(2):342–353, 1981.
12. Marcus ML: *The coronary circulation in health and disease*, New York, 1983, McGraw-Hill.
13. Suga H, Sagawa K, Shoukas AA: Load independence of the instantaneous pressure-volume ratio of the canine left ventricle and effects of epinephrine and heart rate on the ratio. *Circ Res* 32(3):314–322, 1973.
14. Burkhoff D: Pressure-volume loops in clinical research: a contemporary view. *J Am Coll Cardiol* 62(13):1173–1176, 2013. doi:10.1016/j.jacc.2013.05.049.
15. Mendoza DD, Cooper HA, Panza JA: Cardiac power output predicts mortality across a broad spectrum of patients with acute cardiac disease. *Am Heart J* 153(3):366–370, 2007. doi:10.1016/j.ahj.2006.11.014.
16. Burkhoff D, Naidu SS: The science behind percutaneous hemodynamic support: a review and comparison of support strategies. *Catheter Cardiovasc Interv* 80(5):816–829, 2012. doi:10.1002/ccd.24421.
17. Williams DO, Korr KS, Gewirtz H, et al: The effect of intraaortic balloon counterpulsation on regional myocardial blood flow and oxygen consumption in the presence of coronary artery stenosis in patients with unstable angina. *Circulation* 66(3):593–597, 1982.
18. Yoshitani H, Akasaka T, Kaji S, et al: Effects of intra-aortic balloon counterpulsation on coronary pressure in patients with stenotic coronary arteries. *Am Heart J* 154(4):725–731, 2007. doi:10.1016/j.ahj.2007.05.019.
19. Kern MJ, Aguirre FV, Tatineni S, et al: Enhanced coronary blood flow velocity during intraaortic balloon counterpulsation in critically ill patients. *J Am Coll Cardiol* 21(2):359–368, 1993.
20. Kern MJ, Aguirre F, Bach R, et al: Augmentation of coronary blood flow by intra-aortic balloon pumping in patients after coronary angioplasty. *Circulation* 87(2):500–511, 1993.
21. Burkhoff D, Cohen H, Brunckhorst C, et al: A randomized multicenter clinical study to evaluate the safety and efficacy of the TandemHeart percutaneous ventricular assist device versus conventional therapy with intraaortic balloon pumping for treatment of cardiogenic shock. *Am Heart J* 152(3):469 e461–e468, 2006. doi:10.1016/j.ahj.2006.05.031.
22. Kent KM, Bentivoglio LG, Block PC, et al: Percutaneous transluminal coronary angioplasty: report from the Registry of the National Heart, Lung, and Blood Institute. *Am J Cardiol* 49(8):2011–2020, 1982.
23. Laird JD, Madras PN, Jones RT, et al: Theoretical and experimental analysis of the intra-aortic balloon pump. *Trans Am Soc Artif Intern Organs* 14:338–343, 1968.
24. Voudris V, Marco J, Morice MC, et al: "High-risk" percutaneous transluminal coronary angioplasty with preventive intra-aortic balloon counterpulsation. *Cathet Cardiovasc Diagn* 19(3):160–164, 1990.
25. Kahn JK, Rutherford BD, McConahay DR, et al: Supported "high risk" coronary angioplasty using intraaortic balloon pump counterpulsation. *J Am Coll Cardiol* 15(5):1151–1155, 1990.
26. Hartzler GD: Percutaneous transluminal coronary angioplasty in multivessel disease. *Cathet Cardiovasc Diagn* 9(6):537–541, 1983.
27. Holmes DR, Jr, Detre KM, Williams DO, et al: Long-term outcome of patients with depressed left ventricular function undergoing percutaneous transluminal coronary angioplasty. The NHLBI PTCA Registry. *Circulation* 87(1):21–29, 1993.
28. Briguori C, Airoldi F, Chieffo A, et al: Elective versus provisional intraaortic balloon pumping in unprotected left main stenting. *Am Heart J* 152(3):565–572, 2006. doi:10.1016/j.ahj.2006.02.024.
29. Mishra S, Chu WW, Torguson R, et al: Role of prophylactic intra-aortic balloon pump in high-risk patients undergoing percutaneous coronary intervention. *Am J Cardiol* 98(5):608–612, 2006. doi:10.1016/j.amjcard.2006.03.036.
30. Curtis JP, Rathore SS, Wang Y, et al: Use and effectiveness of intra-aortic balloon pumps among patients undergoing high risk percutaneous coronary intervention: insights from the National Cardiovascular Data Registry. *Circ Cardiovasc Qual Outcomes* 5(1):21–30, 2012. doi:10.1161/CIRCOUTCOMES.110.960385.
31. Perera D, Stables R, Clayton T, et al: Long-term mortality data from the balloon pump-assisted coronary intervention study (BCIS-1): a randomized, controlled trial of elective balloon counterpulsation during high-risk percutaneous coronary intervention. *Circulation* 127(2):207–212, 2013. doi:10.1161/CIRCULATIONAHA.112.132209.
32. Hochman JS, Sleeper LA, Webb JG, et al: Early revascularization in acute myocardial infarction complicated by cardiogenic shock. SHOCK Investigators. Should We Emergently Revascularize

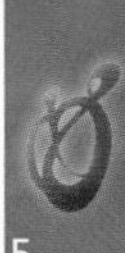

Occluded Coronaries for Cardiogenic Shock. *N Engl J Med* 341(9):625–634, 1999. doi:10.1056/NEJM199908263410901.

33. Shawl FA, Domanski MJ, Wish MH, et al: Percutaneous cardiopulmonary bypass support in the catheterization laboratory: technique and complications. *Am Heart J* 120(1):195–203, 1990.
34. Schreiber TL, Kodali UR, O'Neill WW, et al: Comparison of acute results of prophylactic intraaortic balloon pumping with cardiopulmonary support for percutaneous transluminal coronary angioplasty (PCTA). *Cathet Cardiovasc Diagn* 45(2):115–119, 1998.
35. Stack RK, Pavlides GS, Miller R, et al: Hemodynamic and metabolic effects of venoarterial cardiopulmonary support in coronary artery disease. *Am J Cardiol* 67(16):1344–1348, 1991.
36. Pavlides GS, Hauser AM, Stack RK, et al: Effect of peripheral cardiopulmonary bypass on left ventricular size, afterload and myocardial function during elective supported coronary angioplasty. *J Am Coll Cardiol* 18(2):499–505, 1991.
37. Thiele H, Lauer B, Hambrecht R, et al: Reversal of cardiogenic shock by percutaneous left atrial-to-femoral arterial bypass assistance. *Circulation* 104(24):2917–2922, 2001.
38. Vranckx P, Otten A, Schultz C, et al: Assisted circulation using the TandemHeart, percutaneous transseptal left ventricular assist device, during percutaneous aortic valve implantation: the Rotterdam experience. *EuroIntervention* 5(4):465–469, 2009.
39. Brinkman WT, Rosenthal JE, Eichhorn E, et al: Role of a percutaneous ventricular assist device in decision making for a cardiac transplant program. *Ann Thorac Surg* 88(5):1462–1466, 2009. doi:10.1016/j.athoracsur.2009.07.015.
40. Bruckner BA, Jacob LP, Gregoric ID, et al: Clinical experience with the TandemHeart percutaneous ventricular assist device as a bridge to cardiac transplantation. *Tex Heart Inst J* 35(4):447–450, 2008.
41. Chandra D, Kar B, Idelchik G, et al: Usefulness of percutaneous left ventricular assist device as a bridge to recovery from myocarditis. *Am J Cardiol* 99(12):1755–1756, 2007. doi:10.1016/j.amjcard.2007.01.067.
42. Giesler GM, Gomez JS, Letsou G, et al: Initial report of percutaneous right ventricular assist for right ventricular shock secondary to right ventricular infarction. *Catheter Cardiovasc Interv* 68(2):263–266, 2006. doi:10.1002/ccd.20846.
43. Thiele H, Sick P, Boudriot E, et al: Randomized comparison of intra-aortic balloon support with a percutaneous left ventricular assist device in patients with revascularized acute myocardial infarction complicated by cardiogenic shock. *Eur Heart J* 26(13):1276–1283, 2005. doi:10.1093/eurheartj/ehi161.
44. Kar B, Gregoric ID, Basra SS, et al: The percutaneous ventricular assist device in severe refractory cardiogenic shock. *J Am Coll Cardiol* 57(6):688–696, 2011. doi:10.1016/j.jacc.2010.08.613.
45. Aragon J, Lee MS, Kar S, et al: Percutaneous left ventricular assist device: "TandemHeart" for high-risk coronary intervention. *Catheter Cardiovasc Interv* 65(3):346–352, 2005. doi:10.1002/ccd.20339.
46. Kovacic JC, Nguyen HT, Karajgikar R, et al: The Impella Recover 2.5 and TandemHeart ventricular assist devices are safe and associated with equivalent clinical outcomes in patients undergoing high-risk percutaneous coronary intervention. *Catheter Cardiovasc Interv* 82(1):E28–E37, 2013. doi:10.1002/Ccd.22929.
47. Scholz KH, Figulla HR, Schweda F, et al: Mechanical left ventricular unloading during high risk coronary angioplasty: first use of a new percutaneous transvalvular left ventricular assist device. *Cathet Cardiovasc Diagn* 31(1):61–69, 1994.
48. Frazier OH, Wampler RK, Duncan JM, et al: First human use of the Hemopump, a catheter-mounted ventricular assist device. *Ann Thorac Surg* 49(2):299–304, 1990.
49. Panos A, Kalangos A, Urban P: High-risk PTCA assisted by the Hemopump 14F: the Geneva experience. *Schweiz Med Wochenschr* 129(42):1529–1534, 1999.
50. Dubois-Rande JL, Teiger E, Garot J, et al: Effects of the 14F hemopump on coronary hemodynamics in patients undergoing high-risk coronary angioplasty. *Am Heart J* 135(5 Pt 1):844–849, 1998.
51. Vercaemst L, Vandezande E, Janssens P, et al: Impella: a miniaturized cardiac support system in an era of minimal invasive cardiac surgery. *J Extra Corpor Technol* 34(2):92–100, 2002.
52. Meyns B, Dens J, Sergeant P, et al: Initial experiences with the Impella device in patients with cardiogenic shock—Impella support for cardiogenic shock. *Thorac Cardiovasc Surg* 51(6):312–317, 2003. doi:10.1055/s-2003-45422.
53. Jurmann MJ, Siniawski H, Erb M, et al: Initial experience with miniature axial flow ventricular assist devices for postcardiotomy heart failure. *Ann Thorac Surg* 77(5):1642–1647, 2004. doi:10.1016/j.athoracsur.2003.10.013.
54. Garatti A, Colombo T, Russo C, et al: Different applications for left ventricular mechanical support with the Impella Recover 100 microaxial blood pump. *J Heart Lung Transplant* 24(4):481–485, 2005. doi:10.1016/j.healun.2004.02.002.
55. Dens J, Meyns B, Hilgers RD, et al: First experience with the Impella Recover(R) LP 2.5 micro axial pump in patients with cardiogenic shock or undergoing high-risk revascularisation. *EuroIntervention* 2(1):84–90, 2006.
56. Valgimigli M, Steendijk P, Sianos G, et al: Left ventricular unloading and concomitant total cardiac output increase by the use of percutaneous Impella Recover LP 2.5 assist device during high-risk coronary intervention. *Catheter Cardiovasc Interv* 65(2):263–267, 2005. doi:10.1002/ccd.20380.
57. Remmelink M, Sjauw KD, Henriques JP, et al: Effects of left ventricular unloading by Impella Recover LP2.5 on coronary hemodynamics. *Catheter Cardiovasc Interv* 70(4):532–537, 2007. doi:10.1002/ccd.21160.
58. Remmelink M, Sjauw KD, Henriques JP, et al: Effects of mechanical left ventricular unloading by Impella on left ventricular dynamics in high-risk and primary percutaneous coronary intervention patients. *Catheter Cardiovasc Interv* 75(2):187–194, 2010. doi:10.1002/ccd.22263.
59. Henriques JP, Remmelink M, Baan J, Jr, et al: Safety and feasibility of elective high-risk percutaneous coronary intervention procedures with left ventricular support of the Impella Recover LP 2.5. *Am J Cardiol* 97(7):990–992, 2006. doi:10.1016/j.amjcard.2005.10.037.
60. Dangas GD, Kini AS, Sharma SK, et al: Impact of hemodynamic support with Impella 2.5 versus intra-aortic balloon pump on prognostically important clinical outcomes in patients undergoing high-risk percutaneous coronary intervention (from the PROTECT II randomized trial). *Am J Cardiol* 113(2):222–228, 2014. doi:10.1016/j.amjcard.2013.09.008.
61. Sjauw KD, Konorza T, Erbel R, et al: Supported high-risk percutaneous coronary intervention with the Impella 2.5 device the Europella registry. *J Am Coll Cardiol* 54(25):2430–2434, 2009. doi:10.1016/j.jacc.2009.09.018.
62. Dixon SR, Henriques JP, Mauri L, et al: A prospective feasibility trial investigating the use of the Impella 2.5 system in patients undergoing high-risk percutaneous coronary intervention (The PROTECT I Trial): initial U.S. experience. *JACC Cardiovasc Interv* 2(2):91–96, 2009. doi:10.1016/j.jcin.2008.11.005.
63. Alasnag MA, Gardi DO, Elder M, et al: Use of the Impella 2.5 for prophylactic circulatory support during elective high-risk percutaneous coronary intervention. *Cardiovasc Revasc Med* 12(5):299–303, 2011. doi:10.1016/j.carrev.2011.02.002.
64. Maini B, Naidu SS, Mulukutla S, et al: Real-world use of the Impella 2.5 circulatory support system in complex high-risk percutaneous coronary intervention: the USpella Registry. *Catheter Cardiovasc Interv* 80(5):717–725, 2012. doi:10.1002/ccd.23403.
65. Cohen MG, Ghatak A, Kleiman NS, et al: Optimizing rotational atherectomy in high-risk percutaneous coronary interventions: insights from the PROTECT Iotalota study. *Catheter Cardiovasc Interv* 2013. doi:10.1002/ccd.25277.
66. Henriques PS, Ouweneel D, Naidu S, et al (2014) How can we best observe a learning curve in an ongoing clinical trial of percutaneous left ventricular support system? *Am Heart J* (In Press).
67. Stone GW, Mehran R, Dangas G, et al: Differential impact on survival of electrocardiographic Q-wave versus enzymatic myocardial infarction after percutaneous intervention: a device-specific analysis of 7147 patients. *Circulation* 104(6):642–647, 2001.
68. Kovacic J, Kini A, Banerjee S, et al: TCT-445 patients with 3-vessel coronary artery disease and impaired LVEF undergoing PCI with Impella 2.5 hemodynamic support have improved 90-day outcomes compared to intra-aortic balloon pump: a substudy of the PROTECT II trial. *J Am Coll Cardiol* 2013;62(18_S1):B137-B137 doi:10.1016/j.jacc.2013.08.1187.
69. Hochman JS, Sleeper LA, White HD, et al: One-year survival following early revascularization for cardiogenic shock. *JAMA* 285(2):190–192, 2001.
70. Kumpati GS, Tandar A, Patel A, et al: Impella 5.0 support in severe peripheral vascular disease via iliac artery approach. *Innovations (Phila)* 7(5):379–381, 2012. doi:10.1097/IMI.0b013e31827e3c0b.
71. Lotun K, Shetty R, Patel M, et al: Percutaneous left axillary artery approach for Impella 2.5 liter circulatory support for patients with severe aortoiliac arterial disease undergoing high-risk percutaneous coronary intervention. *J Interv Cardiol* 25(2):210–213, 2012. doi:10.1111/j.1540-8183.2011.00696.x.
72. Greenbaum A, O'Neill WW, Paone G, et al: Caval aortic access to allow transcatheter aortic valve replacement in patients otherwise ineligible: initial human experience. *JACC* 2014 (In Press).
73. Tanawuttiwat T, Chaparro SV: An unexpected cause of massive hemolysis in percutaneous left ventricular assist device. *Cardiovasc Revasc Med* 14(1):66–67, 2013. doi:10.1016/j.carrev.2012.10.011.
74. Elhussein TA, Hutchison SJ: Acute mitral regurgitation: unforeseen new complication of the Impella LP 5.0 ventricular assist device and review of literature. *Heart Lung Circ* 23(3):e100–e104, 2014. doi:10.1016/j.hlc.2013.10.098.
75. Toggweiler S, Jamshidi P, Erne P: Functional mitral stenosis: a rare complication of the Impella assist device. *Eur J Echocardiogr* 9(3):412–413, 2008. doi:10.1093/ejechocard/jen029.
76. Ranc S, Sibellas F, Green L: Acute intraventricular thrombosis of an Impella LP 5.0 device in an ST-elevated myocardial infarction complicated by cardiogenic shock. *J Invasive Cardiol* 25(1):E1–E3, 2013.
77. Garatti A, Colombo T, Russo C, et al: Impella Recover 100 microaxial left ventricular assist device: the Niguarda experience. *Transplant Proc* 36(3):623–626, 2004. doi:10.1016/j.transproceed.2004.02.051.
78. Cheng A, Swartz MF, Massey HT: Impella to unload the left ventricle during peripheral extracorporeal membrane oxygenation. *ASAIO J* 59(5):533–536, 2013. doi:10.1097/MAT.0b013e31829f0e52.
79. Vlasselaers D, Desmet M, Desmet L, et al: Ventricular unloading with a miniature axial flow pump in combination with extracorporeal membrane oxygenation. *Intensive Care Med* 32(2):329–333, 2006. doi:10.1007/s00134-005-0016-2.
80. Koeckert MS, Jorde UP, Naka Y, et al: Impella LP 2.5 for left ventricular unloading during venoarterial extracorporeal membrane oxygenation support. *J Card Surg* 26(6):666–668, 2011. doi:10.1111/j.1540-8191.2011.01338.x.
81. Chaparro SV, Badheka A, Marzouka GR, et al: Combined use of Impella left ventricular assist device and extracorporeal membrane oxygenation as a bridge to recovery in fulminant myocarditis. *ASAIO J* 58(3):285–287, 2012. doi:10.1097/MAT.0b013e31824b1f70.
82. Pozzi M, Quessard A, Nguyen A, et al: Using the Impella 5.0 with a right axillary artery approach as bridge to long-term mechanical circulatory assistance. *Int J Artif Organs* 36(9):605–611, 2013. doi:10.5301/ijao.5000237.
83. Patane F, Grassi R, Zucchetti MC, et al: The use of Impella Recover in the treatment of post-infarction ventricular septal defect: a new case report. *Int J Cardiol* 144(2):313–315, 2010. doi:10.1016/j.ijcard.2009.03.042.
84. La Torre MW, Centofanti P, Attisani M, et al: Posterior ventricular septal defect in presence of cardiogenic shock: early implantation of the Impella Recover LP 5.0 as a bridge to surgery. *Tex Heart Inst J* 38(1):42–49, 2011.
85. Londono JC, Martinez CA, Singh V, et al: Hemodynamic support with Impella 2.5 during balloon aortic valvuloplasty in a high-risk patient. *J Interv Cardiol* 24(2):193–197, 2011. doi:10.1111/j.1540-8183.2010.00625.x.
86. Martinez CA, Singh V, Londono JC, et al: Percutaneous retrograde left ventricular assist support for interventions in patients with aortic stenosis and left ventricular dysfunction. *Catheter Cardiovasc Interv* 80(7):1201–1209, 2012. doi:10.1002/ccd.24303.
87. Miller MA, Dukkipati SR, Chinitz JS, et al: Percutaneous hemodynamic support with Impella 2.5 during scar-related ventricular tachycardia ablation (PERMIT 1). *Circ Arrhythm Electrophysiol* 6(1):151–159, 2013. doi:10.1161/CIRCEP.112.975888.
88. Lu F, Eckman PM, Liao KK, et al: Catheter ablation of hemodynamically unstable ventricular tachycardia with mechanical circulatory support. *Int J Cardiol* 168(4):3859–3865, 2013. doi:10.1016/j.ijcard.2013.06.035.
89. Margey R, Chamakura S, Siddiqi S, et al: First experience with implantation of a percutaneous right ventricular Impella right side percutaneous support device as a bridge to recovery in acute right ventricular infarction complicated by cardiogenic shock in the United States. *Circ Cardiovasc Interv* 6(3):e37–e38, 2013. doi:10.1161/CIRCINTERVENTIONS.113.000283.

6 Radiation Safety in the Cardiac Catheterization Laboratory

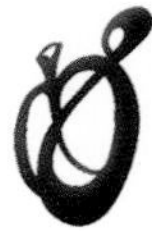

Frederick A. Heupler, Jr., Kevin Wunderle, Nicholas Shkumat, Robert Cecil, and Samir R. Kapadia

INTRODUCTION

Over the past few decades, major technological improvements in Cardiac Catheterization Laboratory (CCL) equipment have enabled acquisition of images with better quality at a potentially lower radiation dose. Concurrently, the number and complexity of angiographic procedures have been increasing, creating the risk of greater radiation exposure to angiographers, patients, and lab personnel. Angiographers have a responsibility to assure appropriate and safe use of radiographic equipment (**Table 6-1**).

Understanding of the following principles is crucial:

- Fluoroscopic equipment function
- Terminology of fluoroscopic modes, radiation doses
- Radiation-induced injuries
- Fluoroscopic image quality
- Minimization of procedural radiation exposure

This chapter provides an overview of these five topics with respect to cardiovascular angiography and intervention. Several excellent reviews on this subject are available.[1-5]

FLUOROSCOPIC EQUIPMENT FUNCTION

A fluoroscope is an x-ray–generating device that provides real-time radiographic imaging. Fluoroscopic equipment in the CCL characteristically consists of a large **c-arm, x-ray tube, image detector, generator,** and **operating console.** The radiographic images are subsequently processed and displayed on a high-performance **image display monitor.**[3]

C-Arm

The x-ray tube and image detector are affixed to opposite ends of the c-arm. The tube is mounted in a fixed orientation with respect to the detector on the c-arm typically positioned below the procedure table. The detector is mounted on a movable suspension above the table. This suspension permits the operator to raise or lower the detector in relation to the patient. The entire c-arm support system may be mounted directly on the floor, ceiling, or a robotically controlled device.

Most c-arms are capable of rotation speeds of up to 35 degrees/second and up to 100 degrees/second for CT-angiography and rotational angiography. Movement of the c-arm is commonly limited by proximity sensors that slow or stop rotation at a certain distance from the patient or the x-ray table.

X-Ray Tube

The x-ray tube consists of an evacuated glass or metal-enclosed assembly that contains a circular anode (positive electrode) and a cathode with one or more filaments (negative electrode). When an electric current is passed through the filament, its temperature increases and electrons are released through thermionic emission. These electrons are accelerated through a potential difference, focused on a small area of the rapidly rotating anode known as the focal spot track. The x-rays produced have a heterogeneous energy distribution dependent on the anode material and tube voltage. Typically, less than 1% of the energy applied to the x-ray tube is converted into x-rays; the majority is lost to heat. Management of this heat production is a major consideration in the design of x-ray tubes.

Characteristics of the x-ray tube include the following:

1. **MA (milliamperes):** The tube current or the number of electrons traveling across the anode-cathode gap per second. The x-ray output is linearly proportional to the tube current.

TABLE 6-1 Physician Responsibilities in the Cath Lab

• You control the radiation dose.
• You are responsible for radiation-induced injuries.
• You must learn how to limit the radiation dose.

2. **Pulse width:** The duration of time that x-rays are used to create a single fluoroscopic image. A shorter pulse width can better capture an image of a moving object. The pulse width for cardiac angiographic procedures varies from approximately 6 msec to 10 msec. X-ray output is linearly proportional to pulse width.
3. **MAs (milliamperes*sec):** The measure of the total charge, the product of the mA, and the pulse width (in seconds) for a given fluoroscopic image. X-ray output is linearly proportional to mAs.
4. **KVp (peak kilovoltage):** The measure of voltage applied across the anode-cathode gap that characterizes the distribution of photon energies within the x-ray beam. Increasing the kVp increases the mean photon energy of the x-ray spectrum, resulting in a more penetrating beam. The tube voltage has a complex relationship to x-ray output, which can be approximated as a power $\left[\frac{kVp_{final}}{kVp_{initial}}\right]^2$ relationship. For example, doubling the peak kilovoltage approximately quadruples the x-ray output.
5. **Focal spot:** A well-defined region on the anode where the accelerated electrons are focused and x-rays are produced. Most x-ray tubes have two or more focal spots, each paired with a dedicated cathode filament. The focal spot size can vary from approximately 0.3 mm to 1.0 mm for cardiac angiographic systems. The limited heat capacity of the anode dictates that when the total heat deposited exceeds a certain threshold, the focal spot must change to a larger size to distribute the electrons over a larger area to prevent anode damage.
6. **X-ray filtration:** The x-ray beam passes through numerous materials prior to reaching the patient. These include substances inherent to the tube (glass/metal assembly, oil, exit port) and those added for spectral shaping (aluminum and/or copper sheets) contained within the collimator. Modern systems allow for variable filtration that can be changed within a procedure or between protocols. This added filtration disproportionately reduces the number of lower energy photons, thereby increasing the average photon energy. This process is referred to as "beam hardening," which can reduce the skin entrance dose for a given detector dose.

Image Detector

Digital flat-panel detectors have replaced the older image intensifier technology in virtually all modern CCL equipment. The vast majority of these detectors uses an amorphous silicon detector coupled with a two-dimensional thin-film transistor (TFT) array. The physical size of detector elements (pixels) ranges from 80 to 200 microns, or one twelfth to one fifth of a millimeter.

1. **Image detector function:** Digital flat panel detectors convert x-ray energy into a digital signal via a process that converts the x-rays into light, which is then converted into an electric signal via photodiodes. Once the x-ray pulse has terminated, the stored information is sampled, amplified, digitized, and transmitted to the nearby workstation. The resulting data then undergo image processing prior to display.
2. **Automatic dose rate control (or automatic brightness control):** In all fluoroscopy systems, the detector acts as the critical component of a feedback loop that regulates the output of x-rays (mA, kVp, pulse width, filtration, and focal spot size). Automatic dose rate control (ADRC) ensures that the dose to the detector is sufficient to provide adequate image quality, accounting for changes in patient size, thickness, and presence of highly attenuating structures. For instance, changing from narrow to steep angulations increases the effective patient thickness. The ADRC increases output parameters to ensure that the image quality is similar to previously obtained images.

Operator Consoles

The angiographer employs the bedside console to control movements of the c-arm and table, field of view, magnification mode, and clinical protocol/techniques. A foot pedal is used to control the duration of x-ray exposure and the type of image that is desired (fluoroscopy/acquisition). The operating console in the nearby control room provides the interface between the operator and the imaging and EKG/hemodynamic systems. It communicates with the image display system, the PACS (Picture Archiving and Communication System), and the EMR (Electronic Medical Record).

Image Display Monitor

Visualization of images on the overhead monitor is an integral part of all angiographic procedures. Monitors vary in size from 17 to 60 inches and should be routinely evaluated to ensure appropriate luminance, grayscale performance, contrast, resolution, spatial linearity, and absence of artifacts. Any issue that impairs the ability of the angiographer to evaluate fluoroscopic images may prolong the procedure and unnecessarily increase the radiation dose. It is not only the monitor that is important but also the display environment, where important variables include the following:

- **Distance:** The optimal viewing distance between the angiographer to the monitor is a factor of 1.5 to 2.0 of the diagonal. For instance, with a 19-inch display, this distance is about 2½ to 3 feet or slightly more than an arm's length.
- **Viewing conditions:** Bright ambient lights within the angiographic suite increase glare on the image monitors, which decreases the ability of the angiographer to visualize differences in shades of gray. Also, glare and reflections from spot lighting near the operator have the potential to interfere with image evaluation.

TERMINOLOGY OF FLUOROSCOPIC MODES, RADIATION DOSES

There is wide variability in the terms describing fluoroscopic operational modes and radiation doses. To minimize confusion, the following terminology is used in this chapter.

Terminology of Fluoroscopic Modes

Historically, the terms "fluoro" and "cine" have been used to denote two different modes of radiographic image observation and/or recording. Fluoro has been used to describe real-time observation of lower dose radiographic temporal

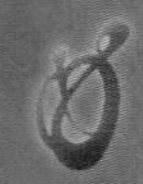

imaging without recording. Cine has been used to describe the recording of higher dose and image quality radiographic temporal imaging. However, the term cine implies the use of motion picture film in the recording of the radiographically produced images. Modern systems no longer employ film; recording is exclusively digital and available for all operational modes, including fluoroscopy.

These two modes of operation shall be defined for this chapter as follows:

1. **Fluoro** (or **fluoroscopic observation)** describes the real-time temporal imaging performed at or below radiation output limits established by regulatory agencies. Fluoro typically defaults to nonrecorded imaging; however, an operator can choose to save either a single fluoro image or image sequence at the operator controls.
2. **Acquisition** describes the mode of operation that requires recording of the real-time imaging, employing increased radiation output that is needed for high-quality images. This mode of imaging is *not* governed by regulatory limits, and it is limited only by hardware capability or by design parameters established by the vendor not typically accessible to the end user without service support.

Within the fluoroscopic mode of operation there are typically three radiation output/image quality levels selectable by the operator. These settings are customizable and can vary greatly between fluoroscopic units. Generally there is a "low dose" fluoro level that is nominally set at 50% of the "standard dose" and a "high dose" level set at 200% of the standard dose level. In the United States, federal regulations pertaining to manufacturers limit the radiation output for the fluoroscopic imaging modes under specific conditions. For the standard and low dose fluoroscopic imaging modes, the air kerma limit is 88 mGy/min (10 R/min in traditional units). The high dose fluoro mode may, given certain additional requirements, extend the air kerma limit to 176 mGy/min (20 R/min). For c-arm fluoroscopes these limitations are defined at 30 cm from the face of the image receptor, regardless of the source to image distance (SID). Again, the acquisition imaging mode of operation does not include regulatory radiation output limitations. Acquisition rates can range from approximately 10 mGy/min to 3000 mGy/min and under most circumstances fall between 100 mGy/min to 300 mGy/min.

Terminology of Radiation Doses

It is important for angiographers to become familiar with the nomenclature of radiation doses to understand basic concepts of radiation dose reduction. This nomenclature is complicated due to different aspects of a "dose" and the proliferation of different systems for naming dose quantities. Dosimetric units within this chapter follow the S.I. standard (Système International)[1,5,6] (**Table 6-2**).

TABLE 6-2 Terminology of Radiation Doses

TYPE OF DOSE	S.I. UNIT	DEFINITION/PURPOSE
Kerma (K)	Gray (Gy)	Sum of initial kinetic energies released in material per unit mass
Air kerma at IRP ($K_{a,r}$)	Gray (Gy)	Kerma in air at the IRP
Air kerma rate at IRP ($\dot{K}_{a,r}$)	Gray/sec (Gy/s)	Instantaneous rate of air kerma at IRP
Air kerma area product (KAP or DAP)	Gy* cm^2	Air kerma × field size; indicative of stochastic risk
Absorbed dose (D)	Gray (Gy)	Mean energy/unit mass by ionizing radiation to a material
Peak skin dose ($D_{skin,max}$)	Gray (Gy)	Maximum absorbed dose at one skin area; indicates skin injury risk
Effective dose (ED)	Sievert (Sv)	Estimate of stochastic risk due to x-ray exposure

1. **Absorbed Dose/Peak Skin Dose ($D_{skin,max}$)**
   Absorbed dose is defined as the amount of energy absorbed per unit mass in units of gray (Gy). This quantity does not reflect the total amount of energy deposited because it is normalized to mass. Since dose in fluoroscopic cases is distributed, it is the peak skin dose ($D_{skin,max}$), which is the best indicator of radiation-induced cutaneous injury. $D_{skin,max}$ is defined as the maximum radiation dose to any one area of skin at the entrance of the x-ray beam into the body during a fluoroscopic exam. This dose estimate is not displayed on current fluoroscopic equipment because there is no convenient method for its measurement. One method that can provide $D_{skin,max}$ in delayed fashion is radiochromic film dosimetry. A thin sheet of this film can be placed between the source and the patient's skin in the direct path of the primary x-ray beam. At the end of the procedure, the film will reveal the two-dimensional radiation dose distribution, including backscatter.[4] With appropriate calibration curves applied, the scanned film can be used to determine the $D_{skin,max}$. A similar result can be obtained by using multiple small calibrated thermoluminescent dosimeters applied at the anticipated location(s) of maximal dose.
2. **Kerma/Air Kerma at the Reference Plane ($K_{a,r}$)**
   Kerma (K) is defined as the kinetic energy released in matter, which is expressed in units of Gy. The displayed quantity $K_{a,r}$, refers to the kerma in the air at the interventional reference plane (IRP) expressed in units of Gy. The IRP was defined by the International Electrotechnical Commission (IEC) as the plane located 15 cm below the isocenter of the c-arm in the direction of the focal spot. This plane is irrespective of the table height, source to image distance, or c-arm positioning. This location puts the patient's skin surface at or near the IRP for a 30-cm thick patient with the axial center of the body at isocenter of the c-arm. Since there is no convenient way to directly measure $D_{skin,max}$, $K_{a,r}$ is commonly used as a surrogate.[4,6]

   There are several reasons why $K_{a,r}$ does not always accurately reflect the $D_{skin,max}$:

   a. The IRP and the plane of the skin entrance commonly differ, depending on the rotation and angulation of the c-arm, the distance from the x-ray tube to the patient, the thickness of the patient, and the height of the table used for the procedure. Two examples illustrate the problems with using $K_{a,r}$ as a direct surrogate for $D_{skin,max}$:
      1. In a scenario where the patient is thin (20 cm thick), the table is maximally elevated, the x-ray tube is located as far as possible from the patient, the image detector is close to the patient's chest, and two views are acquired at two very shallow, nonoverlapping fields: the displayed $K_{a,r}$ may overestimate the $D_{skin,max}$ by a factor of 3.

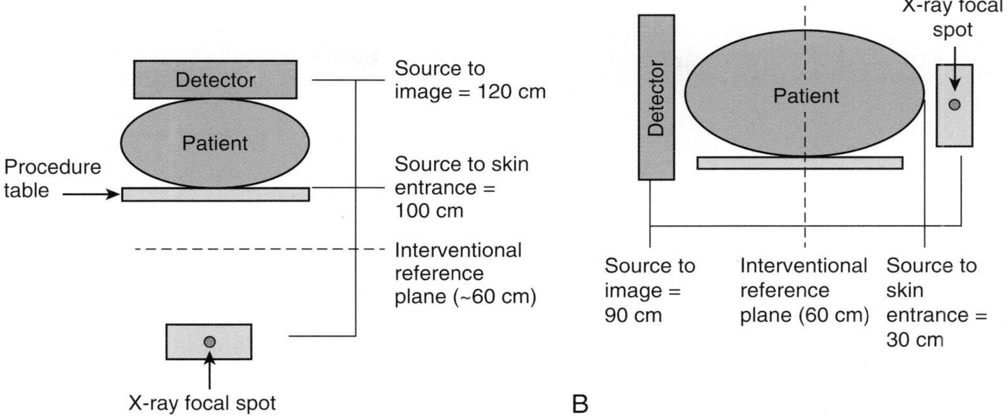

FIGURE 6-1 Relation of IRP to skin entrance site. A, Scenario 1: The x-ray source is far from the thin patient. In PA projection, a thin adult is located far from the x-ray tube. The source to image distance is 120 cm; the source to skin entrance is 100 cm; IRP is 60 cm above the x-ray source. The air kerma at the IRP overestimates the air kerma at the skin entrance. **B,** Scenario 2: The x-ray source is close to the thick patient. In lateral projection, a thick adult is located close to the x-ray tube. The source to image detector distance is 90 cm; the source to skin entrance distance is 30 cm; IRP is 60 cm above the x-ray source. The air kerma at the reference plane underestimates the air kerma at the skin entrance. *(Reused with permission. From Griffin et al. The Cleveland Clinic Cardiology Board Review, 2e. LWW.)*

2. In a scenario where the patient is thick (50 cm in lateral dimension), the x-ray tube is close to the patient, and one lateral view is obtained, the $K_{a,r}$ may underestimate the $D_{skin,max}$, giving a displayed estimate of skin dose that is less than half of the actual dose (**Figure 6-1**).

b. Angiographers commonly employ multiple angulations during fluoro and acquisitions, which results in spreading the skin dose over a wide area, often with no consistent overlap of one area of skin. However, the $K_{a,r}$ includes the contributions of all fluoro and acquisitions as if they had overlapped. The result is that $K_{a,r}$ will overestimate the $D_{skin,max}$ when there is no consistent overlap.

c. The quantity air kerma is defined only in air, whereas skin dose refers to an absorbed dose that is affected by the absorption characteristics of skin.

d. $D_{skin,max}$ includes backscattered radiation from within the body, but $K_{a,r}$ does not. Backscatter may increase the $D_{skin,max}$ by 10% to 40%, depending on beam area and energy.

e. The current requirement for accuracy of the displayed air kerma is ±35% (IEC standard). This means that a procedure in one CCL vs. the same procedure on the same patient in another laboratory may potentially result in a difference of 70% in the displayed air kerma. The accuracy of these quantities should be evaluated annually by a qualified medical physicist and included in any formal radiation dose evaluation.

f. The procedure table and cushion are usually in the path of the primary x-ray beam before the patient's skin entrance. These objects may attenuate the beam by approximately 20% to 40%, depending on photon energy and other secondary factors. This attenuation is not accounted for in the displayed $K_{a,r}$.

As a result of the above reasons, $K_{a,r}$ may overestimate or underestimate the $D_{skin,max}$ by as much as a factor of 4.[1,2,5]

Air Kerma Rate at the Reference Plane ($\dot{K}_{a,r}$)

$\dot{K}_{a,r}$ is the air kerma at the IRP per unit time. It is generally displayed in units of mGy/min. Since it is an instantaneous measurement, it is usually displayed only during x-ray generation. The air kerma rate is a convenient way for an angiographer to instantaneously detect a change in radiation output with changes in c-arm angulation.

3. **Air Kerma Area Product ($P_{k,a}$) or Dose Area Product (DAP)**
Air kerma area product, $P_{k,a}$ (or DAP), is the product of the $K_{a,r}$ and the area of the x-ray beam at the reference plane. It is generally displayed in units of Gy*cm^2. (When $P_{k,a}$ is expressed in μGy*m^2, divide by 100 to convert to Gy*cm^2.) Since the $P_{k,a}$ is the sum of $K_{a,r}$ over the x-ray beam area, it reflects the total amount of energy impinging on the patient's body. $P_{k,a}$ is typically measured in the laboratory by a "DAP meter," a large ionization chamber within the x-ray collimator housing. DAP is independent of the plane of measurement: The DAP near the patient is the same as the DAP near the x-ray tube.

4. **Effective Dose (ED)**
Effective dose (ED) expressed in milliSieverts (mSv) is a value that relates a radiation absorbed dose and radiobiological significance to a stochastic risk such as carcinogenesis. The ED may be estimated by multiplying the DAP by a conversion factor, based on a specific type of procedure and the type of irradiated tissue. This factor may be approximated as 0.12 mSv/Gy*cm^2 for diagnostic coronary angiography and 0.18 to 0.28 for coronary intervention procedures. ED is not provided by the fluoroscopic equipment. Typical EDs for CCL procedures follow: approximately 4 mSv to 8 mSv for diagnostic cases and 8 mSv to 15 mSv for coronary intervention cases.[7-10]

RADIATION-INDUCED INJURIES

Deterministic Risk of Radiation

Deterministic effects of radiation are those in which the severity of the injury increases with an increasing radiation dose and in which there is a threshold dose for onset of injury. Typical examples of deterministic injury are erythema of the skin, localized hair loss, pigmentation changes, cataracts, and, in severe cases, skin necrosis and ulceration[5,11] (**Table 6-3**).

Multiple factors may affect the sensitivity of the skin to radiation-induced injury, including fair skin, collagen

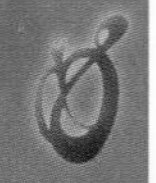

TABLE 6-3 Skin Injury and Radiation Doses

EFFECT	ABSORBED DOSE (GY)	ONSET
Transient erythema, hair loss	2-3	Hours/weeks
Persistent erythema, hair loss	6-7	1-3 weeks
Skin fibrosis, atrophy	10-11	1-3 months
Wet skin loss	15	1 month
Skin necrosis, ulceration	18+	2-5 months

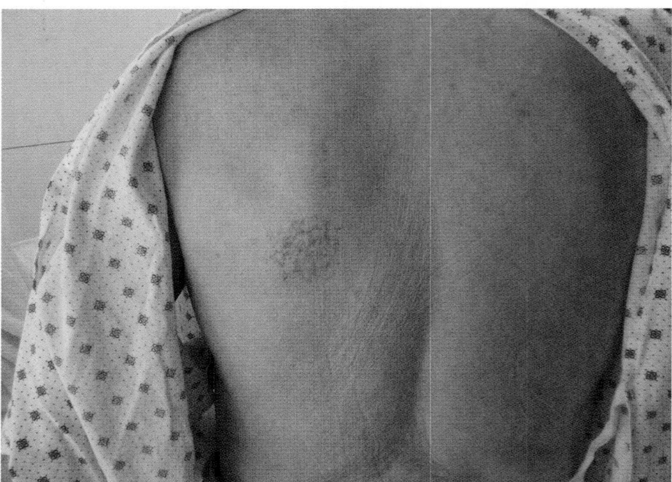

FIGURE 6-2 Radiation-induced skin injury. Left infrascapular telangiectases and skin induration. Mildly pruritic, indurated skin with telangiectases following five left coronary artery percutaneous intervention procedures. Another percutaneous intervention on the left coronary artery would carry significant risk of severe skin injury in this area.

diseases, malnutrition, steroids, diabetes mellitus, chemotherapeutics, and previous radiation exposure at the same site. Predicting the likelihood of radiation-induced skin injury with repeated subsequent exposures is complex, and it depends on the cumulative dose received and the length of time between exposures. As long as permanent skin injury was not induced with a previous exposure, it is likely that the exposed skin will recover completely, but this process occurs over a period of at least 6 months or more.

Minor transient skin erythema is not likely to occur until the $D_{skin,max}$ exceeds about 2 Gy. Persistent or permanent hair loss or pigmentary changes are likely to occur only after $D_{skin,max}$ exceeds 5 Gy (**Figure 6-2**). Telangiectases, dermal atrophy, and skin induration occur only after $D_{skin,max}$ exceeds about 10 Gy. Skin necrosis and ulceration typically do not occur in healthy patients until the peak skin dose has exceeded about 15 Gy.[11]

These estimates of dose-related injury apply only to the **localized area of skin that has received total absorbed doses of radiation exceeding these quantities**. This is best demonstrated by the map of overlapping patterns of peak dose demonstrated on a radiochromic film. Diagnostic coronary angiography typically involves multiple cranial, caudal, RAO, and LAO projections, which distribute the radiation dose over multiple areas of skin. Coronary intervention cases typically involve the same or similar fields of view for each lesion treated (**Table 6-4**).

There are no official limits on the $D_{skin,max}$ that a patient may receive during coronary diagnostic or interventional

TABLE 6-4 Typical Radiation Doses per Procedure

DOSE	COR ANGIO	PCI
$K_{a,r}$ (mGy)	400-800	800-1500
KAP (Gy*cm^2)	30-60	60-120

procedures. However, the Joint Commission (JC) has defined a "sentinel event" for fluoroscopy resulting from cumulative skin dose exceeding 15 Gy to a single field, which requires reporting to the institution's Quality Review Board. The term "cumulative" has not been defined explicitly by the JC; however, it has recommended inclusion of all fluoroscopic exams within a 6- to 12-month period. If a patient undergoes multiple high-dose angiographic procedures within this time frame, it is advisable to consult with a qualified medical physicist regarding the likelihood of radiation-induced skin injury before proceeding with another elective high-dose procedure.

Stochastic Risk of Radiation

A stochastic (or probabilistic) risk of radiation exposure is one in which the likelihood of injury occurs on the basis of statistical probability. The **likelihood** of stochastic injury is proportional to the radiation dose magnitude, but the **severity** of a stochastic injury is not. It is generally accepted that stochastic risk has no dose threshold for injury, although this is controversial. The currently accepted model of stochastic injury is the "linear no-threshold" (LNT) model, which theorizes that risk is linearly proportional to dose. The LNT model indicates that there is no dose at which risk is not present.[8,10,12,13]

Stochastic effects of radiation include malignancy and birth defects. Certain tissues are particularly sensitive to radiation-induced malignancy, including colon, stomach, breast, lung, and bone marrow. The latency period between radiation exposure and detection of malignancy varies greatly among different tissues and different patients: as little as 7 years for leukemia to 20 years or more for other malignancies.

The lifetime risk for radiation-induced malignancy is related not only to radiation dose but also to age at exposure. Younger age is associated with an increased lifetime risk of radiation-induced malignancy.[13]

The "average" lifetime risk of malignancy from all causes is 30%, and the risk of death due to malignancy is 15%. The contribution of radiation exposure to this risk is small. There is approximately a 1% increased lifetime risk of malignancy for every 100 mSv of acute effective dose. The average effective dose from natural background radiation exposure is approximately 3 mSv/yr. For comparison, typical effective doses for various medical radiographic procedures are summarized in **Table 6-5.** Please note that dose ranges for radiographic procedures are a moving target, because they have generally been decreasing over the years[10,12,14] (**Table 6-5**).

FLUOROSCOPIC IMAGE QUALITY

The basic purpose of fluoroscopic imaging is to obtain adequate image quality to make a diagnosis or conduct an intervention. Reductions in the radiation dose have the potential to decrease image quality. Therefore, we cannot institute broad measures to reduce radiation doses without taking into account the effects that these changes will have

TABLE 6-5 Typical Effective Doses for X-Ray Exposure

PROCEDURE	EFFECTIVE DOSE (M-SV)
Background dose/yr (E. Coast/Denver, Col.)	2.5/9
PA/Lat chest x-ray	0.1
Diagnostic coronary angiogram	4-8
Coronary CT angiogram	8-12
PCI	8-15
Interventional cardiologist/year	3

on image quality.[3] The following are key characteristics of fluoroscopic image quality.

Spatial Resolution

Spatial resolution refers to the ability to differentiate fine detail within an image. The "limiting" spatial resolution is the smallest distance in space that two objects can be separated and still appear distinct. This is important in cardiac angiography for the perception and delineation of small vessels, fine wires, and anatomic boundaries. Factors that can significantly influence the achievable spatial resolution include the focal spot size, geometric magnification, and presence of motion. Since the focal spot has a finite size, it causes the edges of objects to appear blurred within a projected image. This phenomenon, called a "penumbra," is linearly proportional to the size of the focal spot. The penumbra is also influenced by the location of the imaged object, relative to the tube and detector. As the geometric magnification increases (object moved closer to the source), the blur increases. An object moving within the duration of a single pulse width will also appear blurred; this is referred to as motion blur.[3]

Contrast Resolution

Contrast resolution is the ability of a system to resolve differences in signal intensity (pixel values) or shades of gray. Contrast resolution is important in cardiac angiography for detecting small differences in attenuation, for instance, a contrast-filled artery overlying the spine or diaphragm. Contrast can be divided into three categories: subject, detector, and display. Subject contrast is dependent on the object being imaged (composition, size) and the x-ray beam quality (kVp, filtration). Detector contrast is dependent on the type of detector and its response to radiation. Display contrast is influenced by ambient lighting, monitor brightness and linearity, matrix size, and bit depth. Typically, cardiovascular images are displayed in 256 shades of gray.

Temporal Resolution

Temporal resolution is the ability to resolve two events separated in time. This is directly dependent on fluoroscopic pulse width and the time **between** pulses, as temporal resolution is assessed over multiple images. For instance, an acquisition acquired at 3 frames/s will have a temporal resolution 10 times poorer than one acquired at 30 frames/s. This is irrespective of spatial resolution, which occurs **within** a pulse width and is assessed in a single image. To reduce noise and/or dose, frame averaging is often utilized, at the cost of temporal resolution.

Noise

Noise is broadly defined as information contained within an image that is not useful or interferes with the clinical task. Typically it is divided into three main categories: quantum, detector, and anatomic noise.

1. **Quantum Noise:** The most familiar form of noise, quantum noise or "mottle," is an inherent property of x-ray imaging. This type of noise is proportional to the number of quanta (x-rays) used to form the image and decreases as the dose to the detector is increased. The relationship between relative image noise and detector dose is approximately a square root. To reduce the proportion of noise by a factor of 2, the detector dose must be increased by a factor of 4. Image processing techniques such as spatial and temporal filtering can be used to reduce quantum noise in an image; however, these may decrease spatial and temporal resolution.
2. **Detector Noise:** Flat-panel detectors are not flawless, and they contain various nonuniformities. Unlike quantum noise, these nonuniformities are both structured and random in nature. Structured noise is due to fixed nonuniformities in detector response, variation in sensitivity, and linearity. Random noise includes electronic noise as well as sporadic malfunctioning individual detector elements or electronics. Structured detector noise can be addressed through calibration and image processing, whereas random noise cannot.
3. **Anatomic Noise:** Anatomic noise is radiographic information that is unimportant for the diagnostic or therapeutic task. In cardiac interventions, the most common form of anatomic noise is the presence of bony anatomy. At very high detector doses, anatomic noise dominates over quantum and detector noise.
4. **Subtraction Angiography:** Subtraction angiography creates a special situation with respect to noise. The process of subtracting one image from another can significantly reduce anatomic noise and some forms of detector noise. However, subtraction angiography does not decrease quantum mottle, because this form of noise is randomly distributed in both images. This produces increased noise in the subtracted image if standard radiation doses are used. To maintain similar noise characteristics, subtracted images require an increased detector dose compared to unsubtracted images. This increase may be as much as 10 to 20 times the dose/frame of standard-dose acquisition images. Angiographers usually employ low frame rates with subtraction angiography to conserve the radiation dose.

Summary of Fluoroscopic Image Quality Characteristics

Fluoroscopic image quality is unavoidably affected by the interaction among spatial resolution, temporal resolution, contrast resolution, and noise. Any modification to improve one has the potential to adversely affect another. It is the responsibility of the angiographer to understand the interaction among these image quality characteristics.

MINIMIZATION OF PROCEDURAL RADIATION EXPOSURE

Angiographers who operate fluoroscopic equipment in the CCL have a responsibility to minimize radiation exposure while obtaining sufficient imaging information. The **ALARA**

TABLE 6-6 Minimizing Radiation Exposure to the Patient

1. Decrease the number and duration of acquisitions and fluoroscopy time.
2. Decrease the fluoro and acquisition frame rates.
3. Decrease the dose per the fluoro and acquisition frames.
4. Substitute the fluoroscopic recording for the standard dose acquisition.
5. Decrease the patient to image detector distance.
6. Increase the source to skin distance.
7. Minimize the c-arm angulation.
8. Vary the c-arm angulation to minimize repetitive exposure.
9. Exclude body parts outside the area of interest.
10. Use low-dose acquisition software or hardware.
11. Limit the use of digital magnification.
12. Apply collimation where appropriate.
13. Minimize the use of subtraction angiography.
14. Apply the "frequent flyer" rule for repeat interventions.

principle establishes that radiation exposure to the patient, angiographer, and CCL personnel should be maintained **As Low As Reasonably Achievable.** This principle encourages angiographers to aim for the lowest radiation dose that will produce image quality that is adequate for the goal of the study, not for a dose that will produce optimal image quality. In addition to maintaining a low radiation dose to the patient, it is important to assure proper protection of the angiographer and lab personnel. Both of these aspects of radiation protection are discussed below.

Radiation Exposure to the Patient

Every angiographer should be familiar with specific methods for reducing patient radiation exposure. These are summarized in **Table 6-6** and discussed in detail below.

1. **Decrease the Number and Duration of Acquisitions and Fluoroscopy Time:** The need to limit the number of acquisitions must be weighed against the need to obtain adequate information regarding angiographic anatomy, especially the origins and bifurcations of blood vessels. The length of acquisition runs should be limited, while long enough to see collaterals. The angiographer should never press the fluoro pedal when not observing the monitor. The modality can be programmed to limit the duration of acquisition runs to prevent overheating the x-ray tube. Although the default maximum acquisition run length may be 30 seconds, it is usually preferable to decrease this to no more than 15 or 20 seconds. It is rarely necessary to continue acquisition runs longer than this. The angiographer should minimize the number and duration of acquisition runs and the duration of fluoroscopy.
2. **Decrease Frame Rates for Fluoro and Acquisition:** Most CCL angiographic systems offer choices to select fluoroscopic and acquisition frame rates. Typically, these frame rates are set as low as 7.5 to 10 pulses per second. Acquisition frame rates may be increased to 15 frames per second or more to capture additional information when overlapping coronary arteries move back and forth across each other in certain views or to improve visualization of flow-related phenomena. The angiographer should employ the lowest fluoroscopy pulse rates and the lowest acquisition frame rates compatible with obtaining adequate information.
3. **Decrease Dose per Frame for Fluoro and Acquisition:** Pulsed fluoroscopy is universally employed in modern fluoroscopy systems. Nearly all systems offer a choice of detector dose per frame for fluoroscopy and acquisition. The angiographer should start with the lowest dose and then increase as needed. These settings may require the assistance of vendor service or application support. The angiographer should use the lowest dose per frame for fluoroscopy and acquisition, consistent with obtaining adequate diagnostic information.
4. **Substitute Fluoroscopic Recording for Standard Dose Acquisition:** Some angiographic systems permit the recording of fluoroscopic images with doses that are one fifth to one tenth of standard higher dose acquisitions. The fluoroscopic recording mode should be employed instead of standard dose acquisitions when the fluoro recording provides adequate image quality.
5. **Decrease Patient to Image Detector Distance:** When the image detector is not positioned as close as reasonably possible to the patient, several effects occur:
   a. The patient dose increases.
   b. Scattered radiation increases, resulting in a higher occupational dose.
   c. Geometric magnification increases image blurring.

   In summary, when the angiographer positions the image detector farther away from the patient, there is a double penalty: image quality is degraded, and the radiation dose is increased[1] (**Figure 6-3**). The angiographer should position the image detector as close as possible to the surface of the patient's chest during radiographic imaging.
6. **Increase Source to Skin Distance:** The closer the x-ray tube is to the patient's skin, the greater the peak skin dose and the scattered dose. The source to skin distance is increased by raising the table, because the x-ray tube is in a fixed position on the c-arm below the table. Tall angiographers have an advantage over their shorter colleagues because they may more easily perform catheter manipulation with the table elevated. Some state laws require a cone to be placed above the x-ray tube to act as a "spacer" to ensure a minimum distance between the tube and the patient (see **Figure 6-3**).[1] The operator should try to keep the patient as far away from the x-ray source as possible to limit the radiation dose.
7. **Minimize C-arm Angulation:** When the c-arm is positioned in steep RAO/LAO and/or cranial/caudal angulations, the length of the x-ray path through the patient increases, compared to the PA projection. This causes an increase in the peak skin dose for two reasons:
   a. The source to skin distance is decreased.
   b. The ADRC increases radiation output to maintain a constant detector dose. As a rule of thumb, approximately 25% of the x-ray beam intensity is attenuated for each 1 cm of soft tissue. After traversing an additional 4 cm of additional soft tissue, the x-ray beam is attenuated to about one third of the original beam intensity. An increase in patient body thickness requires an increase in the x-ray dose, similar to the effect of increasing angulation. This means the x-ray beam must increase in intensity by about three times to compensate for the added attenuation.

   As the c-arm rotates into the cranial, caudal, or lateral projection, the radiation dose increases approximately as the square of the angle. This means that small increases in angulation below 30 degrees produce only small increases in the dose, but the same small

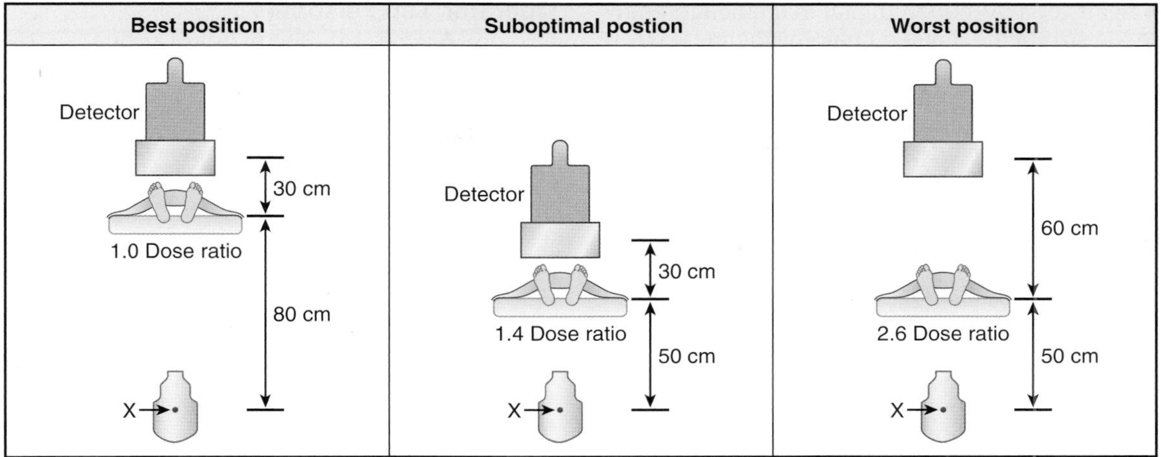

FIGURE 6-3 Relation of table height to skin entrance dose. BEST position: The patient is located far from the x-ray source; the image detector is close to the patient. This position maximizes the skin entrance dose. SUBOPTIMAL position: The patient is closer to the x-ray source; the image detector remains close to the patient. Proximity of the patient to the x-ray source increases the skin entrance dose by about 40%. WORST position: The patient remains closer to the x-ray source; the image detector is now elevated away from the patient. The combination of the patient proximity to the x-ray source and increased distance of the image detector from the patient results in a skin entrance dose that is more than 2½ times the dose in the "BEST" position.

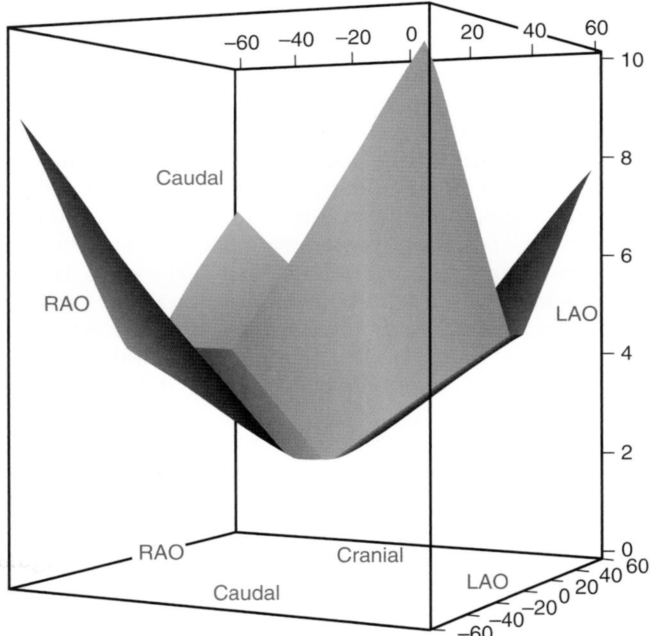

FIGURE 6-4 Air kerma rates and c-arm angulation. Three-dimensional representation of air kerma rates (mGy/sec on the ordinate) in relation to c-arm angulation during coronary angiographic acquisitions. Data are derived from more than 35,000 acquisitions at the Cleveland Clinic. LAO angulations were associated with higher air kerma rates per degree of angulation rather than RAO and caudal angulations with higher air kerma rather than cranial. *(Courtesy of Samir Kapadia, MD.)*

increases in angulation between 30 and 60 degrees produce disproportionately large increases in the dose[1,15] (**Figure 6-4**).

At high doses, overheating of the anode may be prevented by increasing either focal spot size, pulse width, or both. A larger focal spot produces a larger penumbra on the image receptor, which accounts for "focal spot blurring," decreased spatial resolution, and degraded image quality. A longer pulse width increases motion blur in rapidly moving structures.

The angiographer should limit RAO/LAO and cranial/caudal angulation of the c-arm to the minimum necessary to obtain the required information.

8. **Vary C-arm Angulation to Minimize Repetitive Exposure:** With subsequent acquisitions, angiographers commonly vary c-arm angulations during diagnostic angiography, less so during coronary intervention procedures. This variation in c-arm angulations minimizes the number of repetitive exposures of the same radiation entry site, thereby decreasing the skin dose at that site. Although this variation is easy to achieve in diagnostic cases, it is more difficult in coronary intervention cases, because of the need to repeatedly visualize a single area of interest.[1]

   The angiographer should attempt to vary the c-arm angulation to avoid repetitive radiation exposure of the same area of skin.
9. **Exclude Body Parts Outside the Area of Interest:** With steep angulations, it is common for the patient's arm to appear in the field of view, overlapping the arteries being visualized. When this occurs, the angiographer should move the patient's arm outward to avoid the higher radiation dose and unnecessary exposure of the arm to radiation.[3]

   The angiographer should reposition body parts that inappropriately overlap the vessels being visualized angiographically.
10. **Use Low Dose Acquisition Software or Hardware:** Some fluoroscopic systems offer a separate "low dose acquisition" pedal or selectable protocol that can lower the standard acquisition dose. The dose per frame with low dose acquisition can generally be lowered about 50% compared to the standard dose acquisition. Although low dose acquisition may not be suitable for obese patients or steeply angulated views, it is commonly useful for other situations.

    When low dose acquisition is available, it should be used if it produces adequate image quality.
11. **Limit the Use of Digital Magnification:** Magnification of a digital flat panel image, e.g., from 22 cm field of view

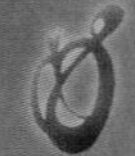

(7 inches) to 16 cm (5 inches), can increase peak skin dose by nearly 50%. Although digital magnification may increase the size of the imaged anatomy, the increase in dose may require the use of a larger focal spot, which decreases spatial resolution.

Angiographers should limit the use of digital magnification provided that adequate information can be obtained at the larger field of view.

12. **Apply Collimation Where Appropriate:** Collimation reduces the x-ray field of view, thereby decreasing radiation dose to tissue outside the area of interest. This reduces scattered radiation, which improves image quality and reduces occupational exposure. Collimation reduces the dose area product; however, it does not reduce the peak skin dose in the area being irradiated.

    Appropriate collimation can reduce the effective dose to the patient but not the peak skin dose.
13. **Minimize the Use of Subtraction Angiography:** Although subtraction angiography provides the advantages of removing anatomical noise, such as bony structures, it requires a marked increase in dose per frame. This is why subtracted images are characteristically obtained at low frame rates of 3 to 4 frames/sec.[1,3] Angiographers should restrict subtraction angiography to situations where it is necessary, because of the markedly increased radiation dose per frame.
14. **Apply the "Frequent Flyer" Rule for Repeat Interventions:** Patients who have had previous coronary intervention procedures may present a challenge with regard to evaluating the risk of skin injury with a subsequent procedure. This is especially true if the patient has had multiple interventional procedures on the same obstruction or has had one or more prolonged procedures, such as a chronic total occlusion. The risk of serious skin injury is greatly magnified if even mild permanent skin injury has occurred as a result of previous procedures (see **Figure 6-2**). In questionable cases, the interventionist should consult with a qualified medical physicist for advice about the risk of another procedure in the same location.

    Interventionists should evaluate and examine patients who have had previous intervention procedures to assess the risk of skin injury before performing additional procedures.

Radiation Exposure to Operator and Lab Personnel

The National Council on Radiation Protection and Measurements (NCRP) recommends an effective dose limit of 50 mSv per year and a cumulative lifetime of 10 mSv multiplied by age for radiation workers and 1 mSv per year for members of the general public. Occupational dose is determined through the use of personal radiation dosimeters. Common dosimeters include film, thermoluminescent dosimeters (TLDs), optically stimulated luminescent dosimeters (OSL), and solid state electronic dosimeters. These are worn by radiation workers and typically placed at the level of the neck, on the outside of any lead apparel.

Any efforts that reduce the radiation dose to the patient are likely to also reduce the dose to the operator and lab personnel. Beyond patient dose reduction, there are three primary approaches that can reduce occupational exposure: decrease time near a radiation source, increase distance from a radiation source, and maximize the amount of shielding (**Table 6-7**).

TABLE 6-7 Minimizing Radiation Exposure to the Operator, Lab Personnel

1. Reduce time near the source of radiation.
2. Increase the distance of the operator and lab personnel from the x-ray source.
3. Maximize shielding during radiation exposure.
4. Avoid direct radiation exposure.
5. Minimize c-arm angulations with the x-ray tube near the operator.

1. **Reduce Time Near Sources of Radiation:**
    a. Limit in-lab personnel to only those necessary during the procedure.
    b. Limit the number and duration of acquisition runs and fluoroscopic time.
2. **Increase Distance from Radiation Sources:** Scattered radiation from the patient is the primary source of radiation to the operator and lab personnel. An additional source of exposure to personnel is leakage radiation emanating from the x-ray tube. The intensity of radiation decreases by the square of the distance from a point source. Therefore, increasing the distance from 1 meter to 2 meters away from the source reduces the intensity of radiation by a factor of 4. Individuals who work in the cath lab should maintain the greatest possible distance from all radiation sources, consistent with their responsibilities.
3. **Maximize Shielding during Radiation Exposure:** Various types of shielding provide radiation protection for the angiographer and others at the side of the cath table. The radiation protective effect of shielding is expressed in "lead equivalents." For instance, a leaded glass shield with a lead equivalent value of 1.0 provides the same radiation protection as 1 mm of lead. Three major types of radiation shielding are standard in the catheterization laboratory: personal, tableside, and movable.
    a. Personal shielding includes leaded apron, thyroid collar, and an option of leaded glasses.
    b. Leaded drapes suspended from the side of the cath table provide protection below the table.
    c. An overhead movable leaded glass shield has the capacity to reduce radiation in the shielded area, including the operator's head, thyroid, eyes and chest, by at least 95%, depending on the lead-equivalent value of the shield and its placement. The proper position of this shield is close to the patient and between the operator and the entry site of the x-ray beam into the patient. Protection provided by the leaded glass shield is in addition to that provided by the leaded apron and thyroid shield.

    Various types of ancillary shielding are available, such as radio-opaque pads placed on the patient. These have the capacity to reduce scatter radiation as long as the x-ray beam never passes through the pads. If the beam passes through the pads, the radiation doses to both the patient and the operator are increased. This type of ancillary shielding generally offers little additional radiation protection for the operator who properly utilizes the three major types of shielding listed above. Ancillary shielding should never be considered as a substitute for standard radiation shielding. Additionally, routine use of sterile

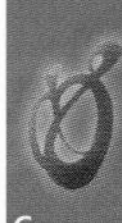

disposable radio-opaque drapes has the potential to add considerable additional expense to the procedure, with little benefit to the operator. The same logic applies to radio-opaque caps worn on the operator's head during procedures, with the added discomfort of the heavy cap.

Ancillary shielding may be appropriate for the following:

a. Extremely obese patients, in whom scatter radiation is likely to be high.
b. Operators who frequently reach or exceed monthly radiation limits on their badges because of a high volume of procedures or multiple cases requiring higher radiation doses.
c. Radial artery procedures: All major types of radiation shielding should be used routinely to ensure radiation protection for the angiographer and other personnel in the cath lab. Ancillary shielding may be appropriate in special circumstances.

4. **Avoid Direct Radiation Exposure:** Angiographers should assiduously avoid placing their hands in the direct x-ray beam. Although leaded gloves protect the angiographer's hands when placed near the direct beam, they may actually increase x-ray output when the hands are placed directly in the beam. The attenuation due to double layers of lead on the fingers will result in an increased dose to the patient and angiographer. The angiographer must avoid placing his or her hands in the direct x-ray beam.
5. **Minimize Projections with the X-ray Tube Near the Operator:** The spatial distribution of scattered radiation is asymmetrical. Maximum scattered radiation to the angiographer occurs when standing on the x-ray tube side of the patient during the lateral or oblique view, for instance, standing at the patient's right side when the c-arm is in the LAO projection. The angiographer should minimize projections that place the x-ray tube near his or her body.

FUTURE CARDIAC CATH LAB TECHNOLOGY

Future developments in cardiac catheterization laboratory technology promise a reduction in radiation doses and improvement in image quality. Three major areas of technology advances include the following.

X-ray Generation

Recent developments in the x-ray tube and generator permit increased power delivery, improved cooling processes, and greater anode heat capacity. These enhancements allow for greater maximum tube current (mA) during image acquisition, which, combined with increased radiation filtering, results in a decreased skin dose. The increased current permits a decrease in pulse width, resulting in improved spatial resolution through a reduction of motion blur. These advances also ensure that x-ray tube heating is less of a concern during prolonged procedures and that smaller focal spots can be utilized, which improves spatial resolution.

A new flat emitter cathode technology allows for improved focal spot performance. This technology produces focal spots that are square rather than rectangular, have a more uniform temperature distribution, improved cooling characteristics, and smaller overall size than conventional filament-generated focal spots. This can produce sharper images at a potentially lower radiation dose.

X-ray Detection

New generations of x-ray detectors improve the conversion of x-ray energy into digital information, and this can directly lower the radiation dose. This improvement is accomplished by more efficient conversion materials, methods to reduce electronic noise, and technology to achieve faster readout rates. Crystalline silicon detectors, compared to amorphous silicon detectors, reduce electronic noise, improve spatial resolution, and permit a decrease in the radiation dose. Improved readout rates permit higher frame rates, which is important especially for 2-D biplane and 3-D acquisition, resulting in improved spatial and temporal resolution.

Image Processing

Innovative image processing techniques are being developed for real-time application during image acquisition and fluoroscopy. Advanced image processing methods can result in noise reduction and in improved contrast, spatial, and temporal resolution. These improvements have the potential to reduce the detector dose without degrading overall image quality.

Radiation Dose Tracking

New technology is available that provides more sophisticated and useful skin dose mapping during interventional procedures. The approximate skin dose can be calculated from geometric and dose parameters to produce a 3-D color-coded graphical display of the skin dose in real time. Although this calculated dose is typically not as accurate as an actual dose measurement with radiochromic film, it can help guide the interventionist in selecting angulations and procedure duration.

Summary of Cath Lab Innovations

Each of these forthcoming technological innovations has the potential to improve image quality and reduce radiation exposure in the cardiac catheterization laboratory. Individually and in combination, these advancements must be integrated into the cardiac interventional suite in the future, with the interventionist being assisted by the institutional physicist and the manufacturer in their proper utilization.

CONCLUSIONS

Greater attention is being placed on cumulative radiation exposure to patients from medical imaging and procedures. Newer imaging systems have been designed with much greater consideration given to reduce radiation exposure to the patient, as well as to the operator. Nevertheless, the key remains operator knowledge of the basic principles of balancing image acquisition and optimization with radiation safety. Future research will need to identify additional approaches to reduce the risks of radiation to everyone in the interventional suite.

References

1. Hirshfeld JW, Balter S, Brinker JA, et al: ACCF/AHA/HRS/SCAI clinical competence statement on physician knowledge to optimize patient safety and image quality in fluoroscopically guided invasive cardiovascular procedures. A report of the American College of Cardiology Foundation/ American Heart Association/American College of Physicians task force on clinical competence and training. *J Am Coll Cardiol* 44:2259–2282, 2004.
2. Balter S, Moses J: Managing patient dose in interventional cardiology. *Catheter Cardiovasc Interv* 70:244–249, 2007.
3. Balter S: Interventional fluoroscopy. In *Physics, technology and safety*, New York, 2001, Wiley-Liss.
4. International Atomic Energy Agency (IAEA). Patient Dose Optimization in Fluoroscopically Guided Interventional Procedures. Final report of a coordinated research project. IAEA TEC DOC-1641. Vienna, 2010.
5. Stecker MS, Balter S, Towbin RB, et al: Guidelines for patient radiation dose management. *J Vasc Interv Radiol* 20:S263–S273, 2009.

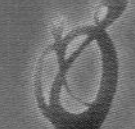

6. Balter S: Capturing patient doses from fluoroscopically based diagnostic and interventional systems. *Health Phys* 95:535–540, 2008.
7. National Council on Radiation Protection and Measurements, 2007. Ionizing Radiation Exposure of the Population of the United States, Report 160, Bethesda, MD (2009).
8. IAEA. Radiation Protection of Patients (RPOP). Patient and staff dose in fluoroscopy. 2014. https://rpop.iaea.org/RPOP/RPoP/Content/InformationFor/HealthProfessionals/4_InterventionalRadiology/patient-staff-dose-fluoroscopy.htm (Accessed on August 22, 2014.).
9. Padovani R, Vano E, Trianni A, et al: Reference levels at European level for cardiac interventional procedures. *Radiat Prot Dosimetry* 129:104–107, 2008.
10. Picano E, Vañó E, Rehani MM, et al: The appropriate and justified use of medical radiation in cardiovascular imaging: a position document of the ESC associations of cardiovascular imaging, percutaneous cardiovascular interventions and electrophysiology. *Eur Heart J* 35:665–672, 2014. Advance Access January 8, 2014.
11. Balter S, Hopewell JW, Miller DL, et al: Fluoroscopically guided interventional procedures: a review of radiation effects on patients' skin and hair. *Radiology* 254:326–341, 2010.
12. Einstein AJ: Effects of radiation exposure from cardiac imaging. how good are the data? *J Am Coll Cardiol* 59:553–564, 2012.
13. Foffa I, Cresci M, Andreassi MG: Health risk and biological effects of cardiac ionising imaging: from epidemiology to genes. *Int J Environ Res Public Health* 6:1882–1893, 2009.
14. Ron E: Ionizing radiation and cancer risk: evidence from epidemiology. *Radiat Res* 150:S30–S41, 1998.
15. Kuon E, Dahm JB, Empen K, et al: Identification of less-irradiating tube angulations in invasive cardiology. *J Am Coll Cardiol* 44:1420–1428, 2004.

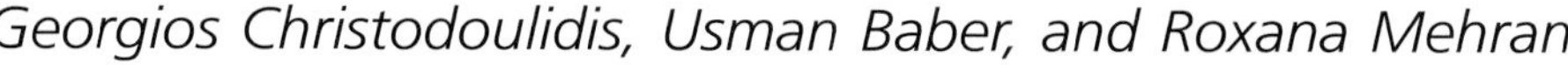

7 Contrast Selection

Georgios Christodoulidis, Usman Baber, and Roxana Mehran

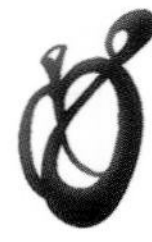

INTRODUCTION

Iodinated contrast media (CM) are widely used in interventional cardiology. Efficacy is predicated on the capacity to opacify intravascular structures; however, when selecting a CM, other important properties should be considered. Most notably, chemical properties such as ionicity, osmolality, and viscosity, as well as the potential for adverse effects, should be incorporated in the decision for CM selection. This chapter aims to provide a comprehensive review of various CM used in interventional cardiology in regard to their structure and properties. Special consideration is given to potential adverse effects, with evidence-based suggestions for prevention and management.

CHEMICAL STRUCTURE

CM consist of an organic carrier molecule (benzene ring) with iodine located at the 2, 4, and 6 positions and organic side chains at the 1, 3, and 5 positions. They are traditionally classified based on their structure, ionicity, osmolality, and viscosity; however, it needs to be stressed that these properties are interconnected.

Structure refers to the number of benzene rings per molecule. Monomers consist of a single tri-iodinated benzene ring, whereas dimers consist of two bound tri-iodinated benzene rings. Depending on the side chain, CM can be ionic or nonionic. Ionic CM are substituted by a carboxyl side chain (anion), which conjugates with a cation (usually sodium), resulting in a water-soluble compound. In contrast, nonionic side chains consist of hydrophilic hydroxyl groups and hence do not ionize in solution. **Figure 7-1** illustrates different CM according to structure and ionicity.

Osmolality refers to the number of osmotically active molecules per fluid mass. As noted above, ionic CM dissociate when placed in a solution and therefore are expected to have higher osmolality. The nomenclature regarding osmolality is based on normal blood osmolality (280 mOsm/kg H_2O).

Viscosity represents the intrinsic resistance of a fluid to flow and is primarily determined by the other properties of the CM and is influenced by temperature. As a general rule, viscosity is directly related to particle size, inversely related to osmolality, and decreases with warming. It is important to note that by definition, agents with lower viscosity maintain flow rates at lower injection pressures.[1]

CLASSIFICATION

The first generation of CM were high osmolality CM (HOCM) with an osmolality of >1400 mOsm/kg. This class is composed of ionic monomers and includes diatrizoate, metrizoate, and iothalamate (**Figure 7-2**). The hyperosmolality of these agents contributes to significant fluid shifts, whereas ionicity and the additives that they contain promote cardiotoxic and arrythmogenic effects.[2]

The next generation of low osmolality CM (LOCM) was characterized by an osmolality between 600 mOsm/kg and 850 mOsm/kg. First in this class was the ionic dimer ioxaglate with an osmolality of 600 mOsm/kg (**Figure 7-3**). Subsequently, monomeric, nonionic LOCM were developed with osmolalities varying between 500 mOsm/kg and 850 mOsm/kg. Included in this class are some of the most commonly used agents, such as iopamidol, iohexol, iopromide, ioxilan, and ioversol (see **Figure 7-2**). Early studies showed a significantly improved safety profile of LOCM compared to HOCM in regard to arrythmogenic potential, hemodynamic abnormalities, and contrast-induced nephropathy (CIN), resulting in a substantial decrease in HOCM use.[3,4]

The last class of agents has an osmolality similar to plasma (290 mOsm/kg) and is therefore classified as iso-osmolar CM (IOCM). This class only includes the nonionic dimer iodixanol, which is unique among contrast agents for its high viscosity[1] (see **Figure 7-2**).

PROPERTIES OF CM

CM are known to have several properties that are clinically significant in the setting of percutaneous coronary intervention (PCI). These include hematologic, hemodynamic, and electrophysiological effects.

Hematologic Effects

The potential effects of CM on coagulation were first suspected after an observation that thrombus formed more rapidly in angiographic catheters filled with blood when mixed with nonionic CM.[5] Subsequent studies suggested that CM exert various effects on the clotting cascade, including the intrinsic and extrinsic coagulation pathways, platelets, and fibrinolysis.[6]

In vitro studies showed that the ionic LOCM ioxaglate exerts prominent anticoagulant effects by inhibiting the activation of factors V and VIII and by decreasing thrombin-induced fibrin polymerization.[7,8] Further in vitro studies showed that all CM have an intrinsic anticoagulant effect; however, more prominent inhibition was noted when the ionic agent ioxaglate was used compared to other nonionic media.[9,10] Of note, however, the clinical significance of the above observations is controversial, especially when considering that the difference in anticoagulant effect observed with the nonionic agents is equalized with the use of heparin.[11]

The effect of CM on platelets also differs between ionic and nonionic agents. In a study evaluating the in vitro effects of different classes of contrast media on platelet function as measured by the release of platelet factor-4 (PF4), serotonin, and platelet-derived growth factor-AB (PDGF-AB), ioxaglate had no effect on platelet function, whereas iodixanol and iohexol showed moderate and major degrees of platelet activation, respectively.[9]

Since CM carry both prothrombotic (via platelet activation) and anticoagulant properties, the net effect on thrombus formation and fibrinolysis was further evaluated. In an in vitro study, the ionic agent ioxaglate was not associated with thrombus formation, whereas the nonionic agents iohexol and iodixanol were associated with a tenfold increase in thrombus formation compared to saline controls, and the thrombi formed were more resistant to fibrinolysis.[12]

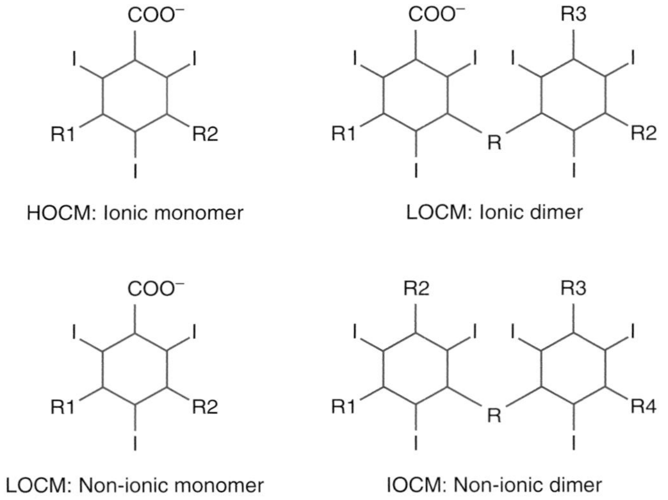

HOCM: Ionic monomer

LOCM: Ionic dimer

LOCM: Non-ionic monomer

IOCM: Non-ionic dimer

FIGURE 7-1 Prototypic structure of different classes of contrast media.

Hemodynamic Effects

CM are also associated with several hemodynamic effects, such as fluid shifts, peripheral vasodilation, and changes in cardiac contractility.

Most of the agents used are hyperosmolar to plasma (with the exception of iodixanol, which is iso-osmolar); therefore rapid infusion of a large amount of CM can cause fluid shifts from the extracellular to the intravascular compartment and can lead to fluid overload and even pulmonary edema.

Additionally, CM are associated with systemic vasodilation and subsequent hypotension. Hyperosmolality is again a potential explanation for this phenomenon,[13] but histamine release from basophils has also been proposed as a possible explanation.[14] Hypotension can also be attributed to the direct effect of the CM to the myocardium, causing a transient decrease in cardiac contractility and a subsequent decrease in cardiac output.[1]

Finally, CM may exert several effects, ranging from common vasovagal responses to rare ventricular arrhythmias. Within seconds after coronary injection, transient sinus bradycardia and atrioventricular conduction delay occur, likely secondary to a vasovagal response.[15] This type of reaction does not prohibit further injection but is

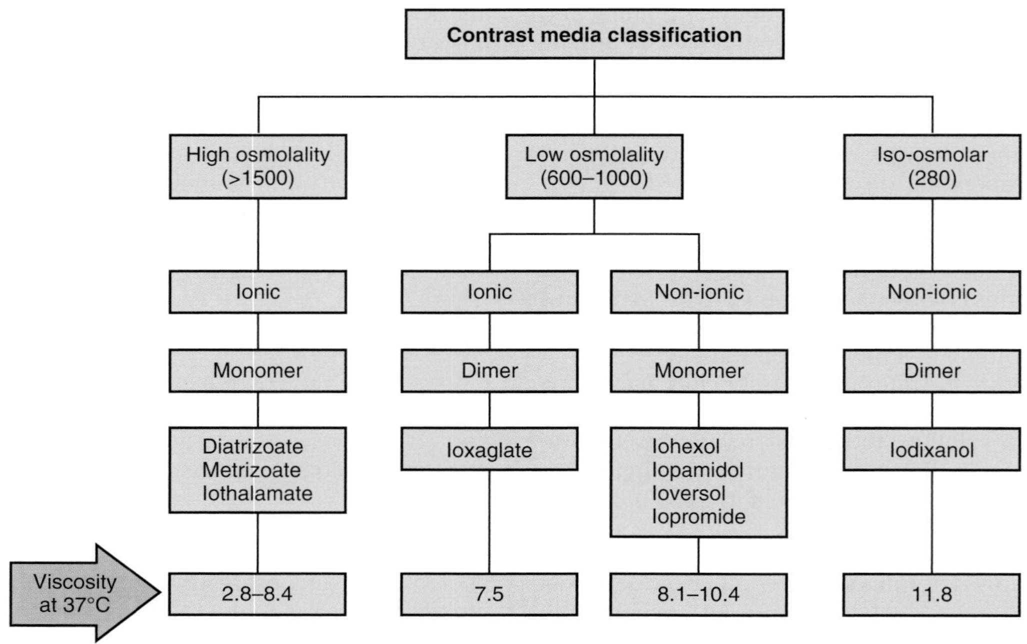

FIGURE 7-2 Contrast media classification.

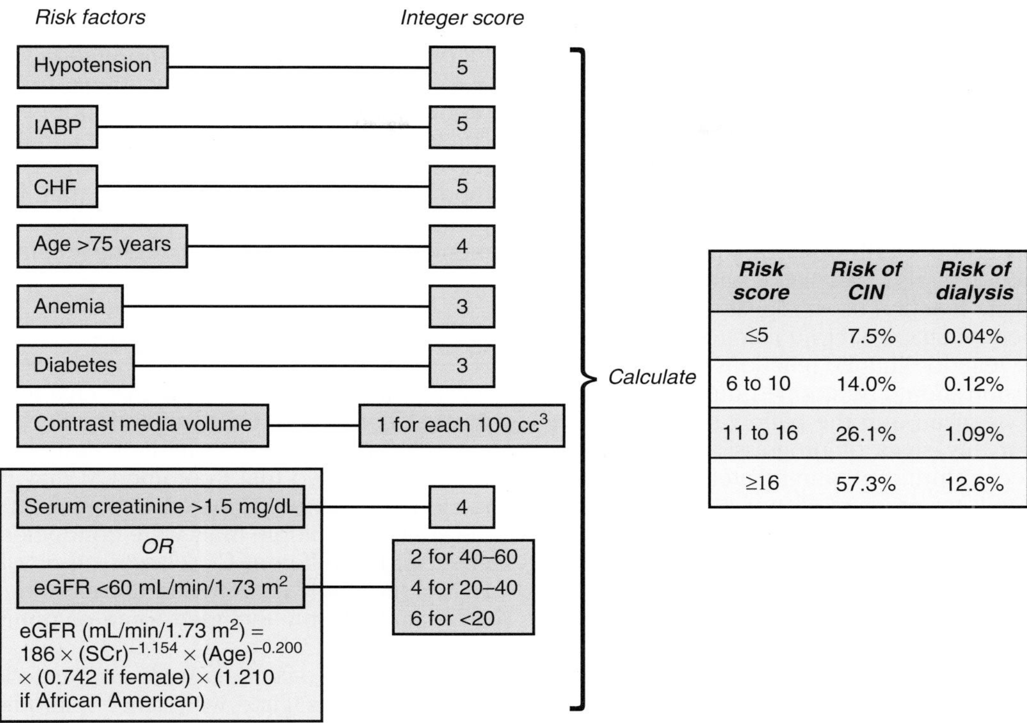

Risk score	Risk of CIN	Risk of dialysis
≤5	7.5%	0.04%
6 to 10	14.0%	0.12%
11 to 16	26.1%	1.09%
≥16	57.3%	12.6%

FIGURE 7-3 Algorithm for CIN risk assessment.*CHF*, Congestive heart failure class III-IV by the New York Heart Association or history of pulmonary edema; *CIN*, contrast-induced nephropathy; *eGFR*, estimated glomerular filtration rate; *SCr*, serum creatinine. Anemia: baseline hematocrit value <39% for men and <36% for women. Hypotension: systolic blood pressure <80 mm Hg for at least 1 hour requiring inotropic support or intra-aortic balloon pump (IABP) within 24 hours periprocedurally.

reasonable to slow the rate of injection, as this may mitigate the response.

Electrophysiologic Effects

Changes in the cardiac cell membrane excitability can also occur, resulting in a decrease in the ventricular fibrillation threshold and predisposition to ventricular arrhythmias. The incidence of ventricular arrhythmias decreases significantly if calcium cations are added, indicating that calcium chelation by anions dissociated from ionic CM is at least partially responsible for this effect.[16] Additionally, these types of arrhythmias are more common with the HOCM, suggesting a role of hyperosmolality in their pathogenesis.[17]

ADVERSE EFFECTS RELATED TO CM ADMINISTRATION

Hypersensitivity Reactions

Hypersensitivity reactions are fairly common with an incidence that varies depending on the type of CM used. Sutton et al., in a study comparing the most commonly used CM, reported that early reactions (within 24 hours) occurred in 22.2%, 7.6%, and 8.8% of those receiving ioxaglate, iodixanol, and iopamidol, respectively, whereas late skin reactions (>24 hours to 7 days) occurred in 12.2% of those receiving iodixanol, 4.3% of those receiving ioxaglate, and 4.2% of those receiving iopamidol.[18]

The pathophysiology of CM reactions remains disputed. Although clinically similar to anaphylaxis, it is rarely IgE mediated.[19] The most possible explanation is of an anaphylactoid reaction in which the CM directly activates the mast cells and basophills with a subsequent release of histamine.[20]

Several factors have been associated with increased risk for contrast reactions, including the type of media used, the history of previous reactions, the history of atopy, and β-blocker use.

The class of media used correlates strongly with the propensity for a CM reaction. In general, HOCM are associated with a higher incidence of reactions compared to LOCM.[21] Additionally, there is evidence to suggest that the nonionic iso-osmolar agent iodixanol might be the safer agent to use in terms of hypersensitivity reactions.[18]

A personal history of an anaphylactoid reaction is probably the most important risk factor for it.[21] Moreover, any personal history of atopy doubles the risk for developing an adverse reaction to CM.[22] Also, the use of β-blockers has been associated with an increased risk for anaphylactoid reaction.[23,24]

A common misconception is that contrast allergy is related to the iodine in the contrast media. However, the antigenic epitope is actually on the organic compound. Iodine is present throughout the body and a true allergy to iodine would be incompatible with life. It also needs to be clarified that patients with shellfish allergy are not at high risk for contrast reaction.[25] Notably, the specific antigen responsible for shellfish allergy is a shellfish-specific tropomyosin.[25]

Clinical manifestations of hypersensitivity reactions can be broadly categorized in immediate reactions that happen within minutes to 1 hour and delayed reactions that occur within 1 hour to 1 week after.

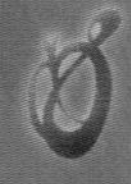

Immediate reactions usually manifest as urticarial rash and pruritus. On rare occasions, a more dramatic picture occurs, with angioedema, laryngospasm, and bronchospasm causing stridor, wheezing, and respiratory distress. Also, circulatory collapse may occur with hypotension and tachycardia, leading to death.

Delayed reactions usually occur within 2 days (although, as mentioned above, delayed reactions were described as late as 1 week after). Common manifestations include skin rash, fatigue, fever, congestion, abdominal pain, diarrhea, constipation, and polyarthropathy.[6] A personal history of a delayed reaction is also associated with an increased risk of an immediate reaction upon repeat exposure to CM.

The management of anaphylactoid reactions depends on the severity of the reaction. In mild reactions (urticarial rash, pruritus), the infusion should be stopped, diphenhydramine 50 mg IV should be given, and the patient should be carefully observed for any signs of progression.[26] In general, reactions that occur during or immediately after the CM administration tend to progress if not treated, whereas reactions occurring 5 minutes or more after tend to be self-limiting.

The management of severe reactions is identical to that of anaphylaxis. The first step is to immediately stop the infusion of the contrast and give 0.3 mg to 0.5 mg IM epinephrine. Intubation should be performed if clinically indicated and supplemental oxygen should be given. Normal saline boluses should be given as needed for hypotension. Additionally, 125 mg of methyl prednisone should be given to prevent recurrent reactions, as well as 50 mg IV of diphenhydramine and 50 mg of ranitidine. If the patient is not responding to the above measures, an epinephrine drip should be started at a rate of 2 to 10 mcg/min and titrated according to blood pressure, and if needed, a second vasopressor can be started. Patients on β-blockers can be given glucagon 1 mg to 5 mg IV over 5 minutes, followed by infusion of 5 to 15 mcg/min.[26] **Table 7-1** summarizes the treatment of hypersensitivity reactions.

TABLE 7-1 Presentation and Treatment of Hypersensitivity Reactions

SEVERITY	SYMPTOMS	MANAGEMENT
Mild	Urticarial rash Pruritus	Stop infusion Diphenhydramine 50 mg IV Observe for progression to severe
Severe	Hives Angioedema Laryngospasm causing stridor Bronchospasm with wheezing Respiratory distress Circulatory collapse (hypotension and tachycardia)	Stop CM infusion IM epinephrine 0.3 to 0.5 mg Intubation if clinically indicated Supplemental oxygen (at least 8-10 L) Normal saline boluses for hypotension Methyl prednisone 125 mg IV Diphenhydramine 50 mg IV Ranitidine 50 mg IV
Refractory symptoms	Patients with inadequate response to IM epinephrine and IV saline	Epinephrine continuous infusion, 2 to 10 micrograms per minute Additional pressor if needed If patient on β-blockers and not responding to epinephrine: glucagon 1 to 5 mg IV over 5 minutes

Another important consideration is prevention in patients with a previous history of hypersensitivity reaction to CM. Multiple protocols have been proposed, but a validated protocol includes 50 mg of prednisone orally, 13 hours, 7 hours, and 1 hour prior to the procedure, in combination with diphenhydramine 50 mg IV, 1 hour prior to the procedure.[27] For emergency procedure recommendations, include the use of LOCM or IOCM, hydrocortisone 200 mg IV once, and diphenhydramine 50 mg IV. Note that premedication in patients with no history of adverse reaction is not recommended. **Table 7-2** summarizes the recommended premedication protocols.

ISCHEMIC COMPLICATIONS

As mentioned previously in this chapter, in vitro studies illustrated that CM exert multiple effects on the clotting cascade, platelets, and fibrinolysis. Furthermore, early observations suggested that nonionic CM may promote clot formation in excess compared to ionic CM.[5] Following this observation, multiple trials were conducted to evaluate the effect of the different CM classes on clot formation. Since HOCM are rarely if ever used in the modern era, we focus on trials that only included ionic or nonionic LOCM and IOCM.

In the 1990s, six trials were conducted comparing the ionic LOCM ioxaglate with other nonionic LOCM among patients undergoing PCI.[28-33] In all of these trials, thrombotic events and subacute recoil were more common among patients receiving nonionic CM. Of note, the aforementioned studies were performed in the prestent era and prior to the routine use of glycoprotein IIb-IIIa inhibitors.

Schrader et al. were the first to compare the thrombogenic potential of ionic versus nonanionic CM in the stent era in a randomized controlled trial of 2000 patients.[34] In this study, the incidence of reocclusion necessitating repeat angioplasty occurred in 2.9% of the patients receiving the nonionic iomeprol versus 3.0% of the patients receiving the ionic ioxaglate. Moreover, there were no significant differences in the rate of major ischemic complications between iomeprol and ioxaglate (emergency bypass surgery: 0.8% vs. 0.7%, MI: 1.8 vs. 2.0%, cardiac death during hospital stay: 0.2% vs. 0.2%, respectively).[34]

Studies comparing the nonionic IOCM iodixanol with ionic LOCM ioxaglate have been controversial. The multicenter VIP trial (Visipaque in percutaneous transluminal coronary angioplasty [PTCA]) compared iodixanol with ioxaglate in 1411 patients undergoing coronary intervention.[35] In the 2-day period post-PCI, major adverse cardiac events (a composite of death, stroke, MI, coronary artery

TABLE 7-2 Prevention from CM Reactions

PATIENT STATUS	RECOMMENDED PROTOCOL
No previous history of CM reaction	Premedication is not recommended
Previous history of adverse reaction (elective procedure)	Prednisone 50 mg orally 13 hours, 7 hours, and 1 hour prior to procedure Diphenhydramine 50 mg PO 1 hour prior to procedure
Previous history of adverse reaction (emergent procedure)	Hydrocortisone 200 mg IV once Diphenhydramine 50 mg IV

bypass grafting, and revascularization) were comparable between groups (4.7% vs. 3.9% for iodixanol vs. ioxaglate, respectively, $p = 0.45$). Similarly, at the 1-month follow-up, no significant difference was noted between the groups in the rates of rehospitalization secondary to MACE ($p = 0.27$).[35]

In contrast to the VIP trial, the COURT trial (randomized trial of contrast media utilization in high-risk PTCA), which was also reported at about the same period, showed improved ischemic outcomes with iodixanol compared to ioxaglate.[36] More specifically, the incidence of in-hospital MACE was decreased in those receiving iodixanol compared to those receiving ioxaglate (5.4% versus 9.5%, respectively, $p = 0.027$). However, this difference was attenuated and was no longer significant at 30 days (9.1% versus 13.2% for iodixanol vs. ioxaglate, respectively, $p = 0.07$).[36] Additionally, in the subgroup of patients who were treated with glycoprotein IIb-IIIa inhibitors, the in-hospital difference in MACE rates was no longer present.

Subsequently, Le Feuvre et al. compared ioxaglate and iodixanol in a single center prospective study, which included 498 consecutive patients.[37] Of note, more contemporary techniques were used, including clopidogrel, enoxaparin, glycoprotein IIb-IIIa inhibitors, and drug-eluting stents. In contrast to previous reports, results were in favor of ioxaglate, with the in-hospital MACE shown to be significantly lower in the ioxaglate group compared to the iodixanol group (0.3% vs. 4.8%, respectively, $p < 0.005$).[37]

Moreover, there is a paucity of data comparing iodixanol to nonionic LOCM in regard to ischemic complications. Only reported in the form of an abstract, the VICC trial (Visipaque vs. Isovue in Cardiac Catheterization) compared iodixanol with the nonionic LOCM iopamidol in 1276 patients undergoing PCI.[38] The incidence of in-hospital MACE was higher in the iopamidol group, a result that was primarily driven by a higher incidence of periprocedural MI diagnosed by elevated biomarkers.[38] However, the study was heavily criticized because baseline biomarker tests were not mandatory and hence the biomarker elevation that was used for the MI diagnosis might have been present even prior to the procedure.

In summary, whether differences exist in the thrombogenic potential of the various classes of CM remains controversial. It appears that in the prestent era, the ionic LOCM ioxaglate was associated with decreased ischemic complications compared to the nonanionic LOCM. However, these differences are completely attenuated in the modern era with the use of more potent antiplatelet and anticoagulant medications. Further studies are needed comparing the nonionic IOCM iodixanol with the nonionic LOCM.

CONTRAST-INDUCED NEPHROPATHY (CIN)

Definition and Clinical Course

CIN frequently complicates the use of radiographic CM and constitutes the third leading cause of hospital-acquired acute renal failure (ARF).[39]

CIN is defined as the deterioration of renal function following the administration of contrast agents in the absence of other causes. The exact definition of CIN varies within the literature, but it is most commonly defined as an absolute rise in serum creatinine of greater than 0.5 mg/dL or a 25% increase from baseline within 48 hours from contrast administration.[6]

The typical course of CIN includes an elevation of serum creatinine within 24 to 48 hours of contrast administration and a peak within 3 to 5 days, with a gradual resolution within 1 to 2 weeks following exposure.[40] Permanent renal impairment is rare and occurs only in a few cases.[40]

Incidence

The incidence of CIN varies within studies, depending on the definition used and the characteristics of the population studied. In a retrospective analysis of an unselected registry of patients undergoing PCI, CIN (defined as a rise in creatinine of >0.5 mg/dL) was reported to be 3.3%.[41] However, the presence of underlying chronic kidney disease (CKD) and other risk factors can raise the incidence of CIN to as high as 50%.[42]

Of note, the incidence of CIN is lower in patients undergoing computed tomography compared to patients undergoing PCI (likely secondary to the lower amount of CM used), and it has been reported to be 2% to 9%, depending on underlying predisposing conditions.[43,44]

Risk Factors

Predisposing conditions to CIN can be broadly categorized to patient-related conditions and to the ones related to extrinsic factors.

The most important patient-related risk factor is preexisting renal insufficiency.[41,42,44,45] In a prospective study that included 222 patients undergoing angiographic procedures, CIN occurred in 2%, 10.4%, and 62% of patients with baseline serum creatinine levels of ≤1.2 mg/dL, 1.3-1.9 mg/dL, and ≥2 mg/dL, respectively.[46] The detrimental effects of CKD in the incidence of CIN become even more prominent when the underlying reason for CKD is diabetes.[42]

Age has also been shown to be an independent predictor of CIN.[47] Possible explanations for this observation could be the gradual decline of renal function that naturally happens with aging as well as the multiple comorbidities that are found in the elderly population.

Any condition associated with inadequate renal perfusion can be a major risk factor. Specifically, the presence of heart failure, hypovolemia, hemodynamic instability, and the use of an intraaortic balloon pump have been shown to increase the incidence of CIN.[48]

The presence of anemia is an additional well-described but underappreciated risk factor. In a study of 6773 patients treated with PCI, Nikolsky et al. showed an inverse association between the incidence of CIN and baseline hematocrit.[49] The presence of multiple comorbidities in the anemic patients partially explains this association, and hypoxic renal injury may offer an additional explanation.

Procedure-related factors such as the type and volume of CM used can also influence the incidence of CIN. The importance of contrast volume was first shown by McCullough et al. in a cohort of 1826 consecutive patients undergoing coronary intervention.[50] In this study, increasing contrast volume was a major risk factor for CIN, and the risk of CIN was minimal in patients receiving less than 100 mL of CM. Subsequently, Freeman et al. developed a formula for calculating the maximum radiographic contrast dose (MRCD) aloud to avoid nephropathy requiring dialysis.[51] According to this study, MRCD = 5 mL × body weight (kg)/serum creatinine (mg/dL), and the authors demonstrated that after multivariable adjustment, overpassing the MRCD was the strongest independent predictor for dialysis.[51]

The type of CM used also influences the risk for CIN. Multiple studies in the 1990s showed that in patients with underlying renal impairment, the use of HOCM is associated with a higher incidence of CIN when compared to LOCM.[52,53] Studies comparing the nonanionic IOCM iodixanol with various LOCM have had various results. In general, it appears to be a benefit of the IOCM iodixanol over the ionic LOCM ioxaglate and the nonionic LOCM iohexol.[54,55] However, when comparing iodixanol to the nonanionic LOCM, iopamidol, or ioversol, no significant differences were observed.[56,57]

To assess the cumulative risk of the aforementioned risk factors, Mehran et al. developed a simple risk score for predicting CIN after PCI using easily available information[48] (see **Figure 7-3**). More recently, Gurm et al., using data from 68,573 PCI performed in Michigan, developed a computational tool for predicting the risk of CIN.[58] The calculator for this model can be found at https://bmc2.org/calculators/cin.

Pathophysiology

The exact mechanisms leading to the development of CIN remain unclear. A modest decline in renal blood flow has been described after administration of CM.[59] These modest changes though, are unlikely to account for the substantial changes in renal function that are often noticed with CIN.

Based on normal physiology, the outer medulla is more susceptible to hypoxia and is likely differentially affected by CM administration and decreased perfusion.[60] More specifically, CM have been shown to disrupt the fine balance between local vasodilators (NO, PGE2, dopamine) and vasoconstrictors (angiotensin II, endothelin, adenosine) in the renal medulla and cause hypoxia.[61]

Moreover, the anatomy of the vasculature in the renal medulla may offer an additional explanation. The vasa recta that supply the renal medulla are long, narrow, caliber vessels, so further reduction in medullary blood flow may occur due to changes in viscosity, especially when the high-viscosity IOCM are used.[62]

Additionally, CM administration appears to increase the formation of reactive oxygen species.[63] High oxidative stress may further decrease the formation of NO, thereby promoting vasoconstriction.[64]

Finally, there is some evidence to suggest that CM have direct cytotoxic effects. In vitro studies showed that different CM augment apoptosis of cultured renal mesangial and tubular cells.[65] These toxic effects are mediated via induction of cellular energy failure, disruption of calcium homeostasis, and disturbance of tubular cell polarity, ultimately leading to apoptosis.[66]

Preventive Strategies

Periprocedural Hydration

Volume expansion with intravenous fluids (IVF) has been the cornerstone for CIN prevention. The first to show the beneficial effects of hydration was Solomon et al. in a prospective study of 78 patients randomized to receive 0.45% saline versus a combination of 0.45% saline plus mannitol or furosemide.[67] In this study, simple hydration provided better protection against CIN than hydration plus mannitol or furosemide (10.7% vs. 28.0% vs. 40.0%, respectively, $p = 0.02$).[67]

Subsequent studies proved the superiority of isotonic saline over half normal saline in preventing CIN,[68] but studies comparing different modes of fluid administration (intravenous vs. oral) have been controversial.[69,70]

Controversy also exists regarding the optimal amount of fluids as well as the duration of the hydration protocol. Overall, for hospitalized patients, the CIN Consensus Working Panel recommends 1 mL/kg to 1.5 mL/kg per hour of intravenous 0.9% saline, initiated 12 hours before the procedure and continued for 6 to 24 hours afterward. For practical reasons, the recommendations for outpatients change to intravenous 0.9% saline for up to 3 hours before the procedure and for up to 12 hours afterward.[71]

Isotonic Sodium Bicarbonate

Administration of sodium bicarbonate can cause alkalization of the urine and thus decrease free radical formation and possibly ameliorate the risk for CIN. On that theoretical basis, various studies evaluated an alternative hydration protocol with sodium bicarbonate, but results have been controversial.

Results from three randomized trials showed that a hydration protocol with sodium bicarbonate was superior from an alternative saline hydration irrespective of other concomitant administration of other prophylactic medications.[72-74] In contrast, three subsequent trials failed to show any additional benefit from sodium bicarbonate administration.[75-77] Moreover, a retrospective cohort study from Mayo Clinic, which included 7977 patients, showed that the use of intravenous sodium bicarbonate was associated with an increased incidence of CIN.[78]

Finally, Brar et al. reported a metaanalysis regarding the role of sodium bicarbonate versus normal saline administration for CIN prevention, which included 3 large trials and 12 small trials.[79] Analysis from the 3 large trials illustrated no significant benefit from sodium bicarbonate (relative risk 0.85, 95% confidence interval 0.63-1.16), whereas pooled results from the 12 small, less methodologically rigorous trials showed evidence of benefit with sodium bicarbonate.[79]

RenalGuard System

As mentioned above, hydration with normal saline has been shown to be beneficial in the prevention of CIN. However, concerns surrounding excessive hydration have led investigators toward alternative strategies, which included the concomitant use of fluids with diuretics. Theoretically, apart from protecting from overhydration, the increased urine flow promotes contrast dilution with subsequent decrease in the direct toxicity on tubular cells.[80] However, early studies testing this hypothesis have been disappointing, possibly as a result of overdiuresis.[67]

More recently, the RenalGuard System was developed to achieve balanced hydration and diuresis via a computerized infusion system that balances the fluid administration rate with real-time diuresis. The safety and performance of the RenalGuard System were first shown in a phase II feasibility study by Dorval et al.[81] Subsequently, the REMEDIAL II investigators tested this system in 194 patients with severe CKD undergoing PCI.[82] CIN (defined as an increase in creatinine ≥0.3 mg/dL) occurred in 16 of 146 patients in the RenalGuard group, compared to 30 of 146 patients in the control group (odds ratio, 0.47; 95% confidence interval, 0.24-0.92).[82] Similar results were reported later by

Marenzi et al. in the MYTHOS (Induced Diuresis with Matched Hydration Compared to Standard Hydration for Contrast Induced Nephropathy Prevention) trial.[83]

Currently, the U.S. Pivotal Trial for the RenalGuard System is actively enrolling patients and is aiming to include at least 326 individuals in whom to compare the efficacy of the RenalGuard System with the current standard of care (ClinicalTrials.gov Identifier: NCT01456013).

Removal of CM by Extracorporeal Therapies

Since CM are primarily removed from the body via the kidneys, it was reasonable to assume that different modes of extracorporeal therapies may protect from CIN.

However, hemodialysis performed immediately after CM administration failed to protect from CIN in patients with preexisting renal impairment despite effective elimination of the CM.[84,85] In contrast, periprocedural continuous venovenous hemofiltration (CVVH) was shown to be protective from CIN in CKD patients undergoing PCI, but the cost-effectiveness of this method raises concerns.[86]

Renal Artery Vasodilation

Fenoldopam is a selective D-1 receptor agonist, so theoretically it could ameliorate the CM effects to the kidney via induction of renal artery vasodilation. However, in the CONTRAST (Fenoldopam Mesylate for the Prevention of Contrast-Induced Nephropathy) trial, the systemic infusion of fenoldopam in addition to hydration failed to decrease the incidence of CIN.[87] Subsequently, selective intrarenal fenoldopam using a dedicated catheter infusion system was tested in a pilot study, showing promising results in increasing renal plasma flow with less systemic hypotension.[88] Notably, however, a randomized controlled study comparing intrarenal fenoldopam with a placebo is lacking.

Theophylline is an adenosine receptor antagonist and can cause local renal vasodilation and thus ameliorate the effects of CM to the kidney. However, results from randomized trials testing the efficacy of theophylline in reducing the incidence of CIN have been controversial.[89,90]

Antioxidant Therapy

Since oxidative kidney injury is implicated in the pathophysiology of CIN, antioxidants such as *N*-acetylcysteine (NAC) and ascorbic acid have been tested for CIN prevention.

Early trials evaluating the use of NAC in CIN prevention showed promising results.[91,92] However, in the largest randomized controlled study to date, the use of NAC was ineffective in preventing CIN in high-risk patients.[93] Specifically, patients with CKD undergoing cardiac catheterization were randomly assigned to intravenous NAC 500 mg or placebo in addition to a fluid hydration protocol. After enrolling 487 patients, the Data Safety Monitoring Committee determined futility and the study was terminated.[93]

The use of ascorbic acid for CIN prevention was evaluated by Briguory et al. in a cohort of 326 patients with CKD undergoing angiography.[73] In this study, the addition of ascorbic acid in a preventive strategy that included hydration with normal saline and NAC provided no additional protection from CIN.[73]

Statins

Results from several observational studies suggested a beneficial role of statins in preventing contrast-induced nephropathy possibly via their antioxidant and antiinflammatory effects. However, subsequent randomized studies have been controversial. A metaanalysis that included eight clinical trials with a total of 1423 patients showed that short-term high-dose statin treatment can decrease the occurrence of CIN compared to conventional dose statin or placebo (risk ratio 0.51, $p = 0.001$).[94]

Since the aforementioned metaanalysis, two additional randomized trials have been conducted. Han et al. randomized 2998 patients with type 2 DM and concomitant CKD who were undergoing angiography, to rosuvastatin for 2 days before and 3 days after the procedure or no statin.[95] Prophylactic hydration was given at the discretion of the treating physician. In this study, the incidence of CIN was significantly lower among patients in the rosuvastatin group compared to controls (2.3% vs. 3.9%, OR = 0.58, $p = 0.01$).[95] Similarly, Leoncini et al. studied the effect of rosuvastatin in the incidence of CIN in non-ST-elevation ACS.[96] Patients were randomly assigned to receive rosuvastatin or no statin in addition to hydration and NAC. The incidence of CIN was significantly lower among patients treated with rosuvastatin compared to the control group (6.7% vs. 15.1%; adjusted odds ratio, $p = 0.003$).[96]

Overall, it appears that statins may play a role in CIN prevention. However, further studies are needed to define their role in different patient subgroups (most notably CKD patients) as well as to compare the effect of different statin regimens.

The different preventive strategies for CIN and our recommendations for their use are summarized in **Table 7-3**.

Prognosis

Typically, CIN is a self-limited condition and only rarely progresses to end-stage renal disease requiring dialysis.[40] However, multiple observational studies illustrate that the

TABLE 7-3 Preventive Strategies for CIN

PREVENTIVE STRATEGY	RECOMMENDATION
Hydration with normal saline	Strongly recommended for all patients
Hydration with sodium bicarbonate	No additional benefit over normal saline
RenalGuard system	Investigational device—Not available for commercial use
Minimize amount of CM	Strongly recommended for all patients
Use of nonionic LOCM or IOCM	Recommended for all patients, especially if renal impairment is present
Hemodialysis	Not recommended
Continuous veno-venous hemofiltration	Likely beneficial but not cost-effective
Systemic fenoldopam	Not recommended
Intrarenal fenoldopam	Further studies are required to establish effectiveness
Theophylline	Controversial—Currently not recommended
N-acetylcysteine	No proven benefit Considering that it is safe and inexpensive we do not recommend against its use
Ascorbic acid	Not recommended
Statins	Likely beneficial—Further studies are required

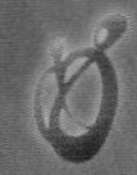

development of CIN is associated with increased length of hospital stay, adverse cardiovascular outcomes, and higher mortality.

A recent systematic review and metaanalysis, which included 34 studies, provided further input in the deleterious effects of CIN.[97] With respect to mortality, 11 studies that did not adjust for confounding features illustrated that CIN was associated with an eightfold increase in the risk of mortality (pooled RR, 8.19; 95% CI, 4.30-15.60). Importantly, this association remained significant after adjusting for potential confounders (pooled RR, 2.39; 95% CI, 1.98-2.90).[97]

The risk for adverse cardiovascular events was increased in patients with CIN in all 14 studies (70,031 participants) reporting on cardiovascular events. Specifically, RR from these studies was 2.42 (95% CI, 1.62-3.64) and was not significantly different between studies adjusting or not adjusting for confounders.[97]

Finally, 10 studies with a total of 19,674 participants reported an additional unadjusted mean hospitalization length that ranged from 0.5 to 8.3 days in patients with CIN, with significant heterogeneity in the size of this difference (Q statistic $p < 0.001$; $I2 = 99.2\%$). Only one study adjusted for baseline clinical characteristics, reporting 1.6 additional days of hospitalization attributable to CIN ($p = 0.005$).[97]

Overall, CIN has been associated with increased morbidity and mortality as well as prolonged hospital stay. However, it remains unclear whether the association between CIN and adverse events is causal or just identifying a subgroup of very high-risk patients.

OVERALL CONSIDERATIONS

The final decision for CM selection ideally should be individualized. Important factors to consider could be broadly categorized into patient characteristics and procedural factors. When considering patient characteristics, special attention should be paid to the various risk factors for CIN (most notably history of CKD), history of previous reaction to CM, and atopy.

Procedure-related factors such as the location of the intervention should also be considered. Carbon dioxide (CO_2) is an alternative CM that can be used in interventions in the arterial circulation and is completely safe in regard to CIN and allergic reactions.[98] However, CO_2 is contraindicated in procedures above the diaphragm, including the thoracic aorta, coronaries, and carotids, due to the risk for embolization.[98] This limits the use of CO_2 in peripheral procedures and procedures within the venous circulation.

Finally, in the absence of a clearly superior agent, cost should also be considered. Notably, the newer agent iodixanol is considerably more expensive compared to the most commonly used nonionic LOCM.

CONCLUSIONS

Iodinated CM are usually classified based on their osmolality into HOCM, LOCM, and IOCM and further categorized to ionic and nonionic. HOCM have fallen out of favor secondary to overall increased potential for adverse reactions. Ionic CM are more likely to be associated with hypersensitivity reactions whereas some evidence postulates that IOCM might be the safer class in terms of hypersensitivity reactions. In the current era, with the use of potent antiplatelet and anticoagulant medications, the rate of thrombotic complications is similar within the different classes of CM. CIN is the most common adverse reaction associated with the use of CM, especially in patients with underlying risk factors, and it has been shown to adversely affect morbidity and mortality. Evidence-based approaches to prevent CIN are periprocedural hydration with NS, use of nonionic LOCM or IOCM, and minimization of the amount of CM used.

References

1. Voeltz MD, Nelson MA, McDaniel MC, et al: The important properties of contrast media: focus on viscosity. *J Invasive Cardiol* 19:1A–9A, 2007.
2. Zukerman LS, Friehling TD, Wolf NM, et al: Effect of calcium-binding additives on ventricular fibrillation and repolarization changes during coronary angiography. *J Am Coll Cardiol* 10:1249–1253, 1987.
3. Piao ZE, Murdock DK, Hwang MH, et al: Hemodynamic abnormalities during coronary angiography: comparison of Hypaque-76, Hexabrix, and Omnipaque-350. *Cathet Cardiovasc Diagn* 16:149–154, 1989.
4. Barrett BJ, Carlisle EJ: Metaanalysis of the relative nephrotoxicity of high- and low-osmolality iodinated contrast media. *Radiology* 188:171–178, 1993.
5. Robertson HJ: Blood clot formation in angiographic syringes containing nonionic contrast media. *Radiology* 162:621–622, 1987.
6. Klein LW, Sheldon MW, Brinker J, et al: The use of radiographic contrast media during PCI: a focused review: a position statement of the Society of Cardiovascular Angiography and Interventions. *Catheter Cardiovasc Interv* 74:728–746, 2009.
7. Al Dieri R, Beguin S, Hemker HC: The ionic contrast medium ioxaglate interferes with thrombin-mediated feedback activation of factor V, factor VIII and platelets. *J Thromb Haemost: JTH* 1:269–274, 2003.
8. Brass O, Belleville J, Sabattier V, et al: Effect of ioxaglate—an ionic low osmolar contrast medium—on fibrin polymerization in vitro. *Blood Coagul Fibrinolysis* 4:689–697, 1993.
9. Corot C, Chronos N, Sabattier V: In vitro comparison of the effects of contrast media on coagulation and platelet activation. *Blood Coagul Fibrinolysis* 7:602–608, 1996.
10. Grabowski EF, Kaplan KL, Halpern EF: Anticoagulant effects of nonionic versus ionic contrast media in angiography syringes. *Invest Radiol* 26:417–421, 1991.
11. Mukherjee M, Scully MF, Thomas M, et al: The potential thrombogenic action of a nonionic radiographic contrast medium used during coronary angiography is offset by heparin during coronary angioplasty. *Thromb Haemost* 76:679–681, 1996.
12. Jones CI, Goodall AH: Differential effects of the iodinated contrast agents ioxaglate, iohexol and iodixanol on thrombus formation and fibrinolysis. *Thromb Res* 112:65–71, 2003.
13. Dawson P, Grainger RG, Pitfield J: The new low-osmolar contrast media: a simple guide. *Clin Radiol* 34:221–226, 1983.
14. Assem ES, Bray K, Dawson P: The release of histamine from human basophils by radiological contrast agents. *Br J Radiol* 56:647–652, 1983.
15. Kyriakidis M, Jackson G, Jewitt D: Contrast media during coronary arteriography: electrocardiographic changes in the presence of normal coronary arteries. *Br J Radiol* 51:799–801, 1978.
16. Thomson KR, Violante MR, Kenyon T, et al: Reduction in ventricular fibrillation using calcium-enriched Renografin 76. *Invest Radiol* 13:238–240, 1978.
17. Wolf GL, Mulry CS, Kilzer K, et al: New angiographic agents with less fibrillatory propensity. *Invest Radiol* 16:320–323, 1981.
18. Sutton AG, Finn P, Grech ED, et al: Early and late reactions after the use of iopamidol 340, ioxaglate 320, and iodixanol 320 in cardiac catheterization. *Am Heart J* 141:677–683, 2001.
19. Brockow K, Ring J: Anaphylaxis to radiographic contrast media. *Curr Opin Allergy Clin Immunol* 11:326–331, 2011.
20. Idee JM, Pines E, Prigent P, et al: Allergy-like reactions to iodinated contrast agents. A critical analysis. *Fundam Clin Pharmacol* 19:263–281, 2005.
21. Katayama H, Yamaguchi K, Kozuka T, et al: Adverse reactions to ionic and nonionic contrast media. A report from the Japanese Committee on the Safety of Contrast Media. *Radiology* 175:621–628, 1990.
22. Enright T, Chua-Lim A, Duda E, et al: The role of a documented allergic profile as a risk factor for radiographic contrast media reaction. *Ann Allergy* 62:302–305, 1989.
23. Lang DM, Alpern MB, Visintainer PF, et al: Elevated risk of anaphylactoid reaction from radiographic contrast media is associated with both beta-blocker exposure and cardiovascular disorders. *Arch Intern Med* 153:2033–2040, 1993.
24. Lang DM, Alpern MB, Visintainer PF, et al: Increased risk for anaphylactoid reaction from contrast media in patients on beta-adrenergic blockers or with asthma. *Ann Intern Med* 115:270–276, 1991.
25. Huang SW: Seafood and iodine: an analysis of a medical myth. *Allergy Asthma Proc* 26:468–469, 2005.
26. Goss JE, Chambers CE, Heupler FA, Jr: Systemic anaphylactoid reactions to iodinated contrast media during cardiac catheterization procedures: guidelines for prevention, diagnosis, and treatment. Laboratory Performance Standards Committee of the Society for Cardiac Angiography and Interventions. *Cathet Cardiovasc Diagn* 34:99–104, discussion 105, 1995.
27. Greenberger PA, Patterson R: The prevention of immediate generalized reactions to radiocontrast media in high-risk patients. *J Allergy Clin Immunol* 87:867–872, 1991.
28. Esplugas E, Cequier A, Jara F, et al: Risk of thrombosis during coronary angioplasty with low osmolality contrast media. *Am J Cardiol* 68:1020–1024, 1991.
29. Piessens JH, Stammen F, Vrolix MC, et al: Effects of an ionic versus a nonionic low osmolar contrast agent on the thrombotic complications of coronary angioplasty. *Cathet Cardiovasc Diagn* 28:99–105, 1993.
30. Lefevre T, Bernard A, Bertrand M, et al: [Electron microscopic comparison of the antithrombotic potential of 2 low osmolality iodine contrast media in percutaneous transluminal coronary angioplasty]. *Arch Mal Coeur Vaiss* 87:225–233, 1994.
31. Grines CL, Schreiber TL, Savas V, et al: A randomized trial of low osmolar ionic versus nonionic contrast media in patients with myocardial infarction or unstable angina undergoing percutaneous transluminal coronary angioplasty. *J Am Coll Cardiol* 27:1381–1386, 1996.
32. Qureshi NR, den Heijer P, Crijns HJ: Percutaneous coronary angioscopic comparison of thrombus formation during percutaneous coronary angioplasty with ionic and nonionic low osmolality contrast media in unstable angina. *Am J Cardiol* 80:700–704, 1997.
33. Malekianpour M, Bonan R, Lesperance J, et al: Comparison of ionic and nonionic low osmolar contrast media in relation to thrombotic complications of angioplasty in patients with unstable angina. *Am Heart J* 135:1067–1075, 1998.
34. Schrader R, Esch I, Ensslen R, et al: A randomized trial comparing the impact of a nonionic (iomeprol) versus an ionic (ioxaglate) low osmolar contrast medium on abrupt vessel closure and ischemic complications after coronary angioplasty. *J Am Coll Cardiol* 33:395–402, 1999.
35. Bertrand ME, Esplugas E, Piessens J, et al: Influence of a nonionic, iso-osmolar contrast medium (iodixanol) versus an ionic, low-osmolar contrast medium (ioxaglate) on major adverse cardiac

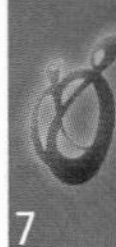

events in patients undergoing percutaneous transluminal coronary angioplasty: a multicenter, randomized, double-blind study. Visipaque in Percutaneous Transluminal Coronary Angioplasty [VIP] Trial Investigators. *Circulation* 101:131–136, 2000.

36. Davidson CJ, Laskey WK, Hermiller JB, et al Randomized trial of contrast media utilization in high-risk PTCA: the COURT trial. *Circulation* 2000;101:2172-2177.
37. Le Feuvre C, Batisse A, Collet JP, et al: Cardiac events after low osmolar ionic or isosmolar non-ionic contrast media utilization in the current era of coronary angioplasty. *Catheter Cardiovasc Interv* 67:852–858, 2006.
38. Harrison KJHJ, Vetrovec GW, et al: A randomized study of 1276 patients undergoing PCI using iodixanol (Visipaque) vs. iopamidol (Isovue): comparison of in-hospital and 30 day major adverse cardiac events. The results of the VICC trial. *Circulation* 108(Suppl IV):IV354–IV355, 2003.
39. Nash K, Hafeez A, Hou S: Hospital-acquired renal insufficiency. *Am J Kidney Dis* 39:930–936, 2002.
40. Thomsen HS, Morcos SK: Contrast media and the kidney: European Society of Urogenital Radiology (ESUR) guidelines. *Br J Radiol* 76:513–518, 2003.
41. Rihal CS, Textor SC, Grill DE, et al: Incidence and prognostic importance of acute renal failure after percutaneous coronary intervention. *Circulation* 105:2259–2264, 2002.
42. Manske CL, Sprafka JM, Strony JT, et al: Contrast nephropathy in azotemic diabetic patients undergoing coronary angiography. *Am J Med* 89:615–620, 1990.
43. Dittrich R, Akdeniz S, Kloska SP, et al: Low rate of contrast-induced nephropathy after CT perfusion and CT angiography in acute stroke patients. *J Neurol* 254:1491–1497, 2007.
44. Cheruvu B, Henning K, Mulligan J, et al: Iodixanol: risk of subsequent contrast nephropathy in cancer patients with underlying renal insufficiency undergoing diagnostic computed tomography examinations. *J Comput Assist Tomogr* 31:493–498, 2007.
45. Rich MW, Crecelius CA: Incidence, risk factors, and clinical course of acute renal insufficiency after cardiac catheterization in patients 70 years of age or older. A prospective study. *Arch Intern Med* 150:1237–1242, 1990.
46. Hall KA, Wong RW, Hunter GC, et al: Contrast-induced nephrotoxicity: the effects of vasodilator therapy. *J Surg Res* 53:317–320, 1992.
47. Gussenhoven MJ, Ravensbergen J, van Bockel JH, et al: Renal dysfunction after angiography; a risk factor analysis in patients with peripheral vascular disease. *J Cardiovasc Surg (Torino)* 32:81–86, 1991.
48. Mehran R, Aymong ED, Nikolsky E, et al: A simple risk score for prediction of contrast-induced nephropathy after percutaneous coronary intervention: development and initial validation. *J Am Coll Cardiol* 44:1393–1399, 2004.
49. Nikolsky E, Mehran R, Lasic Z, et al: Low hematocrit predicts contrast-induced nephropathy after percutaneous coronary interventions. *Kidney Int* 67:706–713, 2005.
50. McCullough PA, Wolyn R, Rocher LL, et al: Acute renal failure after coronary intervention: incidence, risk factors, and relationship to mortality. *Am J Med* 103:368–375, 1997.
51. Freeman RV, O'Donnell M, Share D, et al: Nephropathy requiring dialysis after percutaneous coronary intervention and the critical role of an adjusted contrast dose. *Am J Cardiol* 90:1068–1073, 2002.
52. Taliercio CP, Vlietstra RE, Ilstrup DM, et al: A randomized comparison of the nephrotoxicity of iopamidol and diatrizoate in high risk patients undergoing cardiac angiography. *J Am Coll Cardiol* 17:384–390, 1991.
53. Rudnick MR, Goldfarb S, Wexler L, et al: Nephrotoxicity of ionic and nonionic contrast media in 1196 patients: a randomized trial. The Iohexol Cooperative Study. *Kidney Int* 47:254–261, 1995.
54. Jo SH, Youn TJ, Koo BK, et al: Renal toxicity evaluation and comparison between Visipaque (iodixanol) and Hexabrix (ioxaglate) in patients with renal insufficiency undergoing coronary angiography: the RECOVER study: a randomized controlled trial. *J Am Coll Cardiol* 48:924–930, 2006.
55. Aspelin P, Aubry P, Fransson SG, et al: Nephrotoxic effects in high-risk patients undergoing angiography. *N Engl J Med* 348:491–499, 2003.
56. Solomon RJ, Natarajan MK, Doucet S, et al: Cardiac angiography in renally impaired patients (CARE) study: a randomized double-blind trial of contrast-induced nephropathy in patients with chronic kidney disease. *Circulation* 115:3189–3196, 2007.
57. Rudnick MR, Davidson C, Laskey W, et al: Nephrotoxicity of iodixanol versus ioversol in patients with chronic kidney disease: the Visipaque Angiography/Interventions with Laboratory Outcomes in Renal Insufficiency (VALOR) Trial. *Am Heart J* 156:776–782, 2008.
58. Gurm HS, Seth M, Kooiman J, et al: A novel tool for reliable and accurate prediction of renal complications in patients undergoing percutaneous coronary intervention. *J Am Coll Cardiol* 61:2242–2248, 2013.
59. Mockel M, Radovic M, Kuhnle Y, et al: Acute renal haemodynamic effects of radiocontrast media in patients undergoing left ventricular and coronary angiography. *Nephrol Dial Transplant* 23:1588–1594, 2008.
60. Brezis M, Rosen S: Hypoxia of the renal medulla—its implications for disease. *N Engl J Med* 332:647–655, 1995.
61. Heyman SN, Brezis M, Epstein FH, et al: Early renal medullary hypoxic injury from radiocontrast and indomethacin. *Kidney Int* 40:632–642, 1991.
62. Persson PB, Hansell P, Liss P: Pathophysiology of contrast medium-induced nephropathy. *Kidney Int* 68:14–22, 2005.
63. Bakris GL, Lass N, Gaber AO, et al: Radiocontrast medium-induced declines in renal function: a role for oxygen free radicals. *Am J Physiol* 258:F115–F120, 1990.
64. Araujo M, Welch WJ: Oxidative stress and nitric oxide in kidney function. *Curr Opin Nephrol Hypertens* 15:72–77, 2006.
65. Peer A, Averbukh Z, Berman S, et al: Contrast media augmented apoptosis of cultured renal mesangial, tubular, epithelial, endothelial, and hepatic cells. *Invest Radiol* 38:177–182, 2003.
66. Haller C, Hizoh I: The cytotoxicity of iodinated radiocontrast agents on renal cells in vitro. *Invest Radiol* 39:149–154, 2004.
67. Solomon R, Werner C, Mann D, et al: Effects of saline, mannitol, and furosemide to prevent acute decreases in renal function induced by radiocontrast agents. *N Engl J Med* 331:1416–1420, 1994.
68. Mueller C, Buerkle G, Buettner HJ, et al: Prevention of contrast media-associated nephropathy: randomized comparison of 2 hydration regimens in 1620 patients undergoing coronary angioplasty. *Arch Intern Med* 162:329–336, 2002.
69. Taylor AJ, Hotchkiss D, Morse RW, et al: PREPARED: preparation for angiography in renal dysfunction: a randomized trial of inpatient vs outpatient hydration protocols for cardiac catheterization in mild-to-moderate renal dysfunction. *Chest* 114:1570–1574, 1998.
70. Trivedi HS, Moore H, Nasr S, et al: A randomized prospective trial to assess the role of saline hydration on the development of contrast nephrotoxicity. *Nephron Clin Pract* 93:C29–C34, 2003.
71. Stacul F, Adam A, Becker CR, et al: Strategies to reduce the risk of contrast-induced nephropathy. *Am J Cardiol* 98:59K–77K, 2006.
72. Merten GJ, Burgess WP, Gray LV, et al: Prevention of contrast-induced nephropathy with sodium bicarbonate: a randomized controlled trial. *JAMA* 291:2328–2334, 2004.
73. Briguori C, Airoldi F, D'Andrea D, et al: Renal Insufficiency Following Contrast Media Administration Trial (REMEDIAL): a randomized comparison of 3 preventive strategies. *Circulation* 115:1211–1217, 2007.
74. Ozcan EE, Guneri S, Akdeniz B, et al: Sodium bicarbonate, N-acetylcysteine, and saline for prevention of radiocontrast-induced nephropathy. A comparison of 3 regimens for protecting contrast-induced nephropathy in patients undergoing coronary procedures. A single-center prospective controlled trial. *Am Heart J* 154:539–544, 2007.
75. Brar SS, Shen AY, Jorgensen MB, et al: Sodium bicarbonate vs sodium chloride for the prevention of contrast medium-induced nephropathy in patients undergoing coronary angiography: a randomized trial. *JAMA* 300:1038–1046, 2008.
76. Adolph E, Holdt-Lehmann B, Chatterjee T, et al: Renal Insufficiency Following Radiocontrast Exposure Trial (REINFORCE): a randomized comparison of sodium bicarbonate versus sodium chloride hydration for the prevention of contrast-induced nephropathy. *Coron Artery Dis* 19:413–419, 2008.
77. Maioli M, Toso A, Leoncini M, et al: Sodium bicarbonate versus saline for the prevention of contrast-induced nephropathy in patients with renal dysfunction undergoing coronary angiography or intervention. *J Am Coll Cardiol* 52:599–604, 2008.
78. From AM, Bartholmai BJ, Williams AW, et al: Sodium bicarbonate is associated with an increased incidence of contrast nephropathy: a retrospective cohort study of 7977 patients at Mayo Clinic. *Clin J Am Soc Nephrol* 3:10–18, 2008.
79. Brar SS, Hiremath S, Dangas G, et al: Sodium bicarbonate for the prevention of contrast-induced acute kidney injury: a systematic review and meta-analysis. *Clin J Am Soc Nephrol* 4:1584–1592, 2009.
80. Liss P, Nygren A, Ulfendahl HR, et al: Effect of furosemide or mannitol before injection of a non-ionic contrast medium on intrarenal oxygen tension. *Adv Exp Med Biol* 471:353–359, 1999.
81. Dorval JF, Dixon SR, Zelman RB, et al: Feasibility study of the RenalGuard balanced hydration system: a novel strategy for the prevention of contrast-induced nephropathy in high risk patients. *Int J Cardiol* 166:482–486, 2013.
82. Briguori C, Visconti G, Focaccio A, et al: Renal Insufficiency After Contrast Media Administration Trial II (REMEDIAL II): RenalGuard System in high-risk patients for contrast-induced acute kidney injury. *Circulation* 124:1260–1269, 2011.
83. Marenzi G, Ferrari C, Marana I, et al: Prevention of contrast nephropathy by furosemide with matched hydration: the MYTHOS (Induced Diuresis With Matched Hydration Compared to Standard Hydration for Contrast Induced Nephropathy Prevention) trial. *JACC Cardiovasc Interv* 5:90–97, 2012.
84. Lehnert T, Keller E, Gondolf K, et al: Effect of hemodialysis after contrast medium administration in patients with renal insufficiency. *Nephrol Dial Transplant* 13:358–362, 1998.
85. Sterner G, Frennby B, Kurkus J, et al: Does post-angiographic hemodialysis reduce the risk of contrast-medium nephropathy? *Scand J Urol Nephrol* 34:323–326, 2000.
86. Marenzi G, Marana I, Lauri G, et al: The prevention of radiocontrast-agent-induced nephropathy by hemofiltration. *N Engl J Med* 349:1333–1340, 2003.
87. Stone GW, McCullough PA, Tumlin JA, et al: Fenoldopam mesylate for the prevention of contrast-induced nephropathy: a randomized controlled trial. *JAMA* 290:2284–2291, 2003.
88. Teirstein PS, Price MJ, Mathur VS, et al: Differential effects between intravenous and targeted renal delivery of fenoldopam on renal function and blood pressure in patients undergoing cardiac catheterization. *Am J Cardiol* 97:1076–1081, 2006.
89. Huber W, Ilgmann K, Page M, et al: Effect of theophylline on contrast material-nephropathy in patients with chronic renal insufficiency: controlled, randomized, double-blinded study. *Radiology* 223:772–779, 2002.
90. Erley CM, Duda SH, Rehfuss D, et al: Prevention of radiocontrast-media-induced nephropathy in patients with pre-existing renal insufficiency by hydration in combination with the adenosine antagonist theophylline. *Nephrol Dial Transplant* 14:1146–1149, 1999.
91. Tepel M, van der Giet M, Schwarzfeld C, et al: Prevention of radiographic-contrast-agent-induced reductions in renal function by acetylcysteine. *N Engl J Med* 343:180–184, 2000.
92. Marenzi G, Assanelli E, Marana I, et al: N-acetylcysteine and contrast-induced nephropathy in primary angioplasty. *N Engl J Med* 354:2773–2782, 2006.
93. Webb JG, Pate GE, Humphries KH, et al: A randomized controlled trial of intravenous N-acetylcysteine for the prevention of contrast-induced nephropathy after cardiac catheterization: lack of effect. *Am Heart J* 148:422–429, 2004.
94. Zhang BC, Li WM, Xu YW: High-dose statin pretreatment for the prevention of contrast-induced nephropathy: a meta-analysis. *Can J Cardiol* 27:851–858, 2011.
95. Han Y, Zhu G, Han L, et al: Short-term rosuvastatin therapy for prevention of contrast-induced acute kidney injury in patients with diabetes and chronic kidney disease. *J Am Coll Cardiol* 25:5353–5359, 2013.
96. Leoncini M, Toso A, Maioli M, et al: Early high-dose rosuvastatin for contrast-induced nephropathy prevention in acute coronary syndrome. Results from Protective effect of Rosuvastatin and Antiplatelet Therapy On contrast-induced acute kidney injury and myocardial damage in patients with Acute Coronary Syndrome (PRATO-ACS Study). *J Am Coll Cardiol* 63:71–79, 2014.
97. James MT, Samuel SM, Manning MA, et al: Contrast-induced acute kidney injury and risk of adverse clinical outcomes after coronary angiography: a systematic review and meta-analysis. *Circ Cardiovasc Interv* 6:37–43, 2013.
98. Back MR, Caridi JG, Hawkins IF, Jr, et al: Angiography with carbon dioxide (CO_2). *Surg Clin North Am* 78:575–591, 1998.

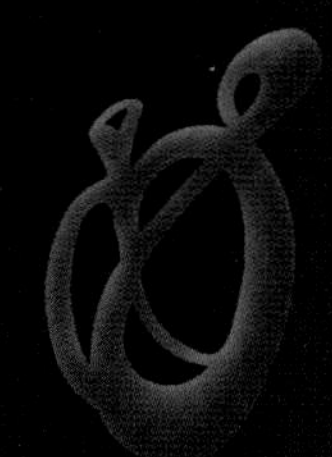

PART II

CORONARY ARTERY INTERVENTION

8 Percutaneous Coronary Intervention for Unprotected Left Main Disease

Philippe Généreux and Gregg W. Stone

INTRODUCTION

Left main (LM) coronary artery disease, defined by a visually estimated diameter stenosis of at least 50%, is present in approximately 3% to 5% of patients undergoing coronary angiography.[1-4] Without revascularization, mortality is as high as 50% within 3 years of follow-up.[5-10] Current treatment guidelines recommend coronary artery bypass grafting (CABG) for most patients with unprotected LM disease[11,12]; however, significant advances in stent technology, revascularization techniques, and antithrombotic therapies have made percutaneous coronary intervention (PCI) a safe, feasible, and effective method of revascularization in many patients with LM disease. The present chapter will review the current evidence related to LM PCI and describe PCI techniques to manage diverse LM disease anatomy.

Philippe Généreux has received speaker fees from Abbott Vascular and is a consultant for Cardiovascular System, Inc.

RANDOMIZED CONTROLLED TRIALS

To date, there have been four randomized controlled trials (RCTs) comparing PCI with CABG for LM intervention (**Table 8-1**). The Study of Unprotected Left Main Stenting versus Bypass Surgery (LE MANS) was the first RCT to compare the safety and efficacy of PCI with CABG.[13] LE MANS enrolled 105 symptomatic patients with >50% diameter stenosis in the LM with or without concomitant multivessel coronary artery disease (CAD) to revascularization with either PCI or CABG. The primary endpoint was the change in left ventricular ejection fraction (LVEF) at 12 months as measured by two-dimensional echocardiography. The secondary endpoint was major adverse cardiac and cerebrovascular events (MACCE), the composite of all-cause death, myocardial infarction (MI), stroke, or target vessel revascularization (TVR). At 30 days, PCI was associated with a significantly lower rate of MACCE (2% vs. 13%; p = 0.03) and shorter duration of hospitalization (6.8 ± 3.7 vs. 12.0 ± 9.6 days; p = 0.0007). At 1 year, LVEF improved to a significantly greater degree with PCI than with CABG (3.3 ± 6.7% vs. 0.5 ± 0.8%; p = 0.047), resulting in greater LVEF in the PCI

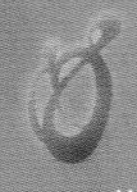

TABLE 8-1 Randomized Controlled Trials and Metaanalyses Comparing PCI and CABG in Patients with Left Main Disease

STUDIES	YEAR	N	FOLLOW-UP	POPULATION/ STUDIES	PRIMARY ENDPOINTS	PCI %	CABG %	P VALUE
Randomized Trials								
LE MANS[13]	2008	105	1 yr	Stable and unstable angina	% Change in LVEF	3.3 ± 6.7	0.5 ± 0.8	0.047
SYNTAX[14-16]	2009	705	5 yr	Stable and unstable angina	MACCE	36.9	31.0	0.12
PRECOMBAT[17]	2011	600	1 yr	Angina, NSTE-ACS	MACCE	8.7	6.7	0.01
Boudriot et al.[18]	2011	201	1 yr	Stable and unstable angina	MACE	19	13.9	0.19
Metaanalyses								
Capodanno et al.[19]	2011	1611	1 yr	RCTs	MACCE	14.5	11.8	0.11
Athappan et al.[20]	2013	14,203	5 yr	RCTs, registries	MACCE*	—	—	NS

*Primary outcome not mentioned and outcomes were reported as odds ratios.

CABG, Coronary artery bypass graft; *LVEF,* left ventricular ejection fraction; *MACCE,* major adverse cardiac and cerebrovascular events; *MACE,* major adverse cardiac events; *NS,* not significant; *NSTE-ACS,* non-ST-segment elevation acute coronary syndrome; *PCI,* percutaneous coronary; intervention; *RCT,* randomized controlled trials.

group (58.0 ± 6.8% vs. 54.1 ± 8.9%; p = 0.01). Angina status and treadmill exercise performance were comparable in the two groups. There was no difference in all-cause mortality, and 1-year MACCE rates were also similar in both groups (relative risk [RR], 1.09; 95% confidence interval [CI], 0.85 to 1.38). At 28 ± 9.9 months of follow-up, MACCE-free survival was comparable in both groups, but there was a trend of fewer deaths in the PCI group (p = 0.08). The major limitations of this trial were its small size, a relatively low rate (72%) of internal mammary artery graft use in the surgical cohort, and a high rate of bare-metal stent use (65%), with mainly first-generation drug-eluting stents (DES) in the remainder.

The Synergy Between PCI with Taxus and Cardiac Surgery (SYNTAX) trial is the largest RCT to date to evaluate optimal revascularization strategy (PCI vs. CABG) in patients with LM disease.[14] SYNTAX randomized 1800 patients with three-vessel or LM disease to PCI with first-generation TAXUS paclitaxel-eluting stents (PES) or CABG, stratified by the presence of LM disease and medically treated diabetes. The primary endpoint was 1-year rate of MACCE (death from any cause, stroke, MI, or repeat revascularization), and patients were followed up to 5 years. The study used a hierarchical statistical approach that prespecified statistical testing on the LM subgroup only after the demonstration of noninferiority between PCI and CABG in the overall population for the primary endpoint of 1-year MACCE. Since PCI was not shown to be noninferior to CABG in the trial (1-year MACCE: 17.8% for PCI vs. 12.4% for CABG; p = 0.002), the findings of the LM subgroup are considered hypothesis-generating.

A total of 705 patients were enrolled with LM disease. The mean EuroSCORE of the LM cohort was 3.8, and the mean SYNTAX score was 30, consistent with complex and extensive CAD. The 1-year rate of MACCE in the LM subgroup was similar in the two groups (15.8% PCI vs. 13.7% for CABG; p = 0.44).[15] The 1-year rate of TVR was significantly greater in the PCI group (11.8% vs. 6.5%; p = 0.02); however, the rate of stroke was significantly greater in the CABG group (2.7% vs. 0.3%; p = 0.009). There were no differences in the rates of all-cause death or MI between the two groups. Comparing PCI to CABG, the 1-year MACCE rate was greater in the CABG group in patients with isolated LM or LM + one-vessel CAD (7.5% vs. 13.2%, respectively) but was greater in the PCI group in patients with LM + two-vessel or LM + three-vessel CAD (19.8% vs. 14.4% and 19.3% vs. 15.4%, respectively). When stratified by SYNTAX score tertiles (0-22, 23-32, >32), the MACCE rates in the lower two tertiles were similar between PCI and CABG; however, the highest tertile had a significantly greater MACCE rate with PCI compared with CABG.

The final 5-year results of the SYNTAX trial have been recently published.[16] The MACCE rate did not differ significantly between the two treatment groups (36.9% for PCI vs. 31.0% for CABG; p = 0.12). When stratified by SYNTAX tertiles (0-22, 22-32, >32), the MACCE rates were similar between PCI and CABG in the lower two tertiles; however, in the highest tertile, PCI had a significantly higher rate of MACCE compared with CABG (**Figure 8-1**). While these data suggest that PCI with TAXUS stents may be a reasonable alternative to CABG in patients with low and intermediate SYNTAX scores, given the small sample sizes of these subsets, prospective trials are required for confirmation before such an approach is widely adopted.

The Premier of Randomized Comparison of Bypass Surgery versus Angioplasty Using Sirolimus-Eluting Stent in Patients with Left Main Coronary Artery Disease (PRECOMBAT) randomized 600 patients with LM disease to first-generation Cypher sirolimus-eluting stents (SES) versus CABG.[17] The primary endpoint was MACCE (the composite of death from any cause, MI, stroke, or ischemia-driven TVR) at 1 year, powered for noninferiority. The mean EuroScore was 2.7, and the mean SYNTAX score was 25. At 1 year, PCI was shown to be noninferior to CABG (8.7% for PCI vs. 6.7% for CABG; p = 0.01 for noninferiority) for MACCE. Additionally, there were no differences at 1 year in any of the individual components of the composite endpoint. At 2 years the rate of MACCE was also not significantly different between the groups (12.2% for PCI vs. 8.1% for CABG; p = 0.12), although ischemia-driven TVR was significantly more common in the PCI group (9.0% vs. 4.2%; p = 0.02). The main limitations of this trial were the modest number of patients enrolled, the wide margin for noninferiority, and the low event rates in both groups, making these results hypothesis-generating rather than conclusive.

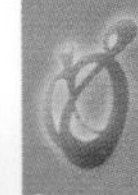

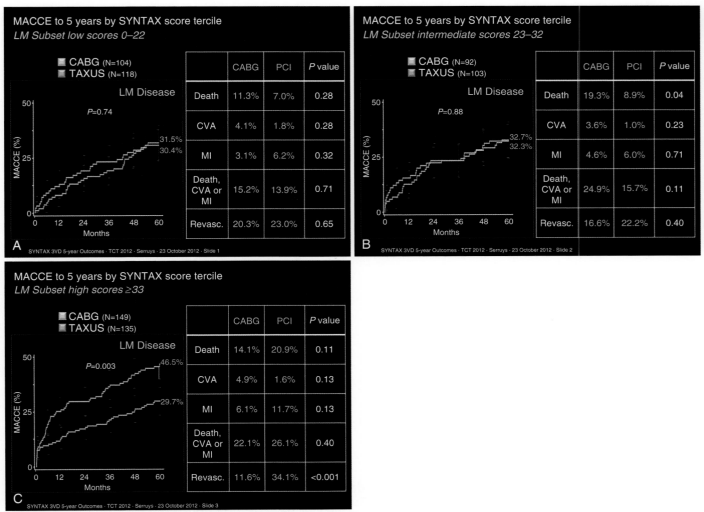

MACCE to 5 years by SYNTAX score tercile
LM Subset low scores 0–22

CABG (N=104)
TAXUS (N=118)

LM Disease
P=0.74
31.5%
30.4%
MACCE (%)
Months

	CABG	PCI	*P* value
Death	11.3%	7.0%	0.28
CVA	4.1%	1.8%	0.28
MI	3.1%	6.2%	0.32
Death, CVA or MI	15.2%	13.9%	0.71
Revasc.	20.3%	23.0%	0.65

A
SYNTAX 3VD 5-year Outcomes · TCT 2012 · Serruys · 23 October 2012 · Slide 1

MACCE to 5 years by SYNTAX score tercile
LM Subset intermediate scores 23–32

CABG (N=92)
TAXUS (N=103)

LM Disease
P=0.88
32.7%
32.3%
MACCE (%)
Months

	CABG	PCI	*P* value
Death	19.3%	8.9%	0.04
CVA	3.6%	1.0%	0.23
MI	4.6%	6.0%	0.71
Death, CVA or MI	24.9%	15.7%	0.11
Revasc.	16.6%	22.2%	0.40

B
SYNTAX 3VD 5-year Outcomes · TCT 2012 · Serruys · 23 October 2012 · Slide 2

MACCE to 5 years by SYNTAX score tercile
LM Subset high scores ≥33

CABG (N=149)
TAXUS (N=135)

LM Disease
P=0.003
46.5%
29.7%
MACCE (%)
Months

	CABG	PCI	*P* value
Death	14.1%	20.9%	0.11
CVA	4.9%	1.6%	0.13
MI	6.1%	11.7%	0.13
Death, CVA or MI	22.1%	26.1%	0.40
Revasc.	11.6%	34.1%	<0.001

C
SYNTAX 3VD 5-year Outcomes · TCT 2012 · Serruys · 23 October 2012 · Slide 3

FIGURE 8-1 Final 5-year results of the SYNTAX trial in the subgroup of patients with left main disease (n = 705) stratified by baseline SYNTAX score. MACCE rates did not significantly differ between CABG and PCI revascularization in patients with low **(A)** or intermediate **(B)** SYNTAX scores. However, among patients with high SYNTAX scores, MACCE was substantially higher with PCI compared with CABG **(C)**.

The fourth RCT comparing PCI with CABG in unprotected LM disease is a small study from Boudriot et al.[18] This trial enrolled 201 patients with documented ischemia and LM diameter stenosis >50% with or without multivessel disease. The primary clinical endpoint was the composite rate of major adverse cardiac events (MACE) at 1 year, including cardiac death, MI, or TVR, powered for noninferiority. PCI failed to reach noninferiority compared with CABG for 1-year MACE (19% PCI vs. 13.9% CABG; p = 0.19 for noninferiority), driven by greater TVR after PCI. The overall results remained unchanged at extended 3-year follow-up. Major limitations of this study included a small sample size, the noninclusion of stroke as an endpoint, and use of first-generation DES.

METAANALYSES

Several metaanalyses of observational registries and RCTs have been conducted comparing PCI and CABG for LM revascularization. In a recent metaanalysis, Athappan and colleagues compared the long-term outcomes between PCI using first-generation DES and CABG in unprotected LM patients.[20] This analysis included 21 observational studies and three RCTs, for a total of 14,203 patients. At 5 years, there were no significant differences between PCI and CABG in all-cause death (odds ratio [OR] = .0.79; 95% CI, 0.57 to 1.08), cardiac death (OR = 0.95; 95% CI, 0.36 to 2.50), or nonfatal MI (OR = 1.38; 95% CI, 0.71 to 2.70). PCI was associated with significantly lower 5-year rates of stroke (OR = 0.27; 95% CI, 0.13 to 0.55) and cumulative MACCE (OR = 0.64; 95% CI, 0.51 to 0.80) but a greater rate of TVR (OR = 3.77; 95% CI, 2.43 to 5.87) compared with CABG. When stratifying patients by complexity and extent of baseline coronary disease by SYNTAX score assessment (reported in only three studies), PCI and CABG had nonsignificantly different rates of all-cause mortality, MI, and MACCE in the lower two tertiles of the SYNTAX score (<32); however, with more complex disease (SYNTAX score >32), CABG was associated with significantly better outcomes at 3 years. The combination of randomized trials and registries (which dominated the numbers of patients) limits the interpretation of this metaanalysis.

Capodanno and colleagues performed a metaanalysis of the four RCTs of PCI with first-generation DES versus CABG for unprotected LM disease (total 1611 patients).[19] The 1-year rate of MACCE was nonsignificantly different between

PCI and CABG (14.5% vs. 11.8%; OR = 1.28; 95% CI, 0.95 to 1.72; p = 0.11), although TVR was greater after PCI (11.4% vs. 5.4%; OR = 2.25; 95% CI, 1.54 to 3.29; p = 0.001). Conversely, stroke occurred less frequently with PCI (0.1% vs. 1.7%; OR = 0.15; 95% CI, 0.03 to 0.67; p = 0.013). There were no significant differences in the rates of all-cause death (3.0% vs. 4.1%; OR = 0.74; 95% CI, 0.43 to 1.29; p = 0.29) or MI (2.8% vs. 2.9%; OR = 0.98; 95% CI, 0.54 to 1.78; p = 0.95) between the two groups. Long-term outcomes were not reported.

ONGOING TRIALS

On the basis of these data, two large-scale trials are ongoing which will importantly inform the relative risks and benefits of PCI with contemporary DES versus CABG. Both trials are based on the observations that in the trials completed to date, PCI with first-generation DES appeared comparable to CABG in patients with low or intermediate anatomic disease complexity, but not in those with concomitant extensive multivessel CAD. Both trials are also utilizing second-generation DES for which outcomes have been shown to be improved compared with first-generation devices used in the earlier studies. The Evaluation of XIENCE Prime or XIENCE V versus CABG for Effectiveness of Left Main Revascularization (EXCEL) trial (NCT01205776) is a prospective, randomized multicenter trial in which 1905 patients with significant LM CAD and a SYNTAX score of ≤32 have been enrolled at 148 international sites and randomized 1:1 to either PCI using XIENCE everolimus-eluting stents or CABG. The primary endpoint, powered for sequential noninferiority and superiority testing, is the composite rate of all-cause death, MI, or stroke at median 3-year follow-up. Follow-up for all randomized subjects is planned for at least 5 years with an option for additional follow-up to 10 years. A second RCT is enrolling at 126 European sites and is comparing PCI using the bioabsorbable polymer biolimus-eluting BIOMATRIX stent (n = 600) with CABG (n = 600) in approximately 1200 patients with LM CAD with ≤3 additional noncomplex lesions (excluding lesions with length >25 mm, chronic total occlusions, bifurcation lesions requiring two stents, and calcified or tortuous vessels) (NCT01496651). The primary endpoint is the composite endpoint of death, stroke, nonindex treatment related MI or repeat revascularization, with follow-up for 5 years.

CURRENT GUIDELINES AND APPROPRIATE USE CRITERIA

Pending the results of EXCEL and Nordic-Baltic-British Left Main Revascularization (NOBLE), the evidence from the randomized trials of first-generation DES versus CABG has been reflected in the current guidelines (**Tables 8-2 and 8-3**). In the American College of Cardiology/American Heart Association/Society of Cardiovascular Angiography and Interventions guidelines (ACC/AHA/SCAI), LM PCI has been upgraded from a Class III indication in 2006 to a Class IIb indication in 2009 and to a Class IIa indication in 2011 for selected patients in whom the coronary anatomy is deemed suitable for PCI and surgical risk is high (**Table 8-2**).[11] To guide selection of the most appropriate revascularization modality for significant unprotected LM disease, these guidelines recommend the following:

TABLE 8-2 The American College of Cardiology Foundation/American Heart Association/Society of Cardiovascular Angiography and Interventions 2011 Guidelines for PCI in Unprotected Left Main Disease

COR	LOE	RECOMMENDATION
I	C	Heart Team approach to revascularization is recommended in patients with unprotected LM or complex CAD
IIa	B	Calculation of STS and SYNTAX scores is reasonable in patients with unprotected LM and complex CAD
IIa	B	PCI to improve survival is reasonable as an alternative to CABG in selected stable patients with significant (>50% diameter stenosis) unprotected LM CAD with the following: • anatomic conditions associated with a low risk of PCI procedural complications and a high likelihood of good long-term outcome (e.g., a low SYNTAX score [<22], ostial or trunk LM CAD); • clinical characteristics that predict a significantly increased risk of adverse surgical outcomes (e.g., STS-predicted risk of operative mortality >5%)
IIa	B	PCI to improve survival is reasonable in patients with UA/NSTEMI when an unprotected LM coronary artery is the culprit lesion and the patient is not a candidate for CABG
IIa	B	IVUS is reasonable for the assessment of angiographically indeterminate LM CAD
IIa	C	PCI to improve survival is reasonable in patients with acute STEMI when an unprotected LM coronary artery is the culprit lesion, distal coronary flow is less than TIMI Grade 3, and PCI can be performed more rapidly and safely than CABG
IIb	B	PCI to improve survival may be reasonable as an alternative to CABG in selected stable patients with significant (>50% diameter stenosis) unprotected LM CAD with the following: • anatomic conditions associated with a low to intermediate risk of PCI procedural complications and an intermediate to high likelihood of good long-term outcome (e.g., low-intermediate SYNTAX score of <33, bifurcation left main CAD) • clinical characteristics that predict an increased risk of adverse surgical outcomes (e.g., moderate-severe chronic obstructive pulmonary disease, disability from previous stroke, or previous cardiac surgery; STS-predicted risk of operative mortality >2%)
IIb	C	IVUS may be considered for guidance of coronary stent implantation, particularly in cases of LM coronary artery stenting
III	B	PCI to improve survival should not be performed in stable patients with significant (>50% diameter stenosis) unprotected LM CAD who have unfavorable anatomy for PCI and who are good candidates for CABG

CABG, Coronary artery bypass graft; *CAD,* coronary artery disease; *COR,* class of recommendation; *IVUS,* intravascular ultrasound; *LM,* left main; *LOE,* level of evidence; *PCI,* percutaneous coronary intervention; *STS,* Society of Thoracic Surgeons; *SYNTAX,* Synergy Between Percutaneous Coronary Intervention with TAXUS and Cardiac Surgery; *TIMI,* thrombolysis in myocardial infarction; *UA/STEMI,* unstable angina/ ST-segment-elevation myocardial infarction.
Adapted from Levine GN, Bates ER, Blankenship JC, et al: 2011. ACCF/AHA/SCAI Guideline for Percutaneous Coronary Intervention. A report of the American College of Cardiology Foundation/American Heart Association Task Force on Practice Guidelines and the Society for Cardiovascular Angiography and Interventions. J Am Coll Cardiol 58:e44–e122, 2011.

1. A heart team approach to decision making involving at least one interventional cardiologist and one cardiothoracic surgeon (Class 1, level of evidence [LOE] C)
2. Utilization of angiographic risk stratification by the SYNTAX score and clinical risk stratification by the Society of Thoracic Surgeons (STS) score (Class IIa, level of evidence B)

PCI is considered a reasonable alternative to CABG in patients with stable ischemic heart disease having a SYNTAX score <22 and ostial/shaft LM disease with STS predicted operative mortality >5% (Class IIa, LOE B) and in patients with SYNTAX score <32 and LM bifurcation disease with STS predicted operative mortality >2% (Class IIb, LOE B). It is important to note that most of the RCTs comparing PCI and CABG enrolled patients who could undergo equivalent revascularization with either modality.

TABLE 8-3 Appropriate Use Criteria for Coronary Revascularization of Unprotected Left Main Disease

	Appropriate Use Score (1-9)	
	PCI	**CABG**
Isolated left main stenosis	Uncertain (6)	Appropriate (9)
Left main stenosis and additional CAD with low CAD burden (i.e., 1- to 2-vessel additional involvement, low SYNTAX score)	Uncertain (5)	Appropriate (9)
Left main stenosis and additional CAD with intermediate to high CAD burden (i.e., 3-vessel involvement, presence of CTO, or high SYNTAX score)	Inappropriate (3)	Appropriate (9)

Method of revascularization in presence of multivessel coronary artery disease, Canadian Class Society angina ≥III, and/or evidence of intermediate- to high-risk findings on noninvasive testing.
CABG, Coronary artery bypass graft; *CAD,* coronary artery disease; *CTO,* chronic total occlusion; *PCI,* percutaneous coronary intervention.
Adapted from Patel MR, Dehmer GJ, Hirshfeld JW, et al: ACCF/SCAI/STS/AATS/AHA/ASNC/HFSA/SCCT 2012. Appropriate use criteria for coronary revascularization focused update: a report of the American College of Cardiology Foundation Appropriate Use Criteria Task Force, Society for Cardiovascular Angiography and Interventions, Society of Thoracic Surgeons, American Association for Thoracic Surgery, American Heart Association, American Society of Nuclear Cardiology, and the Society of Cardiovascular Computed Tomography. J Am Coll Cardiol 59:857–881, 2012.

The Appropriate Use Criteria (AUC) recommendations have also evolved to incorporate the long-term evidence from randomized clinical trial data.[21] **Table 8-3** summarizes their recommendations.

The European Society of Cardiology and the European Association for Cardio-Thoracic Surgery (ESC/EACTS) 2014 guidelines for myocardial revascularization have recently upgraded the status of PCI for LM revascularization.[12] LM with SYNTAX score ≤22 has been given a Class I recommendation (LOE B), while LM with SYNTAX score 22-32 was given a Class IIa recommendation (LOE B). LM with SYNTAX score >32 was given a Class III recommendation (LOE B). The ESC/EACTS also focused on the central importance of the multidisciplinary heart team discussion in all scenarios involving complex multivessel CAD and unprotected LM disease.

SCORING ALGORITHMS

Scoring algorithms to assess clinical risk and anatomic disease complexity bring objectivity to risk stratification and, paired with clinical judgment, can guide the decision-making process to select the most appropriate revascularization strategy for a given patient. ESC/EACTS recommendations for various scores are shown in **Table 8-4**. The clinical STS and EuroSCORE II are recommended to assess suitability for CABG (Class I, LOE B, and Class IIa, LOE B, respectively), whereas the anatomic SYNTAX score is useful to discriminate relative outcomes between PCI and CABG (Class I, LOE B).

The SYNTAX score, first developed and evaluated in the SYNTAX trial,[14,22] was subsequently validated and studied in many unprotected LM studies.[15,23-28] In most of these studies, rates of composite ischemic endpoints (death, MI, target lesion revascularization [TLR], or TVR) were significantly greater after PCI in the highest tertile of SYNTAX score than in the lower two tertiles. Capodanno et al. demonstrated that a SYNTAX score >34 was associated with significantly higher rates of ischemic events in patients with LM CAD undergoing PCI than in those undergoing CABG.[23] Of note, only the baseline SYNTAX score had prognostic value; the lesion location in the LM (ostial, shaft, or bifurcation) and number of stents implanted were not predictive of clinical outcomes. Similarly, analysis from the ISAR-Left Main trial also showed

TABLE 8-4 European Society of Cardiology and the European Association for Cardio-Thoracic Surgery Recommendations for Risk Stratification for PCI and CABG

	Number of Variables			*Class (LOE)*	
SCORE	**CLINICAL**	**ANATOMICAL**	**OUTCOME MEASURE**	**PCI**	**CABG**
EuroSCORE	17	0	Operative mortality	III (C)	III (B)
EuroSCORE II	18	0	In-hospital mortality	IIb (C)	IIa (B)
SYNTAX Score	0	11	MACCE	I (B)	I (B)
NCDR Cath PCI	8	0	In-hospital mortality	IIb (B)	—
STS Score	40	2	In-hospital or 30-day mortality, and in-hospital morbidity (permanent stroke, renal failure, prolonged ventilation, deep sternal wound infection, re-operation, length of stay, 6 or 14 days)	—	I (B)
ACEF Score	3	0	In-hospital or 30-day mortality	IIb (C)	IIb (C)

ACEF, Age, creatinine, ejection fraction; *CABG,* coronary artery bypass grafting; *class,* class of recommendation; *LOE,* level of evidence; *MACCE,* major adverse cardiac and cerebrovascular events; *NCDR,* National Cardiovascular Database Registry; *PCI,* percutaneous coronary intervention; *STS,* Society of Thoracic Surgeons.
Adapted from Authors/Task Force members, Windecker S, Kolh P, et al: 2014. ESC/EACTS Guidelines on myocardial revascularization: the Task Force on Myocardial Revascularization of the European Society of Cardiology (ESC) and the European Association for Cardio-Thoracic Surgery (EACTS). Developed with the special contribution of the European Association of Percutaneous Cardiovascular Interventions (EAPCI). Eur Heart J 35(37):2541–2619, 2014.

a clear association between the overall burden and complexity of CAD, as assessed by SYNTAX score, and the rate of TLR and MACE at 3 years.[29]

By combining clinical variables and the angiographic SYNTAX score, several other scores have been created and studied in an attempt to improve the predictive capability of the solely anatomic SYNTAX score. Of note, the Global Risk Classification, which is a combination of the SYNTAX score and EuroSCORE, showed the best calibration and discrimination in the prediction of adverse events such as mortality after LM PCI.[30] Additionally, the Global Risk Classification identified a low-risk cohort of patients (low SYNTAX score) who could be safely treated with PCI.[31]

The recently developed SYNTAX Score II combines the SYNTAX score with anatomical and clinical variables that were shown to alter the threshold value at which equipoise was achieved between CABG and PCI for long-term mortality.[32] The variables included are age, creatinine clearance, LVEF, presence of unprotected LM disease (vs. three-vessel CAD), peripheral vascular disease, female sex, and chronic obstructive pulmonary disease. This score may be used to identify some patients considered low-risk by the anatomic SYNTAX score who might preferentially benefit by CABG, and some patients considered high-risk by the anatomic SYNTAX score who might preferentially benefit by PCI (**Figure 8-2**). Further validation of the SYNTAX Score II (including assessment of endpoints other than mortality) is required prior to its widespread adoption.[33]

IMPACT OF STENT CHOICE

Given the fact that ≥70% of the myocardial mass is typically perfused by the LM, stent failure, such as restenosis and stent thrombosis, may have potentially catastrophic consequences.[34] Despite its large diameter, disease involving the LM frequently involves the distal bifurcation and side branches (SBs). **Table 8-5** presents data from observational registries and trials comparing different stent types for LM PCI. A metaanalysis of observational studies and RCTs involving 10,342 patients demonstrated lower event rates for DES than BMS for mortality, repeat revascularization, and MACE at 6 to 12 months, 2 years, and 3 years. Adjusted analyses among 5081 patients demonstrated a significantly lower risk of mortality with DES at 2-year (OR = 0.42; 95% CI, 0.28 to 0.62; $p < 0.001$) and 3-year (OR = 0.70; 95% CI, 0.53 to 0.92; $p < 0.01$) follow-up. Although these analyses should be seen as hypothesis-generating, given their retrospective nature, these data support a default strategy of DES for LM PCI in most cases unless long-term dual antiplatelet therapy is contraindicated.[35]

To date, only two RCTs have compared different DES in LM PCI.[38,39] In ISAR-Left Main, no significant difference in the 1-year composite endpoint of death, MI, or TLR was present between Cypher SES and Taxus PES (both first-generation DES).[38] Similarly, no difference in the same endpoint was observed in ISAR-Left Main II between slow-release resolute zotarolimus-eluting stents (ZES) and everolimus-eluting stents (EES) (both second-generation DES).[39] The modest number of patients included in these studies (~600), however, precludes definitive conclusions. Recently, a retrospective study demonstrated better mid-term (2-year) outcomes when comparing a first-generation DES (PES) to a second-generation DES (EES) in terms of target vessel failure (a composite of cardiac death, target vessel MI, or TLR).[41] Once again, given the small number of patients included in this study (n = 344) and the retrospective nature of the analysis, these results are hypothesis-generating. That being said, in light of the important burden of evidence supporting the improved safety and efficacy of second-generation DES compared with both first-generation DES and bare-metal stent (BMS),[42,43] second-generation DES should be the default platform when performing unprotected LM PCI, assuming the absence of contraindication to their use.[11,12]

IN-STENT RESTENOSIS

No dedicated RCTs examining treatment options of LM in-stent restenosis (ISR) have been conducted so far, and most of the current evidence has originated from registry data and observational series. In the CORPAL (Córdoba and Las Palmas) registry, 7% of patients who underwent PCI with DES in unprotected LM disease developed ISR at a median follow-up of 9 months.[44] The location of restenosis was divided equally among the main vessel (MV) (LM/left anterior descending artery [LAD]) or isolated to the ostium of circumflex or both arteries. Angiographically, ISR lesions were divided equally between focal (47%) and diffuse (51%). Intravascular ultrasound (IVUS) was conducted in 79% of ISR patients and demonstrated that stent under expansion was present in 14% of the cases. All patients except four were treated with repeat PCI with DES—58% with provisional stenting and 42% with a two-stent approach. During a follow-up period of 4 years, the overall recurrent MACE rate was 22%, with the provisional approach having a significantly higher MACE-free survival compared with the two-stent approach (85% vs. 53%; $p < 0.05$). Similarly, patients with ISR involving only one bifurcation segment had better MACE-free survival compared with patients with more than one segment involved (84% vs. 47%; $p < 0.05$) at 4 years.

In the MITO (Milan and New-Tokyo) registry, 92 out of 474 (19%) unprotected LM patients undergoing PCI with DES developed ISR, and 84 (19%) were treated with repeat PCI (43 with balloon angioplasty alone and 41 with further DES implantation).[45] Of note, patients with focal left circumflex (LCX) stenosis were frequently asymptomatic and were discovered only on angiographic follow-up. During a follow-up period of 2 years, the patients undergoing POBA had significantly greater MACE rates compared with repeat PCI with DES (higher risk [HR], 2.75; 95% CI, 1.26 to 5.98; p = 0.01).

One of the important independent predictors of LM ISR is the final minimum stent area as determined by IVUS.[46] Post-PCI optimal values for the MV, both branches, and the polygon of confluence (POC) have been established and were shown to be associated with significantly improved outcomes (**Figure 8-3**).

DISEASE LOCATION: OSTIAL/MID-SHAFT VERSUS DISTAL LM

PCI of the distal LM bifurcation has been associated with higher follow-up MACE rates than PCI limited to the LM ostium or mid-shaft in most, but not all, studies. The Drug-Eluting Stent for Left Main Coronary Artery Disease (DELTA) registry is the largest study to examine this issue.[47] A total of 1612 LM PCI patients were included in the study, including 1130 patients with distal bifurcation lesions. During a median follow-up of 3.4 years, patients with distal bifurcation disease had a greater rate of MACE (a composite endpoint of death,

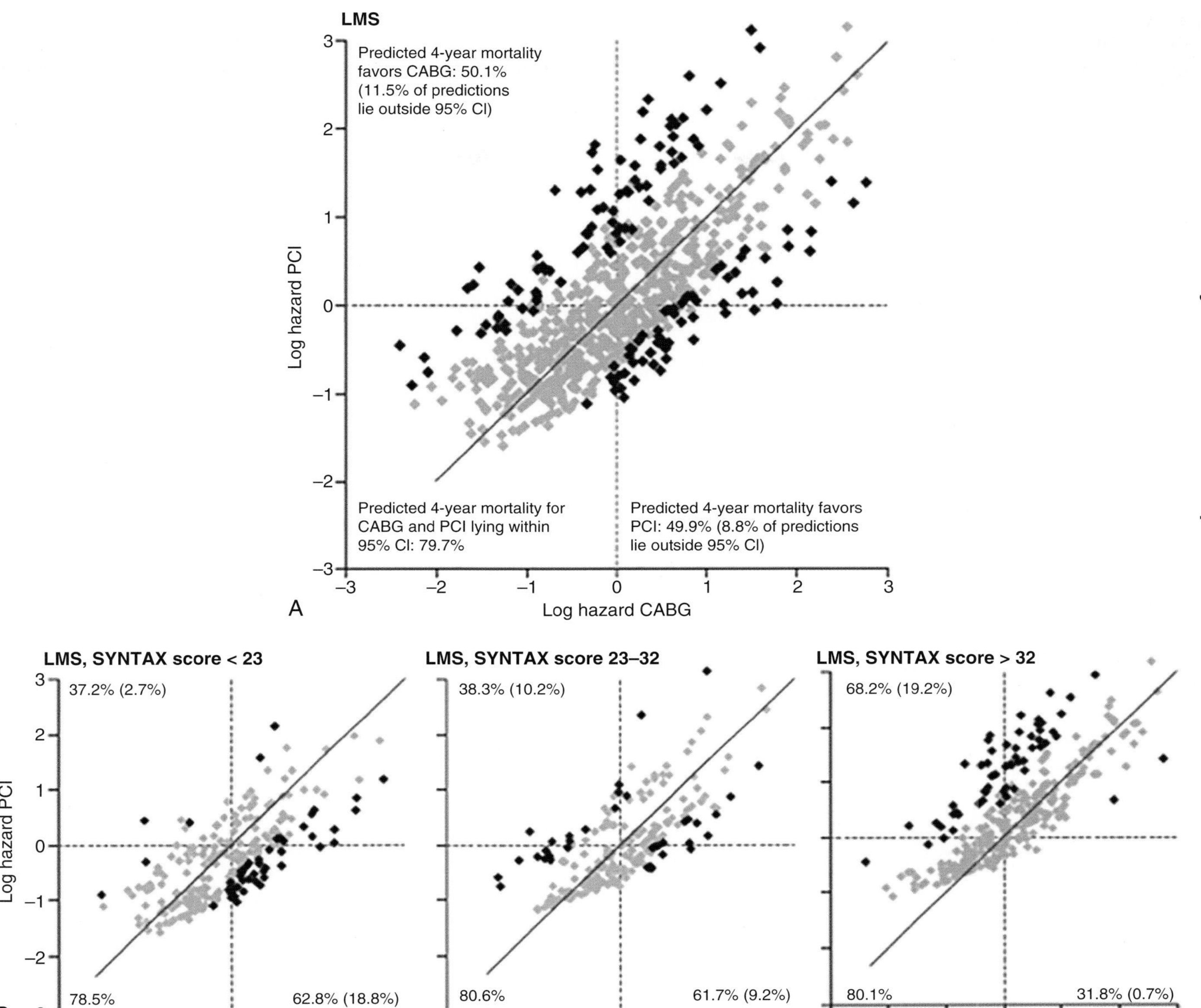

FIGURE 8-2 Predicted 4-year mortality rates after CABG and PCI for individual patients with left main disease in the SYNTAX trial according to the SYNTAX score II. The top graph **(A)** is the entire left main cohort, while the bottom three graphs **(B)** are the left main cohort separated by low, intermediate, and high SYNTAX score tertiles. The diagonal line represents identical mortality predictions for CABG and PCI. Patients to the left of the diagonal line favor CABG (actual percentages shown in top left corner), and to the right favor PCI (actual percentages shown in bottom right corner). Individual mortality predictions for CABG or PCI that could be separated with 95% confidence interval (CI) (p <0.05) are colored black (actual percentages shown in parentheses in respective corners). Mortality predictions that could not be separated with 95% CI (p >0.05) are highlighted in gray, and identify patients with similar 4-year mortality. Percentages of patients in each category are shown. *CABG,* Coronary artery bypass surgery; *LMS,* left main stem; *PCI,* percutaneous coronary intervention. *(Adapted from Farooq V, van Klaveren D, Steyerberg EW, et al: Anatomical and clinical characteristics to guide decision making between coronary artery bypass surgery and percutaneous coronary intervention for individual patients: development and validation of SYNTAX score II. Lancet 381:639–650, 2013.)*

MI, or TVR) compared with ostial/mid-shaft lesions (propensity-score adjusted HR, 1.48; 95% CI, 1.16 to 1.89; p = 0.001), primarily driven by a higher rate of TVR (propensity-score adjusted HR, 1.68; 95% CI, 1.19 to 2.38; p = 0.003). Similar findings have been reported by other groups.[29]

In another registry analysis of 1111 patients with 2 years of follow-up, Palmerini et al. showed that distal bifurcation lesions had a lower freedom from MACE compared with ostial/mid-shaft lesions (72% vs. 80%; p = 0.03).[48] However, whereas patients with distal bifurcation lesions treated with a two-stent strategy had worse outcomes, patients with distal bifurcation lesions treated with a one-stent (provisional) approach had clinical outcomes similar to those with ostial and mid-shaft LM lesions. Given the difference in outcomes after PCI of distal bifurcation LM and nonbifurcation LM lesions, the ACC/AHA guidelines recommend PCI as a Class IIb recommendation for distal bifurcation lesions and Class IIa for ostial/mid-shaft lesions.

ONE-STENT VERSUS TWO-STENT APPROACH FOR LM BIFURCATION DISEASE

Bifurcation lesions represent >50% of all LM PCIs.[15] True distal bifurcation lesions may be treated by either a single-stent or a two-stent strategy. Choice of strategy is based on vessel and lesion characteristics (plaque distribution,

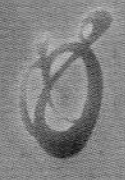

TABLE 8-5 Randomized Trials and Large Observational Studies Comparing Stent Types in Left Main Percutaneous Coronary Intervention

STUDY	YEAR	N	TYPE	F/U	STENT TYPE	PRIMARY OUTCOME	PRIMARY OUTCOME	TVR/TLR	STENT THROMBOSIS
BMS vs. DES									
Erglis et al.[36]	2007	103	RCT	6 mo	BMS vs. PES	Freedom from death/MI/TLR	70.0% vs. 86.8% p = 0.036	16.0% vs. 2.0% p = 0.014	—
Palmerini et al.[34]	2008	1453	NR	2 yr	BMS vs. DES	Freedom from cardiac death	82.4% vs. 93.1% p = 0.00001	—	—
Kim et al.[37]	2009	1217	NR	3 yr	BMS vs. DES	Death/MI	14.9% vs. 14.3% p = 0.85	12.1% vs. 5.4% p < 0.001	—
Onuma et al.[25]	2010	227	NR	4 yr	BMS vs. SES/PES	Death/MI/TVR	53.2% vs. 51.4% p = 0.9	13.9% vs. 16.2% p = 0.7	—
Brennan et al.[4]	2012	2765	NR	2.5 yr	BMS vs. DES	Death	52.7% vs. 39.6% p = significant	—	—
DES vs. DES									
ISAR-LM[38]	2009	607	RCT	1 yr	PES vs. SES	Death/MI/TLR	13.6% vs. 15.8% p = 0.44	6.5% vs. 7.8% p = 0.49	0.3% vs. 0.7% p = 0.57
ISAR-LM II[39]	2013	650	RCT	1 yr	ZES vs. EES	Death/MI/TLR	17.5% vs. 14.3% p = 0.25	11.7% vs. 9.4% p = 0.35	0.9% vs. 0.6% p = 0.99
PRECOMBAT II[40]	2012	661	NR	1.5 yr	EES vs. SES	Death/MI/stroke/ TVR	8.9% vs. 10.8% p = 0.51	6.5% vs. 8.2% p = 0.65	0% vs. 0.3% p = 0.11
LEMAX[41]	2013	344	NR	2 yr	EES vs. PES	TLF	7.6% vs. 16.3% p = 0.01	—	*1.7% vs. 7.0% p = 0.01

BMS, Bare-metal stent; *EES,* everolimus-eluting stent; *F/U,* follow-up; *ISAR,* intracoronary stenting and angiographic results; *LEMAX,* left main XIENCE; *LM,* left main; *MI,* myocardial infarction; *NR,* nonrandomized; *PCI,* percutaneous coronary intervention; *PES,* paclitaxel-eluting stent; *PRECOMBAT,* premier of randomized comparison of bypass surgery versus angioplasty using sirolimus-eluting stent in patients with left main coronary artery disease; *RCT,* randomized control trial; *SES,* sirolimus-eluting stent; *ST,* stent thrombosis; *TLF,* target lesion failure (cardiac death, target vessel MI, and target lesion revascularization); *TLR,* target lesion revascularization; *TVR,* target vessel revascularization; *ZES,* resolute zotarolimus-eluting stent.
*Reported as definite, probable, or possible stent thrombosis.

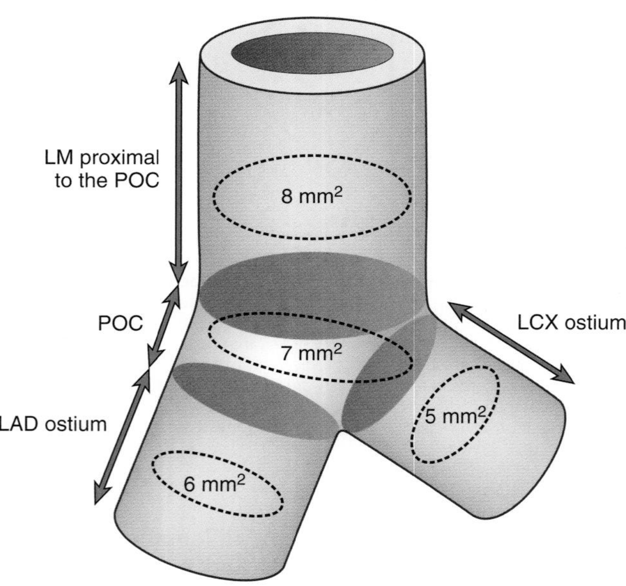

FIGURE 8-3 Approximate values for the intravascular ultrasound-derived minimal lumen area (MLA) for different coronary segments associated with freedom from restenosis and major adverse ischemic events at 2 years after LM stenting in Korea. *LAD,* Left anterior descending; *LCX,* left circumflex; *LM,* left main; *POC,* polygon of confluence. *(Adapted from Kang SJ, Ahn JM, Song H, et al: Comprehensive intravascular ultrasound assessment of stent area and its impact on restenosis and adverse cardiac events in 403 patients with unprotected left main disease. Circ Cardiovasc Interv 4:562–569, 2011.)*

diameter of the branches and the angle between them, anatomy of the SB) in addition to operator experience and expertise.

Few dedicated RCTs have compared stenting strategies in LM bifurcation lesions. Most bifurcation studies have been performed in populations that include both non-LM and LM bifurcation, with the latter usually representing only 2% to 10% of all bifurcation lesions. Nevertheless, outcomes from these studies may be extrapolated to LM patients, although the results of adverse outcomes can be more severe in the LM cohort. Nearly all RCTs in non-LM bifurcations have demonstrated that a routine two-stent approach (stenting both the MV and SB) offers no angiographic or clinical benefits compared with a provisional stenting strategy (stenting the MV only, with stenting of the SB reserved for suboptimal balloon angioplasty results).[49-54] One trial did report lower rates of angiographic and clinical restenosis with a routine two-stent approach,[55] whereas another trial demonstrated an increase in adverse ischemic events, mainly periprocedural MI, with the two-stent approach.[56] All of these studies were, however, limited by modest sample size, heterogeneity in SB lesion severity and length, and diversity in the two-stent technique.

From a registry report of 782 LM bifurcation patients undergoing PCI with DES, provisional stenting resulted in significantly higher MACE-free survival at 2-year follow-up compared with a routine two-stent approach (75% vs. 67%; p = 0.02). The lower MACE in the provisional group was primarily driven by greater TLR-free survival (87% vs. 73%; p = 0.00001).[48] Thus, most experts agree that the provisional approach should be the default LM bifurcation treatment strategy for most cases. Exceptions include severe disease in both the LAD and LCX, and/or a sharply angulated SB entry.

TWO-STENT TECHNIQUES

While many techniques have been described for a two-stent approach (a comprehensive description of which is beyond the scope of this chapter), only a few have been compared in RCTs. The Nordic Stent Technique Study randomized 424 patients undergoing PCI for bifurcation lesions to either the crush or culotte technique.[36] Only 10% were LM bifurcation lesions. The primary outcome was MACE, a composite of cardiac death, MI, TVR, or stent thrombosis. At 6 months, there was no significant difference between the two groups (4.3% for crush vs. 3.7% for culotte; p = 0.87); however, the rate of procedure-related increase in biomarkers of myocardial injury was 15.5% with the crush technique versus 8.8% with the culotte (p = 0.08). At 8 months there was a trend toward less in-segment restenosis (12.1% vs. 6.6%; p = 0.10) and significantly reduced ISR (10.5% vs. 4.5%; p = 0.046) following culotte stenting.

In the only dedicated LM bifurcation two-stent technique trial, the DK Crush Versus Culotte Stenting for the Treatment of Unprotected Distal Left Main Bifurcation Lesions (DKCRUSH) III study compared the double-kissing crush (DK) technique versus culotte stenting among 450 unprotected LM patients.[57] The culotte group had a significantly greater 12-month MACE rate (the primary endpoint) compared with the DK group (16.3% vs. 6.6%; p = 0.001), which was mainly driven by increased TVR (11.0% vs. 4.3%; p = 0.016). Notably, SB ISR was also significantly higher in the culotte group compared with the DK group (12.6% vs. 6.8%; p = 0.037). The DK group compared with the culotte group also had lower MACE rates among patients with bifurcation angle >70° (3.8% vs. 16.5%; p < 0.001) and patients with a SYNTAX score ≥23 (7.1% vs. 18.9%; p = 0.006). However, highly angulated bifurcation lesions may be most optimally (and simply) treated with a modified T-stent or T-stenting and small protrusion (TAP) technique, which was not tested in this study. However, in a post hoc analysis of the ISAR-Left Main study, culotte stenting had lower rates of 6- to 9-month ISR (21% vs. 56%; p = 0.02) and 1-year TLR (15% vs. 56%; p < 0.001) than T-stenting, although routine angiographic follow-up complicates interpretation of these results.[29]

DEDICATED BIFURCATION STENTS

Patients in whom a two-stent approach is planned may be candidates for dedicated bifurcation stents. In the recently reported TRYTON randomized trial in non-LM bifurcation lesions, the bare-metal Tryton Side Branch Stent (Tryton Medical, Durham, NC), which facilitates culotte stenting, compared with a provisional approach, did not meet the 9-month primary noninferiority endpoint, a composite of cardiac death, target vessel MI, and target vessel failure (12.9% with a provisional approach vs. 17.4% with the Tryton; p = 0.11), mainly due to a higher rate of periprocedural MI (13.6% vs. 10.1%; p = 0.19).[58] However, the trial did meet the 9-month angiographic secondary superiority endpoint of reduced SB percent diameter stenosis (38.6% with a provisional approach vs. 31.6% with the Tryton; p = 0.002). These findings highlight that SB angiographic restenosis, especially

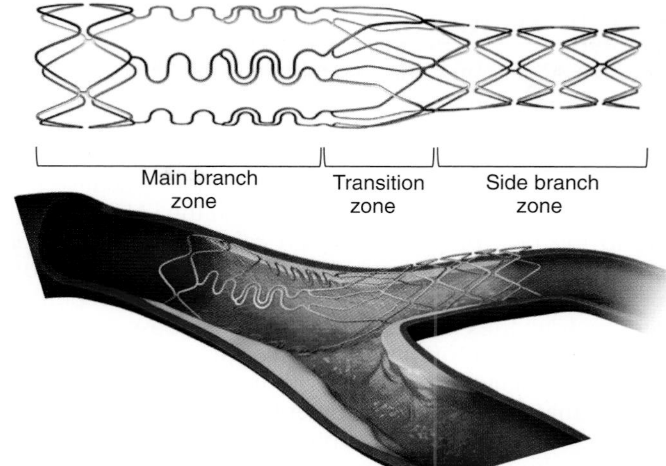

FIGURE 8-4 Dedicated-bifurcation Tryton stent. The *Tryton Side Branch Stent* consists of a bare-metal stent made of three zones: (1) side branch (SB) zone, (2) transition zone, and (3) main branch (MB) zone. The side branch zone is a typical slotted tube designed for insertion into the side branch; the transition zone is composed of undulating struts designed to provide adequate radial strength and coverage throughout the carina; and the main branch zone has a minimal metal-to-artery ratio intended as an open path for a main branch stent. The implantation technique involves lesion preparation (predilatation of both MB and SB), placement of the Tryton Side Branch Stent into the SB, and placement of a standard metallic drug-eluting stent (or bioresorbable scaffold) within the MB. Simultaneous or sequential final kissing balloon inflations are then performed.

in smaller SBs, is uncommonly expressed clinically. Use of the Tryton for true bifurcation lesions involving the LM has been described and appears to be safe[58a,59] (**Figure 8-4**). There are other dedicated bifurcation stents in various stages of evaluation, including the Nile PAX (Minvasys SAS, Gennevilliers, France) and AXXESS-LMTM (AXXESS, Biosensors, Singapore) stents.[60,61] Additional studies are required to examine the potential role of dedicated bifurcation stents in LM (and non-LM) disease.

IMPORTANCE OF FINAL KISSING BALLOON INFLATION

While final kissing balloon is considered a mandatory step when using a two-stent strategy,[62,63] it is still a matter of debate whether routine kissing should be systematically performed with provisional stenting, especially when a satisfactory final result in the SB is achieved with balloon angioplasty only.[64] The NORDIC III trial compared a routine strategy of final kissing with no final kissing in patients undergoing a provisional stenting approach. Despite a reduction in angiographic SB restenosis at 8-month follow-up in true (non-LM) bifurcations, no differences in clinical endpoints were apparent (6-month MACE 2.1% vs. 2.5%; p = 1.00), and procedural duration, contrast use, and fluoroscopy times were greater with final kissing balloon inflations.[65] That being said, whether routine postdilatation after provisional stenting involving true LM bifurcation lesions should be performed routinely within the nonstented SB has never been studied. It is, however, generally accepted that in cases of LM PCI involving true bifurcations, routine kissing should be performed when a significant (>75% diameter stenosis) lesion is present, if the coronary flow of the SB is compromised, or if pressure-wire assessment demonstrates significant ischemia by fractional flow reserve (FFR).[64,66]

ROLE OF IMAGING

Although angiography has long been considered the gold standard for coronary evaluation, important limitations that are relevant to LM evaluation and revascularization have been described. Angiographic assessment of lesion severity involving the LM is often challenging, in part because the detection of diffuse, concentric disease in the LM is difficult due to the lack of a nondiseased reference segment for comparison. Moreover, vessel overlap, ostial angulation and deformity, foreshortening, and streaming of contrast medium from the catheter tip make accurate assessment of the LM segment notoriously difficult even by the most experienced clinicians (**Figure 8-5**). Studies have shown significant mismatch between angiography and both IVUS[67] and FFR,[68] particularly in angiographically intermediate lesions. Therefore, the final decision regarding whether to revascularize intermediate LM lesions should not be based on coronary angiogram alone. Adequate knowledge of the strengths and weaknesses of IVUS and FFR are mandatory for proper LM assessment. Additional evaluation with IVUS/FFR may avoid revascularization of functionally insignificant lesions and the associated complications and costs.

INTRAVASCULAR ULTRASOUND

IVUS has an important role both before and after PCI of LM lesions. Prior to PCI, IVUS may be used to objectively assess stenosis severity, lesion extent (including SB involvement), lumen dimensions, plaque distribution, and calcification. Abizaid et al. were among the first to highlight the important lack of correlation between angiographic and IVUS assessment of lesion severity.[69] They also demonstrated the importance of the minimal lumen diameter (MLD) in prediction of future ischemic adverse events. Jasti et al. identified an LM MLD <2.8 mm and a minimum lumen area (MLA) <5.9 mm^2 as being the most predictive of an FFR value of <0.75.[70] In a patient cohort with a smaller body surface area, Kang et al. reported that the only independent predictor of FFR <0.80 was the LM MLA value on IVUS, with a value <4.8 mm^2 being the most accurate correlate.[71]

Subsequent studies have attempted to identify an IVUS MLA cutoff to safely guide the LM revascularization decision-making process. LITRO was a multicenter prospective study validating the IVUS-derived cutoff value of 6 mm^2 as a safe MLA parameter to guide revascularization of intermediate LM lesions.[67] A total of 354 patients were enrolled, among

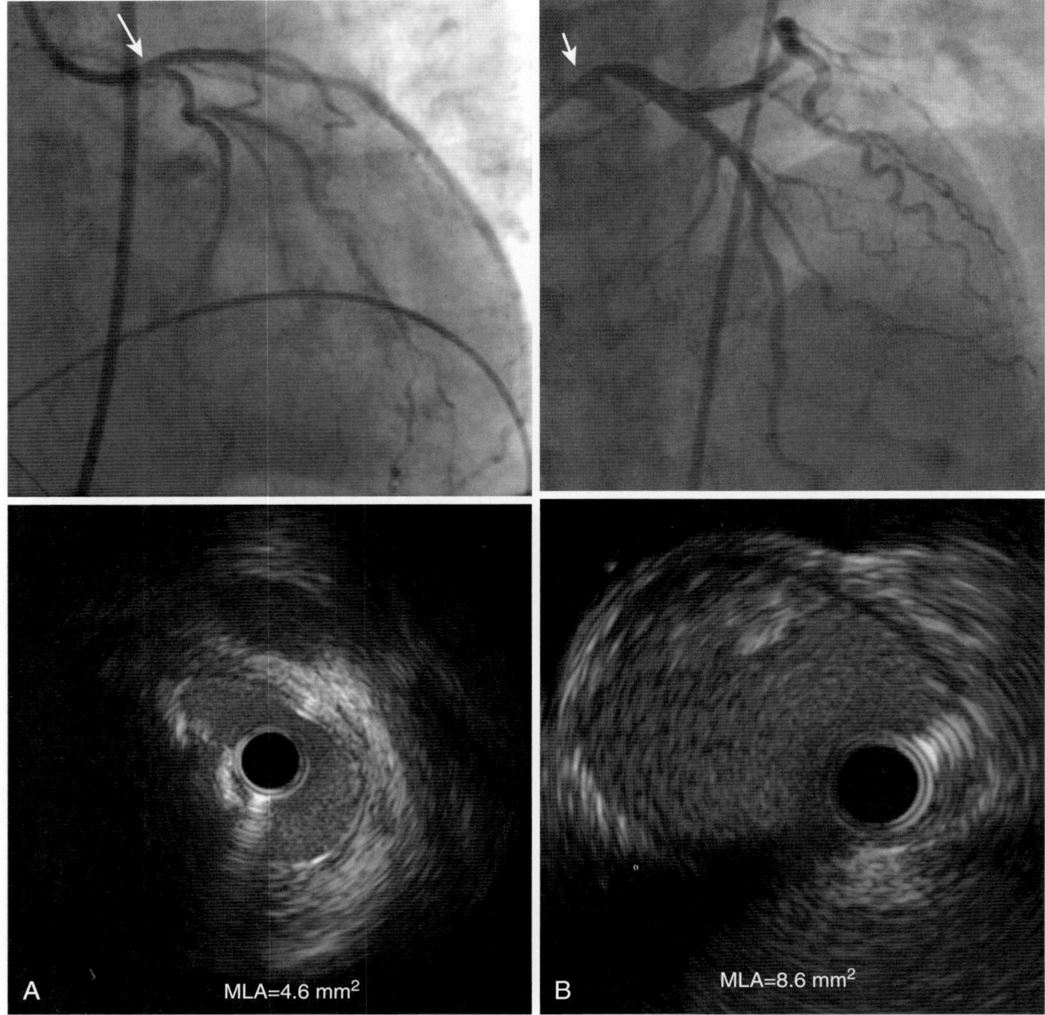

FIGURE 8-5 Discrepancy between angiography and intravascular ultrasound. A, Coronary angiogram showing haziness in the shaft of the LM, with no obvious stenosis. Intravascular ultrasound assessment demonstrated a significant stenosis (MLA 4.6 mm^2). **B,** Coronary angiogram showing a potential ostial lesion. Intravascular ultrasound assessment demonstrated the absence of a significant lesion (MLA 8.6 mm^2). *(Courtesy Akiko Maehara.)*

whom 179 with an LM MLA of ≥6 mm^2 were treated medically and 152 with an LM MLA <6 mm^2 were revascularized (45% with PCI and 55% with CABG). No difference in the 2-year rate of cardiac death and MI was observed between the two groups. While the 6 mm^2 MLA value is widely accepted as the IVUS threshold at which revascularization may be safely deferred, the optimal MLA cutoff still remains a matter of debate, with the 4.8 mm^2 value also shown as having clinical utility in an Asian cohort.[71]

In addition to assessing intermediate lesions, IVUS plays an important role in interventional guidance of LM procedures, including choice of stent diameter and length, need for debulking, and technique selection (e.g., provisional vs. planned two-stent approach). After LM stenting IVUS is useful in assessing plaque versus carinal shift, geometric changes in the polygon of confluence (POC), and optimization of MLA (stent expansion).[72] Suboptimal stent expansion is the single most important factor which has most strongly been associated with stent thrombosis and restenosis after LM PCI.[46] Stent underexpansion is more common with a two-stent approach, particularly at the ostium of the LCX, partially explaining the higher rates of ISR in that location. The proposed MSA cutoff values are shown in **Figure 8-3**, although as a general rule the larger the MSA, the lower the adverse event rates. Kang et al. have evaluated the optimal IVUS stent area to predict angiographic ISR after SES implantation for LM disease.[46] The MSA values post-PCI that best predicted ISR on a segmental basis were 8.2 mm^2 for the LM shaft, 7.2 mm^2 for the POC, 6.3 mm^2 for the ostial LAD, and 5.0 mm^2 for the ostial LCX (or 4.0 mm^2 if the ostial LCX was not stented). Stent underexpansion at any of these locations was an independent predictor for 2-year MACE, especially repeat revascularization, while stent malapposition did not predict ISR or MACE. Park et al. have reported that long-term mortality in patients undergoing IVUS-guided LM stenting may be lower than in those undergoing LM stenting with angiographic guidance alone.[73]

Finally, optical coherence tomography (OCT) is a novel intracoronary imaging modality with higher resolution than IVUS and offers a more detailed assessment of the lumen and intima. Drawbacks of OCT for LM assessment include its reduced depth of penetration compared with IVUS and difficulty in clearing the LM lumen with an adequate flush. While interesting observations have recently been presented regarding OCT optimization of bifurcation LM PCI,[74-78] further data are needed before this technique can be widely recommended to guide LM decision making.

FRACTIONAL FLOW RESERVE

Pressure-wire derived FFR is the gold standard for the physiological assessment of coronary artery stenosis,[11,12,79-82] and it may be useful in the management of bifurcation lesions.[66,83] Data from the randomized DEFER, FAME I, and FAME II trials in non-LM CAD have demonstrated that an FFR-guided revascularization strategy is associated with improved outcomes compared with a purely angiographic strategy when managing single or multivessel CAD.[79,80,82] Subsequently, several investigators have demonstrated the potential utility of pressure-wire assessment in the assessment of LM lesions with PCI.[68,70,84-89]

Hamilos and colleagues evaluated the long-term clinical outcomes of an LM revascularization strategy based on FFR in 215 patients with an angiographically indeterminate LM coronary artery stenosis.[68] Patients with an FFR ≥0.80 were treated medically (nonsurgical group; n = 138), while patients with an FFR <0.80 where treated with CABG (surgical group; n = 75). The 5-year survival estimates were similar in both groups (89.8% in the nonsurgical group and 85.4% in the surgical group; p = 0.48). The 5-year event-free survival (a composite of death, MI, or revascularization) estimates were 74.2% and 82.8% in the nonsurgical and surgical groups, respectively (p = 0.50). In 23% of patients with a diameter stenosis <50%, the LM coronary artery stenosis was hemodynamically significant by FFR. This study illustrates the value of an FFR-guided strategy when the severity of the LM stenosis is uncertain by angiography.

While FFR is useful to assess the physiologic significance of the isolated LM lesion, several theoretical limitations of FFR in patients with LM plus concomitant multivessel CAD should be appreciated. Since FFR readings across the LM segment may be influenced by the presence of disease within any of the distal coronary segments, high-grade stenoses within the LAD or LCX territories may artificially increase the FFR measured across the LM if the transducer is placed distally.[89] In this situation, an FFR pullback should be undertaken starting within both daughter branches to localize the most significant distribution of disease across the region bordering the distal LM segment and ostia of both daughter branches.[89,90] Alternatively, FFR across the LM segment may be artificially low in the setting of severe downstream disease if the transducer is placed in a branch without severe disease. PCI of functionally significant distal lesions may be required to unmask the true hemodynamic significance of the diseased LM segment. FFR may also be useful in determining the functional significance of an angiographically narrowed LCX ostium after provisional stenting, specifically when ostial stenosis is >75%.[83]

Other issues to consider when using FFR to assess intermediate LM lesions are as follows:

1. There is no definite consensus related to the exact FFR cutoff for LM. While an FFR of ≤0.80 is usually considered appropriate to initiate revascularization, some argue that an FFR value between 0.80 and 0.85 should be repeated and complemented with an IVUS assessment.
2. Special attention should be deployed to avoid deep engagement of the guiding catheter (pressure damping) while performing the FFR measurement, which may falsely increase the FFR value.
3. Given the large myocardium mass deserved by the LM, adenosine doses should be increased to ensure maximal hyperemia if the FFR is borderline (e.g., <0.85 but >0.80).

In summary, improvement in procedural and clinical outcomes with the use IVUS- and FFR-guided LM PCI have been demonstrated in several moderate-sized nonrandomized studies. Nevertheless, given the potential dramatic clinical consequences of stent failure (thrombosis or restenosis) within the LM segment, IVUS and/or FFR guidance are strongly recommended during LM PCI to optimize acute and long-term outcomes.

MYOCARDIAL INFARCTION DUE TO LM THROMBOSIS

Most LM revascularization studies have excluded patients presenting with ST-segment elevation MI (STEMI). Though primary PCI is the preferred revascularization strategy in patients with STEMI, limited data are available in those presenting with LM thrombosis. In a metaanalysis including a total of 977 patients, 26% of patients presenting to a hospital with STEMI involving the LM were in cardiogenic shock; these patients had significantly higher 30-day all-cause mortality compared with those presenting without shock (55% vs. 15%; $p < 0.001$).[91] Similarly, in the Acute Myocardial Infarction in Switzerland (AMIS) Plus Registry in which 348 patients undergoing LM primary PCI were compared with 6318 patients undergoing primary PCI of a non-LM vessel, LM patients presented more frequently with cardiogenic shock (12.2% vs. 3.5%; $p = 0.001$) and had higher mortality, especially when concomitant non-LM CAD was present.[92] Finally, Patel and colleagues, using the British Cardiovascular Intervention Society database, compared the 3-year clinical outcomes of 568 patients presenting with STEMI with unprotected occlusive LM (TIMI [thrombolysis in myocardial infarction] flow grade 0/1 and diameter stenosis >75%) with 1045 emergency patients treated with non-occlusive LM disease.[93] Compared with nonocclusive LM disease, occlusive LM disease in patients with STEMI was associated with a doubling in the likelihood of periprocedural shock (57.9% vs. 27.9%; $p < 0.001$) and/or intra-aortic balloon pump support (52.5% vs. 27.2%; $p < 0.001$). In-hospital (43.3% vs. 20.6%; $p < 0.001$), 1-year (52.8% vs. 32.4%; $p < 0.001$), and 3-year (73.9% vs. 52.3%; $p < 0.001$) mortality rates were also markedly higher in patients with occlusive LM disease.

HEMODYNAMIC SUPPORT

The routine use of hemodynamic support devices such as intra-aortic balloon counterpulsation or left ventricular support (e.g., microaxial propelling pump, etc.) has been advocated in specific patients undergoing PL PCI to reduce periprocedural risks.[94-97] The PROTECT II trial, in which 452 high-risk patients undergoing PCI were randomized to hemodynamic support with the Impella 2.5 versus intra-aortic balloon counterpulsation, failed to demonstrate reductions in mortality or adverse events at 30 and 90 days.[98] Among 107 patients undergoing PCI for unprotected LM disease, the relative risk (95% CI) for major adverse events at 30 days (1.02 [0.65-1.60]) and 90 days (0.88 [0.59-1.33]) were also nonsignificantly different with the two support devices, respectively. While it is generally accepted that routine use of hemodynamic support devices in LM PCI is not required, the use of such devices to decrease procedural risk may be reasonable in some clinical situations (**Table 8-6**).

DUAL ANTIPLATELET THERAPY SELECTION AND DURATION

In the SYNTAX trial, stent thrombosis with TAXUS PES occurred in ~10% of patients at 5 years, significantly contributing to MACE among the randomized PCI cohort.[99] Of note, 19.4% of all stent thromboses in SYNTAX occurred in the LM segment. Premature discontinuation of dual antiplatelet therapy (DAPT) is an important predictor of stent thrombosis.[100] Most of the episodes of death or MI occurred among patients treated with DAPT for less than 6 months in the GISE survey, especially in the setting of an acute coronary syndrome.[101] Given the potential dramatic consequences of DAPT discontinuation after LM PCI, every effort should be made to ensure patient medication compliance. Despite the newer generation of DES showing an improved safety profile,[42] the optimal duration of DAPT after PCI using DES placement still remains a matter of active debate.[102-104] In the absence of compelling data, it seems reasonable to recommend DAPT for at least 1 year after LM PCI.[11,12]

Migliorini et al. showed that in patients who underwent LM PCI, high residual platelet reactivity after a loading dose of 600 mg clopidogrel was associated with a fourfold increase in the risk of stent thrombosis and cardiac death.[105] High residual platelet reactivity was the only independent predictor of both stent thrombosis and cardiac death in this study. The more potent P2Y12 inhibitors ticagrelor and prasugrel have been shown to reduce stent thrombosis in a large cross section of patients with acute coronary syndromes undergoing PCI,[106,107] although few patients in these studies had LM disease. Although there are no conclusive studies to date demonstrating the utility of ticagrelor or prasugrel in patients with LM disease, the use of these agents may be reasonable in such patients who are at high risk of thrombosis (e.g., suboptimal two-stent bifurcation treatment of multiple stents for complex CAD) and low risk of bleeding.

TABLE 8-6 Clinical Scenarios in Which Hemodynamic Support May Be Beneficial During Left Main PCI

Cardiogenic shock
Refractory or decompensated heart failure
Low left ventricular ejection fraction (<40%)
Concomitant critical disease of the right coronary artery
Severe multivessel disease
Use of rotational atherectomy
High thrombotic burden or otherwise high-risk for no or slow reflow phenomenon
Left dominance

FOLLOW-UP AFTER LEFT MAIN PCI

In light of the results of the SYNTAX trial, demonstrating the relative safety of LM-DES PCI, and according to the most recent published guidelines,[11] routine angiographic follow-up is not recommended (previously Class IIa) following unprotected LM PCI. The role of routine or selective computed tomography (with or without physiological assessment) after LM PCI remains to be defined.

LEFT MAIN BIFURCATION PCI TECHNIQUES

Distal bifurcation lesions involving only one SB should usually be approached with a provisional technique (planned one-stent, with or without SB balloon angioplasty, and with or without final kissing). For true bifurcations involving the distal LM bifurcation and the need for a two-stent approach, a variety of techniques have been described. With this approach, a final kissing balloon inflation is mandatory to optimize long-term outcomes and preserve future accessibility to the SBs. The choice of the most appropriate two-stent LM PCI technique varies according to factors such as plaque distribution (Medina classification), lesion location (ostium, mid-shaft, or distal involving bifurcation), LM bifurcation angulation, and operator experience and expertise.

PROVISIONAL STENT TECHNIQUE (Figure 8-6 AND Video 8-1)

The provisional stent technique involves the initial placement of a single stent in the LM and LAD (or rarely the

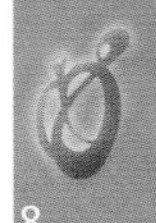

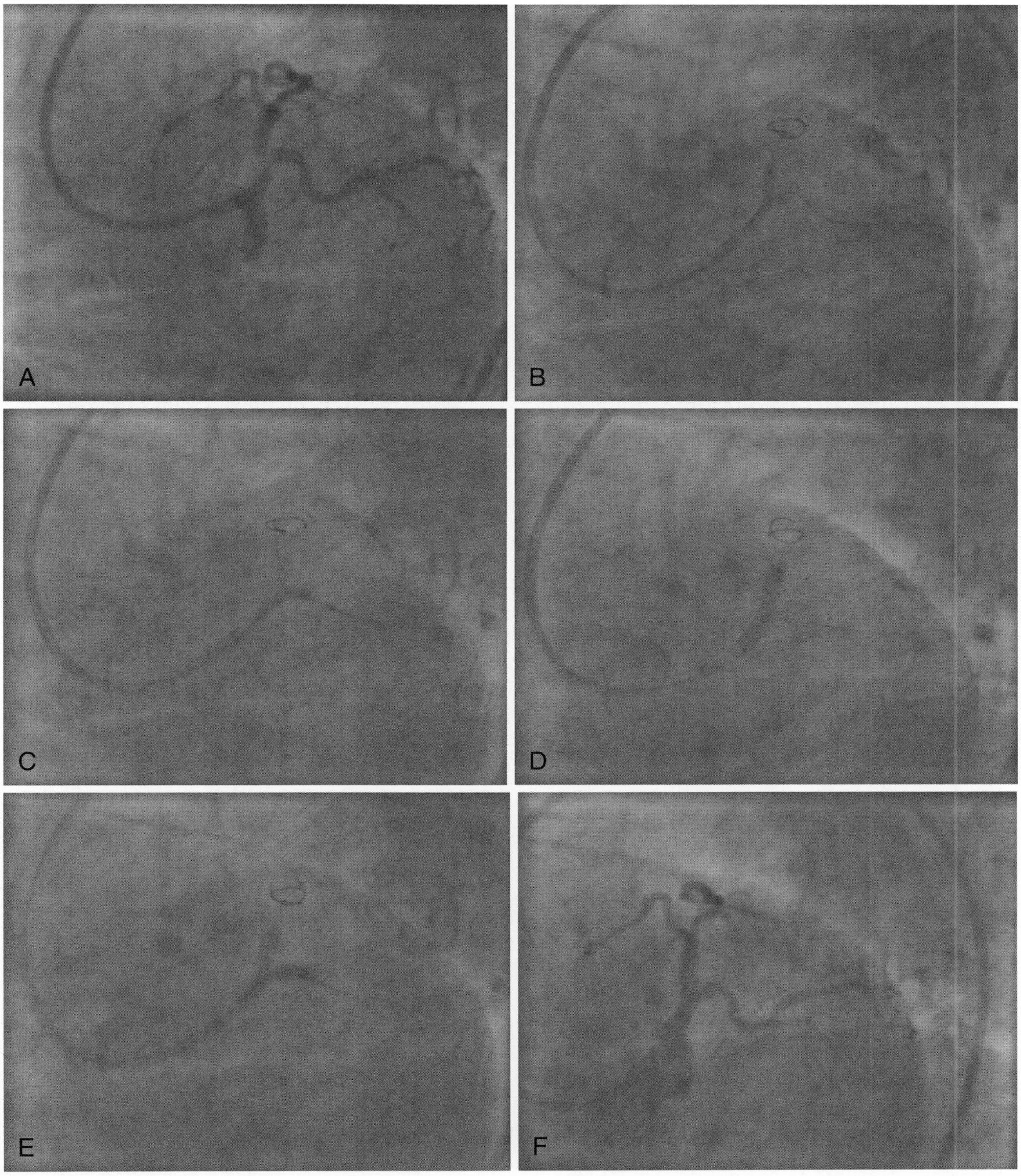

FIGURE 8-6 LM PCI using a one-stent provisional approach with final kissing (see also Video 8-1). A, Baseline angiogram showing severe distal LM disease with involvement of the proximal LAD and an intermediate lesion of the LCX. **B,** Predilatation of LM and LAD. **C,** Predilatation of LCX. **D,** Stent implantation in the LM-LAD axis. **E,** After removal and rewiring of the LCX, simultaneous final kissing. **F,** Final angiogram showing an excellent result.

LCX) with crossover of the other SB. The steps are as follows:

1. Wiring the MV and SB.
2. Balloon predilatation of MV and the SB (SB optional).
3. Stenting MV with both wires in place.
4. Assessment of SB integrity: Consider whether balloon angioplasty or stenting is required. If the stenosis is <50%, without good flow and without dissection, SB treatment may be deferred. Otherwise intervention is usually performed, most frequently balloon angioplasty first to achieve an acceptable result. Stenting may be required in ~20% of cases (although the threshold varies by operator from <10% to >30%) if TIMI flow <3, severe ostial compromise (>80% stenosis), threatened SB closure, dissection ≥type B, or FFR <0.75. Placement of a second stent in the SB may be done by T-stent, TAP, reverse crush, or culotte approach.
5. Rewiring the SB and final kissing balloon inflation (per operator discretion if an SB stent is not placed; mandatory if two-stent approach).

Positioning of a wire in the SB until MV stenting and/or postdilatation is complete, especially in the presence of complex anatomy (tortuosity, acute angle, severe stenosis, presence of heavy calcification), is an important step and facilitates SB access in case of SB closure or significant compromise. The temporary jailed wire can usually be retrieved easily. A jacketed polymer-coated wire should not be used for this purpose, however, as the polymer may be stripped off during retrieval of the jailed wire. Polymer-coated wires may be used effectively, however, for re-crossing the stent into the SB. Postdilatation of the proximal MV stent after LM stent implantation before kissing balloon inflation of placement of a second stent (the proximal optimization technique, or POT) is strongly recommended to optimize

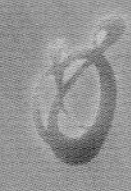

final geometry of the bifurcation and facilitates SB accessibility through the distal side cell of the MV stent.[64,108,109]

TWO-STENT TECHNIQUES

Various two-stent techniques have been described. Selection of a particular technique should be based on bifurcation characteristics, operator preference, and experience. The following general principles should be considered when selecting the most appropriate technique for a given patient:

1. **Size of SB.** In LM PCI, the SB, which is most frequently the LCX artery, may supply a relatively large amount of myocardium (especially in case of left dominancy). Preserving its patency and integrity is important. If a significant discrepancy in vessel diameter exists between the SB and the LM body (i.e., SB considerably smaller than MV), the culotte stenting technique may be problematic and should be avoided. T-stenting, the crush technique, or a double-kissing crush (DK-crush) technique should be favored in this situation.
2. **Lesion length in SB.** Focal lesions <5 mm, even if angiographically severe, are rarely physiologically significant and should usually be treated initially with a provisional approach, followed by a FFR-guided assessment and management, and optimized with or without final kissing inflation. However, if a significant lesion extends several millimeters (>5 mm) into the SB, especially if angulated or calcified, a two-stent approach should be considered.
3. **Bifurcation angulation.** For angles <70° or Y-shaped morphology, SB access may be more easily performed; however, plaque shift (or carina shift) may still occur and be severe. In lesions with angles ≥70° or T-shaped morphology, SB access is difficult but plaque shift is less pronounced. For LM bifurcation lesions requiring a two-stent technique with SB angulation ≥70°, a T-stent, modified T-stent, or TAP technique is usually performed.[110] If the SB angulation is <70°, the crush, DK-crush, or culotte techniques are usually preferred.
4. **Calcification severity and extent.** Calcification extent and severity is underestimated by angiography compared with IVUS. If at least moderate calcification is present, plaque modification with either a cutting or scoring balloon or atherectomy is recommended. While the necessity to perform atherectomy does not mandate a two-stent technique, such patients often have diffuse atherosclerotic disease, increasing the likelihood to benefit from an upfront two-stent approach.

Description of Techniques

Culotte Technique (Figure 8-7 and Video 8-2)

This technique uses two stents and results in full coverage of the bifurcation area (especially the carina and SB ostium), though with two layers of metal in the proximal MV. The

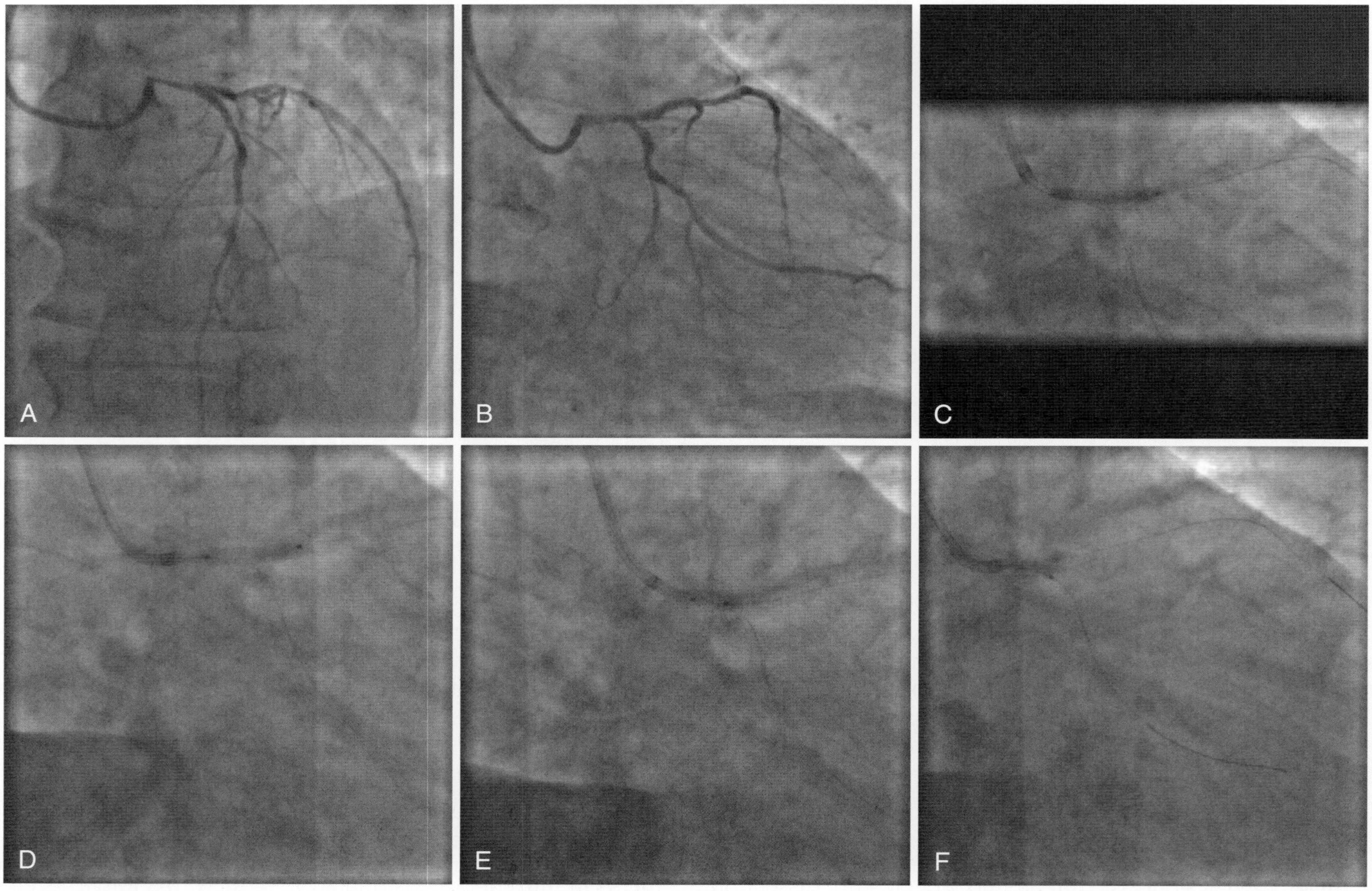

FIGURE 8-7 LM PCI using a two-stent culotte technique with final kissing (see also Video 8-2). A, Baseline angiogram showing severe LM disease with involvement of the proximal LAD. **B,** An intermediate lesion of the ostial LCX and more severe lesion of the proximal LCX. **C,** Predilatation of the LM and LAD. **D,** Stent implantation in the LM-LAD axis. **E,** Balloon inflation of the LM segment of the previously deployed stent, just proximal to the LCX ostium, using a short noncompliant balloon (proximal optimization technique [POT]). **F,** After removal of the LCX wire and rewiring of the LCX, predilatation of the ostial LCX through the LM stent.

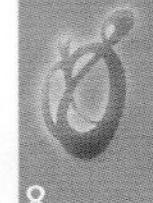

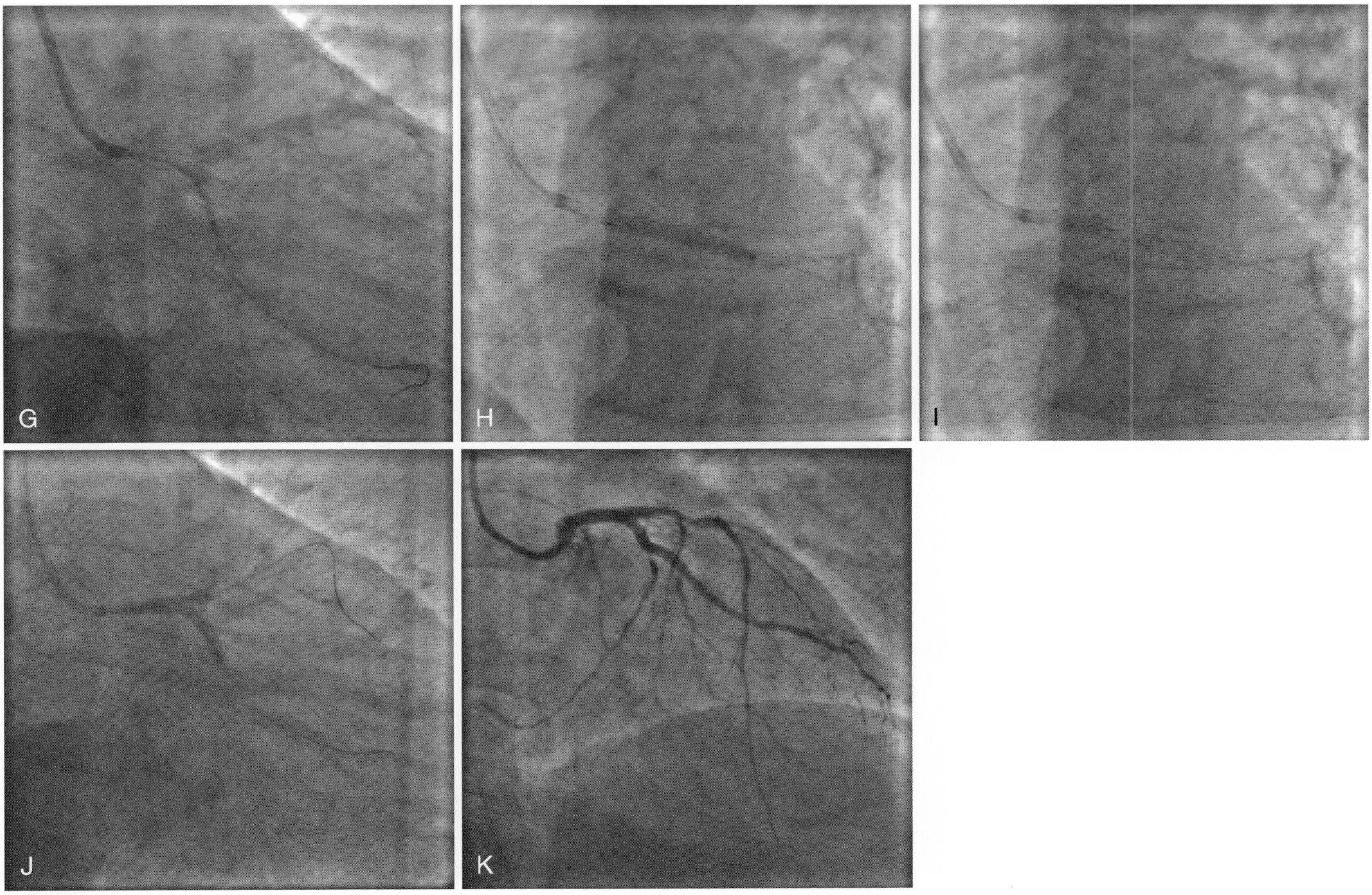

FIGURE 8-7, cont'd **G,** After removal of the wire in the LAD, placement of the LM-LCX stent, through the first deployed LM-LAD stent. **H,** Stent implantation in the LM-LCX axis. **I,** Balloon inflation of the LM segment of the previously deployed stent, just proximal to the LAD ostium, using a short noncompliant balloon (POT). **J,** After rewiring of the LAD, simultaneous final kissing. **K,** Final angiogram showing an excellent result.

steps described here were used in the Nordic Stent Technique Study[36]:

1. Wiring of both MV and SB.
2. Predilatation of MV and/or SB (optional but recommended).
3. Stenting of the MV.
4. Rewiring SB through MV stent and removal of jailed wire in SB.
5. Dilatation of SB through MV stent.
6. Stenting proximal MV and SB through MV stent.
7. Rewiring MV through SB stent.
8. Final kissing balloon inflation.

Typically, the first stent should be placed in the branch with the most angulated entry, whether the MB or SB. To allow full opening of the SB and preservation of the SB stent architecture, an open cell design stent, rather than a closed cell design, should be used when performing culotte stenting. Also, this technique should not be used if a large difference (≥1.5 mm) in vessel diameter between the MV and SB exists.[111]

Crush Techniques (Figure 8-8 and Video 8-3)

This technique was first described by Colombo et al.,[112,113] and it has undergone a few iterations over time:

1. Wiring of both MV and SB.
2. Predilatation of MV and/or SB (optional but recommended).
3. Stenting of the SB first, with an uninflated stent (or balloon) positioned in the MV. The proximal end of the SB stent should be several millimeters in the MV, but the proximal edge of the uninflated MV stent (or balloon) must be proximal to the proximal edge of the SB stent.
4. Assess patency and flow in the SB to ensure an additional SB stent or immediate balloon angioplasty is not required.
5. SB wire and stent balloon are removed.
6. Crushing the SB stent with MV stent or balloon inflation (followed by MV stent).
7. Rewiring the SB through MV stent.
8. High-pressure inflation of SB (optional).
9. Final kissing balloon inflation (mandatory).

Some variants of this technique have been described. Today, most operators try to minimize the length (2-3 mm) of the SB stent within the MV to reduce the multiple layers of crumpled stent (minicrush technique).[110,114] If the SB stent is crushed within the MV stent, it is called the internal or reverse crush technique. In another variant, the MV stent is crushed by the SB stent (inverted crush technique).[115] Another variant was developed to make this technique feasible by radial approach using a 6 Fr catheter. In this technique, the balloon is used to crush the SB stent, and the two stents are advanced and deployed sequentially (step crush or modified balloon crush technique). Disadvantages of the crush technique include difficulty in SB rewiring for final kissing inflation and the presence of multiple layers of

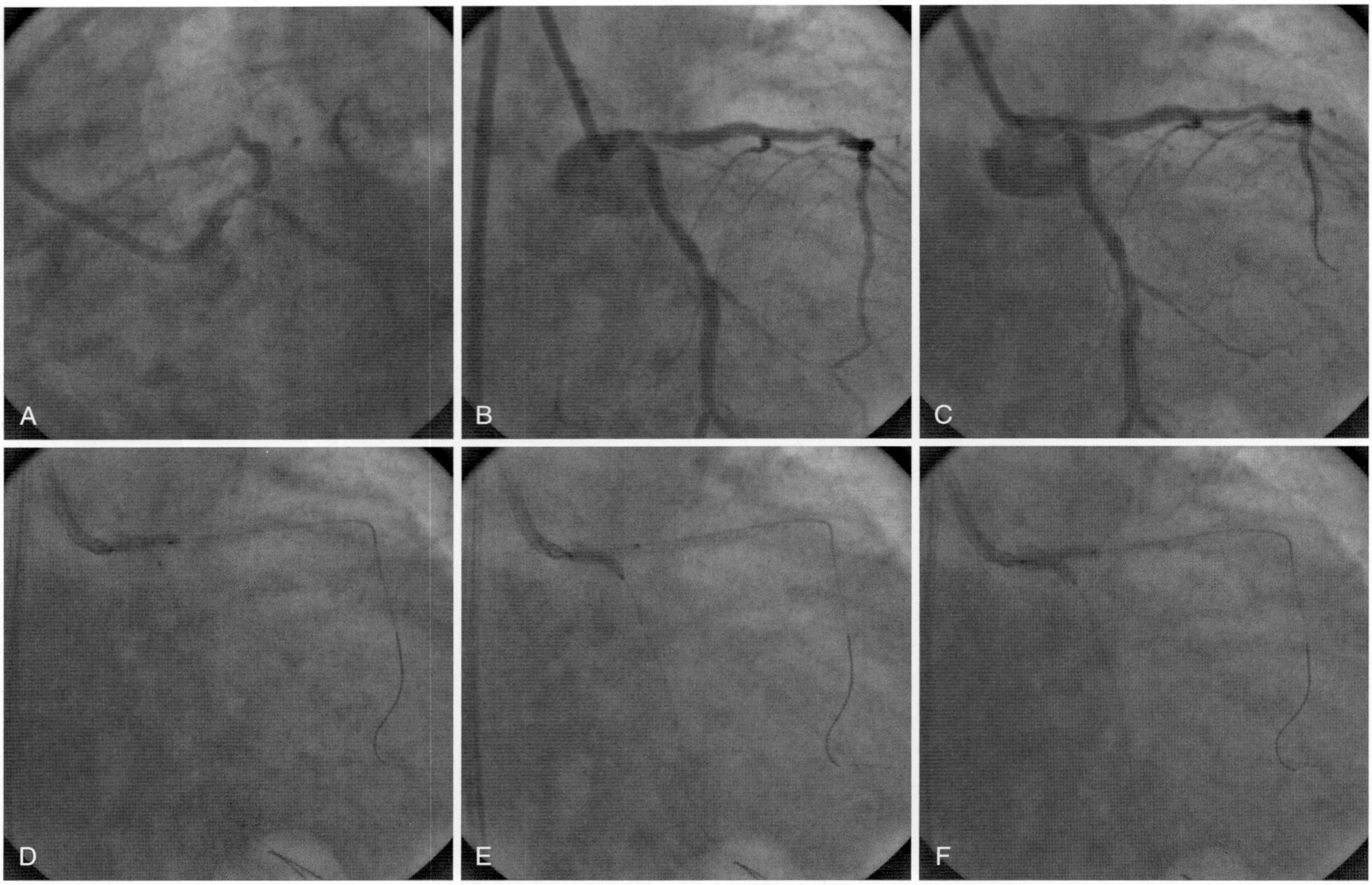

FIGURE 8-8 LM PCI using a two-stent crush technique with final kissing (see also Video 8-3). A and B, Baseline angiogram showing severe lesions involving the distal LM, the ostial LAD, and the ostial LCX (Medina 1-1-1 bifurcation). C, Wiring of the two branches. D, Predilatation of the LAD. E, Predilatation of the LCX. F, Simultaneous kissing predilatation.

crumpled stent at the SB ostium, substantially increasing the rate of SB ostial ISR. In cases of difficult rewiring with conventional wire, a hydrophilic wire may be helpful in crossing into the SB. The most recent iteration of this technique is the double-kissing crush (DK crush),[57,116] which involves two instances of balloon kissing, the first after the SB stent is crushed (facilitating rewiring for final kissing), and the second (final kiss) after deployment of the MV stent (**Figure 8-9**, Video 8-4).

T-Stent Techniques (Figure 8-10 and Video 8-5)

T-stent techniques are used when SB stenting is required after a suboptimal result with provisional stenting, or in a planned two-stent approach when the angle into the SB is ≥70° but ≤100°.

1. Wiring of MV and SB.
2. MV and/or SB dilatation (recommended but optional).
3. Stenting MV with wire in place in SB (alternatively, SB may be stented first).
4. Rewiring SB and removal of jailed wire.
5. Dilatation of SB through MV stent.
6. Stenting SB through MV stent with no stent protrusion in MV (or placement of the MV stent if the SB was stented first).
7. Final kissing balloon inflation.

The main disadvantage of this technique is the high rate of ostial restenosis of the SB due to suboptimal stent coverage in the bifurcation area, particularly the ostium. However, full coverage is possible with this technique if the angle into the SB from the MV is near 90°. Alternatively, the TAP technique, with intentional minimal protrusion of the SB stent within the MV, may be performed when dealing with bifurcation angle >70°. After stenting of the main vessel, the SB stent is positioned in the SB with minimal protrusion in the MV, with a deflated balloon concurrently positioned in the main vessel. After inflation of the SB stent, the stent balloon is removed from the SB and the MV balloon is inflated. After rewiring of the SB, a final kissing inflation is performed. If performed correctly, this technique increases the likelihood of complete coverage of the ostium without deformation of the stent or malapposed struts.

V-Stent Technique (Figure 8-11 and Video 8-6)

In this technique both MV and SB are stented simultaneously. It is mainly used for distal disease in bifurcation (Medina 0,1,1).

1. Wiring of MV and SB.
2. Predilatation of MV and SB.
3. Placement of stents in both branches with minimal proximal protrusion in MV.
4. Placement of balloons in both branches and simultaneous (or sequential) deployment of stents.
5. Final kissing balloon inflation.

In cases with proximal disease (Medina 1,1,1), both stents are lined up in the LM shaft, creating a new carina—this approach is called the Y technique, simultaneous kissing

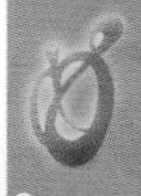

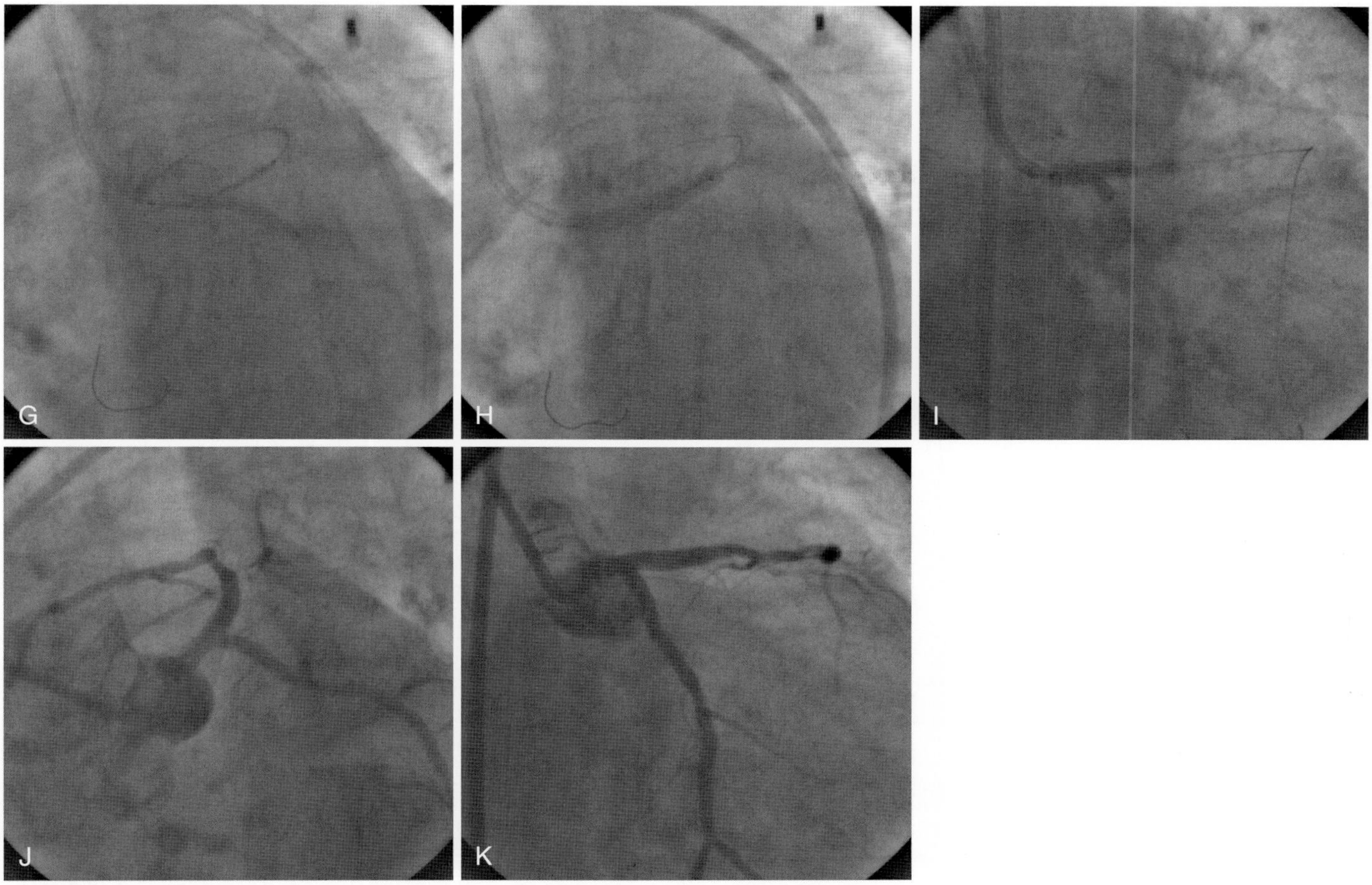

FIGURE 8-8, cont'd **G,** Two stents are simultaneously positioned in the bifurcation lesion: the eventually crushed stent (LCX) is positioned in the LCX, with minimal (~2-3 mm) protrusion in the LM; the "crushing" stent is positioned in the LM-LAD axis. The LCX stent is deployed first, with the LM-LAD stent in place but not deployed. **H,** After removal of the LCX stent balloon and wire, deployment of the LM-LAD stent, crushing the LM and carina portion of the previously deployed LCX stent. **I,** After rewiring of the LCX through the crushed stent, final kissing inflation. **J** and **K** show an excellent final result.

stents (SKS), or double barrel technique. In another variant of this technique for cases of extensive proximal disease in the MV, a proximal stent is first implanted before the bifurcation stenting—this is termed the Skirt or extended Y technique. Y-stenting is rarely used as the new carina is often eccentric and difficult to rewire in cases of ISR, and if a proximal dissection develops it must be converted into a crush or culotte, a complex procedure. MACE rates have also been reported to be high after Y-stenting.[117,118] Y-stenting may be useful, however, in a patient with hemodynamic instability in whom rapid stabilization of a high-grade LM stenosis is the main priority.

OSTIAL LM PCI

When the LM length allows for a single stent implantation, PCI of the LM ostium is usually straightforward. Challenges related to this ostial LM stenting include proper assessment of the stenosis (spasm, angulation, severity), the potential for guide catheter-induced stent damage (longitudinal compression), systemic stent embolization if a short stent is deployed (an 8 mm stent should rarely be deployed in the ostial LM), retrograde sinus or aortic dissection, and difficulty to subsequently re-engage the LM ostium in case of excessive stent protrusion into the aorta (**Figure 8-12**). Dedicated devices exist to help and guide more precise stent deployment in case of ostial lesion (e.g., Ostial Pro, Merit Medical Systems, Inc, South Jordan, Utah).

CONCLUSIONS

Revascularization decisions for patients with LM CAD are complex, requiring appropriate lesion assessment from noninvasive and invasive testing, and risk stratification with prognostic instruments such the anatomic SYNTAX score and the clinical/anatomic SYNTAX score II, paired with a formal multidisciplinary Heart Team discussion. LM patients with extensive multivessel CAD are best managed by CABG. However, current evidence from RCTs suggests that PCI may provide at least equivalent results to CABG in selected LM patients with simple or moderately complex coronary anatomy. Given the large amount of myocardium supplied, LM PCI is inherently high-risk, and the results are dependent on operator expertise and experience, a factor which must be taken into account in Heart Team discussions. However, all RCTs completed to date have been underpowered to be conclusive, and registry reports are limited by selection bias and confounding. The ongoing EXCEL and NOBLE trials will provide important data regarding the safety and efficacy of LM PCI with contemporary DES

Text continued on p. 136

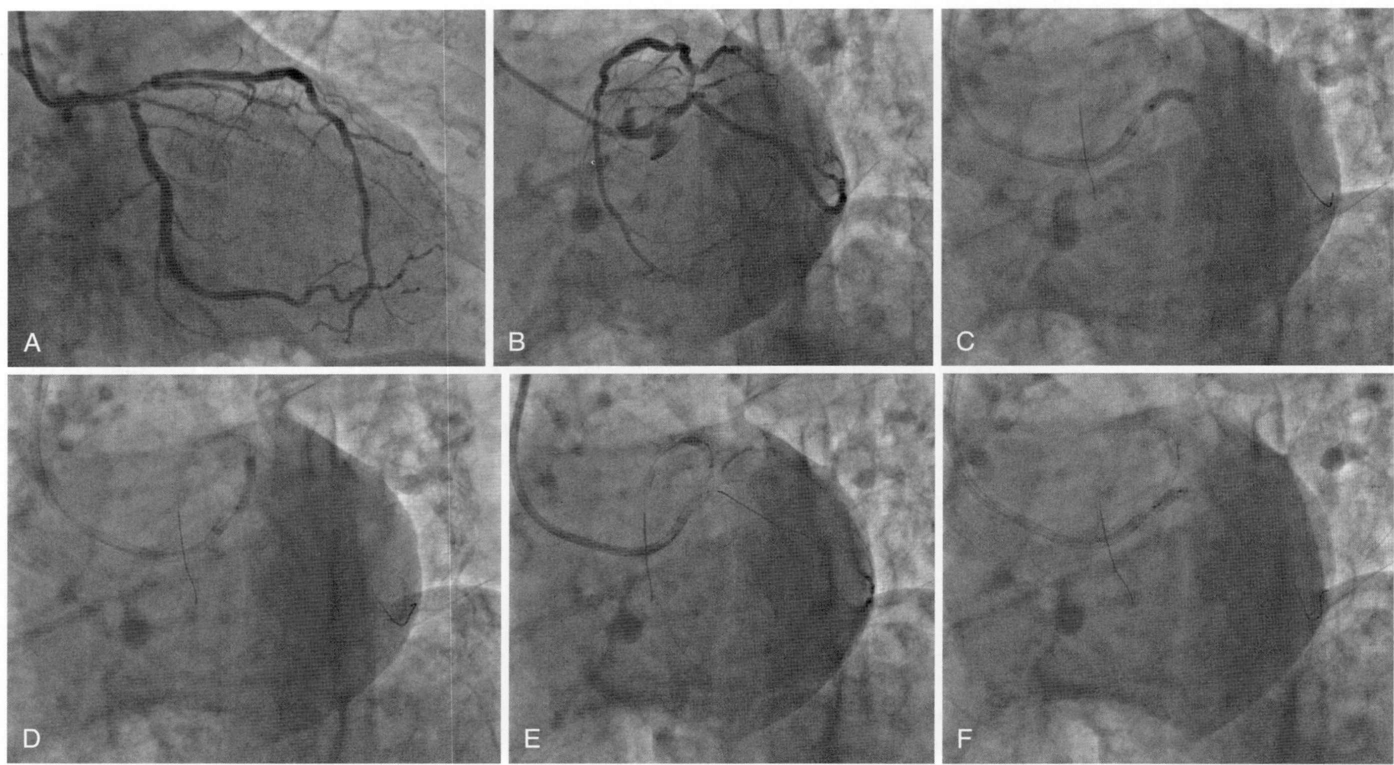

FIGURE 8-9 LM PCI using DK-crush technique (see also Video 8-4). A and **B,** Baseline angiograms showing LM bifurcation (1-1-1 Medina classification) with involvement of LAD (distal main branch) and LCX (side branch; SB). **C,** After predilatation of both branches, implantation of the first stent in the SB (LCX) with a balloon already in place in the distal main branch (LAD). **D,** After removal of the stent balloon in the LCX, inflation of the balloon in the LM-LAD to "crush" the portion of LCX stent protruding in the LM. **E,** After removal of the LAD balloon, removal of the LCX guidewire and rewire of the LCX. Performance of the first kissing inflation with **(F)** dilatation of the ostium of the LCX followed by **(G)** the simultaneous kissing.

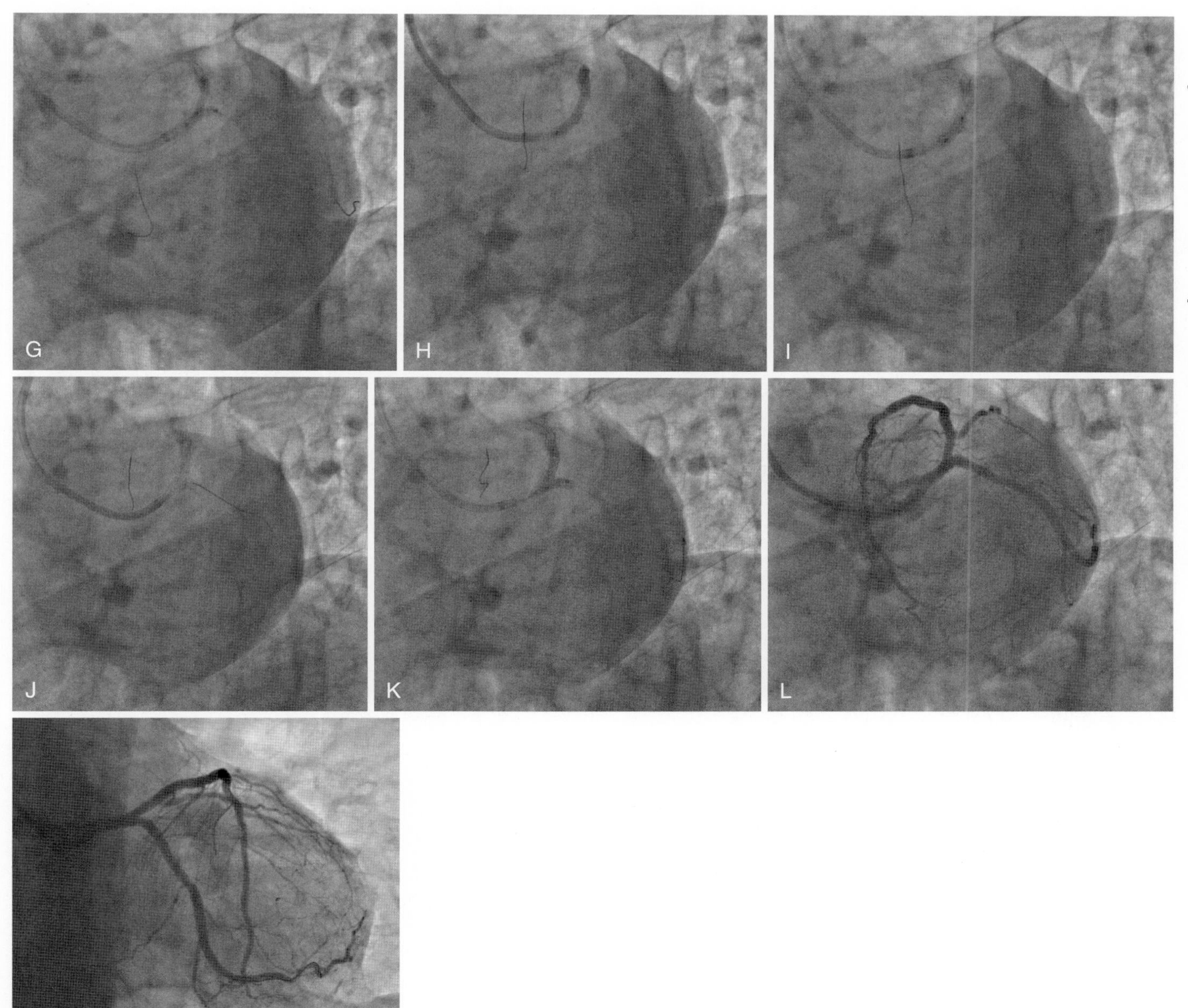

FIGURE 8-9, cont'd **H,** Stenting of the LM-LAD followed by **(I)** postdilatation of the proximal LM stent, with the distal portion of the balloon in front of the LCX ostium (proximal optimization technique; POT). **J,** Removal of the guidewire in the LCX and rewire of the LCX. **K,** Second kissing simultaneous inflation. **L** and **M,** Angiogram of the final result.

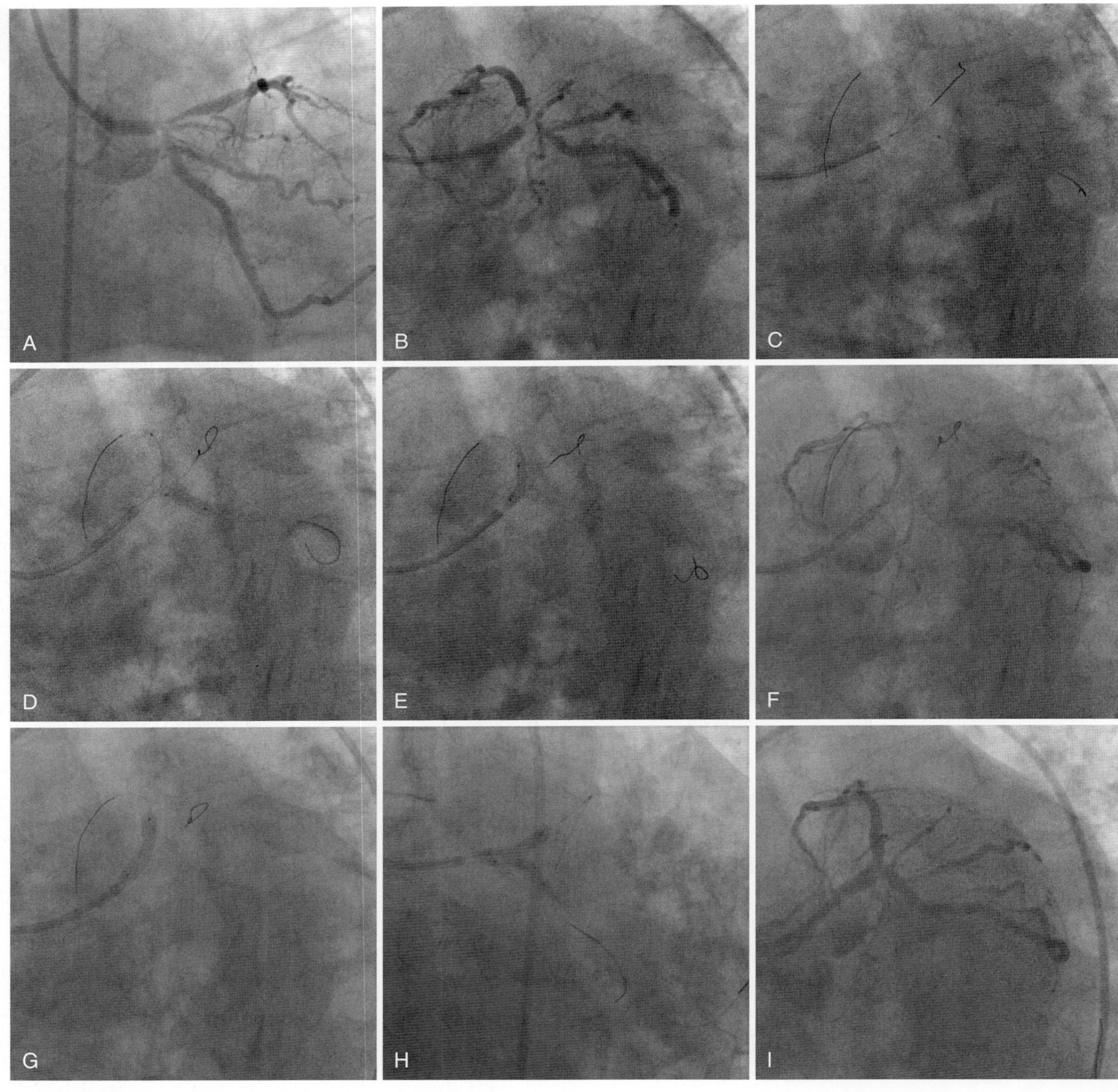

FIGURE 8-10 **LM PCI using a two-stent T-stent technique (see also Video 8-5). A** and **B,** Baseline angiogram showing a trifurcation lesion involving the distal LM, LAD, LCX, and ramus. A sharp angle (~90°) is present between the LM and the LCX, making this favorable for a T-stent technique. **C,** Predilatation of the LCX. **D,** Stent implantation in the LCX, with minimal protrusion of the LCX stent in the LM. Note the wire in the LAD and ramus helping to position the stent in the LCX. **E,** Predilatation of the LAD after LCX stent deployment. If LCX struts were protruding in the LM, they would have been crushed, facilitating stent passage into the LAD. **F,** Stent placement in the LM-LAD axis. **G,** Stent deployment in the LM-LAD axis. **H,** After removal and rewiring of the LCX, final kissing inflation. **I,** Final angiogram showing an excellent result.

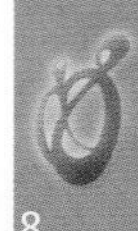

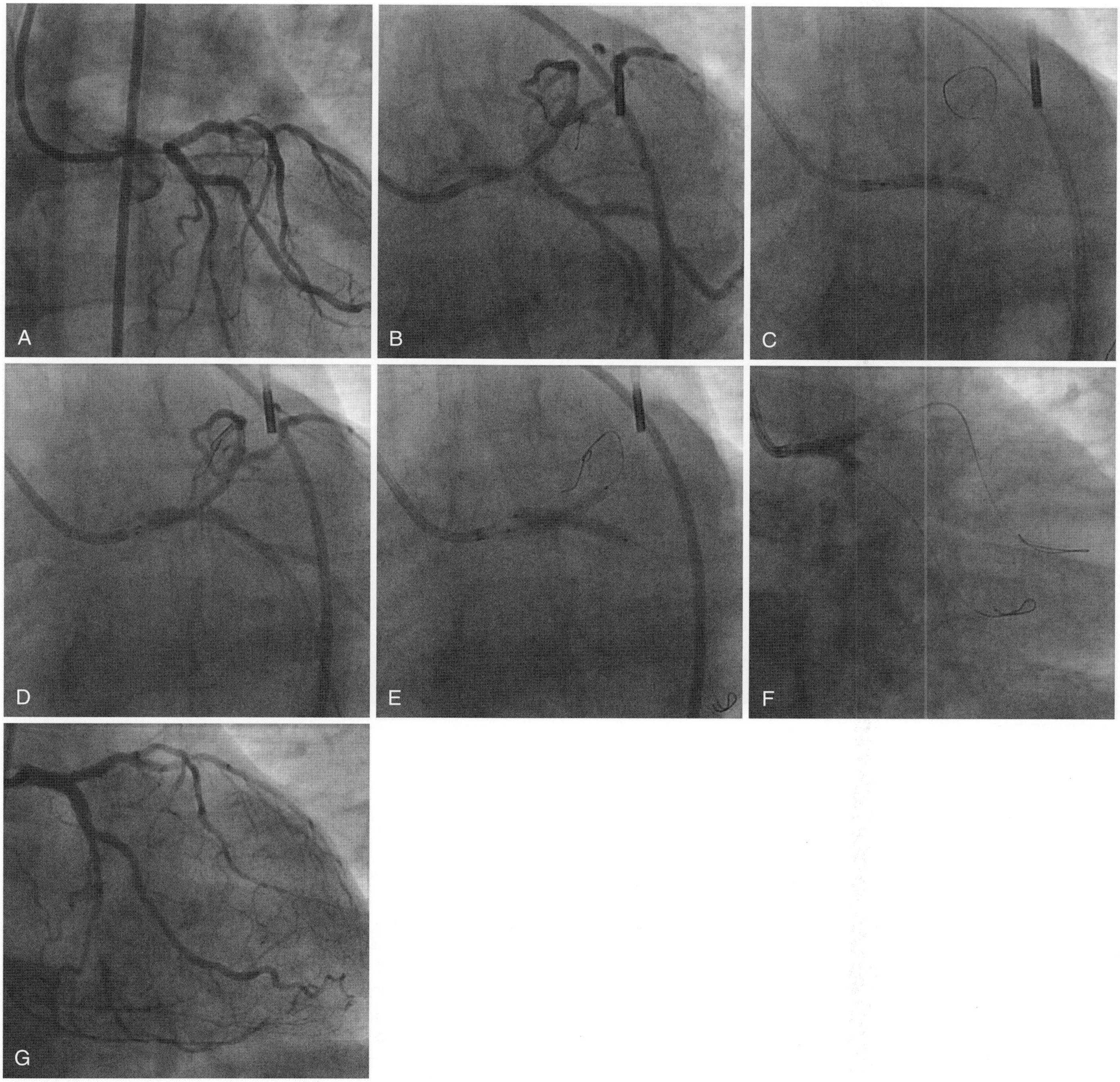

FIGURE 8-11 **LM PCI using a two-stent V stenting (double-barrel) technique (see also Video 8-6). A** and **B,** Baseline angiogram showing a bifurcation lesion involving the distal LM, the ostial LAD, and the ostial LCX (Medina bifurcation 1-1-1). **C,** Balloon predilatation of the LCX. **D,** Simultaneous stent placement. **E,** Simultaneous stent deployment. **F,** Simultaneous postdilatation (without removing the wires). **G,** Final angiogram showing an excellent result.

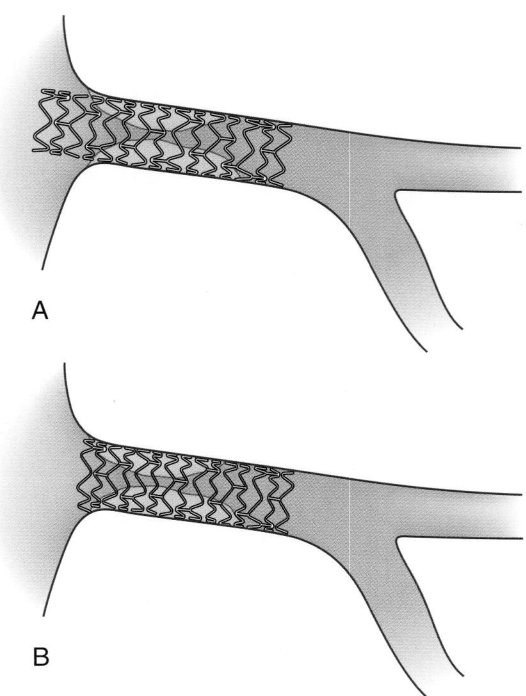

FIGURE 8-12 PCI of an ostial LM lesion. A, Stenting of LM with significant stent protrusion into the aorta. **B,** More desirable stenting of LM ostium with minimal stent protrusion into the aorta. *(Modified from SJ Park's presentation "Left Main CTO Summit 2013," New York.)*

compared with CABG in patients suitable for either treatment strategy.

References

1. DeMots H, Rosch J, McAnulty JH, et al: Left main coronary artery disease. *Cardiovasc Clin* 8:201–211, 1977.
2. Ragosta M, Dee S, Sarembock IJ, et al: Prevalence of unfavorable angiographic characteristics for percutaneous intervention in patients with unprotected left main coronary artery disease. *Catheter Cardiovasc Interv* 68:357–362, 2006.
3. Cohen MV, Cohn PF, Herman MV, et al: Diagnosis and prognosis of main left coronary artery obstruction. *Circulation* 45:I57–I65, 1972.
4. Brennan JM, Dai D, Patel MR, et al: Characteristics and long-term outcomes of percutaneous revascularization of unprotected left main coronary artery stenosis in the United States: a report from the National Cardiovascular Data Registry, 2004 to 2008. *J Am Coll Cardiol* 59:648–654, 2012.
5. Taylor HA, Deumite NJ, Chaitman BR, et al: Asymptomatic left main coronary artery disease in the Coronary Artery Surgery Study (CASS) registry. *Circulation* 79:1171–1179, 1989.
6. Chaitman BR, Fisher LD, Bourassa MG, et al: Effect of coronary bypass surgery on survival patterns in subsets of patients with left main coronary artery disease. Report of the Collaborative Study in Coronary Artery Surgery (CASS). *Am J Cardiol* 48:765–777, 1981.
7. Cohen MV, Gorlin R: Main left coronary artery disease. Clinical experience from 1964-1974. *Circulation* 52:275–285, 1975.
8. Yusuf S, Zucker D, Peduzzi P, et al: Effect of coronary artery bypass graft surgery on survival: overview of 10-year results from randomised trials by the Coronary Artery Bypass Graft Surgery Trialists Collaboration. *Lancet* 344:563–570, 1994.
9. Caracciolo EA, Davis KB, Sopko G, et al: Comparison of surgical and medical group survival in patients with left main equivalent coronary artery disease. Long-term CASS experience. *Circulation* 91:2335–2344, 1995.
10. Takaro T, Peduzzi P, Detre KM, et al: Survival in subgroups of patients with left main coronary artery disease. Veterans Administration Cooperative Study of Surgery for Coronary Arterial Occlusive Disease. *Circulation* 66:14–22, 1982.
11. Levine GN, Bates ER, Blankenship JC, et al: 2011 ACCF/AHA/SCAI Guideline for Percutaneous Coronary Intervention. A report of the American College of Cardiology Foundation/American Heart Association Task Force on Practice Guidelines and the Society for Cardiovascular Angiography and Interventions. *J Am Coll Cardiol* 58:e44–e122, 2011.
12. Task Force members, Windecker S, Kolh P, et al: 2014 ESC/EACTS Guidelines on myocardial revascularization: the Task Force on Myocardial Revascularization of the European Society of Cardiology (ESC) and the European Association for Cardio-Thoracic Surgery (EACTS) Developed with the special contribution of the European Association of Percutaneous Cardiovascular Interventions (EAPCI). *Eur Heart J* 35(37):2541–2619, 2014.
13. Buszman PE, Kiesz SR, Bochenek A, et al: Acute and late outcomes of unprotected left main stenting in comparison with surgical revascularization. *J Am Coll Cardiol* 51:538–545, 2008.
14. Serruys PW, Morice MC, Kappetein AP, et al: Percutaneous coronary intervention versus coronary-artery bypass grafting for severe coronary artery disease. *N Engl J Med* 360:961–972, 2009.
15. Morice MC, Serruys PW, Kappetein AP, et al: Outcomes in patients with de novo left main disease treated with either percutaneous coronary intervention using paclitaxel-eluting stents or coronary artery bypass graft treatment in the Synergy Between Percutaneous Coronary Intervention with TAXUS and Cardiac Surgery (SYNTAX) trial. *Circulation* 121:2645–2653, 2010.
16. Mohr FW, Morice MC, Kappetein AP, et al: Coronary artery bypass graft surgery versus percutaneous coronary intervention in patients with three-vessel disease and left main coronary disease: 5-year follow-up of the randomised, clinical SYNTAX trial. *Lancet* 381:629–638, 2013.
17. Park SJ, Kim YH, Park DW, et al: Randomized trial of stents versus bypass surgery for left main coronary artery disease. *N Engl J Med* 364:1718–1727, 2011.
18. Boudriot E, Thiele H, Walther T, et al: Randomized comparison of percutaneous coronary intervention with sirolimus-eluting stents versus coronary artery bypass grafting in unprotected left main stem stenosis. *J Am Coll Cardiol* 57:538–545, 2011.
19. Capodanno D, Stone GW, Morice MC, et al: Percutaneous coronary intervention versus coronary artery bypass graft surgery in left main coronary artery disease: a meta-analysis of randomized clinical data. *J Am Coll Cardiol* 58:1426–1432, 2011.
20. Athappan G, Patvardhan E, Tuzcu ME, et al: Left main coronary artery stenosis: a meta-analysis of drug-eluting stents versus coronary artery bypass grafting. *JACC Cardiovasc Interv* 6:1219–1230, 2013.
21. Patel MR, Dehmer GJ, Hirshfeld JW, et al: ACCF/SCAI/STS/AATS/AHA/ASNC/HFSA/SCCT 2012 Appropriate use criteria for coronary revascularization focused update: a report of the American College of Cardiology Foundation Appropriate Use Criteria Task Force, Society for Cardiovascular Angiography and Interventions, Society of Thoracic Surgeons, American Association for Thoracic Surgery, American Heart Association, American Society of Nuclear Cardiology, and the Society of Cardiovascular Computed Tomography. *J Am Coll Cardiol* 59:857–881, 2012.
22. Yadav M, Palmerini T, Caixeta A, et al: Prediction of coronary risk by SYNTAX and derived scores: synergy between percutaneous coronary intervention with taxus and cardiac surgery. *J Am Coll Cardiol* 62:1219–1230, 2013.
23. Capodanno D, Capranzano P, Di Salvo ME, et al: Usefulness of SYNTAX score to select patients with left main coronary artery disease to be treated with coronary artery bypass graft. *JACC Cardiovasc Interv* 2:731–738, 2009.
24. Kim YH, Park DW, Kim WJ, et al: Validation of SYNTAX (Synergy between PCI with Taxus and Cardiac Surgery) score for prediction of outcomes after unprotected left main coronary revascularization. *JACC Cardiovasc Interv* 3:612–623, 2010.
25. Onuma Y, Girasis C, Piazza N, et al: Long-term clinical results following stenting of the left main stem: insights from RESEARCH (Rapamycin-Eluting Stent Evaluated at Rotterdam Cardiology Hospital) and T-SEARCH (Taxus-Stent Evaluated at Rotterdam Cardiology Hospital) Registries. *JACC Cardiovasc Interv* 3:584–594, 2010.
26. Capodanno D, Caggegi A, Capranzano P, et al: Validating the EXCEL hypothesis: a propensity score matched 3-year comparison of percutaneous coronary intervention versus coronary artery bypass graft in left main patients with SYNTAX score </= 32. *Catheter Cardiovasc Interv* 77:936–943, 2011.
27. Chakravarty T, Buch MH, Naik H, et al: Predictive accuracy of SYNTAX score for predicting long-term outcomes of unprotected left main coronary artery revascularization. *Am J Cardiol* 107:360–366, 2011.
28. Shiomi H, Morimoto T, Hayano M, et al: Comparison of long-term outcome after percutaneous coronary intervention versus coronary artery bypass grafting in patients with unprotected left main coronary artery disease (from the CREDO-Kyoto PCI/CABG Registry Cohort-2). *Am J Cardiol* 110:924–932, 2012.
29. Tiroch K, Mehilli J, Byrne RA, et al: Impact of coronary anatomy and stenting technique on long-term outcome after drug-eluting stent implantation for unprotected left main coronary artery disease. *JACC Cardiovasc Interv* 7:29–36, 2014.
30. Capodanno D, Miano M, Cincotta G, et al: EuroSCORE refines the predictive ability of SYNTAX score in patients undergoing left main percutaneous coronary intervention. *Am Heart J* 159:103–109, 2010.
31. Serruys PW, Farooq V, Vranckx P, et al: A global risk approach to identify patients with left main or 3-vessel disease who could safely and efficaciously be treated with percutaneous coronary intervention: the SYNTAX Trial at 3 years. *JACC Cardiovasc Interv* 5:606–617, 2012.
32. Farooq V, van Klaveren D, Steyerberg EW, et al: Anatomical and clinical characteristics to guide decision making between coronary artery bypass surgery and percutaneous coronary intervention for individual patients: development and validation of SYNTAX score II. *Lancet* 381:639–650, 2013.
33. Xu B, Genereux P, Yang Y, et al: Validation and comparison of the long-term prognostic capability of the SYNTAX score II among 1,528 consecutive patients who underwent left main percutaneous coronary intervention. *JACC Cardiovasc Interv* 7(10):1128–1137, 2014.
34. Palmerini T, Marzocchi A, Tamburino C, et al: Two-year clinical outcome with drug-eluting stents versus bare-metal stents in a real-world registry of unprotected left main coronary artery stenosis from the Italian Society of Invasive Cardiology. *Am J Cardiol* 102:1463–1468, 2008.
35. Pandya SB, Kim YH, Meyers SN, et al: Drug-eluting versus bare-metal stents in unprotected left main coronary artery stenosis: a meta-analysis. *JACC Cardiovasc Interv* 3:602–611, 2010.
36. Erglis A, Kumsars I, Niemela M, et al: Randomized comparison of coronary bifurcation stenting with the crush versus the culotte technique using sirolimus eluting stents: the Nordic stent technique study. *Circ Cardiovasc Interv* 2:27–34, 2009.
37. Kim YH, Park DW, Lee SW, et al: Long-term safety and effectiveness of unprotected left main coronary stenting with drug-eluting stents compared with bare-metal stents. *Circulation* 120:400–407, 2009.
38. Mehilli J, Kastrati A, Byrne RA, et al: Paclitaxel versus sirolimus-eluting stents for unprotected left main coronary artery disease. *J Am Coll Cardiol* 53:1760–1768, 2009.
39. Mehilli J, Richardt G, Valgimigli M, et al: Zotarolimus versus everolimus-eluting stents for unprotected left main coronary artery disease. *J Am Coll Cardiol* 62:2075–2082, 2013.
40. Kim YH, Park DW, Ahn JM, et al: Everolimus-eluting stent implantation for unprotected left main coronary artery stenosis. The PRECOMBAT-2 (Premier of Randomized Comparison of Bypass Surgery versus Angioplasty Using Sirolimus-Eluting Stent in Patients with Left Main Coronary Artery Disease) study. *JACC Cardiovasc Interv* 5:708–717, 2012.
41. Moynagh A, Salvatella N, Harb T, et al: Two-year outcomes of everolimus vs. paclitaxel-eluting stent for the treatment of unprotected left main lesions: a propensity score matching comparison of patients included in the French Left Main Taxus (FLM Taxus) and the LEft MAin Xience (LEMAX) registries. *EuroIntervention* 9:452–462, 2013.
42. Palmerini T, Biondi-Zoccai G, Della Riva D, et al: Stent thrombosis with drug-eluting and bare-metal stents: evidence from a comprehensive network meta-analysis. *Lancet* 379:1393–1402, 2012.
43. Bangalore S, Kumar S, Fusaro M, et al: Short- and long-term outcomes with drug-eluting and bare-metal coronary stents: a mixed-treatment comparison analysis of 117,762 patient-years of follow-up from randomized trials. *Circulation* 125:2873–2891, 2012.
44. Ojeda S, Pan M, Martin P, et al: Immediate results and long-term clinical outcome of patients with unprotected distal left main restenosis: the CORPAL (cordoba and las palmas) registry. *JACC Cardiovasc Interv* 7(2):212–221, 2014.
45. Ielasi A, Takagi K, Latib A, et al: Long-term clinical outcomes following drug-eluting stent implantation for unprotected distal trifurcation left main disease: the Milan-New TOkyo (MITO) registry. *Catheter Cardiovasc Interv* 83(4):530–538, 2013.
46. Kang SJ, Ahn JM, Song H, et al: Comprehensive intravascular ultrasound assessment of stent area and its impact on restenosis and adverse cardiac events in 403 patients with unprotected left main disease. *Circ Cardiovasc Interv* 4:562–569, 2011.
47. Naganuma T, Chieffo A, Meliga E, et al: Long-term clinical outcomes after percutaneous coronary intervention for ostial/mid-shaft lesions versus distal bifurcation lesions in unprotected left main coronary artery: the DELTA Registry (Drug-Eluting Stent for Left Main Coronary Artery Disease): a multicenter registry evaluating percutaneous coronary intervention versus coronary artery bypass grafting for left main treatment. *JACC Cardiovasc Interv* 6:1242–1249, 2013.
48. Palmerini T, Sangiorgi D, Marzocchi A, et al: Ostial and midshaft lesions vs. bifurcation lesions in 1111 patients with unprotected left main coronary artery stenosis treated with drug-eluting

stents: results of the survey from the Italian Society of Invasive Cardiology. *Eur Heart J* 30:2087–2094, 2009.
49. Colombo A, Moses JW, Morice MC, et al: Randomized study to evaluate sirolimus-eluting stents implanted at coronary bifurcation lesions. *Circulation* 109:1244–1249, 2004.
50. Pan M, de Lezo JS, Medina A, et al: Rapamycin-eluting stents for the treatment of bifurcated coronary lesions: a randomized comparison of a simple versus complex strategy. *Am Heart J* 148:857–864, 2004.
51. Steigen TK, Maeng M, Wiseth R, et al: Randomized study on simple versus complex stenting of coronary artery bifurcation lesions: the Nordic bifurcation study. *Circulation* 114:1955–1961, 2006.
52. Ferenc M, Gick M, Kienzle RP, et al: Randomized trial on routine vs. provisional T-stenting in the treatment of de novo coronary bifurcation lesions. *Eur Heart J* 29:2859–2867, 2008.
53. Colombo A, Bramucci E, Sacca S, et al: Randomized study of the crush technique versus provisional side-branch stenting in true coronary bifurcations: the CACTUS (Coronary Bifurcations: Application of the Crushing Technique Using Sirolimus-Eluting Stents) Study. *Circulation* 119:71–78, 2009.
54. Song YB, Hahn JY, Song PS, et al: Randomized comparison of conservative versus aggressive strategy for provisional side branch intervention in coronary bifurcation lesions: results from the SMART-STRATEGY (Smart Angioplasty Research Team-Optimal Strategy for Side Branch Intervention in Coronary Bifurcation Lesions) randomized trial. *JACC Cardiovasc Interv* 5:1133–1140, 2012.
55. Chen SL, Santoso T, Zhang JJ, et al: A randomized clinical study comparing double kissing crush with provisional stenting for treatment of coronary bifurcation lesions: results from the DKCRUSH-II (Double Kissing Crush versus Provisional Stenting Technique for Treatment of Coronary Bifurcation Lesions) trial. *J Am Coll Cardiol* 57:914–920, 2011.
56. Hildick-Smith D, de Belder AJ, Cooter N, et al: Randomized trial of simple versus complex drug-eluting stenting for bifurcation lesions: the British Bifurcation Coronary Study: old, new, and evolving strategies. *Circulation* 121:1235–1243, 2010.
57. Chen SL, Xu B, Han YL, et al: Comparison of double kissing crush versus Culotte stenting for unprotected distal left main bifurcation lesions: results from a multicenter, randomized, prospective DKCRUSH-III study. *J Am Coll Cardiol* 61:1482–1488, 2013.
58. Genereux P, Kumsars I, Lesiak M: A randomized trial of a dedicated bifurcation stent versus provisional stenting in the treatment of coronary bifurcation lesions. *J Am Coll Cardiol* 2015. In press.
58a. Magro M, Girasis C, Bartorelli AL, et al: Acute procedural and six-month clinical outcome in patients treated with a dedicated bifurcation stent for left main stem disease: the TRYTON LM multicentre registry. *EuroIntervention* 8:1259–1269, 2013.
59. Grundeken MJ, Asgedom S, Damman P, et al: Six-month and one-year clinical outcomes after placement of a dedicated coronary bifurcation stent: a patient-level pooled analysis of eight registry studies. *EuroIntervention* 9:195–203, 2013.
60. Hasegawa T, Ako J, Koo BK, et al: Analysis of left main coronary artery bifurcation lesions treated with biolimus-eluting DEVAX AXXESS plus nitinol self-expanding stent: intravascular ultrasound results of the AXXENT trial. *Catheter Cardiovasc Interv* 73:34–41, 2009.
61. Costa RA, Abizaid A, Abizaid AS, et al: Procedural and early clinical outcomes of patients with de novo coronary bifurcation lesions treated with the novel Nile PAX dedicated bifurcation polymer-free paclitaxel coated stents: results from the prospective, multicentre, non-randomised BIPAX clinical trial. *EuroIntervention* 7:1301–1309, 2012.
62. Ge L, Airoldi F, Iakovou I, et al: Clinical and angiographic outcome after implantation of drug-eluting stents in bifurcation lesions with the crush stent technique: importance of final kissing balloon post-dilation. *J Am Coll Cardiol* 46:613–620, 2005.
63. Chen SL, Zhang JJ, Ye F, et al: Effect of coronary bifurcation angle on clinical outcomes in Chinese patients treated with crush stenting: a subgroup analysis from DKCRUSH-1 bifurcation study. *Chin Med J* 122:396–402, 2009.
64. Hildick-Smith D, Lassen JF, Albiero R, et al: Consensus from the 5th European Bifurcation Club meeting. *EuroIntervention* 6:34–38, 2010.
65. Niemela M, Kervinen K, Erglis A, et al: Randomized comparison of final kissing balloon dilatation versus no final kissing balloon dilatation in patients with coronary bifurcation lesions treated with main vessel stenting: the Nordic-Baltic Bifurcation Study III. *Circulation* 123:79–86, 2011.
66. Koo BK, Park KW, Kang HJ, et al: Physiological evaluation of the provisional side-branch intervention strategy for bifurcation lesions using fractional flow reserve. *Eur Heart J* 29:726–732, 2008.
67. de la Torre Hernandez JM, Hernandez Hernandez F, Alfonso F, et al: Prospective application of pre-defined intravascular ultrasound criteria for assessment of intermediate left main coronary artery lesions results from the multicenter LITRO study. *J Am Coll Cardiol* 58:351–358, 2011.
68. Hamilos M, Muller O, Cuisset T, et al: Long-term clinical outcome after fractional flow reserve-guided treatment in patients with angiographically equivocal left main coronary artery stenosis. *Circulation* 120:1505–1512, 2009.
69. Abizaid AS, Mintz GS, Abizaid A, et al: One-year follow-up after intravascular ultrasound assessment of moderate left main coronary artery disease in patients with ambiguous angiograms. *J Am Coll Cardiol* 34:707–715, 1999.
70. Jasti V, Ivan E, Yalamanchili V, et al: Correlations between fractional flow reserve and intravascular ultrasound in patients with an ambiguous left main coronary artery stenosis. *Circulation* 110:2831–2836, 2004.
71. Kang SJ, Lee JY, Ahn JM, et al: Intravascular ultrasound-derived predictors for fractional flow reserve in intermediate left main disease. *JACC Cardiovasc Interv* 4:1168–1174, 2011.
72. Park SJ, Ahn JM, Kang SJ: Unprotected left main percutaneous coronary intervention: integrated use of fractional flow reserve and intravascular ultrasound. *J Am Heart Assoc* 1:e004556, 2012.
73. Park SJ, Kim YH, Park DW, et al: Impact of intravascular ultrasound guidance on long-term mortality in stenting for unprotected left main coronary artery stenosis. *Circ Cardiovasc Interv* 2:167–177, 2009.
74. Kubo T, Akasaka T, Shite J, et al: OCT compared with IVUS in a coronary lesion assessment: the OPUS-CLASS study. *JACC Cardiovasc Imaging* 6:1095–1104, 2013.
75. Di Mario C, Iakovou I, van der Giessen WJ, et al: Optical coherence tomography for guidance in bifurcation lesion treatment. *EuroIntervention* 6(Suppl J):J99–J106, 2010.
76. Okamura T, Onuma Y, Yamada J, et al: 3D optical coherence tomography: new insights into the process of optimal rewiring of side branches during bifurcational stenting. *EuroIntervention* 2014.
77. Fujino Y, Attizzani GF, Bezerra HG, et al: Serial assessment of vessel interactions after drug-eluting stent implantation in unprotected distal left main coronary artery disease using frequency-domain optical coherence tomography. *JACC Cardiovasc Interv* 6:1035–1045, 2013.
78. Fujino Y, Bezerra HG, Attizzani GF, et al: Frequency-domain optical coherence tomography assessment of unprotected left main coronary artery disease—a comparison with intravascular ultrasound. *Catheter Cardiovasc Interv* 82:E173–E183, 2013.
79. Tonino PA, De Bruyne B, Pijls NH, et al: Fractional flow reserve versus angiography for guiding percutaneous coronary intervention. *N Engl J Med* 360:213–224, 2009.
80. De Bruyne B, Pijls NH, Kalesan B, et al: Fractional flow reserve-guided PCI versus medical therapy in stable coronary disease. *N Engl J Med* 367:991–1001, 2012.
81. Melikian N, De Bondt P, Tonino P, et al: Fractional flow reserve and myocardial perfusion imaging in patients with angiographic multivessel coronary artery disease. *JACC Cardiovasc Interv* 3:307–314, 2010.
82. Pijls NH, De Bruyne B, Peels K, et al: Measurement of fractional flow reserve to assess the functional severity of coronary-artery stenoses. *N Engl J Med* 334:1703–1708, 1996.
83. Koo BK, Kang HJ, Youn TJ, et al: Physiologic assessment of jailed side branch lesions using fractional flow reserve. *J Am Coll Cardiol* 46:633–637, 2005.
84. Bech GJ, Droste H, Pijls NH, et al: Value of fractional flow reserve in making decisions about bypass surgery for equivocal left main coronary artery disease. *Heart* 86:547–552, 2001.
85. Jimenez-Navarro M, Hernandez-Garcia JM, Alonso-Briales JH, et al: Should we treat patients with moderately severe stenosis of the left main coronary artery and negative FFR results? *J Invasive Cardiol* 16:398–400, 2004.
86. Legutko J, Dudek D, Rzeszutko L, et al: Fractional flow reserve assessment to determine the indications for myocardial revascularisation in patients with borderline stenosis of the left main coronary artery. *Kardiol Pol* 63:499–506, discussion 507–508, 2005.
87. Suemaru S, Iwasaki K, Yamamoto K, et al: Coronary pressure measurement to determine treatment strategy for equivocal left main coronary artery lesions. *Heart Vessels* 20:271–277, 2005.
88. Lindstaedt M, Yazar A, Germing A, et al: Clinical outcome in patients with intermediate or equivocal left main coronary artery disease after deferral of surgical revascularization on the basis of fractional flow reserve measurements. *Am Heart J* 152(156):e1–e9, 2006.
89. Puri R, Kapadia SR, Nicholls SJ, et al: Optimizing outcomes during left main percutaneous coronary intervention with intravascular ultrasound and fractional flow reserve: the current state of evidence. *JACC Cardiovasc Interv* 5:697–707, 2012.
90. Pijls NH, De Bruyne B, Bech GJ, et al: Coronary pressure measurement to assess the hemodynamic significance of serial stenoses within one coronary artery: validation in humans. *Circulation* 102:2371–2377, 2000.
91. Vis MM, Beijk MA, Grundeken MJ, et al: A systematic review and meta-analysis on primary percutaneous coronary intervention of an unprotected left main coronary artery culprit lesion in the setting of acute myocardial infarction. *JACC Cardiovasc Interv* 6:317–324, 2013.
92. Pedrazzini GB, Radovanovic D, Vassalli G, et al: Primary percutaneous coronary intervention for unprotected left main disease in patients with acute ST-segment elevation myocardial infarction: the AMIS (Acute Myocardial Infarction in Switzerland) Plus registry experience. *JACC Cardiovasc Interv* 4:627–633, 2011.
93. Patel N, De Maria GL, Kassimis G, et al: Outcomes after emergency percutaneous coronary intervention in patients with unprotected left main stem occlusion: the BCIS national audit of percutaneous coronary intervention 6-year experience. *JACC Cardiovasc Interv* 7:969–980, 2014.
94. Briguori C, Airoldi F, Chieffo A, et al: Elective versus provisional intraaortic balloon pumping in unprotected left main stenting. *Am Heart J* 152:565–572, 2006.
95. Mishra S, Chu WW, Torguson R, et al: Role of prophylactic intra-aortic balloon pump in high-risk patients undergoing percutaneous coronary intervention. *Am J Cardiol* 98:608–612, 2006.
96. Briguori C, Sarais C, Pagnotta P, et al: Elective versus provisional intra-aortic balloon pumping in high-risk percutaneous transluminal coronary angioplasty. *Am Heart J* 145:700–707, 2003.
97. Dixon SR, Henriques JP, Mauri L, et al: A prospective feasibility trial investigating the use of the Impella 2.5 system in patients undergoing high-risk percutaneous coronary intervention (The PROTECT I Trial): initial U.S. experience. *JACC Cardiovasc Interv* 2:91–96, 2009.
98. O'Neill WW, Kleiman NS, Moses J, et al: A prospective, randomized clinical trial of hemodynamic support with Impella 2.5 versus intra-aortic balloon pump in patients undergoing high-risk percutaneous coronary intervention: the PROTECT II study. *Circulation* 126:1717–1727, 2012.
99. Farooq V, Serruys PW, Zhang Y, et al: Short-term and long-term clinical impact of stent thrombosis and graft occlusion in the SYNTAX trial at 5 years: synergy between Percutaneous Coronary Intervention with Taxus and Cardiac Surgery trial. *J Am Coll Cardiol* 62:2360–2369, 2013.
100. Iakovou I, Schmidt T, Bonizzoni E, et al: Incidence, predictors, and outcome of thrombosis after successful implantation of drug-eluting stents. *JAMA* 293:2126–2130, 2005.
101. Palmerini T, Marzocchi A, Tamburino C, et al: Temporal pattern of ischemic events in relation to dual antiplatelet therapy in patients with unprotected left main coronary artery stenosis undergoing percutaneous coronary intervention. *J Am Coll Cardiol* 53:1176–1181, 2009.
102. Airoldi F, Colombo A, Morici N, et al: Incidence and predictors of drug-eluting stent thrombosis during and after discontinuation of thienopyridine treatment. *Circulation* 116:745–754, 2007.
103. Park DW, Yun SC, Lee SW, et al: Stent thrombosis, clinical events, and influence of prolonged clopidogrel use after placement of drug-eluting stent data from an observational cohort study of drug-eluting versus bare-metal stents. *JACC Cardiovasc Interv* 1:494–503, 2008.
104. Schulz S, Schuster T, Mehilli J, et al: Stent thrombosis after drug-eluting stent implantation: incidence, timing, and relation to discontinuation of clopidogrel therapy over a 4-year period. *Eur Heart J* 30:2714–2721, 2009.
105. Migliorini A, Valenti R, Marcucci R, et al: High residual platelet reactivity after clopidogrel loading and long-term clinical outcome after drug-eluting stenting for unprotected left main coronary disease. *Circulation* 120:2214–2221, 2009.
106. Wallentin L, Becker RC, Budaj A, et al: Ticagrelor versus clopidogrel in patients with acute coronary syndromes. *N Engl J Med* 361:1045–1057, 2009.
107. Wiviott SD, Braunwald E, McCabe CH, et al: Prasugrel versus clopidogrel in patients with acute coronary syndromes. *N Engl J Med* 357:2001–2015, 2007.
108. Mylotte D, Routledge H, Harb T, et al: Provisional side branch-stenting for coronary bifurcation lesions: evidence of improving procedural and clinical outcomes with contemporary techniques. *Catheter Cardiovasc Interv* 82:E437–E445, 2013.
109. Stankovic G, Lefevre T, Chieffo A, et al: Consensus from the 7th European Bifurcation Club meeting. *EuroIntervention* 9:36–45, 2013.
110. Burzotta F, Gwon HC, Hahn JY, et al: Modified T-stenting with intentional protrusion of the side-branch stent within the main vessel stent to ensure ostial coverage and facilitate final kissing balloon: the T-stenting and small protrusion technique (TAP-stenting). Report of bench testing and first clinical Italian-Korean two-centre experience. *Catheter Cardiovasc Interv* 70:75–82, 2007.
111. Foin N, Sen S, Allegria E, et al: Maximal expansion capacity with current DES platforms: a critical factor for stent selection in the treatment of left main bifurcations? *EuroIntervention* 8:1315–1325, 2013.
112. Colombo A: Balloon crush: new tool in bifurcation treatment armamentarium. *Catheter Cardiovasc Interv* 63:417–418, 2004.
113. Colombo A, Stankovic G, Orlic D, et al: Modified T-stenting technique with crushing for bifurcation lesions: immediate results and 30-day outcome. *Catheter Cardiovasc Interv* 60:145–151, 2003.
114. Galassi AR, Colombo A, Buchbinder M, et al: Long-term outcomes of bifurcation lesions after implantation of drug-eluting stents with the "mini-crush technique." *Catheter Cardiovasc Interv* 69:976–983, 2007.
115. Furuichi S, Airoldi F, Colombo A: Rescue inverse crush: a way of get out of trouble. *Catheter Cardiovasc Interv* 70:708–712, 2007.
116. Chen S, Zhang J, Ye F, et al: DK crush (double-kissing and double-crush) technique for treatment of true coronary bifurcation lesions: illustration and comparison with classic crush. *J Invasive Cardiol* 19:189–193, 2007.
117. Siotia A, Morton AC, Malkin CJ, et al: Simultaneous kissing drug-eluting stents to treat unprotected left main stem bifurcation disease: medium term outcome in 150 consecutive patients. *EuroIntervention* 8:691–700, 2012.
118. Stinis CT, Hu SP, Price MJ, et al: Three-year outcome of drug-eluting stent implantation for coronary artery bifurcation lesions. *Catheter Cardiovasc Interv* 75:309–314, 2010.

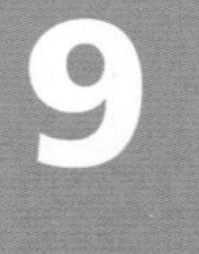

Chronic Total Coronary Occlusions: Rationale, Technique, and Clinical Outcomes

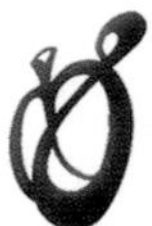

David E. Kandzari

INTRODUCTION

Despite remarkable advances in the procedural and clinical outcomes of percutaneous revascularization, chronically occluded coronary arteries represent persistent technical challenges and unresolved clinical dilemmas in interventional cardiology. Although a coronary chronic total occlusion (CTO) is identified in approximately one in every three to five diagnostic cardiac catheterizations, revascularization is attempted in fewer than 10% of instances and overall accounts for less than 8% of all percutaneous coronary interventions (PCI) (**Figure 9-1**).[1,2] Such a disparity between their frequency and treatment not only underscores the technical and procedural frustrations associated with these complex lesions but also the clinical uncertainties regarding which patients may benefit from CTO revascularization. Chronic occlusions remain the single most important reason not to attempt PCI in favor of bypass surgery or medical treatment.[3] As an example, in the multivessel PCI versus coronary artery bypass graft (CABG) surgery SYNTAX (SYNergy Between PCI with TAXUS and Cardiac Surgery) study, the prevalence of CTO in the randomized arm was only 10%, yet it was 40% in the CABG registry arm.[4]

Unlike catheter-based revascularization of nonocclusive coronary disease, much of our understanding regarding total occlusions has been further limited by relatively few studies describing the procedural and clinical outcomes among patients undergoing attempted revascularization. Moreover, these investigations are limited by their retrospective, observational design, variability in operator skills, inconsistencies regarding the definition of total occlusions, and bias regarding patient selection. Since the duration of an occluded artery is an independent predictor of procedural outcome,[5-7] an inability to date these lesions, in addition to their heterogeneous composition, have restricted the evaluation of novel revascularization technologies. Until recently, many of the technologies promoted for the treatment of total occlusions were simply modeled after devices applied to nonocclusive disease, erroneously assuming that the pathophysiology between these lesion subsets was similar.

ANATOMIC CONSIDERATIONS

The definition of a coronary CTO is reflective of the degree of lumen stenosis, the extent of antegrade blood flow, and the age of the occlusion. In general, a CTO is defined as a high-grade coronary occlusion with reduced antegrade flow (Thrombolysis in Myocardial Infarction [TIMI] grade 0 or 1 flow) with estimated duration of at least 3 months. Without serial angiograms, however, the duration of coronary occlusion is difficult to specify with any certainty and must be estimated from available clinical information related to the timing of the event that caused the occlusion, for example, clinical history of myocardial infarction or a sudden change in angina pattern with electrocardiographic changes consistent with the location of the occlusion. In addition, despite presenting with such advanced disease, less than half of the patients demonstrate a clinical history or electrocardiogram suggestive of prior myocardial infarction.[2] In most patients, the age of the CTO cannot be determined with confidence. Furthermore, the temporal criterion used to define a CTO has varied among registries, trials, and

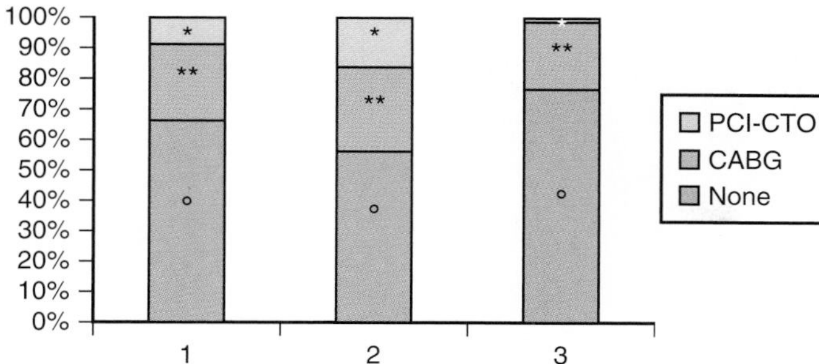

- CTO identified in 18.4% of 1,697 pts
- Only 40% had history of prior MI, 26% had Q waves in CTO distribution
- Attempt rate varied among 3 hospitals from 1% to 16%
- CTO PCI attempted in only 10% of patients with 70% success

FIGURE 9-1 **Prevalence of and variability in treatment of coronary CTOs.** Despite a high prevalence of CTOs among patients undergoing diagnostic coronary angiography at three hospitals, PCI accounted for only 10% of treatment strategies. *(Reproduced with permission from Fefer P, Knudtson ML, Cheema AN, et al: Current perspectives on coronary chronic total occlusions: the Canadian Multicenter Chronic Total Occlusions Registry. J Am Coll Cardiol 59:991–997, 2012.)*

databases, ranging from >2 weeks to >3 months, which in part explains interstudy differences in lesion characteristics and procedural success.

Histopathology of CTOs

Chronic coronary occlusions most often arise from thrombotic occlusion, followed by thrombus organization and tissue aging. Particularly relevant to PCI strategies for CTO recanalization is the histological finding that approximately half of all CTOs are <99% stenotic when observed by histopathology, despite the angiographic appearance of total occlusion with TIMI grade 0 antegrade flow.[8] Moreover, little to no relationship exists between the severity of the histopathological lumen stenosis and either plaque composition or lesion age.[8]

The typical atherosclerotic plaque of a CTO consists of intracellular and extracellular lipids, smooth muscle cells, extracellular matrix, and calcium.[9] Collagens are the major structural components of the extracellular matrix, with predominance of types I and III (and minor amounts of IV, V, and VI) in the fibrous stroma of atherosclerotic plaques. The concentration of collagen-rich fibrous tissue is particularly dense at the proximal and distal ends of the lesion, contributing to a column-like lesion of calcified, resistant fibrous tissue surrounding a softer core of organized thrombus and lipids.

Key histopathological attributes of CTOs include calcification extent, inflammation, and neovascularization. The typical CTO may be classified as "soft," "hard," or a mixture of both. Soft plaque consists of cholesterol-laden cells and foam cells with loose fibrous tissue and neovascular channels and is more frequent in younger occlusions (<1 year old). Soft plaque is more likely to allow wire passage either directly through tissue planes or via neovascular channels into the distal lumen. Conversely, hard plaque is characterized by dense fibrous tissue and often contains large fibrocalcific regions without neovascular channels. During percutaneous revascularization, these occlusions are thus more likely to deflect coronary guidewires into the subintimal area, thereby creating dissection planes. Hard plaque is more prevalent with increasing CTO age (>1 year old). Of note, however, areas of calcification frequently occur even in CTOs <3 months of age, although the extent and severity of calcification increase with occlusion duration. This age-related increase in calcium and collagen content of CTOs in part underlies the progressive difficulty during PCI in crossing older occlusions.

Inflammatory cell infiltrates in CTOs consist of macrophages, foam cells, and lymphocytes. Inflammation may exist in the intima, media, and adventitia of CTOs, although it is most predominant in the intima. As fibrotic CTO lesions age, the vessels typically undergo negative remodeling with a decreasing dimension of the external elastic membrane, a phenomenon due to adventitial vascular responses. Less commonly, plaque hemorrhage and inflammation may result in positive remodeling. Notably, although negative remodeling may be initially observed following successful CTO recanalization, serial angiographic surveillance may reveal temporal recovery of normal vessel dimensions.[10]

Another observation common to CTOs is the presence of extensive neovascularization that occurs throughout the extent of the vessel wall. Capillary density and angiogenesis increase with increasing occlusion age. In CTOs <1 year old, new capillary formation is greatest in the adventitia. In CTOs of more advanced duration, the number and size of capillaries in the intima have increased to a similar or greater extent than those present in the adventitia. Relatively large (>250 μm) capillaries are frequently present throughout the CTO vessel wall, even in young occlusions, suggesting that angiogenesis within the CTO is an early event. Frequent co-localization of inflammation and neovascularization within the intimal plaque and adventitia suggests that these findings are closely related, although it is unclear whether inflammation is a cause or an effect of neovascularization in CTOs.

A rich neovasculature network often traverses the CTO vessel wall, arising from the adventitial vasa vasorum across the media and into the lesion intima, suggesting that vessel in-growth proceeds from the adventitia in younger lesions. An autopsy study of subtotal atherosclerotic lesions demonstrated that new intimal vessels originate in the adventitial vasa vasorum of lesions with >70% stenosis but rarely from the coronary lumen.[11] Such microchannels, which can recanalize the distal lumen, may result from thrombus-derived angiogenic stimuli and are suggested on an angiogram of an old CTO without a well-defined proximal cap or stump. In this regard, the distinction should be made between ipsilateral epicardial angiographic "bridging" collateral vessels and true microvascular collaterals. Neochannels may also develop with organization of thrombus, connecting the proximal and distal lumens; this is suggested by a tapered CTO proximal cap on an angiogram. Such channels may serve as a route for a guidewire to reach the distal vessel and hence may have therapeutic value.

Collaterals and CTOs

Collaterals preserve myocardial function and avoid cardiac myocyte death in the distribution of the occluded artery. The most widely used angiographic grading system for collaterals described by Rentrop does not actually characterize the collaterals themselves but rather their contribution to filling the occluded arterial segment.[12] Recently, a grading of collateral connections was introduced specifically for CTOs that may assist in interventional decision making regarding retrograde strategies[13] (**Figure 9-2**).

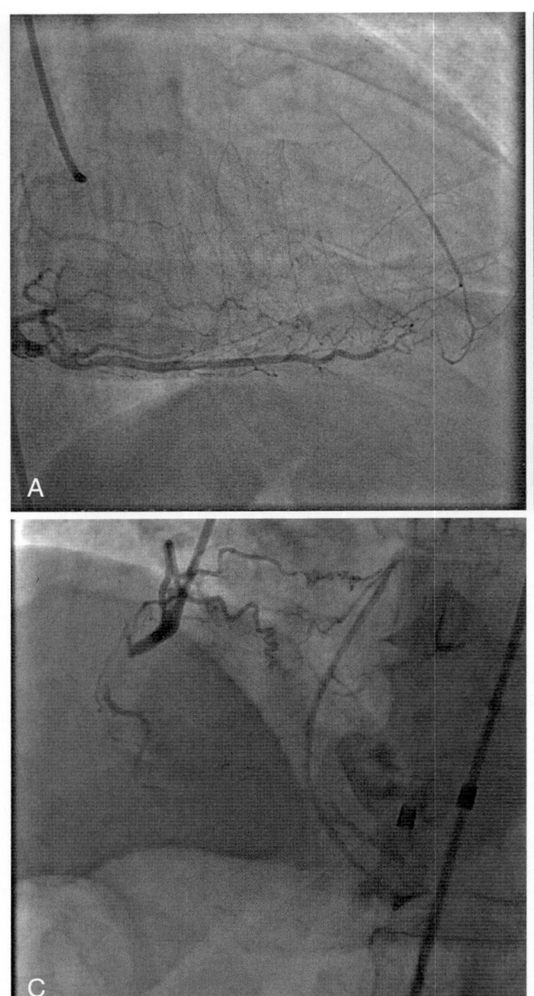

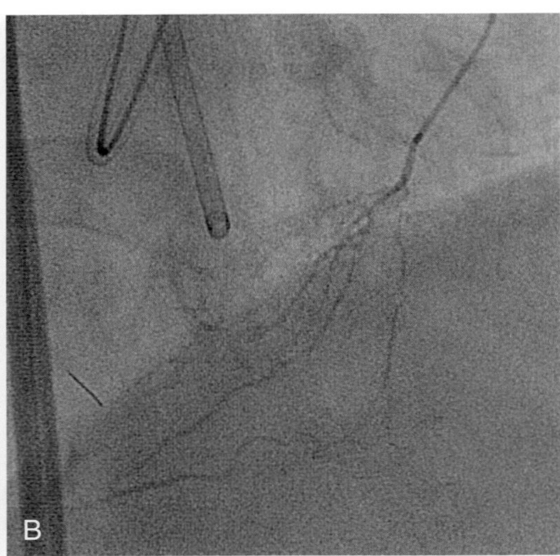

FIGURE 9-2 Coronary collateral circulation to CTOs. Angiographic examples of septal (panels **A** and **B**) and epicardial (panel **C**) collateral circulation. Panel B depicts microcatheter selective contrast injection into a septal collateral to the distal right coronary artery. Collaterals may be graded as grade 0, no continuous connection between donor and recipient artery; grade 1, continuous, thread-like connection; and grade 2, continuous, small, side branch-like size of the collateral throughout its course. *(Reproduced with permission from Surmely JF, Katoh O, Tsuchikane E, et al: Coronary septal collaterals as an access for the retrograde approach in the percutaneous treatment of coronary chronic total occlusions. Catheter Cardiovasc Interv 69:826–832, 2007.)*

Importantly, a common misperception is the unawareness that even well-developed collaterals do not prevent ischemia during exercise.[14] A total occlusion that is well collateralized is functionally equivalent to a 90% stenosis in a non-CTO vessel.[15] When FFR is performed following initial CTO recanalization, the FFR value is persistently ischemic (Pd/Pa < 0.80), and resting ischemia was present in 78% of instances.[16] Ischemia was demonstrated in all CTO cases independent of collateral development or presence of severe regional left ventricular dysfunction. The myocardium remains viable but produces ischemia during periods of increased oxygen demand, and thus patients with these lesions are likely to have exertional angina. Although the risk of a spontaneous acute coronary syndrome due to a chronically occluded lesion is unlikely, infarction in distribution of the CTO may result during instances of increased demand or if the arteries supplying the collaterals become compromised in any way.

Target Vessel

Very little data exist regarding the potential for differential benefit of CTO recanalization depending on the target vessel (e.g., left anterior descending [LAD], left circumflex [LCX], or right coronary artery [RCA]). In a large, single-center registry, PCI for CTO of the LAD, but not LCX or RCA, was associated with improved long-term survival.[17] There were 2608 patients included, and the LAD was the target vessel in 936 (36%), the LCX in 682 (26%), and the RCA in 990 (38%) patients. The angiographic success rates were similar across coronary artery distributions (LAD, 77%; LCX, 76%; RCA, 72%). Procedural success compared with failure was associated with improved 5-year survival in the LAD (88.9% vs. 80.2%, $p < 0.001$) group but not in the LCX (86.1% vs. 82.1%, $p = 0.21$) and RCA (87.7% vs. 84.9%, $p = 0.23$) groups. In multivariable analysis, CTO PCI success in the LAD group remained associated with decreased mortality risk (hazard ratio [HR] 0.61; 95% confidence interval [CI], 0.42 to 0.89). In addition to other clinical characteristics, this information may assist in selecting patients for attempted CTO PCI.

INDICATIONS

In general, when the CTO represents the only significant lesion in the coronary tree, PCI is warranted when the following three conditions are all present: (1) the occluded vessel is responsible for the patient's symptoms of chest pain or heart failure, or the vessel is responsible for a reduced ventricular function (PCI may also be considered in selected cases of silent ischemia if a large myocardial territory at risk is demonstrable); (2) the myocardial territory supplanted by the occluded artery is viable; and (3) the likelihood of success is moderate to high (>60%), with an anticipated major complication rate of death <1% and myocardial infarction <5%.[18] If the PCI attempt is unsuccessful, further management will depend on the symptomatic status and the extent of jeopardized ischemic myocardium. Repeated PCI following initial failure (typically with an allowance of several weeks for vessel healing in the case of dissection) or surgical revascularization may be warranted if a large myocardial territory is ischemic or the patient is very symptomatic. Alternatively, conservative therapy may be appropriate if repeated PCI is unlikely to be successful and the patient's symptoms can be controlled with antianginal medications.

Despite the intuitive benefit of an open artery, the rationale for CTO PCI is mistakenly challenged by a singular trial demonstrating no clinical benefit with revascularization of *subacute* total occlusions following recent myocardial infarction.[19] Differences in the indication and pathophysiology notwithstanding, it is noteworthy that unlike the clinical characteristics of patients included in the Occluded Artery Trial (OAT), CTO patients selected for attempted PCI often represent a very different patient population characterized by features systematically excluded from the OAT trial, including symptoms refractory to medical therapy, abnormal left ventricular function, multivessel coronary disease, and/or extensive ischemia demonstrated by noninvasive testing. Performance of CTO revascularization based on these indications is also in accord with recent multidisciplinary committee recommendations regarding appropriateness of PCI in specific patient and lesion subsets.[20,21]

Recently, consensus recommendations regarding appropriateness of PCI in general have highlighted disparate conclusions related to percutaneous revascularization depending on the stenosis severity.[22] The 2011 American College of Cardiology/American Heart Association PCI guidelines endorse CTO PCI with a class IIA recommendation, citing that PCI of a CTO in patients with appropriate clinical indications and suitable anatomy is reasonable when performed by operators with appropriate expertise.[20] Similarly, the 2010 European Society of Cardiology states that similar to nonchronically occluded vessels, revascularization of a CTO may be considered in the presence of angina or ischemia related to the corresponding territory.[21] In contrast, the 2012 statement on Appropriate Use Criteria for Coronary Revascularization provided a lower level recommendation for CTO PCI compared with patients having one- or two-vessel coronary disease and without a CTO in 10 of 36 clinical scenarios assessed.[22] In particular, for both symptomatic and asymptomatic patients, several instances exist for which PCI may be considered "appropriate" or "uncertain" for a non-CTO lesion but downgraded for the same respective indications to "uncertain" or "inappropriate" for a CTO lesion. Although it is likely that such endorsements are based on both evidence and opinion, the reasons for differing recommendations are not provided. Further, establishing unconditional treatment recommendations regarding CTO revascularization for any individual patient is especially challenging given that the risk/benefit balance may vary considerably depending on the symptoms, the extent of ischemia or left ventricular dysfunction, the presence of multivessel disease, or additional comorbidities that increase procedural risk (e.g., chronic kidney disease). Therefore, for consideration of CTO PCI, the document should be considered a guideline for treatment rather than an absolute standard, and the presence of a CTO should not have an impact on revascularization decision making with the caveat that appropriate expertise in CTO PCI is locally available.

Angina and Quality of Life

Stress-induced ischemia can typically be elicited in patients with a CTO, especially in the absence of a history of prior myocardial infarction and irrespective of collateral development.[23,24] The temporal changes in contractility and hyperemic and resting myocardial blood flow in dependent and remote myocardium after PCI of CTOs have been further characterized using cardiovascular magnetic resonance imaging.[25] Three groups were prospectively studied: 17 patients scheduled for CTO PCI, 17 scheduled for PCI of a stenosed but nonoccluded coronary artery (non-CTO), and 6 patients with CTO who were not scheduled for revascularization. Contractility in treated segments was improved at 24 hours and 6 months after CTO PCI but only at 6 months after non-CTO PCI. In both intervention groups, treated segments no longer had reduced myocardial blood flow or contractility compared with remote segments (**Figure 9-3A**). In patients with nonrevascularized CTO segments and treated with medical therapy alone, myocardial blood flow and wall thickening did not improve at follow-up (**Figure 9-3B**).

The majority of patients undergoing CTO PCI have stable or progressive angina, whereas many asymptomatic patients with CTO and minimal or no ischemia by noninvasive imaging are managed medically. In several large databases, only 10% to 15% of patients undergoing angioplasty for CTO were asymptomatic. Conversely, the proportion of patients presenting with unstable angina due to a CTO is also fairly low and of similar prevalence to asymptomatic patients. Patients with medically refractory angina or a moderate to large ischemic burden deserve consideration for percutaneous revascularization, particularly if the symptoms or territory are enough to warrant surgical revascularization as an option. The presence of moderate or severe ischemia is associated with worse clinical outcomes in patients with CTO.[26] In a study of 301 patients who underwent myocardial perfusion imaging before and after CTO PCI, a baseline ischemic burden of >12.5% identified patients most likely to have a significant decrease in ischemic burden post-CTO PCI, indicating that the highest benefit of CTO revascularization is likely to be achieved in patients with a significant baseline ischemic burden.[27]

In a metaanalysis of six observational studies evaluating angina following CTO PCI, patients undergoing successful revascularization experienced a significant reduction in recurrent angina during a 6-year follow-up compared with patients undergoing unsuccessful PCI (odds ratio [OR], 0.45; 95% CI, 0.30 to 0.67).[28] In the Flowcardia's Approach to Chronic Total Occlusion Recanalization (FACTOR) trial,[29] among patients referred for the CTO PCI (which per protocol required symptoms and/or abnormal stress testing), two thirds of the patients had angina, and one third had no angina. Presence of angina was objectively assessed using the Seattle Angina Questionnaire (SAQ) and defined as angina frequency scores of less than 90. Among those with angina at baseline, the impairment in angina-associated quality of life was significant, and CTO PCI was associated with significant improvement in self-reported angina measures.

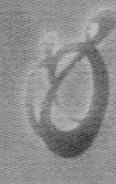

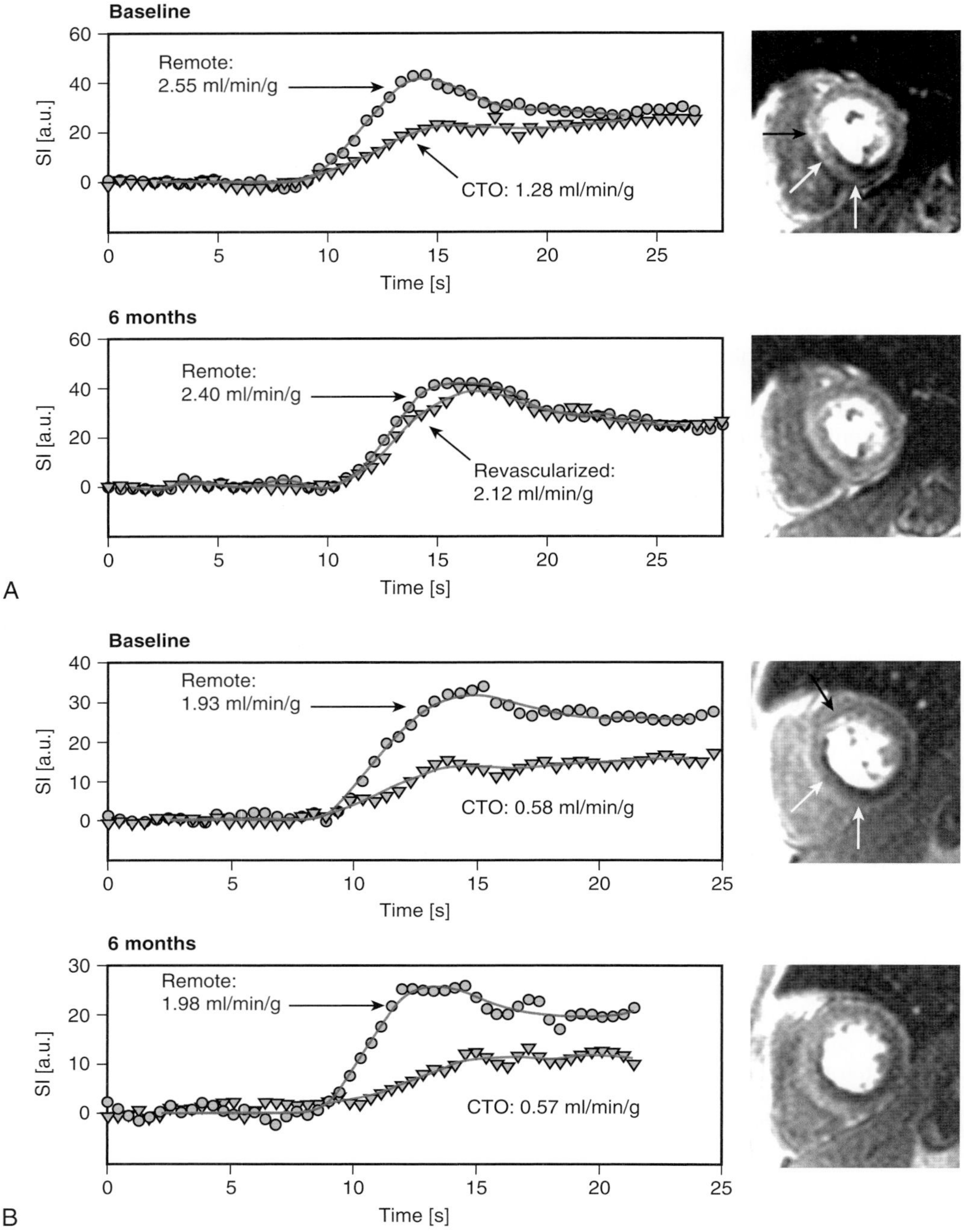

FIGURE 9-3 Impact of CTO revascularization on regional myocardial blood flow. Following CTO PCI, treated segments no longer had reduced myocardial blood flow or impaired contractility compared with remote myocardial regions with no coronary disease (panel **A**). In contrast, among patients with nonrevascularized CTO segments and treated with medical therapy alone, myocardial blood flow and wall thickening did not improve at follow-up (panel **B**). *(Adapted with permission from Cheng AS, Selvanayagam JB, Jerosch-Herold M, et al: Percutaneous treatment of chronic total coronary occlusions improves regional hyperemic myocardial blood flow and contractility: insights from quantitative cardiovascular magnetic resonance imaging. J Am Coll Cardiovasc Interv 1:44–53, 2008.)*

The first assessment of the most common angina equivalent (dyspnea) among patients with CTO was reported by Safley and colleagues.[30] In this study, 98 patients with single-vessel CTO were matched with 687 patients undergoing non-CTO PCI. Baseline and post-PCI SAQ and Rose dyspnea scale scores were compared. Dyspnea was present among both CTO and non-CTO patients as reflected in baseline Rose dyspnea scale scores of 1.9 versus 1.7, $p = 0.21$ (higher scores indicating more dyspnea), in the CTO and non-CTO groups, respectively. Percutaneous CTO revascularization was statistically noninferior to non-CTO PCI in alleviating both dyspnea and angina ($p < 0.02$ for all domains), suggesting that the clinical benefit was of at least a similar magnitude for both CTO and non-CTO PCI.

Improvement in Left Ventricular Dysfunction

Regional left ventricular systolic function has been demonstrated to improve after CTO PCI.[25,31-37] The degree of improvement is especially evident in patients with decreased left ventricular systolic function at baseline, while no change in ejection fraction can be expected when the baseline

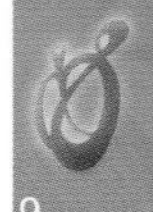

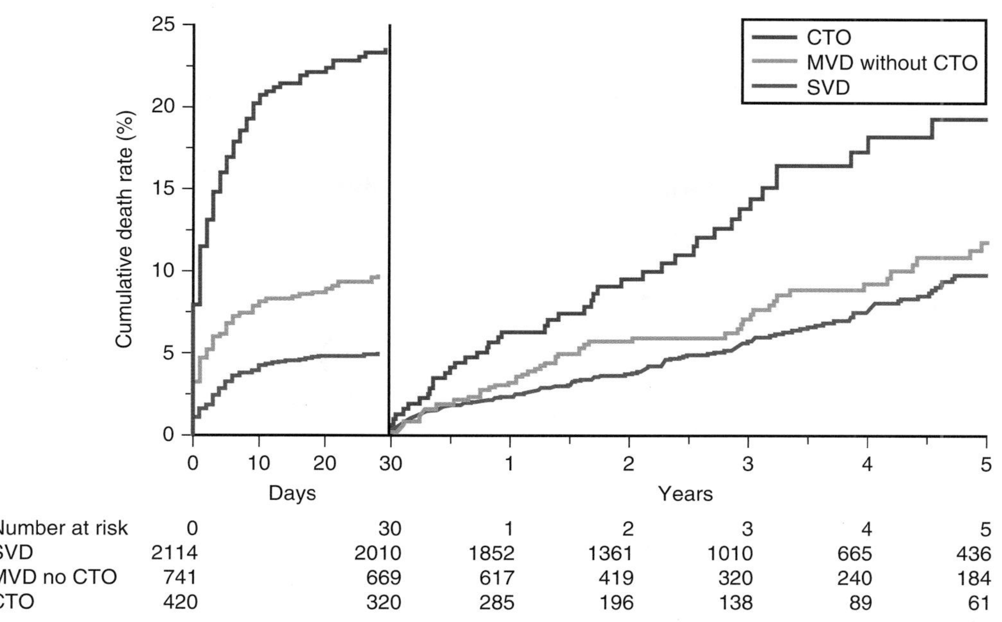

FIGURE 9-4 Impact of CTO on survival following acute myocardial infarction in a non–CTO-related artery. Among patients with ST-segment elevation acute myocardial infarction treated with primary PCI, the presence of a CTO was a stronger and independent predictor for 30-day mortality than the presence of multivessel disease without a CTO.[39] In a landmark analysis from 30 days to 5 years, the presence of a CTO remained an independent predictor of mortality that exceeded the risk associated with single-vessel or multivessel disease without CTO.

function is normal.[25,37] Improvement in left ventricular function is not predicted by a history of myocardial infarction or the duration of occlusion.[37] Further, recovery of impaired ventricular function after revascularization of a CTO is not directly related to the quality of collateral function, as collateral development does not appear to require the presence of viable myocardium.[37] Left ventricular function improvement is dependent on maintenance of CTO target vessel patency and on viability of the perfused myocardial territory.[34-37]

Reduction in Arrhythmic Events

Although no study has documented a reduction in ventricular arrhythmic events with CTO PCI, the contribution of CTOs to either ischemia-driven or scar-related arrhythmic events has been recently characterized. In the Ventricular Arrhythmia Chronic Total Occlusion (VACTO) study, among 162 patients with ischemic cardiomyopathy who received an implantable cardioverter defibrillator, 44% had at least one CTO.[38] During a median follow-up of 26 months, the presence of CTO was associated with higher ventricular arrhythmia and mortality rates compared with patients without a CTO. In particular, the occurrence of appropriate defibrillator therapy was significantly more common in comparison with patients having multivessel disease but without a CTO.

Improved Tolerance of Ischemic Events

A consistent finding among patients presenting with high-risk acute coronary syndromes has been the association of a CTO with adverse short- and late-term outcome. Potential mechanisms include preexisting left ventricular function, poor tolerance of ischemia secondary to limited collateral supply, and a "double jeopardy" phenomenon associated with simultaneous acute and chronic coronary occlusion in separate coronary artery territories.

Among 3277 patients with ST-segment elevation acute myocardial infarction treated with primary PCI, the presence of a CTO was a stronger and independent predictor for 30-day mortality (HR 3.6; 95% CI, 2.6 to 4.7; $p < 0.01$) than the presence of multivessel disease without a CTO (HR 1.6; 95% CI, 1.2 to 2.2; $p = 0.01$) (**Figure 9-4**).[39] Only presentation of shock was a greater predictor of mortality than presence of a CTO. In a landmark analysis that included surviving patients from 30 days to 5 years, the presence of a CTO remained an independent predictor of mortality that exceeded the risk associated with single-vessel or multivessel disease without CTO (**Figure 9-4**).

Similarly, in 3283 patients participating in the Harmonizing Outcomes with Revascularization and Stents in Acute Myocardial Infarction (HORIZONS-AMI) study, a CTO in a non–infarct-related artery was identified in 8.6% of patients.[40] As with the prior study, CTO in a non–infarct-related artery was an independent predictor of both 30-day mortality (HR 2.88; 95% CI, 1.41 to 5.88, $p = 0.004$) and day 30 to 3-year mortality (HR 1.98; 95% CI, 1.19 to 3.29; $p = 0.009$). In comparison, multivessel disease without a CTO was associated with higher 30-day mortality (HR 2.20; 95% CI, 1.00 to 3.06; $p = 0.049$) but not late (day 30 to 3 years) mortality. Finally, the Thrombus Aspiration in Percutaneous Coronary Intervention in Acute Myocardial Infarction (TAPAS) trial also reported a higher mortality risk among CTO patients presenting with acute myocardial infarction (8% of 1071 total); over a median follow-up period of 2.1 years, mortality was twofold greater for CTO compared with non-CTO patients (HR 2.41; 95% CI, 1.26 to 4.61; $p = 0.008$).[41]

Despite the consistent association of CTOs with higher risk following presentation with an acute coronary syndrome, limited evidence exists to support a routine strategy of attempted CTO revascularization following myocardial infarction related to a non-CTO target vessel. One small retrospective study demonstrated improved outcomes for patients who underwent successful versus failed CTO PCI after primary PCI for ST-segment elevation acute myocardial infarction.[42] The ongoing EXPLORE (Evaluating Xience V and Left Ventricular Function in Percutaneous Coronary Intervention on Occlusions After ST-Elevation Myocardial Infarction) trial is examining whether PCI of a CTO in a non–infarct-related artery within 1 week after primary PCI can improve left ventricular dimensions and function.[43]

Survival and Completeness of Revascularization

There are no published randomized controlled trials comparing CTO PCI with medical therapy or with surgical revascularization, although comparative study is ongoing (**www.clinicaltrials.gov**, identifiers NCT01760083 and NCT01078051). Nevertheless, several issues related to CTO revascularization challenge the conduct of a randomized trial, for example, variability in operator experience, selection and treatment biases, and management of patient crossover and intention to treat. Moreover, although all-cause mortality has been proposed as a singular trial endpoint,[44] the appropriateness of requiring CTO revascularization to achieve a different standard than non-CTO PCI is debated.

Nevertheless, several observational studies have compared late-term survival among patients undergoing successful versus failed CTO PCI.[45-50] Despite limitations in study design, a remarkable consistency across such studies is the association of improved survival with successful CTO revascularization. For example, in a single-center observational study of 6996 patients undergoing elective PCI, 836 (11.9%) CTO procedures were attempted, of which 69.6% were successful.[50] Baseline characteristics were similar between cohorts except for a higher frequency of prior revascularization in failed CTO PCI cases. Intraprocedural complications were also more common in unsuccessful cases but did not influence in-hospital major adverse cardiac events. Through 5 years, all-cause mortality was 17.2% for unsuccessful CTO patients and 4.5% for successful CTO patients ($p < 0.0001$; **Figure 9-5A**). Also, the need for coronary bypass surgery was reduced following successful CTO PCI (3.1% versus 22.1%; $p < 0.0001$; **Figure 9-5B**). Multivariate analysis demonstrated that procedural success was independently predictive of reduced mortality (HR 0.32; 95% CI, 0.18 to 0.58), which persisted following propensity score adjustment (HR 0.28; 95% CI, 0.15 to 0.52). In a metaanalysis of 13 observational studies, mortality over a weighted average follow-up of 6 years was 14.3% among 5056 patients with successful CTO recanalization compared with 17.5% among 2232 patients with failed CTO recanalization (OR 0.56; 95% CI, 0.43 to 0.72).[28]

Whether following bypass surgery or PCI, incomplete coronary revascularization has been associated with worse clinical outcomes compared to complete revascularization, and the presence of a CTO is one of the major reasons for incomplete revascularization.[51,52] While such observations are suggestive but do not establish that CTO revascularization improves patient outcome, it is notable that as angiographic disease complexity increases, completeness of revascularization measured by the residual SYNTAX score paradoxically decreases.[52] Among patients with multivessel coronary disease including a CTO, complete revascularization (i.e., that included successful CTO PCI) was associated with improved cardiovascular survival compared with incomplete revascularization.[48] Recently, the impact of CTOs on incomplete revascularization and its clinical implications were described from the SYNTAX trial.[53] In this study, the prevalence of a CTO was 26.3% and 36.4% in the PCI and bypass surgery groups, respectively. Nearly 70% of all CTOs were localized to the proximal or midsegment of a major coronary artery, indicating at least moderate territory at ischemic risk, and the CTO PCI success rate was low in this trial (49.4%). The presence of a CTO was the most significant predictor of incomplete revascularization after PCI (HR 2.70; 95% CI, 1.98 to 3.67; $p < 0.001$). At 4-year follow-up, incomplete revascularization was associated with significantly higher mortality and major adverse cardiac and cerebrovascular events independent of treatment assignment to PCI or bypass surgery.

PROCEDURAL OUTCOMES AND FUNDAMENTALS

In parallel with outcomes data indicating benefit following CTO revascularization and the successes of drug-eluting stents (DES) in maintaining target-vessel patency is the stark reality that any potential advantage of CTO PCI is handicapped from the outset by the commonality of procedural failure. The technical and procedural success rates of PCI in CTOs have steadily increased over the last 20 years because of greater operator experience and improvements in equipment and procedural techniques. Despite this observation, CTOs remain the lesion subtype in which angioplasty is most likely to fail, and until recently, both attempt and procedural success rates remained relatively stagnant.[54] In recent contemporary series, procedural success rates have ranged from approximately 50% to more than 80%, with the variability reflecting differences in operator technique and experience, availability of advanced guidewires, CTO definition, and case selection. The most common PCI failure mode for CTOs is inability to successfully pass a guidewire across the lesion into the true lumen of the distal vessel.

Predictors of Procedural Outcome

Most historical studies have consistently reported that increasing age of the occlusion, greater lesion length, presence of a nontapered proximal stump, origin of a side branch at the occlusion site, excessive vessel and lesion tortuosity, calcification, ostial occlusion, and lack of visibility of the distal vessel course negatively affect the ability to successfully cross a CTO.[55] However, performance of advanced methods, with newer guidewire developments, has in many instances overcome the historical predictors associated with CTO procedural failure (e.g., CTO length, calcification, side branch involvement). In a more contemporary series, selected clinical and angiographic variables have been incorporated into a model to predict procedural time and success rates. Specifically, the multicenter Japanese CTO (J-CTO) registry surveyed approximately 500 CTO PCI attempts, identifying five independent predictors of crossing time within 30 minutes and overall procedural success[56]: (1) calcification, (2) bending >45° in the CTO segment, (3) a blunt proximal cap, (4) the length of the occluded segment >20 mm, and (5) a previously failed attempt. A scoring model was developed applying 1 point for each of these independent variables when present. The CTO case complexity was further stratified into easy (J-CTO score = 0), intermediate (score = 1), difficult (score = 2), and

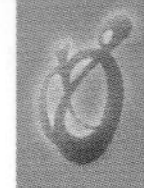

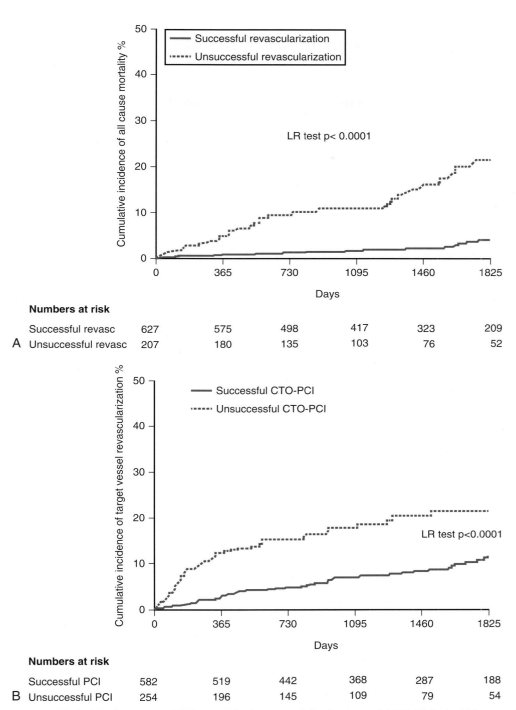

Successful revascularization
Unsuccessful revascularization
Cumulative incidence of all cause mortality %
LR test p< 0.0001
Days

Numbers at risk

	0	365	730	1095	1460	1825
Successful revasc	627	575	498	417	323	209
A Unsuccessful revasc	207	180	135	103	76	52

Successful CTO-PCI
Unsuccessful CTO-PCI
Cumulative incidence of target vessel revascularization %
LR test p<0.0001
Days

Numbers at risk

	0	365	730	1095	1460	1825
Successful PCI	582	519	442	368	287	188
B Unsuccessful PCI	254	196	145	109	79	54

FIGURE 9-5 Long-term survival and need for repeat revascularization following successful and unsuccessful CTO PCI. Kaplan Meier curves demonstrating cumulative probability of late-term survival (panel **A**) and need for target vessel revascularization following successful and unsuccessful CTO PCI (panel **B**). *(Reproduced with permission from Jones DA, Weerackody R, Rathod K, et al: Successful recanalization of chronic total occlusions is associated with improved long-term survival. J Am Coll Cardiol Interv 5:380–388, 2012.)*

very difficult (score = 3-5). However, more advanced techniques including retrograde and hybrid strategies were underrepresented in the J-CTO registry. In a more recent evaluation to externally validate the J-CTO model that included such methods, a single-center study reported that the J-CTO score demonstrated excellent discrimination for predicting crossing time within 30 minutes;[57] however, using a hybrid antegrade and retrograde approach and dissection reentry techniques, the overall angiographic recanalization success rate was not affected by the score.

Vascular Access, Equipment Selection, and Angiography

Decisions regarding femoral or radial vascular access are generally, according to operator's preference notwithstanding, patient-specific factors that may mandate one or the other method. In general, the relative merits of accommodating larger and possibly more supportive guiding catheters with femoral access can be weighed against the reduction in vascular complications and improved patient comfort with a radial approach. Importantly, among experienced radial CTO operators, procedural success rates applying complex antegrade and retrograde techniques have been demonstrated similar to other contemporary studies employing more traditional femoral access.[58] A guiding principle of vascular access is that operators should utilize access routes that support their typical and optimal technique.

In part based on the vascular access method, selection of the guiding catheter size is commonly limited to 6 Fr (or occasionally sheathless 7 Fr) from the radial approach, compared with 6 Fr to 8 Fr caliber sheaths and guides used in transfemoral CTO PCI. When femoral access is selected, the use of long (45 cm) sheaths is recommended for increased passive support. Guide catheter support and coaxial alignment are essential from the outset, and it is therefore important to avoid accepting satisfactory backup rather than achieving optimal support prior to guidewire engagement in the CTO. In addition, CTO operators should be familiar with adjunctive catheter support methods including balloon anchoring and mother-and-child techniques.

A fundamental of successful CTO PCI is the expert ability to perform diagnostic angiography and its interpretation. Only in rare, selected instances is the performance of contralateral angiography not indicated prior to attempted CTO revascularization. Even in instances in which only ipsilateral collateral supply exists, impaired antegrade flow following the creation of dissections and shearing of vascular tissue planes may result in a preferential collateral shift to retrograde channels otherwise initially inapparent. The performance of the diagnostic angiogram is an opportunity for the CTO operator to delineate collateral supply, identify the proximal and distal CTO cap, and troubleshoot challenges to successful recanalization prior to attempted revascularization. Ad hoc CTO PCI is strongly discouraged; instead, the diagnostic angiogram provides imaging in multiple views and oftentimes with simultaneous contralateral angiography to fully evaluate the coronary anatomy without expenditure of contrast and radiation exposure during the CTO procedure itself.

Guidewires and Microcatheters

Crossing the CTO with a guidewire is the most important and challenging step of the procedure, and it is the most frequent cause for failed PCI of a CTO. There are three separate steps to crossing a CTO: (1) penetrating the proximal fibrous cap, (2) traversing the body of the CTO to reach the distal fibrous cap, and (3) penetrating the distal fibrous cap. Wires designed particularly for treating CTOs can be broadly divided into two major groups: (1) polymer-coated (hydrophilic or lubricious) guidewires and (2) stiffer, nonpolymer (nonhydrophilic, hydrophobic, or nonlubricious) guidewires. The stiffer, nonhydrophilic guidewires are typically more controllable, provide better tactile feel, and are less likely to cause vessel dissection. Hydrophilic wires offer maneuverability in tortuous vessels and may be steered more easily in a true lumen immediately after sharp bends. On the other hand, they are more likely to penetrate beneath plaque and cause subintimal dissections than noncoated wires. Several dedicated CTO guidewires are also designed with a tapered (e.g., 0.009 to 0.010 inch) tip to permit engagement in microchannels and facilitate crossing. Once a specialized CTO guidewire has crossed the occlusion and passed into the distal lumen, the wire should be exchanged with a soft, floppy-tipped wire to minimize the risk of distal wire perforation or dissection.

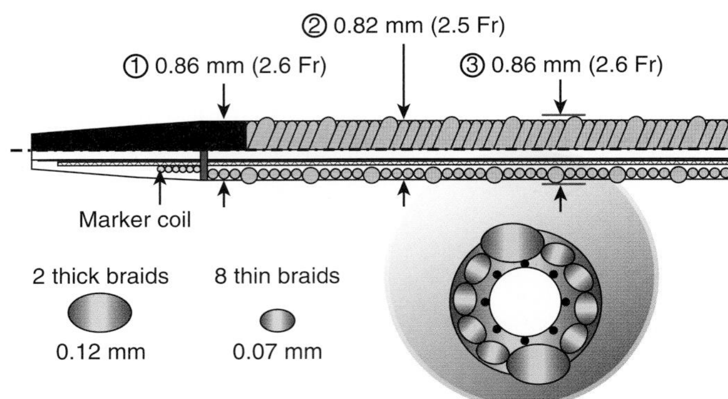

FIGURE 9-6 The Corsair channel dilator catheter. The Corsair catheter, also known as a channel dilator catheter, is most commonly used in retrograde CTO PCI given its ability to navigate through very angulated and small-caliber collateral channels.

A microcatheter or an over-the-wire low-profile (e.g., 1.2 or 1.25 mm) balloon catheter can be used for support as well as access for ease of exchanging wires. A balloon catheter also offers the option of treatment with dilation of the vessel as well as added support by using it as an anchor. Several devices are available to create a larger lumen when a balloon catheter is unable to cross expand the lesion. These include the braided stainless steal Tornus catheter (Asahi Intecc, Inc., Nagoya, Japan) and the Corsair catheter (Asahi Intecc, Inc.). The Corsair catheter (**Figure 9-6**), also known as a channel dilator catheter, is most commonly used in retrograde CTO PCI given its ability to navigate through very angulated and small-caliber collateral channels.

Procedural Antithrombotic Therapy

Unfractionated heparin is the preferred antithrombin therapy during a CTO PCI procedure. In the rare instance of hemodynamically significant perforation, the drug can be reversed with protamine. Although case series using bivalirudin have been reported in CTO PCI,[59] anecdotal reports of donor vessel thrombosis during retrograde PCI and the inability of immediate reversal of the anticoagulant effect have discouraged the use of direct thrombin inhibitors and low molecular weight heparins. Compared with alternative antithrombin therapy, unfractionated heparin is also advantageous given that it permits a more precise assessment and titration of the antithrombin effect during the procedure. For antegrade and retrograde CTO procedures, an activated clotting time of >300 and >350 seconds, respectively, is recommended. In the case of retrograde CTO PCI, more intensive anticoagulation is required to prevent donor vessel and collateral thrombosis, especially considering the longer dwell time of the equipment in the artery. Frequent (e.g., at least every 30 minutes) measurement of the activated clotting time is advocated.

Similar to non-CTO PCI, preprocedural administration of aspirin and thienopyridine therapy is recommended; in particular, attempted CTO PCI should not be avoided in instances of prior treatment with aspirin and thienopyridine therapy. Excepting rare instances of coronary thrombosis refractory to therapeutic antithrombin therapy, treatment with glycoprotein IIb/IIIa inhibition is rarely indicated.

Technical Strategies

Apart from a variety of novel but ultimately disappointing technologies for crossing occluded coronary segments,[60-62] specialized coronary guidewires remain the mainstay instruments in the CTO toolbox.[63] In parallel with considerable advancements in CTO-specific guidewire technology, a more revolutionary advancement relates to the technical skills and strategies regarding how these tools are used. In particular, the performance of sophisticated antegrade and retrograde guidewire manipulations in addition to dissection reentry methods[64-67] have informed procedural technique and contributed to improved clinical outcome.

Traditional Antegrade Techniques

The antegrade approach is the most common initial strategy for attempting to recanalize a CTO. Starting equipment can vary depending on lesion characteristics and anatomy. A support catheter (over-the-wire balloon or microcatheter) with either a stiff, nonhydrophillic guidewire or a tapered/nontapered hydrophilic wire is used to drill and probe the lesion initially. If the proximal cap cannot be penetrated or the wire is unable to be advanced within the lesion, progressively stiffer wires can be used. Wire shaping for the antegrade approach of CTOs is markedly different than for nonocclusive disease. In general, the initial wire should have a bend with an angle <30° approximately 1 mm from the tip. If more angulated bends are required to access the CTO, this should be done with a soft, floppy wire and then exchanged for a CTO wire to avoid proximal vessel trauma associated with free passage of the CTO wire.

Two specialized techniques for recanalization of CTOs with an antegrade approach have evolved from failure after initial wire entry in the lesion. The parallel wire technique is an increasingly less common method to approach CTO PCI with the advent of dissection reentry technology but remains a traditional method for luminal reentry. Occasionally a guidewire may exit the true lumen of the occluded vessel and enter a subintimal dissection plane. In this instance, the wire is left in place as a visual landmark, to avoid further vessel trauma and to obstruct entry into the false lumen. A second wire (stiff or hydrophilic, depending on the lesion) is advanced to the point of the first wire's exit and then redirected toward the true lumen. An alternative method is the subintimal tracking and reentry (STAR) technique.[68] This is a method of intentional subintimal dissection using a hydrophilic wire typically shaped with a prolapsed tip. The wire is advanced beyond the occlusion adjacent to the distal lumen. The looped "knuckle wire" follows the subintimal path to a point where the dissection can no longer be propagated and may spontaneously reenter the true lumen in the main vessel or more commonly in side branches. Ultimately, an extensive dissection is created that needs to be treated with several stents or alternatively with angioplasty alone to permit more rapid vessel healing followed by more selective stent placement weeks later. This method can result in pruning and occlusion of side branches and should be reserved as a bailout technique for highly symptomatic patients refractory to medical therapy.

Antegrade Device-Assisted Dissection Reentry Technique

The primary mode of failure to recanalize a chronically occluded vessel is entrapment of the guidewire within the subintimal space and inability to access the distal true lumen. Recent technological developments have enabled more predictable lumen reentry, reduced the need for retrograde bailout methods, and increased procedural success. The system consists of the Crossboss support catheter, Stingray balloon, and Stingray reentry guidewire (Bridgepoint Medical/Boston Scientific, Plymouth, Minnesota) (**Figure 9-7**).[69] The Crossboss catheter is a metal-braided, over-the-wire support catheter with a 1 mm rounded distal tip that can support standard guidewire manipulation or can be advanced using rapid rotation with or without the wire leading. Without the wire leading, this catheter may cross independently into the distal true lumen or enter the subintimal space, permitting setup of the Stingray system (below).

If the Crossboss catheter or a guidewire remains trapped in the subintimal space but distal to the occluded segment, further advancement is not indicated given the creation of a larger dissection and hematoma formation that will compress the distal lumen. Instead, coronary reentry can be systematically achieved with the Stingray system. The Stingray balloon is a 1 mm thick, over-the-wire balloon catheter with three exit ports (one distal and two 180-degree diametrically opposed sideports; **Figure 9-7**). When the balloon is inflated, it contours the artery with one exit port always directed to the adventitia and one always directed toward the lumen. Using fluoroscopy, the operator can select the lumen port with the dedicated Stingray reentry wire, pierce the thin intimal tissue, and gain entry to the distal lumen. Importantly, this method should not be equated to guidewire-based methods of dissection (e.g., STAR) given that targeted reentry intends to limit the extent of dissection and preserve side branches.

Retrograde Techniques: CART and Reverse CART

More advanced techniques for difficult CTOs include the retrograde approach as well as the controlled antegrade and retrograde subintimal tracking (CART) and reverse CART methods[64-67,70] (**Figure 9-8**). In 2006, Katoh and colleagues pioneered the modern era of retrograde CTO recanalization.[71] The novelties introduced in this procedure were targeted septal or epicardial collateral crossing, retrograde lesion crossing, and management of the subintimal space by using balloon dilation to connect antegrade and retrograde channels. Currently, retrograde procedures account for 15% to 35% of all CTO PCI procedures in CTO registries.[72,73] All of these methods require access into the distal CTO vessel from a septal or epicardial collateral (or occasionally bypass graft) vessel with successful placement of a support catheter. Because the collaterals often originate from the contralateral coronary artery, dual arterial catheter access is required, and shortened guiding catheters (85 to 90 cm) are essential (at least for the retrograde "donor" catheter) to enable appropriate working length. Selective angiograms of the collaterals are required to define the location, size, and tortuosity of the vessels. Once localized, the collateral can be crossed with a soft, nontraumatic wire (Sion, Fielder [Asahi-Intecc, Inc.] or Pilot 50 [Abbott Vascular, Santa Clara, California]) and Corsair microcatheter.

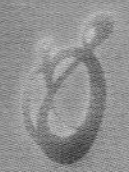

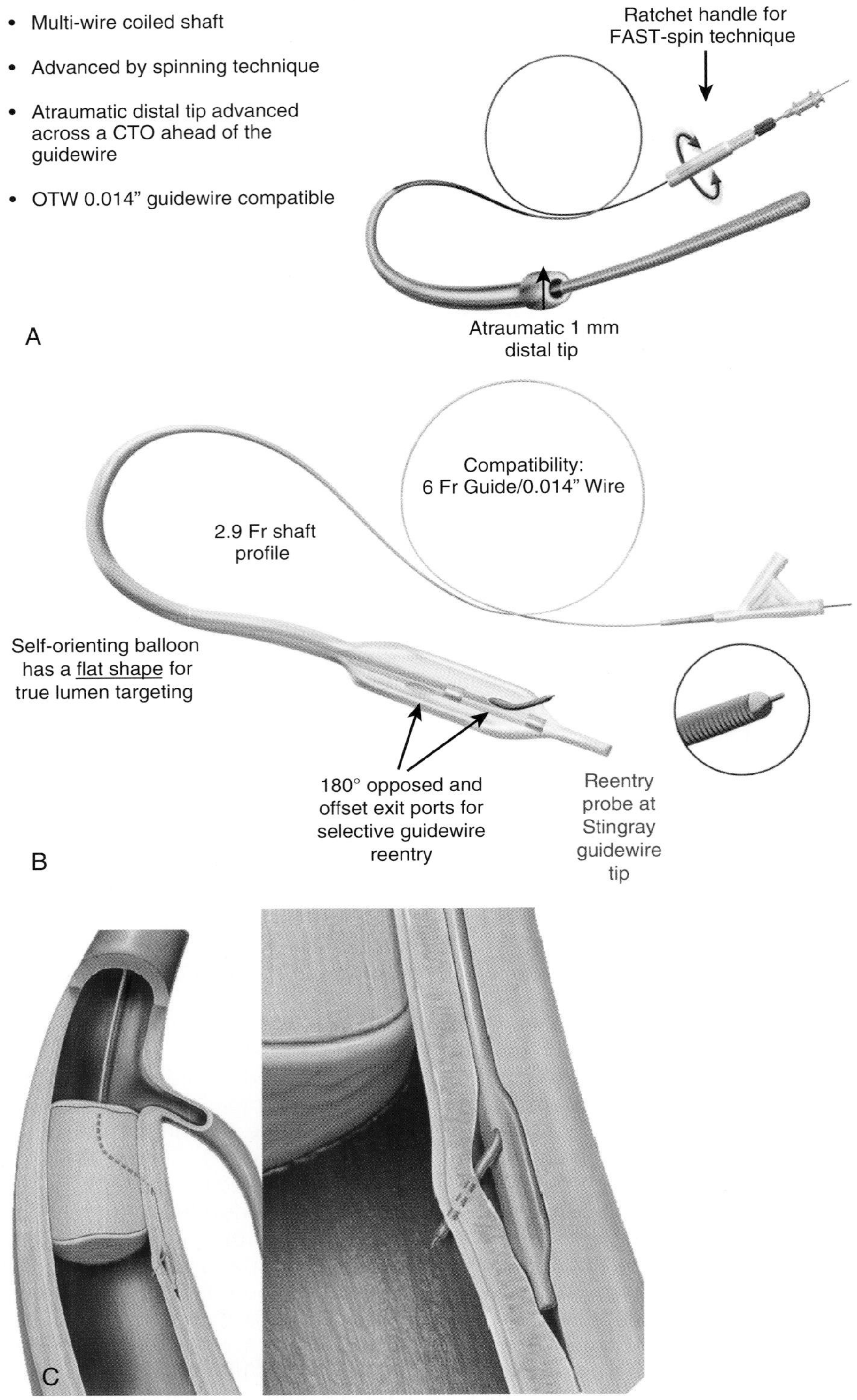

FIGURE 9-7 Stingray balloon and Stingray reentry guidewire. The Crossboss catheter (panel **A**) is a metal-braided, over-the-wire support catheter with a 1 mm rounded distal tip that can support standard guidewire manipulation or can be advanced using rapid rotation with or without the wire leading. The Stingray balloon (panel **B**) is an over-the-wire balloon catheter with three exit ports (one distal and two 180-degree diametrically opposed sideports). When the balloon is inflated, it contours the artery with one exit port always directed to the adventitia (panel **C**) and one always directed toward the lumen, permitting advancement of a specialized guidewire to enter into the true lumen space.

Occasionally, direct luminal crossing is achieved with the retrograde wire. Intravascular ultrasound from the proximal portion of the CTO may also assist in guiding the wire into the true lumen. In cases of direct luminal crossing, a specialized long (325 cm) retrograde guidewire may be externalized through the antegrade guiding catheter followed by antegrade PCI over the externalized guidewire.

Primary retrograde crossing is successful in <70% of attempts without additional controlled dissection and/or antegrade wire techniques.[73,74] When primary retrograde crossing failure occurs, variations on the retrograde approach include controlled dissection techniques termed CART and reverse CART. When antegrade and retrograde guidewires are used to cross a CTO, the guidewires typically

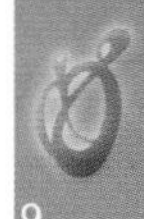

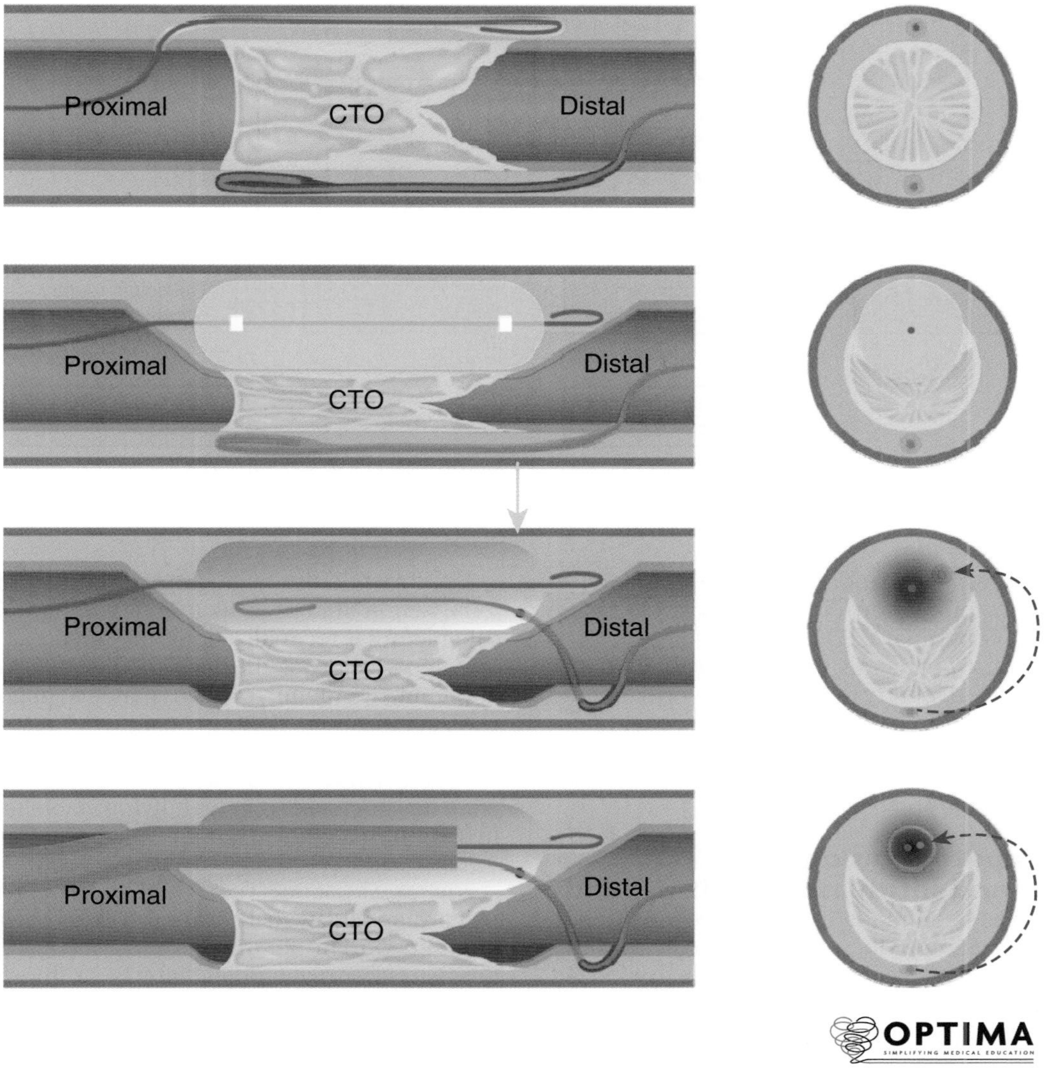

FIGURE 9-8 Reverse CART method. The reverse CART method is the most commonly used technique for retrograde dissection reentry. An angioplasty balloon catheter is advanced over the antegrade wire and then advanced to the reentry zone. The balloon is inflated to create a larger subintimal space, and the retrograde wire is then used to advance into this space, thereby establishing a connection between the anterograde and retrograde spaces. The retrograde microcatheter is then advanced into the antegrade guide catheter, and the procedure is completed in an antegrade fashion over the externalized wire. *(Images courtesy Dr. James Spratt/Optima Education.)*

will reside with four locations relative to one another: (1) antegrade intraplaque/retrograde intraplaque, (2) antegrade intraplaque/retrograde false lumen, (3) antegrade false lumen/retrograde intraplaque, and (4) antegrade false lumen/retrograde false lumen. The reverse CART method is more commonly used as it avoids delivery of balloon catheters through collateral channels. With reverse CART, a balloon is inflated in the proximal segment of the CTO over the antegrade wire that is located in the false lumen. A retrograde guidewire is introduced past the distal cap of the CTO and into the subintimal space. When the antegrade balloon is inflated, expanding the subintimal space, intentional dissection that leads proximally to the true lumen is created. The retrograde wire is then directed toward the antegrade balloon, and once the retrograde wire enters the space occupied by the balloon, it may then be advanced proximally into the true lumen parallel to the path taken by the antegrade guidewire and balloon. Intravascular ultrasound (IVUS) to identify the relationships of the guidewires and to facilitate luminal entry is more conveniently utilized in reverse CART.[74] The CART is the same concept, although the roles are reversed; specifically, a balloon is inflated in the distal portion of the CTO on the retrograde wire, and the antegrade wire is advanced into the subintimal space. They require dedicated equipment and unique skills learned from extensive training, separate from most other interventional procedures.

Hybrid Technique

Not all CTO procedures are successful. Using the retrograde technique, still only approximately 75% of collateral channels may be traversed with a guidewire,[73] and failure to do so is expectedly the greatest determinant of failure. Moreover, antegrade methods remain the most common methods of CTO revascularization. Therefore, to become a proficient CTO operator, the clinician must develop skill sets for both antegrade and retrograde methods. To this purpose, the hybrid method was proposed to explore sequential options through an algorithm-based approach to shorten procedure time, minimize contrast and radiation use, and improve procedural success (**Figure 9-9**).[75] In particular, the hybrid method limits variability among operators regarding

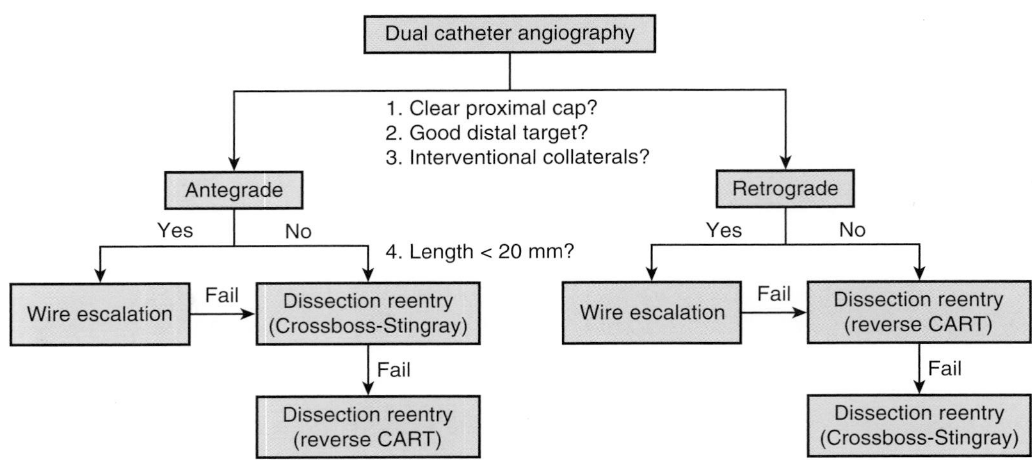

FIGURE 9-9 Hybrid strategy for CTO PCI. The hybrid strategy incorporates antegrade, retrograde, and dissection/reentry techniques into an algorithm based on angiographic characteristics of the CTO.

technique and strategy by standardizing the approach to CTO PCI based on four lesion characteristics: (1) lesion length >20 mm, (2) proximal CTO cap ambiguity, (3) presence of interventional collaterals, and (4) suitability of the distal vessel for targeted reentry. Recently, the hybrid method has been demonstrated to achieve CTO PCI success rates that exceed 90% overall and may be associated with higher success than more traditional methods in more complex (e.g., J-CTO score ≥ 3) lesions.[76]

Imaging: Computed Tomographic Angiography and Intravascular Ultrasound

Once a decision has been made to attempt recanalization of a CTO, characterization of the plaque (i.e., calcification) and visualization of the distal vessel must be optimized. This can usually be done with invasive angiography utilizing contralateral injection of contrast into the artery supplying collaterals the distal vessel. However, if there is doubt regarding the location of vessel anatomy, especially within the occluded segment, a computed tomographic (CT) angiogram with three-dimensional reconstruction can be very helpful. Futhermore, when indicated, a CT angiogram may improve patient selection for CTO recanalization, decrease the time and contrast needed for the procedure, decrease complications, and ultimately improve outcomes.[77] Recent developments with coregistration algorithms that integrate the three-dimensional CT and two-dimensional fluoroscopy images may also facilitate the CTO procedural success by identifying the best angiographic projection and providing a directional guide through the occluded segment not visible by conventional fluoroscopy.[78]

IVUS has become a routine imaging modality in interventional cardiology and can be very useful in the evaluation and treatment of CTOs (see Chapter 16). Using an antegrade approach to the lesion, IVUS can be used to (1) identify the proximal cap location using the IVUS catheter in the side branch, (2) confirm the wire penetration into the proximal cap, (3) redirect the wire into the true lumen after penetrating the subintimal space, and (4) optimize stent placement, expansion, and apposition. When performing a retrograde approach, IVUS can be used to help guide the retrograde wire into the proximal lumen of the CTO.[74]

Finally, while the angiographic results of intended revascularization are unmistakable (i.e., either failed or successful epicardial recanalization), the effects of total occlusion and reperfusion at the level of the myocardium are less apparent. To identify which patients might benefit from revascularization, contrast magnetic resonance imaging (MRI) may be useful for the identification of viable and ischemic myocardium subtended by a CTO. Clinical experience has been useful in identifying viable myocardial tissue in spite of matched, regional wall motion abnormalities by other imaging methods.[79] Among 44 patients with 58 CTO segments, 37 patients (64%) had ≤50% transmural infarction by cardiac MRI, with 12 patients (21%) having no evidence of infarction. Further, the presence of collateral flow did not predict either myocardial viability or improvement following revascularization. Territories without extensive infarction at baseline demonstrated significant regional wall motion improvement following revascularization, and more recent evaluations with an adenosine stress MRI following percutaneous revascularization have demonstrated a resolution of ischemia.[25]

STENT SELECTION FOR CTO REVASCULARIZATION

Clinical Rationale for Drug-Eluting Stents in Percutaneous Revascularization of Coronary Occlusions

The appeal of DES to improve long-term vessel patency following CTO recanalization is related not only to the successes of DES in other complex lesion morphologies but also to the clinical inadequacies of bare-metal stents to sustain restenosis-free patency in this particular lesion subset. As an example, in the Total Occlusion Study of Canada 1 (TOSCA-1) trial, 6-month rates of restenosis and reocclusion following bare-metal stent revascularization exceeded 50% and 10%, respectively (**Table 9-1**).[80]

Altogether, failure to achieve or sustain patency after CTO recanalization has been associated with impairment in regional and global left ventricular systolic function, recurrent angina and target vessel revascularization, and a greater need for late bypass surgery. At 3-year follow-up in the TOSCA-1 trial, reocclusion was associated with higher

TABLE 9-1 Evolution of Stent Trials in CTO Revascularization: Timeline of Stent Trials in CTO PCI Highlight Advancement of DES in Reducing Rates of Angiographic Restenosis, Repeat Revascularization, and Reocclusion

ERA	TRIALS	COMPARISON	REOCCLUSION %, RR	RESTENOSIS %, RR	REPEAT REVASCULARIZATION %, RR
1996-1999	GISSOC, TOSCA, STOP, SPACTO, SICCO	PTCA vs. BMS, Randomized	22 vs. 9, ↓59%	67 vs. 37, ↓45%	35 vs. 19, ↓46%
2003-2009	ACROSS, ASIAN, RESEARCH, etc.	DES, Observational	2	8	8
2006	PRISON II, GISSOC II	BMS vs. DES, Randomized	15 vs. 2, ↓87%	52 vs. 9, ↓83%	33 vs. 7, ↓79%
2005-2007	ASIAN, RESEARCH, etc.	PES vs. SES, Observational	—	18 vs. 7, ↓61%	6 vs. 4, ↓33%
2010	Meta-analyses	BMS vs. DES	10 vs. 5, ↓50%	37 vs. 10, ↓73%	30 vs. 5, ↓83%
2011	PRISON III, CIBELES	SES vs. ZES/EES, Randomized	3.2 SES vs. 1 EES	10.5 SES vs. 9.1 EES	11.6 SES vs. 7.9 EES
2011	EXPERT CTO, ACE CTO, Florence Registry	EES, Observational	—	Florence 3.0%, ACE CTO 45%	Florence 10.5% (MACE)

mortality and a significant increase in the need for repeat revascularization. Therefore, the implications of improving long-term restenosis-free patency in coronary occlusions have potentially significant clinical impact.

Contemporary DES Trials in CTO Revascularization

In the randomized Primary Stenting of Totally Occluded Native Coronary Arteries (PRISON) II trial (N = 200), treatment with sirolimus-eluting stents (SES) was associated with statistically significant reductions in 6-month angiographic restenosis (in-stent, 36% versus 7%, $p < 0.0001$), reocclusion (13% versus 4%, $p < 0.04$), and 1-year repeat revascularization (21% versus 5%, $p < 0.0001$).[81] At 5 years, the benefit of SES was sustained, demonstrating significant reductions in target lesion revascularization (TLR, 30% versus 12%, $p = 0.001$) and major adverse cardiac events despite numerically higher definite or probable stent thrombosis (ST).[82] Similar clinical and angiographic benefit with first-generation DES has been supported in nonrandomized studies (**Table 9-1**).[83-87] Among 200 CTO patients treated with SES in the prospective Approaches to Chronic Occlusions With Sirolimus-Eluting Stents/Total Occlusion Study of Coronary Arteries-4 (ACROSS/TOSCA-4) trial, the 3-year rate of TLR and ST remained favorable at 10.9% and 1.0%, respectively, with no occurrences of ST beyond 1 year.

Increasing clinical trial experience with DES in CTO revascularization has also permitted metaanalysis of angiographic and clinical outcomes.[88,89] Among 17 studies evaluating SES and/or paclitaxel-eluting stents (PES) against bare-metal stents in CTO revascularization, treatment with DES was associated with a significant reduction in angiographic restenosis (OR 0.15, 95% CI, 0.08 to 0.26) and repeat revascularization (OR 0.13, 95% CI, 0.06 to 0.26) with similar long-term incidence of death, myocardial infarction, or ST.[89]

While these findings further support the safety and efficacy of DES in following CTO recanalization, they also have implications regarding procedural technique. For example, given that restenosis in the entire treated segment after recanalization occurs nearly twice as common beyond the stent margins than in-stent, DES treatment of the entire segment exposed to predilatation angioplasty may yield further reductions in restenosis and subsequent TLR than balloon angioplasty alone or in combination with bare-metal stents.[80,90] Nevertheless, considering that percutaneous revascularization of CTOs is routinely associated with more extensive stent placement, whether the improvement in restenosis is offset by a potentially higher risk of thrombotic occlusion or complications associated with stent fracture or acquired late malapposition is uncertain.[80]

Whether disparities in angiographic and clinical outcome emerge in more complex lesion morphologies is an issue of ongoing study and is especially relevant to coronary total occlusions. At least five comparative trials of SES and PES in CTOs have been performed. In general, these studies have been restricted by their small study populations that limit statistical comparisons, variability in trial design, and clinical and angiographic follow-up; demonstration of differences in clinical outcome across individual trials has been less consistent. More recently, the PRISON III trial randomized 300 CTO patients to receive either SES or two different zotarolimus-eluting stents (Endeavor and Resolute, Medtronic CardioVascular, Santa Rosa, California).[91] Compared with SES, the primary endpoint of in-segment late lumen loss at 8-month angiographic follow-up was significantly higher with Endeavor but similar to Resolute. Given the overall small sample size, clinical outcomes did not statistically vary according to DES assignment.

Additional studies have evaluated everolimus-eluting stents (EES) compared with PES,[92-94] reporting lower angiographic and clinical restenosis with EES. In the Non-acute Coronary OcclusIon Treated By Everolimus Eluting Stent (CIBELES) randomized trial comparing SES with EES (N = 207), 9-month in-stent late loss (primary endpoint, 0.13 ± 0.69 mm EES versus 0.29 ± 0.60 mm SES, $p = 0.12$) and angiographic restenosis were similar between stent types.[94] At 12 months, TLR and ST were numerically but not significantly higher among SES-treated patients. In a single-center registry comprising 1035 patients for whom successful CTO PCI occurred in 77% (N = 802), 66% of the patients received first-generation SES or PES, and 34% of the patients were treated with EES.[92] Follow-up angiography was performed at

6 to 9 months following successful revascularization in 82% of the patients. Reocclusion was identified in 3% of the patients receiving EES compared with 10.1% of the patients with alternative DES ($p = 0.001$). In multivariable analysis, predictors of reocclusion were subintimal tracking and reentry technique (OR 29.5, $p < 0.001$). Importantly, the subintimal tracking methods applied in this case series should not be equated with more contemporary targeted reentry methods as detailed previously. Additional studies evaluating EES in CTO revascularization are forthcoming (Evaluation of the XIENCE PRIME LL and XIENCE Nano Everolimus Eluting Coronary Stent Coronary Stents, Performance, and Technique in Chronic Total Occlusions [EXPERT CTO], **www.clinicaltrials.gov**, identifier NCT01435031).

LIMITATIONS

CTO Complications

Angioplasty of the CTO has traditionally been considered benign, with the presupposition that because the artery is already occluded with collateral circulation, no harm can be done. However, research has demonstrated that CTO angioplasty carries much the same risk as conventional PCI.[95,96] Although coronary perforations are common in CTO PCI (27.6% in one series[97]), most perforations are related to localized wire exit from the vessel architecture and are limited to angiographic evidence of contrast staining. As most perforations do not have serious clinical consequences, the risk of tamponade is low (0.3%).[95] However, clinically significant coronary perforation can be associated with significant morbidity and mortality, with reported rates of death of 42%, emergency surgery of 39%, myocardial infarction of 29%, and transfusion of 65% in one case series not limited to CTO PCI.[98] Management of perforations includes the following: (1) prolonged inflation across the perforation with an occluding balloon or perfusion balloon catheter; (2) reversal of anticoagulation; (3) covered stent placement, emergency surgery, or embolization; and (4) pericardiocentesis. To avoid target and donor vessel thrombosis, reversal of anticoagulation is generally not recommended, provided that hemostasis can be achieved by mechanical means.

The operator needs to be vigilant if a perforation is suspected. It is important to recognize that perforation often may not occur at the occluded segment or be related to the guidewire itself but instead adjunctive devices (e.g., balloon or stent inflation, atherectomy). Further, perforation is not always manifest during the procedure, with 45% of 31 events diagnosed after leaving the catheterization laboratory in another series of nonselected CTO and non-CTO PCI.[98] Angiography of the contralateral vessel must be performed to exclude the possibility of extravasation via the collaterals. Close monitoring with a Swan-Ganz catheter and serial echocardiograms may be necessary. If development of an effusion occurs without tamponade, many instances may be managed conservatively without pericardiocentesis. If a pericardial effusion is identified but there is uncertainty whether ongoing extravasation is present, administration of echocardiographic contrast may be useful;[99] if contrast is not visualized in the pericardial space, conservative therapy (i.e., no pericardiocentesis) may be sufficient. Other procedural-related complications include thrombus formation, coronary dissection, and side branch or collateral occlusion, leading to periprocedural myocardial infarction. Catheter entrapment is also an uncommon but reported complication.

Two additional complications not specific to CTO PCI but associated with more complex, longer duration procedures are contrast nephropathy and radiation injury. Contrast-induced nephropathy is a complication that is dose dependent to contrast exposure with increasing risk relative to baseline renal impairment. Similarly, radiation-induced dermal injury is dose dependent and requires careful surveillance in patients who receive significant radiation exposure.[100] Fluoroscopic time is inadequate for measuring radiation exposure, but instead total air kerma at the interventional reference point is the procedural cumulative air kerma (x-ray energy delivered to air) at the interventional reference point and should be used to monitor deterministic skin effects. Measures to reduce focal radiation exposure include collimation, frequent changing of viewing projections, and reduction in fluoroscopic frame rates.

CONCLUSIONS

The implications of improving early procedural and long-term clinical outcomes among patients with CTOs are considerable. Until recently, however, our knowledge of procedural, angiographic, and clinical outcomes following PCI for CTOs was limited by the systematic or preferential exclusion of patients with CTO target lesions from major interventional cardiology clinical trials. Further, no technology is presently available to reliably predict procedural success in patients considered for CTO revascularization. In comparison to revascularization for nonocclusive lesions, the complexity of CTOs is reflected in differences regarding lesion length, plaque burden, negative vascular remodeling, thrombus, and calcification.

While the challenges associated with CTOs may seem formidable, it is equally clear that our evolving understanding of the benefits of revascularization has contributed to increasing interest in CTOs, reflected in an increasing number of CTO procedures, the development of novel technologies, and the design of trials dedicated to CTO revascularization. Over the past decade alone, a number of alternative technologies and techniques have been advanced, including sophisticated antegrade and retrograde guidewire methods, microdissection, and device-assisted luminal reentry. Noninvasive imaging has further enhanced patient candidacy for CTO PCI through assessment of myocardial viability and clarification of ambiguous coronary anatomy. Recent reports have also demonstrated that despite greater resource utilization, CTO PCI is not an economic disincentive.[95] Altogether, the learning curve for advanced CTO techniques has never been more abbreviated through expansion of clinical trials, regional and international educational sessions, online didactic programs, and direct proctoring.

Thus, while CTOs reflect the current inadequacies in PCI methods for achieving initial procedural success and for sustaining restenosis-free patency following initial success, they also represent a very unique opportunity to conquer perhaps the most difficult and yet one of the most common lesion subsets in interventional cardiology. While there remains opportunity for improvement, the advancement of innovative techniques and technologies that may safely improve outcome in a lesion complexity termed the "last great barrier to PCI success" is welcomed.

References

1. Srinivas V, Borrks MM, Detre KM, et al: Contemporary percutaneous coronary intervention versus balloon angioplasty for multivessel coronary artery disease. A comparison of the National Heart, Lung, and Blood Institute Dynamic Registry and the Bypass Angioplasty Revascularization Investigation (BARI) study. *Circulation* 106:1627–1633, 2002.
2. Fefer P, Knudtson ML, Cheema AN, et al: Current perspectives on coronary chronic total occlusions: the Canadian Multicenter Chronic Total Occlusions Registry. *J Am Coll Cardiol* 59:991–997, 2012.
3. King SB, Lembo NJ, Weintraub WS, et al., for the Emory Angioplasty versus Surgery Trial Investigators: A randomized trial comparing coronary angioplasty with coronary bypass surgery. *N Engl J Med* 331:1044–1050, 1994.
4. Serruys PW: *SYNTAX trial: chronic total occlusion subsets*. Presented at Cardiovascular Research Technologies 2009, Washington, D.C., March 4, 2009.
5. Serruys PW, van Geuns RJ: Arguments for recanalization of chronic total occlusions. *J Am Coll Cardiol Intv* 1:54–55, 2008.
6. Bell MR, Berger PB, Bresnahan JF, et al: Initial and long-term outcome of 345 patients after coronary balloon angioplasty of total coronary artery occlusions. *Circulation* 85:1003–1011, 1992.
7. Noguchi T, Miyazaki S, Morii I, et al: Percutaneous transluminal coronary angioplasty of chronic total occlusions: determinants of primary success and long-term outcome. *Cathet Cardiovasc Interv* 49:258–264, 2000.
8. Srivatsa SS, Edwards WD, Boos CM, et al: Histologic correlates of angiographic chronic total coronary artery occlusions influence of occlusion duration on neovascular channel patterns and intimal plaque composition. *J Am Coll Cardiol* 29:955–963, 1997.
9. Katsuragawa M, Fujiwara H, Miyamae M, et al: Histologic studies in percutaneous transluminal coronary angioplasty for chronic total occlusion: comparison of tapering and abrupt types of occlusion and short and long occluded segments. *J Am Coll Cardiol* 21:604–611, 1993.
10. Galassi AR, Tomasello SD, Crea F, et al: Transient impairment of vasomotion function after successful chronic total occlusion recanalization. *J Am Coll Cardiol* 59:711–718, 2012.
11. Kumamoto M, Nakashima Y, Sueishi K: Intimal neovascularization in human coronary atherosclerosis: its origin and pathophysiological significance. *Hum Patho* 26:450–456, 1995.
12. Rentrop KP, Cohen M, Blanke H, et al: Changes in collateral channel filling immediately after controlled coronary artery occlusion by an angioplasty balloon in human subjects. *J Am Coll Cardiol* 5:587–592, 1985.
13. Surmely JF, Katoh O, Tsuchikane E, et al: Coronary septal collaterals as an access for the retrograde approach in the percutaneous treatment of coronary chronic total occlusions. *Catheter Cardiovasc Interv* 69:826–832, 2007.
14. Werner GS, Figulla HR: Direct assessment of coronary steal and associated changes of collateral hemodynamics in chronic total coronary occlusions. *Circulation* 106:435–440, 2002.
15. Puma JA, Sketch MH, Jr, Thompson TD, et al: Support for the open artery hypothesis in survivors of acute myocardial infarction: analysis of 11,228 patients treated with thrombolytic therapy. *Am J Cardiol* 83:482–487, 1999.
16. Sachdeva R, Agrawal M, Flynn SE, et al: The myocardium supplied by a chronic total occlusion is a persistently ischemic zone. *Catheter Cardiovasc Interv* 83:9–16, 2014.
17. Safley DM, House JA, Marso SP, et al: Improvement in survival following successful percutaneous coronary intervention of chronic total occlusion: variability by target vessel. *J Am Coll Cardiol Intv* 1:295–302, 2008.
18. Stone GW, Kandzari DE, Mehran R: Percutaneous recanalization of chronically occluded coronary arteries: a consensus document: part I. *Circulation* 112:2364–2372, 2005.
19. Hochman JS, Lamas GA, Buller CE, et al: Coronary intervention for persistent occlusion after myocardial infarction. *N Engl J Med* 355:2395–2407, 2006.
20. Levine GN, Bates ER, Blankenship JC, et al: 2011 ACCF/AHA/SCAI Guideline for Percutaneous Coronary Intervention. A report of the American College of Cardiology Foundation/American Heart Association Task Force on Practice Guidelines and the Society for Cardiovascular Angiography and Interventions. *J Am Coll Cardiol* 58:e44–e122, 2011.
21. Wijns W, Kolh P, Danchin N, et al: Guidelines on myocardial revascularization: The Task Force on Myocardial Revascularization of the European Society of Cardiology (ESC) and the European Association for Cardio-Thoracic Surgery (EACTS). *Eur Heart J* 31:2501–2555, 2010.
22. Patel MR, Dehmer GJ, Hirshfeld JW, et al., for the Coronary Revascularization Writing Group: ACCF/SCAI/STS/AATS/AHA/ASNC 2009 Appropriateness Criteria for Coronary Revascularization: a Report by the American College of Cardiology Foundation Appropriateness Criteria Task Force, Society for Cardiovascular Angiography and Interventions, Society of Thoracic Surgeons, American Association for Thoracic Surgery, American Heart Association, and the American Society of Nuclear Cardiology. *J Am Coll Cardiol* 53:530–553, 2009.
23. He ZX, Mahmarian JJ, Verani MS: Myocardial perfusion in patients with total occlusion of a single coronary artery with and without collateral circulation. *J Nucl Cardiol* 8:452–457, 2001.
24. Aboul-Enein F, Kar S, Hayes SW, et al: Influence of angiographic collateral circulation on myocardial perfusion in patients with chronic total occlusion of a single coronary artery and no prior myocardial infarction. *J Nucl Med* 45:950–955, 2004.
25. Cheng AS, Selvanayagam JB, Jerosch-Herold M, et al: Percutaneous treatment of chronic total coronary occlusions improves regional hyperemic myocardial blood flow and contractility: insights from quantitative cardiovascular magnetic resonance imaging. *J Am Coll Cardiovasc Interv* 1:44–53, 2008.
26. Galassi AR, Werner GS, Tomasello SD, et al: Prognostic value of exercise myocardial scintigraphy in patients with coronary chronic total occlusions. *J Interv Cardiol* 23:139–148, 2010.
27. Safley DM, Koshy S, Grantham JA, et al: Changes in myocardial ischemic burden following percutaneous coronary intervention of chronic total occlusions. *Catheter Cardiovasc Interv* 78:337–343, 2011.
28. Joyal D, Afilalo J, Rinfret S: Effectiveness of recanalization of chronic total occlusions: a systematic review and meta-analysis. *Am Heart J* 160:179–187, 2010.
29. Grantham JA, Jones PG, Cannon L, et al: Quantifying the early health status benefits of successful chronic total occlusion recanalization: results from the FlowCardia's Approach to Chronic Total Occlusion Recanalization (FACTOR) Trial. *Circ Cardiovasc Qual Outcomes* 3:284–290, 2010.
30. Safley DM, Grantham J, Jones PG, et al: Health status benefits of angioplasty for chronic total occlusions; an analysis from the OPS/PRISM studies. *J Am Coll Cardiol* 59:E101, 2012.
31. Danchin N, Angioi M, Cador R, et al: Effect of late percutaneous angioplasty recanalization of total coronary artery occlusion on left ventricular remodeling, ejection fraction, and regional wall motion. *Am J Cardiol* 78:729–735, 1996.
32. Van Belle E, Blouard P, McFadden EP, et al: Effects of stenting of recent or chronic coronary occlusions on late vessel patency and left ventricular function. *Am J Cardiol* 80:1150–1154, 1997.
33. Sirnes PA, Myreng Y, Molstad P, et al: Improvement in left ventricular ejection fraction and wall motion after successful recanalization of chronic coronary occlusions. *Eur Heart J* 19:273–281, 1998.
34. Piscione F, Galasso G, De Luca G, et al: Late reopening of an occluded infarct related artery improves left ventricular function and long term clinical outcome. *Heart* 91:646–651, 2005.
35. Baks T, van Geuns RJ, Duncker DJ, et al: Prediction of left ventricular function after drug-eluting stent implantation for chronic total coronary occlusions. *J Am Coll Cardiol* 47:721–725, 2006.
36. Kirschbaum SW, Baks T, van den Ent M, et al: Evaluation of left ventricular function three years after percutaneous recanalization of chronic total coronary occlusions. *Am J Cardiol* 101:179–185, 2008.
37. Werner GS, Surber R, Kuethe F, et al: Collaterals and the recovery of left ventricular function after recanalization of a chronic total coronary occlusion. *Am Heart J* 149:129–137, 2005.
38. Nombela-Franco L, Mitroi CD, Fernandez-Lozano I, et al: Ventricular arrhythmias among implantable cardioverter-defibrillator recipients for primary prevention: impact of chronic total coronary occlusion (VACTO Primary Study). *Circ Arrhythm Electrophysiol* 5:147–154, 2012.
39. Claessen BE, van der Schaaf RJ, Verouden NJ, et al: Evaluation of the effect of a concurrent chronic total occlusion on long-term mortality and left ventricular function in patients after primary percutaneous coronary intervention. *J Am Coll Cardiol Intv* 2:1128–1134, 2009.
40. Claessen BE, Dangas GD, Weisz G, et al: Prognostic impact of a chronic total occlusion in a non-infarct-related artery in patients with ST-segment elevation myocardial infarction: 3-year results from the HORIZONS-AMI trial. *Eur Heart J* 33:768–775, 2012.
41. Lexis CP, van der Horst IC, Rahel BM, et al: Impact of chronic total occlusions on markers of reperfusion, infarct size, and long-term mortality: a substudy from the TAPAS-trial. *Catheter Cardiovasc Interv* 77(4):484–491, 2011.
42. Yang ZK, Zhang RY, Hu J, et al: Impact of successful staged revascularization of a chronic total occlusion in the non-infarct-related artery on long-term outcome in patients with acute ST-segment elevation myocardial infarction. *Int J Cardiol* 165:76–79, 2013.
43. van der Scaaf RJ, Claessen BE, Hoebers LP, et al: Rationale and design of EXPLORE: a randomized, prospective, multicenter trial investigating the impact of recanalization of a chronic total occlusion on left ventricular function in patients after primary percutaneous coronary intervention for acute ST-elevation myocardial infarction. *Trials* 11:89, 2010.
44. Whitlow P, Muhammed K: Chronic total coronary occlusion percutaneous revascularization: the case for randomized trials. *J Am Coll Cardiol Intv* 4:962–964, 2011.
45. Suero JA, Marso SP, Jones PG, et al: Procedural outcomes and long-term survival among patients undergoing percutaneous coronary intervention of a chronic total occlusion in native coronary arteries: a 20-year experience. *J Am Coll Cardiol* 38:409–414, 2001.
46. Olivari Z, Rubartelli P, Piscione F, et al: Immediate results and one-year clinical outcome after percutaneous coronary interventions in chronic total occlusions: data from a multicenter, prospective, observational study (TOAST-GISE). *J Am Coll Cardiol* 41:1672–1678, 2003.
47. Hoye A, van Domburg RT, Sonnenschein K, et al: Percutaneous coronary intervention for chronic total occlusions: the Thoraxcenter experience 1992-2002. *Eur Heart J* 26:2630–2636, 2005.
48. Valenti R, Migliorini A, Signorini U, et al: Impact of complete revascularization with percutaneous coronary intervention on survival in patients with at least one chronic total occlusion. *Eur Heart J* 29:2336–2342, 2008.
49. Mehran R, Claessen BE, Godino C, et al: Long-term outcome of percutaneous coronary intervention for chronic total occlusions. *J Am Coll Cardiol Intv* 4:952–961, 2011.
50. Jones DA, Weerackody R, Rathod K, et al: Successful recanalization of chronic total occlusions is associated with improved long-term survival. *J Am Coll Cardiol Intv* 5:380–388, 2012.
51. Hannan EL, Wu C, Walford G, et al: Incomplete revascularization in the era of drug-eluting stents: impact on adverse outcomes. *J Am Coll Cardiol Intv* 2:17–25, 2009.
52. Genereux P, Palmerini T, Caixeta A, et al: Quantification and impact of untreated coronary artery disease after percutaneous coronary intervention: the residual SYNTAX (Synergy Between PCI with Taxus and Cardiac Surgery) score. *J Am Coll Cardiol* 59:2165–2174, 2012.
53. Farooq V, Serruys PW, Garcia-Garcia HM, et al: The negative impact of incomplete angiographic revascularization on clinical outcomes and its association with total occlusions: the SYNTAX (Synergy Between Percutaneous Coronary Intervention with Taxus and Cardiac Surgery) Trial. *J Am Coll Cardiol* 61:282–294, 2013.
54. Grantham JA, Marso SP, Spertus J, et al: Chronic total occlusion angioplasty in the United States. *J Am Coll Cardiol Intv* 2:479–486, 2009.
55. Stone GW, Reifard NJ, Moussa I, et al: Percutaneous recanalization of chronically occluded coronary arteries: a consensus document part II. *Circulation* 112:2530–2537, 2005.
56. Morino Y, Abe M, Morimoto T, et al., for the J-CTO Registry Investigators: Predicting successful guidewire crossing through chronic total occlusion of native coronary lesions within 30 minutes: the J-CTO (Multicenter CTO Registry in Japan) score as a difficulty grading and time assessment tool. *J Am Coll Cardiol Intv* 4:213–221, 2011.
57. Nombela-Franco L, Urena M, et al: Validation of the J-chronic total occlusion score for chronic total occlusion percutaneous coronary intervention in an independent contemporary cohort. *Circ Cardiovasc Interv* 6:635–643, 2013.
58. Rinfret S, Joyal D, Nguyen CM, et al: Retrograde recanalization of chronic total occlusions from the transradial approach; early Canadian experience. *Catheter Cardiovasc Interv* 78:366–374, 2011.
59. Kini AS, Rafael OC, Sarkar K, et al: Changing outcomes and treatment strategies for wire induced coronary perforations in the era of bivalirudin use. *Catheter Cardiovasc Interv* 74:700–707, 2009.
60. Baim DS, Baden G, Heuser R, et al: Utility of the Safe-Cross–guided radiofrequency total occlusion crossing system in chronic coronary total occlusions. *Am J Cardiol* 94:853–858, 2004.
61. Serruys PW, Hamburger JN, Koolen JJ, et al: Total occlusion trial with angioplasty by using laser guidewire: the TOTAL trial. *Eur Heart J* 21:1797–1805, 2000.
62. Cannon LA, John J, LaLonde J: Therapeutic ultrasound for chronic total coronary artery occlusions. *Echocardiography* 18:219–223, 2001.
63. Sumitsuji S, Inoue K, Ochiai O, et al: Fundamental wire technique and current standard strategy of percutaneous intervention for chronic total occlusion with histopathological insights. *J Am Coll Cardiol Intv* 4:941–951, 2011.
64. Surmely JF, Katoh O, Tsuchikane E, et al: Coronary septal collaterals as an access for the retrograde approach in the percutaneous treatment of coronary chronic total occlusions. *Cathet Cardiovasc Interv* 69:826–832, 2007.
65. Rathore S, Katoh O, Matsuo H, et al: Retrograde percutaneous recanalization of chronic total occlusion of the coronary arteries: procedural outcomes and predictors of success in contemporary practice. *Circ Cardiovasc Interv* 2:124–132, 2009.
66. Saito S: Different strategies of retrograde approach in coronary angioplasty for chronic total occlusion. *Cathet Cardiovasc Interv* 71:8–19, 2008.
67. Thompson CA, Jayne JE, Robb JF, et al: Retrograde techniques and the impact of operator volume on percutaneous intervention for coronary chronic total occlusions: an early United States experience. *J Am Coll Cardiol Intv* 9:834–842, 2009.
68. Colombo A, Mikhail GW, Michev I, et al: Treating chronic total occlusions using subintimal tracking and reentry: the STAR technique. *Cathet Cardiovasc Interv* 64:407–411, 2005.
69. Whitlow PL, Burke MN, Lombardi WL, et al: Use of a novel crossing and re-entry system in coronary chronic total occlusions that have failed standard crossing techniques: results of the FAST-CTOs (Facilitated Antegrade Steering Technique in Chronic Total Occlusions) Trial. *JACC Cardiovasc Interv* 5:393–401, 2012.
70. Joyal D, Thompson CA, Grantham JA, et al: The retrograde technique for recanalization of chronic total occlusions: a step-by-step approach. *J Am Coll Cardiol Intv* 5:1–11, 2012.
71. Surmely JF, Tsuchikane E, Katoh O, et al: New concept for CTO recanalization using controlled antegrade and retrograde subintimal tracking: the CART technique. *J Invasive Cardiol* 18:334–338, 2006.
72. Galassi AR, Tomasello SD, Reifart N, et al: In-hospital outcomes of percutaneous coronary intervention in patients with chronic total occlusion: insights from the ERCTO (European Registry of Chronic Total Occlusion) registry. *EuroIntervention* 7:472–479, 2011.
73. Karmpaliotis D, Michael T, Brilakis ES, et al: Retrograde coronary chronic total occlusion revascularization: procedural and in-hospital procedural outcomes from a multicenter registry in the United States. *J Am Coll Cardiol Intv* 5:1273–1279, 2012.

74. Rathore S, Katoh O, Tuschikane E, et al: A novel modification of the retrograde approach for the recanalization of chronic total occlusion of the coronary arteries intravascular ultrasound-guided reverse controlled antegrade and retrograde tracking. *J Am Coll Cardiol Intv* 3:155–164, 2010.
75. Brilakis ES, Grantham JA, Rinfret S, et al: A percutaneous treatment algorithm for crossing coronary chronic total occlusions. *J Am Coll Cardiol Intv* 5:367–379, 2012.
76. Karmpaliotis D, Michael TT, Brilakis ES, et al: Coronary chronic total occlusion revascularization: procedural outcomes from a multicenter United States registry. *Am J Cardiol* 112:488–492, 2013.
77. Mollet NR, Hoye A, Lemos PA, et al: Value of preprocedure multislice computed tomographic coronary angiography to predict the outcome of percutaneous recanalization of chronic total occlusions. *Americ J Cardiol* 95:240–243, 2005.
78. Magro M, Schultz C, Simsek C, et al: Computed tomography as a tool for percutaneous coronary intervention of chronic total occlusions. *EuroIntervention* 6(Suppl G):G123–G131, 2010.
79. Kim HW, Shah D, Patel M, et al: Assessment of viability in patients with chronic total occlusions. *Circulation* 108:IV–698, 2003.
80. Kandzari DE, Rao SV, Moses JW, et al: Clinical and angiographic outcomes with sirolimus-eluting stents in total coronary occlusions: the ACROSS/TOSCA-4 (Approaches to Chronic Occlusions With Sirolimus-Eluting Stents/Total Occlusion Study of Coronary Arteries-4) trial. *J Am Coll Cardiol Intv* 2:97–106, 2009.
81. Suttorp MJ, Laarman GJ, Rahel BM, et al: Primary stenting of totally occluded native coronary arteries II (PRISON II): a randomized comparison of bare metal stent implantation with sirolimus-eluting stent implantation for the treatment of total coronary occlusions. *Circulation* 114:921–928, 2006.
82. Van den Branden BJ, Rahel BM, Laarman GJ, et al: Five-year clinical outcome after primary stenting of totally occluded native coronary arteries: a randomised comparison of bare metal stent implantation with sirolimus-eluting stent implantation for the treatment of total coronary occlusions (PRISON II study). *EuroIntervention* 7:1189–1196, 2012.
83. Ge L, Iakovou I, Cosgrave J, et al: Immediate and mid-term outcomes of sirolimus-eluting stent implantation for chronic total occlusions. *Eur Heart J* 26:1056–1062, 2005.
84. Hoye A, Tanabe K, Lemos PA, et al: Significant reduction in restenosis after the use of sirolimus-eluting stents in the treatment of chronic total occlusions. *J Am Coll Cardiol* 43:1954–1958, 2004.
85. Werner GS, Krack A, Schwarz G, et al: Prevention of lesion recurrence in chronic total coronary occlusions by paclitaxel-eluting stents. *J Am Coll Cardiol* 44:2301–2306, 2004.
86. Nakamura S, Muthusamy TS, Bae JH, et al: Impact of sirolimus-eluting stent on the outcome of patients with chronic total occlusions. *Am J Cardiol* 95:161–166, 2005.
87. Lotan C, Almagor Y, Kuiper K, et al: Sirolimus-eluting stent in chronic total occlusion: the SICTO study. *J Interv Cardiol* 19:307–312, 2006.
88. Colmenarez HJ, Escaned J, Fernandez C, et al: Efficacy and safety of drug-eluting stents in chronic total coronary occlusion recanalization: a systematic review and meta-analysis. *J Am Coll Cardiol* 55:1854–1866, 2010.
89. Saeed B, Kandzari DE, Agostoni P, et al: Use of drug-eluting stents for chronic total occlusions: a systematic review and meta-analysis. *Catheter Cardiovasc Interv* 77:315–332, 2011.
90. Werner GS, Schwarz G, Prochnau D, et al: Paclitaxel-eluting stents for the treatment of chronic total coronary occlusions: a strategy of extensive lesion coverage with drug-eluting stents. *Catheter Cardiovasc Interv* 67:1–9, 2006.
91. Suttorp MJ, Laarman GJ: A randomized comparison of sirolimus-eluting stent implantation with zotarolimus-eluting stent implantation for the treatment of total coronary occlusions: rationale and design of the Primary Stenting of Occluded Native coronary arteries III (PRISON III) study. *Am Heart J* 154:432–435, 2007.
92. Valenti R, Vergara R, Migliorini A, et al: Predictors of reocclusion after successful drug-eluting stent-supported percutaneous coronary intervention of chronic total occlusion. *J Am Coll Cardiol* 61:545–550, 2013.
93. Valenti R, Vergara R, Migliorini A, et al: Comparison of everolimus-eluting stent with paclitaxel-eluting stent in long chronic total occlusions. *Am J Cardiol* 107:1768–1771, 2011.
94. Moreno R, García E, Teles R, et al., for the CIBELES Investigators: Randomized comparison of sirolimus-eluting and everolimus-eluting coronary stents in the treatment of total coronary occlusions: results from the chronic coronary occlusion treated by everolimus-eluting stent randomized trial. *Circ Cardiovasc Interv* 6:21–28, 2013.
95. Karmpaliotis D, Lembo N, Kalynych A, et al: Development of a high-volume, multiple-operator program for percutaneous chronic total coronary occlusion revascularization: procedural, clinical and cost-utilization outcomes. *Catheter Cardiovasc Interv* 82:1–8, 2013.
96. Patel VG, Brayton KM, Tamayo A, et al: Incidence of angiographic success and procedural complications in patients undergoing percutaneous coronary chronic total occlusion interventions: a weighted meta-analysis of 18,061 patients from 65 studies. *J Am Coll Cardiol Intv* 6:128–136, 2013.
97. Rathore S, Matsuo H, Terashima M, et al: Procedural and in-hospital outcomes after percutaneous coronary intervention for chronic total occlusions of coronary arteries 2002 to 2008: impact of novel guidewire techniques. *J Am Coll Cardiol Intv* 2:489–497, 2009.
98. Fejka M, Dixon SR, Safian RD, et al: Diagnosis, management, and clinical outcome of cardiac tamponade complicating percutaneous coronary intervention. *Am J Cardiol* 90:1183–1186, 2002.
99. Bagur R, Bernier M, Kandzari DE, et al: A novel application of contrast echocardiography to exclude active coronary perforation bleeding in patients with pericardial effusion. *Cathet Cardiovasc Interv* 82:221–229, 2013.
100. Chambers CE, Fetterly KA, Holzer R, et al: Radiation safety program for the cardiac catheterization laboratory. *Catheter Cardiovasc Interv* 77:546–556, 2011.

10 Bifurcations

Antonio Colombo and Azeem Latib

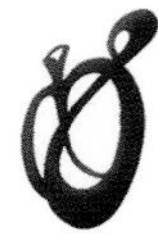

INTRODUCTION

A bifurcation coronary lesion is a stenosis involving or adjacent to the origin of an arterial side branch ≥2 mm in diameter. The stenosis can involve the large branch (main branch, MB), the smaller branch (side branch, SB), or both. Coronary bifurcation lesions have been the subject of several classifications. However, attempts to classify bifurcation lesions suffer all the limitations of coronary angiography (different plaque distribution and extent of disease when evaluated by intravascular ultrasound).[1] Furthermore, these classifications are all anatomical and do not per se dictate the treatment strategy or prognosis of a specific bifurcation lesion. There are currently eight different classifications of bifurcation lesions (**Figure 10-1**).[2-9] The most important distinction is to divide bifurcation lesions into "true" bifurcations, where the MB and SB are both significantly narrowed (>50% diameter stenosis), and "nontrue" bifurcations, which include all the other lesions involving a bifurcation. Other important elements to consider that are not inherent in the bifurcation classifications include the extent of disease on the SB (limited to the ostium or involving the vessel beyond the ostium), its size (over 2.5 mm in reference diameter), bifurcation angle, and disease distribution. In routine practice, the "Medina" classification is still the most simplified and widely used approach to classify the distribution of atherosclerotic plaque at the bifurcation site.[7] However, as mentioned, the Medina classification does not take into account the size, area of distribution, and lesion length of the branches, which are the most important features in decision making. The best way to summarize these three features is to measure FFR (physiological summary of the three features).

Approximately 15% to 20% of percutaneous coronary interventions (PCI) are performed to treat coronary bifurcations.[10-13] However, PCI for bifurcation disease continues to remain a lesion subset of great interest for interventional cardiologists because it is known to be technically challenging and has historically been associated with lower procedural success rates and worse clinical outcomes than nonbifurcation lesions.[12] This is predominantly related to the variability in anatomy (plaque burden, location of plaque, angle between branches, diameter of branches, bifurcation site), the technical challenges of treating two vessels at the same time where intervention in one of the vessels can negatively impact the other, the numerous technical approaches that could potentially be applied, and the challenges in individualizing the treatment to a specific bifurcation anatomy and patient. The trend and much of the available data support simplifying the treatment of bifurcations to that of treating a nonbifurcated segment of the coronary artery. Attempts to reduce the complexity of bifurcation PCI should not be interpreted as a one-technique approach (i.e., single MB stent provisional approach) that can be applied to all bifurcations but rather that simple techniques should be used for noncomplex bifurcations and complex techniques should be reserved for complex bifurcations or as a bail-out for failure or complications during a provisional approach.

It should be remembered that procedural complications and challenges could also occur when performing a simple approach mainly due to acute closure or severe stenosis of the SB. In fact, the complexity of treating bifurcations relates predominantly to understanding and choosing the correct strategy of managing the SB. It is the size, anatomy, extent of disease, distribution, and importance of the SB that dictate the approach. In some cases, PCI may be avoided completely or contraindicated if the SB cannot be protected. An important point to stress is that the implantation of one single stent on the MB is the most widely used approach and should be considered the default approach in most bifurcations. The presence of SB disease extending beyond the ostium, the larger the size of the SB, and the larger the territory the SB supplies may necessitate the implantation of two stents as intention to treat.

In this chapter, we summarize the important clinical data and give a detailed explanation of the technical aspects of bifurcation PCI.

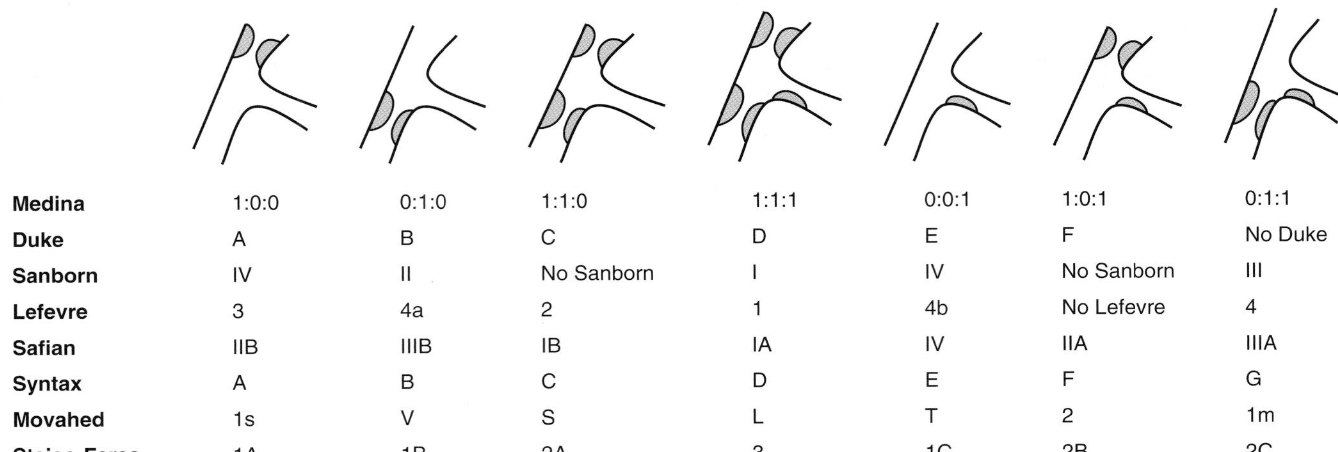

Medina	1:0:0	0:1:0	1:1:0	1:1:1	0:0:1	1:0:1	0:1:1
Duke	A	B	C	D	E	F	No Duke
Sanborn	IV	II	No Sanborn	I	IV	No Sanborn	III
Lefevre	3	4a	2	1	4b	No Lefevre	4
Safian	IIB	IIIB	IB	IA	IV	IIA	IIIA
Syntax	A	B	C	D	E	F	G
Movahed	1s	V	S	L	T	2	1m
Staico-Feres	1A	1B	2A	3	1C	2B	2C

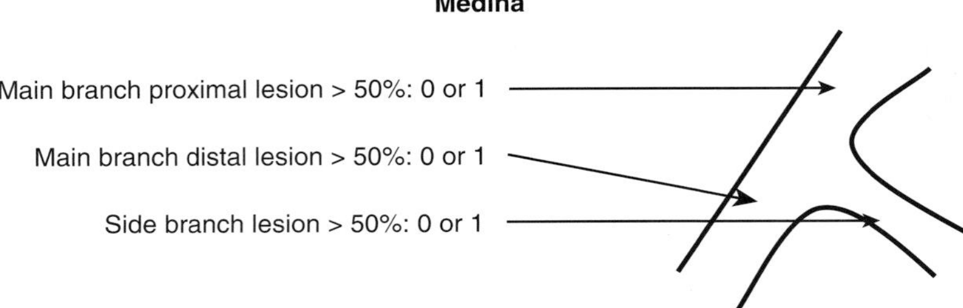

FIGURE 10-1 Classifications of bifurcations according to plaque distribution: Medina,[7] Duke,[2] Sanborn,[5] Lefevre,[3] Safian,[4] SYNTAX,[9] Movahed,[8] Staico-Feres.

SIMPLIFIED GUIDELINES AFTER 10 YEARS OF BIFURCATION STUDIES

Bifurcations have become an area of increased research over the past 10 years. This was spurred by the advent of drug-eluting stents (DESs) and their effectiveness in reducing restenosis, particularly in complex lesions such as bifurcations that led to numerous bifurcation-specific randomized trials being performed. However, the superiority of DESs over bare-metal stents (BMSs) was not evaluated in a specific randomized trial, which seemed unnecessary and unethical because restenosis and revascularization rates were dramatically lower than those seen when bifurcations were treated with BMSs.[14,15] The only randomized data comparing DESs and BMSs come from a subanalysis of the SCANDSTENT (Stenting Coronary Arteries in Non-Stress/Benestent Disease) trial, which examined a total of 126 patients with bifurcation lesions treated with sirolimus-eluting stents (SESs) or BMSs.[16] In 55% of the SES cohort and 53% of the BMS cohort, stents were implanted in both branches of the bifurcation. SES implantation was associated with significant reductions in restenosis rates at the MB (4.9% vs. 28.3%, $p < 0.001$) and SB (14.8% vs. 43.4%, $p < 0.001$), as well as major adverse cardiac events (MACE) (9% vs. 28%, $p = 0.009$) during the 7-month follow-up period. Similarly, registry studies have shown marked reductions in MACE and target lesion revascularization (TLR) rates, compared with historical BMS controls. These reductions occurred irrespective of whether a one-stent (MACE: 5.4% vs. 38%; TLR: 5.4% vs. 36%) or two-stent (MACE: 13.3% vs. 51%; TLR: 8.9% vs. 38%) strategy was employed.[15,17] As a result, DESs are the preferred stent platform for the treatment of coronary bifurcations, and outcomes related to DESs in bifurcations are discussed henceforth. However, BMSs may still be indicated when there are contraindications to prolonged dual antiplatelet therapy, in the setting of bifurcation stenting in acute myocardial infarction due to concerns about a higher risk of stent thrombosis (ST),[18] or in short lesions in large MBs of nontrue bifurcations.

Provisional Approach Is the Default Strategy

There are now seven randomized studies[10,19-24] available comparing a provisional approach of implanting one DES (1S) in the MB only versus a two-DES (2S) approach of implanting a DES on both the MB and SB of the bifurcation, the results of which are summarized in **Table 10-1 and Figure 10-2**. It is apparent from these data that routine stenting of both branches offers no clear advantage over a provisional strategy of stenting the MB only with balloon angioplasty of the SB, with regard to restenosis in the main or side branches or in repeat bifurcation revascularization. A 2S approach is associated with procedures that are longer, with more fluoroscopy time and contrast volumes and a higher rate of procedure-related biomarker release.[10] Importantly, none of these studies showed that elective double stenting of the bifurcation is associated with higher revascularization, follow-up MI, or stent thrombosis rates. Interestingly, the most recent of these studies (DKCRUSH-II) is the first and only randomized trial to suggest that double stenting may be superior to provisional stenting and associated with a lower rate of restenosis and repeat revascularization.[23] In this study, 370 true bifurcations were randomly assigned to treatment with either provisional stenting or a modification of the crush technique, the DK (double-kissing) crush. The DK crush was associated with a reduction in

TABLE 10-1 Randomized Studies Comparing Provisional Stenting to Elective Double Stenting with DES in Coronary Bifurcations

				One-Stent Group								*Two-Stent Group*									
					SIDE BRANCH			RESTENOSIS %					SIDE BRANCH			RESTENOSIS %					
AUTHOR	AIM	NO	FOLLOW-UP	ANGIO FU, %	RVD mm	DS%	Lesion Length mm	MB	SB	TLR %	*ST %	ANGIO FU, %	RVD mm	DS%	Lesion Length mm	MB	SB	TLR %	*ST %	CROSS-OVER FROM ONE STENT TO TWO STENTS	SB STENTED IF:
Colombo et al 2004[19]	Both branches vs. provisional	85	6 months	84	2.1	46.2	5.1	4.8	14.2	4.5	0	95	2.1	56.8	5.5	5.7	21.8	9.5	4.7	51.2%	>50% residual stenosis in SB
Pan et al 2004[20]	Both branches vs. provisional	91	6 months	87	2.5	64	N/A	2.4	4.9	2.1	0	89	2.5	65	N/A	10.3	15.4	4.5	2.2	2.1%	>50% residual stenosis and TIMI flow <3
Steigen et al 2006[10]	Crush, culotte, Y vs. provisional	413	6 months	73	2.6	46	6.0	4.6	19.2	1.9	0.5	76	2.6	47	6.4	5.1	11.5	1	0	4.3%	TIMI flow = 0 after SB dilatation
Ferenc et al 2007[21]	Reverse crush vs. provisional	202	12 months	95	2.39	53.1	10.4	7.3	9.4	10.9	1.0	95	2.38	54.4	9.9	3.1	12.5	8.9	2.0	18.8%	>60% stenosis and/or flow-limiting dissection
Hildick-Smith et al 2010[24]	Crush, culotte vs. provisional	500	6 months	13	N/A	63	N/A	2.8	2.8	5.6	0.4	17	N/A	68	N/A	4	3.6	7.2	2	3%	>70% stenosis, or flow-limiting dissection or TIMI flow <3
Colombo et al 2009[22]	Crush vs. provisional	350	6 months	86	2.16	61	5.7	6.7	14.7	6.3	1.1	86	2.30	63	5.9	4.6	13.2	7.3	1.7	31%	>50% stenosis and/or flow-limiting dissection
Chen et al 2013[25]	DK Crush vs. provisional	370	12 months	92	2.29	63.4	14.9	9.7	22.2	13	0.5	92	2.29	62.8	15.4	3.8	4.9	4.3	2.2	28.6%	>50% stenosis, or flow-limiting dissection or TIMI flow <3
Kumsars et al 2013[26]	Culotte, crush, T-stenting vs. provisional in large SBs	450	6 months	N/A	2.9	N/A	7.4	N/A	N/A	3.2	0.9	N/A	2.9	N/A	8	N/A	N/A	1.3	0.4	3.7%	TIMI flow <3

MB, Main branch of the bifurcation; *SB,* side branch of the bifurcation; one-stent group, bifurcation lesions treated with provisional stent technique; two-stent group, bifurcation lesions treated with both branch stenting technique; *N/A,* not available or not applicable; *ST,* stent thrombosis; *TLR,* target lesion revascularization.
*Stent thrombosis defined as per definition in study.

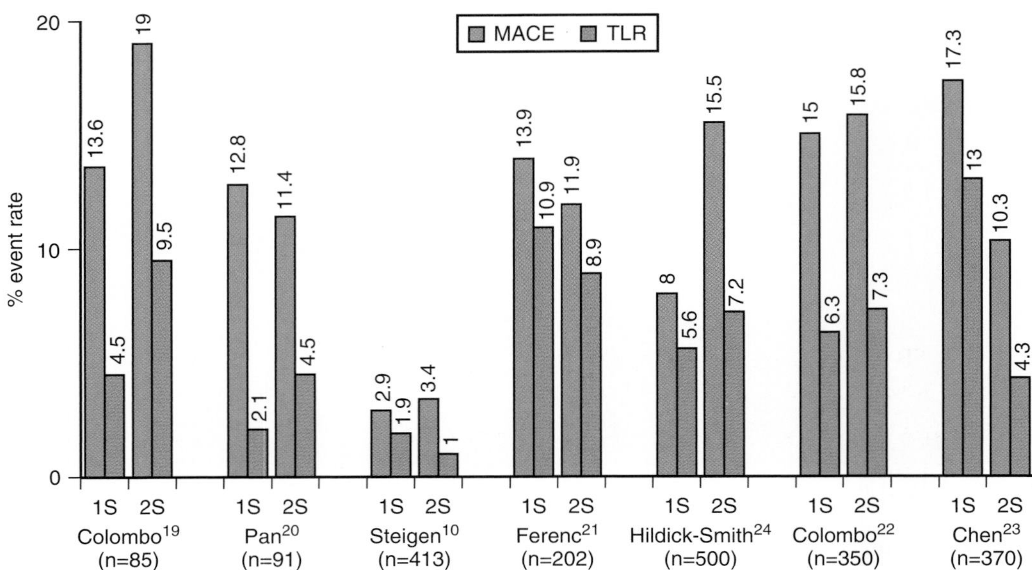

FIGURE 10-2 Clinical outcomes in the seven randomized trials comparing one- versus two-stent strategy, utilizing drug-eluting stents. *1S*, Single stent; *2S*, two stents; *MACE*, major adverse cardiac events; *TLR*, target lesion revascularization.

restenosis, especially of the SB (4.9% vs. 22.2%, $p < 0.001$) and TLR (4.3% vs. 13%, $p = 0.005$) but not in MACE (10.3% vs. 17.3%, $p = 0.07$). How do we reconcile the contradictory findings of the DKCRUSH-II study with those of the other six bifurcation studies? In our opinion, this study reconfirms the importance of the bifurcation technique, and optimization of the final result (in this case, a refinement of the standard crush technique) with a 2S approach is directly related to long-term outcomes. Nevertheless, we see no rationale to make a procedure more complex when similar immediate and medium-term follow-up results can be obtained with a simpler approach.

These randomized bifurcation studies provide us with the evidence that the provisional approach should be the default strategy in most bifurcations. However, we should not incorrectly interpret them as stating that **all** bifurcations must be treated with a provisional approach, as complex or high-risk bifurcations were not well represented in these trials. As seen in **Table 10-1**, patients included in these RCTs had moderately sized SBs with focal ostial lesions of moderate severity, and patients with long and/or severe SB stenoses or large SBs were largely excluded. Also, other important anatomic features, such as the myocardial territory supplied by the SB, the angle of the SB, and the presence or absence of distal SB disease, were not provided in these trials. In an attempt to resolve these shortcomings, there are two other randomized trials about to be published or near completion. In the Nordic-Baltic Bifurcation Study IV, Kumsars randomized true bifurcations with large SBs (≥2.75 mm) to provisional SB stenting or a 2S approach.[26] A 2S approach was associated with a longer procedure and a nonsignificantly lower rate of MACE (1.8% vs. 4.6%, $p = 0.09$) and TLR (1.3% vs. 3.2%) as compared to the provisional approach. However, once again these data may not be applicable to more complex bifurcations, as SBs with lesions >15 mm were excluded. Hopefully, the European Bifurcation Club Two (EBC-TWO) trial that has randomized true bifurcations (with SBs of >2.5 mm and lesion length >5 mm) to provisional or culotte stenting will provide us better data in regard to more complex bifurcations (ClinicalTrials.gov Identifier: NCT01560455).

Thus, although the default strategy for most bifurcations should be the provisional approach, we should continue to individualize decision making based on the patient's individual anatomy, as there are bifurcation lesions where two stents (main and side branch stenting) need to be implanted as intention to treat due to the characteristics of the lesion and the distribution of the SB. Not all bifurcations can be treated with one technique, but rather the technique should be matched to the individual bifurcation anatomy, guided by the available data as well as by personal experience.

Two Stents Can Be Selectively Implanted As Intention to Treat or Crossover from Provisional

The distinction between a provisional approach and electively implanting two stents is that, in the 1S approach, the operator may be willing to accept a suboptimal result in the SB, provided TIMI (thrombolysis in myocardial infarction) flow is normal and the SB has limited clinical relevance regarding territory of distribution. However, how do we define a suboptimal result in the SB? It is important to note that a major difference among the eight randomized trials in **Table 10-1** was the definition of a suboptimal result in the SB. This definition has a major impact on both the crossover rate from a 1S to 2S strategy and the restenosis rate in SBs treated with a provisional strategy. In the Sirius Bifurcation study,[19] a residual stenosis of >50% in the SB was considered unacceptable, which explains the very high crossover rate of 51.2%. In contrast, in the Nordic study,[10] the residual SB stenosis was irrelevant and the SB had to remain open with TIMI >0 flow. This clarifies why the highest (19.2%) SB restenosis rate with a 1S approach was observed in this study. Although it may be satisfactory to accept a suboptimal result with TIMI 1 flow in a small obtuse marginal branch, such a result is not acceptable when treating a distal left main bifurcation or a bifurcation involving a large diagonal branch. In examining the recent CACTUS,[27] Bad Krozingen,[21] and DKCRUSH-II[23] bifurcation studies, a more realistic figure is that in about 20% of bifurcations treated with a provisional strategy, a second stent will have to be implanted on the SB.

The major difference between an elective 2S approach and crossover to 2S from a 1S approach is that in the former, the SB is stented first. This may be appropriate in complex bifurcations where the risk of SB occlusion with MB stenting is high, such as those with more severe disease, longer lesions, wider angles that are difficult to rewire or that have a dissection after predilatation. Although the presence of a large plaque burden at the bifurcation can be associated with SB ostial deterioration or occlusion after MB stent implantation, even in the absence of baseline SB ostial disease, the presence of SB disease increases this risk. A number of studies have shown that the risk of SB occlusion increases with the severity of SB disease. Aliabadi et al. showed that the risk of SB occlusion was 14% to 27% for SBs with ostial stenosis >50% as compared to 1% to 4% in SBs with minimal or no disease.[28] Furukawa et al. showed that the risk of SB deterioration (final TIMI ≤2) was more common in SBs with ostial disease ≥50% (20.8% vs. 6.1%, $p = 0.049$) and in longer lesions.[29] Similarly, Chaudhry et al. demonstrated that the risk of SB compromise increased with increased SB ostial stenosis severity (for every 10% increase in SB stenosis severity, the risk of SB compromise increased by 23%) and calcification (46% vs. 26%, $p = 0.06$).[30] A criticism of these studies is that they are old and may not reflect current advances in techniques and devices. However, Hahn et al. recently studied the predictors of SB occlusion that occurred in 187 (8.4%) of 2227 bifurcation lesions.[31] On multivariable analysis, independent predictors of SB occlusion were preprocedural percentage diameter stenosis of the SB ≥50% and proximal MV >50%, SB lesion length, and acute coronary syndromes. Of 187 occluded SBs, flow was restored spontaneously in 26 (13.9%) and by SB intervention in 103 (55.1%) but not in 58 (31.0%).

However, an important change that has occurred in clinical practice is the understanding that in SBs without high-risk features, the operator could cross over to 2S if necessary (i.e., significant residual stenosis or flow-limiting dissection). The reasons for crossover depend on the size, the severity of residual disease, and the myocardial territory of the SB. All of these features are best assessed by a physiological evaluation as discussed in the next section. There are a number of bifurcation techniques that can be performed as crossover as discussed later in the chapter, but we prefer the T-stenting and small protrusion (TAP) technique because of its simplicity and that it is associated with excellent long-term outcomes. We evaluated the long-term outcomes of this technique in 95 patients who underwent SB stenting with the TAP as a crossover from the provisional approach. TAP stenting was successful in all patients and was associated with a TLR rate of 5.1% and no stent thrombosis at 3-year follow-up.[32]

Residual SB Stenosis After the Provisional Approach Is Often Not Significant

As the provisional approach has now become the gold standard, important questions are the cause, significance, and management of a residual stenosis at the ostium of the SB. There has been considerable debate as to whether the appearance of a new stenosis or aggravation of an existing stenosis at the SB ostium after MB stenting is due to plaque shift or carina shift. Historically, it has been suggested that SB compromise during PCI is the result of snowplowing of plaque over the SB ostium, that is, plaque shift, especially in bifurcations with a shallow SB angle. However, pathologic evaluation and IVUS studies have shown that although atherosclerosis develops frequently at the bifurcation, it is often located opposite to the flow divider, that is, opposite to the origin of the SB. This led to the hypothesis that has subsequently been demonstrated on IVUS that SB compromise after MB stenting may be due to carina shift rather than plaque shift (see **Figure 10-3** for an example of carina shift).

A recent study by Koo et al.[33] of IVUS evaluation after MB stent implantation showed the following: (1) a significant increase in the vessel and lumen volume index in both the proximal and distal segments of the MB, (2) a significant decrease in the plaque volume index in the proximal segment of the MB, and (3) no change in the plaque volume index in the distal segment of the MB after stenting. These results suggest that the lumen increase in the distal MB is primarily due to enlargement of the vessel and not plaque shift, supporting the concept that part of the luminal narrowing of an SB after stenting the MB is explained by carina shift. However, in the proximal MB, the plaque area changed significantly after stent implantation, particularly in the region closest to the ostium of the SB. Although plaque shift to the SB ostium was not observed directly, these data provide indirect evidence of plaque shift from the proximal segment of the MB into the SB ostium after main vessel stent implantation. Thus both plaque shift from the MB and carina shift contribute to the creation and aggravation of an SB ostial lesion after main vessel stent implantation. Carina shift will occur if the bifurcation angle is less than 90° when full MB dilatation is performed. Although carina shift may be prevented by selecting the MB stent diameter according to the distal MB diameter, the operator should not compromise optimal MB dilatation to avoid carina shift.

Additionally, there appears to be increasing evidence that trying to get an optimal angiographic result with minimal residual stenosis in the SB may not be physiologically important. This concept is especially important in smaller SBs, where the majority of angiographically significant SB lesions have been demonstrated to be not functionally significant by fractional flow reserve (FFR) analysis.[34] Koo et al. performed FFR measurements on 94 jailed SB lesions after stent implantation on the MB. No lesion with a ≥50% and <75% stenosis had an FFR <0.75. Among 73 lesions with >75% stenosis, only 20 lesions were functionally significant, and among those with >95% stenosis, only 14 out of 25 had FFR values <0.75.[34] Furthermore, smaller SBs are less likely to result in angina if a residual stenosis is left untreated or if restenosis occurs.[35,36] Indeed, FFR may be the most physiological and evidence-based method to guide the decision as to whether a jailed SB with a residual stenosis should be treated. Koo et al. evaluated the FFR in 91 jailed SBs (RVD: 2.3 ± 0.3) after MB stenting and if treatment based on whether the FFR was functionally significant would impact clinical outcomes. Only 30% of all jailed SB lesions had an FFR <0.75, with 96% of all SBs successfully accessed with pressure wire. The functionally significant SB lesions were treated with kissing balloon inflation, which resulted in 92% (23/25) of these lesions having an FFR >0.75. At 6-month follow-up, 48% of SB lesions had a stenosis >75% but only 8% had a functionally significant FFR. However, this approach

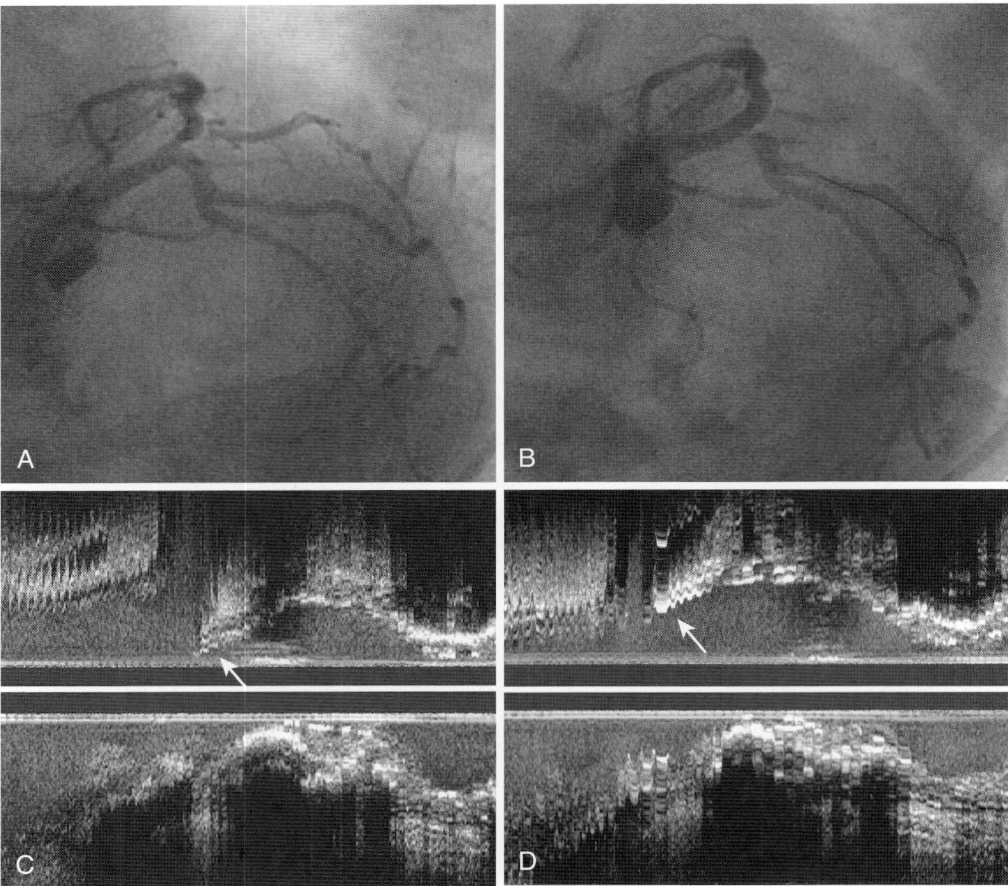

FIGURE 10-3 Example of carina shift. Angiographic and IVUS images of an LMCA bifurcation showing an unobstructed circumflex ostium **(A)** before stenting and an ostial narrowing **(B)** after stent implantation from the LMCA to the LAD. The IVUS images **(C)** demonstrate there is an alteration in the location and geometry of the carina *(arrow)*. The carina is shifted toward the side branch, and this shift results in an eccentric luminal narrowing of the SB ostium **(D)**; a three-dimensional image such as with optical coherence tomography will probably show that this narrowing occurs only in one single plane while the total lumen dimensions remain functionally adequate.

is more time consuming, costly, at times technically challenging (rewiring the jailed SB with a pressure wire), and not associated with better clinical outcomes than an angiography-guided approach (MACE: 4.6% vs. 3.7%, p = 0.7). Nevertheless, this study does confirm that kissing inflation is effective in treating functionally significant SB stenoses caused by carina or plaque shift and that many moderately sized jailed SBs with a residual stenosis may be treated conservatively or only with kissing inflation rather than stenting.

Kissing Balloon Inflation or High-Pressure Individual (SB & MB) Postdilatation Should Always Be Used When Implanting Two Stents and Optionally When Implanting One Stent

Final kissing balloon inflation (FKBI) allows SB ostium treatment and apposition of the MB stent struts on the SB ostium. It also enables correction of stent distortion and inadequate apposition in the MB.[37,38] However, FKBI increases procedural complexity and may result in stent ovalization, proximal dissection when balloons are inadequately positioned, and even suboptimal deployment of the proximal stent segment. There is uncertainty as to whether FKBI is mandatory when a provisional approach is used. Theoretically, and from benchmark studies, FKBI has the advantage of opening stent struts that potentially can scaffold the SB ostium, correcting MB stent distortion and proximal expansion caused by SB balloon dilatation through the MB struts, and facilitate future access to the SB. There is also concern that stenting across a bifurcation without opening the stent struts into the SB results in "malapposed" struts across the SB ostium that are not endothelialized. There are now two clinical studies that address whether FKBI should be routinely performed after the provisional approach. In the Nordic-Baltic Bifurcation Study III, 477 patients with bifurcation lesions undergoing main vessel stenting were randomized to FKBI (n = 238) or no FKBI (n = 239).[39] The 6-month MACE rates were 2.1% and 2.5% (p = 1.0) in the final kissing and no-final kissing groups, respectively. At 8 months, the rate of angiographic restenosis of the entire bifurcation lesion was 11.0% versus 17.3% (p = 0.11), 3.1% versus 2.5% in the MB (p = 0.68), and 7.9% versus 15.4% in the SB (p = 0.039), in the final kissing versus no-final kissing groups, respectively. The lower restenosis rate in the SB was due to the efficacy of FKBI in reducing angiographic restenosis in true bifurcation lesions, where the SB restenosis rate was 7.6% versus 20.0% (p = 0.024) in the final kissing and no-final kissing groups, respectively. Similar results were obtained in the CORPAL-KISS study that compared the incidence of 1-year clinical events in patients with bifurcation lesions that had been treated with a simple approach who were randomized to either a simultaneous FKBI or an isolated SB balloon postdilation.[40] The angiographic data and immediate results were also similar in both groups. Target lesion revascularization was required in 7 patients (3%): 5 from the FKBI group and 2 from the non-FKBI group. The incidence of MACE at 1 year (death, TLR, or acute myocardial infarction) was similar in both groups: 11 (9%) from the FKBI group and 7 (6%) from the non-FKBI group (p = NS). These studies support the simple approach of only MB stenting without routine FKBI in nontrue bifurcation lesions. However, in true bifurcation lesions that are treated with the provisional approach, FKBI should be considered, as it is associated with improved angiographic outcomes in the SB. Also, as previously mentioned, FKBI is very effective in improving the FFR in functionally significant SB lesions. Finally, it should be remembered that FKBI should only be performed in bifurcations in which the SB is suitable for stenting should dissection occur. Indeed, to reduce the risk of SB injury, compliant balloons should be avoided, as they may result in underexpansion of the MB stent and significant overexpansion of the SB ostium.[41] Indeed, in a study by Mylotte et al., systematic kissing balloon postdilatation with noncompliant balloons was associated with favorable procedural results, a low (6%) rate of crossover to SB stenting, and a promising 12-month MACE rate of 4%.[41]

In contrast to the provisional approach, FKBI has been repeatedly demonstrated to reduce late loss and restenosis, especially at the SB ostium, and it has now become standard in the performance of all double stenting techniques.[22,42-44] FKBI is not only important in correcting stent distortion and expansion[37,38] but is especially significant in fully expanding the proximal stent, in particular when treating the LMCA bifurcation where the diameter of the distal LMCA is usually much larger than the diameters of the LAD and LCX. The initial data supporting the importance of FKBI with a 2S approach come from bench-testing by Ormiston with three different stent platforms (BX Velocity, Cordis, a Johnson & Johnson Company, Miami Lakes, Florida; Express II, Boston Scientific, Natick, Massachusetts; and Driver, Medtronic, Minneapolis, Minnesota) utilizing the crush technique.[37,45] FKBI with appropriately sized SB and MB postdilatation was needed to fully expand the stent at the SB ostium, to widen gaps between stent struts overlying the SB (facilitating subsequent access), and to minimize stent distortion. The importance of FKBI with the crush technique has also been confirmed in a clinical study that demonstrated significant reductions in restenosis (11.1% vs. 37.9%) and late loss (0.32 mm vs. 0.52 mm) of the SB in the group treated with FKBI.[43] Similarly, a subanalysis of the CACTUS trial showed that FKBI was associated with better angiographic results and lower MACE rates when complex stenting was performed, and similar results were observed when using a simpler provisional SB stenting technique.[22]

However, it is imperative that FKBI with a 2S approach be performed with an optimal technique for it to be effective, including the use of adequately sized noncompliant balloons (i.e., a diameter equal to greater than the implanted stent), high pressure inflation, two-step kissing inflation, and correction of proximal distortion by the overlapping balloons with a short, noncompliant balloon. The two-step kissing inflation consists of high-pressure balloon inflation in the SB before performing the true FKBI at medium pressures and is particularly important when performing the crush technique. Ormiston et al. recently demonstrated through imaging of bench deployments that (1) recrossing the crushed stent for kissing postdilation, the most difficult part of the procedure, is technically easier with minicrush than with classical crush; (2) traditional one-step FKBI leaves considerable residual metallic stenosis that may not be visible on angiography and may predispose to thrombosis because of eddy currents, stasis, altered shear stress, and foreign body presence; and (3) SB ostial coverage and residual stenosis by metal struts are significantly reduced by two-step FKBI (**Figure 10-4**).[46]

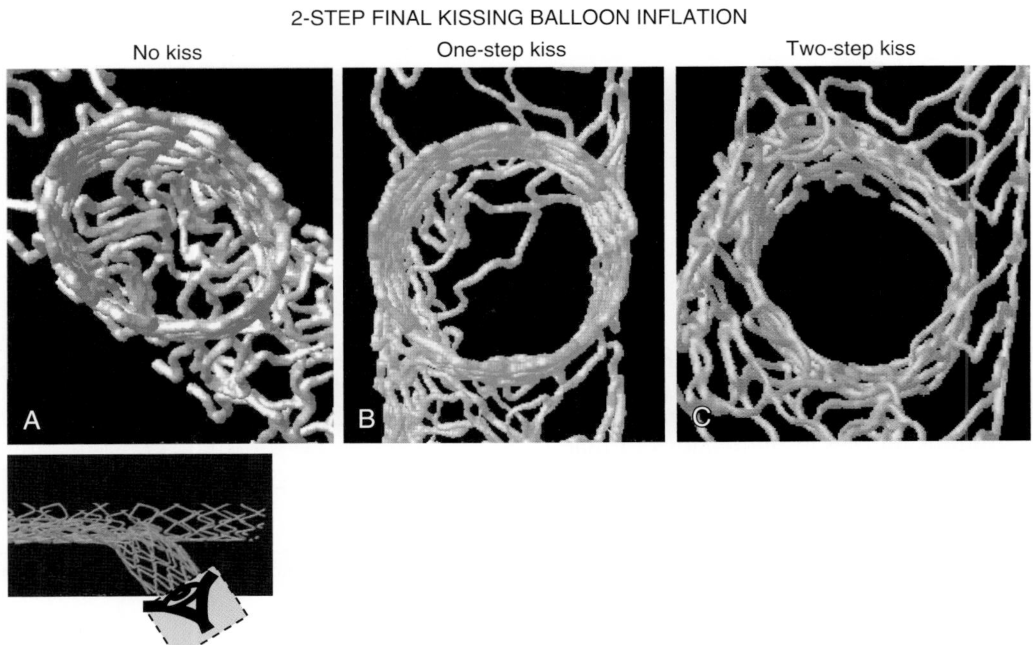

FIGURE 10-4 Bench-top imaging of the ostium of the SB after the crush technique with no FKBI **(A)**, classical one-step FKBI **(B)**, and the recommended two-step FKBI **(C)** that results in the best opening of struts toward the SB. *(Images provided courtesy Dr. John Ormiston.)*

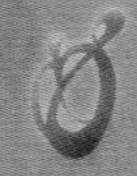

Optimal Technique Is a Must, Especially When Two Stents Have Been Implanted

The requirement for double stenting is dependent on the complexity of the bifurcation that the interventional cardiologist is willing to treat, the importance of the bifurcation to that patient, and the willingness to accept a suboptimal angiographic result in the SB. Thus, in treating simple bifurcations with small to moderately sized SBs, the rate of double stenting may be as low as 5% to 10%. In more complex bifurcations with large and extensively diseased SBs, this may be as high as 15% to 20%, with the highest rate of double stenting in the LMCA bifurcation (up to 30%). Thus, there will still be situations where the operator needs to implant a stent in both branches of the bifurcation electively or as a crossover from the provisional approach. If properly performed, there appears to be no evidence of harm to the patient and there may even be an advantage over the provisional approach in certain situations. However, when implanting two stents, the operator takes on the responsibility to ensure optimal performance of the technique, as a 2S approach is less forgiving to a suboptimal result, which may result in restenosis or stent thrombosis. In this regard, there are a number of important technical factors that may contribute to optimizing outcomes when performing 2S techniques such as high-pressure SB inflation, the use of noncompliant balloons, selection of the correct balloon size for FKBI, the double-kissing crush technique, and the use of intravascular imaging.[12] Despite the absence of a dedicated IVUS study, we strongly favor utilizing IVUS to evaluate and improve the final result when implanting two stents. An exception to this approach is present when the TAP technique is utilized. This approach may make IVUS evaluation difficult to perform.

Stent Thrombosis After Bifurcation PCI

Stenting bifurcation lesions with DES have been identified as a risk factor for stent thrombosis (ST).[47] However, data from the individual randomized trials discussed above have not demonstrated an increased risk when utilizing two stents versus one stent.[10,19-23] Similarly, two metaanalyses of the randomized trials performed have not demonstrated an increased risk of ST with double stenting techniques.[48,49] Finally, long-term data from the Nordic Bifurcation Study have shown similar rates of definite ST with provisional and double stenting (3% vs. 1.5%, $p = 0.31$) at 5 years.[50] However, the usage of two stents may be associated with an increased risk of ST in the setting of acute myocardial infarction.[51] Furthermore, it would appear that ST at coronary bifurcations is associated with a higher in-hospital and long-term mortality rate than ST at nonbifurcation lesions.[52] This higher mortality rate is at least partly explained by a larger area of myocardium at risk among subjects with bifurcation ST. There is currently no convincing evidence to suggest that we should refrain from using DES in bifurcations or that a 2S strategy is associated with a greater risk of ST. However, we should make every attempt to prevent ST when DESs are implanted in bifurcations. This requires attention to the technical aspects of the procedure, optimization of stent implantation, and dual antiplatelet therapy for at least 12 months. Despite these statements, we should take into consideration the fact that implanting two stents always demands more attention and expertise to obtain the best result in both the MB and SB.

AN INDIVIDUALIZED APPROACH TO BIFURCATIONS

The objective of bifurcation PCI is to end the procedure with both branches open and an optimal result in the MB. However, bifurcations vary not only in anatomy (plaque burden, location of plaque, angle between branches, diameter of branches, bifurcation site) but also in the dynamic changes in anatomy during treatment (plaque shift, carina shift, dissection). As a result, no two bifurcations are identical and there is no single strategy that can be applied to every bifurcation. Thus, the more important issue in bifurcation PCI is selecting the most appropriate strategy for an individual bifurcation and optimizing the performance of this technique.

Selection of the best strategy requires accurate assessment of lesion severity, distribution, extension, and presence of concomitant disease by the combination of clinical characteristics, angiography, intravascular imaging, and functional evaluation. This will result not only in the appropriate patients being selected for double stenting, which is more complex, time consuming, and labor intensive than provisional stenting, but also reduces the risk of complications. The major factors that need to be assessed and taken into account, when the operator is deciding between provisional stenting and elective double stenting, are described below. Although each of these factors is discussed separately, there is usually a combination of these factors present.

An individualized approach to treating a bifurcation (**Figure 10-5**) is dictated by the SB through evaluating the following factors:

1. Importance of SB for that patient and for that specific anatomy
   The territory of viable myocardium supplied by the SB and risk of SB occlusion is usually the most important factor when evaluating the bifurcation approach.

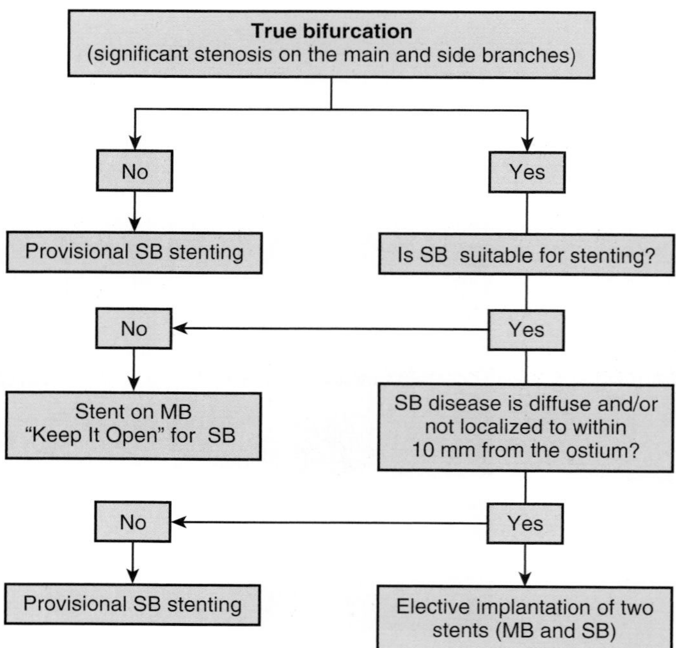

FIGURE 10-5 A proposed algorithm for treating coronary bifurcations. This approach to bifurcation stenting is based on whether both branches have significant disease, the diameter of the SB, and the extent of disease in the SB. *MB,* Main branch; *SB,* side branch.

2. Distribution of disease
   An important distinction is whether the disease at the bifurcation only involves one branch of the bifurcation or if it extends into both branches.
3. Size and territory of distribution
   The size of the branch is not considered in isolation but in combination with the severity and length of disease. In general, we would not stent SBs that are <2.5 mm unless they are long with a somewhat large territory of distribution or the branch is in danger of occlusion.
4. Extent of SB disease
   The severity and length of disease in the SB are probably the most common reasons for performing double stenting rather than provisional SB stenting. Focal ostial SB disease should be treated with a provisional approach. However, if the SB is large (≥2.5 mm), supplies a relatively large territory of myocardium, and has significant disease that extends 10 mm to 20 mm or more from the ostium, we would favor a double stenting technique from the outset.
5. Bifurcation angle
   The bifurcation angle is the angle between the MB and SB distal to the bifurcation. The bifurcation angle has an influence on the accessibility of the SB and may frequently be a reason for initially stenting the SB. A wide angle may make initial wiring of the SB difficult and may also impede recrossing into the SB with a wire, balloon, or stent after MB stenting. However, the decision to electively implant a stent on the SB should be made only after wire insertion, which may favorably modify this angle. An acute bifurcation angle is a predictor of SB occlusion during MB stenting, that is, the more acute the angle, the higher the risk of plaque shift, compromise of the ostium, and SB occlusion.[6,53,54]
6. Presence of concomitant distal disease in the SB
   If the ostium is nondiseased but there is distal disease close to it that can be covered by a long stent from the MB, we would prefer double stenting. However, if the distal disease cannot be treated with the MB stent and requires a second stent to be implanted distally, we prefer implanting the distal stent first if possible and then treating the bifurcation. This approach avoids difficulty later in passing a stent through stent struts at the bifurcation.

TECHNICAL ASPECTS OF BIFURCATION PCI

General Aspects

Guide Catheter

Most bifurcation lesions should be treated via a 6 Fr guide catheter because a provisional strategy will be utilized most of the time. Furthermore, crossover to a 2S approach from provisional and most elective double stenting techniques can also be performed with a 6 Fr guide catheter. However, in very complex bifurcation or trifurcation lesions where multiple (>2) guidewires will be placed or a 2S technique such as the classical crush or V-stenting is required, we recommend placing a 7 Fr or 8 Fr guide catheter. If two stents are needed and a 6 Fr guide catheter is employed, some limitations need to be known: (1) The two stents can only be inserted and deployed sequentially; (2) when performing T-balloon stenting, step-crush, or TAP, the stent should be advanced into the SB first and then the balloon to the MB; and (3) the standard crush, V, or kissing stents technique cannot be performed unless a guide catheter of 7 Fr or 8 Fr is utilized.

Vascular Access

We have no preference as regard to femoral or radial access for treating bifurcations. Even complex bifurcations can be treated via the radial approach providing that guide catheter support is adequate.[55] In cases where large guide catheters are required, a 7 Fr guide catheter can usually be inserted in males or sheathless guide catheters can be utilized.

Wiring Both Branches of the Bifurcation and Jailed Guidewires

Two wires should be placed in most bifurcations and the SB wire should be "jailed" in the majority, following deployment of the stent on the MB. This approach of wiring both branches during bifurcation stenting is important in protecting the SB from closure due to plaque shift, carina shift, and/or stent struts during MB stenting. Even SBs with minimal disease may occlude during MB stenting (**Figure 10-6A-B**, Videos 10-1 and 10-2). There has been some debate as to whether placing a wire in the SB can protect it from closure

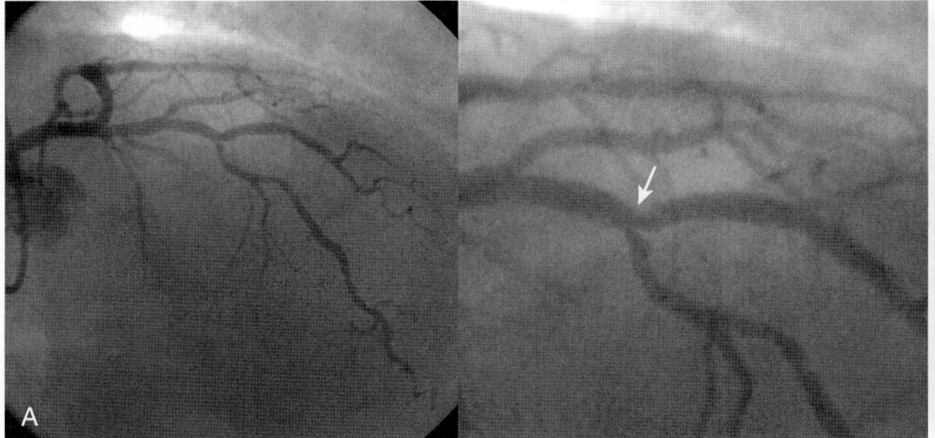

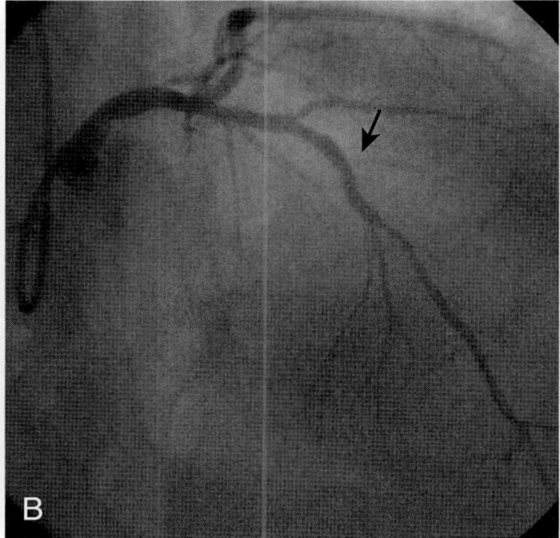

FIGURE 10-6 Demonstrates a critical stenosis on the mid-LAD with minimal disease of the diagonal ostium **(6A, Video 10-1)**. The operator placed a wire in the LAD only and stented across the diagonal ostium, which, despite minimal disease, occluded **(6B, Video 10-2)**. An SB wire may have prevented closure or at least facilitated reopening of the vessel.

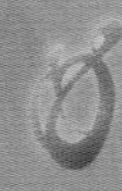

after MB stenting. A recent study has finally confirmed that the jailed wire in the SB is associated with flow recovery of SBs that occlude after MB stenting (74.8% vs. 57.8%, $p = 0.02$). Protecting SBs with guidewires to prevent their closure is important, as SB compromise may not be inconsequential. Occlusion of SBs >1 mm can be associated with a 14% incidence of myocardial infarction,[56] and SB (≥2 mm) compromise during a provisional approach can be associated with a large periprocedural myocardial infarct.[30] The jailed SB wire not only protects it from closure but also facilitates rewiring of the SB (if SB postdilatation-stenting or final kissing inflation is needed or if the side branch occludes) by[38,57] widening the angle between the MB and SB, acting as a marker for the SB ostium, and changing the angle of SB takeoff.[37,56] Finally, in the case of SB occlusion, the jailed wire can be used to reopen the SB by pushing a small balloon between the stent and the wall of the vessel. There is no need to remove the jailed wire during high-pressure stent dilatation in the MB. It is preferable to avoid jailing hydrophilic guidewires, as there is a risk of removing the polymer coating. Accurate handling of the guide catheter to prevent migration into the ostium of the coronary vessel will allow removal of the jailed wire.

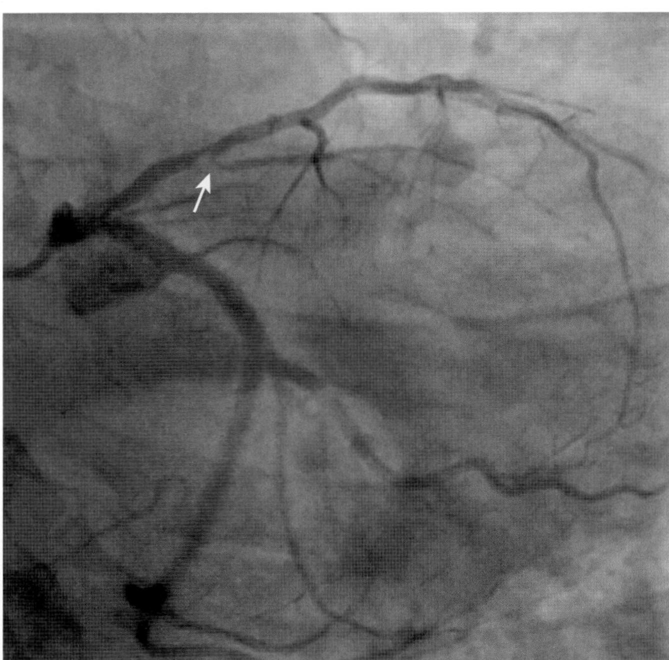

FIGURE 10-7 Angiography demonstrating a severe stenosis of the proximal LAD involving the diagonal ostium that has a hairpin bend origin **(Video 10-3)** and was very difficult to wire with standard techniques. A pullback wiring technique as demonstrated in **Video 10-4** was utilized to wire this angulated SB.

Difficult SB Access

Safe guidewire placement in the MB and SB is the first step to a successful bifurcation PCI procedure. In some cases of complex bifurcation anatomy with wide SB takeoff angles (≥90°) and/or severe disease at the bifurcation, wiring the SB may be extremely challenging, and if not properly performed, it could result in dissection of the SB ostium and acute closure. An inability to wire the SB may be a reason not to perform bifurcation PCI or to abort the procedure because the risk of losing the SB will be too high considering the size and distribution of the branch (typically an angulated circumflex artery). There are a number of technical tips that may help in the situation when the SB cannot be wired with a workhorse coronary guidewire:[58]

1. Antegrade wiring with a change of guidewire to a stiffer or hydrophilic polymer-coated wire, making a single wide bend or double bend shape, with the support of a microcatheter. Stiffer wires enhance precision and torque control and are usually our first option when a workhorse wire fails. Hydrophilic or polymer-jacket wires are usually our last option because although they may shorten and facilitate SB wiring, they have a greater risk of wire perforation or subintimal navigation (especially if the SB has been injured by balloon dilatation).
2. Pullback wiring technique (**Figure 10-7**, Videos 10-3 and 10-4): A guidewire with a smooth, large, distal bend or loop is advanced into the distal MB and pulled back to the bifurcation; because of the hook-like bend, the distal tip of the guidewire engages the SB ostium; gentle counterclockwise rotation advances the wire in the SB.
3. Reverse wire technique: A polymer-jacket hydrophilic guidewire with a round shape (reverse bend) at about 3 cm from the distal tip is advanced distal to the bifurcation; the guidewire is pulled back to the bifurcation and owing to the hairpin bend, the distal tip engages the SB; a gentle counterclockwise rotation advances the guidewire in the SB; at this stage, the reverse guidewire is usually exchanged for a conventional wire using a microcatheter.
4. A Venture wire control catheter or SuperCross angled tip microcatheter (Vascular Solutions, Inc., Minneapolis, Minnesota) enables the guidewire to be directed toward the SB after active or passive deflection of the catheter tip. The deflectable catheter is tracked over a guidewire just distal to the SB ostium; the guidewire is withdrawn into the deflectable catheter; the SuperCross catheter tip changes from a straight tip to its preformed curve (45, 90, or 120, depending on which catheter is selected), whereas the Venture catheter is actively deflected to the required angulation; once the catheter is adequately oriented to the SB ostium, the guidewire can be easily advanced.
5. Rotational atherectomy on the MB with the intent to remove the plaque that prevents entry toward the SB and facilitate SB wiring.
6. MB predilatation with the rationale that the plaque modification and a favorable plaque shift will facilitate access toward the SB. This is usually a last resort, as it may result in occlusion of the SB.

Each of these options has its rationale and specific anatomical indication. The operator's experience and the clinical scenario will direct the selection of the best strategy. Usually the final option is the one frequently employed when wiring has failed and is effective most of the time.

Provisional Approach

We divide the provisional approach into two different strategies depending on the size, extent of disease, and importance of the SB. Making this distinction at the outset saves time and clarifies the operator's objective regarding the expected final result, especially if the stenosis of the SB is aggravated by MB stenting. A 6 Fr guide catheter is usually preferred for the provisional approach.

1. **The SB is not suitable (too small) for stenting or clinically irrelevant AND has ostial or diffuse disease.**

In these bifurcations, the ***Keep It Open*** strategy is utilized, which is performed as follows:

1. Wire both branches.
2. Dilate the MB if needed but not the SB.
3. Stent the MB and leave the wire in the SB.
4. Perform postdilatation of the MB with a jailed wire in the SB.
5. Do not rewire the SB or postdilate the SB.

This "jailed wire" strategy allows protection of an SB that may not require treatment but where the need to maintain patency is important. This strategy can be utilized as a standalone technique or as part of the provisional strategy when the operator may need to eventually dilate or stent the SB. This approach of just "keep it open" for the SB was the strategy used in the provisional stenting group of the Nordic Study.[10]

2. **The SB is suitable for stenting AND it has minimal disease or disease at the ostium only.**

In these bifurcations, the ***Provisional*** strategy is utilized. This strategy is quick, safe, easy to perform, and has been shown to be associated with results comparable to a more complex approach. The provisional approach is performed as follows:

1. Wire both branches.
2. Predilate the MB and the SB as required; many SBs without significant disease or calcification do not require predilatation.
3. Stent the MB and perform a proximal optimization technique (POT), leaving the SB wire in place. If the angiographic results in the MB and SB are satisfactory, the procedure is complete and the SB wire jailed behind the MB stent struts can be gently removed.
4. Rewire the SB and then remove the jailed wire. Recrossing through the distal strut ("carina strut") following the MB stenting is strongly recommended because it creates better SB scaffolding as opposed to proximal crossing. In our experience, recrossing into the SB through the MB stent struts is usually possible using a conventional guidewire or the Rinato-Prowater wire (Asahi Intecc Co Ltd, Nagoya, Japan). The recommended technique for wire recrossing is to first advance the guidewire distally through the MB, preferably with a curve, to avoid passing under the MB stent struts; the wire is then pulled back with the tip facing the SB ostium and grating the stent struts; when the tip reaches the first cell covering the ostium, it engages the SB and with a gentle rotation is advanced into the SB. The jailed wire in the SB should always be left in place as a marker until complete recrossing has been done or MB stenting has been completed, including high-pressure stent deployment or postdilatation. The operator should refrain from removing the jailed wire when difficulties are encountered to rewire the side branch. The POT should be liberally utilized to facilitate rewiring of the SB.
5. Perform SB balloon dilatation and FKBI with moderate pressure (8 atm) in the SB, until the balloon is fully expanded. FKBI is mandatory if the SB is dilated through the MB stent struts to correct MB stent distortion and expansion.[37,38] FKBI should only be performed in bifurcations in which the SB is suitable for stenting should dissection occur.
6. If the result remains unsatisfactory (suboptimal result, FFR <0.75, plaque or carina shift with >75% residual stenosis or TIMI <3; in an SB ≥2.5 mm) or SB balloon dilatation is complicated by a flow-limiting SB dissection, perform SB stenting.

Proximal Optimization Technique (POT)

To prevent carina shift, the MB stent diameter should be selected according to the diameter of the distal MB. Inflation of a short, bigger balloon just proximal to the carina corrects the underdeployment of the proximal part of the MB stent. As a result, the original anatomical configuration of the bifurcation is restored in compliance with the Murray's and Finet's law.[59] The POT also changes the orientation of the SB ostium and the projection of struts in the SB ostium, thus facilitating wire recrossing into the most distal strut, balloon crossing, and if necessary, a stent in the SB. The POT is especially useful in bifurcation lesions with a large SB because a marked difference in the diameter of the proximal and distal MB is observed.

Final Kissing Balloon Inflation (FKBI)

The selection of appropriately sized noncompliant balloons for FKBI is crucial. The diameter must match that of the two distal branches. The balloons must be sufficiently short to avoid inflation outside the stent in the MB and in disease-free areas in the SB. The use of noncompliant balloons prevents overexpansion at the SB ostium, vessel injury, and dissection, while ensuring adequate MB stent expansion.[41] In cases where POT has not been performed, FKBI may optimize the proximal segment of the MB. During FKBI, we inflate a balloon in the MB first and then the SB balloon to achieve strut projection in the ostium. The pressure applied depends on the persistence of a waist on the balloon. In bifurcations with a large proximal MB, some operators prefer reperforming the POT to correct ovalization of the proximal MB stent caused by the kissing balloons. Sequential balloon inflation (side, main, side or only side, main) has also been proposed as an alternative to FKBI.[60]

Technical Tips for Provisional Approach

1. Always wire both branches.
2. Predilate the SB only if there is severe disease and/or the patient is at risk of occlusion after MB stenting.
3. The MB stent is selected according to the distal MB diameter.
4. The SB wire should be jailed behind the MB stent.
5. Use the POT to optimize proximal MB stent deployment and facilitate wire recrossing.
6. Recross the MB through the distal strut.
7. Do not remove the jailed wire until recrossing or MB stent optimization has been performed.
8. FKBI is not mandatory but probably advantageous in true bifurcations with significant residual SB stenosis (>70%) and/or an FFR <0.75.
9. High pressure proximal stent inflation using a short, noncompliant balloon should be considered for correction of possible proximal stent distortion after FKBI.

Crossover to Double Stenting from a Provisional Approach

If the SB result remains unsatisfactory after MB stenting and balloon dilatation of the SB (>75% residual stenosis,

1. Wire both branches and predilate if needed.

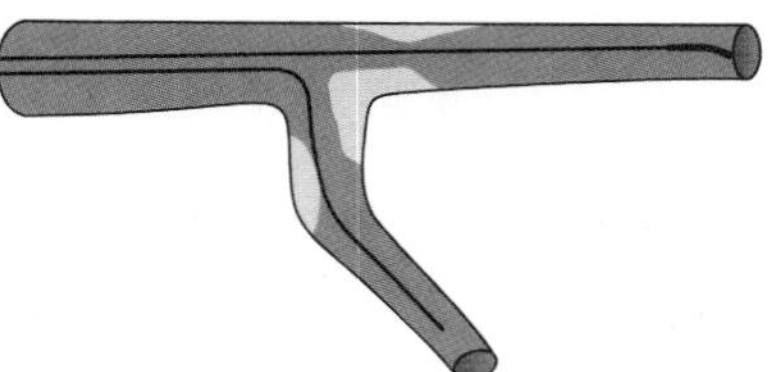

2. Stent the MB leaving a wire in the SB. The stent in the MB can be deployed at high pressure.

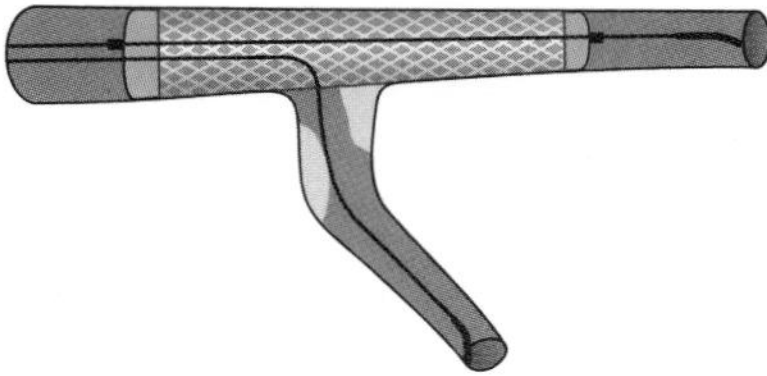

3. Rewire the SB passing through the struts of the MB stent, remove the jailed wire, dilate toward SB, and perform final kissing inflation.

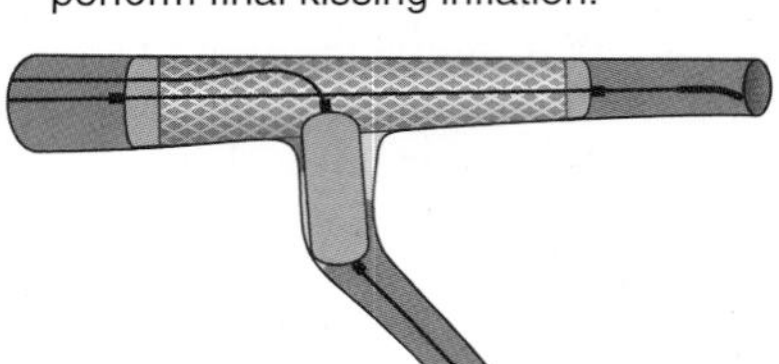

Assuming that the result is suboptimal

4. Advance stent into the SB with no MB protrusion and deploy the stent.

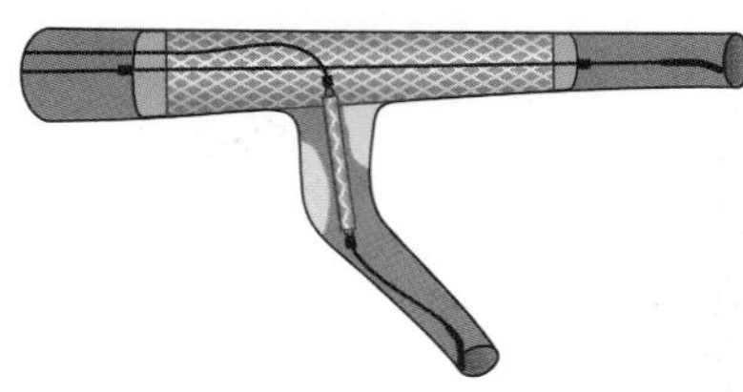

5. Perform final kissing inflation following advancement of a balloon in the MB. If needed use a new balloon for the SB.

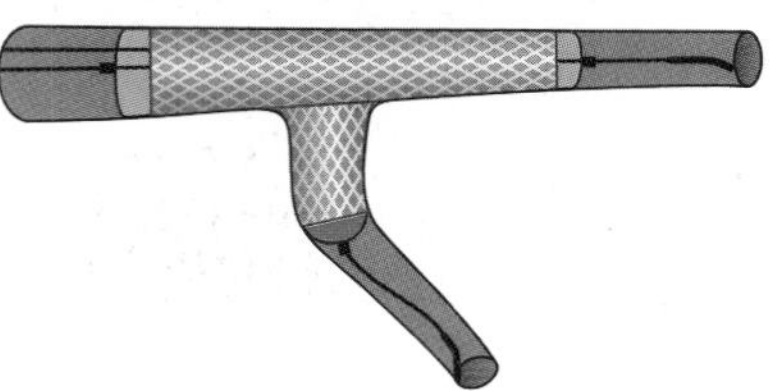

FIGURE 10-8 A schematic representation of the provisional T-stenting technique.

dissection, TIMI flow grade <3 or FFR <0.75 in an SB ≥2.5 mm), SB stenting should be performed. SB stenting can be performed with the TAP, reverse crush, or culotte techniques, followed by kissing balloon inflation.

T Technique

This technique (**Figure 10-8**) is the one most frequently utilized to shift from provisional stenting to stenting the SB. The T technique consists of advancing a second stent into the SB (following adequate dilatation of the MB stent struts). The stent is positioned at the ostium of the SB in an attempt to minimize any possible gap. A second kissing balloon inflation is also performed. The T technique is best suited when the angle between the MB and the SB is close to 90° because in narrow angles it is impossible to fully cover the ostium without protruding into the MB. Thus we have replaced this technique with the TAP.

T-Stenting and Small Protrusion (TAP)

The TAP technique (**Figure 10-9**) is a modification of the T-stenting technique and is based on an intentional minimal protrusion of the SB stent within the MB.[32] This technique can be described as follows:

1. A second stent is positioned in the SB with the aim to protrude as minimally as possible into the MB (1 or 2 mm), thus ensuring complete coverage of the ostium of the SB.
2. A balloon is advanced in the MB.
3. The SB stent is deployed as usual (12 atm or more), while the uninflated balloon remains parked in the MB at the bifurcation.
4. The SB stent balloon is pulled backward slightly, ensuring that it is still within the MB stent. Subsequently, simultaneous FKBI is performed using the SB balloon and the previously positioned MB balloon at high pressure.
5. The SB is deflated last and both balloons are deflated and removed.

The SB stent now completely covers the ostium. Despite some concerns about stent protrusion in the MB, in our experience we have been able to perform IVUS in the MB and SB and, when needed, to advance additional stents distally in the MB and in the SB. The TAP has become our preferred technique when we need to implant a stent in the SB during a provisional approach because it is easy to perform, does not require recrossing of the SB struts to perform FKBI, and appears to be associated with good long-term outcomes.[32]

Reverse Crush

This technique (**Figure 10-10**) should be used as a crossover approach with the intent to minimize any possible

1. Leave a wire in the SB and deploy a stent in the MB.

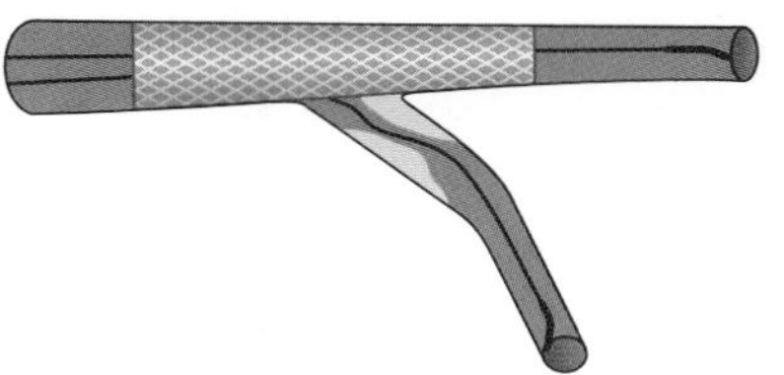

2. Rewire the SB passing through the struts of the MB stent, remove the jailed wire, dilate toward SB, and perform final kissing inflation.

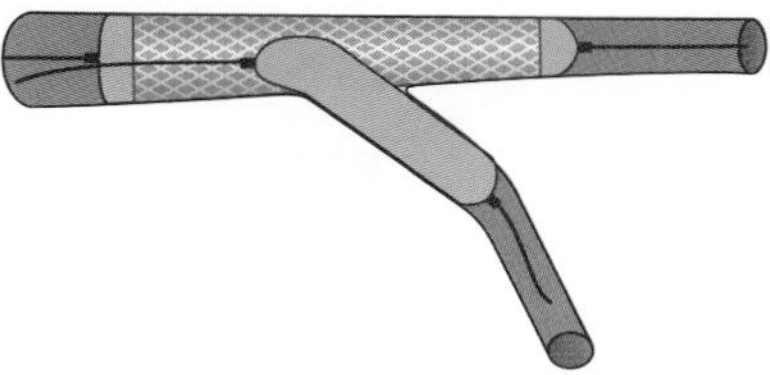

Assuming that the result is suboptimal

3. Advance stent into SB ensuring coverage of ostium with minimal protrusion (1–2 mm) into MB and place non-compliant balloon in MB stent.

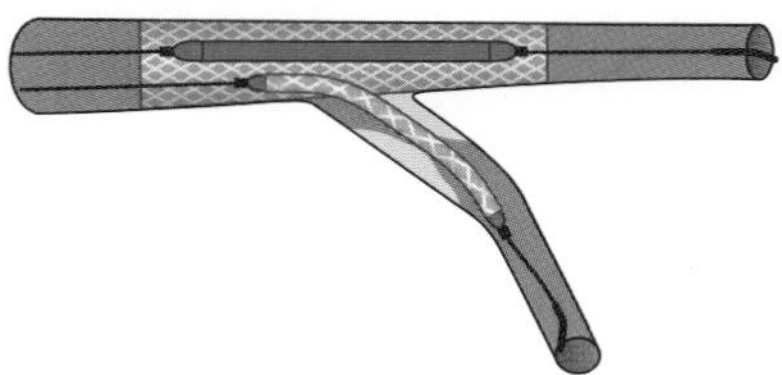

4. Deploy SB stent as usual while MB balloon remains uninflated.

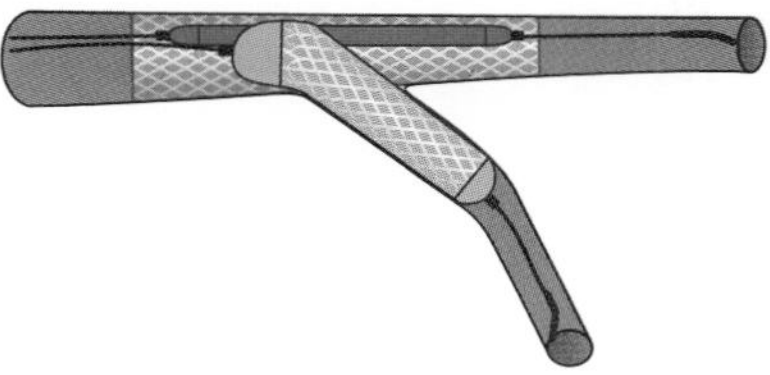

5. Pull back SB balloon and simultaneously inflate both balloons to perform final kissing.

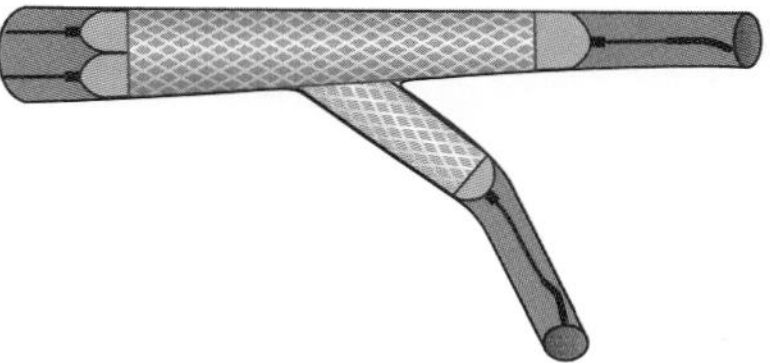

6. To ensure optimal final results at SB ostium, SB balloon must be deflated last when kissing inflation is finished.

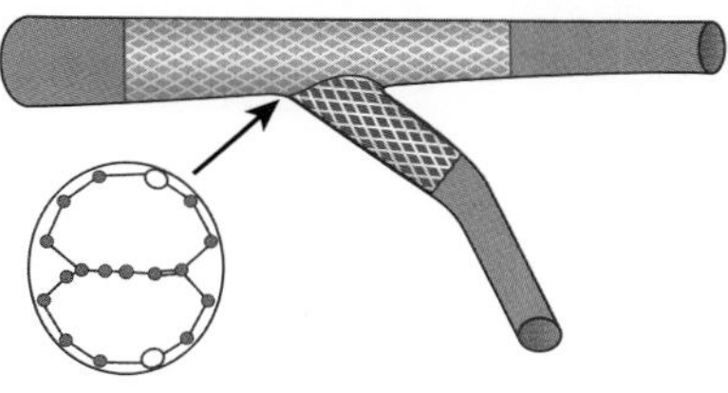

FIGURE 10-9 A schematic representation of the T-stenting and small Protrusion (TAP) technique.

stent gap between the MB and SB stents, in conditions where the angle between the MB and the SB is acute (usually less than 60°). In this situation, the TAP technique may result in excessive protrusion when attempting to fully cover the ostium of the SB. The reverse crush can be performed utilizing a 6 Fr guide catheter according to the following steps:

1. A second stent is advanced into the SB and left in position without being deployed.
2. A balloon sized according to the diameter of the MB and shorter than the stent already deployed is advanced in the MB and positioned at the level of the bifurcation; be sure to stay inside the stent previously deployed in the MB.
3. The stent in the SB is retracted about 1 mm to 2 mm into the MB and deployed. The deploying balloon is removed and an angiogram is obtained to verify the absence of any distal dissection and the need for an additional stent. If such is the case, the wire from the SB is removed and the balloon in the MB is inflated at high pressure (12 atm or more).
4. SB struts are recrossed with a wire and a balloon. The balloon is sized to the SB reference diameter and inflated at high pressure (12-20 atm), and final kissing inflation is performed (i.e., two-step kissing balloon inflation).

Provisional Culotte

The provisional culotte technique (**Figure 10-11**) can be proposed as a provisional SB stenting strategy in Y-shaped angulated bifurcation lesions without a large discrepancy in size between the MB and SB.[61] This technique can be described as follows:

1. After MB stenting, a second stent is advanced in the SB, protruding into the MB to overlap with the proximal part of the MB stent and expanded.
2. The MB is rewired through the protruding SB stent struts, the jailed MB wire is removed, and a balloon is advanced into the MB across the protruding struts and dilated.
3. Kissing balloon inflation is performed.

Both the reverse crush and culotte require a second recrossing of stent struts; as a result, they have been superseded by the TAP when the bifurcation angle is unfavorable.

Elective Double Stenting

Correct patient selection for elective double stenting requires an accurate assessment of lesion severity, distribution, extension, and presence of concomitant disease.[12,62,63] The decision to perform double stenting depends predominantly on the SB and should generally be reserved for true bifurcations with SBs that (**Figure 10-12**):

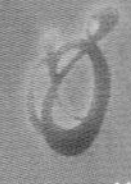

1. Leave a wire in the SB and deploy a stent in the MB.

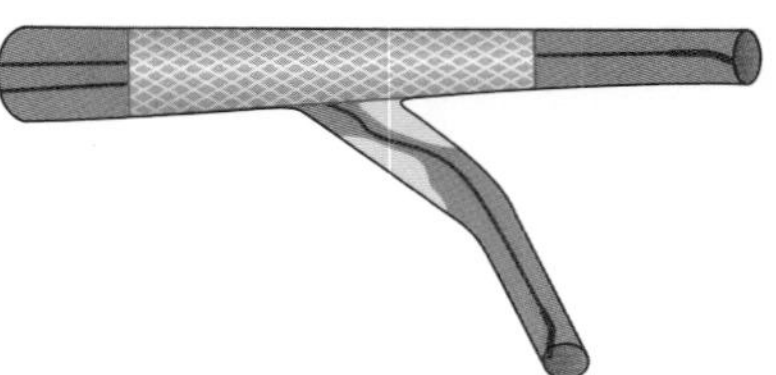

2. Rewire the SB passing through the struts of the MB stent, remove the jailed wire, dilate toward SB, and perform final kissing inflation.

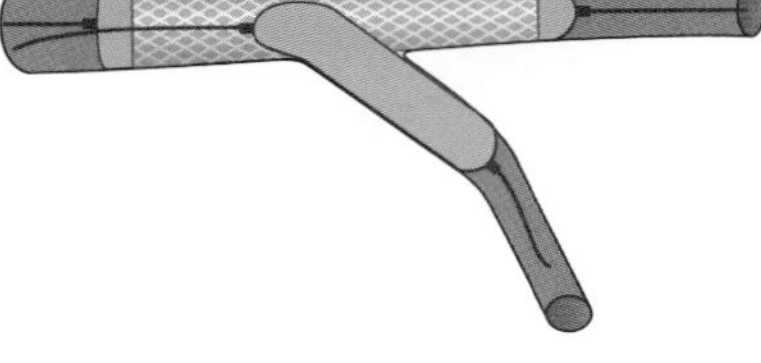

Assuming that the result is suboptimal

3. Advance stent into SB ensuring coverage of ostium with minimal protrusion (1–2 mm) into MB and place non-compliant balloon in MB stent.

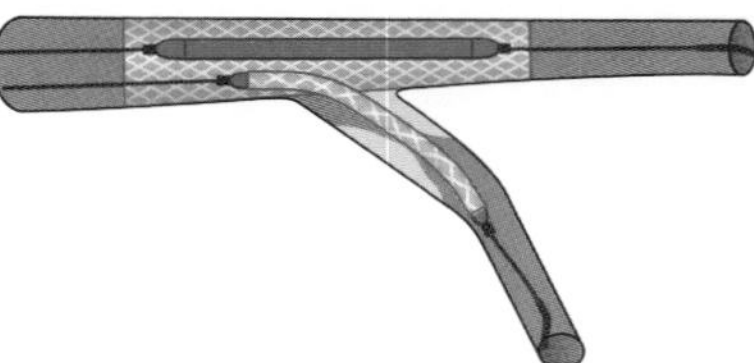

4. Deploy SB stent as usual while MB balloon remains uninflated.

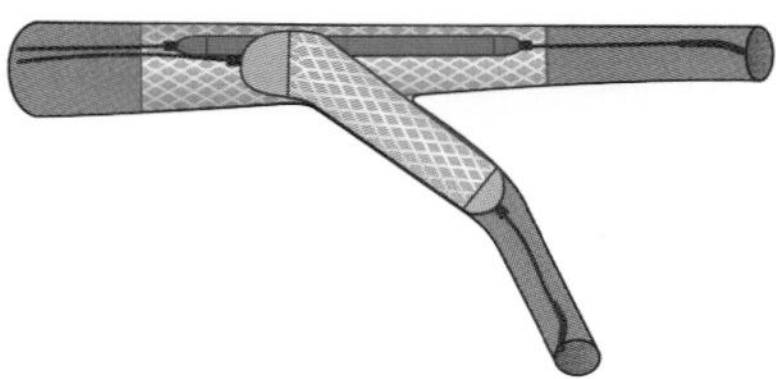

5. Remove SB balloon and ensure that no distal dissection is present before removing SB wire. Inflate MB at high pressure to crush SB stent.

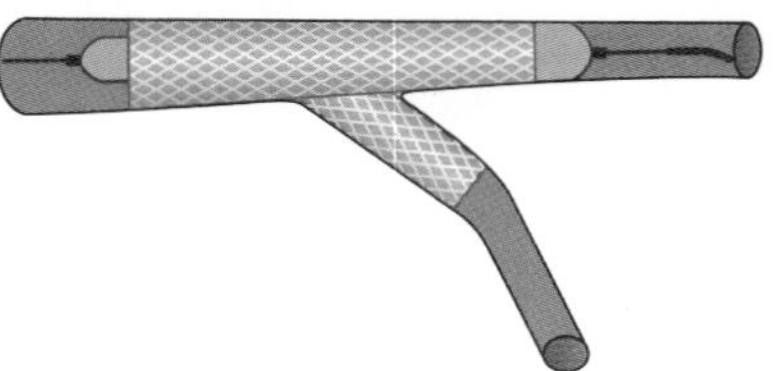

6. To ensure optimal final results at SB ostium, SB balloon must be deflated last when kissing inflation is finished.

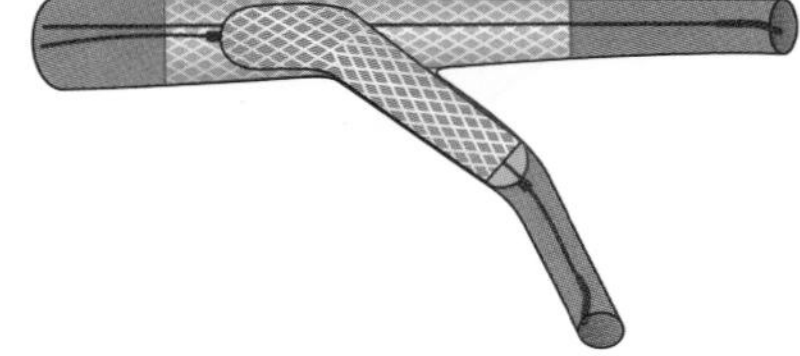

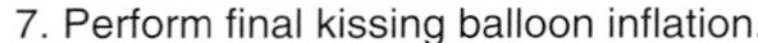

7. Perform final kissing balloon inflation.

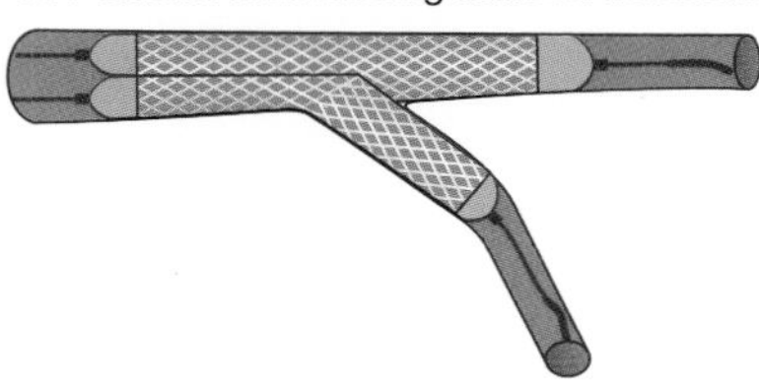

FIGURE 10-10 A schematic representation of the reverse crush technique.

1. Are relatively large in diameter (≥2.5 mm) and have a large territory of distribution (**Figure 10-13**).
2. Have severe disease that extends well beyond the ostium, that is, 10 mm to 20 mm or more (**Figure 10-14**).
3. Have an unfavorable angle for recrossing after MB stent implantation (**Figure 10-15**).

We do not consider these variables in isolation, but there is usually a combination of these factors present that dictates the decision to electively perform double stenting. The only situation in which we would perform double stenting as intention to treat for a nontrue bifurcation with a nondiseased ostium is if there is distal disease close to the ostium that can be covered by a long stent from the MB. We should emphasize that the decision to implant a second stent may also be made at an intermediate time, such as after wire insertion that may favorably modify the bifurcation angle or following predilatation of the MB and SB. However, a timely taken action will affect the result, help save time and cost, and lower the risk of complications.

Selecting a Double Stenting Technique

There are limited data comparing different double stenting bifurcation techniques and there is no unequivocal evidence demonstrating the superiority of one technique over others. The Nordic Stent Technique Study was the first randomized trial comparing two different double stent techniques that result in complete coverage of the SB ostium. In this study, 424 patients were randomized to either crush or culotte stenting utilizing sirolimus-eluting stents (77% of which were true bifurcation lesions).[64] At 6-month clinical follow-up, there were no significant differences between the two groups in terms of death, myocardial infarction, or revascularization (crush 4.3% vs. culotte 3.7%, p = 0.87). Procedure and fluoroscopy times and contrast volumes were also

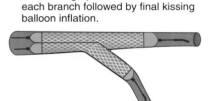

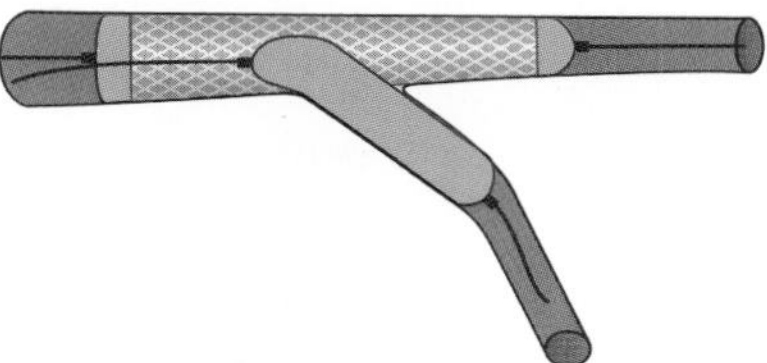

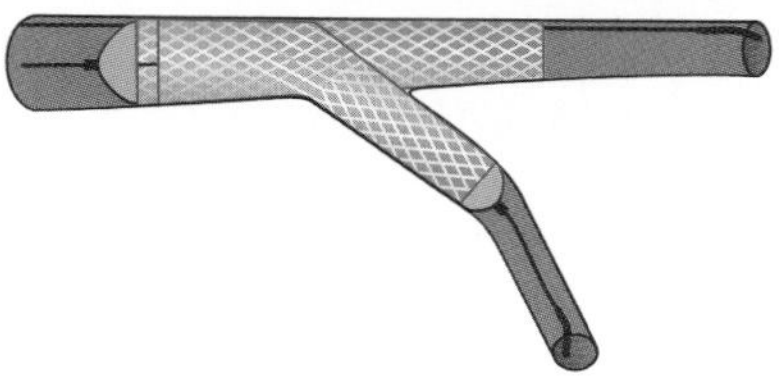

3. Advance stent into SB to overlap with the proximal part of the MB stent and deploy.

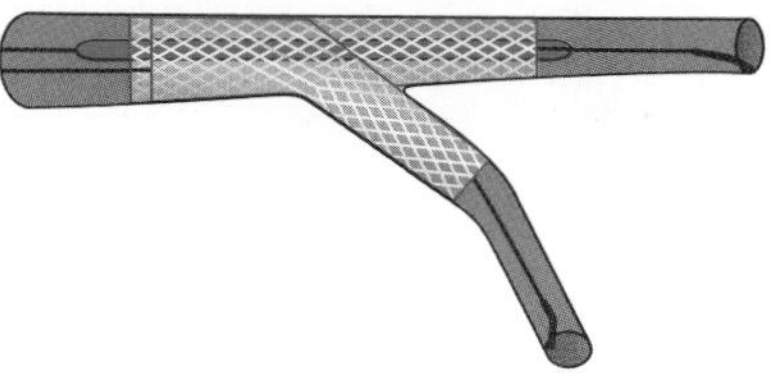

4. Rewire the MB, remove jailed MB wire, and advance a balloon in the MB.

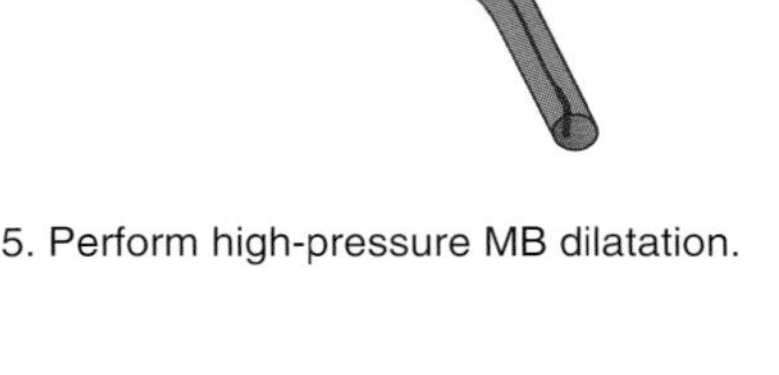

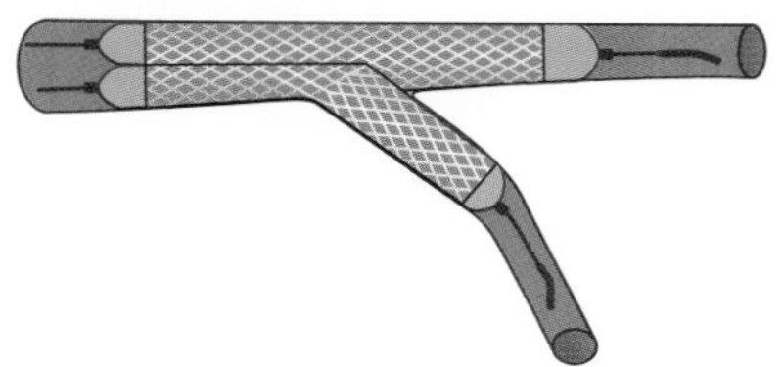

6. Perform high-pressure inflation toward each branch followed by final kissing balloon inflation.

FIGURE 10-11 A schematic representation of the reverse culotte technique.

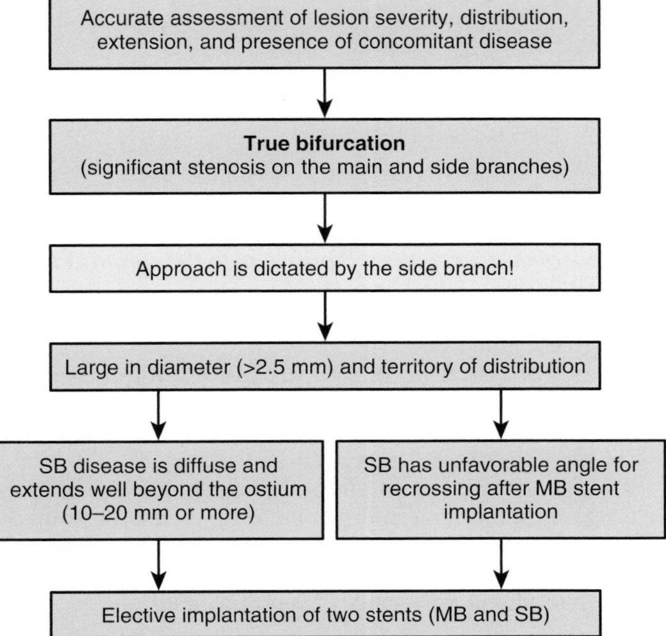

FIGURE 10-12 A proposed algorithm for when to perform elective double stenting. The approach is dictated by the size, angle, and severity of disease of the SB. *MB*, Main branch; *SB*, side branch.

similar in the two groups. However, there was a trend toward a higher incidence of periprocedural MI (crush 15.5% vs. culotte 8.8%, p = 0.08). Angiographically, there was a trend toward less in-segment restenosis (6.6% vs. 12.1%, p = 0.10) and significantly reduced in-stent restenosis following culotte stenting (4.5% vs. 10.5%, p = 0.046). The relevance of this angiographic finding is unclear and may be explained by the lower rate of FKBI in the crush group (85% vs. 92%, p = 0.03) as well as the lack of a two-step FKBI when performing crush stenting. Chen et al. randomized 419 distal left main bifurcation lesions to double stenting with the DK crush or culotte techniques in the DKCRUSH-III study.[25] Only true bifurcation lesions were treated and FKBI was performed in 99.5% of both groups. Procedural and fluoroscopy times were similar but contrast volume was higher in the DK crush group. At 12-month follow-up, the culotte group had a significantly higher MACE rate (16.3% vs. 6.2%, p = 0.001), mainly driven by increased TVR (11% vs. 4.3%, p = 0.016) and TLR (6.7% vs. 2.4%, p = 0.037), compared with the DK group. Also, restenosis in the SB was higher after culotte stenting (12.6% vs. 6.8%, p = 0.037). A definite ST rate was 1.0% in the culotte group and 0% in the DK group (p = 0.248).

As a result of these contradictory findings and other large RCTs, we cannot recommend one technique over another, and certainly not all bifurcations can be treated with a single technique. As summarized in **Figure 10-16**, the

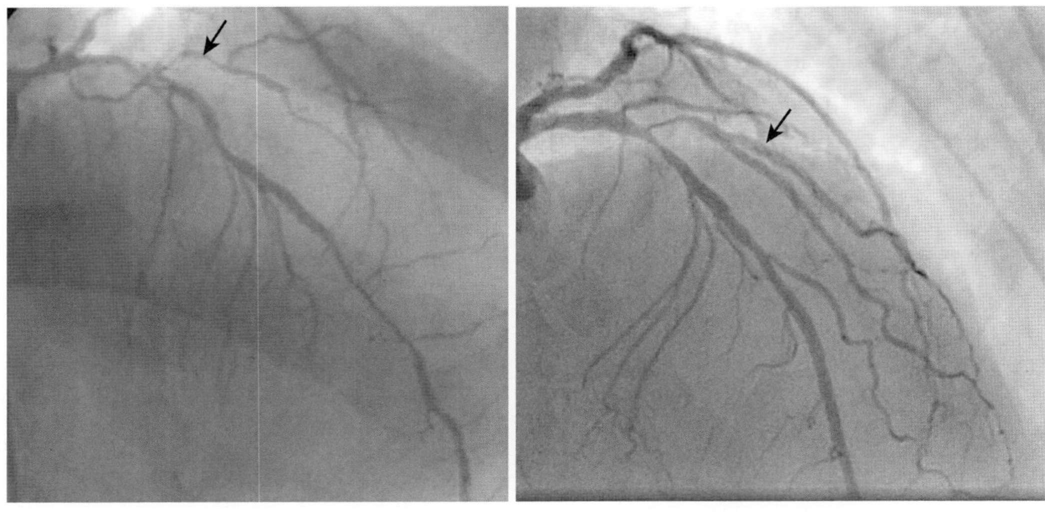

FIGURE 10-13 Angiographic examples of two LAD-diagonal bifurcations showing SBs of different size and territory of distribution.

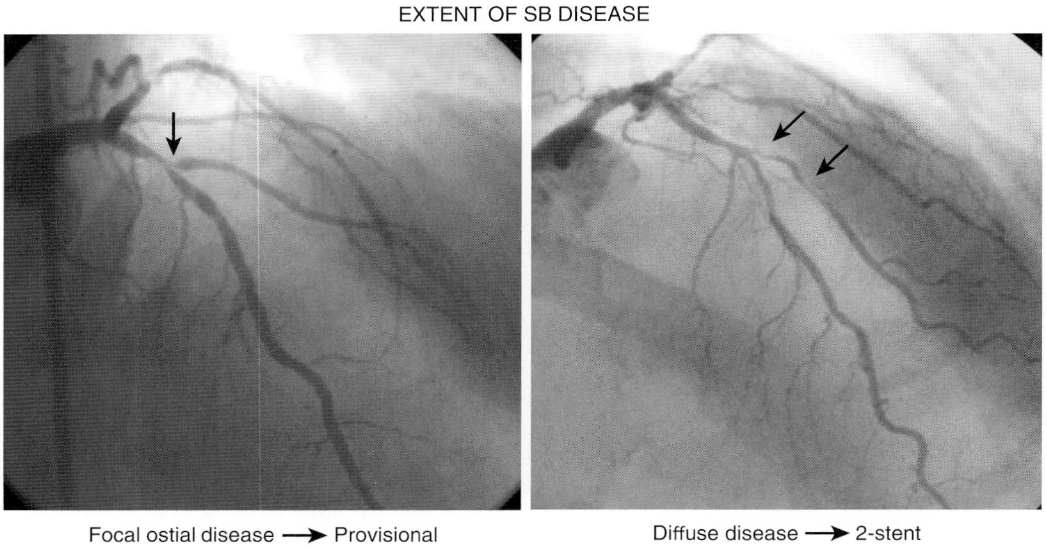

EXTENT OF SB DISEASE

Focal ostial disease → Provisional

Diffuse disease → 2-stent

FIGURE 10-14 Angiographic examples of two LAD-diagonal bifurcations demonstrating SBs with different severity and extent of disease.

selection of the double stenting technique is based on the stability of the patient, the anatomy of the bifurcation, and the familiarity and competence of the operator with a specific technique. Important anatomical factors that need to be considered include the following:

1. *Diameter of the two branches* (**Figure 10-17A-B**; Videos 10-5 through 10-8)
   If similar, use the culotte or minicrush techniques, but if there is a large discrepancy between the proximal MB and SB, the minicrush is preferred.
2. *Bifurcation angle* (**Figure 10-18A-B**; Videos 10-9 through 10-12)
   T-stenting and culotte are preferred when the angle is >70° because the crush technique is associated with a high risk of stent malapposition in the SB. Culotte or crush are preferred with angles <70° and T-stenting should be avoided because it does not provide complete coverage of the SB ostium.
3. *Extent of disease in the MB proximal to the carina* (**Figure 10-19**; Videos 10-13 and 10-14)
   If minimal, V-stenting may be preferred, especially in large proximal SBs.
4. *Severity of the ostial SB stenosis* (does it require aggressive predilatation?)
5. *Presence of dissection in the MB and SB after predilatation* (**Figure 10-20A-B**; Videos 10-15 through 10-17)
   If a dissection is present in both branches of the bifurcation, we prefer the minicrush because it ensures immediate patency of both branches as compared to the culotte, where recrossing stent struts into a dissected branch may be challenging and result in vessel closure.
6. *Complex bifurcations involving large territories or emergencies* (**Figure 10-21A-C**; Videos 10-18 through 10-23)
   In situations where it is crucial to maintain optimal patency of both branches, we recommend the V-stenting or minicrush techniques.

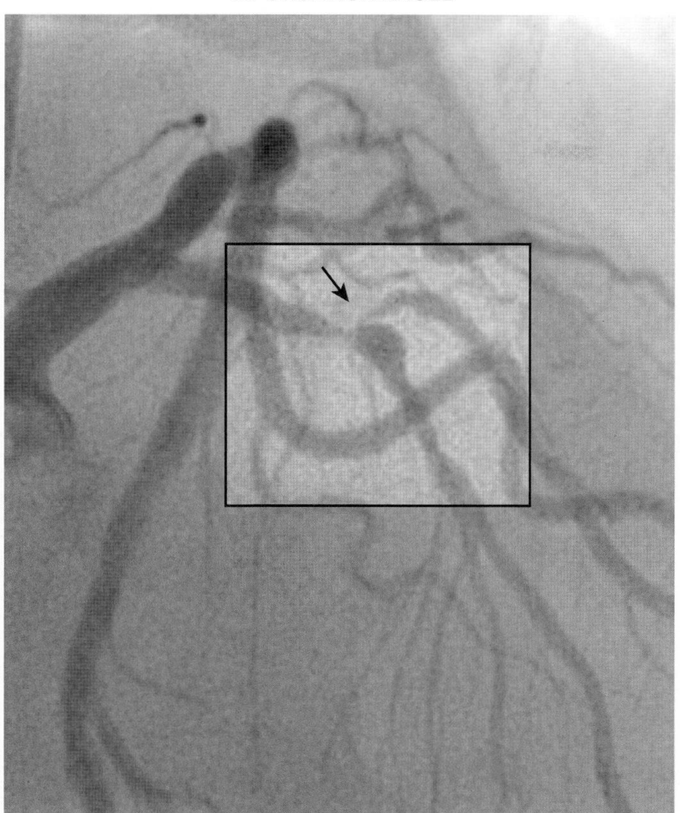

BIFURCATION ANGLE
Difficult to access SB. Access may be even more challenging or even impossible after MB stenting

FIGURE 10-15 Angiographic example of an unfavorable bifurcation angle where elective double stenting would be indicated.

When dealing with complex bifurcations involving large territories or during emergency situations where it is crucial to maintain optimal patency of both branches, we recommend the V-stenting or minicrush techniques. We strongly believe that optimal performance of a double stenting technique and optimization of the final result are more important than which technique is selected and is what determines clinical outcomes. Important technical factors that may contribute to optimizing outcomes when performing two stent techniques include FKBI, high-pressure SB inflation, the use of noncompliant balloons, the selection of the correct balloon size for FKI, and the use of IVUS.[12]

Double Stenting Technique Description

In this section, we describe how to perform and select patients for all of the currently utilized techniques for elective double stenting. We would once again stress that it is not only the specific technique but rather meticulous attention to performing the procedure that is important in ensuring success and improving long-term results.

The Culotte Technique

The culotte technique provides near-perfect coverage of the carina and SB ostium at the expense of an excess of metal covering the proximal end.[61] It gives the best immediate angiographic result, and theoretically, it may guarantee a more homogeneous distribution of struts and drugs at the site of the bifurcation. This technique can be used in almost all true bifurcation lesions irrespective of the bifurcation angle. The only anatomic limitation to the culotte technique is when there is a large mismatch between the proximal MB and SB diameters due to the risk of incomplete SB stent apposition to the proximal MB. The main disadvantage of the technique

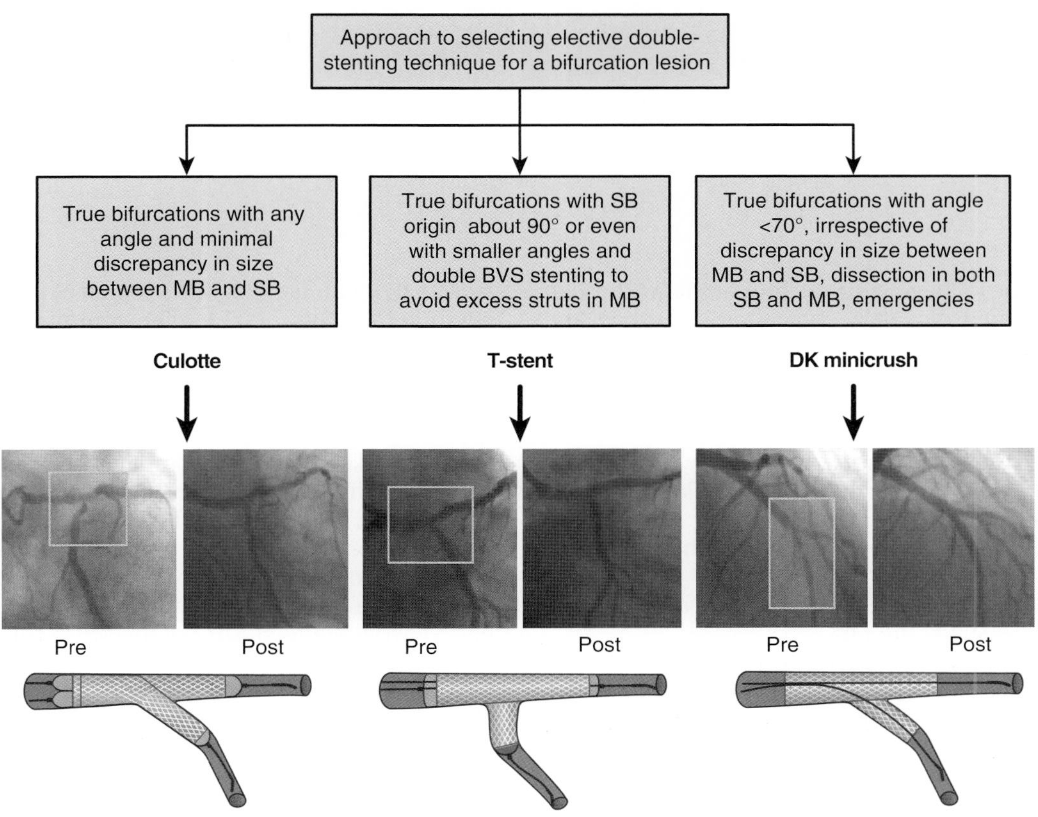

FIGURE 10-16 Algorithm summarizing how to select a double-stenting technique based on anatomy.

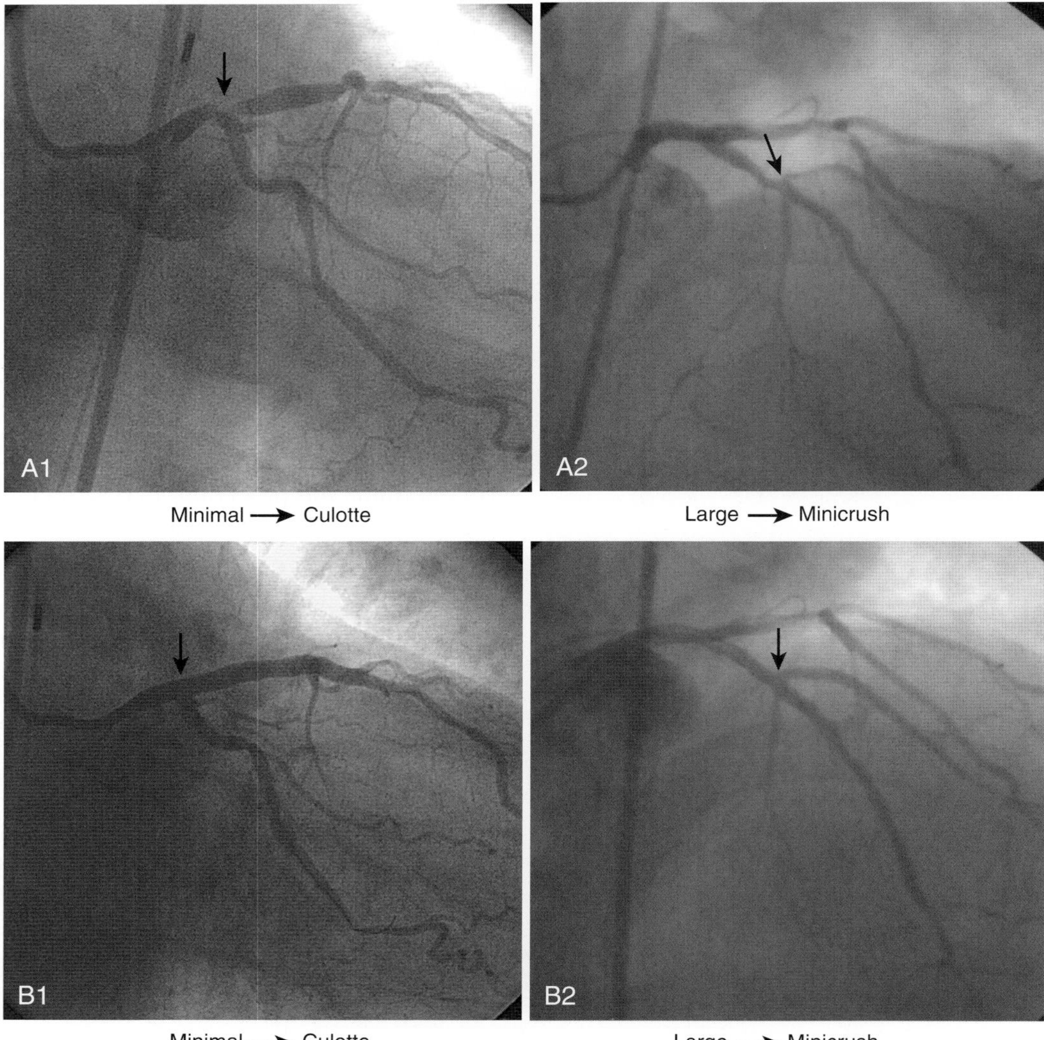

FIGURE 10-17 Angiography demonstrating an LMCA bifurcation with minimal discrepancy between distal left main and circumflex **(A1, Video 10-5)** that would be suitable for culotte stenting **(B1, Video 10-6)** as compared to an LAD-diagonal bifurcation with a large discrepancy between the LAD and diagonal **(A2, Video 10-7)** that would not be suitable for culotte stenting but should rather be treated with a minicrush technique **(B2, Video 10-8)**.

is its complexity due to the rewiring of both branches through the stent struts, which can be technically demanding and time consuming; thus we do not suggest this technique if both branches are dissected after predilatation.

The culotte technique can be performed with a 6 Fr guide catheter (see **Figure 10-22**):

1. Both branches are wired and predilated.
2. A stent is deployed across the most angulated branch, usually the SB.
3. The nonstented branch is rewired through the stent struts and dilated.
4. A second stent is advanced and expanded into the nonstented branch, usually the MB.
5. Kissing balloon inflation is performed. When performing the kissing inflation, we prefer using noncompliant balloons and dilating each limb of the culotte at high pressure (≥16 atm) individually before simultaneously inflating both balloons at 8 atm to 12 atm.

Although the culotte technique may be technically more challenging than other techniques, there are a number of factors that can facilitate its successful performance. When rewiring the other branch after stent placement, we always first place the guidewire distal into the stented branch to be sure that we have not passed under the stent struts before recrossing into the branch. In performing the culotte technique, we recommend stenting the branch with the sharpest angle first. This has the advantage in that recrossing stent struts into the less angulated branch will be easier as will passing the second stent through stent struts into a less angulated branch. However, this conventional practice has recently been challenged in the Nordic Stent Technique Study, where the authors recommended stenting of the MB first to avoid acute closure of the MB.[64] This approach guarantees patency of the MB and may avoid one of the potential problems of performing the culotte technique, where we always need to remove the wire from one of the two branches and patency of this branch is not guaranteed. It is for this reason we prefer not to perform the culotte technique if there is a dissection in both branches after predilatation.

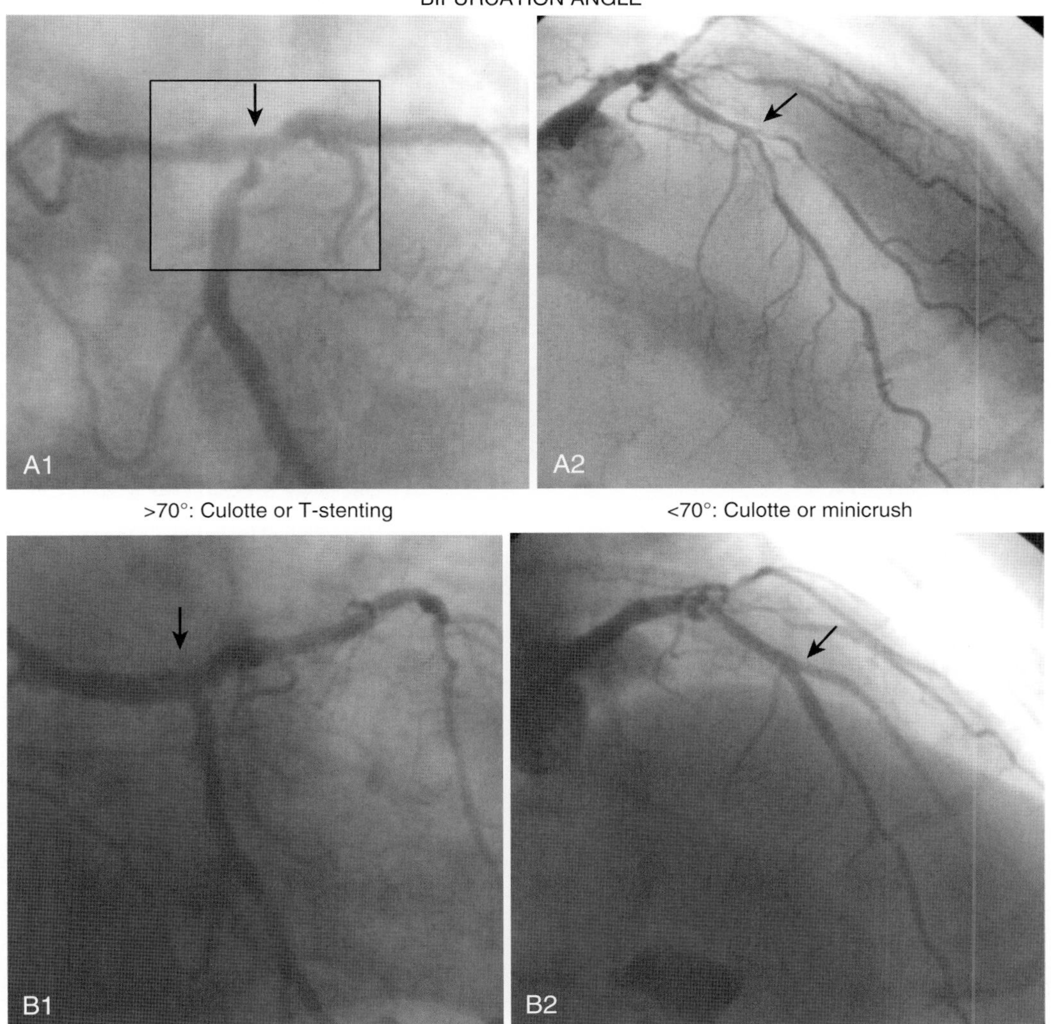

FIGURE 10-18 Angiography demonstrating an LMCA bifurcation with an angle between distal LAD and circumflex >70° **(A1, Video 10-9)** where culotte or T-stenting would be preferred over the crush **(B1, Video 10-10)** as compared to an LAD-diagonal bifurcation with an angle <70° between distal LAD and diagonal **(A2, Video 10-11)** that would not be suitable for T-stenting but should rather be treated with a minicrush or culotte technique **(B2, Video 10-12)**.

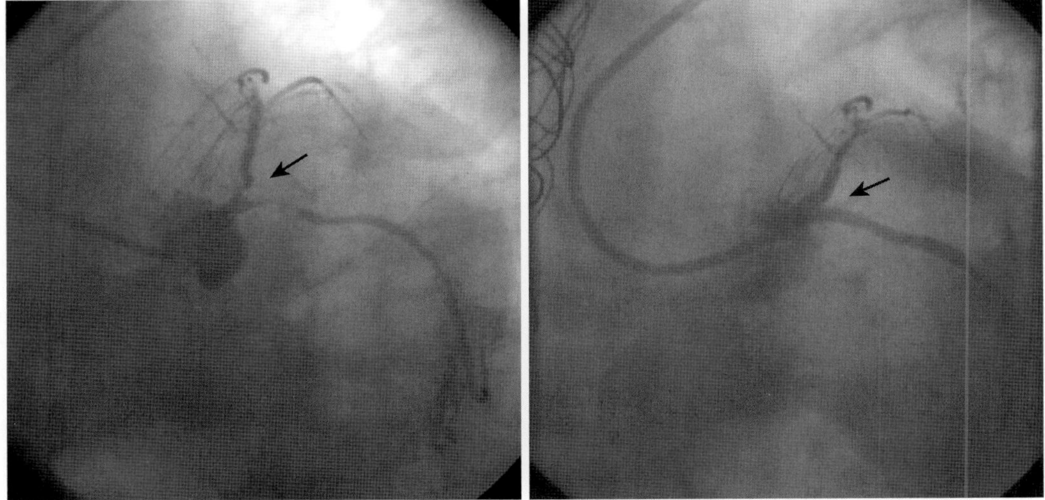

FIGURE 10-19 Angiography showing a Medina 0.1.1 bifurcation with minimal disease in the proximal MB that would be suitable for V-stenting (**Videos 10-13 and 10-14**).

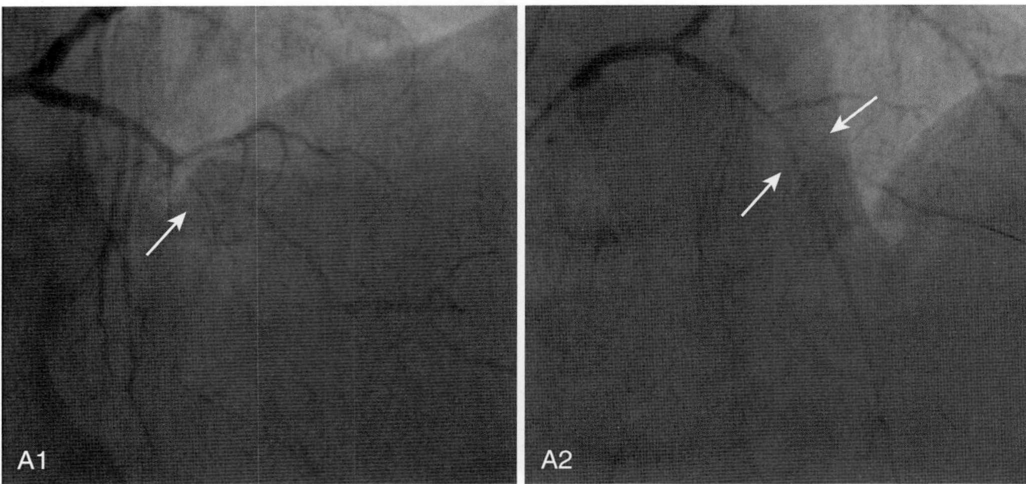

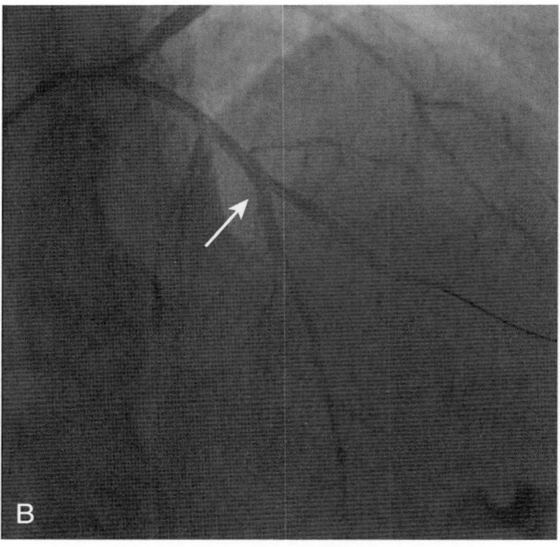

FIGURE 10-20 Angiography showing a chronic total occlusion of an LAD-diagonal bifurcation **(A1, Video 10-15)** that, after wire passage and predilatation, shows a dissection of both branches **(A2, Video 10-16).** The bifurcation was treated with the double-kissing minicrush technique because it guarantees patency of both branches and avoids having to recross stent struts into a dissected branch **(B, Video 10-17).**

The Minicrush Technique (SB Stent Crushed by the MB Stent)

The main advantage of the crush technique is that immediate patency of both branches is assured and therefore it should be applied in conditions of instability or when the anatomy appears complex.[22] This objective is notably important when the SB is functionally relevant or difficult to be wired. In addition, this technique provides excellent coverage of the ostium of the SB. It can be used in almost all true bifurcation lesions but should be avoided in wide-angle bifurcations. The main disadvantage is that to perform FKBI, there is the need to recross multiple struts with a wire and a balloon. However, only the SB has to be rewired and not both branches as in the culotte technique. The crush technique has evolved and is presently performed with less stent protrusion into the MB (i.e., minicrush) and mandatory two-step FKI.[65,66]

The minicrush technique requires at least a 7 Fr guide catheter (see **Figure 10-23**):

1. Both branches are wired and fully dilated.
2. The SB stent is positioned in the SB and then the MB stent is advanced.
3. The SB stent is pulled back into the MB about 1 mm to 2 mm and is verified in at least two projections.
4. The SB stent is deployed at least at 12 atm. The balloon is deflated and removed from the guide catheter. An angiogram is taken to verify that the SB has an appropriate lumen and normal flow and that no distal dissection or residual lesions are present. If an additional stent is needed in the SB, this is the time to implant it. Following this check, the stent in the MB is fully deployed at high pressure, usually above 12 atm. An angiogram is taken following removal of the balloon from the MB. When we use this technique, we keep only a single indeflator on the table that is connected to the SB stent. This will prevent inadvertent deployment of the MB stent first, thereby crushing the undeployed SB stent.

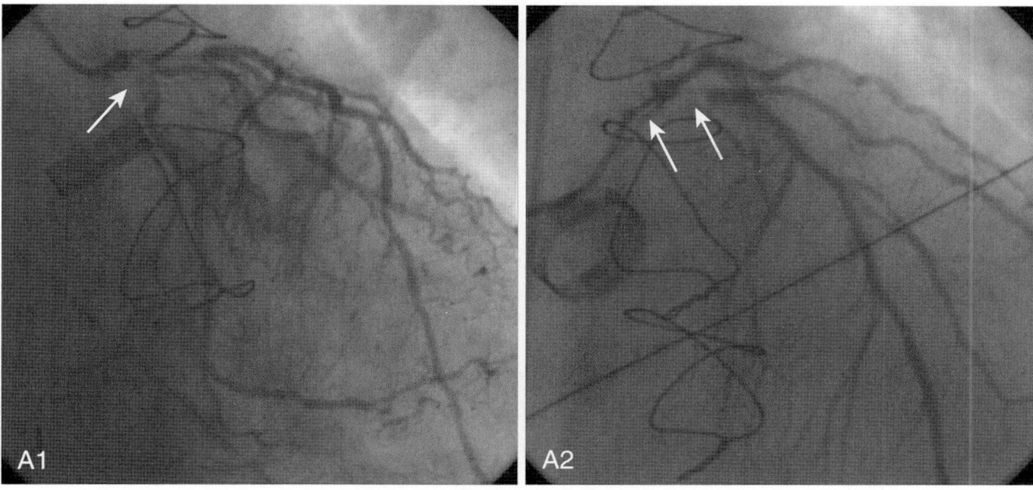

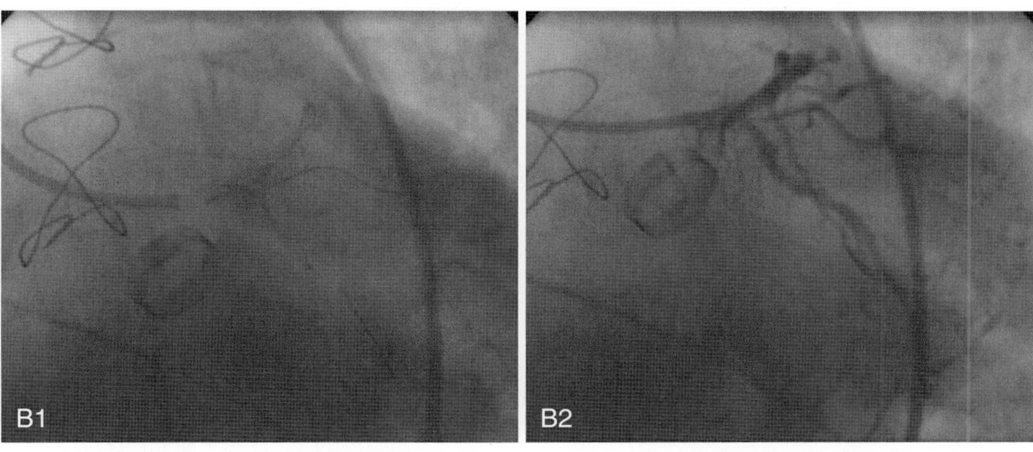

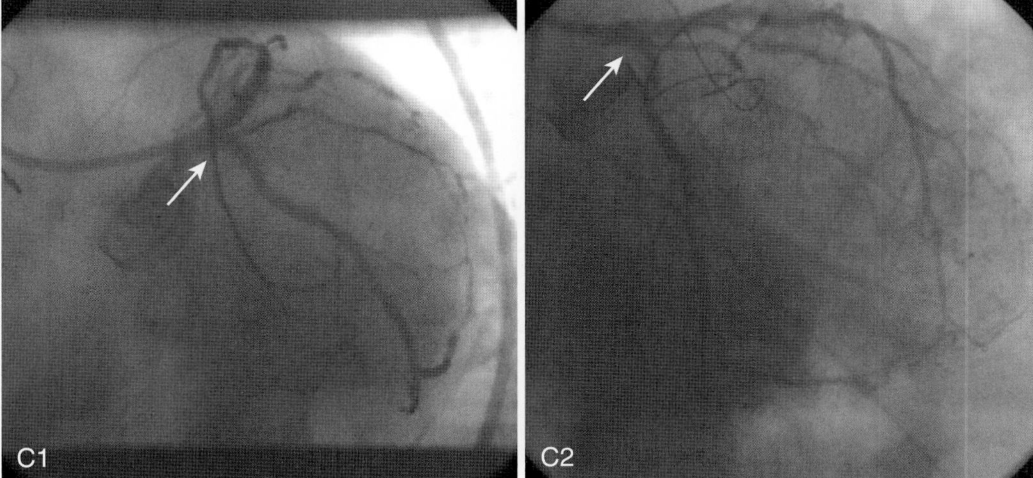

FIGURE 10-21 Baseline angiography in a patient presenting with a STEMI and cardiogenic shock showing severe thrombotic occlusion of the distal left main involving the proximal LAD and circumflex **(A1, A2, Videos 10-18 and 10-19).** In this emergency situation, where rapid and immediate patency of both branches needs to be guaranteed, the V-stenting and classical minicrush techniques are preferred. The procedure was performed with an 8Fr guide catheter, and both stents were placed at the same time with the SB stent protruding minimally into the MB **(B1, Video 10-20);** the SB stent was inflated first and the stent delivery balloon removed, followed by inflation of the MB stent. Angiography immediately after stent implantation confirmed patency of both branches **(B2, Video 10-21),** and the final result after optimization with a two-step FKBI is shown in **C1** and **C2** and **Videos 10-22 and 10-23**.

1. Wire both branches and predilate if needed.

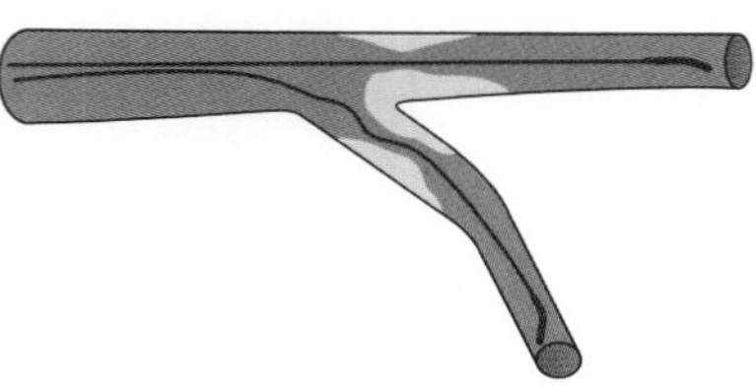

2. Leave the wire in the more straight branch (MB) and deploy a stent in the more angulated branch (SB).

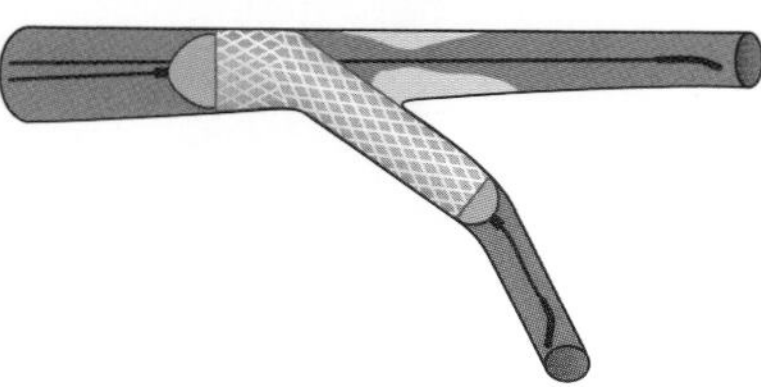

3. Rewire the unstented branch and dilate the stent struts to unjail the branch (MB).

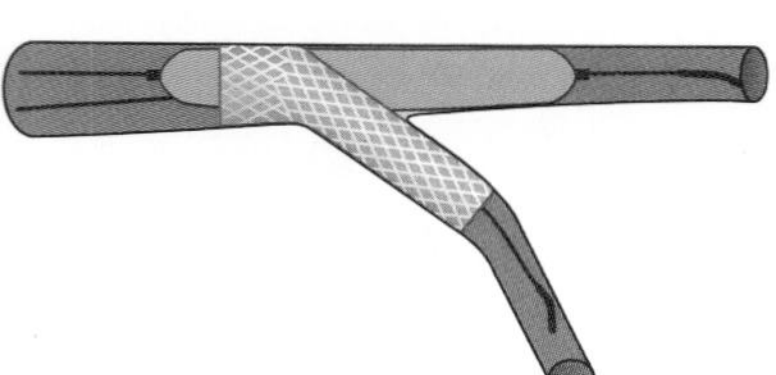

4. Place a second stent into the unstented branch (MB) and expand the stent leaving some proximal overlap.

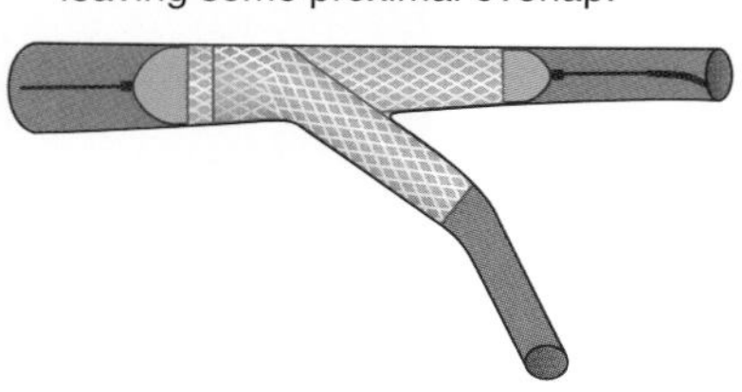

5. Re-cross the 2nd stent's (MB) struts into the 1st stent (SB) with a wire and perform kissing balloon inflation.

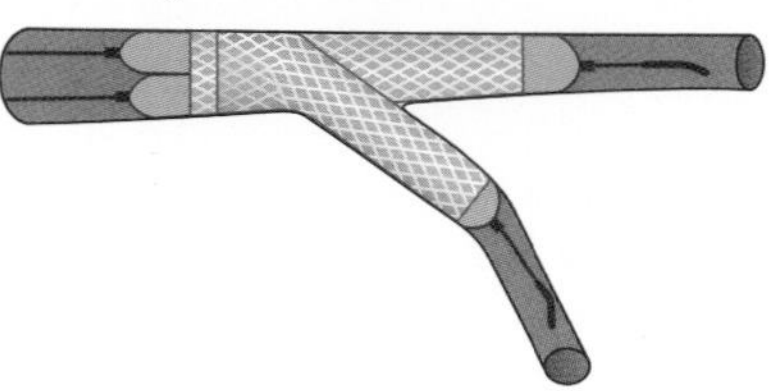

FIGURE 10-22 A schematic representation of the culotte technique.

1. Wire both branches and predilate if needed.

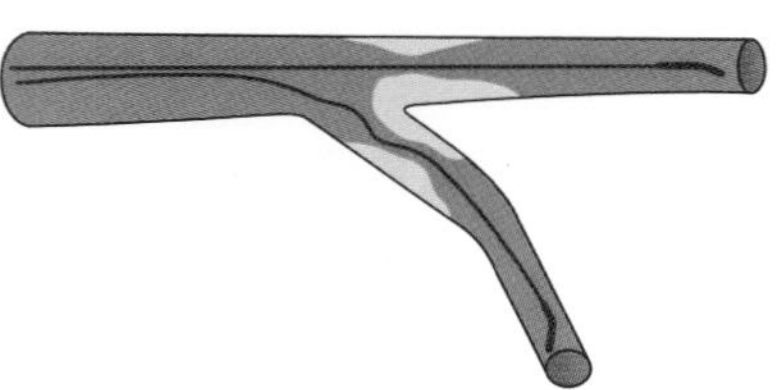

2. Advance the 2 stents. MB stent positioned proximally. SB stent will protrude only minimally into MB.

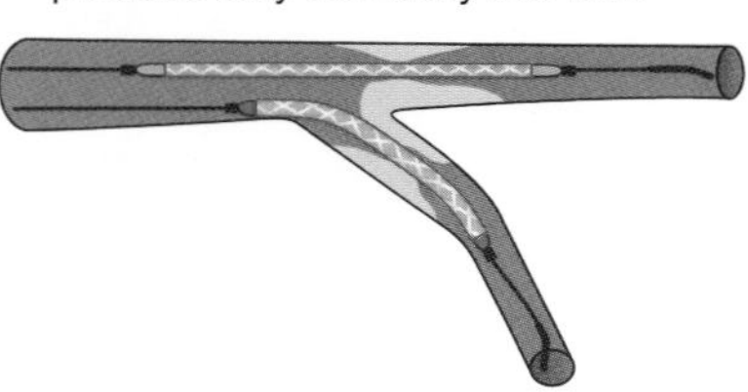

3. Deploy the SB stent.

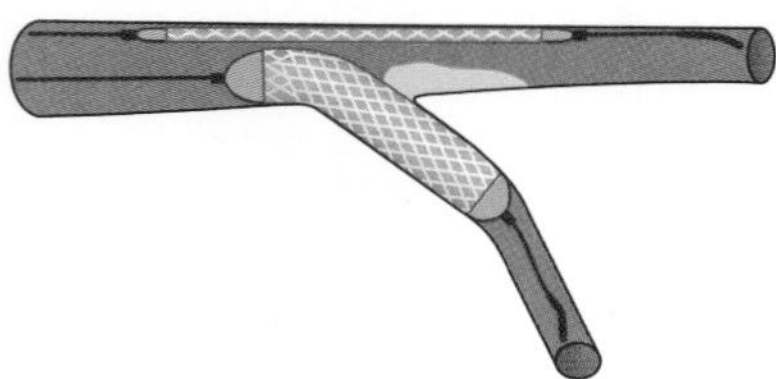

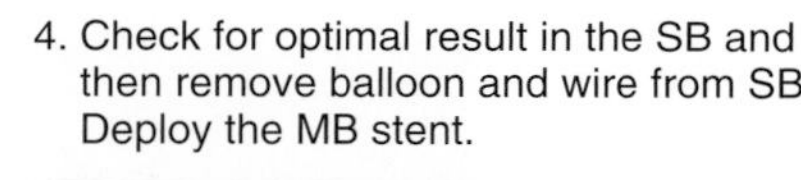

4. Check for optimal result in the SB and then remove balloon and wire from SB. Deploy the MB stent.

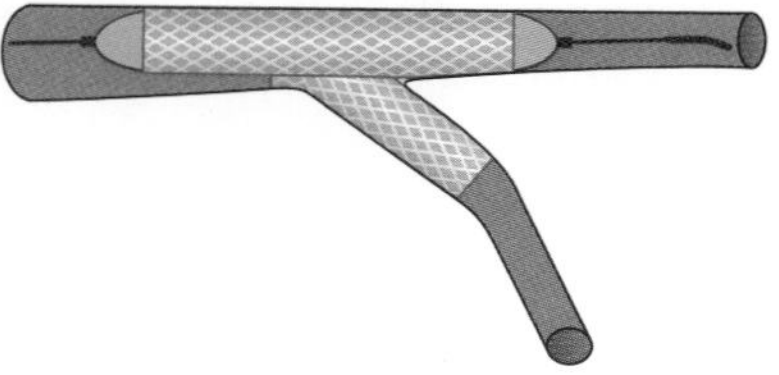

5. Rewire the SB and perform high-pressure dilatation.

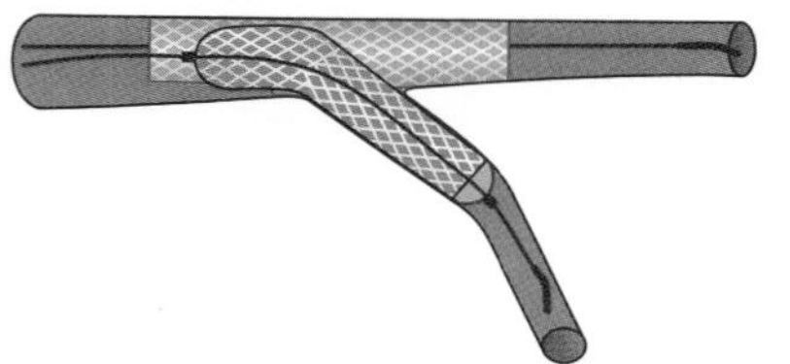

6. Perform final kissing balloon inflation.

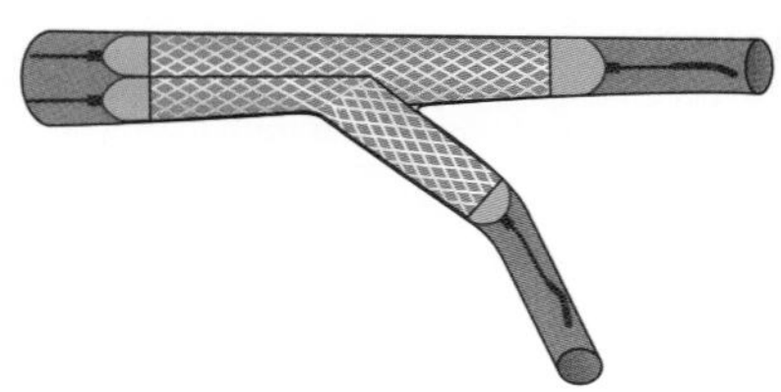

FIGURE 10-23 A schematic representation of the classical minicrush technique.

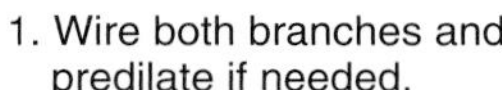
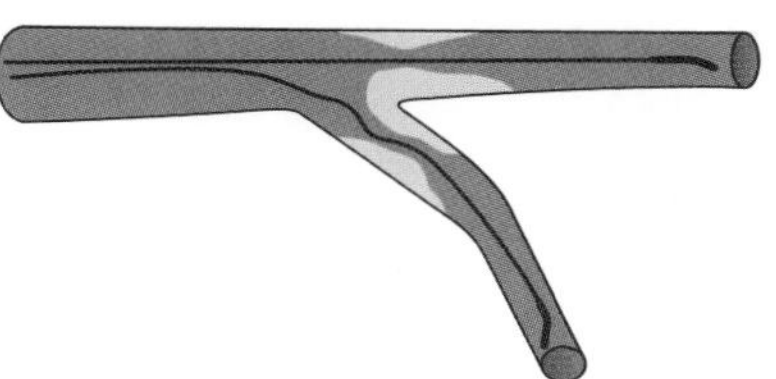
1. Wire both branches and predilate if needed.

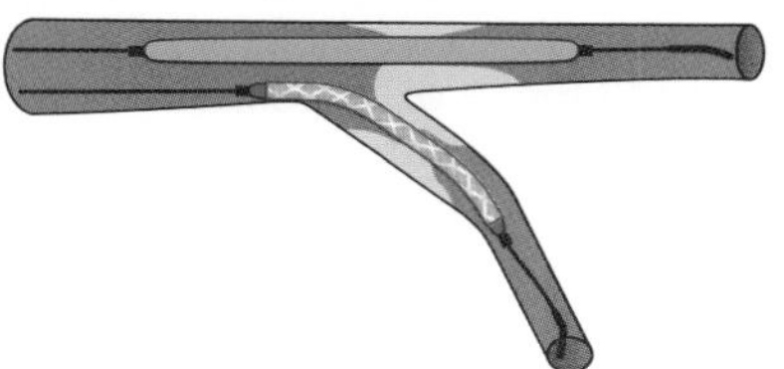
2. Advance the SB stent with only minimal protrusion in MB and place non-compliant balloon in MB stent.

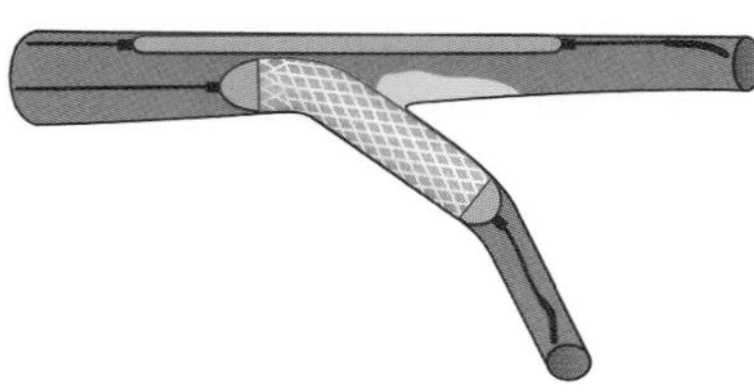
3. Deploy the SB stent.

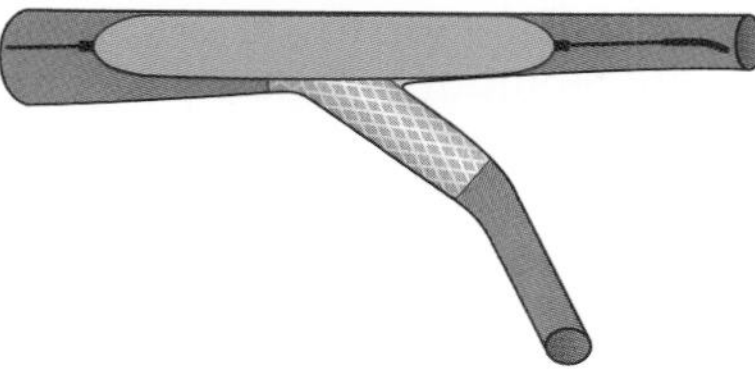
4. Check for optimal result in the SB and then remove balloon and wire from SB.

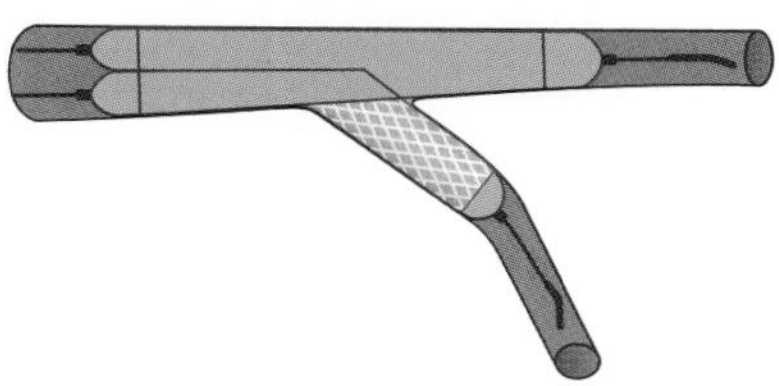
5. Rewire SB, dilate SB struts, and perform the first kissing balloon inflation.

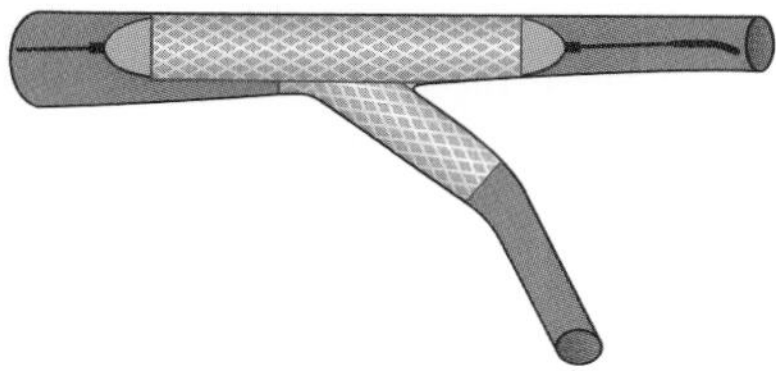
6. Advance stent in MB and deploy.

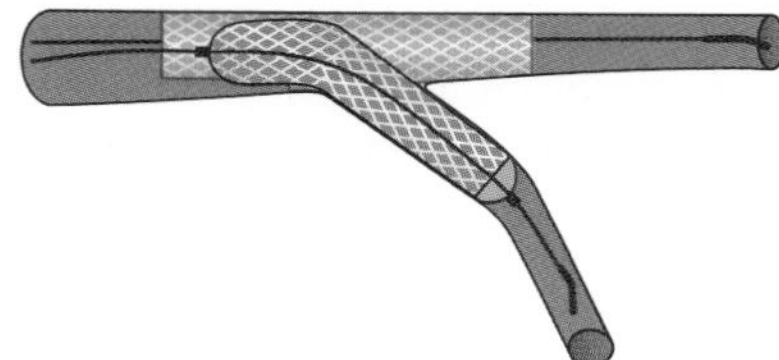
7. Rewire the SB and perform high-pressure dilatation.

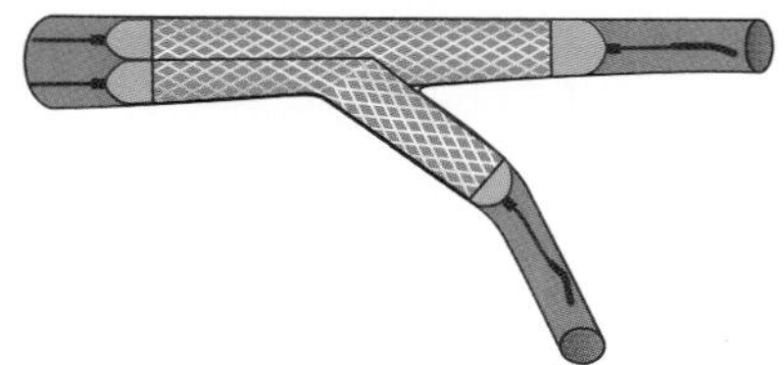
8. Perform final kissing inflation.

FIGURE 10-24 A schematic representation of the double-kissing minicrush technique.

5. Rewire the SB. It is important to perform a two-step FKI. First, we suggest a dilatation of the stent toward the SB with a balloon appropriately sized to the diameter of this branch and inflated at high pressure (16 atm or more). Then we suggest FKI with a second balloon in the MB with an inflation pressure approximately 8 atm to 14 atm in both balloons.

Double-Kissing Minicrush (DK Crush)

When there is the need to perform the minicrush technique and a 6 Fr guide catheter is the only available approach (radial approach), the "step crush" or "the modified balloon crush" technique can be used. The final result is basically similar to that obtained with the standard crush technique, with the only difference being that each stent is advanced and deployed separately. We now routinely perform the double-kissing (DK) crush technique. This technique is a modification of the step crush where kissing balloon inflation is performed twice: first after the SB stent is crushed by the MB balloon and then the routine FKBI at the end of the procedure. DK crush may result in less stent distortion and improved stent apposition and facilitate FKI. This technique may be superior to the classic crush technique in optimizing acute procedural results and possibly also improves clinical outcomes by facilitating FKBI in all patients.[67] Unless there is a compelling reason to obtain immediate patency of the MB and the SB (need for the standard minicrush technique with a 7 Fr or 8 Fr guide catheter), we recommend that the DK crush be the default two-stent technique, when this approach is selected as intention to treat.

The double-kissing minicrush technique can be performed with a 6 Fr guide catheter (see **Figure 10-24**):

1. Both branches are wired and fully dilated.
2. The stent is advanced in the SB, protruding a few millimeters into the MB. A balloon is advanced in the MB over the bifurcation.
3. The stent in the SB is deployed, the balloon is removed, an angiogram is performed, and if the result is adequate, the wire is also removed.
4. The MB balloon is then inflated (to crush the protruding SB stent) and removed.

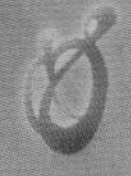

5. The crushed SB stent is then recrossed and a two-step kissing balloon inflation is performed.
6. A second stent is advanced in the MB and deployed (usually at 12 atm or more).
7. The next steps are similar to those of the classical crush technique and involve recrossing into the SB, SB stent dilatation, and a two-step final kissing balloon inflation.

An important change in the classical crush technique is that we now try to limit the area of crush stenting and multiple layering of stent struts by performing a minicrush. The minicrush may be associated with more complete endothelialization (and theoretically less stent thrombosis) and easier recrossing of the crushed stent. Finally, the bifurcation angle may be an important factor to be considered when performing the crush technique. When the angle between the MB and SB is close to 90°, it is possible to minimize the gap even without crushing the SB stent and utilizing the modified T technique. Furthermore, a bifurcation angle B ≥ 50° between the two branches has been suggested as an independent predictor of MACE after crush stenting.[68]

T and Modified T Techniques

The T technique is the most frequently utilized to cross over from provisional stenting to stenting the SB and is most suited to bifurcations where the angle between the branches is close to 90°. This technique is less laborious than the crush or culotte techniques. In our view, the T technique is associated with the risk to leave a small gap between the stent implanted in the MB and the one implanted in the SB. This gap may be a factor contributing to an uneven distribution of the drugs, leading to ostial restenosis at the SB. For this reason, this technique has largely been replaced by the modified T-stenting technique. Currently, we rarely perform the classical T technique in our practice; in our opinion, there are two reasons to perform the classical T technique: The first reason is to place a stent at the ostium of an SB after placement of a stent in the MB, because the result at the SB ostium was unsatisfactory (provisional SB stenting). In this situation, we have replaced the classical T technique with the TAP (T and Protrusion). The second reason is to perform stenting at the ostium of the SB when there is isolated SB ostial stenosis (e.g., T-balloon stenting).

The classical T technique requires a 6 Fr guide catheter:

1. Position a stent first at the ostium of the SB, being careful to avoid stent protrusion into the MB while trying to minimize any possible gap.
2. Deploy the stent and remove the balloon from the SB (keep the wire in the SB).
3. Advance and deploy the MB stent.
4. Rewire the SB and remove the jailed wire.
5. Perform SB balloon dilatation and FKI.

The above description of T-stenting describes the situation in which the operator decides to stent the SB first. However, in the majority of cases, the T-stenting technique is performed after MB and provisional SB stenting for a suboptimal result of flow-limiting dissection.

Modified T Technique

Modified T-stenting is a variation performed by simultaneously positioning stents at the SB and MB (requires at least a 7 Fr guide catheter), with the SB stent minimally protruding into the MB when the angle between the branches is close to 90° (**Figure 10-25**). The SB stent is deployed first, and then after wire and balloon removal from the SB, the MB stent is deployed. The procedure is completed with FKBI.

The V and the Simultaneous Kissing Stent (SKS) Techniques

The V and the SKS techniques are performed by delivering and implanting two stents together.[69,70] One stent is advanced into the SB and the other into the MB. Both stents are pulled back to create a neocarina as close as possible to the original one. When the two stents protrude into the MB with the creation of a double barrel and a very proximal carina, the technique is called SKS.[70] The main advantage of these techniques is that access to both branches is always preserved during the procedure with no need for rewiring any of the branches. V-stenting is relatively easy and fast and thus ideal in emergencies. In addition, when FKI is performed, there is no need to recross the SB stent. V-stenting is ideal for Medina 0:1:1 bifurcations with a large proximal MB that is relatively free from disease and with a <90° angle between both branches. We reserve this technique for patients with a short LMCA free from disease and critical disease of both the LAD and LCX ostia. Interestingly, a modified V-technique (Y or Skirt technique) with two stents deployed together on the SB and distal MB and a stent (manually crimped onto two balloons) placed in the proximal MB was the first double stenting technique utilized for coronary bifurcations and to be demonstrated in a live case course.[71]

The V and Simultaneous Kissing Stent techniques require at least a 7 Fr guide catheter (see **Figure 10-26**):

1. Both branches are wired and fully predilated.
2. Two stents are positioned into the branches with a slight protrusion of both stents into the proximal MB. Different operators allow a variable amount of protrusion creating sometimes a rather long (5 or more mm) double barrel in the proximal MB (SKS). While we recognize that it is impossible to be so accurate in positioning the stents exactly at the ostium of each branch, we generally try to limit the length of the new carina to less than 5 mm. Sometimes it is necessary to advance the first stent more distally into the vessel to facilitate the advancement of the second stent. This maneuver is essential when the kissing stent technique is used to stent a trifurcation using three kissing stents (need of a 9 Fr guide catheter). Following accurate stent positioning, it is important to verify their correct placement in two projections before deploying the stents.
3. Each stent is deployed individually at high pressure of 12 atm or more. Some operators prefer deploying the stents simultaneously. When the stents are deployed simultaneously, the operator needs to be aware of the risk of proximal MB dissection. This can be avoided by using lower deployment pressure.
4. Perform high-pressure sequential single stent postdilatation followed by medium-pressure FKI with short and noncompliant balloons. Balloon sizes are chosen according to the diameter of the treated vessels. In the event that the reference vessel size proximal to the bifurcation is relatively small, FKBI should be performed using low-pressure inflation to avoid proximal dissection.

There are several limitations for this technique that need to be considered: (a) There is a possibility of balloon barotrauma to the proximal MB during stent deployment or postdilatation, which can lead to dissection, progression of disease, or proximal edge restenosis; (b) if a proximal stent

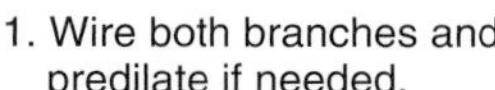

1. Wire both branches and predilate if needed.

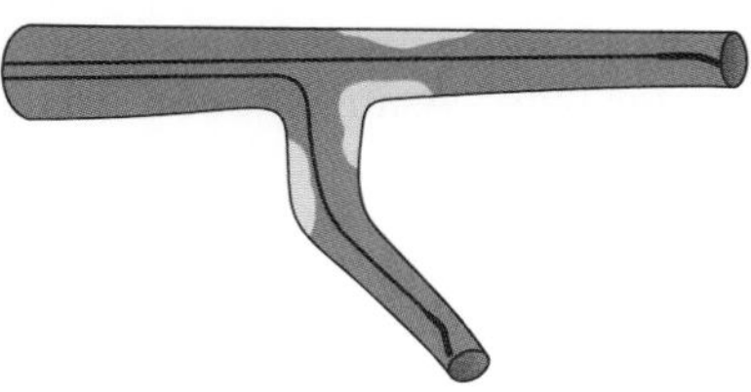

2. Advance the 2 stents. SB stent positioned with minimal protrusion into MB.

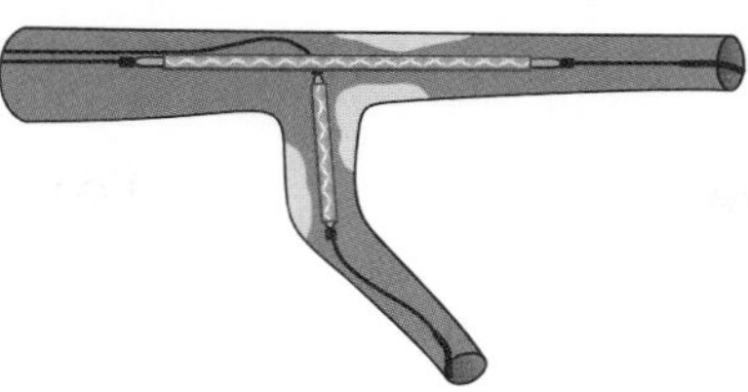

3. SB stent deployed at nominal pressure.

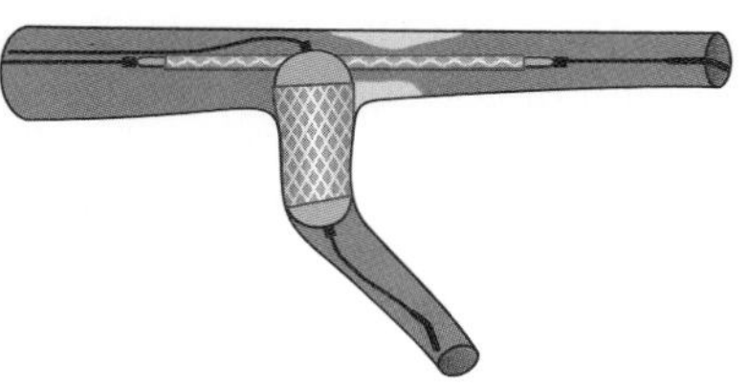

4. Check for optimal result in the SB and then remove balloon and wire from SB. Deploy the MB stent at high pressure.

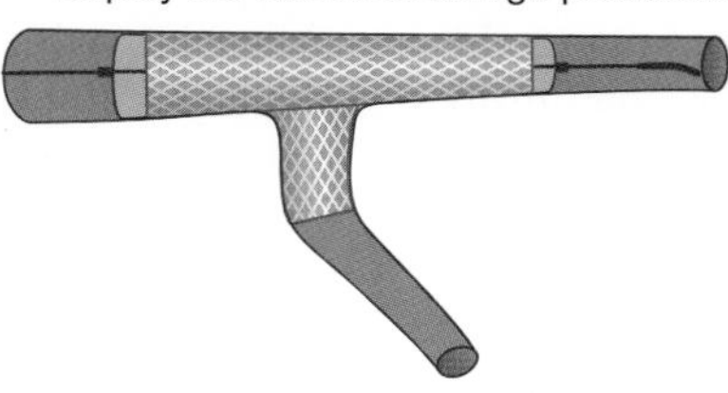

5. Rewire the SB and perform high-pressure dilatation.

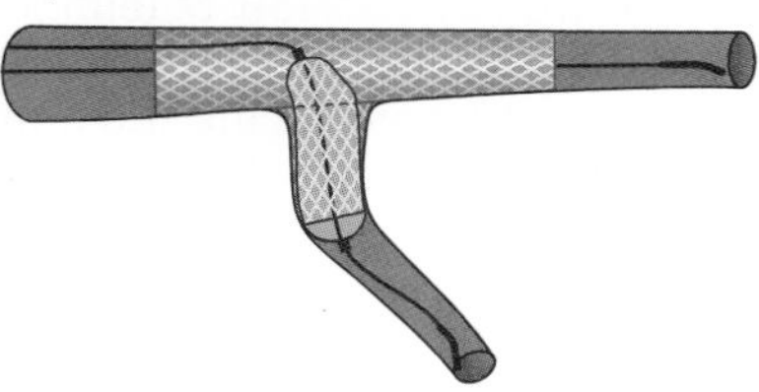

6. Perform final kissing inflation following advancement of a balloon into the MB.

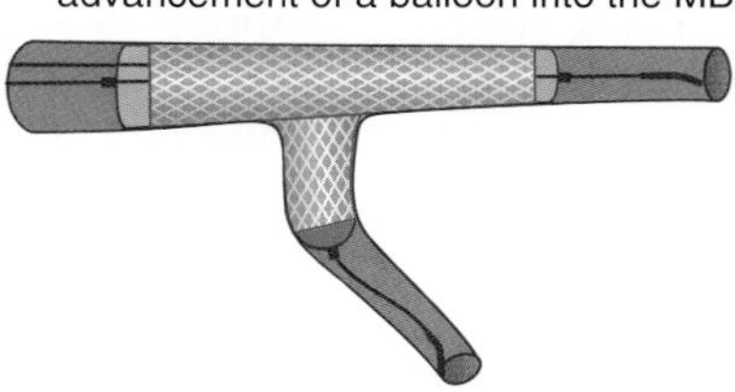

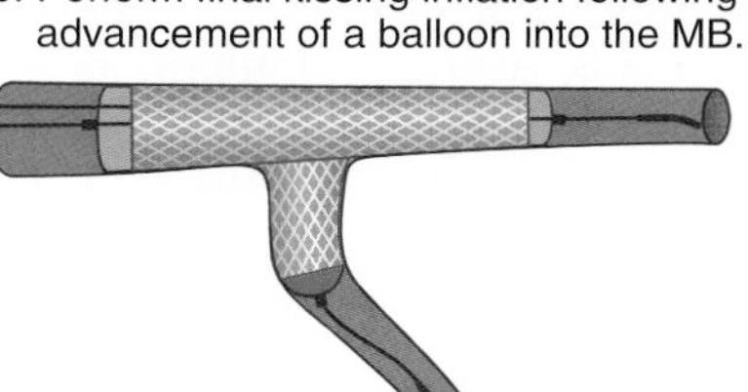

FIGURE 10-25 A schematic representation of the modified T-stenting technique.

1. Wire both branches and predilate if needed.

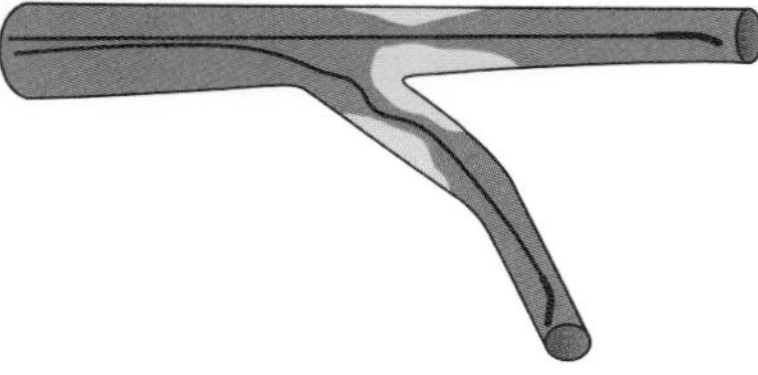

2. Position two parallel stents covering both branches and extending into the MB.
V: minimal protrusion into MB.
SKS: double barrel into the MB.

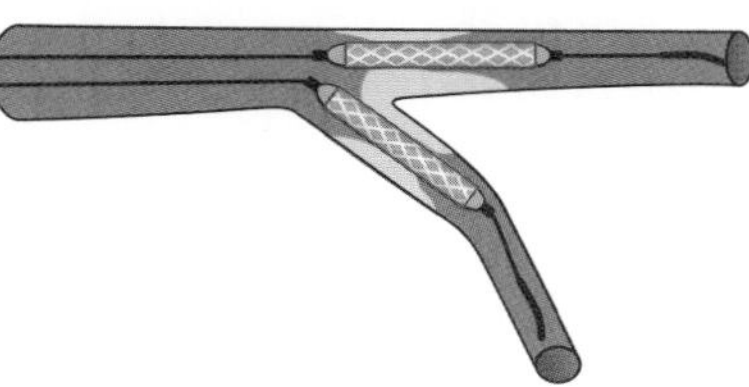

3. Deploy one stent.

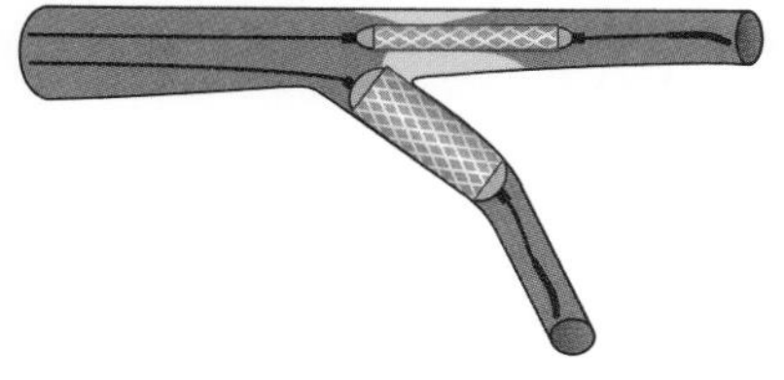

4. Deploy the second stent.

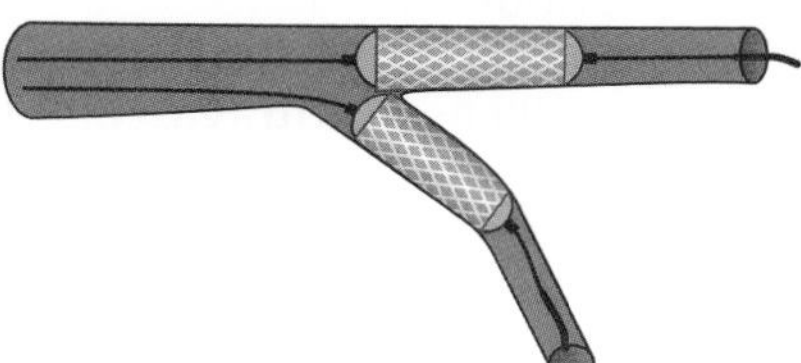

Some operators deploy the two stents simultaneously

5. Perform high-pressure single stent postdilatation and medium-pressure kissing inflation with short and non-compliant balloons.

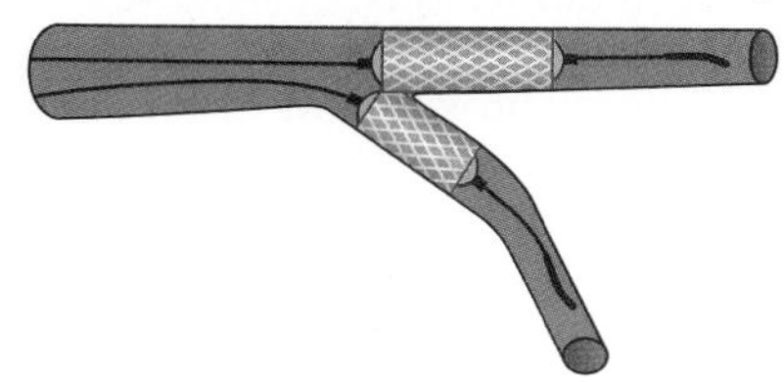

FIGURE 10-26 A schematic representation of the V-stenting technique.

becomes necessary to treat a proximal dissection, there is almost always the risk of leaving a small gap, and the stent needs to be directed toward one of the two arms of the V; (c) if restenosis occurs in the neocarina or at the proximal stent edge, it would require converting to the crush technique for treatment, which would make recrossing into the branch covered by the crushed stent potentially challenging, as four layers of stent struts would need to be traversed; (d) if disease distal to the V-stenting or SKS site needs to be treated at follow-up, rewiring the stented vessels may be complicated by the wire passage behind the stent struts. If additional guidewires need to be inserted during the procedure to treat distal disease, we recommend using a dual access catheter such as the Twin-Pass catheter (Vascular Solutions, Minnesota). When previous V-stenting or SKS needs traversing at another PCI, we suggest passing through the stent with a loop on the radiopaque part of the guidewire to prevent the guidewire from passing through the stent struts.

The SKS technique results in a new metallic carina quite proximally into the LMCA. We do not know what the long-term outcome risks are of leaving this exposed double stent layer in a vessel when utilizing DES. There have been case reports describing a thin diaphragmatic membranous structure at the new carina (at the level of the kissing struts) resulting in an angiographic filling defect. Other than producing a very distressing angiographic appearance, the exact long-term significance and relation to adverse advents of this membrane are not known.[63]

Final Kissing Inflation (FKBI) after Double Stenting

FKBI for carina reconstruction is mandatory in two-stent techniques. A special mention needs to be made of the importance of FKI when implanting two stents in LMCA bifurcations. FKI is not only important in correcting stent distortion and expansion[37,38] but is especially significant in fully expanding the stent in the distal LMCA, where the diameter is usually much larger than the diameters of the LAD and LCX. The effective balloon diameter in the distal LMCA (which we calculate as the MB balloon diameter plus one third of the SB balloon diameter) from the two balloons used for FKBI is essential to fully expand the stent(s). In performing FKBI, it is critical to choose noncompliant, post-dilatation balloons of appropriate size; that is, the kissing balloons should be the same size or larger than the deploying balloons to prevent stent distortion.[37] As previously mentioned, individual noncompliant, high-pressure "ostial" postinflations are mandatory in complex stenting techniques to achieve full stent expansion. When performing FKBI, we inflate both balloons simultaneously and slowly, which makes "melon seeding" less likely. We also deflate the balloons simultaneously to avoid distortion. High pressure proximal stent inflation using a short, noncompliant balloon should be considered for correction of possible proximal stent distortion after FKBI.

Difficult Access to the SB or MB after Stenting

Access to the SB is one of the greatest challenges in bifurcation PCI. Difficult access to the SB or MB can occur either at the start of the procedure or after SB or MB stenting. Difficulty may occur in recrossing the stent struts with a guidewire or advancing a balloon through the stent struts. We would like to address the problem of rewiring and advancing balloons into one of the branches after having stented the other branch (MB or SB), which is often the greatest difficulty with double stenting techniques, such as the mini-crush or even culotte. In our experience, recrossing into the SB through the MB stent struts or vice versa is usually possible using the Rinato-Prowater wire (Asahi Intecc Co Ltd, Nagoya, Japan). In difficult situations, we have also successfully used the Pilot 50 and 150 (Abbott Vascular Devices, Redwood City, California), Fielder FC, Asahi Intermediate, or Miracle 3/4.5 gm (Asahi Intecc Co Ltd, Nagoya, Japan) wires. However, we are very cautious about using hydrophilic guidewires when recrossing into the SB due to the risk of wire-induced dissection and perforation. If SB rewiring fails despite different wire curves and wires, a possible cause may be the presence of underexpanded stents in the MB impeding wiring of the ostium. Proximal MB stent postdilatation with the POT may be useful in correcting the underexpansion and causing protrusion of MB struts into the SB, even with double stenting techniques. The jailed wire in the branch should always be left in place as a marker until complete recrossing has been done. After having recrossed into the branch with a guidewire, there may subsequently be great difficulty advancing a balloon through the struts to dilate them. We frequently try first to cross through the stent struts with the smallest balloon we have on the table. If this balloon fails, we then use a Maverick (Boston Scientific, Natick, Massachusetts) 1.5-mm-diameter balloon to separate struts and allow a larger balloon to pass. If the 1.5-mm balloon cannot cross, we consider recrossing with a second wire while the first wire remains in place to traverse the stent struts in another spot. If balloon insertion through the strut still proves impossible, the stent should be further dilated. Another attempt should be made with a 1.5-mm coaxial balloon. Another trick that sometimes works is to advance the balloon as close as is possible to the stent struts, inflating the balloon to at least 12 atm to 14 atm for 20 seconds and while deflating the balloon to attempt advancing it further. Repeating this maneuver can often result in the balloon being slowly advanced through the stent struts.[12,63] If it still proves impossible to recross into the branch, another technique that we have used is to try to pass a 1.5-mm balloon over the jailed wire behind the stent struts, to either (a) redilate a subtotally occluded or dissected branch ostium and then try again to pass the stent struts with a guidewire or (b) convert the procedure into a reverse crush.

Ancillary Devices and Procedures

Intravascular Ultrasound (IVUS)

IVUS provides valuable baseline information regarding plaque distribution, especially in relation to the SB ostium, plaque composition, vessel size, and severity of angiographically ambiguous left main lesions. An example is the study by Furukawa et al. that demonstrated that the presence and severity of ostial SB plaque as observed by IVUS is the most important predictor of SB occlusion after bifurcation PCI.[29] IVUS after stent implantation is essential for correct stent optimization, especially in complex bifurcations, left main lesions, or when 2S techniques are applied by evaluating stent expansion and apposition, especially of the SB ostium; proximal or distal dissection; and periadventitial hematoma. Costal et al. demonstrated the importance of IVUS when performing complex techniques such as the crush because incomplete crushing (i.e., incomplete apposition of the three layers of the main and side branch stent struts) and ostial SB stent underexpansion are common and often not suspected angiographically.[72] However, the most important unanswered question that remains is whether routine IVUS usage results in improved clinical outcomes. Regarding bifurcations specifically, Kim et al. performed a retrospective evaluation of 758 patients with de novo nonleft main coronary bifurcation lesions.[73] In patients receiving DES, IVUS-guided stenting significantly reduced the 4-year long-term mortality rate (HR 0.24, 95% CI 0.06 to 0.86, p = 0.03) and late ST (0.4% vs. 2.8%, p = 0.03, log-rank test) as compared to angiographically guided stenting. Similarly, in left main lesions, IVUS guidance was associated with a tendency to a lower risk of 3-year mortality compared with angiography guidance (6.0% vs. 13.6%, log-rank p = 0.063; HR = 0.54, 95% CI 0.28-1.03, p = 0.061) in the MAIN-COMPARE (Revascularization for Unprotected Left Main Coronary Artery Stenosis: Comparison of Percutaneous Coronary Angioplasty versus Surgical Revascularization) registry.[74] IVUS guidance, however, did not modify the risk of MI or repeat revascularization. Similarly, in our multicenter registry evaluating 731 LMCA lesions (76.5% involving the distal left main) undergoing DES implantation, IVUS guidance was associated with reduced cardiac death (OR = 0.93, 95% CI 0.16-0.93, p = 0.03) at univariate exact logistic (unconditional) analysis.[75] Despite the lack of randomized data, the authors strongly believe that IVUS guidance utilizing modern and feasible criteria should be utilized when implanting stents in bifurcation lesions involving a large amount of myocardium at jeopardy or when complex double stenting is performed.

Lesion Preparation: Role of Debulking

Although lesion preparation should not be considered routine, it should be used when (a) there are diffuse and severe calcifications, (b) the predilating balloon does not cross the lesion or fully expand, and (c) it is difficult to cross the lesion with the stent. In these cases we usually perform rotational atherectomy with a 1.25-mm or 1.5-mm burr. However, if the IVUS catheter crosses the lesion, we use information on the plaque morphology to determine our lesion debulking strategy in the following way: (1) Superficial calcium extending more than 180° may demand lesion preparation with rotational atherectomy (Rotablator, Boston Scientific, Natick, Massachusetts) or orbital atherectomy (CSI, St. Paul, Minnesota); (2) severe fibrosis or moderate calcifications may demand a cutting balloon (cutting balloon Ultra and Flextome, Boston Scientific, Natick, Massachusetts), a scoring balloon (AngioSculpt, Angioscore Inc., Fremont, California), or a noncompliant balloon sized to the media diameter; and (3) the presence of soft plaque may permit direct stenting. We generally prefer scoring balloons to cutting balloons as they have a better profile and tend to cause fewer vessel dissections and perforations. We undersize the scoring balloon by 0.5 mm to 0.75 mm less than the reference vessel diameter obtained by IVUS and perform high-pressure inflations >14 atm (usually 18-20 atm).

Drug-Eluting Balloons in Bifurcations

Paclitaxel-coated drug-eluting balloons (DEB) may potentially have a role in bifurcations as part of a provisional strategy of DEB on the SB and a DES on the MB to avoid double stenting in bifurcations with large side branches. Theoretical advantages of this strategy are a reduction of SB restenosis by homogeneous drug delivery, preservation of normal bifurcation anatomy, and the avoidance of excess metal overlap, distortion, malapposition, and underexpansion in the bifurcation. This strategy may be particularly interesting for left circumflex ostium, where the results with DES continue to be disappointing. However, there are limited data available with the only randomized trial evaluating a combination of DEB with BMS, which not surprisingly was negative.[76] Finally, when evaluating the effectiveness of DEB, it should be remembered that there is no class effect with DEB and that different DEBs vary considerably in regard to efficacy.

Dedicated Bifurcation Stents

Several stents have been specifically designed for bifurcations, with particular emphasis on maintaining ease of access to the SB and allowing for optimal coverage of the bifurcation carina. The currently available (or under investigation) dedicated bifurcation stents can be broadly divided into the following: (1) stents that are implanted in both the MB and SB at the same time, (2) stents for provisional SB stenting that facilitate or maintain access to the SB after MB stenting and do not require recrossing of MB stent struts, and (3) stents that usually require another stent implanted in the bifurcation.[77,78] They have undergone a rapid evolution from the pioneering dedicated stents that were bulky and impractical. The new devices have a lower profile, but adequate lesion preparation remains vital to ensuring their implantation success. There are still a number of devices that require two wires to be delivered and wire wrap and bias remain important reasons for failure. Also, there are some devices that have a poor placement tolerance or where accurate placement is vital to the success of the device. Many devices rely on passive rotation for their accurate placement, questioning their utility in highly complex lesions. Drug-eluting versions have been an essential advancement for the future of many of these devices whose first-generation bare-metal versions were hampered by a high degree of restenosis. The promise of dedicated bifurcation stents are procedures that are less complex, with shorter procedural times, less contrast usage, a lower risk of SB closure, and possibly improved angiographic and clinical outcomes. However, these devices have not become widely accepted because none of them has shown significant advantages over current techniques with regard to procedural variables or clinical outcomes. The only randomized controlled trial performed involved 704 bifurcation lesions to a 2S strategy with the Tryton SB stent (Tryton Medical, Newton, Massachusetts) or provisional SB stenting.[79] At 9 months, the primary noninferiority endpoint of target vessel failure (composite of cardiac death, target vessel MI, or target vessel revascularization) was not met (12.8% Provisional vs. 17.4% Tryton). However, the results may have been biased by the fact that only 41% of the SBs were ≥2.25 mm in diameter. Another dedicated stent that should be mentioned is the Axxess stent system (Biosensors Europe SA, Morges, Switzerland), which was the first of these dedicated bifurcation stents designed to elute an antirestenotic drug (biolimus A9). The Axxess stent was evaluated in the large multicenter single-arm DIVERGE (Drug-Eluting Stent Intervention for Treating Side Branches Effectively) Study that enrolled 302 patients with de novo coronary bifurcations.[80] In keeping with the Axxess concept, 88% of patients required an additional stent to the Axxess: 67% in both branches, 17.7% in the distal MB, and 4% only in the SB. The MACE rate was 9.3% at 1 year, 14.0% at 2 years, and 16.1% at 3 years.[81] Ischemia-driven TLR was 4.3% at 9 months and 10.1% at 3 years.

Bioresorbable Scaffolds (BRS) in Bifurcations

Despite the initial hesitancy, real-world experience with BRS has demonstrated that they can be used in bifurcations, but there are currently insufficient data to speculate as to whether BRS will have any advantage over DES in bifurcation lesions.[82] Theoretically, when the scaffolds are resorbed, the normal bifurcation anatomy, flow, and vascular function will be restored while jailed SBs will be liberated. However, dedicated studies are needed and coronary bifurcations are not an absolute contraindication for BRS. Based on our own experience, we can offer the following advice:

1. A provisional approach remains the default. Residual SB stenosis after MB stenting can be treated with gentle SB balloon dilatation (balloon not greater than 2.5 mm), followed by MB postdilatation to correct for MB scaffold distortion.
2. SB wires can be jailed as normal and removed without difficulty.
3. T-kissing balloon dilatation with minimal protrusion of the SB balloon can be performed when necessary. Significant overlapping of the kissing balloons in the MB scaffold should be avoided and can result in scaffold disruption.
4. Crossover from provisional should be performed with the TAP technique. It may be difficult to advance current generation scaffolds through the MB scaffold, and conventional DES can be implanted more easily.
5. Elective double stenting can be performed with two BRS, and the T-stenting technique is preferred.
6. Culotte and crush stenting with BRS should be avoided to prevent overlapping of thick struts and scaffold disruption.

A more detailed discussion of this topic can be found in dedicated review articles.[83,84]

CONCLUSIONS

The introduction of second-generation drug-eluting stents and refinement in the stenting techniques resulted in a remarkable improvement in the treatment of bifurcation lesions. The current appropriate application of provisional stenting and perfecting stent techniques when implanting two stents are improving the acute results and long-term follow-up. Particular attention should be given to dual antiplatelet therapy when treating these lesions, especially when two stents have been implanted.

References

1. Fujii K, Kobayashi Y, Mintz GS, et al: Dominant contribution of negative remodeling to development of significant coronary bifurcation narrowing. *Am J Cardiol* 92:59–61, 2003.
2. Popma J, Leon M, Topol EJ: *Atlas of interventional cardiology*, Philadelphia, PA, 1994, Saunders.
3. Lefevre T, Louvard Y, Morice MC, et al: Stenting of bifurcation lesions: classification, treatments, and results. *Catheter Cardiovasc Interv* 49:274–283, 2000.
4. Safian RD: Bifurcation lesions. In Safian RD, Freed M, editors: *Manual of interventional cardiology*, vol 10, 2001, Royal Oak: Physicians' Press, pp 221–236.
5. Spokojny AM, Sanborn TM: The bifurcation lesion. In Ellis SG, Holmes DR, editors: *Strategic approaches in coronary intervention*, Baltimore, MD, 1996, Williams and Wilkins, p 288.
6. Louvard Y, Lefevre T, Morice MC: Percutaneous coronary intervention for bifurcation coronary disease. *Heart* 90:713–722, 2004.
7. Medina A, Suarez de Lezo J, Pan M: A new classification of coronary bifurcation lesions. *Rev Esp Cardiol* 59:183, 2006.
8. Movahed MR, Stinis CT: A new proposed simplified classification of coronary artery bifurcation lesions and bifurcation interventional techniques. *J Invasive Cardiol* 18:199–204, 2006.
9. Sianos G, Morel MA, Kappetein AP: The SYNTAX score: an angiographic tool grading the complexity of coronary artery disease. *Euro Intervention* 1:219–227, 2005.
10. Steigen TK, Maeng M, Wiseth R, et al: Randomized study on simple versus complex stenting of coronary artery bifurcation lesions: the Nordic bifurcation study. *Circulation* 114:1955–1961, 2006.
11. Myler RK, Shaw RE, Stertzer SH, et al: Lesion morphology and coronary angioplasty: current experience and analysis. *J Am Coll Cardiol* 19:1641–1652, 1992.
12. Latib A, Colombo A: Bifurcation disease: what do we know, what should we do? *J Am Coll Cardiol Interv* 1:218–226, 2008.
13. Iakovou I, Colombo A: Contemporary stent treatment of coronary bifurcations. *J Am Coll Cardiol* 46:1446–1455, 2005.
14. Al Suwaidi J, Berger PB, Rihal CS, et al: Immediate and long-term outcome of intracoronary stent implantation for true bifurcation lesions. *J Am Coll Cardiol* 35:929–936, 2000.
15. Yamashita T, Nishida T, Adamian MG, et al: Bifurcation lesions: two stents versus one stent—immediate and follow-up results. *J Am Coll Cardiol* 35:1145–1151, 2000.
16. Thuesen L, Kelbaek H, Klovgaard L, et al: Comparison of sirolimus-eluting and bare metal stents in coronary bifurcation lesions: subgroup analysis of the Stenting Coronary Arteries in Non-Stress/Benestent Disease Trial (SCANDSTENT). *Am Heart J* 152:1140–1145, 2006.
17. Ge L, Tsagalou E, Iakovou I, et al: In-hospital and nine-month outcome of treatment of coronary bifurcational lesions with sirolimus-eluting stent. *Am J Cardiol* 95:757–760, 2005.
18. Ong AT, Hoye A, Aoki J, et al: Thirty-day incidence and six-month clinical outcome of thrombotic stent occlusion after bare-metal, sirolimus, or paclitaxel stent implantation. *J Am Coll Cardiol* 45:947–953, 2005.
19. Colombo A, Moses JW, Morice MC, et al: Randomized study to evaluate sirolimus-eluting stents implanted at coronary bifurcation lesions. *Circulation* 109:1244–1249, 2004.
20. Pan M, de Lezo JS, Medina A, et al: Rapamycin-eluting stents for the treatment of bifurcated coronary lesions: a randomized comparison of a simple versus complex strategy. *Am Heart J* 148:857–864, 2004.
21. Ferenc M, Gick M, Kienzle RP, et al: Randomized trial on routine vs. provisional T-stenting in the treatment of de novo coronary bifurcation lesions. *Eur Heart J* 29:2859–2867, 2008.
22. Colombo A, Bramucci E, Sacca S, et al: Randomized study of the crush technique versus provisional side-branch stenting in true coronary bifurcations: the CACTUS (Coronary Bifurcations: Application of the Crushing Technique Using Sirolimus-Eluting Stents) Study. *Circulation* 119:71–78, 2009.
23. Chen SL, Santoso T, Zhang JJ, et al: A randomized clinical study comparing double kissing crush with provisional stenting for treatment of coronary bifurcation lesions: results from the DKCRUSH-II (Double Kissing Crush versus Provisional Stenting Technique for Treatment of Coronary Bifurcation Lesions) trial. *J Am Coll Cardiol* 57:914–920, 2011.
24. Hildick-Smith D, de Belder AJ, Cooter N, et al: Randomized trial of simple versus complex drug-eluting stenting for bifurcation lesions: the British Bifurcation Coronary Study: old, new, and evolving strategies. *Circulation* 121:1235–1243, 2010.
25. Chen SL, Xu B, Han YL, et al: Comparison of double kissing crush versus culotte stenting for unprotected distal left main bifurcation lesions: results from a multicenter, randomized, prospective DKCRUSH-III study. *J Am Coll Cardiol* 61:1482–1488, 2013.
26. Kumsars I NORDIC-BALTIC BIFURCATION IV: A Prospective, Randomized Trial of a Two-Stent Strategy vs. a Provisional Stent Strategy in True Coronary Bifurcation Lesions. Presented at Transcatheter Cardiovascular Therapeutics (TCT) 2013 in San Francisco on 30 October 2013. Available at: http://www.tctmd.com/show.aspx?id=121729. Accessed 26 March 2014.
27. Colombo A CACTUS Trial (**C**oronary Bifurcation **A**pplication of the **C**rush **T**echnique **U**sing **S**irolimus-Eluting Stents). Presented at Transcatheter Cardiovascular Therapeutics (TCT) 2007 in Washington, DC, on 24 October 2007.
28. Aliabadi D, Tilli FV, Bowers TR, et al: Incidence and angiographic predictors of side branch occlusion following high-pressure intracoronary stenting. *Am J Cardiol* 80:994–997, 1997.
29. Furukawa E, Hibi K, Kosuge M, et al: Intravascular ultrasound predictors of side branch occlusion in bifurcation lesions after percutaneous coronary intervention. *Circ J* 69:325–330, 2005.
30. Chaudhry EC, Dauerman KP, Sarnoski CL, et al: Percutaneous coronary intervention for major bifurcation lesions using the simple approach: risk of myocardial infarction. *J Thromb Thrombolysis* 2007.
31. Hahn JY, Chun WJ, Kim JH, et al: Predictors and outcomes of side branch occlusion after main vessel stenting in coronary bifurcation lesions: results from the COBIS II Registry (COronary BIfurcation Stenting). *J Am Coll Cardiol* 62:1654–1659, 2013.
32. Naganuma T, Latib A, Basavarajaiah S, et al: The long-term clinical outcome of T-stenting and small protrusion technique for coronary bifurcation lesions. *JACC Cardiovasc Interv* 6:554–561, 2013.
33. Koo BK, Waseda K, Kang HJ, et al: Anatomic and functional evaluation of bifurcation lesions undergoing percutaneous coronary intervention. *Circ Cardiovasc Interv* 3:113–119, 2010.
34. Koo BK, Kang HJ, Youn TJ, et al: Physiologic assessment of jailed side branch lesions using fractional flow reserve. *J Am Coll Cardiol* 46:633–637, 2005.
35. Dauerman HL, Higgins PJ, Sparano AM, et al: Mechanical debulking versus balloon angioplasty for the treatment of true bifurcation lesions. *J Am Coll Cardiol* 32:1845–1852, 1998.
36. Hermiller JB: Bifurcation intervention: keep it simple. *J Invasive Cardiol* 18:43–44, 2006.
37. Ormiston JA, Currie E, Webster MW, et al: Drug-eluting stents for coronary bifurcations: insights into the crush technique. *Catheter Cardiovasc Interv* 63:332–336, 2004.
38. Brunel P, Lefevre T, Darremont O, et al: Provisional T-stenting and kissing balloon in the treatment of coronary bifurcation lesions: results of the French multicenter "TULIPE" study. *Catheter Cardiovasc Interv* 68:67–73, 2006.
39. Niemela M, Kervinen K, Erglis A, et al: Randomized comparison of final kissing balloon dilatation versus no final kissing balloon dilatation in patients with coronary bifurcation lesions treated with main vessel stenting: the Nordic-Baltic Bifurcation Study III. *Circulation* 123:79–86, 2011.
40. Pan M, Medina A, Suarez de Lezo J, et al: Coronary bifurcation lesions treated with simple approach (from the Cordoba & Las Palmas [CORPAL] Kiss Trial). *Am J Cardiol* 107:1460–1465, 2011.
41. Mylotte D, Hovasse T, Ziani A, et al: Non-compliant balloons for final kissing inflation in coronary bifurcation lesions treated with provisional side branch stenting: a pilot study. *Euro Intervention* 7:1162–1169, 2012.
42. Hoye A, Iakovou I, Ge L, et al: Long-term outcomes after stenting of bifurcation lesions with the "crush" technique: predictors of an adverse outcome. *J Am Coll Cardiol* 47:1949–1958, 2006.
43. Ge L, Airoldi F, Iakovou I, et al: Clinical and angiographic outcome after implantation of drug-eluting stents in bifurcation lesions with the crush stent technique: importance of final kissing balloon post-dilation. *J Am Coll Cardiol* 46:613–620, 2005.
44. Adriaenssens T, Byrne RA, Dibra A, et al: Culotte stenting technique in coronary bifurcation disease: angiographic follow-up using dedicated quantitative coronary angiographic analysis and 12-month clinical outcomes. *Eur Heart J* 29:2868–2876, 2008.
45. Ormiston JA: Drug-eluting stents for coronary bifurcations: bench testing of provisional side-branch strategies. *Catheter Cardiovasc Interv* 67:49–55, 2006.
46. Ormiston JA, Webster MWI, Webber B, et al: The "crush" technique for coronary artery bifurcation stenting: insights from micro-computed tomographic imaging of bench deployments. *J Am Coll Cardiol Interv* 1:351–357, 2008.
47. Iakovou I, Schmidt T, Bonizzoni E, et al: Incidence, predictors, and outcome of thrombosis after successful implantation of drug-eluting stents. *JAMA* 293:2126–2130, 2005.
48. Brar SS, Gray WA, Dangas G, et al: Bifurcation stenting with drug-eluting stents: a systematic review and meta-analysis of randomised trials. *Euro Intervention* 5:475–484, 2009.
49. Katritsis DG, Siontis GC, Ioannidis JP: Double versus single stenting for coronary bifurcation lesions: a meta-analysis. *Circ Cardiovasc Interv* 2:409–415, 2009.

50. Maeng M, Holm NR, Erglis A, et al: Nordic-Baltic Percutaneous Coronary Intervention Study G. Long-term results after simple versus complex stenting of coronary artery bifurcation lesions: Nordic Bifurcation Study 5-year follow-up results. *J Am Coll Cardiol* 62:30–34, 2013.
51. Ong AT, Hoye A, Aoki J, et al: Thirty-day incidence and six-month clinical outcome of thrombotic stent occlusion after bare-metal, sirolimus, or paclitaxel stent implantation. *J Am Coll Cardiol* 45:947–953, 2005.
52. Armstrong EJ, Yeo KK, Javed U, et al: Angiographic stent thrombosis at coronary bifurcations: short- and long-term prognosis. *JACC Cardiovasc Interv* 5:57–63, 2012.
53. Louvard Y, Lefevre T: Bifurcation lesion stenting. In Colombo A, Stankovic G, editors: *Problem oriented approaches in interventional cardiology*, 2007, Informa Healthcare, pp 37–57.
54. Louvard Y, Thomas M, Dzavik V, et al: Classification of coronary artery bifurcation lesions and treatments: time for a consensus! *Catheter Cardiovasc Interv* 71:175–183, 2008.
55. Chung S, Her SH, Song PS, et al: Trans-radial versus trans-femoral intervention for the treatment of coronary bifurcations: results from Coronary Bifurcation Stenting Registry. *J Korean Med Sci* 28:388–395, 2013.
56. Arora RR, Raymond RE, Dimas AP, et al: Side branch occlusion during coronary angioplasty: incidence, angiographic characteristics, and outcome. *Cathet Cardiovasc Diagn* 18:210–212, 1989.
57. Weinstein JS, Baim DS, Sipperly ME, et al: Salvage of branch vessels during bifurcation lesion angioplasty: acute and long-term follow-up. *Cathet Cardiovasc Diagn* 22:1–6, 1991.
58. Burzotta F, De Vita M, Sgueglia G, et al: How to solve difficult side branch access? *Euro Intervention* 6(Suppl J):J72–J80, 2010.
59. Lefevre T, Darremont O, Albiero R: Provisional side branch stenting for the treatment of bifurcation lesions. *Euro Intervention* 6(Suppl J):J65–J71, 2010.
60. Foin N, Torii R, Mortier P, et al: Kissing balloon or sequential dilation of the side branch and main vessel for provisional stenting of bifurcations: lessons from micro-computed tomography and computational simulations. *JACC Cardiovasc Interv* 5:47–56, 2012.
61. Chevalier B, Glatt B, Royer T, et al: Placement of coronary stents in bifurcation lesions by the "culotte" technique. *Am J Cardiol* 82:943–949, 1998.
62. Favero L, Pacchioni A, Reimers B: Elective double stenting for non-left main coronary artery bifurcation lesions: patient selection and technique. In Moussa I, Colombo A, editors: *Tips and tricks in interventional therapy of coronary bifurcation lesions*, 2010, Informa Healthcare, pp 83–115.
63. Latib A, Chieffo A, Colombo A: Elective double stenting for left main coronary artery bifurcation lesions: patient selection and technique. In Moussa I, Colombo A, editors: *Tips and tricks in interventional therapy of coronary bifurcation lesions*, 2010, Informa Healthcare, pp 149–192.
64. Erglis A, Kumsars I, Niemela M, et al: For the Nordic PCI Study Group. Randomized comparison of coronary bifurcation stenting with the crush versus the culotte technique using sirolimus eluting stents: the Nordic Stent Technique Study. *Circ Cardiovasc Interv* 27–34, 2009.
65. Colombo A, Stankovic G, Orlic D, et al: Modified T-stenting technique with crushing for bifurcation lesions: immediate results and 30-day outcome. *Catheter Cardiovasc Interv* 60:145–151, 2003.
66. Galassi AR, Colombo A, Buchbinder M, et al: Long-term outcomes of bifurcation lesions after implantation of drug-eluting stents with the "mini-crush" technique. *Catheter Cardiovasc Interv* 69:976–983, 2007.
67. Chen SL, Zhang JJ, Ye F, et al: Study comparing the double kissing (DK) crush with classical crush for the treatment of coronary bifurcation lesions: the DKCRUSH-1 Bifurcation Study with drug-eluting stents. *Eur J Clin Invest* 38:361–371, 2008.
68. Dzavik V, Kharbanda R, Ivanov J, et al: Predictors of long-term outcome after crush stenting of coronary bifurcation lesions: importance of the bifurcation angle. *Am Heart J* 152:762–769, 2006.
69. Schampaert E, Fort S, Adelman AG, et al: The V-stent: a novel technique for coronary bifurcation stenting. *Cathet Cardiovasc Diagn* 39:320–326, 1996.
70. Sharma SK: Simultaneous kissing drug-eluting stent technique for percutaneous treatment of bifurcation lesions in large-size vessels. *Catheter Cardiovasc Interv* 65:10–16, 2005.
71. Baim DS: Editorial comment: is bifurcation stenting the answer? *Cathet Cardiovasc Diagn* 37:314–316, 1996.
72. Costa RA, Mintz GS, Carlier SG, et al: Bifurcation coronary lesions treated with the "crush" technique: an intravascular ultrasound analysis. *J Am Coll Cardiol* 46:599–605, 2005.
73. Kim SH, Kim YH, Kang SJ, et al: Long-term outcomes of intravascular ultrasound-guided stenting in coronary bifurcation lesions. *Am J Cardiol* 106:612–618, 2010.
74. Park SJ, Kim YH, Park DW, et al: Impact of intravascular ultrasound guidance on long-term mortality in stenting for unprotected left main coronary artery stenosis. *Circ Cardiovasc Interv* 2009:CIRCINTERVENTIONS.108.799494.
75. Chieffo A, Park S-J, Meliga E, et al: Late and very late stent thrombosis following drug-eluting stent implantation in unprotected left main coronary artery: a multicentre registry. *Eur Heart J* 29:2108–2115, 2008.
76. Stella PR, Belkacemi A, Dubois C, et al: A multicenter randomized comparison of drug-eluting balloon plus bare-metal stent versus bare-metal stent versus drug-eluting stent in bifurcation lesions treated with a single-stenting technique: six-month angiographic and 12-month clinical results of the drug-eluting balloon in bifurcations trial. *Catheter Cardiovasc Interv* 80:1138–1146, 2012.
77. Latib A, Sangiorgi GM, Colombo A: Current status and future of dedicated bifurcation stent systems. In Moussa I, Colombo A, editors: *Tips and tricks in interventional therapy of coronary bifurcation lesions*, 2010, Informa Healthcare, pp 211–250.
78. Latib A, Colombo A, Sangiorgi GM: Bifurcation stenting: current strategies and new devices. *Heart* 95:495–504, 2009.
79. Leon M: TRYTON: A prospective, randomized trial of a dedicated side branch stent vs. a provisional stent strategy in true coronary bifurcation lesions. Presented at Transcatheter Cardiovascular Therapeutics (TCT) 2013 in San Francisco on 30 October 2013. Available at: http://www.tctmd.com/show.aspx?id=121730. Accessed 26 March 2014.
80. Verheye S, Agostoni P, Dubois CL, et al: 9-month clinical, angiographic, and intravascular ultrasound results of a prospective evaluation of the Axxess self-expanding biolimus A9-eluting stent in coronary bifurcation lesions: the DIVERGE (Drug-Eluting Stent Intervention for Treating Side Branches Effectively) study. *J Am Coll Cardiol* 53:1031–1039, 2009.
81. Buysschaert I, Dubois CL, Dens J, et al: Three-year clinical results of the Axxess Biolimus A9 eluting bifurcation stent system: the DIVERGE study. *Euro Intervention* 9:573–581, 2013.
82. Latib A, Costopoulos C, Naganuma T, et al: Which patients could benefit the most from bioresorbable vascular scaffold implant: from clinical trials to clinical practice. *Minerva Cardioangiol* 61:255–262, 2013.
83. Ormiston JA, Webber B, Ubod B, et al: Absorb everolimus-eluting bioresorbable scaffolds in coronary bifurcations: a bench study of deployment, side branch dilatation and post-dilatation strategies. *Euro Intervention* 2014.
84. Dzavik V, Colombo A: The absorb bioresorbable vascular scaffold in coronary bifurcations: insights from bench testing. *JACC Cardiovasc Interv* 7:81–88, 2014.

Bypass Graft Interventions

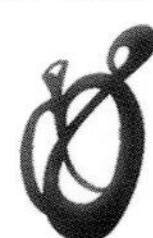

Emmanouil S. Brilakis and Subhash Banerjee

INTRODUCTION

Two types of grafts are currently used for coronary artery bypass graft surgery (CABG): saphenous vein grafts (SVGs) and arterial grafts (internal mammary artery grafts [IMAs], radial artery grafts, and gastroepiploic grafts). IMA grafts have the best long-term patency rates,[1,2] but in most cases, SVGs are still being used to bypass all coronary arteries that need revascularization. SVGs have high rates of failure,[3-5] which increase with increasing time post-CABG (**Figure 11-1**).[2,6]

EPIDEMIOLOGY

Angina in patients with prior CABG can be due to native coronary artery disease progression, bypass graft disease, or proximal subclavian artery stenosis development (**Figure 11-1**). In an analysis from the National Cardiovascular Data Registry (NCDR), between 2004 and 2009, percutaneous coronary intervention (PCI) in prior CABG patients represented 17.5% of the total PCI volume (300,902 of 1,721,046).[6] The PCI target vessel was a native coronary artery in 62.5% and a bypass graft in 37.5% of cases. Bypass graft PCI represented 6.6% of all PCI[6] and consisted mainly of SVG PCI (6.1% of all PCI), followed by arterial graft PCI (0.44% of all PCI), and, rarely, both arterial graft and SVG PCI (0.04% of all PCI). The proportion of SVGs as PCI target vessels increased after 5 years and even more so after 10 years from CABG (**Figure 11-2**). From January 1, 2010, through June 2011, bypass graft and SVG PCI constituted 6.0% and 5.5%, respectively, of the total NCDR PCI volume.[7]

Dr. Brilakis: Research support from the Department of Veterans Affairs (PI of the Drug Eluting Stents in Saphenous Vein Graft Angioplasty—DIVA trial and Merit grant—I01-CX000787-01) and from the National Institutes of Health (1R01HL102442-01A1); consulting fees/speaker honoraria from St. Jude Medical, Boston Scientific, Asahi, Abbott Vascular, Somahlution, Elsevier, and Terumo; research support from Guerbet and InfraRedx; spouse is an employee of Medtronic.

Dr. Banerjee: Research support from the Department of Veterans Affairs (PI of the Plaque Regression and Progenitor Cell Mobilization with Intensive Lipid Elimination Regimen [PREMIER]) trial. Speaker honoraria from Medtronic and Merck; research support from Boston Scientific and InfraRedx; intellectual property in HygeiaTel and MDcare Global..

INDICATIONS FOR BYPASS GRAFT INTERVENTIONS

Patients who present with bypass failure can be treated with redo CABG, medical therapy, PCI of a native coronary artery, or bypass graft PCI.

Redo CABG is infrequently performed due to high morbidity and mortality.[8,9] Redo CABG can also cause injury of patent grafts, which is especially concerning for IMA grafts. In the Angina With Extremely Serious Operative Mortality Evaluation (AWESOME) trial, the risk for subsequent clinical events was similar after redo CABG and after PCI.[10] According to the 2011 American College of Cardiology/American Heart Association (ACC/AHA) PCI guidelines, redo CABG is favored in patients with vessels unsuitable for PCI, multiple diseased bypass grafts, availability of the IMA for grafting chronically occluded coronary arteries, and good distal targets for bypass graft placement.[11] Factors favoring PCI over CABG include limited areas of ischemia causing symptoms, suitable PCI targets, a patent graft to the left anterior descending artery, poor CABG targets, and comorbid conditions.[11]

In patients with SVG lesions, native coronary artery PCI is preferred over SVG PCI, supplying the same territory because of better short-[6] and long-term[12-14] outcomes, especially in diffusely diseased and degenerated SVGs. Indeed, a native coronary artery was the target vessel in the majority of prior CABG patients undergoing PCI in NCDR.[6] However, native coronary arteries supplied by a failing SVG may be chronic total occlusions (CTOs) that can be challenging to recanalize,[15] although the SVG can, at times, be used as a conduit for retrograde native vessel revascularization.[16]

SVG PCI has two major limitations: high rates of distal embolization and in-stent restenosis (**Figure 11-3**), which are discussed in subsequent sections. Patients undergoing SVG PCI are usually older and have more comorbidities compared with patients undergoing native coronary artery PCI,[17] and as a result, they are at high risk for subsequent events, both cardiovascular and noncardiovascular.

DISTAL EMBOLIZATION AND EMBOLIC PROTECTION DEVICES

SVG lesions can have complex morphology (**Figure 11-4**) and friable atheromas[18] that can result in distal embolization

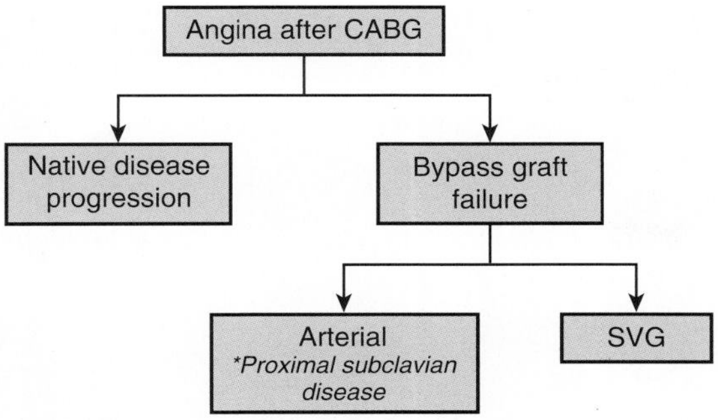

Angina after CABG
- Native disease progression
- Bypass graft failure
  - Arterial *Proximal subclavian disease
  - SVG

FIGURE 11-1 Potential causes of angina in prior CABG patients.

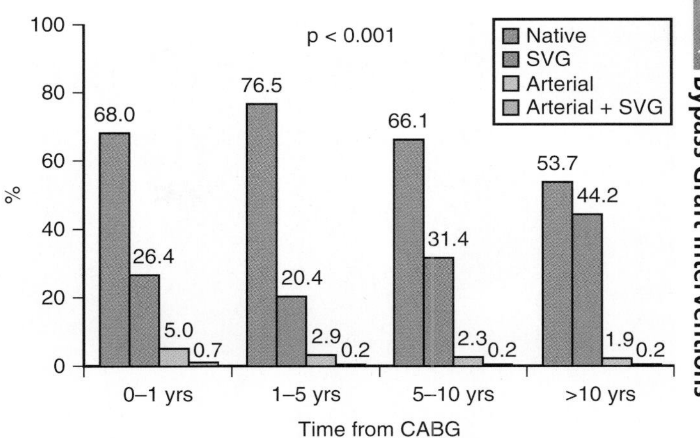

FIGURE 11-2 Comparison of the percutaneous coronary intervention target vessel in patients with prior CABG surgery during different time intervals from CABG, showing a significant increase in the proportion of SVG interventions over time. *CABG*, Coronary artery bypass graft surgery; *SVG*, saphenous vein graft. *(Reproduced with permission from Brilakis ES, Rao SV, Banerjee S, et al: Percutaneous coronary intervention in native arteries versus bypass grafts in prior coronary artery bypass grafting patients: a report from the National Cardiovascular Data Registry. JACC Cardiovasc Interv 4:844–850, 2011.)*

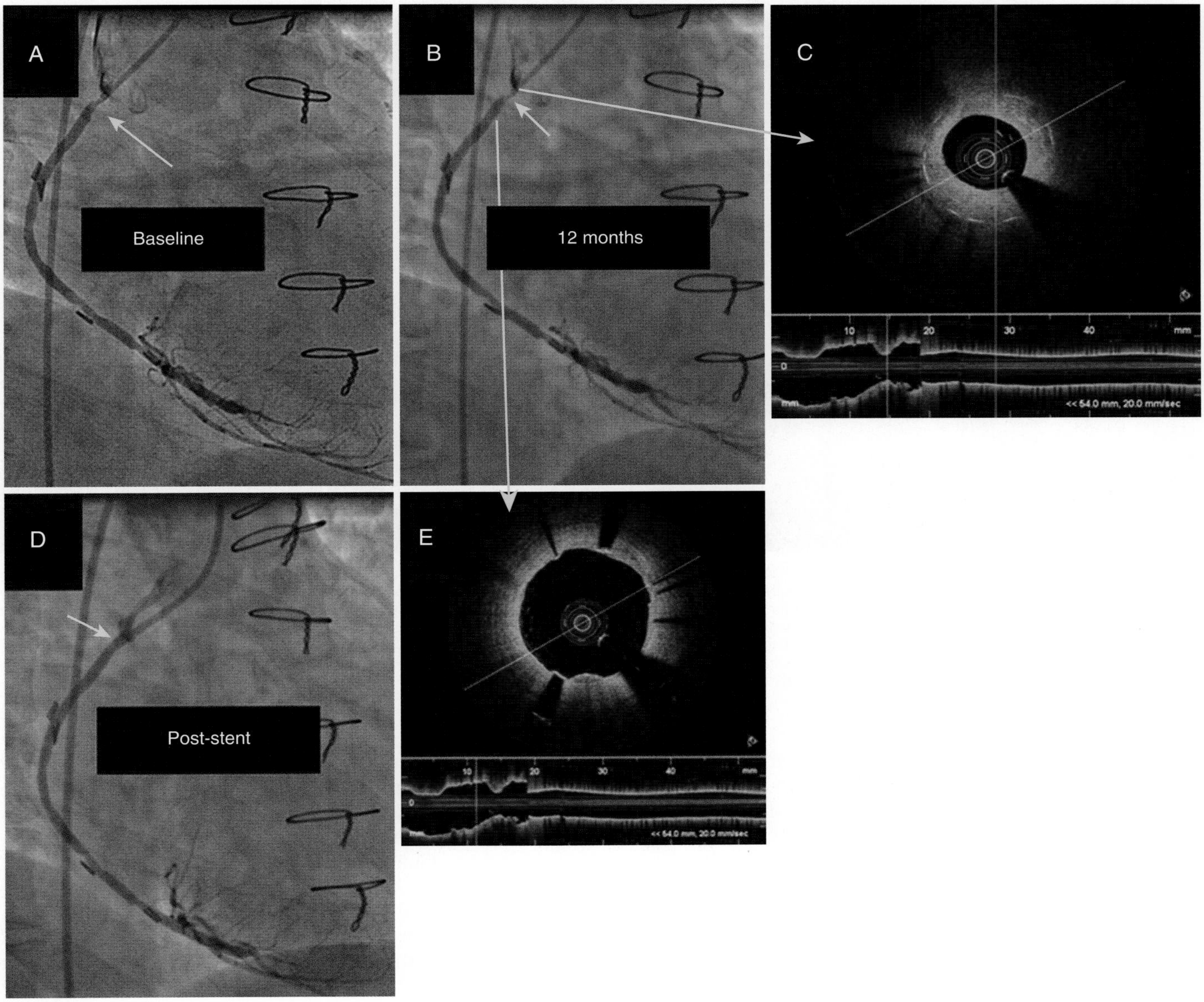

A Baseline

B 12 months

C

D Post-stent

E

FIGURE 11-3 Example of in-stent restenosis of an ostial saphenous vein graft lesion 12 months after stenting (panels **A** and **B**). Optical coherence tomography demonstrated that restenosis was due to neointimal hyperplasia (panels **C** and **E**). After repeat stent implantation, SVG patency was restored (panel **D**).

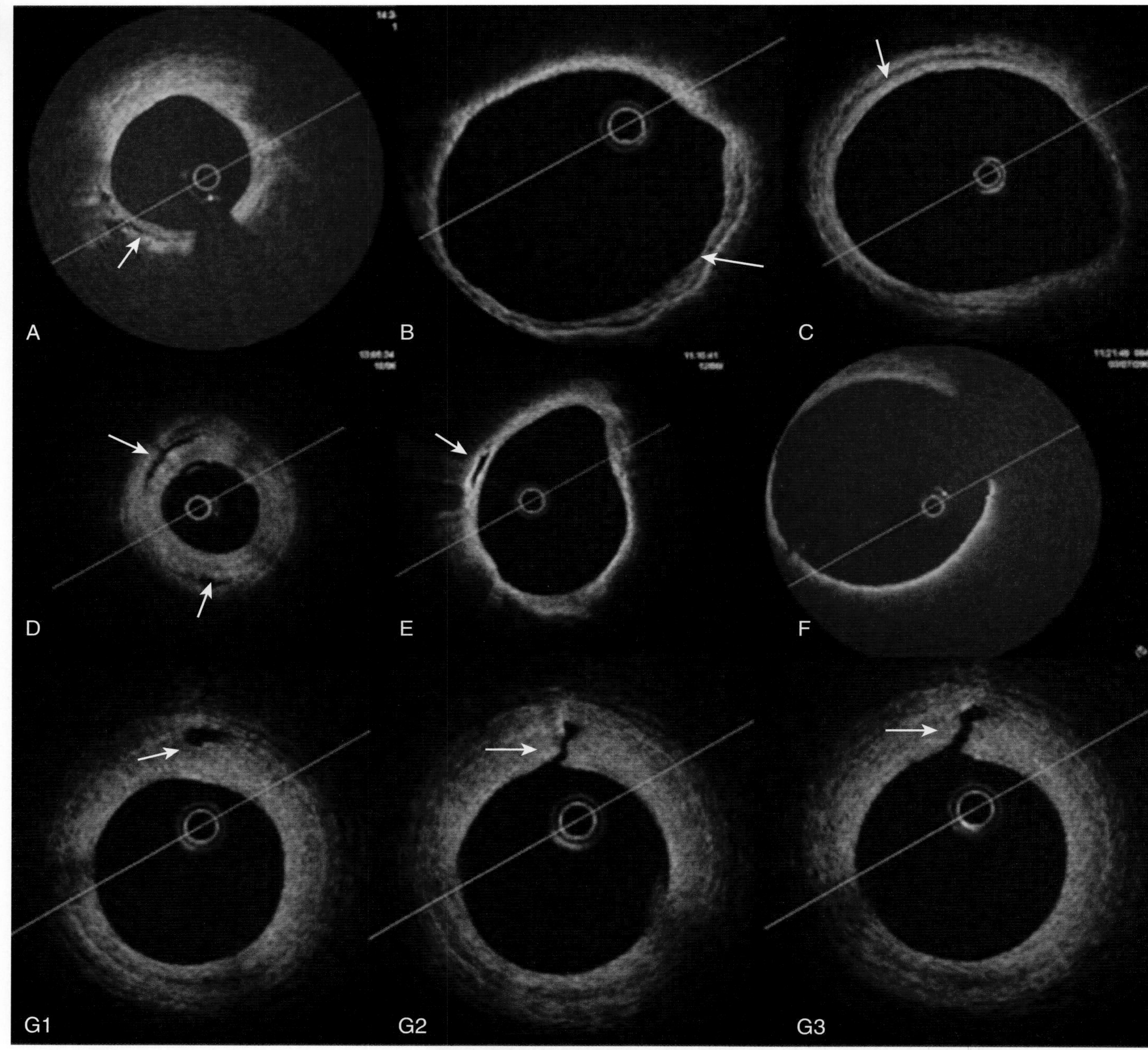

FIGURE 11-4 Optical coherence tomography findings in SVGs from patients presenting with acute coronary syndromes. **A** to **D,** Arrows point to signal-free zones inside the walls of SVGs. Over these zones, signal-rich tissue is loosely adherent to the SVG wall. As such, images corresponded to areas of severe angiographic degeneration; they were considered an indication of SVG friable tissue. **E,** The arrow points to a signal-free "microcavity," which may represent neovascularization or tissue rupture. **G1** to **G3** show three successive OCT frames depicting tissue rupture with communication of a small cavity with the SVG lumen. In **B** and **F,** the wall of the SVG looks very thin with severe circumferential signal attenuation that is probably related to its tissue composition, which was given the name "sun eclipse." *OCT,* Optical coherence tomography. *(Reproduced with permission from Davlouros P, Damelou A, Karantalis V, et al: Evaluation of culprit saphenous vein graft lesions with optical coherence tomography in patients with acute coronary syndromes. JACC Cardiovasc Interv 4:683–693, 2011.)*

during PCI (**Figure 11-5** and Videos 11-1 and 11-2). Distal embolization can cause no reflow and acute ST-segment elevation or present as asymptomatic cardiac biomarker elevation. Cardiac biomarker elevation post-SVG PCI (especially CK-MB increase >5× upper limit of normal) has been associated with increased mortality;[19] hence, it is important to prevent distal embolization or promptly treat it if it occurs.

Use of an embolic protection device (EPD) is the only proven strategy for preventing distal embolization during SVG PCI (**Figure 11-6** and Videos 11-3 and 11-4). EPDs capture debris liberated during PCI before it enters the coronary microcirculation causing injury. As of January 2015, three EPDs are available in the United States (**Figure 11-7**, **Table 11-1**): the FilterWire (Boston Scientific, Natick, Massachusetts), the Spider (Covidien, Mansfield, Massachusetts), and the GuardWire (Medtronic Vascular, Santa Rosa, California).[20] The first two EPDs are filters, whereas the GuardWire is a 0.014 inch guidewire with a distal balloon that when inflated stops antegrade flow; after completion of PCI, any column of blood within the SVG is aspirated with a thrombectomy catheter before restoring antegrade flow (**Figure 11-8**). The GuardWire allows "complete" protection,

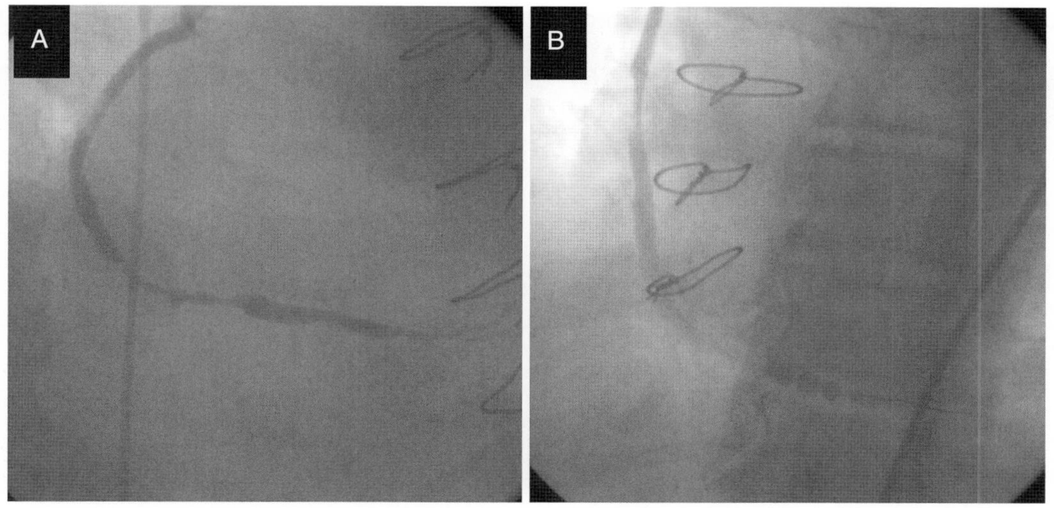

FIGURE 11-5 Example of no reflow during SVG intervention. No reflow with severe chest pain and ST-segment elevation occurred after crossing a degenerated SVG (panel **A** and **Video 11-1**) with a FilterWire (panel **B** and **Video 11-2**).

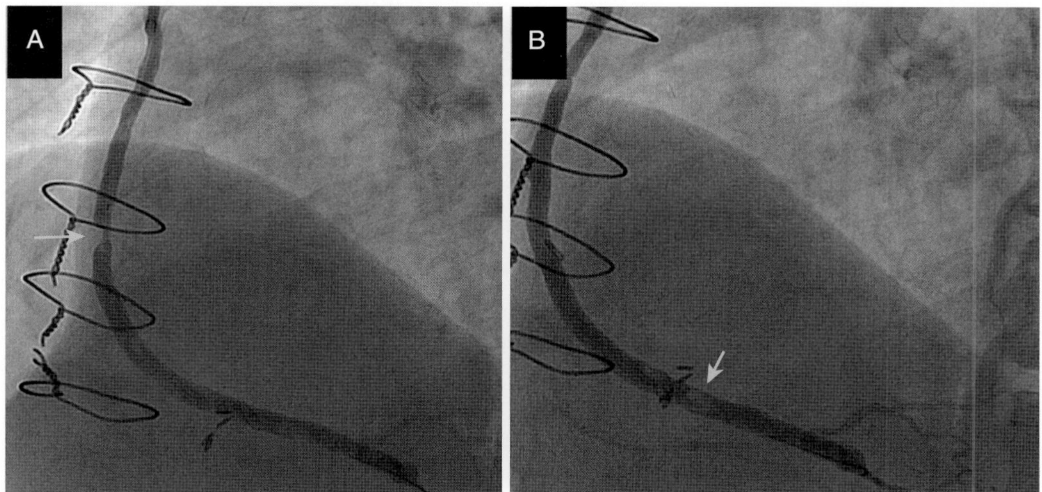

FIGURE 11-6 Example of debris capture by a filter. A FilterWire was placed distally to an eccentric SVG body lesion (panel **A** and **Video 11-3**). During PCI, debris embolized distally and was captured within the filter (panel **B** and **Video 11-4**).

Embolic protection devices available in the US for SVG interventions in 2014

Device	Manufacturer
GuardWire 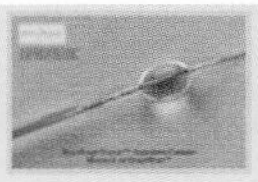	Medtronic
FilterWire 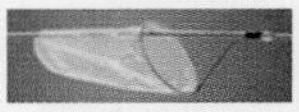	Boston Scientific
Spider 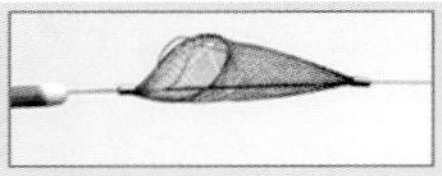	Covidien

FIGURE 11-7 Embolic protection devices available for clinical use in the United States as of January 2014.

that is, capture of all released particles and humoral factors, in contrast to filters that only capture larger size particles. Moreover, it has a lower crossing profile and requires a shorter landing zone (20 mm vs. 25-50 mm for filters). However, the GuardWire can be cumbersome to use and cessation of blood flow may be poorly tolerated by some patients, especially those in whom the SVG supplies a large area of myocardium.

The Saphenous vein graft Angioplasty Free of Emboli Randomized (SAFER) trial randomized 801 patients undergoing SVG PCI to GuardWire or stenting over a standard guidewire.[21] The study's primary endpoint (composite of death, myocardial infarction, emergency CABG, or target lesion revascularization by 30 days) occurred in 65 patients (16.5%) assigned to control versus 39 patients (9.6%) assigned to the GuardWire ($p = 0.004$). This significant 42% relative reduction in the primary endpoint was driven by a reduction in the incidence of myocardial infarction (8.6% vs. 14.7%, $p = 0.008$). No reflow was also less common in the EPD group (3% vs. 9%, $p = 0.02$). Given the significant clinical

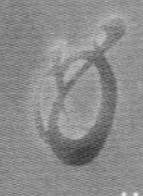

TABLE 11-1 Description of Various Embolic Protection Devices Available for Clinical Use in the United States in 2014

DEVICE	DESIGN	GUIDE CATHETER	PORE SIZE	DIAMETER	CROSSING PROFILE	LANDING ZONE
GuardWire	0.014 inch guidewire with distal balloon	6 Fr	NA	2.5-5.0 and 3.0-6.0 mm	2.1 and 2.7 Fr	≥20 mm
FilterWire	Polyurethane filter basket	6 Fr	110 μm	2.25-3.5 and 3.5-5.5 mm	3.2 Fr	>25 mm (2.25) or >30 mm (3.5)
Spider	Nitinol mesh-filter/ coated with heparin	6 Fr	70 μm distal end, 165 μm mid, 200 μm proximal end	3, 4, 5, 6, 7 mm	3.2 Fr	≥40-50 mm

Fr, French; *NA,* not applicable.

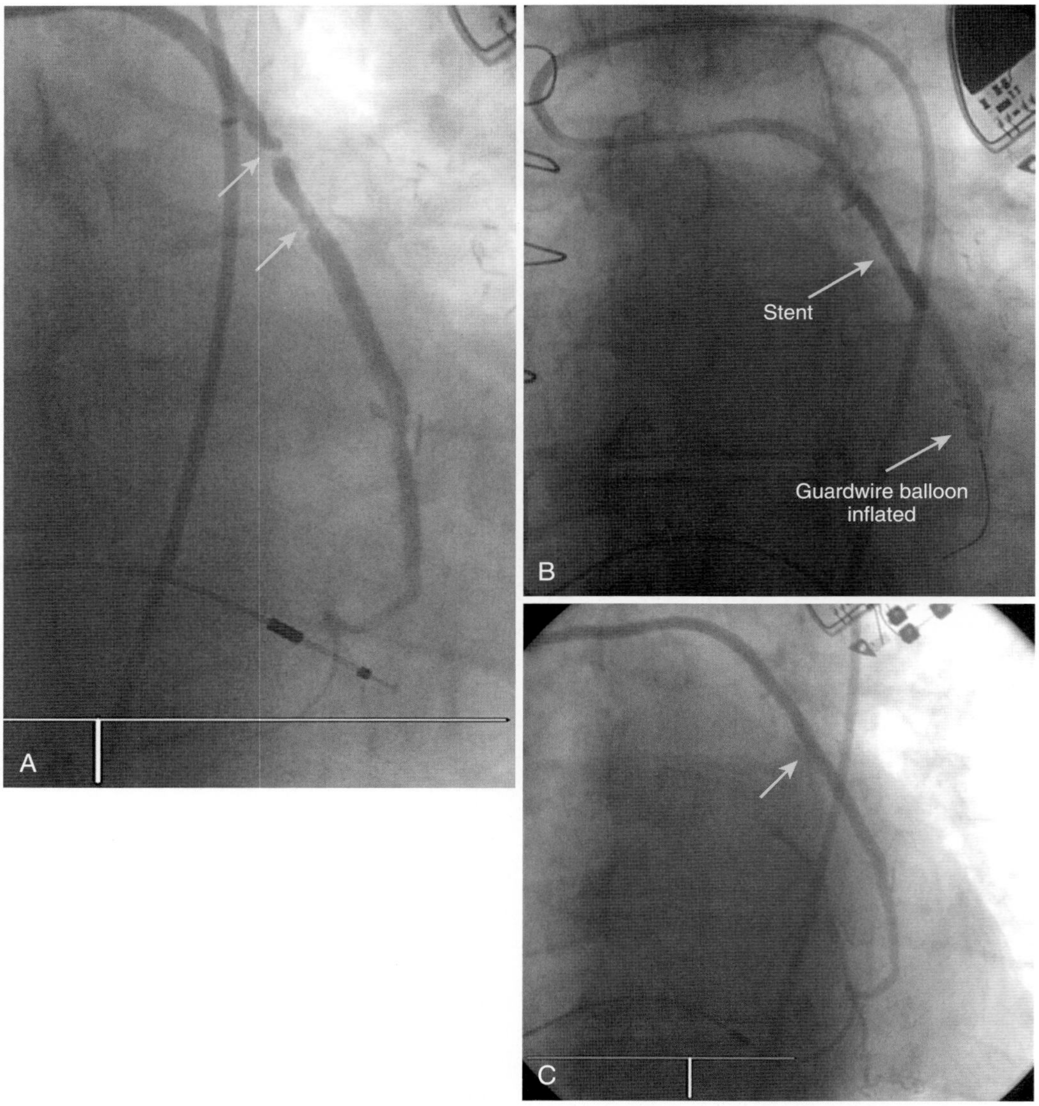

FIGURE 11-8 Saphenous vein graft intervention using the GuardWire (Medtronic Vascular, Santa Rosa, California). Coronary angiography demonstrating a lesion in the body of the saphenous vein graft (arrows, panel **A**). A stent was implanted after inflation of the GuardWire balloon distally (panel **B**), with an excellent final angiographic result (panel **C**). *(Reproduced with permission from Brilakis ES: Chapter 26. Bypass graft intervention and embolic protection. In Kern MJ, editor: SCAI interventional cardiology board review, Philadelphia, 2014, Lippincott Williams & Wilkins.)*

TABLE 11-2 Trials of Embolic Protection Devices in SVG PCI

TRIAL NAME	YEAR	N	PRIMARY ENDPOINT			
EPD vs. no EPD				**EPD event rate (%)**	**Control group event rate (%)**	**P superiority**
SAFER[21]	2002	801	30-day composite of death, MI, emergency CABG, or TLR	(GuardWire) 9.6	16.5	0.004
One EPD vs. another EPD				**Test EPD event rate (%)**	**Control EPD event rate (%)**	**P noninferiority**
FIRE[22]	2003	651	30-day composite of death, MI, or TVR	(FilterWire) 9.9	(GuardWire) 11.6%	0.0008
SPIDER	2005	732	30-day composite of death, MI, urgent CABG, or TVR	(Spider) 9.1	(GuardWire 24% or FilterWire 76%) 8.4	0.012
PRIDE[23]	2005	631	30-day composite of cardiac death, MI, or TLR	(Triactiv) 11.2%	(FilterWire) 10.1%	0.02
CAPTIVE[24]	2006	652	30-day composite of death, MI, or TVR	(Cardioshield) 11.4%	(GuardWire) 9.1%	0.057
PROXIMAL[25]	2007	594	30-day composite of death, MI, or TVR	(Proxis) 9.2%	(GuardWire 19% or FilterWire 81%) 10.0%	0.006
AMETHYST[26]	2008	797	30-day composite of death, MI, or urgent repeat revascularization	(Interceptor Plus) 8.0%	(GuardWire 72% or FilterWire 18%) 7.3%	0.025

AMETHYST, assessment of the Medtronic AVE interceptor saphenous vein graft filter system; *CABG,* coronary artery bypass graft surgery; *CAPTIVE,* CardioShield application protects during transluminal intervention of vein grafts by reducing emboli; *EPD,* embolic protection device; *FIRE,* FilterWire EX randomized evaluation; *MI,* myocardial infarction; *PRIDE,* protection during saphenous vein graft intervention to prevent distal embolization; *PROXIMAL,* proximal protection during saphenous vein graft intervention; *SAFER,* saphenous vein graft angioplasty free of emboli randomized;*SPIDER,* saphenous vein graft protection in a distal embolic protection randomized trial; *TLR,* target lesion revascularization; *TVR,* target vessel revascularization.
GuardWire, Medtronic Vascular, Santa Rosa, California; FilterWire, Boston Scientific, Natick, Massachusetts; SPIDER, ev3, Plymouth, Minnesota; Triactive, Kensey Nash Corp., Exton, Pennsylvania; Cardioshield, MedNova, Galway; Proxis, St. Jude Medical, Minneapolis, Minnesota; Interceptor Plus, Medtronic Vascular.

benefit with EPD use, subsequent SVG PCI studies used a noninferiority design to compare one EPD to another, as summarized in **Table 11-2**.[22-26]

Choosing an EPD for a specific SVG lesion is based on several factors, such as lesion location, device availability, local expertise in EPD use, and the potential hemodynamic consequences of SVG flow cessation (**Figure 11-9**). SVG body lesions can be protected with any EPD, as long as there is an adequate landing zone. Ostial SVG lesions should only be protected with a FilterWire or Spider, since use of the GuardWire could result in debris embolization in the aorta from the stagnant column of blood in the SVG. Although ostial SVG lesions were excluded from the pivotal SVG PCI trials, a recent study showed high success rates with EPD use in ostial lesions at the cost of difficulty retrieving the filter in 11% of the lesions;[27] one of these patients developed acute stent thrombosis causing cardiac arrest[27] (**Figure 11-10**). Moreover, ostial and distal anastomotic lesions are more likely to consist of fibrous tissue and less likely to contain lipid core plaque compared with SVG shaft lesions, and hence may be less likely to embolize.[28] Distal anastomotic lesions (**Figure 11-9**) cannot be protected with any of the currently available EPDs (manufacturing of proximal embolic protection devices stopped in 2012). Distal anastomotic lesions constitute approximately 19% of SVG lesions undergoing PCI.[7] Routine use of EPDs in SVG in lesions due to in-stent restenosis may be unnecessary because these lesions are usually caused by neointimal proliferation, making distal embolization unlikely.[29] Similarly, EPD use may not be necessary for recently implanted (<2 years old) SVGs that have not had enough time to develop significant degeneration predisposing to embolization.

The 2011 ACC/AHA PCI guidelines state that, "EPDs should be used during SVG PCI when technically feasible" (Class I indication, level of evidence B).[11] Yet, EPDs were only used in 23% of SVG PCI between 2004 and 2009 in the NCDR registry,[30] although some studies suggest that up to 77% of SVG lesions are eligible.[31] Potential explanations for EPD underutilization include the following: lack of reimbursement for EPDs; technical difficulties and lack of familiarity with EPD use;[32] fear of EPD-related complications, such as device entrapment[33] and acute vessel occlusion;[27] and uncertainty regarding the magnitude of clinical benefit with EPD use. The SAFER trial was performed before the era of potent ADP P2Y12-receptor inhibitors. In the "Is Drug-Eluting-Stenting Associated with Improved Results in Coronary Artery Bypass Grafts?" (ISAR-CABG) trial in which all patients were pretreated with 600 mg clopidogrel before PCI, despite very infrequent EPD use (in <1% of SVG PCIs), the incidence of myocardial infarction was 6%, which is lower than the incidence of myocardial infarction reported in the control arm of the SAFER trial (14.7%).[21]

When use of an EPD is not feasible (for example, in distal anastomotic lesions, lesions without an adequate landing zone, tight lesions that cannot be crossed with an EPD, or thrombotic lesions in which EPD insertion may cause embolization by itself) (**Figure 11-9**), alternative interventions to reduce distal embolization (or obviate its adverse consequences) include the following: (a) intragraft vasodilator administration (such as adenosine,[34] nitroprusside,[35] nicardipine,[36] and verapamil[37]), (b) use of an excimer laser,[38] (c) implantation of slightly undersized stents[39] (which did not result in higher restenosis rates in one retrospective study[39]), (d) direct stenting without predilation,[40] or (e) use

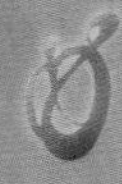

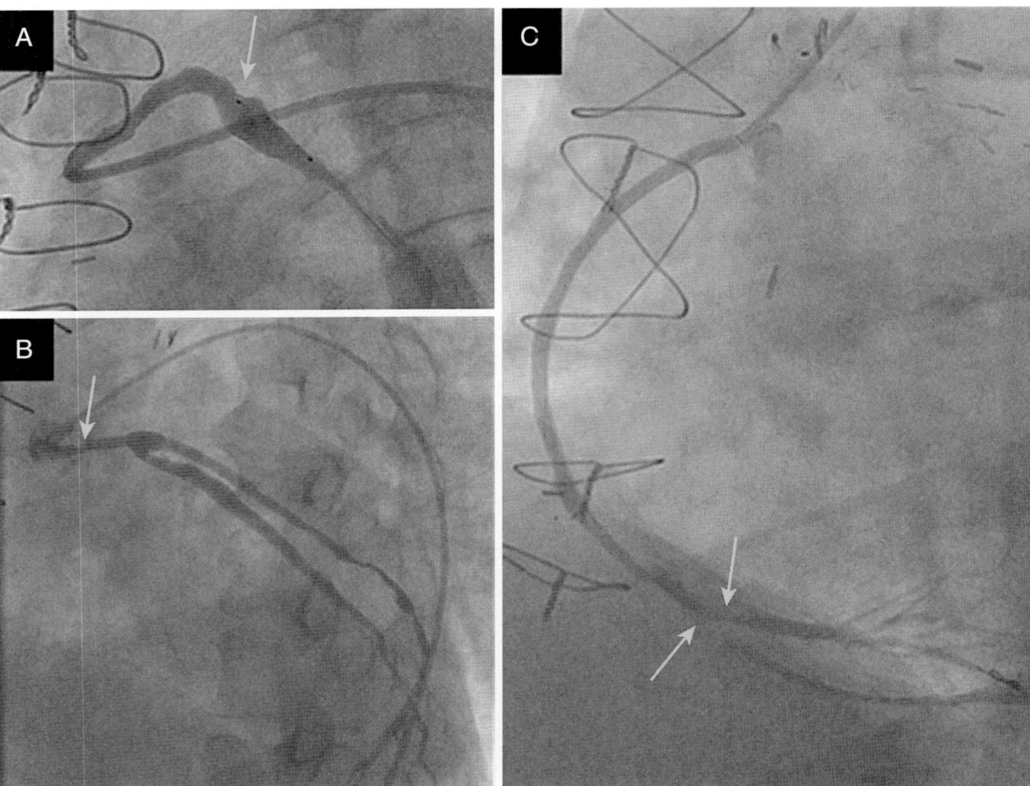

FIGURE 11-9 Saphenous vein graft lesions in which an embolic protection device could not be used because of the large caliber of the graft (panel **A**), the lesion proximal to a Y-graft bifurcation (panel **B**), or the location at the distal SVG anastomosis (panel **C**). *(Reproduced with permission from Brilakis ES: Chapter 26. Bypass graft intervention and embolic protection. In Kern MJ, editor: SCAI interventional cardiology board review, Philadelphia, 2014, Lippincott Williams & Wilkins.)*

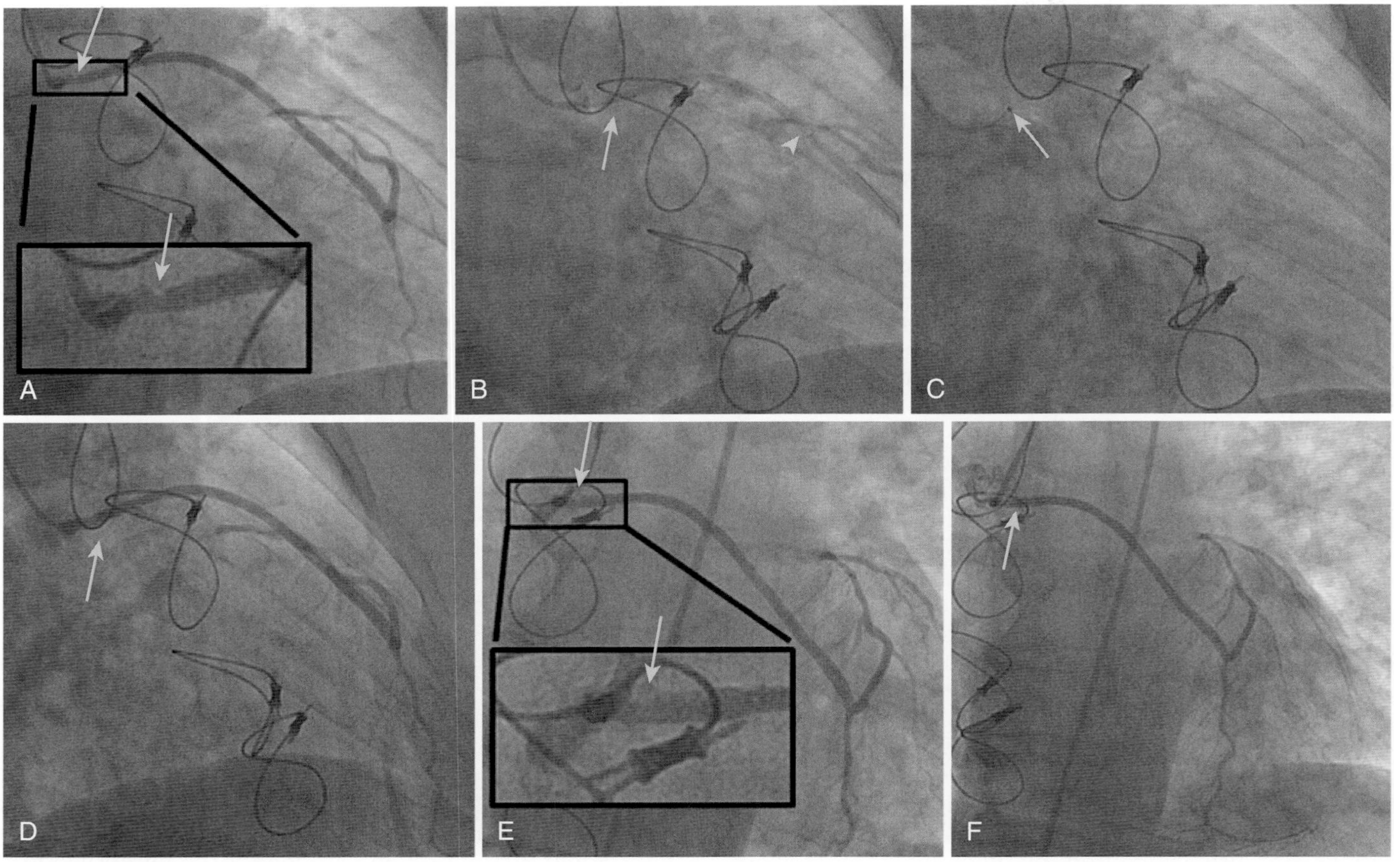

FIGURE 11-10 Complicated treatment of an ostial SVG lesion using an EPD. Coronary angiography demonstrating an ostial lesion in a saphenous vein graft to the left anterior descending artery (arrow, panel **A**) that was successfully treated with implantation of a 3.5 × 15 mm everolimus-eluting stent (arrow, panel **B**) after inserting a FilterWire (Boston Scientific) (arrowhead, panel **C**) for distal embolic protection. Poststenting, the FilterWire retrieval catheter (arrow, panel **C**) could not be advanced through the ostial saphenous vein graft stent, necessitating filter withdrawal through the stent. A satisfactory angiographic result was achieved (arrow, panel **D**). One hour later the patient developed chest pain and cardiac arrest. Emergency angiography during cardiopulmonary resuscitation revealed stent thrombosis of the ostial stent (arrows, panel **E**) that was successfully treated with the implantation of two bare-metal stents (3 × 28 mm and 3.5 × 28 mm) (arrow, panel **F**). *(Reproduced with permission from Abdel-Karim AR, Papayannis AC, Mahmood A, et al: Role of embolic protection devices in ostial saphenous vein graft lesions. Catheter Cardiovasc Interv 80:1120–1126, 2012.)*

TABLE 11-3 Trials of SVG Lesion Stenting

TRIAL NAME	YEAR	N	PRIMARY ENDPOINT	BARE-METAL STENT EVENT RATE (%)	OTHER GROUP EVENT RATE (%)	P
BMS vs. balloon angioplasty						
SAVED[43]	1997	220	6-month angiographic restenosis	37	46	0.24
Venestent[44]	2003	150	6-month angiographic restenosis	19.1	32.8	0.069
BMS vs. covered stents						
RECOVERS[45]	2003	301	6-month angiographic restenosis	24.8	24.2	0.237
STING[46]	2003	211	6-month angiographic restenosis	20	29	0.15
SYMBIOT III[47]	2006	700	8-month angiographic percent diameter stenosis	30.9	31.9	0.80
BARRICADE[48]	2011	243	8-month angiographic restenosis	28.4	31.8	0.63
BMS vs. DES						
RRISC	2006 (49)	75	6-month angiographic restenosis	32.6	13.6	0.031
	2007 (50)		MACE at 32 months	41	58	0.13
SOS	2009 (51)	80	12-month angiographic restenosis	51	9	<0.001
	2010 (52)	80	Target vessel failure at 35 months	72	34	0.001
ISAR-CABG[53]	2011	610	12-month composite of death, MI, and TLR	22	15	0.02

BARRICADE, Barrier approach to restenosis: restrict intima to curtail adverse events trial; *BMS,* bare-metal stent; *DES,* drug-eluting stent; *ISAR-CABG,* Is drug-eluting-stenting associated with improved results in coronary artery bypass grafts? trial; *MACE,* major adverse cardiac events; *MI,* myocardial infarction; *RECOVERS,* European multicenter randomized evaluation of polytetrafluoroethylene COVERed stent in Saphenous vein grafts trial; *RRISC,* reduction of restenosis in saphenous vein grafts with cypher sirolimus-eluting stent trial; *SAVED,* saphenous vein De Novo trial; *SOS,* stenting of saphenous vein grafts trial; *STING,* stents IN grafts trial; *SYMBIOT III,* a prospective, randomized trial of a self-expanding PTFE stent graft during SVG intervention; *TLR,* target lesion revascularization.

of micromesh-covered stents, which are currently not approved for clinical use in the United States.[41,42]

SVG STENTING

Drug-eluting stents (DES) are currently preferred for SVG PCI to reduce the risk for in-stent restenosis (**Figure 11-2**) based on three randomized controlled clinical trials (**Table 11-3**).[43-53]

The Reduction of Restenosis In Saphenous vein grafts with Cypher sirolimus-eluting stent trial (RRISC) compared the sirolimus-eluting stent (SES) Cypher (Cordis, Warren, New Jersey), with a bare-metal stent (BMS) in 75 patients and reported less angiographic restenosis and target lesion revascularization at 6 months.[49,50] During long-term follow-up, the SES group had higher mortality (29% vs. 0%, p = 0.001) rates, and target vessel revascularization was similar in both groups;[50] however, most patients died because of noncardiac causes or cardiac causes unrelated to the target SVG.

The Stenting Of Saphenous Vein Grafts trial (SOS) trial compared a paclitaxel-eluting stent (PES), Taxus (Boston Scientific, Natick, Massachusetts), to a similar BMS in 80 patients and demonstrated less angiographic restenosis and lower incidence of clinical events (both repeat revascularization and myocardial infarction) with PES.[51,52]

The ISAR-CABG study randomized 610 patients to a first-generation DES (SES, PES, or sirolimus-eluting ISAR stent) or a BMS. At 12 months, the DES group had a significantly lower incidence of target lesion revascularization (7% vs. 13%, p = 0.01) compared to BMS, with a similar incidence of all-cause death (5% vs. 5%, p = 0.83), myocardial infarction (5% vs. 6%, p = 0.27), and definite or probable stent thrombosis (1% vs. 1%, p = 0.99).[53] The incidence of occlusive restenosis was 6% with DES and 12% with BMS (p = 0.008).[53] Stent failure in SVG lesions frequently presents with an acute coronary syndrome.[54]

The 2011 ACC/AHA PCI guidelines state, "DES are generally preferred over BMS" for SVG lesions.[11] There is limited data on whether second-generation DES further improve outcomes compared to first-generation DES. In a pilot study use of the second-generation everolimus-eluting stent was associated with high rates of stent strut coverage but also high malapposition rates at 12 months postimplantation.[55] Three retrospective studies have been published, with one showing better (less target vessel revascularization)[56] and two showing similar[57,58] outcomes with second-generation DES. DES with bioabsorbable polymer showed encouraging outcomes in the NOBORI 2 registry, although the risk of death, myocardial infarction, and target vessel revascularization were higher than the corresponding rates of patients undergoing treatment of non-SVG lesions.[59] Preliminary reports have shown promising results with bioabsorbable stents in SVGs, but further study is needed.[60]

BMS implantation should be avoided in distal anastomotic graft lesions due to high rates of in-stent restenosis; DES implantation or balloon angioplasty alone is preferred, and both of these strategies appeared to provide similarly good outcomes in a pilot study.[61] SVG shaft lesions have been associated with a higher risk of distal embolization and long-term adverse clinical events compared to proximal and distal anastomotic lesions.[62]

ADJUNCTIVE PHARMACOTHERAPY

Anticoagulation for SVG PCI can be achieved with unfractionated heparin or bivalirudin. Glycoprotein IIb/IIIa inhibitors are not beneficial[63] and may be harmful[64] in SVG PCI

(Class III, level of evidence B, ACC/AHA guideline recommendation).[11] However, glycoprotein IIb/IIIa inhibitors were used in 40% of SVG PCI in the United States in NCDR between 2004 and 2009.[30]

Prehospital administration of single or dual oral antiplatelet therapy has been associated with better outcomes after SVG PCI compared with no prehospital therapy.[65] After SVG PCI with DES, 12-month duration of dual antiplatelet therapy remains the standard of care;[66] however, high rates of death/myocardial infarction were observed after clopidogrel discontinuation at 12 months in one study,[67] suggesting that prolonged dual antiplatelet therapy might be advantageous. Optimizing the overall medical regimen and aggressively controlling coronary artery disease risk factors are important, given the high risk profile and poor risk factor control of patients undergoing SVG PCI.[17]

TECHNICAL ASPECTS OF SVG PCI

Intravascular Imaging

Intravascular imaging (see **Figures 11-3 and 11-4**) can facilitate SVG PCI by optimal stent size selection and evaluation of the need for pretreatment, for example, in SVGs containing thrombus.[18] Stent undersizing in SVG PCI could result in stent deformation when equipment is advanced through the stent.[68] In a preliminary study, slight undersizing of SVG stents and avoiding postdilation were associated with a lower risk of distal embolization.[39]

SVG Engagement

Bypass graft engagement is significantly facilitated when the CABG anatomy is known;[69] hence, every effort should be made to obtain the CABG surgical report prior to angiography. When such a report cannot be obtained, a systematic approach should be followed with nonselective injections of both subclavian arteries (to identify any IMA grafts), ensuring that the perfusion of each myocardial segment is accounted for. SVG engagement is easier when graft markers are present (**Figure 11-11**), yet such markers are very infrequently inserted at the time of CABG, in part because of concerns about their effect on SVG patency.[70]

The usual location of the SVG proximal anastomosis is shown in **Figure 11-12**. SVGs to the right coronary artery or the right posterior descending artery usually arise from the

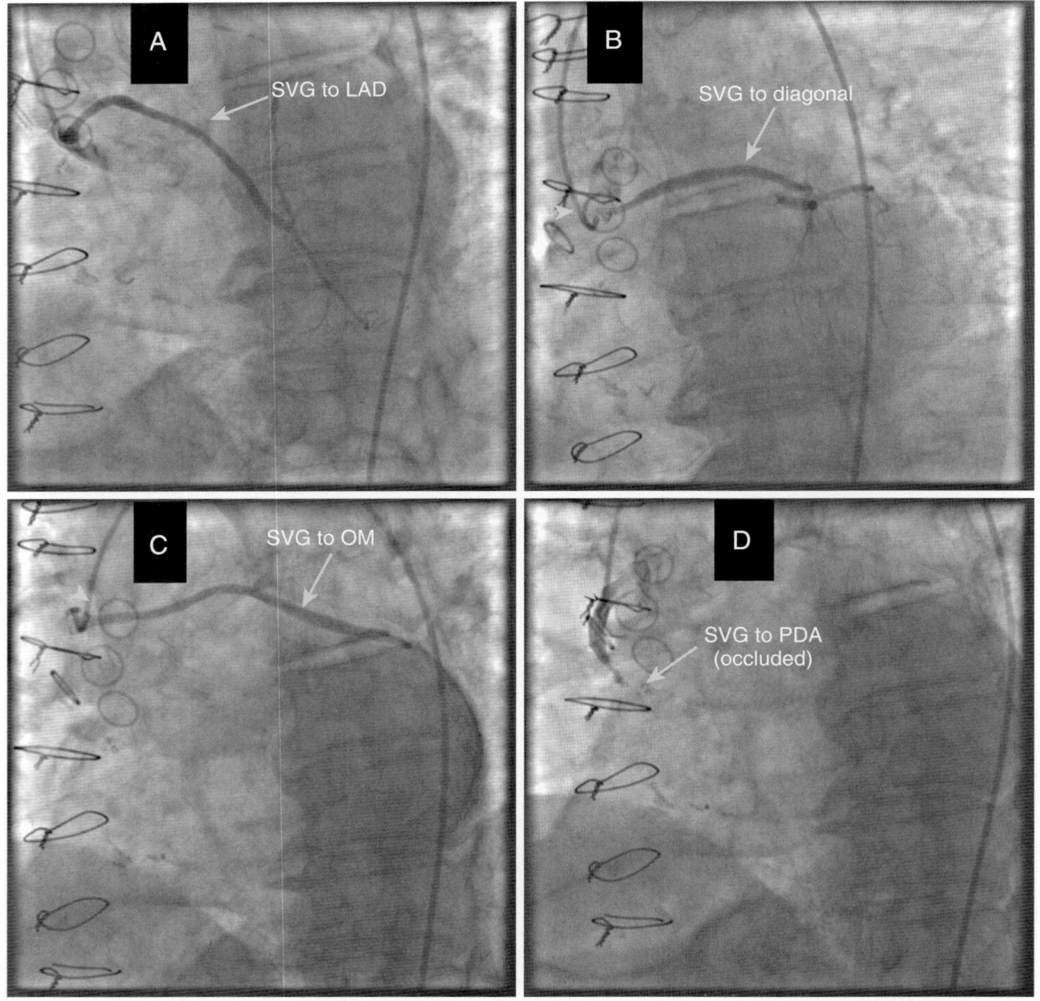

FIGURE 11-11 Example of a patient with bypass graft markers facilitating SVG engagement. The lower left-sided marker marks the ostium of an SVG to the LAD (panel **A**), the mid-left-sided marker marks the ostium of an SVG to a diagonal branch (panel **B**), and the higher left-sided marker marks the ostium of an SVG to an OM branch (panel **C**). The right-sided marker marks the ostium of the SVG to the PDA (this graft is occluded, arrow, panel **D**). *LAD,* Left anterior descending artery; *OM,* obtuse marginal; *PDA,* posterior descending artery; *SVG,* saphenous vein graft.

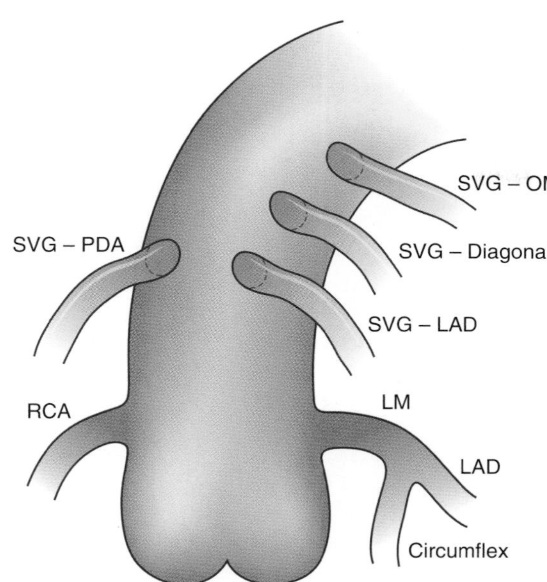

FIGURE 11-12 Usual location of the saphenous vein graft proximal anastomoses. *LAD,* Left anterior descending artery; *LM,* left main; *OM,* obtuse marginal; *PDA,* posterior descending artery; *RCA,* right coronary artery; *SVG,* saphenous vein graft.

right side of the aorta; SVGs to the left coronary artery arise from the left side of the aorta. SVGs to the left anterior descending artery originate lower; SVGs to the diagonal originate higher; and SVGs to the obtuse marginal branches originate even higher in the aorta. A JR4 or 3DRC catheter can usually engage most left- and right-sided grafts. A multipurpose catheter can facilitate cannulation of SVGs to the right coronary/posterior descending artery and an LCB catheter cannulation of left-sided grafts.

In the Randomized Comparison of the Transradial and Transfemoral Approaches for Coronary Artery Bypass Graft Angiography and Intervention (RADIAL-CABG) clinical trial, coronary artery and graft angiography was faster and required less contrast and radiation exposure for both patient and operator when performed using femoral compared to radial access, while the crossover rate from radial to femoral was 17.2%.[71] However, radial access may still play an important role in patients at high risk for vascular access complications and bleeding.[72] Also, occasionally IMA grafts cannot be engaged using femoral access due to subclavian tortuosity, thus requiring radial access. Graft engagement and PCI can be facilitated by guide catheter extensions.[73-75] In rare cases, retrograde SVG wiring can serve as a "last resort" technique for identifying the ostium and cannulating unusual aortocoronary bypass grafts.[76]

Acutely Occluded SVGs

Acutely occluded SVGs may contain a large amount of thrombus, and even when they are successfully recanalized they are at high risk for recurrent failure.[77] Combined use of thrombectomy and an embolic protection device may be advantageous for treating such lesions,[78] and laser also appears promising as an adjunctive modality.[79] Thrombectomy can sometimes be performed by deep SVG intubation with a guide catheter[80] (**Figure 11-13**) or with a guide catheter extension. If thrombectomy fails, dilation with an undersized balloon can be performed to restore TIMI 1-2 flow followed by anticoagulation for 1 to 2 weeks before proceeding with stent implantation.[81] Alternatively, native coronary artery PCI could be performed instead of SVG PCI, if feasible[16] (**Figure 11-14**).

Chronically Occluded SVGs

PCI of SVG CTOs has been given a Class III recommendation (level of evidence C) in the 2011 PCI guidelines[11] due to relatively low success and high restenosis rates.[82,83] SVG CTO PCI is currently reserved for cases in which native vessel PCI cannot be accomplished and can provide significant symptomatic improvement.[84,85]

Intermediate SVG Lesions

Unlike intermediate lesions in native coronary arteries that have low rates of progression,[86] intermediate lesions in SVGs can progress rapidly, often causing acute coronary syndromes[87-89] (**Figure 11-15**). Hence, fractional flow reserve (FFR) has a limited role in intermediate SVG lesions, although it correlated with ischemia in a small pilot study.[90] In the Moderate *VE*in Graft *LE*sion Stenting With the *T*axus Stent and *I*ntravascular Ultrasound (VELETI) pilot trial, patients who underwent intermediate SVG lesion stenting with a PES had a lower rate of SVG disease progression and a trend toward a lower incidence of major adverse cardiac events at 1-year follow-up compared with medical treatment alone.[88] However, more studies are needed before prophylactic SVG stenting becomes a routine clinical strategy.

SVG PCI Complications

Apart from distal embolization and no reflow, SVG PCI can have complications similar to non-SVG PCI. Because of pericardial adhesions, SVG or arterial graft perforation (**Figure 11-16**) may result in localized effusion, although tamponade is still possible and can lead to rapid hemodynamic deterioration and death.[91] Occasionally SVG perforation can cause hemoptysis, likely due to proximity of the SVG with the lung parenchyma.[92] Perforated SVGs are at high risk for subsequent occlusion.[91]

ARTERIAL GRAFT INTERVENTIONS

As described in Part 1, PCI of arterial grafts is significantly less frequent than SVG interventions.[6] PCI of IMA grafts is most commonly needed at the distal anastomotic site and can be hindered by (1) difficulty engaging the graft, especially in the presence of proximal subclavian artery tortuosity; (2) difficulty wiring and delivering equipment through the graft due to "pseudolesion" formation;[93] and (3) difficulty reaching the target lesion, due to long graft length. Specialized catheters have been developed to facilitate IMA engagement (such as the IM VB1 catheter), yet in cases of severe subclavian tortuosity, ipsilateral radial access may be required to achieve IMA engagement. Care should be employed when engaging the IMA ostium to prevent injury.[93] Using soft guidewires may decrease the risk for IMA pseudolesion formation,[94] and occasionally the use of shortened guide catheters may be required to allow balloon or stent delivery to a distal anastomotic lesion (**Figure 11-17**)[95] or to a lesion in the native vessel distal to the IMA anastomosis. In patients with in situ IMA grafts, the proximal subclavian artery should be imaged during diagnostic angiography, because severe proximal subclavian stenosis can present with angina (due to subclavian steal syndrome, **Figure 11-18** and Video 11-5) and even with myocardial infarction.[96]

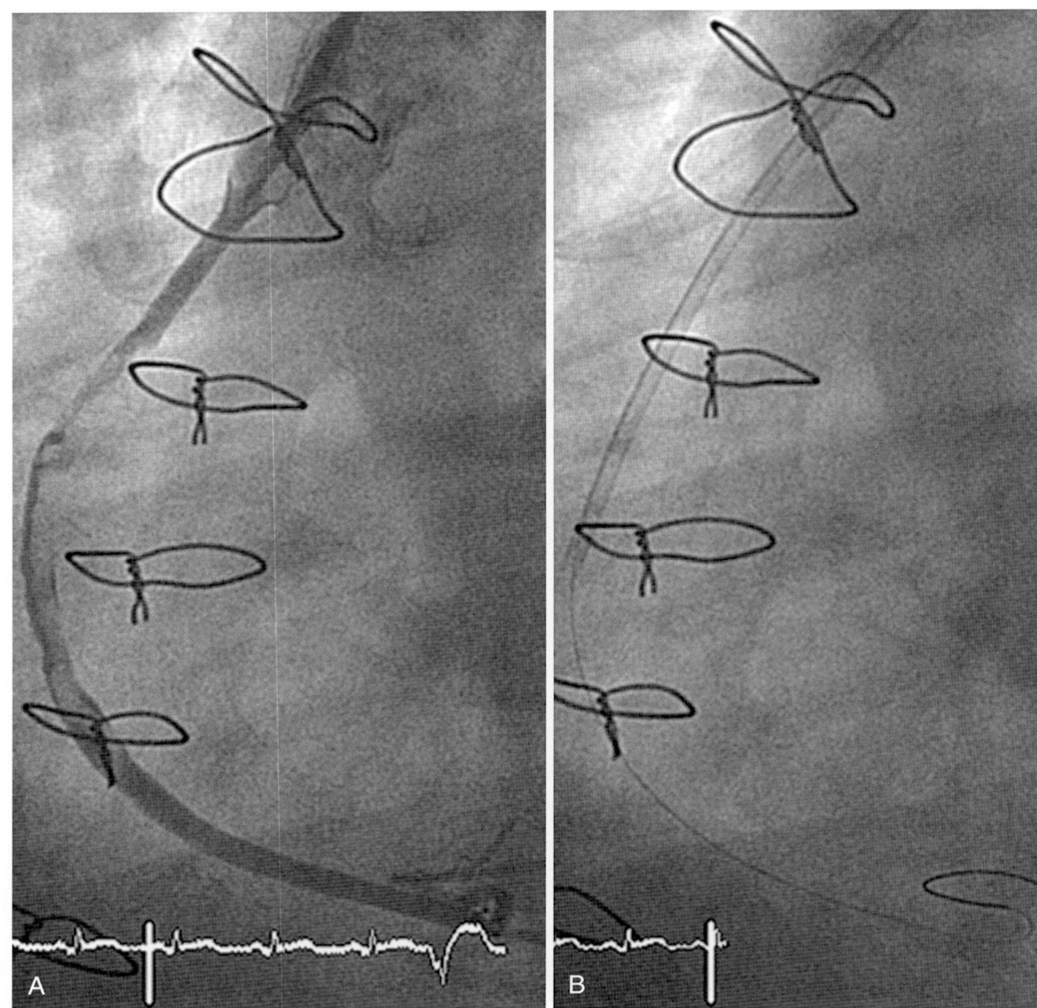

FIGURE 11-13 **A, B,** SVG thrombectomy using deep guide intubation. *(Reproduced with permission from Garcia-Tejada J, Jurado-Roman A, Hernandez F, et al: Guiding-catheter thrombectomy combined with distal protection during primary percutaneous coronary intervention of a saphenous vein graft. Cardiovasc Revasc Med 14:356–358, 2013.)*

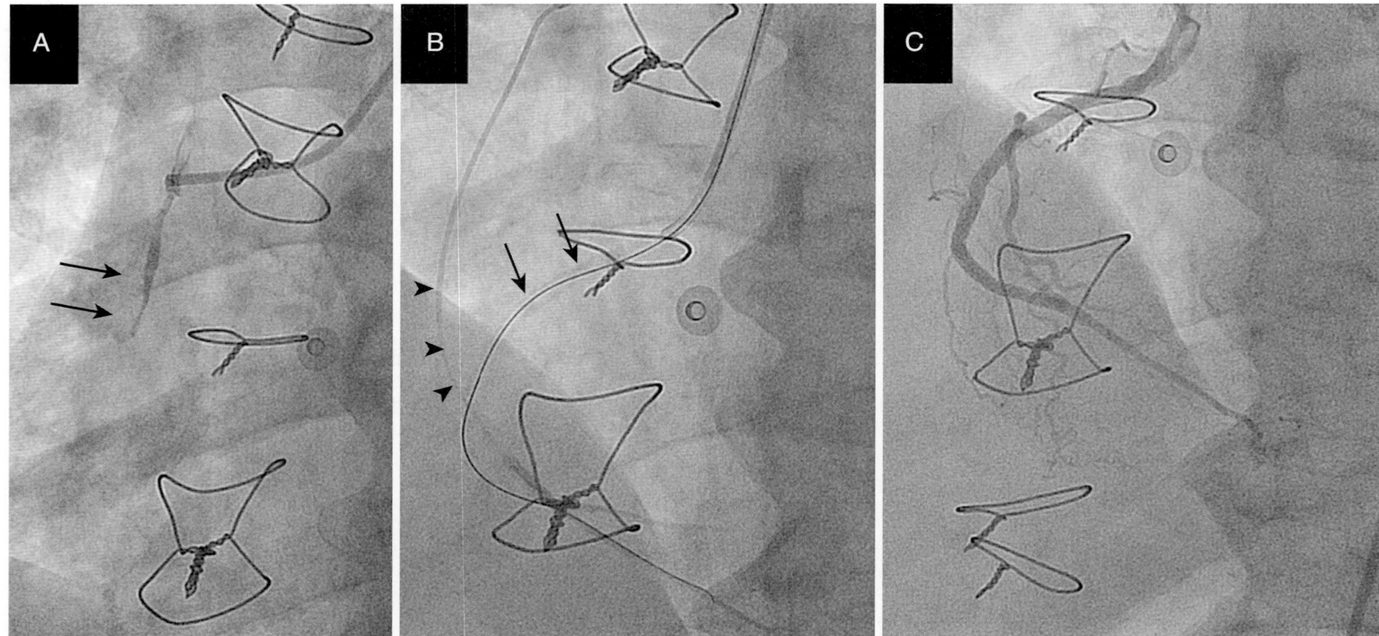

FIGURE 11-14 Treatment of native coronary artery chronic total occlusion after failure to recanalize an acutely occluded SVG. Coronary angiography demonstrating acute thrombotic occlusion of a saphenous vein graft to the right posterior descending artery (arrows, panel **A**). After attempts to intervene on the saphenous vein graft failed, the native right coronary artery chronic total occlusion was successfully crossed (arrows, panel **B**) with visualization via contrast injection through a microcatheter inserted through the occluded saphenous vein graft (arrowheads, panel **B**). After stenting of the native right coronary artery, TIMI 3 flow to the right posterior descending artery was restored (panel **C**). *(Reproduced with permission from Abdel-Karim AR, Banerjee S, Brilakis ES: Percutaneous intervention of acutely occluded saphenous vein grafts: contemporary techniques and outcomes. J Invasive Cardiol 22:253–257, 2010.)*

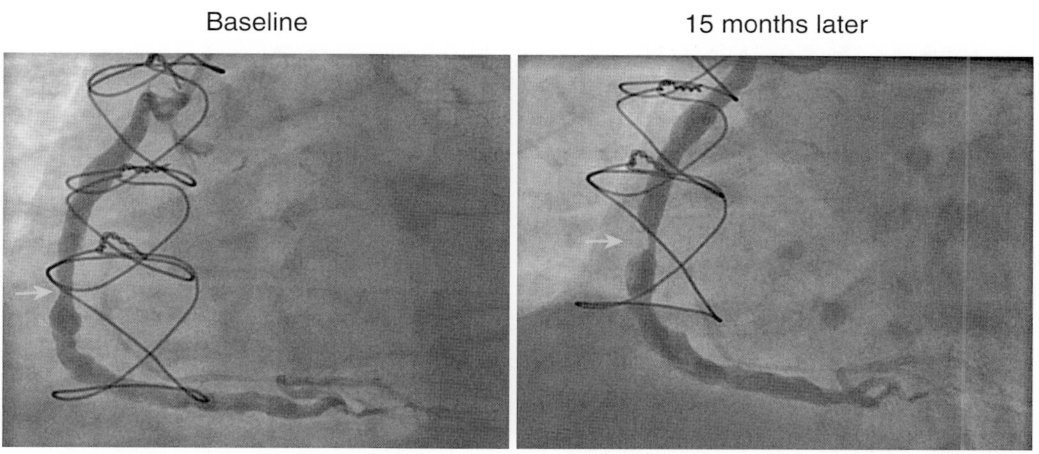

FIGURE 11-15 Rapid progression of an intermediate SVG lesion. *(Reproduced with permission from Abdel-Karim AR, Da Silva M, Lichtenwalter C, et al: Prevalence and outcomes of intermediate saphenous vein graft lesions: findings from the stenting of saphenous vein grafts randomized-controlled trial. Int J Cardiol 168:2468–2473, 2013.)*

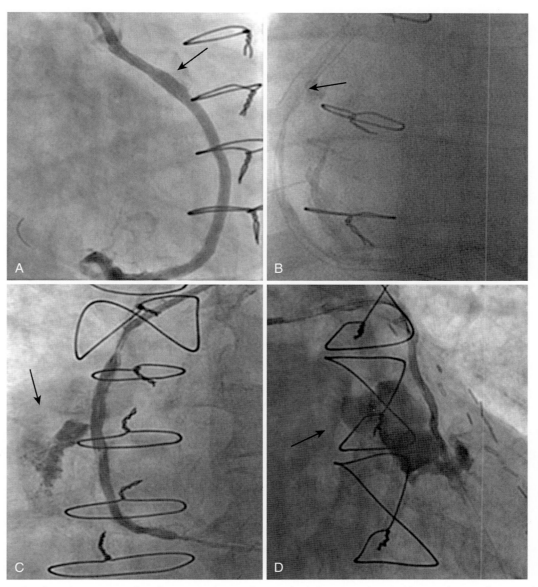

FIGURE 11-16 Examples of a saphenous vein graft perforation. **A,** Class I perforation after balloon angioplasty. **B,** Class II perforation after stent placement. **C,** Class III perforation after postdilation. **D,** Class III perforation with cavity spilling. *(Reproduced with permission from Marmagkiolis K, Brilakis ES, Hakeem A, et al: Saphenous vein graft perforation during percutaneous coronary intervention: a case series. J Invasive Cardiol 25:157–161, 2013.)*

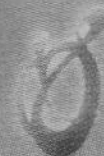

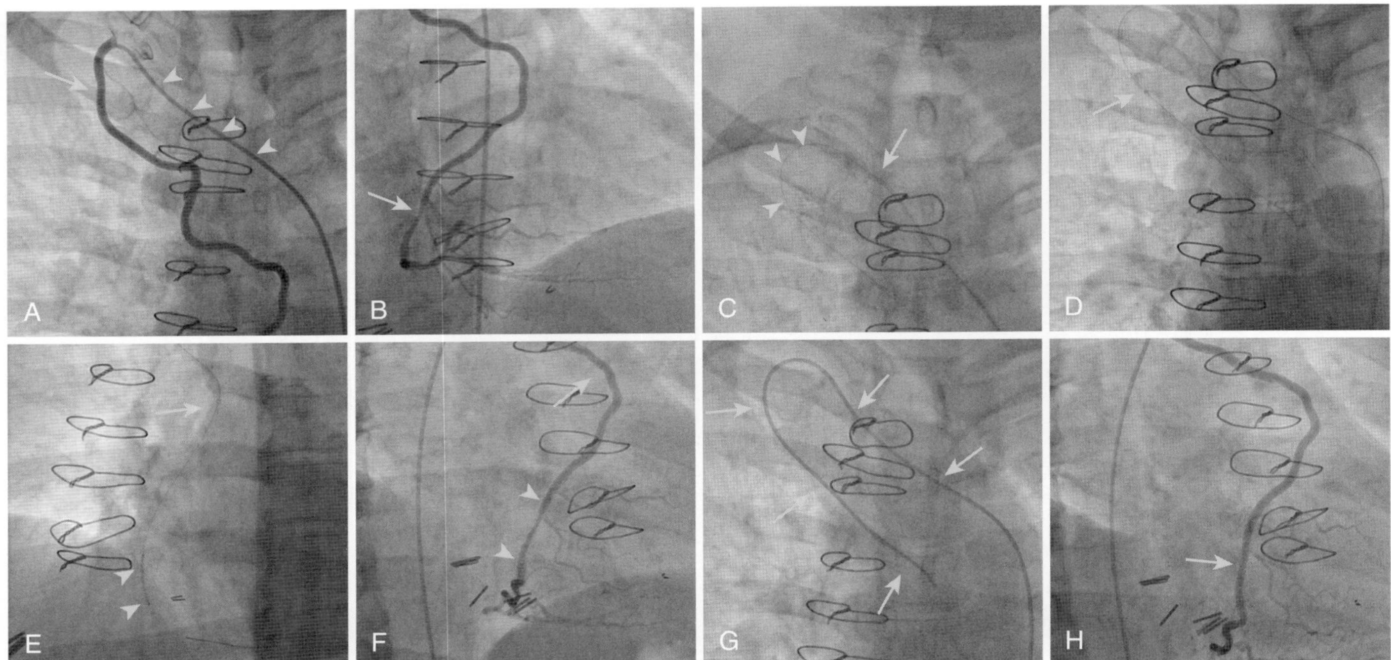

FIGURE 11-17 Treatment of an internal mammary artery distal anastomotic lesion. Diagnostic coronary angiography of the right internal mammary artery (arrowheads, panel **A**) via a 3DRC diagnostic catheter (arrow, panel **A**) demonstrating a distal anastomotic lesion (arrow, panel **B**). The 3DRC diagnostic catheter was removed (arrow, panel **C**) over a Grand Slam (Abbott Vascular) guidewire (arrowheads, panel **C**), and a Proxis catheter (St. Jude Medical) (arrow, panel **D**) was inserted into the RIMA over the guidewire, without using a guide catheter. Injection of contrast via a deep-seated Proxis catheter (arrows, panels **E, F,** and **G**) allowed positioning of a 3.0 × 23 mm sirolimus-eluting stent (arrowheads, panels **E** and **F**) across the distal anastomotic lesion with resolution of the lesion in poststenting angiography (panel **H**). *(Reproduced with permission from Brilakis ES, Banerjee S: Novel uses of the Proxis embolic protection catheter. Catheter Cardiovasc Interv 74:438–445, 2009.)*

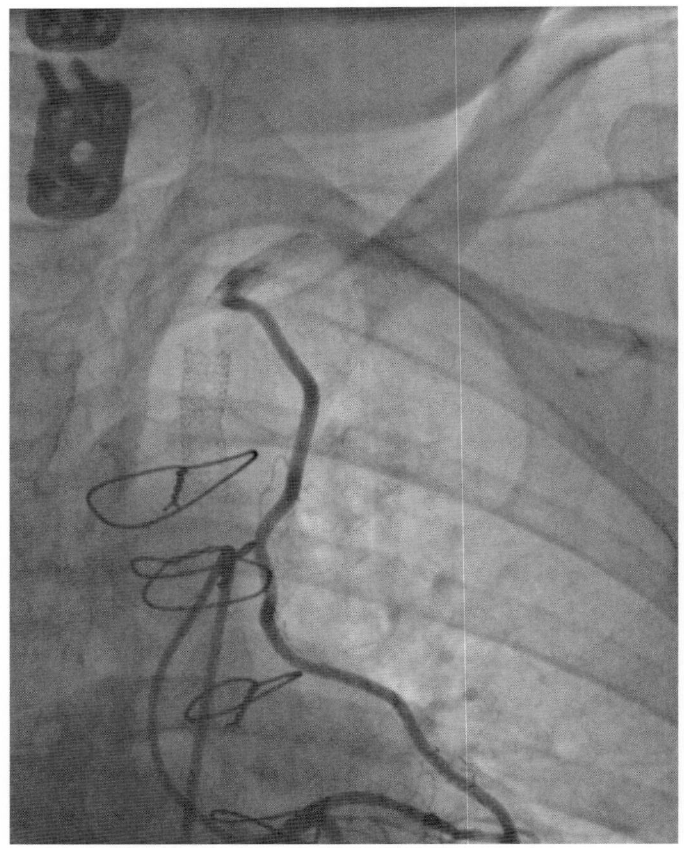

FIGURE 11-18 Example of subclavian steal syndrome. Reversal of flow in the left internal mammary artery graft due to severe proximal left subclavian stenosis **(Video 11-5)**.

CONCLUSIONS

In summary, bypass graft PCI currently accounts for approximately 6% of all PCIs. SVG PCI carries increased risk for distal embolization and subsequent SVG failure compared to native coronary artery PCI. EPDs should be used to prevent distal embolization during SVG PCI when technically feasible. DES should be utilized in SVG PCI if the patients do not have contraindications to long-term antiplatelet therapy. Native coronary arteries should be preferentially treated instead of bypass graft lesions, when technically feasible.

ACKNOWLEDGMENT

We would like to thank Michele Roesle, RN, for expert editorial assistance.

References

1. Loop FD, Lytle BW, Cosgrove DM, et al: Influence of the internal-mammary-artery graft on 10-year survival and other cardiac events. *N Engl J Med* 314:1–6, 1986.
2. Goldman S, Zadina K, Moritz T, et al: Long-term patency of saphenous vein and left internal mammary artery grafts after coronary artery bypass surgery: results from a Department of Veterans Affairs Cooperative Study. *J Am Coll Cardiol* 44:2149–2156, 2004.
3. Widimsky P, Straka Z, Stros P, et al: One-year coronary bypass graft patency: a randomized comparison between off-pump and on-pump surgery angiographic results of the PRAGUE-4 trial. *Circulation* 110:3418–3423, 2004.
4. Alexander JH, Hafley G, Harrington RA, et al: Efficacy and safety of edifoligide, an E2F transcription factor decoy, for prevention of vein graft failure following coronary artery bypass graft surgery: PREVENT IV: a randomized controlled trial. *JAMA* 294:2446–2454, 2005.
5. Morice MC, Feldman TE, Mack MJ, et al: Angiographic outcomes following stenting or coronary artery bypass surgery of the left main coronary artery: fifteen-month outcomes from the synergy between PCI with TAXUS express and cardiac surgery left main angiographic substudy (SYNTAX-LE MANS). *EuroIntervention* 7:670–679, 2011.
6. Brilakis ES, Rao SV, Banerjee S, et al: Percutaneous coronary intervention in native arteries versus bypass grafts in prior coronary artery bypass grafting patients: a report from the National Cardiovascular Data Registry. *JACC Cardiovasc Interv* 4:844–850, 2011.
7. Dehmer GJ, Weaver D, Roe MT, et al: A contemporary view of diagnostic cardiac catheterization and percutaneous coronary intervention in the United States: a report from the CathPCI Registry of the National Cardiovascular Data Registry, 2010 through June 2011. *J Am Coll Cardiol* 60:2017–2031, 2012.

8. Yau TM, Borger MA, Weisel RD, et al: The changing pattern of reoperative coronary surgery: trends in 1230 consecutive reoperations. *J Thorac Cardiovasc Surg* 120:156–163, 2000.
9. Yap CH, Sposato L, Akowuah E, et al: Contemporary results show repeat coronary artery bypass grafting remains a risk factor for operative mortality. *Ann Thorac Surg* 87:1386–1391, 2009.
10. Morrison DA, Sethi G, Sacks J, et al: Percutaneous coronary intervention versus repeat bypass surgery for patients with medically refractory myocardial ischemia: AWESOME randomized trial and registry experience with post-CABG patients. *J Am Coll Cardiol* 40:1951–1954, 2002.
11. Levine GN, Bates ER, Blankenship JC, et al: 2011 ACCF/AHA/SCAI Guideline for Percutaneous Coronary Intervention. A report of the American College of Cardiology Foundation/American Heart Association Task Force on Practice Guidelines and the Society for Cardiovascular Angiography and Interventions. *J Am Coll Cardiol* 58:e44–e122, 2011.
12. Varghese I, Samuel J, Banerjee S, et al: Comparison of percutaneous coronary intervention in native coronary arteries vs. bypass grafts in patients with prior coronary artery bypass graft surgery. *Cardiovasc Revasc Med* 10:103–109, 2009.
13. Bundhoo SS, Kalla M, Anantharaman R, et al: Outcomes following PCI in patients with previous CABG: a multi centre experience. *Catheter Cardiovasc Interv* 78:169–176, 2011.
14. Xanthopoulou I, Davlouros P, Tsigkas G, et al: Long-term clinical outcome after percutaneous coronary intervention in grafts vs native vessels in patients with previous coronary artery bypass grafting. *Can J Cardiol* 27:716–724, 2011.
15. Michael TT, Karmpaliotis D, Brilakis ES, et al: Impact of prior coronary artery bypass graft surgery on chronic total occlusion revascularisation: insights from a multicentre US registry. *Heart* 99:1515–1518, 2013.
16. Brilakis ES, Banerjee S, Lombardi WL: Retrograde recanalization of native coronary artery chronic occlusions via acutely occluded vein grafts. *Catheter Cardiovasc Interv* 75:109–113, 2010.
17. Boatman DM, Saeed B, Varghese I, et al: Prior coronary artery bypass graft surgery patients undergoing diagnostic coronary angiography have multiple uncontrolled coronary artery disease risk factors and high risk for cardiovascular events. *Heart Vessels* 24:241–246, 2009.
18. Davlouros P, Damelou A, Karantalis V, et al: Evaluation of culprit saphenous vein graft lesions with optical coherence tomography in patients with acute coronary syndromes. *JACC Cardiovasc Interv* 4:683–693, 2011.
19. Hong MK, Mehran R, Dangas G, et al: Creatine kinase-MB enzyme elevation following successful saphenous vein graft intervention is associated with late mortality. *Circulation* 100:2400–2405, 1999.
20. Brilakis ES: Chapter 26. Bypass graft intervention and embolic protection. In Kern MJ, editor: *SCAI interventional cardiology board review*, Philadelphia, PA, 2014, Lippincott Williams & Wilkins.
21. Baim DS, Wahr D, George B, et al: Randomized trial of a distal embolic protection device during percutaneous intervention of saphenous vein aorto-coronary bypass grafts. *Circulation* 105:1285–1290, 2002.
22. Stone GW, Rogers C, Hermiller J, et al: Randomized comparison of distal protection with a filter-based catheter and a balloon occlusion and aspiration system during percutaneous intervention of diseased saphenous vein aorto-coronary bypass grafts. *Circulation* 108:548–553, 2003.
23. Carrozza JP, Jr, Mumma M, Breall JA, et al: Randomized evaluation of the TriActiv balloon-protection flush and extraction system for the treatment of saphenous vein graft disease. *J Am Coll Cardiol* 46:1677–1683, 2005.
24. Holmes DR, Coolong A, O'Shaughnessy C, et al: Comparison of the CardioShield filter with the guardwire balloon in the prevention of embolisation during vein graft intervention: results from the CAPTIVE randomised trial. *EuroIntervention* 2:161–168, 2006.
25. Mauri L, Cox D, Hermiller J, et al: The PROXIMAL trial: proximal protection during saphenous vein graft intervention using the Proxis Embolic Protection System: a randomized, prospective, multicenter clinical trial. *J Am Coll Cardiol* 50:1442–1449, 2007.
26. Kereiakes DJ, Turco MA, Breall J, et al: A novel filter-based distal embolic protection device for percutaneous intervention of saphenous vein graft lesions: results of the AMEthyst randomized controlled trial. *JACC Cardiovasc Interv* 1:248–257, 2008.
27. Abdel-Karim AR, Papayannis AC, Mahmood A, et al: Role of embolic protection devices in ostial saphenous vein graft lesions. *Catheter Cardiovasc Interv* 80:1120–1126, 2012.
28. Wood FO, Badhey N, Garcia B, et al: Analysis of saphenous vein graft lesion composition using near-infrared spectroscopy and intravascular ultrasonography with virtual histology. *Atherosclerosis* 212:528–533, 2010.
29. Ashby DT, Dangas G, Aymong EA, et al: Effect of percutaneous coronary interventions for in-stent restenosis in degenerated saphenous vein grafts without distal embolic protection. *J Am Coll Cardiol* 41:749–752, 2003.
30. Brilakis ES, Wang TY, Rao SV, et al: Frequency and predictors of drug-eluting stent use in saphenous vein bypass graft percutaneous coronary interventions: a report from the American College of Cardiology National Cardiovascular Data CathPCI registry. *JACC Cardiovasc Interv* 3:1068–1073, 2010.
31. Webb LA, Dixon SR, Safian RD, et al: Usefulness of embolic protection devices during saphenous vein graft intervention in a nonselected population. *J Interv Cardiol* 18:73–75, 2005.
32. Mahmood A, Khair T, Abdel-Karim AR, et al: Contemporary approaches to saphenous vein graft interventions: a survey of 275 interventional cardiologists. *Catheter Cardiovasc Interv* 79:834–842, 2012.
33. Badhey N, Lichtenwalter C, de Lemos JA, et al: Contemporary use of embolic protection devices in saphenous vein graft interventions: insights from the stenting of saphenous vein grafts trial. *Catheter Cardiovasc Interv* 76:263–269, 2010.
34. Sdringola S, Assali A, Ghani M, et al: Adenosine use during aortocoronary vein graft interventions reverses but does not prevent the slow-no reflow phenomenon. *Catheter Cardiovasc Interv* 51:394–399, 2000.
35. Zoghbi GJ, Goyal M, Hage F, et al: Pretreatment with nitroprusside for microcirculatory protection in saphenous vein graft interventions. *J Invasive Cardiol* 21:34–39, 2009.
36. Fischell TA, Subraya RG, Ashraf K, et al: "Pharmacologic" distal protection using prophylactic, intragraft nicardipine to prevent no-reflow and non-Q-wave myocardial infarction during elective saphenous vein graft intervention. *J Invasive Cardiol* 19:58–62, 2007.
37. Michaels AD, Appleby M, Otten MH, et al: Pretreatment with intragraft verapamil prior to percutaneous coronary intervention of saphenous vein graft lesions: results of the randomized, controlled vasodilator prevention on no-reflow (VAPOR) trial. *J Invasive Cardiol* 14:299–302, 2002.
38. Niccoli G, Belloni F, Cosentino N, et al: Case-control registry of excimer laser coronary angioplasty versus distal protection devices in patients with acute coronary syndromes due to saphenous vein graft disease. *Am J Cardiol* 112:1586–1591, 2013.
39. Hong YJ, Pichard AD, Mintz GS, et al: Outcome of undersized drug-eluting stents for percutaneous coronary intervention of saphenous vein graft lesions. *Am J Cardiol* 105:179–185, 2010.
40. Okabe T, Lindsay J, Torguson R, et al: Can direct stenting in selected saphenous vein graft lesions be considered an alternative to percutaneous intervention with a distal protection device? *Catheter Cardiovasc Interv* 72:799–803, 2008.
41. Maia F, Costa JR, Jr, Abizaid A, et al: Preliminary results of the INSPIRE trial with the novel MGuard stent system containing a protection net to prevent distal embolization. *Catheter Cardiovasc Interv* 76:86–92, 2010.
42. Abizaid A, Weiner B, Bailey SR, et al: Use of a self-expanding super-elastic all-metal endoprosthesis; to treat degenerated SVG lesions: the SESAME first in man trial. *Catheter Cardiovasc Interv* 76:781–786, 2010.
43. Savage MP, Douglas JS, Jr, Fischman DL, et al: Stent placement compared with balloon angioplasty for obstructed coronary bypass grafts. Saphenous Vein De Novo Trial Investigators. *N Engl J Med* 337:740–747, 1997.
44. Hanekamp CE, Koolen JJ, Den Heijer P, et al: Randomized study to compare balloon angioplasty and elective stent implantation in venous bypass grafts: the Venestent study. *Catheter Cardiovasc Interv* 60:452–457, 2003.
45. Stankovic G, Colombo A, Presbitero P, et al: Randomized evaluation of polytetrafluoroethylene-covered stent in saphenous vein grafts: the Randomized Evaluation of polytetrafluoroethylene COVERed stent in Saphenous vein grafts (RECOVERS). *Trial Circulation* 108:37–42, 2003.
46. Schachinger V, Hamm CW, Munzel T, et al: A randomized trial of polytetrafluoroethylene-membrane-covered stents compared with conventional stents in aortocoronary saphenous vein grafts. *J Am Coll Cardiol* 42:1360–1369, 2003.
47. Turco MA, Buchbinder M, Popma JJ, et al: Pivotal, randomized U.S. study of the Symbiot™ covered stent system in patients with saphenous vein graft disease: eight-month angiographic and clinical results from the Symbiot III trial. *Catheter Cardiovasc Interv* 68:379–388, 2006.
48. Stone GW, Goldberg S, O'Shaughnessy C, et al: 5-year follow-up of polytetrafluoroethylene-covered stents compared with bare-metal stents in aortocoronary saphenous vein grafts the randomized BARRICADE (barrier approach to restenosis: restrict intima to curtail adverse events) trial. *JACC Cardiovasc Interv* 4:300–309, 2011.
49. Vermeersch P, Agostoni P, Verheye S, et al: Randomized double-blind comparison of sirolimus-eluting stent versus bare-metal stent implantation in diseased saphenous vein grafts: six-month angiographic, intravascular ultrasound, and clinical follow-up of the RRISC Trial. *J Am Coll Cardiol* 48:2423–2431, 2006.
50. Vermeersch P, Agostoni P, Verheye S, et al: Increased late mortality after sirolimus-eluting stents versus bare-metal stents in diseased saphenous vein grafts: results from the randomized DELAYED RRISC Trial. *J Am Coll Cardiol* 50:261–267, 2007.
51. Brilakis ES, Lichtenwalter C, de Lemos JA, et al: A randomized controlled trial of a paclitaxel-eluting stent versus a similar bare-metal stent in saphenous vein graft lesions: the SOS (Stenting of Saphenous Vein Grafts) trial. *J Am Coll Cardiol* 53:919–928, 2009.
52. Brilakis ES, Lichtenwalter C, Abdel-karim AR, et al: Continued benefit from paclitaxel-eluting compared with bare-metal stent implantation in saphenous vein graft lesions during long-term follow-up of the SOS (Stenting of Saphenous Vein Grafts) trial. *JACC Cardiovasc Interv* 4:176–182, 2011.
53. Mehilli J, Pache J, Abdel-Wahab M, et al: Drug-eluting versus bare-metal stents in saphenous vein graft lesions (ISAR-CABG): a randomised controlled superiority trial. *Lancet* 378:1071–1078, 2011.
54. Lichtenwalter C, de Lemos JA, Roesle M, et al: Clinical presentation and angiographic characteristics of saphenous vein graft failure after stenting: insights from the SOS (stenting of saphenous vein grafts) trial. *JACC Cardiovasc Interv* 2:855–860, 2009.
55. Papayannis AC, Michael TT, Yangirova D, et al: Optical coherence tomography analysis of the stenting of saphenous vein graft (SOS) Xience V Study: use of the everolimus-eluting stent in saphenous vein graft lesions. *J Invasive Cardiol* 24:390–394, 2012.
56. Kitabata H, Loh JP, Pendyala LK, et al: Two-year follow-up of outcomes of second-generation everolimus-eluting stents versus first-generation drug-eluting stents for stenosis of saphenous vein grafts used as aortocoronary conduits. *Am J Cardiol* 112:61–67, 2013.
57. Costopoulos C, Latib A, Naganuma T, et al: Comparison of first- and second-generation drug-eluting stents in saphenous vein grafts used as aorto-coronary conduits. *Am J Cardiol* 112:318–322, 2013.
58. Taniwaki M, Raber L, Magro M, et al: Long-term comparison of everolimus-eluting stents with sirolimus- and paclitaxel-eluting stents for percutaneous coronary intervention of saphenous vein grafts. *EuroIntervention* 2013. published online before print.
59. Wessely R, Marzocchi A, Schwacke H, et al: Long-term follow-up of coronary venous bypass graft lesions treated with a new generation drug-eluting stent with bioabsorbable polymer. *J Interv Cardiol* 26:425–433, 2013.
60. Ong PJ, Jafary FH, Ho HH: "First-in-man" use of bioresorbable vascular scaffold in saphenous vein graft. *EuroIntervention* 9:165, 2013.
61. Badr S, Kitabata H, Dvir D, et al: Optimal revascularization strategies for percutaneous coronary intervention of distal anastomotic lesions after coronary artery bypass surgery. *J Interv Cardiol* 26:366–371, 2013.
62. Hong YJ, Jeong MH, Ahn Y, et al: Impact of lesion location on intravascular ultrasound findings and short-term and five-year long-term clinical outcome after percutaneous coronary intervention for saphenous vein graft lesions. *Int J Cardiol* 167:29–33, 2013.
63. Roffi M, Mukherjee D, Chew DP, et al: Lack of benefit from intravenous platelet glycoprotein IIb/IIIa receptor inhibition as adjunctive treatment for percutaneous interventions of aortocoronary bypass grafts: a pooled analysis of five randomized clinical trials. *Circulation* 106:3063–3067, 2002.
64. Coolong A, Baim DS, Kuntz RE, et al: Saphenous vein graft stenting and major adverse cardiac events: a predictive model derived from a pooled analysis of 3958 patients. *Circulation* 117:790–797, 2008.
65. Harskamp RE, Beijk MA, Damman P, et al: Prehospitalization antiplatelet therapy and outcomes after saphenous vein graft intervention. *Am J Cardiol* 111:153–158, 2013.
66. Brilakis ES, Patel VG, Banerjee S: Medical management after coronary stent implantation: a review. *JAMA* 310:189–198, 2013.
67. Sachdeva A, Bavisetty S, Beckham G, et al: Discontinuation of long-term clopidogrel therapy is associated with death and myocardial infarction after saphenous vein graft percutaneous coronary intervention. *J Am Coll Cardiol* 60:2357–2363, 2012.
68. Sachdeva R, Aleti S, Thai H: Radial stent deformation in saphenous vein graft. *EuroIntervention* 8:876–877, 2012.
69. Varghese I, Boatman DM, Peters CT, et al: Impact on contrast, fluoroscopy, and catheter utilization from knowing the coronary artery bypass graft anatomy before diagnostic coronary angiography. *Am J Cardiol* 101:1729–1732, 2008.
70. Eisenhauer MD, Malik JA, Coyle LC, et al: Impact of aorto-coronary graft markers on subsequent graft patency: a retrospective review. *Cathet Cardiovasc Diagn* 42:259–261, 1997.
71. Michael TT, Alomar M, Papayannis A, et al: A randomized comparison of transradial versus transfemoral approach for coronary artery bypass graft angiography and intervention (the RADIAL CABG trial). *JACC Cardiovasc Interv* 2013. in press.
72. Bundhoo SS, Earp E, Ivanauskiene T, et al: Saphenous vein graft percutaneous coronary intervention via radial artery access: safe and effective with reduced hospital length of stay. *Am Heart J* 164:468–472, 2012.
73. Farooq V, Mamas MA, Fath-Ordoubadi F, et al: The use of a guide catheter extension system as an aid during transradial percutaneous coronary intervention of coronary artery bypass grafts. *Catheter Cardiovasc Interv* 78:847–863, 2011.
74. Michael TT, Brilakis ES: Taming saphenous vein grafts using guide catheter extensions. *Catheter Cardiovasc Interv* 78:864–865, 2011.
75. Banerjee S, Brilakis ES: Use of the Proxis embolic protection device for guide anchoring and stent delivery during complex saphenous vein graft interventions. *Cardiovasc Revasc Med* 10:183–187, 2009.
76. Papayannis AC, Banerjee S, Brilakis ES: Retrograde wiring: a novel technique for identifying the origin of unusual saphenous vein grafts. *Cardiovasc Revasc Med* 13:298–300, 2012.
77. Abdel-Karim AR, Banerjee S, Brilakis ES: Percutaneous intervention of acutely occluded saphenous vein grafts: contemporary techniques and outcomes. *J Invasive Cardiol* 22:253–257, 2010.

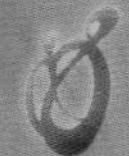

78. Cook J, Uretsky BF, Sachdeva R: Intervention in the occluded vein graft: with high risk can come great reward. Review of techniques with case examples. *J Invasive Cardiol* 24:612–617, 2012.
79. Giugliano GR, Falcone MW, Mego D, et al: A prospective multicenter registry of laser therapy for degenerated saphenous vein graft stenosis: the COronary graft Results following Atherectomy with Laser (CORAL) trial. *Cardiovasc Revasc Med* 13:84–89, 2012.
80. Garcia-Tejada J, Jurado-Roman A, Hernandez F, et al: Guiding-catheter thrombectomy combined with distal protection during primary percutaneous coronary intervention of a saphenous vein graft. *Cardiovasc Revasc Med* 14:356–358, 2013.
81. Fiorina C, Meliga E, Chizzola G, et al: Early experience with a new approach for percutaneous intervention of totally occluded saphenous vein graft: is the flow the best thrombolytic? *EuroIntervention* 6:461–466, 2010.
82. Al-Lamee R, Ielasi A, Latib A, et al: Clinical and angiographic outcomes after percutaneous recanalization of chronic total saphenous vein graft occlusion using modern techniques. *Am J Cardiol* 106:1721–1727, 2010.
83. Jim MH, Ho HH, Ko RL, et al: Paclitaxel-eluting stents for chronically occluded saphenous vein grafts (EOS) study. *J Interv Cardiol* 23:40–45, 2010.
84. Mhatre A, Uretsky BF, Sachdeva R: Substrate for complications. *J Invasive Cardiol* 24:E153–E156, 2012.
85. Garg N, Hakeem A, Gobal F, et al: Outcomes of percutaneous coronary intervention of chronic total saphenous vein graft occlusions in the contemporary era. *Catheter Cardiovasc Interv* 2013. published online before print.
86. Tonino PAL, De Bruyne B, Pijls NHJ, et al: Fractional flow reserve versus angiography for guiding percutaneous coronary intervention. *NEJM* 360:213–224, 2009.
87. Ellis SG, Brener SJ, DeLuca S, et al: Late myocardial ischemic events after saphenous vein graft intervention–importance of initially "nonsignificant" vein graft lesions. *Am J Cardiol* 79:1460–1464, 1997.
88. Rodes-Cabau J, Bertrand OF, Larose E, et al: Comparison of plaque sealing with paclitaxel-eluting stents versus medical therapy for the treatment of moderate nonsignificant saphenous vein graft lesions. The Moderate VEin Graft LEsion Stenting With the Taxus Stent and Intravascular Ultrasound (VELETI) Pilot Trial. *Circulation* 120:1978–1986, 2009.
89. Abdel-Karim AR, Da Silva M, Lichtenwalter C, et al: Prevalence and outcomes of intermediate saphenous vein graft lesions: findings from the stenting of saphenous vein grafts randomized-controlled trial. *Int J Cardiol* 168:2468–2473, 2013.
90. Aqel R, Zoghbi GJ, Hage F, et al: Hemodynamic evaluation of coronary artery bypass graft lesions using fractional flow reserve. *Catheter Cardiovasc Interv* 72:479–485, 2008.
91. Marmagkiolis K, Brilakis ES, Hakeem A, et al: Saphenous vein graft perforation during percutaneous coronary intervention: a case series. *J Invasive Cardiol* 25:157–161, 2013.
92. Chen DY, Chen CC, Hsieh IC: Hemoptysis caused by saphenous vein graft perforation during percutaneous coronary intervention. *J Invasive Cardiol* 25:E8–E10, 2013.
93. Brilakis ES, editor: *Manual of coronary chronic total occlusion interventions. A step-by-step approach*, Waltham, MA, 2013, Elsevier.
94. Lichtenwalter C, Banerjee S, Brilakis ES: Dual guide catheter technique for treating native coronary artery lesions through tortuous internal mammary grafts: separating equipment delivery from target lesion visualization. *J Invasive Cardiol* 22:E78–E81, 2010.
95. Brilakis ES, Banerjee S: Novel uses of the Proxis embolic protection catheter. *Catheter Cardiovasc Interv* 74:438–445, 2009.
96. Dimas B, Lindsey JB, Banerjee S, et al: ST-Segment elevation acute myocardial infarction due to severe hypotension and proximal left subclavian artery stenosis in a prior coronary artery bypass graft patient. *Cardiovasc Revasc Med* 10:191–194, 2009.

12 Calcified Lesions

Amar Krishnaswamy and Patrick L. Whitlow

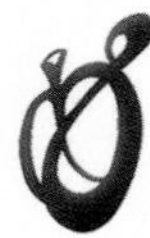

INTRODUCTION

Calcified coronary lesions present an important challenge to interventional cardiologists. Because of the rigidity and noncompliance of a heavily calcified coronary artery segment, heavy calcification was a risk factor for traditional balloon angioplasty failure and remains associated with major adverse cardiac events after stenting lesions with moderate/heavy calcification in patients with acute coronary syndromes and decreased success for chronic total occlusion percutaneous intervention today.[1-3] In the setting of severe luminal narrowing or speculated calcification obstructing the vessel lumen, the operator may be unable to pass balloons or stents. Fibrocalcific plaque is often difficult to dilate, reducing acute luminal gain and therefore limiting stent expansion. This in turn increases the risks of restenosis as well as stent thrombosis.[4,5]

Furthermore, attempts to dilate these lesions with high-pressure balloon inflation increases the risk of extensive dissection and perforation.

It is therefore imperative that contemporary interventionalists are well versed in techniques to modify moderately to heavily calcified segments. These techniques include percutaneous transluminal rotational atherectomy (PTRA), orbital atherectomy (OA), scoring balloon and cutting balloon angioplasty (SBA and CBA), and excimer laser coronary atherectomy (ELCA).

PERCUTANEOUS TRANSLUMINAL ROTATIONAL ATHERECTOMY

High-speed rotational atherectomy was introduced in the 1980s by David Auth as a mechanism to ablate atheromatous plaque by slowly advancing a spinning, diamond-coated burr. PTRA was approved for coronary use by the FDA in 1993. The procedure utilizes the principle of "differential cutting" in which the atherectomy device preferentially ablates inelastic tissue composed of fibrotic or calcific components and is safely deflected by more elastic tissue. The technique was intended to improve acute luminal gain with less deep-wall injury compared with balloon angioplasty alone, which in turn should logically reduce the risk of restenosis. In the contemporary stent era, PTRA was further expected to reduce in-stent restenosis due to a reduction in residual plaque burden and improved apposition between the stent and vessel wall.

Procedural Details

The currently available Rotablator system (Boston Scientific, Natick, Massachusetts) consists of a 4.3 Fr, 135-cm drive shaft through which passes a brass burr coated with small diamond crystals on the leading surface (**Figure 12-1A**). The burr is advanced slowly forward into the lesion and alternatively withdrawn using the Rotalink advancer system (**Figure 12-1B**) to allow forward flow with particle disbursement. Run times are limited to 15 to 30 seconds. During advancement, forward pressure applied to the burr is monitored carefully to minimize RPM drops >5,000 from baseline. Large RPM drops are associated with heat production and an increase in particulate size. After each run, the burr is disengaged from the lesion and forward flow is restored for at least 20 to 30 seconds to allow ST segments to normalize and systemic vasodilation to resolve. Runs are repeated until the lesion is fully crossed and ablated.

The entire system is attached to the Rotablator console that is connected to a tank of compressed nitrogen that is delivered to the console at 90 PSI to 110 PSI to spin the Rotablator turbine and burr (**Figures 12-1C and 12-1D**). The gas tank should contain at least 500 PSI of pressure. Delivery of the compressed gas to the burr is regulated by depression of the operator's foot pedal (**Figure 12-1E**).

The coronary artery is first wired using either the RotaWire Floppy or RotaWire Extra Support guidewire, depending on the characteristics of the vessel and lesion. Both wires consist of a 0.009-inch body and a 0.014-inch tip. The floppy wire is used most commonly, though the extra support wire may be helpful in distal lesions or very heavily calcified lesions. Given the 0.009-inch body and the absence of a lubricious coating, the Rotavirus is difficult to navigate, and a routine coronary wire may be useful to first wire the vessel and exchange for the RotaWire of choice via an over-the-wire balloon or microcatheter.

Prior to insertion of the burr into the back of the guide, the operator should be assured that the rotaflush is seen

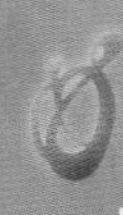

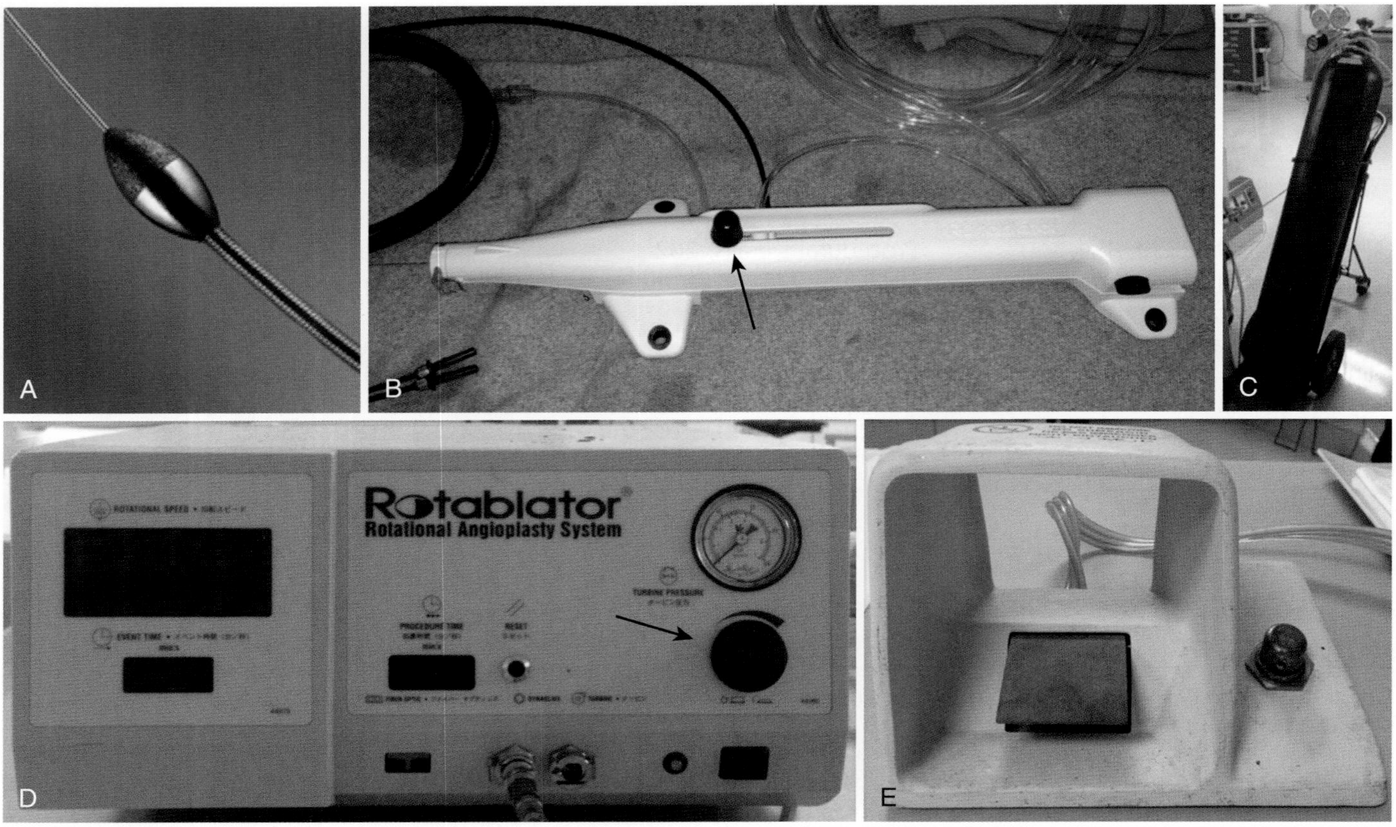

FIGURE 12-1 Rotablator rotational atherectomy system. **(A)** Diamond-coated burr; **(B)** Rotalink advancer system with advancing knob (arrow); **(C)** nitrogen tank; **(D)** Rotablator console (RPM setting knob, arrow); **(E)** foot pedal.

dripping through the drive shaft. The burr should also be tested and intended RPM set on the console, usually 150,000 RPM to 180,000 RPM (**Figure 12-1D**). With the burr held above the patient's drape, the turbine is activated and the nurse/technician should turn the power dial until the desired baseline RPM is achieved. The Rotablator system is then advanced over the wire to a position just proximal of the lesion of interest. It is important that two operators work together in this process; one should "pin" the wire as the other advances the system through the guide (as with an over-the-wire balloon or microcatheter device).

Once the burr is in place, the operator then activates the turbine and advances the burr slowly and steadily back and forth across the lesion. It is imperative that the burr is withdrawn completely from the lesion before stepping off of the pedal, as this can cause the burr to become entrapped in the calcified lesion.

Pushing the burr too firmly or allowing stored tension on the wire to lurch the burr suddenly forward can cause the rotating burr to pass through the lesion without adequate ablation. This operator error may rarely cause the burr to become entrapped distal to the intended lesion. Careful attention to procedural details is necessary to avoid complications.

Once the atherectomy is completed, the DynaGlide should be activated, which provides a 60,000 RPM to 90,000 RPM spin of the burr to facilitate extraction of the system over the wire. Simultaneously, the brake must be disengaged and the entire system smoothly retracted over the wire. Care should be taken at this step to not remove the foot from the pedal or inadvertently reengage the brake, as either could result in pulling the wire out of the vessel along with the burr. This step is most safely performed under continuous fluoroscopy to assure wire position in the vessel.

TABLE 12-1 Guide Catheter Requirement for Intended Rotational Atherectomy Burr Size

ROTABLATOR BURR SIZE	LARGE LUMEN GUIDE SIZE
1.25 mm	5/6 Fr
1.50 mm	6 Fr
1.75 mm	7 Fr
2.00 mm	8 Fr
2.15 mm	8 Fr
2.25 mm	9 Fr
2.38 mm	9 Fr
2.50 mm	9 Fr

The choice of initial burr size is dependent on the lesion and the size of the coronary vessel. To minimize complications such as coronary dissection and perforation, it is recommended that the operator not exceed a burr/artery diameter ratio >0.7. Operators may start with a 1.5-mm or 1.75-mm burr to create a channel and access the passage across the lesion. In patients undergoing PCI of a particularly long or severe lesion, it is occasionally necessary to start with a 1.25-mm burr. The necessary guide catheter size for each burr is given in **Table 12-1**.

The calcified lesion may be considered adequately modified when a 1:1 size balloon can be passed through the lesion and fully inflated without any residual waist at ≤14 atmospheres. If a balloon waist persists, additional rotational atherectomy with a larger burr should be considered.

The burr displaces atheroma and fibrocalcific particles without injuring the normal elastic vessel wall. The microparticles created are generally <5 microns in size and are eventually cleared by the reticuloendothelial system. Nevertheless, some patients do suffer from microvascular occlusion and poor or no reflow. To minimize this risk, the procedure should be conducted with continuous pressurized intracoronary infusion (via the Rotablator catheter) of a "rotaflush" solution. This solution usually consists of the proprietary Rotaglide lubricant to increase passage of the burr and reduce heat generation, as well as a calcium-channel blocker (i.e., verapamil or nicardipine) and nitroglycerin to protect the downstream microvasculature. The Rotaglide should not be used in patients allergic to eggs or olive oil, both of which are constituents of the lubricant. Hemodynamic instability may preclude the use of PTRA as infusion of vasoplegic substances in the Rotaflush solution may induce further hypotension.

In addition to the microvascular debris that may occlude the microvasculature, there is a concern that hemolysis from rotational atherectomy elaborates adenosine and other substances that may be detrimental to proper electrical conduction. In combination with the verapamil that constitutes the flush solution, these factors can induce heart block during the procedure. As a result, operators may consider placement of a temporary pacemaker in the right ventricle prior to rotational atherectomy of the RCA or a dominant left circumflex coronary artery. Alternatively, intravenous infusion of aminophylline ± an atropine bolus during runs may be helpful to minimize conduction block.

A helpful online didactic course in using the Rotablator system is also available at **http://lms.indegene.com/bsc_rotablator/**.

Clinical Studies of Rotational Atherectomy

After a number of nonrandomized trials suggested a benefit of PTRA compared with percutaneous transluminal angioplasty (PTA) alone, Guerin and colleagues published a pilot randomized trial of PTRA.[6] They evaluated 64 patients (32 in each group) with Type B2 coronary lesions randomized to PTA alone versus PTRA followed by balloon angioplasty. There was no significant difference with respect to Q-wave MI (one in each group), numerically greater non–Q-wave MI in the PTRA group (3 vs. 0), and no significant difference in the primary success rate (93.7% vs. 87.5%), defined as a reduction in stenosis by >20% and residual stenosis <50% without a major complication. Angiographic analysis at 6 months demonstrated no significant difference in restenosis between the two groups (39% vs. 42%).

Subsequently, the Excimer Laser, Rotational Atherectomy, and Balloon Angioplasty Comparison (ERBAC) study randomized 685 patients at a single center to one of these three treatment modalities.[7] The primary endpoint of procedural success (final diameter stenosis <50% and no MACE) was significantly greater in the PTRA group compared with the PTA group (89.2% vs. 79.7%, p = 0.0019), in large part due to a higher likelihood of crossing the lesion and achievement of a final diameter stenosis <50%. Despite this encouraging finding, acute gain was relatively similar between the PTRA and PTA groups (1.25 mm vs. 1.19 mm, p = 0.37), as was the postprocedure diameter stenosis (30% vs. 31%, p = 0.68). There was also a nonsignificant trend toward a greater number of patients with restenosis in the PTRA group (57% vs. 47%, p = 0.14) and a significant increase in TVR in the PTRA and laser groups compared with the PTA group (42% vs. 46% vs. 32%, p = 0.013). Furthermore, the incidence of a MACE was significantly greater in the PTRA group (46% vs. 37%, p = 0.04). The authors' statement that the role of PTRA can be viewed "optimistically if restenosis is considered a benign disease" appears to overstate the case, though their assertion that PTRA "provides the means to expand the indication for PCI" is reasonable.

The Comparison of Balloon versus Rotational Angioplasty (COBRA) investigators conducted a randomized trial of 502 patients, 250 of whom received routine PTA alone and 252 of whom received PTRA followed by balloon angioplasty.[8] Despite a greater acute net lumen gain in the PTRA group (0.82 mm vs. 0.64 mm, p = 0.008) and better average final diameter stenosis (46% vs. 52%, p = 0.039), the angiographic restenosis rate was equivalent in the two groups (35% vs. 37%, p = 0.658), as was the rate of TLR (29% vs. 25%, p = 0.43). Notably, the need for stent implantation for inadequate PTRA or PTA lumen gain or for bailout was higher in the PTA alone group (9.6% vs. 2.0%). In the contemporary era where stent implantation is the norm, however, it is difficult to consider less stent placement an advantage.

Rotational atherectomy has also been studied for patients with in-stent restenosis (ISR). The Angioplasty versus Rotational Atherectomy for the Treatment of Diffuse In-Stent Restenosis Trial (ARTIST) randomized patients with diffuse ISR to PTA (n = 146) or PTRA (n = 152).[9] The investigators demonstrated a trend toward more periprocedural complications in the PTRA group (composite of death, MI, CABG, PTCA, tamponade, and puncture site complication: 14% vs. 8%, p = 0.09). Furthermore, at 6 months, event-free survival (defined as freedom from death, MI, or clinically driven TLR) was significantly worse in the PTRA group (79.6% vs. 91.1%, p = 0.005). In addition to greater safety than PTRA, PTA alone also demonstrated better procedural efficacy, with a larger net gain (0.67 mm vs. 0.45 mm, p = 0.0019) and fewer patients with restenosis >50% at 6 months (51% vs. 65%, p = 0.039).

In the contemporary era of routine stent placement, initial PTRA has been studied as a strategy to optimize stent deployment and reduce subsequent ISR. The Rotational Atherectomy Prior to TAXUS Stent Treatment for Complex Native Coronary Artery Disease (ROTAXUS) investigators randomized 240 patients equally to DES placement preceded by PTRA versus PTA followed by DES placement.[10] At the conclusion of the procedure, residual stenosis was less (6% vs. 11%, p = 0.04) and acute gain was greater (1.56 mm vs. 1.44 mm, p = 0.01) in the PTRA group. Nevertheless, at 9 months' angiographic follow-up, there was no significant difference in diameter stenosis or restenosis in the two groups, though in-stent late-lumen loss favored the PTA-alone group (0.31 mm vs. 0.44 mm, p = 0.04). As such, the trial investigators concluded that PTA with provisional PTRA (for uncrossable or undilatable lesions) should remain the default strategy prior to stent placement.

Summary

Despite nonrandomized data and case series that suggest efficacy of PTRA, the totality of clinical trial data does not support the routine use of PTRA compared with PTA either as stand-alone treatment, pretreatment prior to stent

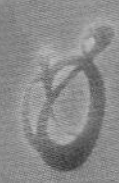

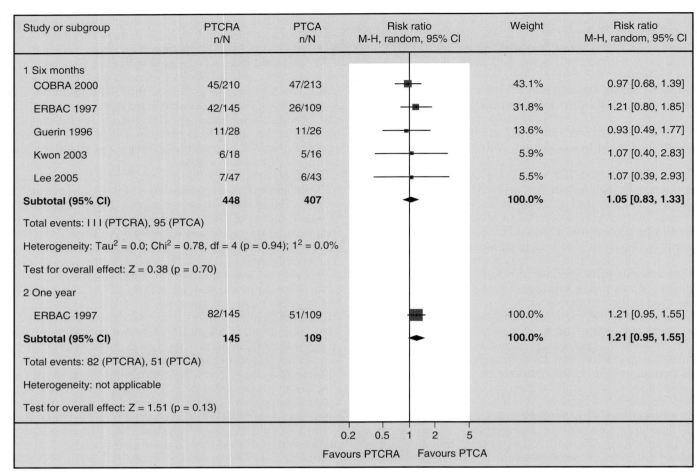

Study or subgroup	PTCRA n/N	PTCA n/N	Risk ratio M-H, random, 95% CI	Weight	Risk ratio M-H, random, 95% CI
1 Six months					
COBRA 2000	45/210	47/213		43.1%	0.97 [0.68, 1.39]
ERBAC 1997	42/145	26/109		31.8%	1.21 [0.80, 1.85]
Guerin 1996	11/28	11/26		13.6%	0.93 [0.49, 1.77]
Kwon 2003	6/18	5/16		5.9%	1.07 [0.40, 2.83]
Lee 2005	7/47	6/43		5.5%	1.07 [0.39, 2.93]
Subtotal (95% CI)	**448**	**407**		**100.0%**	**1.05 [0.83, 1.33]**
Total events: 111 (PTCRA), 95 (PTCA)					
Heterogeneity: $Tau^2 = 0.0$; $Chi^2 = 0.78$, df = 4 (p = 0.94); $I^2 = 0.0\%$					
Test for overall effect: Z = 0.38 (p = 0.70)					
2 One year					
ERBAC 1997	82/145	51/109		100.0%	1.21 [0.95, 1.55]
Subtotal (95% CI)	**145**	**109**		**100.0%**	**1.21 [0.95, 1.55]**
Total events: 82 (PTCRA), 51 (PTCA)					
Heterogeneity: not applicable					
Test for overall effect: Z = 1.51 (p = 0.13)					
			0.2 0.5 1 2 5		
			Favours PTCRA Favours PTCA		

FIGURE 12-2 Metaanalysis of restenosis in complex coronary lesions after percutaneous rotational atherectomy (PTRA) versus angioplasty alone (PTCA). *(Reproduced with permission from Wasiak J, Law J, Watson P, et al: Percutaneous transluminal rotational atherectomy for coronary artery disease. Cochrane Database Syst Rev (12):CD003334, 2012.)*

implantation, or treatment for patients suffering from ISR. This is confirmed by a recent metaanalysis demonstrating that PTRA does not hold a benefit over PTA alone to reduce restenosis in noncomplex lesions, complex lesions, or ISR (**Figure 12-2**).[11] Therefore, PTRA should be reserved for lesions that are severely calcified and for which optimal balloon and stent expansion is not possible without plaque modification (**Figure 12-3**). It may also be necessary for spiculated or severely narrowed lesions that do not allow the passage of balloons and/or stents or lesions that are not dilatable with noncompliant, high-pressure balloons. This is reflected by the 2011 ACC/AHA/SCAI PCI guidelines, which provide a Class IIb recommendation for PTRA in "fibrotic or calcified lesions that might not be crossed by a balloon catheter or adequately dilated before stent implantation" and a Class III recommendation for PTRA "for de novo lesions or in-stent restenosis."[12]

ORBITAL ATHERECTOMY

The Diamondback 360-degree coronary orbital atherectomy system (OAS; Cardiovascular Systems, Inc., St. Paul, Minnesota) was recently approved by the FDA for coronary use. Based on the principles of differential sanding and centrifugal force, the system consists of an eccentrically mounted, diamond-coated "crown" that orbits over a guidewire. A thin layer of plaque is "sanded" off with each pass of the device and elastic tissue flexes away from the crown. Theoretically, the elliptical orbit of the devices allows microdebris to disperse, as opposed to the rota burr, which does not allow blood to flow past. Further, the microparticles elaborated by the OAS average less than 2 microns in size, smaller than those of PTRA.

Procedural Details

The OAS passes over the ViperWire guidewire included in the system. The crown is available in 1.25-mm and 1.5-mm sizes, with a maximum orbit that is influenced by the rotational speed of the crown (1.82 mm and 2.16 mm for each, respectively). Similar to PTRA, a proprietary ViperSlide lubricant is continuously infused in addition to saline to provide lubrication, cooling, and flow of microdebris.

Clinical Studies of Orbital Atherectomy

The ORBIT trial was conducted in 2008 and enrolled 50 patients with mild to severely calcified coronary lesions in a nonrandomized fashion to use the OAS.[13] Complications included in-hospital NSTEMI in two patients (4%), six dissections, and one perforation. Use of the OAS alone proved a reduction in the percentage of diameter stenosis from 85.6% to 40%. Target lesion revascularization was seen in one patient (2%) at 30 days. The trial suggested the safety and efficacy of the OAS, providing a background for a larger study.

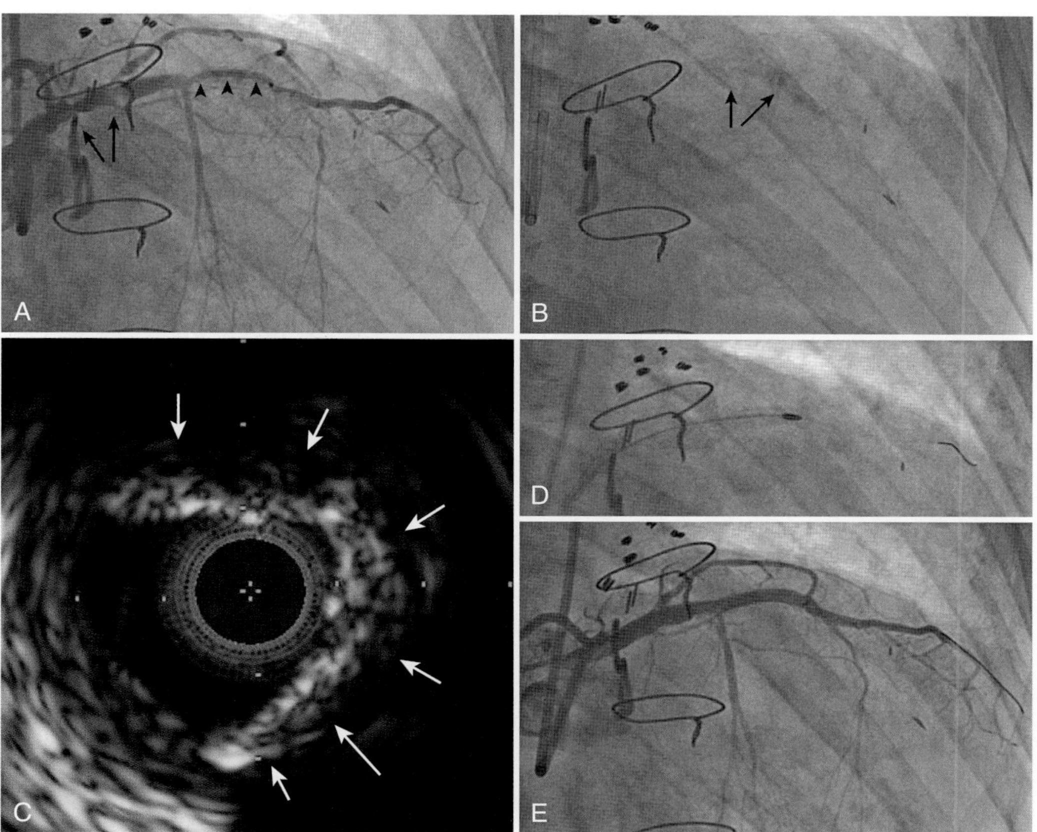

FIGURE 12-3 PTRA of the LAD/Diagonal. **(A)** Initial angiogram demonstrates severe calcified stenosis in the proximal (arrow) and mid LAD (arrowheads) extending to the diagonal. **(B)** Fluoroscopy alone shows the severe calcifications (arrows). **(C)** Intravascular ultrasound demonstrates 270-degree calcification (arrows) with echo dropout behind the calcium. **(D)** Rotaburr in the mid LAD. **(E)** Final angiogram after stent placement.

The ORBIT II trial was recently presented and enrolled 443 patients with severely calcified lesions.[14] With respect to safety, 3.4% demonstrated a significant dissection, 1.8% perforation, 0.9% slow/no reflow, and 1.8% abrupt closure. The composite of Q- and non–Q-wave MI was seen in 9.3% of patients in-hospital. All of these complications are well within the range of those seen in trials of rotational or laser atherectomy, though direct comparisons, of course, cannot be made. The primary efficacy endpoint (stent delivery with residual stenosis <50% and freedom from 30-day MACE) was appreciated by 88.9% of patients, and the primary safety endpoint of freedom from 30-day MACE was appreciated by 89.6% of patients, thereby fulfilling the performance goals of the study.

Summary

Orbital atherectomy in the coronary tree is a recently available and approved modality for the treatment of calcified lesions. Initial trial data are limited but appear promising with respect to safety and efficacy. The optimal utilization of the OAS remains to be defined by accumulating clinical experience and comparative clinical trials.

SCORING BALLOON ANGIOPLASTY (SBA)

Scoring balloon angioplasty is a generic term that refers to inflating a balloon catheter with one or more protruding metallic edges contacting the vessel wall on balloon dilation. The leading metallic edge is designed to cut or score the plaque, causing a cleavage plane that theoretically enhances more controlled lumen dilation than routine balloon angioplasty. The technique is easy to use because no other capital equipment is needed except what is utilized in routine PCI. Two types of scoring balloon systems are currently available for plaque modification.

CBA was developed by Barath et al. in the early 1990s.[15] The balloon material covers three to four longitudinally positioned microsurgical metallic edges. Metal edges are designed to parallel the balloon when the balloon is deflated and then angle outward toward the vessel wall as the balloon expands. These edges are sharp and meant to penetrate the luminal wall in a controlled manner, leading to lumen expansion at lower balloon inflation pressures. On inflation, the blades are deployed at 60 degrees from the balloon to contact the arterial wall to create controlled cuts into the plaque, which should expedite lumen expansion.

This Flextome balloon system is currently distributed by Boston Scientific (Natick, Massachusetts) to dilate coronary lesions. CBA has been utilized to modify fibrotic or mildly to moderately calcified lesions. Clinical experience has shown that cutting balloon inflation sometimes leads to less elastic recoil and more luminal enlargement than dilation with a similar size, noncompliant, high-pressure balloon in ostial or resistant coronary lesions.[16,17]

The AngioSculpt balloon catheter (Angioscore, Fremont, California) was initially developed by Gershony and the first-in-man series published by Fonseca and colleagues in 2008.[18] The device consists of a semicompliant nylon

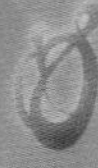

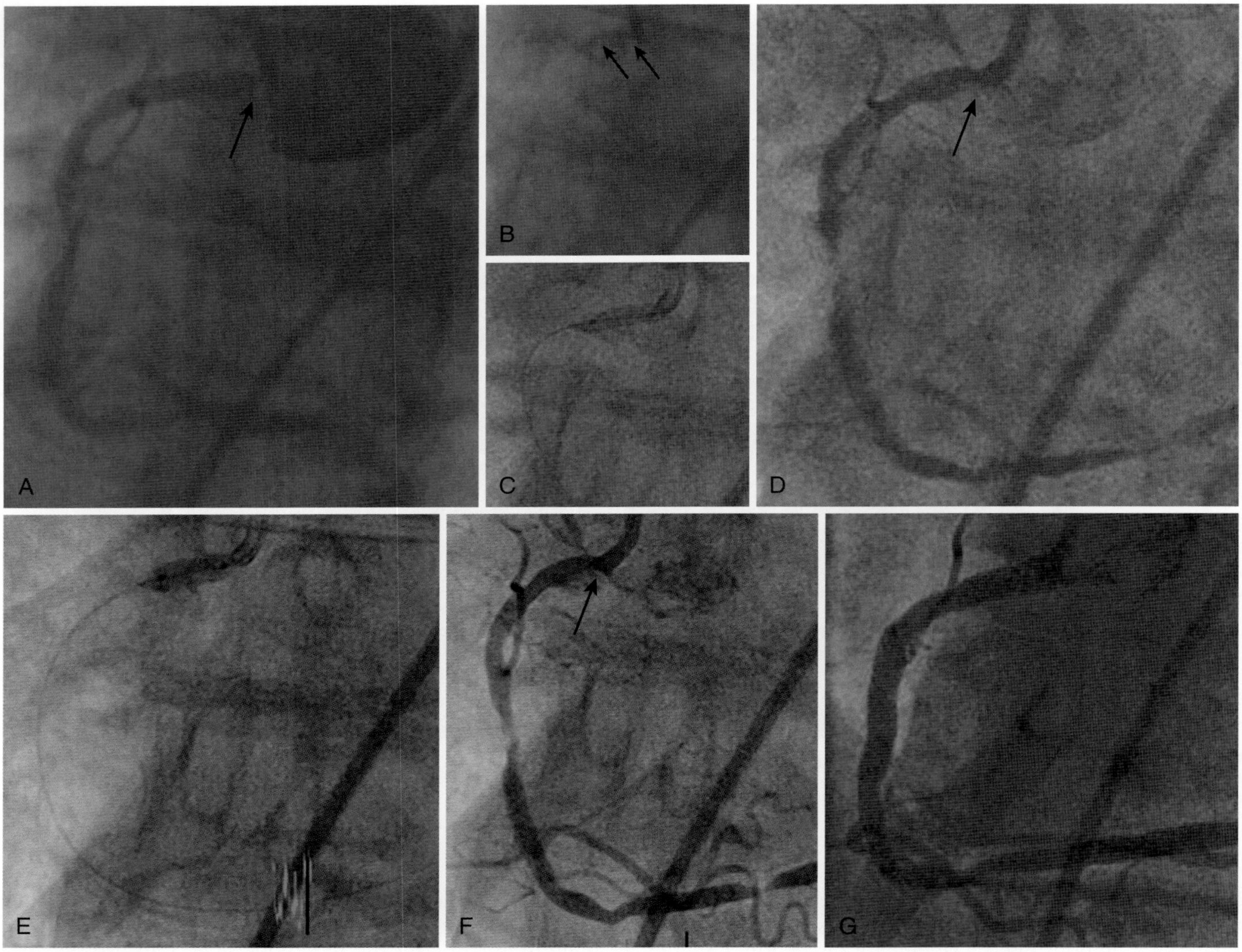

FIGURE 12-4 Scoring balloon angioplasty prior to stent placement. **(A)** Angiography demonstrates a severe ostial RCA (arrow) stenosis with **(B)** severe calcification fluoroscopically. **(C)** Routine balloon angioplasty provided only **(D)** mild improvement in lumen size with difficulty in passing a stent. **(E)** AngioSculpt scoring angioplasty resulted in calcium fracture and **(F)** improved lumen gain, facilitating **(G)** stent placement.

balloon surrounded by an expandable nitinol cage. Upon inflation, the nitinol scoring elements are driven into the arterial wall and concentrate the dilating force to the protruding metallic edges (**Figure 12-4**). Theoretically, the concentration of outward force into the small surface area of the nitinol frame focuses the dilating force and enhances vessel lumen expansion. In addition, the metal surfaces are driven into the arterial wall, expediting lumen expansion. Clinical experience has shown that the AngioSculpt system is useful for dilating resistant lesions, even those with moderate to heavy calcification.

Clinical Studies of Scoring Balloon Angioplasty

The mechanisms involved in lumen expansion with CBA versus PTCA were studied by intravascular ultrasound (IVUS) and QCA in 65 consecutive lesions (40 with CBA, 25 with routine PTCA) by Hara and colleagues.[16] Native de novo lesions <10 mm in length were treated with multiple inflations with the cutting balloon (40 lesions) or conventional balloon angioplasty (25 lesions) at operator discretion. Balloon size (2.8 mm) and balloon/artery ratio were similar for both groups, and procedural success was 100% in both groups. Maximum balloon inflation pressure was significantly higher for PTCA than CBA (10.1 ± 3.5 atm vs. 8.3 ± 2.3 atm, $p < 0.05$). Final MLD was 2.3 mm in both groups.

IVUS confirmed a similar final lumen area in both groups (5.5 ± 1.2 CBA vs. 5.7 ± 1.2 mm^2 PTCA) but more vessel expansion with PTCA (1.3 ± 1.3 vs. 1.8 ± 1.6 mm^2, $p < 0.05$) and more plaque compression with CBA (−1.6 ± 1.4 vs. −0.5 ± 2.1, $p < 0.01$). Therefore, the mechanism of lumen enlargement appears different with CBA than with POBA. Sixty-seven percent of lumen expansion after PTCA appears to be due to vessel area expansion and 33% due to plaque shift or compression. With CBA, 45% of lumen enlargement appears to be due to vessel stretch and 55% due to plaque compression.

Several registries and randomized trials confirmed reasonable clinical results and less bailout stenting with CBA than PTCA.[17,19] However, the largest randomized trial of stand-alone CBA versus PTCA showed no clinical advantage of CBA in angiographic restenosis or TVA but a significant increase in acute vessel perforation and tamponade.[20] Restenosis rates for stand-alone CBA remain in the 30% range, and CBA today is generally used to predilate resistant coronary lesions before stent placement or to dilate in-stent restenosis lesions to prevent balloon slippage. CBA can effectively dilate mild to moderately calcified resistant coronary lesions, but the technique is not considered with dense superficial calcification.

An optical coherence tomography (OCT) examination of coronary lesions after dilation with the AngioSculpt showed clear evidence of plaque scoring with lumen expansion.[21] Three-dimensional stereoscopic reconstruction of a severely calcified coronary lesion treated with the AngioSculpt showed spiral radial scoring of cleavage planes and lumen expansion at sites adjacent to the most severe calcification.[22] These authors concluded that the AngioSculpt might become one of the preferred options for lesion modification for a severely calcified lesion.

De Ribamar Costa and colleagues compared adequacy of DES expansion by IVUS with direct stenting, predilation with a noncompliant balloon, or predilation with the AngioSculpt in 299 consecutive de novo lesions.[23] The minimum stent diameter (2.6 ± 0.4, 2.5 ± 0.4, 2.8 ± 0.4 mm) and minimal stent cross-sectional area (6.0 ± 1.7, 5.9 ± 1.6, 6.8 ± mm^2) were significantly better in the AngioSculpt pretreatment group. In addition, a minimum DES area <5.0 mm^2 (associated with increased restenosis and acute stent thrombosis) was found in only 11% of AngioSculpt pretreated lesions versus 26% of the remaining lesions. The authors concluded that AngioSculpt pretreatment prior to DES placement enhances stent expansion.[24]

Summary

Lesion modification with SBA can often result in successful dilation of a resistant coronary lesion and enhance stent expansion. OCT examination has confirmed radial scoring and lumen expansion of a severely calcified coronary lesion with AngioSculpt treatment. Because of the ease of use and effectiveness of SBA, these devices have become frequently used for lesion modification in our catheterization laboratory.

Because of simplicity of use and cost, SBA is frequently used to dilate ostial lesions, which are traditionally considered as noncompliant, or mild to moderately calcified vessels that would be expected to be difficult to dilate. Furthermore, with increasing clinical experience, the AngioSculpt is being used more often to predilate heavily calcified lesions before stenting. A case example of a very heavily calcified ostial right coronary artery lesion treated with SBA is shown in **Figure 12-4**.

EXCIMER LASER ATHERECTOMY

Laser technology was approved for use in the coronary tree by the FDA in 1992. The contemporary excimer coronary laser operates in the ultraviolet field (λ = 308 nm), which minimizes vapor bubble formation and improves the safety profile of the device in comparison to older generation devices that operated in the infrared field (λ = 2090 nm).[25] The application of laser energy to the vessel results in photochemical, photomechanical, and photothermal interactions that produce gas vapor and acoustic shock waves within the tissue that ultimately provides a debulking effect. Applications of excimer laser coronary atherectomy (ELCA) include uncrossable chronic total occlusions (CTO), balloon-resistant calcified lesions, and underexpanded stent lesions.

Procedural Details

The Spectranetics CVX-300 ELCA system (Spectranetics, Colorado Springs, Colorado) consists of the generator console (**Figure 12-5**), the laser catheter, and the activating pedal. The catheter is available in 0.9-mm, 1.4-mm, 1.7-mm, and 2.0-mm diameters with specifications as provided in **Table 12-2**. Prior to insertion of the laser catheter into the guide, the operator must calibrate the system by aiming the catheter at the energy detector and stepping on the foot switch. Once calibration is complete, the console will state that calibration is "OK" and the system is "Ready."

As with any other catheter, the lesion of interest must first be crossed with a coronary guidewire. A catheter is then chosen, which is optimally two thirds of the size of the target vessel. The laser catheter is then slowly advanced across the lesion. Unlike rotational atherectomy, which debulks only while being advanced, the laser catheter provides energy during advancement and retraction of the catheter, both of which should be performed slowly to optimize energy delivery. Caution should be used to perform continuous saline injection in the guide catheter while

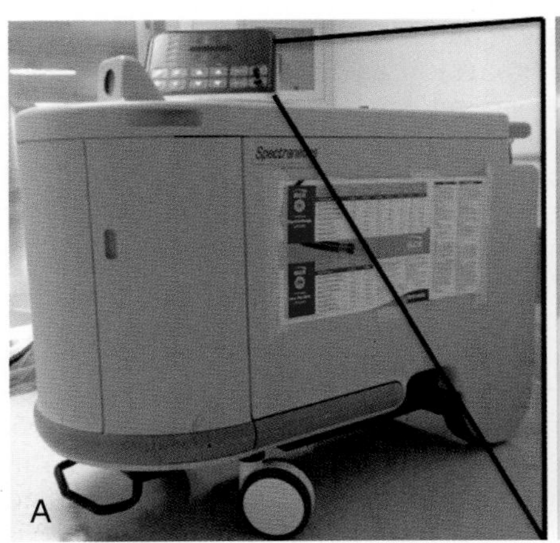

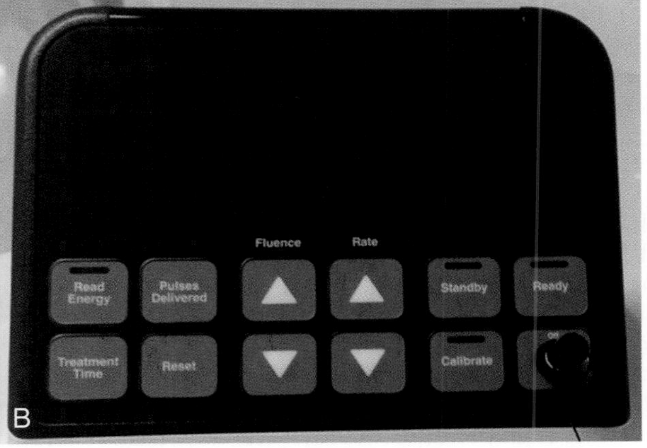

FIGURE 12-5 Spectranetics laser atherectomy console. **(A)** (arrow: energy detector) and main control display **(B)**.

TABLE 12-2 Technical Specifications of the Spectranetics Excimer Laser Coronary Atherectomy Catheter System

LASER CATHETER	0.99 mm	1.4 mm	1.7 mm	2.0 mm	0.9 mm OTW CATHETER
Guide catheter compatibility	6 Fr	7 Fr	7 Fr	8 Fr	6 Fr
Minimum vessel diameter	1.5 mm	2.2 mm	2.5 mm	3.0 mm	1.5 mm
Fluence (mJ/mm²)	30-60	30-60	30-60	30-60	30-60
Repetition rate (Hz)	25-40	25-40	25-40	25-40	25-40

lasing. This reduces the temperature and uncontrolled photomechanical damage in the coronary artery, thereby minimizing complications. The connection of a saline pressurized bag to the guiding catheter via a Tuohy Borst adapter is frequently utilized for this purpose. Specific situations may call for contrast injection at the time of lasing, as discussed below.

Clinical Studies of Excimer Laser Atherectomy

As with PTRA, nonrandomized studies of ELCA provided seemingly hopeful results for atherectomy as an alternative to PTA alone.[26-28] Investigators therefore expected to demonstrate a reduction in restenosis in randomized trials. However, as with PTRA, randomized trials of ELCA versus PTA failed to demonstrate significant benefit.

The multicenter Amsterdam-Rotterdam (AMRO) trial randomized 308 patients with predominantly Type B2 and C lesions, approximately one third of which were classified as calcific, to ELCA followed by PTA (n = 151) or PTA alone (n = 151).[29] There was no difference in the postprocedure diameter stenosis for ELCA versus PTA (37.6% vs. 37.9%, p = 0.76), and despite a borderline significantly larger minimum lumen diameter (1.69 mm vs 1.59 mm, p = 0.05), there was a higher degree of late loss (0.52 mm vs. 0.34 mm, p = 0.04) in the ELCA group, which ultimately resulted in an equivalent MLD at 6-month angiographic follow-up (1.17 mm vs. 1.25 mm, p = 0.34) and a nonsignificant but higher restenosis rate in the ELCA group (51.6% vs. 41.3%, p = 0.13). The rate of periprocedural MI, similar to that in studies of PTRA, was 3.3%.

In the ELCA group of the ERBAC trial discussed above, 18.5% of lesions could not be crossed by the laser catheter and required crossover to PTA.[7] In interpreting these results, it should be noted that at the time of that trial, the 1.4-mm catheter was the smallest available. Nevertheless, procedural success was similar between ELCA and PTA (77% vs. 80%). Postprocedure and 6-month follow-up diameter stenosis was similar in the two groups (31% vs. 30% and 57% vs. 52%, respectively; p = NS), though there was a significantly greater late loss (0.77 mm vs. 0.52 mm, $p < 0.05$) and restenosis rate (59% vs. 47%, p = 0.39) in the ELCA group. As with PTRA, patients treated with ELCA demonstrated a higher incidence of MACE than PTA alone (48% vs. 37%, p = 0.015).

An important use of ELCA today is for patients suffering from ISR associated with an underexpanded stent.[30] In fibrotic or calcified lesions that have not been properly prepared with debulking, predilation, or plaque modification prior to stent placement, achieving appropriate stent expansion even with high-pressure deployment and noncompliant balloon dilation may not be possible. To facilitate adequate stent expansion, ELCA can be used to vaporize and modify the fibrotic/calcified plaque behind the stent, allowing further expansion with noncompliant balloon dilation. **Figure 12-6A** demonstrates severe ISR in the proximal left circumflex (LCS) and proximal ramus intermedius (RI) 8 months after 2.5-mm stent placement in each vessel. The LCX was adequately treated with noncompliant balloon dilation, but severe stenosis remained in the RI even after dilation with a 3.0-mm noncompliant balloon (**Figure 12-6B**). IVUS demonstrated severely calcified atheroma behind the stent and a minimum lumen area (MLA) within the stent of 2.7 mm² (**Figure 12-6C**). After ELCA, the same 3.0-mm noncompliant balloon yielded significantly greater dilation (**Figure 12-6D**) and IVUS demonstrated an MLA of 4.2 mm² (**Figure 12-6E**).

The use of ELCA to treat stent underexpansion was demonstrated in Ellement registry by Latib and colleagues.[31] As stated above, ELCA is routinely performed with simultaneous intracoronary saline infusion or injection to minimize heat generation and vapor bubble formation. However, these investigators instead demonstrated the use of simultaneous contrast injection to essentially create a controlled "explosion" to improve stent expansion. In their series of 28 patients with undilatable stents treated with this method, 27 patients had successful dilation after ELCA (IVUS MSA increased from 3.5 mm to 7.1 mm²). The incidence of periprocedural MI was 3.6%, with a 6-month TLR rate of 3.6%, demonstrating the relative safety of this technique when necessary in appropriately selected patients without other options for further stent expansion.

Summary

Laser atherectomy, similar to PTRA, does not appear to confer any greater benefit than PTA alone in most lesions. However, it does hold an important role in the treatment of severely calcified lesions or for the treatment of stent underexpansion, as demonstrated above. These recommendations are reflected by the 2011 ACC/AHA/SCAI PCI guidelines, which provide a Class IIb recommendation for ELCA in "fibrotic or moderately calcified lesions that cannot be crossed or dilated with conventional balloon angioplasty" and a Class III recommendation for use "routinely during PCI."[12]

CONCLUSIONS

Calcified coronary lesions are an often encountered and challenging situation for interventional cardiologists. Various devices for plaque modification prior to stent deployment have been developed, all with efficacy and safety in appropriate anatomy. These include scoring balloon angioplasty,

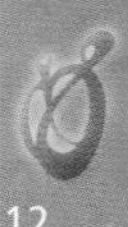

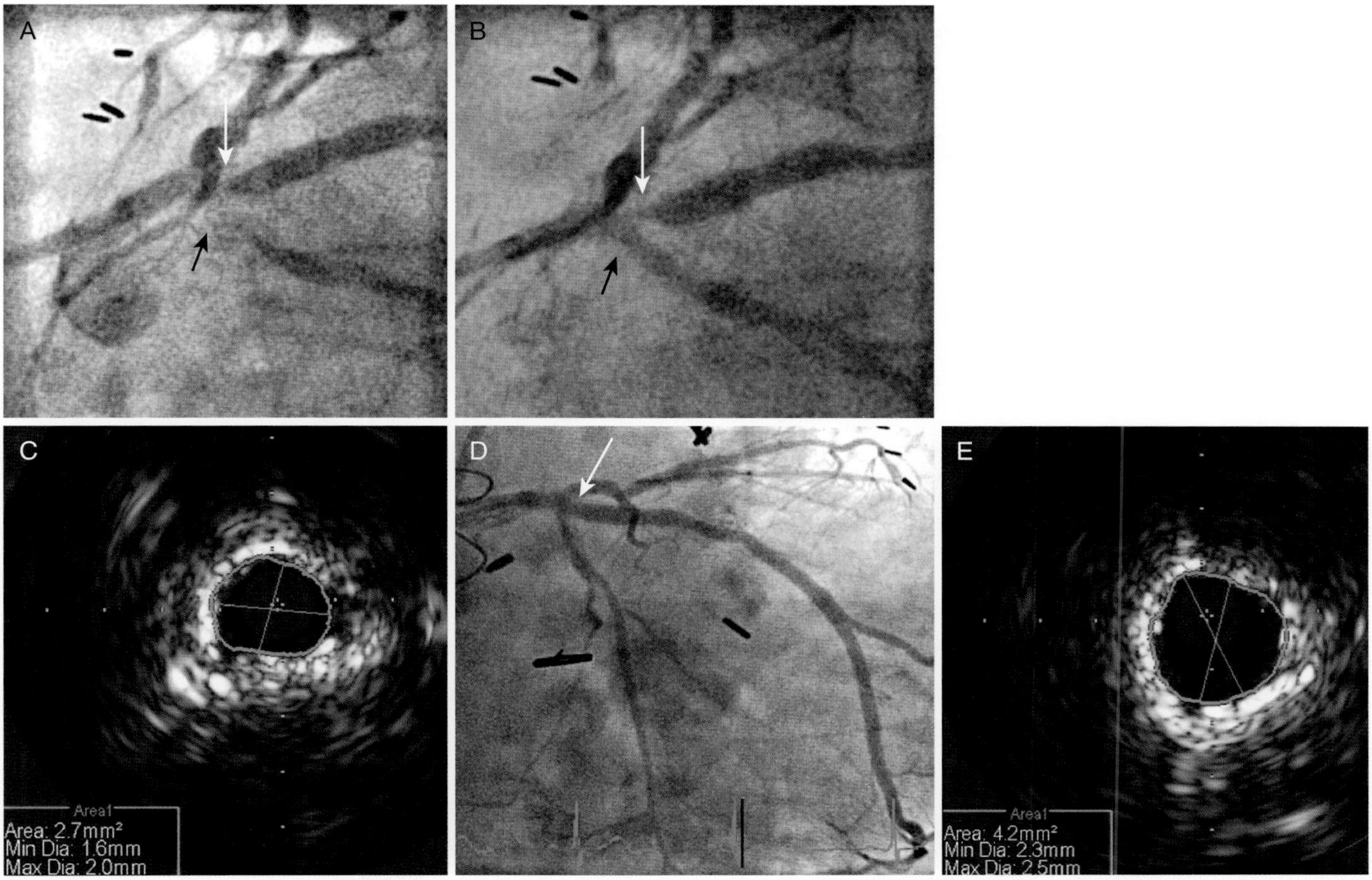

FIGURE 12-6 ELCA to treat ISR associated with stent underexpansion. **(A)** Severe ISR in the proximal ramus (white arrow) and proximal LCX (black arrow). **(B)** Continued severe ISR in the ramus after PTCA (3.0-mm balloon). **(C)** IVUS demonstrates severe calcification and fibrosis behind the stent (MLA 2.7 mm^2). **(D)** Improved expansion after ELCA followed by PTCA (using the same 3.0-mm balloon) of the proximal RI. **(E)** IVUS demonstrates improved stent expansion (MLA 4.2 mm^2).

rotational and orbital atherectomy, and excimer laser atherectomy. The use of a specific modality is chosen based on operator comfort and preference, specific lesion characteristics, and patient-specific factors, including hemodynamic stability. Familiarity with more than one technique is recommended to allow the operator to remain dynamic in the face of varied patient and lesion characteristics. In lesions with the most dense circumferential superficial calcification, rotational atherectomy remains the most reliable tool for plaque modification. However, in less demanding calcified lesions, other approaches are frequently utilized successfully.

References

1. Genereux P, Madhavan MV, Mintz GS, et al: Ischemic outcomes after coronary intervention of calcified vessels in acute coronary syndromes: pooled analysis from the HORIZONS-AMI and ACUITY trials. *J Am Coll Cardiol* 2014.
2. Hsu JT, Kyo E, Chu CM, et al: Impact of calcification length ratio on the intervention for chronic total occlusions. *Int J Cardiol* 150:135–141, 2011.
3. Virmani R, Farb A, Burke AP: Coronary angioplasty from the perspective of atherosclerotic plaque: morphologic predictors of immediate success and restenosis. *Am Heart J* 127:163–179, 1994.
4. Krishnaswamy A: Factors associated with stent thrombosis causing ST-segment elevation myocardial infarction. American Heart Association Scientific Sessions 2013.
5. Kuntz RE, Safian RD, Carrozza JP, et al: The importance of acute luminal diameter in determining restenosis after coronary atherectomy or stenting. *Circulation* 86:1827–1835, 1992.
6. Guerin Y, Spaulding C, Desnos M, et al: Rotational atherectomy with adjunctive balloon angioplasty versus conventional percutaneous transluminal coronary angioplasty in type B2 lesions: results of a randomized study. *Am Heart J* 131:879–883, 1996.
7. Reifart N, Vandormael M, Krajcar M, et al: Randomized comparison of angioplasty of complex coronary lesions at a single center. Excimer Laser, Rotational Atherectomy, and Balloon Angioplasty Comparison (ERBAC) Study. *Circulation* 96:91–98, 1997.
8. Dietz U, Rupprecht HJ, Ekinci O, et al: Angiographic analysis of immediate and long-term results of PTCR vs. PTCA in complex lesions (COBRA study). *Catheter Cardiovasc Interv* 53:359–367, 2001.
9. vom Dahl J, Dietz U, Haager PK, et al: Rotational atherectomy does not reduce recurrent in-stent restenosis: results of the angioplasty versus rotational atherectomy for treatment of diffuse in-stent restenosis trial (ARTIST). *Circulation* 105:583–588, 2002.
10. Abdel-Wahab M, Richardt G, Joachim Buttner H, et al: High-speed rotational atherectomy before paclitaxel-eluting stent implantation in complex calcified coronary lesions: the randomized ROTAXUS (Rotational Atherectomy Prior to Taxus Stent Treatment for Complex Native Coronary Artery Disease) trial. *JACC Cardiovasc Interv* 6:10–19, 2013.
11. Wasiak J, Law J, Watson P, et al: Percutaneous transluminal rotational atherectomy for coronary artery disease. *Cochrane Database Syst Rev* (12):CD003334, 2012.
12. Levine GN, Bates ER, Blankenship JC, et al: 2011 ACCF/AHA/SCAI Guideline for Percutaneous Coronary Intervention: executive summary: a report of the American College of Cardiology Foundation/American Heart Association Task Force on Practice Guidelines and the Society for Cardiovascular Angiography and Interventions. *Circulation* 124:2574–2609, 2011.
13. Parikh K, Chandra P, Choksi N, et al: Safety and feasibility of orbital atherectomy for the treatment of calcified coronary lesions: the ORBIT I trial. *Catheter Cardiovasc Interv* 81:1134–1139, 2013.
14. Chambers JW, Feldman RL, Himmelstein SI, et al: Pivotal trial to evaluate the safety and efficacy of the orbital atherectomy system in treating de novo, severely calcified coronary lesions (ORBIT II). *JACC Cardiovasc Interv* 7:510–518, 2014.
15. Barath P, Fishbein MC, Vari S, et al: Cutting balloon: a novel approach to percutaneous angioplasty. *Am J Cardiol* 68:1249–1252, 1991.
16. Hara H, Nakamura M, Asahara T, et al: Intravascular ultrasonic comparisons of mechanisms of vasodilatation of cutting balloon angioplasty versus conventional balloon angioplasty. *Am J Cardiol* 89:1253–1256, 2002.
17. Yamaguchi T, Nakamura M, Nishida T, et al: Update on cutting balloon angioplasty. *J Interv Cardiol* 11:S114–S119, 1998.
18. Fonseca A, Costa Jde R, Jr, Abizaid A, et al: Intravascular ultrasound assessment of the novel AngioSculpt scoring balloon catheter for the treatment of complex coronary lesions. *J Invasive Cardiol* 20:21–27, 2008.
19. Ergene O, Seyithanoglu BY, Tastan A, et al: Comparison of angiographic and clinical outcome after cutting balloon and conventional balloon angioplasty in vessels smaller than 3 mm in diameter: a randomized trial. *J Invasive Cardiol* 10:70–75, 1998.
20. Mauri L, Bonan R, Weiner BH, et al: Cutting balloon angioplasty for the prevention of restenosis: results of the Cutting Balloon Global Randomized Trial. *Am J Cardiol* 90:1079–1083, 2002.
21. Takano M, Yamamoto M, Murakami D, et al: Optical coherence tomography after new scoring balloon angioplasty for in-stent restenosis and de novo coronary lesions. *Int J Cardiol* 141:e51–e53, 2010.
22. Kanai T, Hiro T, Takayama T, et al: Three-dimensional visualization of scoring mechanism of "AngioSculpt" balloon for calcified coronary lesions using optical coherence tomography. *J Cardiol Cases* 5:e16–e19, 2012.
23. de Ribamar Costa J, Jr, Mintz GS, Carlier SG, et al: Nonrandomized comparison of coronary stenting under intravascular ultrasound guidance of direct stenting without predilation versus conventional predilation with a semi-compliant balloon versus predilation with a new scoring balloon. *Am J Cardiol* 100:812–817, 2007.

24. Sonoda S, Morino Y, Ako J, et al: Impact of final stent dimensions on long-term results following sirolimus-eluting stent implantation: serial intravascular ultrasound analysis from the sirius trial. *J Am Coll Cardiol* 43:1959–1963, 2004.
25. Fracassi F, Roberto M, Niccoli G: Current interventional coronary applications of excimer laser. *Expert Rev Med Devices* 10:541–549, 2013.
26. Ben-Dor I, Maluenda G, Pichard AD, et al: The use of excimer laser for complex coronary artery lesions. *Cardiovasc Revasc Med* 12(69):e1–e8, 2011.
27. Bittl JA, Sanborn TA, Tcheng JE, et al: Clinical success, complications and restenosis rates with excimer laser coronary angioplasty. The Percutaneous Excimer Laser Coronary Angioplasty Registry. *Am J Cardiol* 70:1533–1539, 1992.
28. Bittl JA, Sanborn TA: Excimer laser-facilitated coronary angioplasty. Relative risk analysis of acute and follow-up results in 200 patients. *Circulation* 86:71–80, 1992.
29. Appelman YE, Piek JJ, Strikwerda S, et al: Randomised trial of excimer laser angioplasty versus balloon angioplasty for treatment of obstructive coronary artery disease. *Lancet* 347:79–84, 1996.
30. Noble S, Bilodeau L: High energy excimer laser to treat coronary in-stent restenosis in an under-expanded stent. *Catheter Cardiovasc Interv* 71:803–807, 2008.
31. Latib A, Takagi K, Chizzola G, et al: Excimer Laser LEsion modification to expand non-dilatable stents: the ELLEMENT registry. *Cardiovasc Revasc Med* 15:8–12, 2014.

Treatment of In-Stent Restenosis

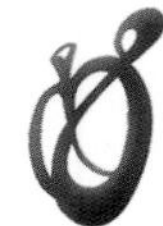

Robert A. Byrne, Michael Joner, Fernando Alfonso, and Adnan Kastrati

INTRODUCTION

The development of percutaneous coronary intervention (PCI) with stent implantation has revolutionized the practice of cardiology over the course of the past decades. However, despite considerable technological advancements, in-stent restenosis (ISR) remains the most common cause of treatment failure after PCI.[1,2] Moreover the high efficacy with contemporary devices—primarily drug-eluting stents (DES)—has facilitated the expansion of PCI to broader and increasingly more complex lesion and patient subsets. Accordingly, despite low rates of ISR in relative terms the absolute numbers of patients presenting with stent failure remain considerable. Importantly the management of this condition remains challenging, with high rates of subsequent events at medium- to long-term follow-up.[3,4]

The term *restenosis* is used in a variety of settings across the field of interventional cardiology. Angiographic restenosis is commonly adjudicated as a binary event defined as a re-narrowing of more than 50% of the vessel diameter as determined by coronary angiography. As this definition is based on two-dimensional parameters accurate measurements are critically dependent on the acquisition of worst-view projections. Typically visual estimation of restenosis is employed in routine clinical practice in the catheterization laboratory. This requires the operator to develop a sense of what comprises a 50% diameter stenosis. In adjudication of ISR the basic frame of reference is the body of the stent—this is known as an in-stent analysis. However, restenosis also shows a predilection for occurrence at stent margins. Accordingly a frame of reference including both the body of the stent and 5-mm margin proximal and distal to the stent edges is also usually assessed—this is known as an in-segment analysis. It is important to recognize that the use of 50% diameter stenosis as a cut-off for determination of restenosis as a binary event is rather arbitrary. For this reason continuous parameters are also commonly employed as surrogate markers of restenosis. These parameters also offer the advantage of superior statistical power for comparison between treatments, which makes them particularly attractive for clinical trials as they reduce the sample size required. The most commonly used continuous parameters are minimal lumen diameter (MLD) or percentage diameter stenosis at follow-up angiography and late lumen loss (which is the difference between the MLD immediately postprocedure and that at follow-up angiography). Of these, percentage diameter stenosis and late loss are the most well-studied markers in clinical trials and mean values of these parameters correlate reliably with incidence of angiographic and clinical restenosis.[5-7]

Intravascular imaging modalities such as intravascular ultrasound (IVUS) or optical coherence tomography (OCT) acquire data in three dimensions. Using these modalities restenosis is defined as a re-narrowing of more than 75% of the reference vessel area in cross-section. Visual estimation of stenosis is not usually employed and rapid online quantitative measurements are routinely available in the catheterization laboratory. Similarly, in autopsy studies restenosis is usually defined as a pathological vessel re-narrowing of more than 75% of the vessel area in cross-section. The term *clinical restenosis* is sometimes used to refer to restenosis of the treated lesion accompanied by requirement for re-treatment, for example, due to symptoms or signs of ischemia. Rates of clinical restenosis are usually considerably lower than rates of restenosis detected by imaging as not all restenotic lesions cause ischemia or elicit symptoms.

The principles underpinning the management of ISR are not dissimilar to those underlying the treatment of de novo coronary atherosclerotic lesions. The basic tenet of interventional treatment is that efficacy is optimized by maximizing acute gain and/or by minimizing late loss (**Figure 13-1**). However, the major difference with restenotic in comparison with de novo lesions is the presence of an existing stent scaffold in the diseased coronary segment. This may offer certain mechanical advantages, if its structural integrity is intact, but also provides a challenge due to the potential disadvantages of implanting multiple stent layers.

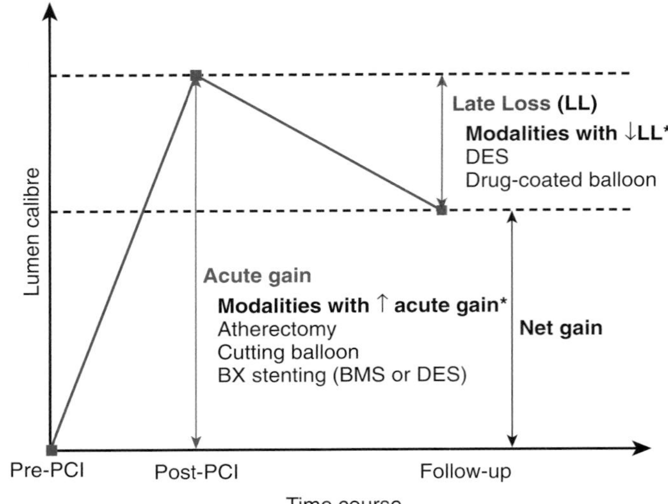

FIGURE 13-1 Schematic of relative contributions of acute gain and late loss to restenosis after coronary intervention. *BMS,* Bare-metal stent; *BX,* balloon expandable; *DES,* drug-eluting stent; *LL,* late loss; *PCI,* percutaneous coronary intervention. *Compared with balloon angioplasty alone.

MECHANISMS OF IN-STENT RESTENOSIS

Restenosis after PCI is well characterized as a distinct pathophysiological process rather than merely an accelerated form of postintervention atherosclerosis.[8] Broadly speaking the contributing factors to restenosis after vascular intervention may be divided into five categories as follows:

1. acute or subacute prolapse of the disrupted plaque
2. elastic recoil of the vessel wall
3. constrictive vascular remodeling
4. neointimal hyperplasia (due to extracellular matrix deposition and smooth muscle cell hyperplasia)
5. de novo in-stent atherosclerosis (so-called neoatherosclerosis)

While implantation of a metal stent after balloon dilatation largely negates the impact of the first three processes on restenosis, the additional vessel injury imposed by stent implantation increases the extent of neointimal tissue formation during vessel healing. Moreover, although DES have reduced the incidence of restenosis dramatically,[9] the delayed vessel healing seen with these stents may contribute to an increased incidence or accelerated course of de novo atherosclerotic disease within the stent in the months and years after intervention.[10] Indeed, from a clinicopathological standpoint it appears that there are considerable differences between the restenosis that occurs after bare-metal versus after drug-eluting stenting (**Table 13-1, Figure 13-2**).[11,12] In addition the availability of high-resolution intravascular imaging modalities such as optical coherence tomography (OCT) permits more detailed characterization of intravascular tissue and recognition of neoatherosclerotic changes in vivo (**Figure 13-3;** Videos 13-1 to 13-4).

In terms of angiographic morphology of restenosis after stenting Mehran et al. developed the most widely accepted classification system for restenosis within bare-metal stents.[13] This scheme is based on stenosis length (≤10 mm is classified as focal, >10 mm as diffuse), geographic localization of the neointima in relation to the stent and whether or not the restenosis is occlusive. Patterns are classified into 4 major groups: type I focal; type II diffuse within stent; type III diffuse within and beyond stent; and type IV occlusive (see case examples Videos 13-5 to 13-19). Importantly the pattern of restenosis at presentation is a predictor of subsequent outcome after re-intervention. In the original study target lesion revascularization rates were 19%, 35%, 50%, and 83% in groups I-IV, respectively ($p < 0.001$). While the majority of restenotic lesions within bare-metal stents are diffuse, in DES the majority are focal (**Table 13-1, Figure 13-4**). This may be because DES are generally very effective at suppressing neointimal overgrowth, which means that focal technical issues (e.g., stent fracture, local underexpansion) may play a relatively more important role in comparison with bare-metal stent restenosis.

The remainder of this chapter summarizes the spectrum of management options for patients presenting with restenosis following bare-metal or drug-eluting stent therapy. The principal randomized trials investigating outcomes of patients treated for ISR are summarized in **E-Table 13-1.**

TABLE 13-1 Comparison of Principle Features of Bare-Metal and Drug-Eluting Stent Restenosis

CHARACTERISTIC	BARE-METAL STENT RESTENOSIS	DRUG-ELUTING STENT RESTENOSIS
Imaging Features		
Angiographic appearance	Diffuse pattern more common	Focal pattern more common
Time course of late luminal loss	Late loss maximal by 6-8 months	Ongoing late loss out to 5 years
Optical coherence tomography tissue properties	Homogeneous, high-signal band typical	Layered structure or heterogeneous typical
Histopathological Features		
Smooth muscle cellularity	Rich	Hypocellular
Proteoglycan content	Moderate	High
Peri-strut fibrin and inflammation	Occasional	Frequent
Complete endothelialization	3-6 months	Up to 48 months
Thrombus present	Occasional	Occasional
Neoatherosclerosis	Relatively infrequent, late after stenting	Relatively frequent, accelerated course

BALLOON ANGIOPLASTY

The earliest approach to the treatment of ISR was with balloon angioplasty. Balloon dilatation directly targets the two principal causes of ISR—namely, neointimal hyperplasia and stent underexpansion. Mechanistically balloon angioplasty compresses and extrudes (axially and longitudinally) neointimal tissue and corrects underlying underexpansion of the stent backbone. One study with intravascular ultrasound (IVUS) suggested that the lumen enlargement with angioplasty was due to additional stent expansion and decrease in neointimal tissue volume in approximately equal measure.[40]

The technical procedure is relatively straightforward and the rate of complications is low. In fact early reports

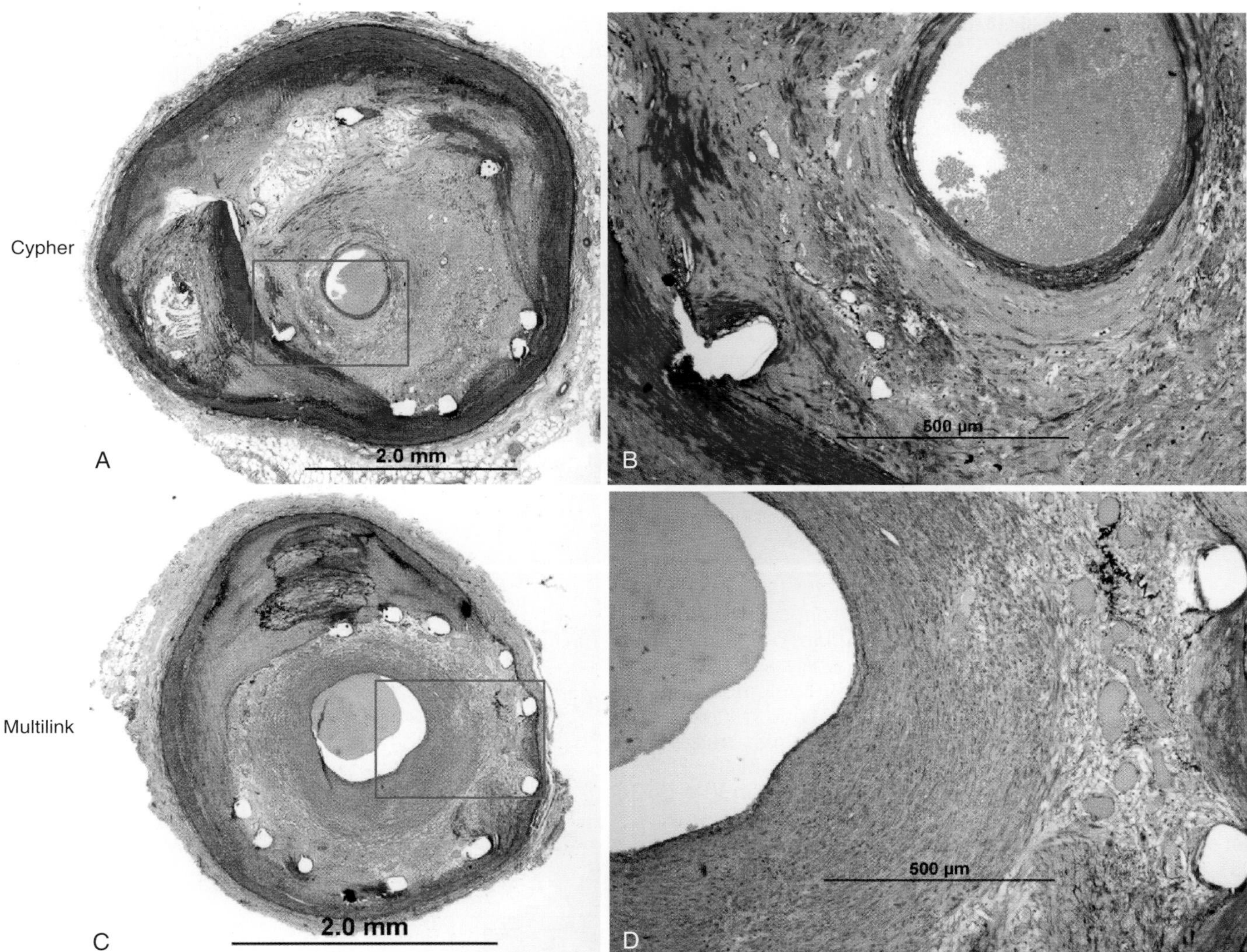

FIGURE 13-2 Histopathology of restenosis after drug-eluting and bare-metal stents. Low-power (2.5×) magnification of a Movat Pentachrome stained section of a Cypher sirolimus-eluting stent **(A)** showing severe in-stent restenosis with almost complete occlusion. There is postmortem clot in the lumen. Higher magnification (10×) section shows a stent strut with surrouding proteoglycan-rich neointimal tissue and presence of foam cells and neovascularization **(B)**. Low-power (2.5×) magnification of a Multilink bare-metal stent **(C)** with severe in-stent restenosis and **(D)** high-power (10×) magnification shows predominance of smooth muscle cells with neovascularization and chronic inflammation in the surrounding stent struts.

suggested that balloon dilatation for ISR entailed less risk than standard angioplasty of de novo coronary lesions.[41] In brief, an angioplasty balloon is advanced to the site of the ISR and expanded to nominal pressure. In general a balloon:vessel ratio of 1.1:1.0 is chosen. The length of balloon is usually targeted to treat only the restenotic segment of the existing stent rather than the entire stented segment. Failure to achieve full expansion of the angioplasty balloon with standard pressures of 8-14 atmospheres is recognized by a "dog-bone"–like appearance of the balloon. This should promote a switch to noncompliant balloons which facilitate high-pressure inflation up to approximately 25 atmospheres. In actual fact some operators recommend systematic use of noncompliant balloons for angioplasty of ISR though in this respect economic considerations may play a role in local practice. In occasional situations dilatation-resistant lesions may be successfully dilated with super-high-pressure balloons using inflation pressures of up to 40 atmospheres, though risk of perforation should be considered.[42]

An important additional technical consideration in angioplasty for ISR is balloon slippage due to "watermelon-seeding."[43] This phenomenon is more often encountered in angioplasty for ISR as compared with de novo disease and occurs when, for example, upon balloon inflation the balloon slips proximally or distally to the intended site of dilatation. This is not just time-consuming but may lead to inadvertent trauma to nontarget regions of the treated vessel, so-called geographic miss, which may increase the risk of subsequent recurrent restenosis. Lesions with higher diameter stenosis and diffuse stenoses are more susceptible. Strategies to anchor the balloon and avoid "watermelon-seeding" include slow step-wise inflation of the balloon, sequential angioplasty starting with smaller balloon sizes and working up, the use of a "buddy wire" to stabilize the balloon, and employment of anti-slip cutting or scoring balloons as an alternative to standard balloons.

Though a limited role for balloon angioplasty alone remains in contemporary practice there are a number of drawbacks that mean that it is no longer the treatment of

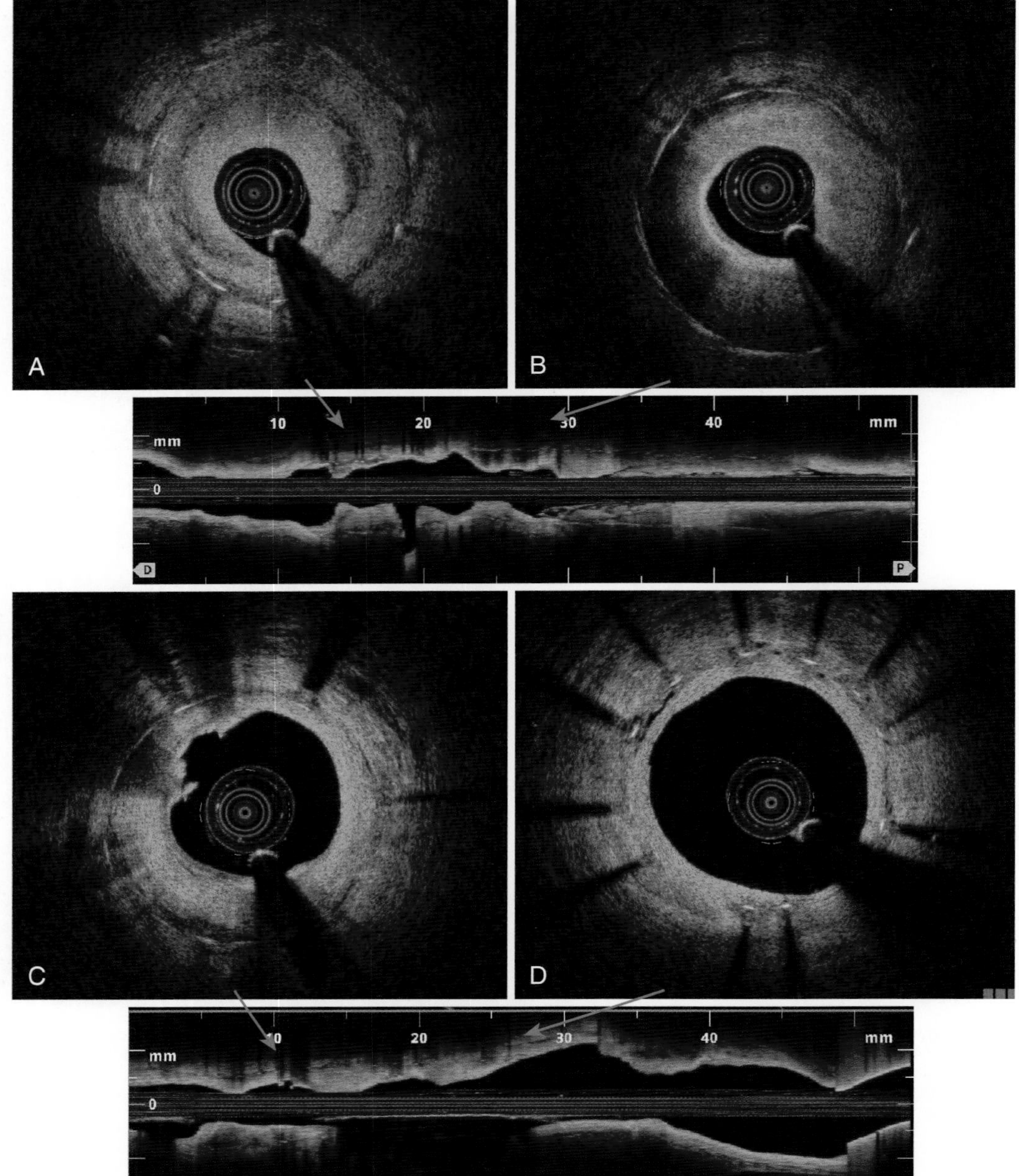

FIGURE 13-3 Diffuse in-stent restenosis showing features of in-stent neoatherosclerosis by optical coherence tomography. In-stent restenosis 9 years after long-segment DES implantation showing features of in-stent neoatherosclerosis. Angiography shows diffuse in-stent restenosis **(Video 13-1)**. Optical coherence tomography shows distal high-grade layered pattern in-stent restenosis **(A)** with an area of attenuated signal intensity 10-15 mm more proximally **(B),** which likely represents lipid-core atherosclerotic plaque. More proximally still an area of possible in-stent plaque erosion/rupture is visible (**C;** at 10 o'clock). The proximal stent edge is free of restenosis with a thin layer of neointima covering stent struts **(D)**. Punctate areas of low signal intensity likely represent neovascularization. Predilatation with noncompliant balloon angioplasty and treatment with drug-coated balloon **(Video 13-2)** and additional distal stent implantation **(Video 13-3)** result in satisfactory acute appearance **(Video 13-4)**.

choice for ISR. First, residual stenosis after the procedure is relatively high (on the order of 20% and more). Second, some studies suggest that further early lumen loss occurs in the initial hours after angioplasty. Indeed, one study that systematically examined patients immediately after intervention and 30-60 minutes later showed a significant reduction in minimal lumen diameter during this time window.[44] This is mainly due to re-intrusion of tissue back into the vessel lumen in the minutes and hours after angioplasty. Moreover higher early lumen loss was associated with subsequent clinical events. Third, randomized trial data have demonstrated superiority of alternative strategies.

PLAQUE DEBULKING WITH ATHERECTOMY

Since the predominant cause of ISR is intimal hyperplasia, debulking techniques were frequently investigated for treatment of this condition. Atherectomy devices relieve coronary stenosis by removing rather than simply compressing coronary plaque. Devices may be broadly characterized as "remove and retrieve" type (e.g., directional atherectomy) or "disrupt and displace" type (e.g., rotational or laser atherectomy). Although initially targeted at primary treatment of de novo disease, their role evolved into that of an adjunctive therapy prior to stent implantation, as well as a useful tool

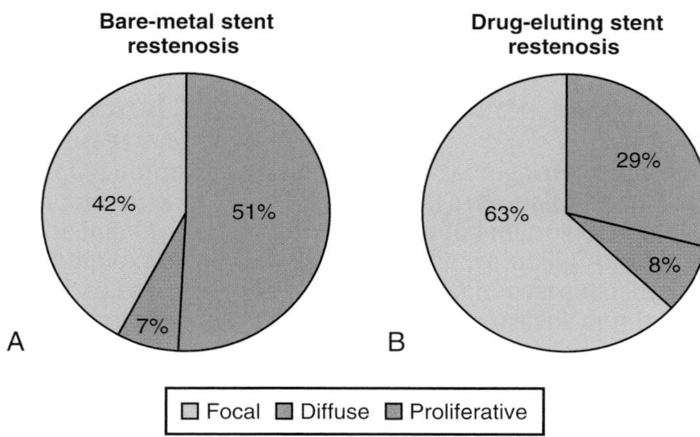

FIGURE 13-4 Angiographic classification of restenosis following bare-metal and drug-eluting stenting. A, Distribution of patterns of restenosis after bare-metal stenting. *(Adapted from Mehran R, Dangas G, Abizaid AS, et al: Angiographic patterns of in-stent restenosis: classification and implications for long-term outcome. Circulation 100:1872–1878, 1999.)* **B,** Distribution of patterns of restenosis after drug-eluting stenting pooling. *(Data from Latib A, Mussardo M, Ielasi A, et al: Long-term outcomes after the percutaneous treatment of drug-eluting stent restenosis. JACC Cardiovasc Interv 4:155–164, 2011; and Mehilli J, Byrne RA, Tiroch K, et al: Randomized trial of paclitaxel- versus sirolimus-eluting stents for treatment of coronary restenosis in sirolimus-eluting stents: the ISAR-DESIRE 2 (intracoronary stenting and angiographic results: drug eluting stents for in-stent restenosis 2) study. J Am Coll Cardiol 55:2710–2716, 2010. Figure adapted from Kastrati A, Byrne R: New roads, new ruts: lessons from drug-eluting stent restenosis. JACC Cardiovasc Interv 4:165–167, 2011.)*

for neointimal tissue removal in ISR. However the passage of time and the advent of newer and more effective devices have seen the use of these modalities decline significantly or in many instances fall completely out of use.

Plaque debulking with rotational atherectomy is done using a metal burr studded with diamonds, which is advanced to the site of the restenosis and rotated at high speed (150,000-200,000 rpm). By pulverizing stenotic plaque to microparticles of 20- to 50-μm diameter (small enough to pass through the coronary microcirculation) additional lumen enlargement is achieved during PCI. Although undoubtedly a useful tool in the armamentarium of the interventionalist performing PCI for ISR, studies investigating a strategy of systematic lesion preparation with atherectomy have yielded mixed results. The initial 200-patient single-center ROSTER randomized trial in patients with ISR was inconclusive. Although rotational atherectomy compared with angioplasty alone showed no evidence of increased acute gain, rates of repeat revascularization were improved at follow-up.[24] On the other hand the 298-patient multicenter Angioplasty versus Rotational Atherectomy for Treatment of Diffuse In-Stent Restenosis Trial (ARTIST) showed higher rates of repeat revascularization with a strategy of rotational atherectomy and adjunctive low-pressure balloon angioplasty compared with standard balloon angioplasty alone.[19] In light of the availability of other high-efficacy devices for the treatment of ISR rotational atherectomy has largely fallen out of use. However, selected cases remain where rotational atherectomy may be required for undilatable ISR due to heavily calcified in-stent plaques or stent underexpansion.[45,46]

Laser atherectomy has also been investigated for the plaque debulking in ISR. Most commonly used catheters were based on XeCl excimer laser ablation using ultraviolet spectrum wavelengths. A multicenter registry study with excimer laser angioplasty and adjunctive balloon angioplasty showed this strategy to be safe and effective.[47] A mechanistic IVUS-based registry examined the use of laser atherectomy followed by angioplasty for ISR. It showed that acute gain was achieved in three almost equal parts: tissue ablation, tissue extrusion by angioplasty, and additional expansion of the underlying stent.[48] Moreover matched to lesions treated with angioplasty alone, laser angioplasty resulted in greater acute lumen gain, and a tendency for less frequent treatment failure. A registry report of laser versus rotational atherectomy with IVUS analysis showed that although significantly greater reduction in intimal hyperplasia volume was seen after rotational atherectomy, both strategies had similar long-term clinical outcomes.[49] Unfortunately, randomized trial data comparing laser atherectomy with standard angioplasty were never published, and this technique is no longer performed.

Finally, directional atherectomy is of interest for being the most potent plaque-debulking technique in use. The basic principle of use is that plaque is removed from the vessel by a cutting device mounted on a positioning balloon catheter. Upon balloon inflation plaque is shaved into the windowed housing of the catheter and removed from the body. The principal scientific interest is the facilitation of histopathological analysis of excised plaque. Small-scale registries showed encouraging results[50] and a comparison against rotational atherectomy suggested more potent and a lower incidence of subsequent target lesion revascularization with directional atherectomy.[51] However, as with other debulking techniques, compelling randomized trial data against standard therapy were not realized and the device is no longer in widespread use, at least in the coronary arena.

CUTTING AND SCORING BALLOON ANGIOPLASTY

Cutting balloons are comprised of standard balloon catheters mounted with lateral metallic blades known as athertomes (**Figure 13-5A**), which on inflation of the balloon incise into the treated stenotic plaque. There are two main advantages to their use:

- the incision of the blades into the stenotic plaque may favor subsequent extrusion
- the interaction of the blades with the plaque anchors the balloon in the plaque and prevents "watermelon-seeding"; this in turn might reduce problems related to geographic miss.

An initial large registry of patients treated with ISR from Lenox Hill, New York, compared outcomes of matched patients according to treatment with cutting balloon, rotational atherectomy, stenting, or plain angioplasty.[52] Results suggested a clear edge for cutting balloon angioplasty in terms of angiographic and clinical outcomes at follow-up. However subsequent results from the restenosis cutting balloon evaluation trial (RESCUT) randomized trial were more disappointing.[20] In 428 patients with restenosis randomized to treatment with cutting balloon versus plain balloon angioplasty, although cutting balloons showed less procedural balloon slippage, no advantage in terms of the primary endpoint of binary angiographic restenosis at 7-month angiographic follow-up was seen (cutting balloon angioplasty 29.8% vs. plain balloon angioplasty 31.4%; $p = 0.82$). Moreover case-control studies in which cutting balloon angioplasty was utilized prior to vascular brachytherapy did not suggest an advantage over standard balloon angioplasty lesion preparation.[53,54]

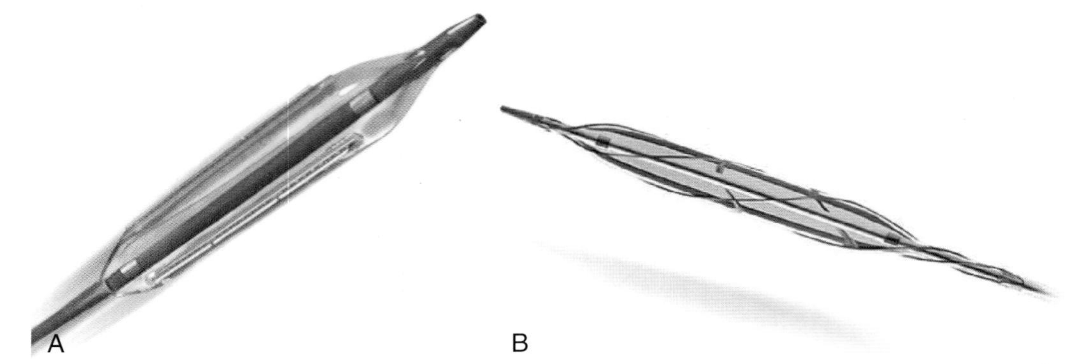

FIGURE 13-5 Cutting and scoring balloon structure. A, Flextome cutting balloon device. The device consists of a balloon catheter mounted with lateral metallic blades known as atherotomes. **B,** Angiosculpt scoring balloon device. The device is comprised of a semi-compliant angioplasty balloon mounted with low-profile nitinol wires in spiral formation. *(**A,** Image downloaded from **www.bostonscientific.com**. **B,** Reused with permission from AngioScore.)*

Scoring balloons have a broadly similar mechanistic basis to cutting balloons. The main difference is that low-profile nitinol wires (on the order of 125 μm) in spiral formation are mounted on the surface of the balloon catheter instead of blades (**Figure 13-5B**). As a result the deliverability and flexibility of the catheters are increased, at the expense of a lesser degree of plaque incision. However, anchoring at the lesion and protection against "watermelon-seeding" are maintained. Although this approach is potentially attractive, published data in ISR are limited at present to case reports,[55] although a randomized trial comparing scoring balloon angioplasty with plain balloon angioplasty is ongoing (ISAR-DESIRE 4; registered at clinicaltrials.gov, identifier: NCT01632371), and a drug-coated scoring balloon device is also being currently tested.[56]

VASCULAR BRACHYTHERAPY

Intracoronary radiation therapy—commonly known as vascular brachytherapy—has also been successfully used to treat ISR. The therapy is delivered at the time of mechanical treatment of the stenosed stent and is termed *brachytherapy* due to the short distance from the radiation source to the target tissue. Radioactive material (typically in the form of seeds, less success with fluids) is delivered to the target lesion inside a specialized catheter, which is left to dwell in the coronary artery for a period of between 2-3 and 30-45 minutes. Both beta and gamma radiation sources have been successfully used. Gamma radiation sources have high energy (roughly 0.2-10 MeV), high tissue penetration, longer dwell times, and requirement for more stringent radiation protection protocols. Beta radiation has lower energy, lesser penetration, shorter dwell times, and a reduced requirement for radiation shielding. Preclinical investigation with both sources showed effective inhibition of neointimal hyperplasia in porcine models of coronary intervention.[57,58]

Initial randomized trials with double-blind, most with sham-catheter, treatments showed improvement in both angiographic and clinical outcomes at 6 to 12 months' follow-up with both gamma and beta radiation sources in comparison with standard balloon angioplasty.[16-18,59,60] There were two chief limitations of vascular brachytherapy, namely, requirement for specialized laboratory equipment with unwieldy treatment protocols and systematic impaired arterial healing following intervention. This latter issue foreshadowed many of the problems observed with early-generation DES technology and was associated with a spectrum of adverse events including geographic miss, edge restenosis, late stent thrombosis, and requirement for prolonged dual antiplatelet therapy and late "catch up" restenosis.[61-63]

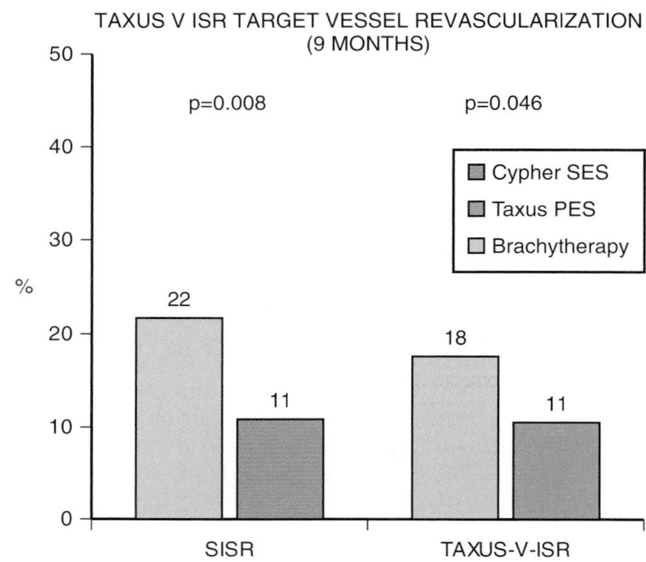

FIGURE 13-6 Outcomes from randomized trials comparing vascular brachytherapy with drug-eluting stent implantation for restenosis within bare-metal stents. Rates of target lesion revascularization in **(A)** SISR trial comparing vascular brachytherapy with sirolimus-eluting stent implantation, and **(B)** TAXUS V ISR comparing vascular brachytherapy with paclitaxel-eluting stent implantation.

In many respects the advent of DES therapy heralded the end of the era of vascular brachytherapy. The combination of high acute gain with low late lumen loss seen with DES was particularly well suited to the challenging condition of ISR. Moreover, although DES therapy was not without its own safety concerns, the overall safety profile and the ease of therapy delivery made DES a superior treatment option in routine clinical practice.

Two important multicenter randomized trials directly compared outcomes of patients with ISR who were allocated to treatment with either vascular brachytherapy or repeat stenting with a DES. In the SISR trial patients treated with sirolimus-eluting Cypher stents had superior outcome to those treated with beta or gamma brachytherapy (see **Figure 13-6A**).[28] Similarly in the Paclitaxel-Eluting Stents versus Brachytherapy for In-stent Restenosis (TAXUS V ISR) trial patients randomized to paclitaxel-eluting Taxus stents had superior angiographic and clinical outcome to beta brachytherapy-treated patients (see **Figure 13-6B**).[29] Subsequent reports from both studies confirmed persistent advantage with DES out to 5 years. Although both studies enrolled only patients with bare-metal stent restenosis, and some encouraging observational data have been reported with brachytherapy for DES restenosis,[64] there is no compelling reason to expect differential findings in patients with DES restenosis. Overall the lack of enthusiasm for brachytherapy coupled with concerns regarding delayed healing and a reduced commercial interest has led to extremely limited use of this treatment modality.

BARE-METAL STENTING

Stent implantation offers considerable advantages over plain balloon angioplasty in terms of prevention of restenosis after intervention. By splinting balloon-disrupted plaque and sealing iatrogenic dissection planes acute results are more stable after stent implantation. In addition, the scaffold properties of stent backbones deliver mechanical advantage and oppose early vessel recoil. This results in greater acute gain in comparison with angioplasty. In addition the radial strength of the stent prevents later-occurring constrictive vessel remodeling. The principal downside is greater vessel injury at the time of PCI and therefore higher levels of neointimal hyperplasia over follow-up. Concerns about long-term adverse effects of bare-metal stents as permanent endovascular prostheses remain poorly defined.

In the specific setting of ISR, however, repeat stent implantation may be undesirable due to the potential disadvantage of two or more layers of metal in the treated vessel segment, the so-called onion-skin effect, which may cause reduction in lumen size or "luminal crowding" (see **Figure 13-7**). Moreover if the structural integrity of the stenosed stent is intact (i.e., the dominant cause of the re-narrowing is neointimal hyperplasia) then there is limited incremental mechanical value of an additional stent layer. On the other hand, if structural discontinuity is present then repeat stenting may be advantageous. Finally, in the case of DES implantation for ISR the additional value of local drug delivery must of course be factored in when assessing the risk-to-benefit ratio of further stent implantation.

In the bare-metal stent era, arguments against repeat stenting were partially tempered by IVUS studies documenting significantly improved acute gain with repeat stenting in comparison with balloon angioplasty.[44] Moreover selected use of repeat stenting in case of significant in-stent dissection after angioplasty seemed feasible and safe[65] though early reports of more widespread use reported mixed results.[66,67] The resultant clinical equipoise was addressed by the RIBS trial that randomized 450 patients presenting with ISR to balloon angioplasty or repeat bare-metal stenting.[21] The main finding was that although acute gain was greater with stenting, this advantage was offset by higher late loss (due to more neointimal hyperplasia) so that the binary restenosis rate at follow-up was similar with the two strategies (angioplasty 39% vs. stenting 38%). This suggests that all things being equal a stent-sparing strategy (i.e., balloon angioplasty) should be preferred. Importantly, however, subgroup analyses of patients with large vessels and edge restenosis suggested benefit with additional stent placement, which intuitively makes sense.[68]

DRUG-ELUTING STENTING

The introduction of polymer-coated drug-eluting coronary stents around the turn of the millennium revolutionized the field of interventional cardiology.[69,70] Adoption into routine practice for the treatment of de novo disease resulted in a

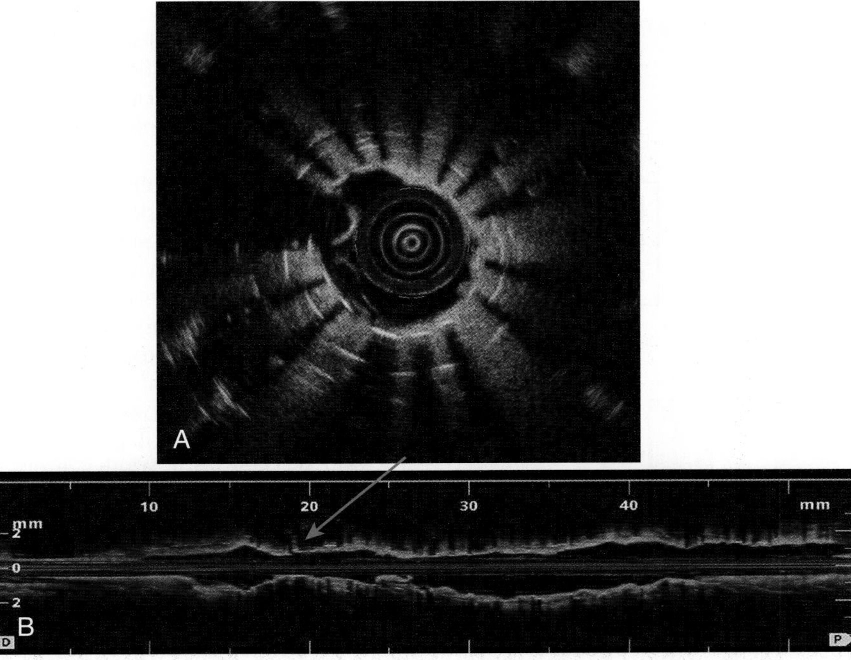

FIGURE 13-7 In-stent restenosis due to severe stent underexpansion imaged by optical coherence tomography. The longitudinal view **(B)** shows focal severe stent underexpansion with evidence of multiple layers of metallic stents—so-called onion skin phenomenon—in the cross-sectional view **(A)**.

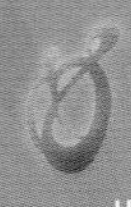

35% to 70% reduction in restenosis in comparison with bare-metal stenting.[9] The uniquely high anti-restenotic efficacy of DES in comparison with foregoing catheter-based interventional modalities is due to the combination of high acute gain with low late loss (see **Figure 13-1**). This high antirestenotic efficacy is particularly important in patients and lesions at high risk for restenosis, including the setting of intervention for ISR.

Restenosis Within Bare-metal Stents

In terms of restenosis within bare-metal stents, early experience with drug-eluting stent implantation from registry reports was encouraging.[71] Moreover, a subsequent retrospective analysis of patients with ISR within bare-metal stents showed significantly better outcomes after repeat stenting with DES versus with bare-metal stents.[72] However, it remained for repeat stenting with DES to be compared with the two most established therapies for ISR, namely, balloon angioplasty and vascular brachytherapy.

The Intracoronary Stenting and Angiographic Results: Drug Eluting Stents for In-Stent Restenosis (ISAR-DESIRE) trial randomized 300 patients with ISR to treatment with either sirolimus-eluting stents (SES; Cypher), paclitaxel-eluting stents (PES; Taxus) or standard balloon angioplasty.[25] The main finding was that in terms of the primary angiographic endpoint of binary restenosis, both drug-eluting stents significantly outperformed balloon angioplasty (SES 14.3%, balloon angioplasty 44.6%, $p < 0.001$; PES 21.7%, $p < 0.001$ vs. balloon angioplasty). Moreover there was a signal that the SES was more efficacious than the PES in this setting. Similar results were observed for need for repeat target lesion revascularization (**Figure 13-8A**). Broadly congruent results were seen in the multicenter Restenosis Intrastent: Balloon Sirolimus-Eluting Stenting (RIBS-II) randomized trial.[27] Patients with ISR treated with sirolimus-eluting stents had significantly better angiographic and clinical outcomes at 9 months in comparison with patients treated with balloon angioplasty (**Figure 13-8B**). Long-term results confirmed durability of efficacy and safety with DES use in this setting.[73]

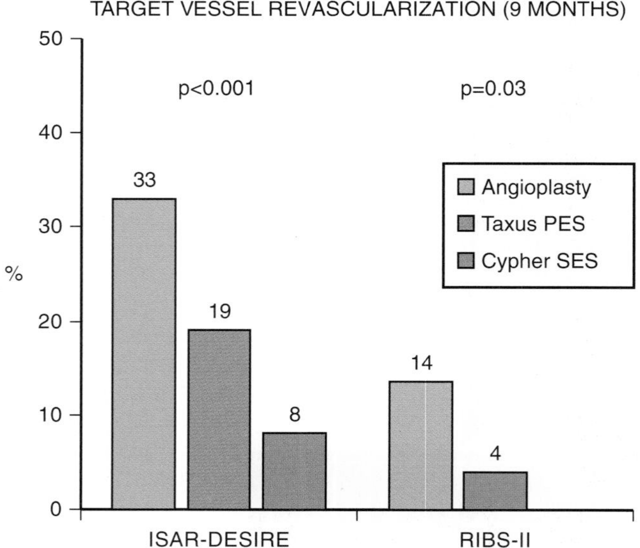

FIGURE 13-8 Outcomes from randomized trials comparing drug-eluting stent implantation with balloon angioplasty for restenosis within bare-metal stents. Rates of target lesion revascularization in **(A)** RIBS-II trial comparing sirolimus-eluting stent implantation with balloon angioplasty and **(B)** ISAR-DESIRE comparing sirolimus-eluting stent and paclitaxel-eluting stent implantation with balloon angioplasty.

In terms of benchmarking against vascular brachytherapy, as mentioned already, the SISR and TAXUS-V-ISR trials demonstrated superior angiographic and clinical outcomes in patients randomized to treatment with SES versus beta or gamma brachytherapy and PES versus beta brachytherapy, respectively (see **Figure 13-6**).[28,29] A subsequent meta-analysis in 2007 supported the impression that DES were markedly superior to both conventional balloon angioplasty and vascular brachytherapy and should be considered as first-line treatment for patients with bare-metal stent restenosis.[74] Metaanalysis of mid-term follow-up data with DES versus brachytherapy confirmed sustained advantage for DES in this indication.[75]

Restenosis Within Drug-Eluting Stents

Although the overall rate of ISR is low after drug-eluting stenting, when it occurs, restenosis can be particularly challenging to treat.[2] Indeed a number of reports suggested poorer clinical outcomes in DES patients who were treated for restenosis within DES as compared with restenosis within bare-metal stents.[76,77] These observations have since been replicated in many registry reports.[78,79] The exact reasons for these findings remain unclear. Certainly there are significant differences between the restenosis that occurs after bare-metal versus after drug-eluting stenting in terms of time course, morphology, and underlying pathophysiology (see **Table 13-1, Figure 13-2**).[11] Moreover recent autopsy studies suggest that in-stent neoatherosclerosis may play a more important role in DES failure.[10] In addition, it may well be that hyporesponsiveness to the drug used for stent coating may play a relevant role.[77]

In terms of initial experience with DES restenosis registry studies from a number of different investigators reported that implantation of another DES seemed to be feasible and safe in both sirolimus- and paclitaxel-eluting stent restenosis.[80-82] Mid- to long-term follow-up of treated patients showed sustained efficacy though overall clinical event rates after intervention for DES restenosis remain high (rates of major adverse cardiac events of around 33% at 3 years).[3,4]

Regarding comparative efficacy data a small randomized trial suggested superiority of DES over cutting balloon angioplasty and no significant differences in outcomes based on whether an early generation or later generation DES was used.[83] However, some debate arises as to whether a strategy of remaining with a DES eluting the same type of drug (same DES or homo-DES strategy) or switching to a DES eluting a different type of drug (switch DES or hetero-DES strategy) is the best approach for these patients. The hypothesis in favor of a switch strategy is that although restenosis is undoubtedly multifactorial hyporesponsiveness or resistance to the eluted drug may play some role in the pathogenesis.[77]

A registry study from Milan including 201 lesions with DES restenosis showed no differences in outcome between patients treated with a same DES strategy versus those treated with a switch DES strategy; about 1 in 4 in both groups showed recurrent restenosis at angiographic surveillance.[84] Similar results were seen in a registry from

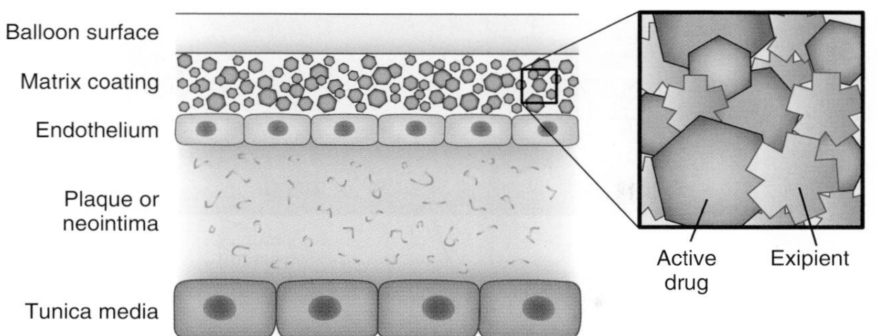

FIGURE 13-9 Drug-coated balloon structure. Drug release is facilitated by a coating that consists of a mixture of lipophilic drug and a hydrophilic spacer or excipient that facilitates faster uptake into the vessel wall. The spacer or excipient combines with the active drug to form a matrix coating that remains on the surface of the balloon catheter.

Washington Hospital Center with clinical follow-up.[85] Against this the multicenter RIBS-III registry from Spain showed better angiographic outcomes and lower rates of clinical events in patients treated with a switch DES versus a no-switch strategy.[86] However, interpretation of the results is complicated as the no-switch (control) group included patients treated with a number of different treatment modalities. Moreover, all of these data are limited by the nonrandomized nature of the treatment comparisons; accordingly it is difficult to fully adjust for treatment selection bias on the part of the operator. Indeed the only randomized trial to examine this issue—the ISAR-DESIRE 2 trial—showed no difference in the primary endpoint of late lumen loss at 6-8 months in patients allocated to treatment with an SES (same DES : late loss 0.40 mm) versus a PES (switch DES : late loss 0.38 mm). Moreover a subsequent metaanalysis also showed no difference between a same DES and a switch DES strategy.[87] Of course all studies must be interpreted against the background that comparisons of same drug versus switch drug strategies usually entail an element of oversimplification, as the compared stents often differ in many characteristics in addition to the type of drug eluted (e.g., polymer, backbone).

BIORESORBABLE STENTS

In general the use of bioresorbable stents has been restricted to relatively straightforward lesion types.[88] Reports of the use of these devices for the treatment of ISR remain preliminary in nature.[89,90] Avoidance of further metallic stent layers is intuitively attractive from a long-term perspective but question marks about acute performance may be particularly relevant for use in the setting of ISR. Further data are needed before recommendations for use can be made.

DRUG-COATED BALLOON ANGIOPLASTY

In general stent-based interventional modalities, in particular DES implantation, tend to have superior antirestenotic efficacy due to the combination of high acute gain and low late loss. However, angioplasty with drug-coated balloons (DCB) has emerged as an attractive therapeutic option in its own right, particularly in situations where implantation of multiple stent layers might be undesirable, for example, at the carina of a bifurcation or in the setting of ISR.[91] Indeed, initial randomized clinical trials with DCB showed most successful results for the indication of ISR.

DCB catheters are comprised of standard angioplasty balloons and a matrix coating that is applied to the surface of the balloon (**Figure 13-9**). The balloon coating is typically comprised of two elements: a lipophilic active drug (to date all commercially available devices use paclitaxel) and a spacer or excipient (which increases the solubility of the active drug and facilitates its transfer from the balloon surface to the vessel wall). Preclinical studies have documented effective drug transfer with evidence of local fibrin deposition in the vessel wall as a signature of therapeutic efficacy.

During DCB angioplasty for ISR, the lesion must first be dilated with a standard or noncompliant balloon in order to extrude and compress neointima and correct stent underexpansion if present. Only after achieving satisfactory initial results should DCB angioplasty be done, typically with a single 30- to 60-second balloon inflation. Transfer of paclitaxel to the vessel wall results in effective suppression of neointimal hyperplasia (**Figure 13-10;** Videos 13-20 to 13-22). In addition, some studies suggest higher acute gain with DCB versus standard angioplasty. This might be simply a manifestation of more assiduous lesion preparation or could also reflect diverging neointimal behaviors after dilation; for example, paclitaxel application might in theory attenuate the acute neointimal recoil reported in some patients after balloon angioplasty by freezing the disrupted neointimal.[92]

Restenosis Within Bare-Metal Stents

Bruno Scheller and colleagues published the proof-of-concept, Treatment of In-Stent Restenosis by Paclitaxel Coated PTCA Balloons (PACCOCATH-ISR), clinical trial with DCB angioplasty in 2006.[26] A total of 52 patients with bare-metal-stent ISR were randomly allocated to DCB angioplasty versus standard angioplasty. The main finding was that DCB therapy significantly reduced late loss at 6 months in comparison with balloon angioplasty (0.03 ± 0.48 mm vs. 0.74 ± 0.86 mm, $p = 0.002$). Subsequently published 5-year results confirmed durability of efficacy over the medium to long term.[93] The chief limitation was that with the advent of DES technology the control treatment of plain angioplasty had been superseded as standard of care. Accordingly in the Paclitaxel-Eluting PTCA-Balloon Catheter in Coronary Artery Disease (PEPCAD-II) study DCB was compared with repeat stenting with paclitaxel-eluting DES.[31] Interestingly, the primary endpoint of in-segment late loss at 6 months was lower with DCB (0.17 ± 0.42 mm vs. 0.38 ± 0.61 mm, p <

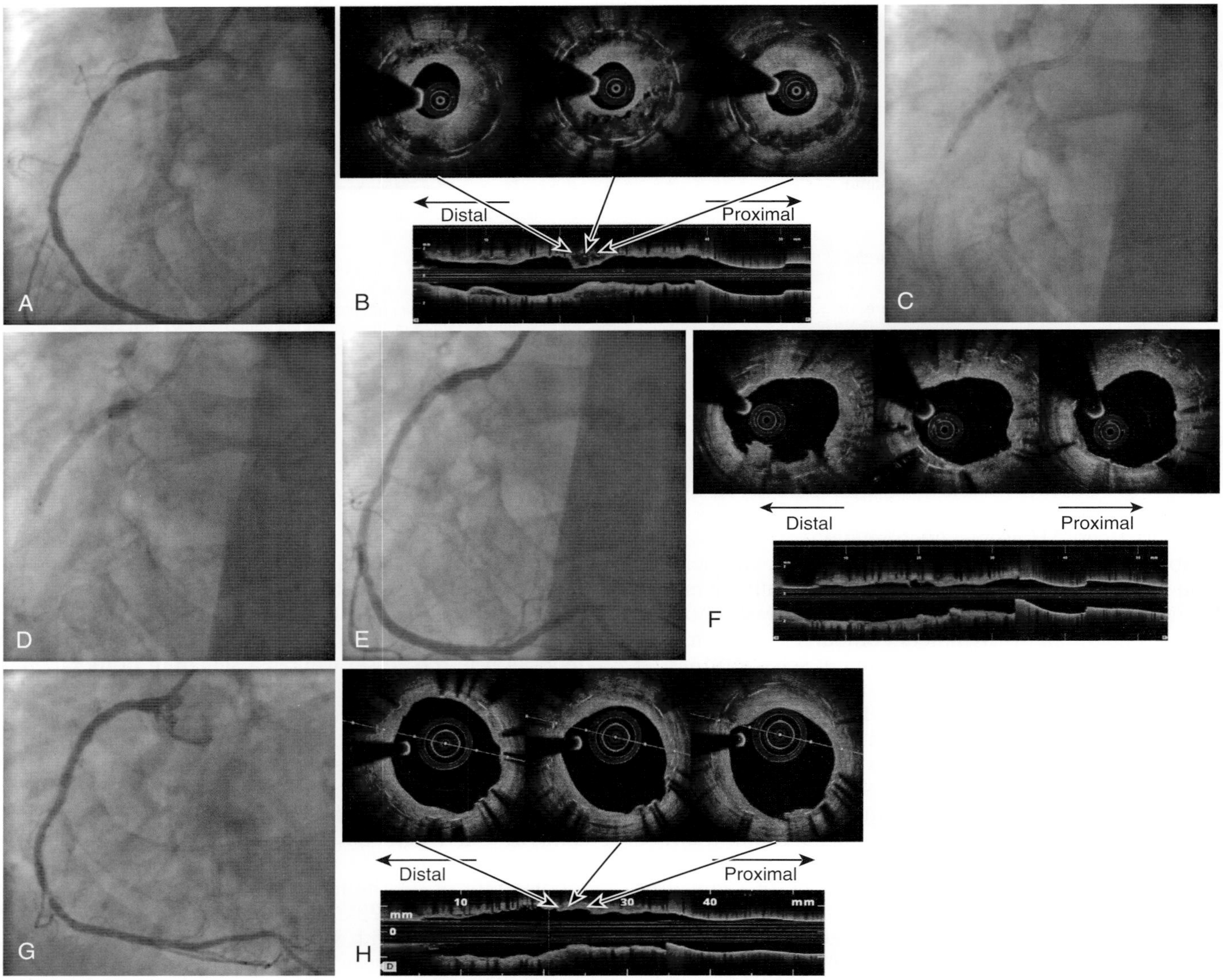

FIGURE 13-10 Treatment of drug-eluting stent in-stent restenosis with drug-coated balloon therapy. Focal recurrent in-stent restenosis 4 years after drug-eluting stent implantation for in-stent restenosis in the proximal RCA (**A; Video 13-20**). Optical coherence tomography (OCT) imaging confirms focal restenosis (**B,** longitudinal view) with heterogeneous and layered pattern tissue (**B,** upper panels). The restenotic lesion was predilated with a noncompliant balloon **(C)** and treated with a 60-second drug-coated balloon inflation **(D)** with good acute angiographic result (**E; Video 13-21**). OCT immediately after the intervention confirms good acute results **(F)** with a small degree of tissue prolapse (**F,** upper left panel). Repeat angiography 7 months later shows an excellent result (**G; Video 13-22**). OCT also shows an excellent result with generally satisfactory vessel healing though with some evidence of uncovered stent struts **(H)**.

0.03). However, in trials comparing angioplasty with stenting, late loss is not a suitable endpoint: modalities with higher acute gain tend to have higher late loss per se ("the more you gain, the more you lose"). Indeed minimal lumen diameter at 6 months was comparable in both groups (DCB: 2.03 ± 0.56 vs. DES: 1.96 ± 0.82, p = 0.60). Nevertheless, while the authors' conclusion of superiority for DCB can be disputed, the achievement of comparable outcomes without requirement for further stent implantation is an important finding.

Early generation paclitaxel-eluting stents have largely fallen out of use due to more effective next generation platforms.[94,95] In the recently published RIBS-IV study DCB angioplasty was compared with repeat stenting with next generation everolimus-eluting stents.[39] The main finding was that the primary endpoint of minimal lumen diameter at follow-up was better after everolimus-eluting DES (DCB: 2.36 mm vs. everolimus-eluting DES: 2.01 mm). However, binary restenosis and clinical events at 1 year were low and similar in both groups. Although further data from larger scale trials are required to provide more definitive evidence, it seems that both DCB angioplasty and repeat stenting with high-efficacy newer generation DES are both good options for patients with bare-metal stent restenosis.

Restenosis Within Drug-Eluting Stents

The first clinical trials of DCB in patients with DES restenosis were encouraging. Habara et al. showed superiority for DCB versus plain angioplasty in terms of angiographic endpoints in 50 patients (late loss, DCB: 0.18 ± 0.45 mm vs. balloon angioplasty 0.72 ± 0.55 mm; p = 0.001)[32] and later extended these findings in a somewhat larger cohort.[38] In addition, the PEPCAD-DES investigators studied 110 patients with broadly

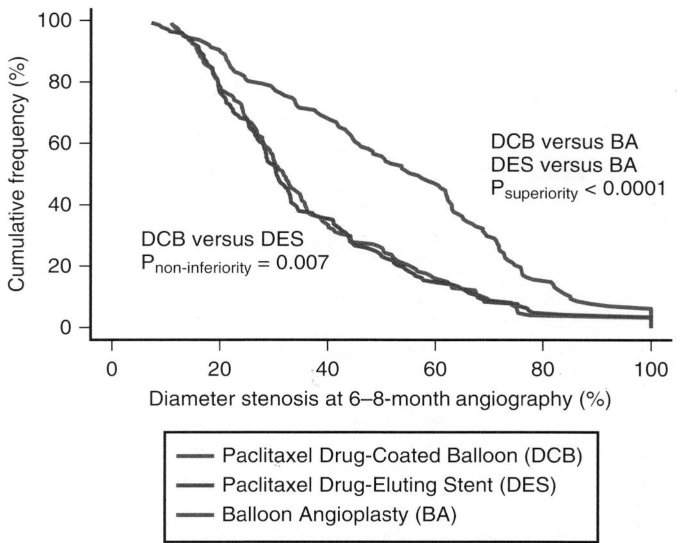

FIGURE 13-11 Comparative efficacy of drug-coated balloon, drug-eluting stent, and balloon angioplasty in the treatment of restenosis within drug-eluting stents. Cumulative frequency distribution curves for percentage diameter stenosis at 6- to 8-month angiographic surveillance in the ISAR-DESIRE 3 randomized trial. *(Adapted from Byrne RA, Neumann FJ, Mehilli J, et al: Paclitaxel-eluting balloons, paclitaxel-eluting stents, and balloon angioplasty in patients with restenosis after implantation of a drug-eluting stent (ISAR-DESIRE 3): a randomised, open-label trial. Lancet 381:461–467, 2013.)*

similar results (late loss, DCB: 0.43 ± 0.61 mm vs. balloon angioplasty 1.03 ± 0.77 mm, $p < 0.001$).[34] However, because in recent years repeat stenting with DES is the established treatment for DES restenosis, balloon angioplasty alone is not a good comparator treatment.

In the ISAR-DESIRE 3 patients with DES restenosis were randomly allocated to treatment with DCB angioplasty, repeat stenting with paclitaxel-eluting DES or plain balloon angioplasty.[37] In terms of the primary endpoint of percentage diameter stenosis at 6-8 months, DCB was comparable to repeat stenting with PES ($P_{noninferiority} = 0.007$; **Figure 13-11**); both DCB and PES were superior to plain balloon angioplasty alone ($P_{superiority} < 0.001$ for both comparisons). Consistent findings were observed for binary restenosis. A number of subsequent metaanalyses confirm superior clinical efficacy for DCB over balloon angioplasty with comparable outcomes for DCB in comparison with repeat stenting with DES.[96,97] Direct randomized trial comparison of DCB angioplasty with next generation DES is outstanding though trials are ongoing. Nevertheless, it seems reasonable to conclude that by obviating the need for repeat stent implantation, DCB angioplasty may be the preferred treatment option for this indication.

CORONARY BYPASS SURGERY

Although the management of ISR remains challenging, it is often focal in nature and lends itself to repeat percutaneous intervention, at least in the first instance.[3,4] The optimal management strategy for recurrent restenosis remains unclear though some reports support the feasibility and safety of repeated percutaneous intervention.[98] Bypass surgery undoubtedly plays an important role in selected patients, particularly if multiple vessels are involved.[99] Systematic evaluation of the role of bypass surgery for ISR is lacking.

ROLE OF INTRAVASCULAR IMAGING

Guidance of percutaneous intervention with intravascular imaging might be a useful adjunct in the treatment of ISR. The principal advantage of intravascular imaging in ISR is that it permits more precise differentiation of the two principal causes of restenosis, namely, neointimal hyperplasia and stent underexpansion (see **Figure 13-7**). This information may be useful to guide therapy: for example, repeat stenting or DCB angioplasty might be preferred for dominant neointimal hyperplasia, aggressive noncompliant balloon angioplasty for stent underexpansion. In addition, intravascular imaging may permit more accurate sizing of the reference vessel, which may guide choice of balloon diameter.

Two types of imaging modalities are widely available: intravascular ultrasound (IVUS; wavelength ca. 50 μm, axial resolution ca. 150 μm) and optical coherence tomography (OCT; wavelength 1.3 μm, axial resolution 12-15 μm). The main advantages of IVUS are deeper tissue penetration, which may facilitate more accurate vessel sizing, and the lack of requirement for a blood-free imaging field. The main advantage of OCT is superior spatial resolution in comparison with IVUS. The main limitation is the requirement for additional contrast agent administration to ensure a blood-free field for image acquisition. In addition, lower tissue penetration means that the external elastic lamina cannot always be well imaged and this makes accurate vessel sizing more difficult.

The higher resolution of OCT imaging permits more detailed characterization of neointimal tissue type (including identification of in-stent neoatherosclerosis; see **Figure 13-3** and Videos 13-1 to 13-4), which might potentially be used to guide therapy. Studies to date have classified restenotic tissue type by OCT into four main groups:

- homogeneous—uniform high signal intensity, low backscatter, typical of areas of high smooth muscle cell content
- heterogeneous—mixed signal intensity, may represent proteoglycan-rich neointimal, granulation tissue, or early neoatherosclerotic plaque
- attenuated—superficial high signal intensity, high backscatter, likely indicative of lipid-core plaque, and
- layered—superficial high signal intensity with deep low signal intensity often in peristrut areas (**Figure 13-12**).

Homogeneous pattern tissue is typical of bare-metal stent restenosis; attenuated, layered, and heterogeneous are more commonly seen in DES restenosis and may represent delayed vessel healing or part of the neoatherosclerotic disease spectrum.

Considerable variation exists in the use of intravascular imaging to guide re-intervention for restenosis. Some centers recommend systemic adjunct imaging, whereas others restrict intravascular imaging to selected cases with challenging diagnostic characteristics. Local factors such as operator experience and reimbursement play an important role. Although its use may be intuitively attractive, clinical trial evidence supporting a clear advantage for systematic intravascular imaging-guided intervention in ISR is lacking.

ADDITIONAL CONSIDERATIONS

Bioresorbable Stent Failure

The recent introduction of fully bioresorbable stents—sometimes known as bioresorbable scaffolds—has represented an important development in clinical practice.[100]

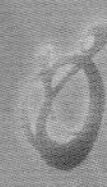

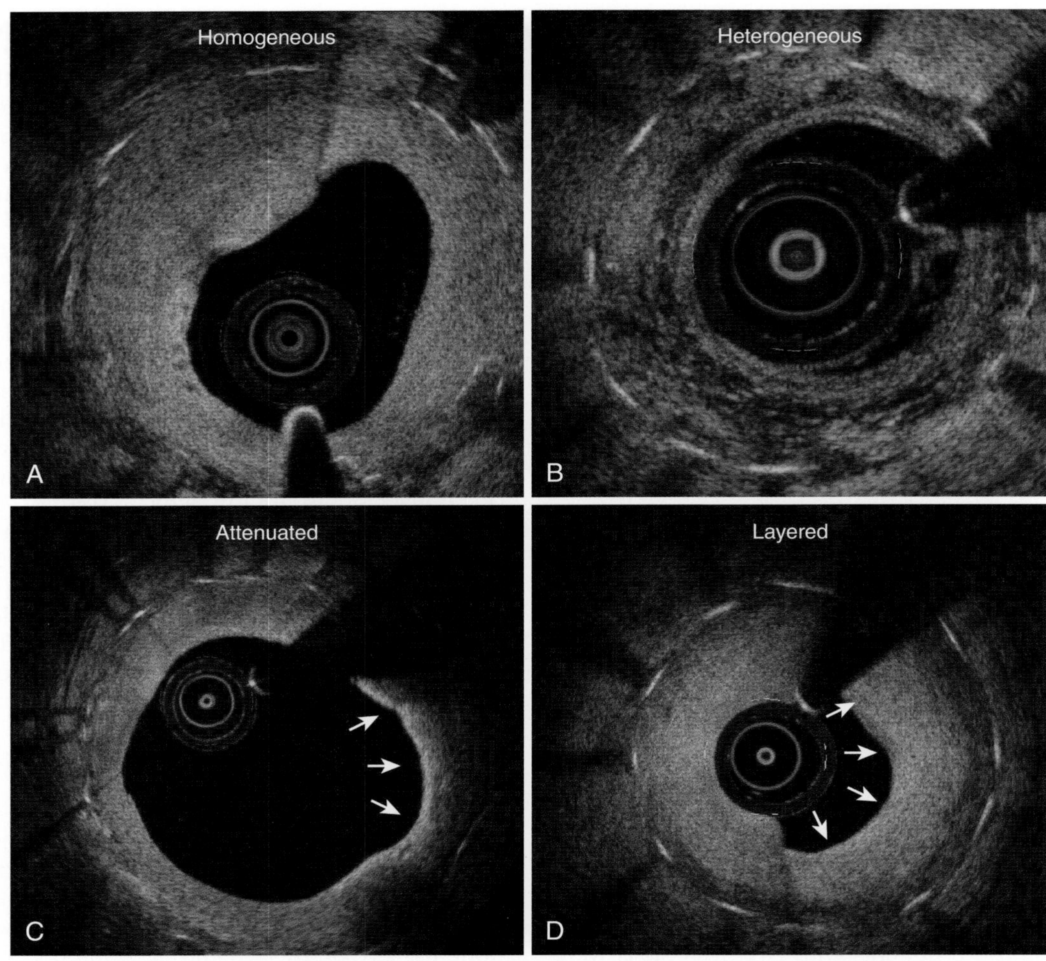

FIGURE 13-12 Classification of tissue types by optical coherence tomography from patients with metallic stent in-stent restenosis. Restenotic tissue types are usually classified into four categories **(A)** homogeneous—uniform high signal intensity; **(B)** heterogeneous—variable signal intensity; **(C)** attenuated—typical features between 2 and 5 o'clock with superficial high signal intensity *(white arrows)*, rapid signal attenuation, and high backscatter; and **(D)** layered—superficial high signal intensity, deep low signal intensity in peristrut areas.

However, these novel devices may present specific challenges in case of stent failure. To date, restenosis after bioresorbable stent implantation remains poorly characterized. Neointimal hyperplasia and premature loss of radial strength may be contributory (**Figure 13-13**). The optimal treatment of these cases remains to be defined.

CONCLUSIONS

In-stent restenosis remains the Achilles' heel of coronary stenting and is the most common cause of stent failure. Although the advent of DES has reduced the incidence of ISR dramatically, the rapid growth in PCI with DES over the past decade means that the absolute number of patients presenting with ISR remains considerable. The substrate of ISR encompasses a pathological spectrum ranging from smooth muscle cell hyperplasia to proteoglycan-rich neointimal to neoatherosclerotic change. Management of this condition remains challenging and optimal treatment algorithms have not been defined. Due to high recurrence rates the use of plain balloon angioplasty has a limited role. In addition atherectomy techniques and vascular brachytherapy have largely fallen out of use. However, repeat stenting with DES has shown good results in clinical trials. More recently use of drug-coated balloons has shown outcomes comparable to those seen with repeat stenting with DES; this approach is attractive as it obviates the need for implantation of further stent layers. Intracoronary imaging provides unique insights on the underlying etiology of ISR but the value of its systematic use in guiding re-interventions remains unsettled. Further studies are required to identify patient-specific characteristics that may help to tailor treatment selection in order to improve clinical outcomes.

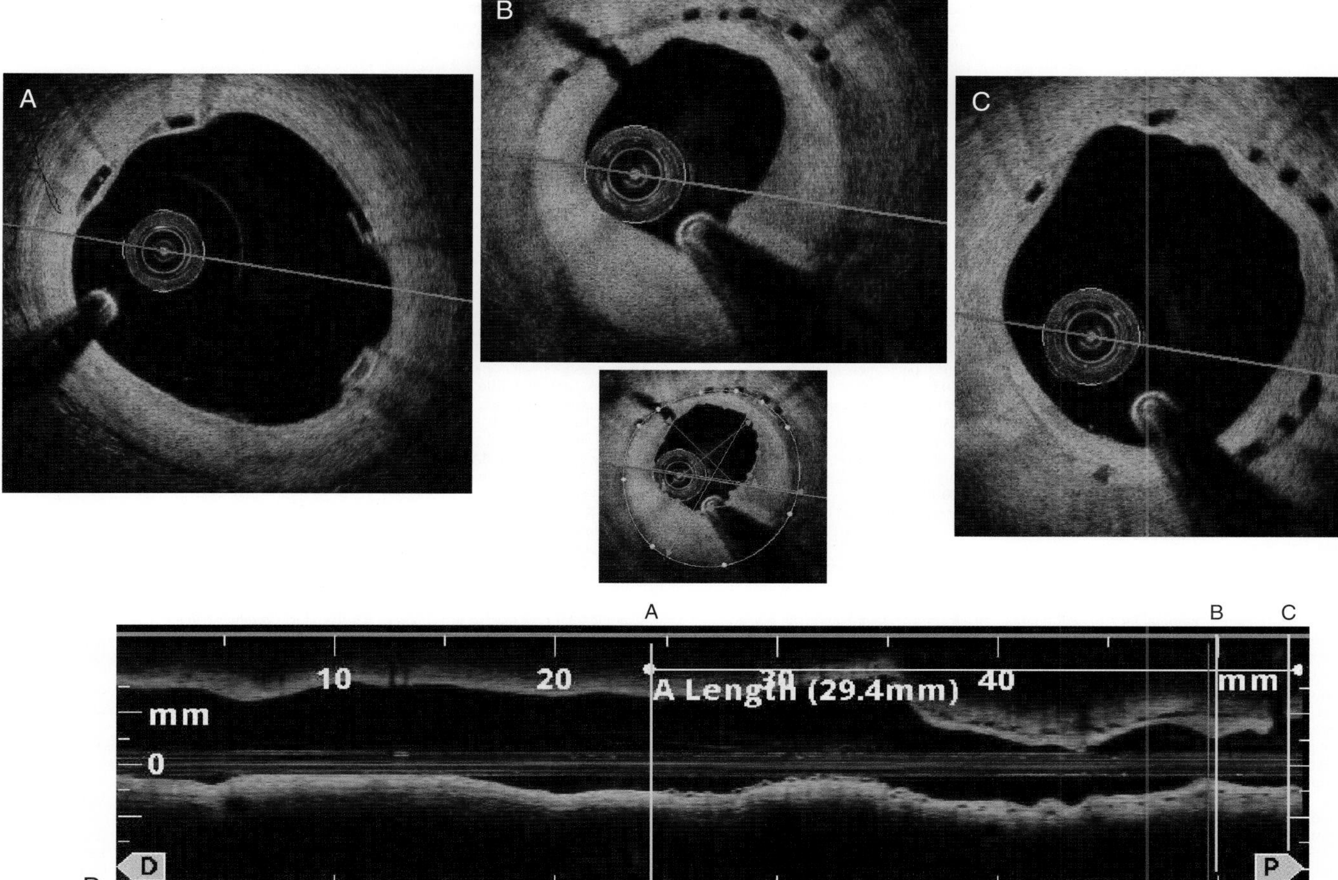

FIGURE 13-13 In-stent restenosis after fully bioresorbable stent implantation imaged by optical coherence tomography. Focal in-stent restenosis 6 months after implantation of overlapping fully bioresorbable everolimus-eluting stents. The longitudinal view **(D)** shows some stent underexpansion with reduced lumen caliber in comparison with both the proximal **(C)** and distal stent **(A)** and the distal native vessel segment. In addition the region of maximal restenosis **(B)** shows eccentric high signal tissue (between 3 and 9 o'clock) with some attenuation of signal intensity (stent struts behind tissue not clearly delineated). *D,* Distal; *P,* proximal.

References

1. Dangas GD, Claessen BE, Caixeta A, et al: In-stent restenosis in the drug-eluting stent era. *J Am Coll Cardiol* 56:1897–1907, 2010.
2. Alfonso F, Byrne RA, Rivero F, et al: Current treatment of in-stent restenosis. *J Am Coll Cardiol* 63:2659–2673, 2014.
3. Kastrati A, Byrne R: New roads, new ruts: lessons from drug-eluting stent restenosis. *JACC Cardiovasc Interv* 4:165–167, 2011.
4. Latib A, Mussardo M, Ielasi A, et al: Long-term outcomes following the percutaneous treatment of drug-eluting stent restenosis. *JACC Cardiovasc Interv* 4:155–164, 2011.
5. Mauri L, Orav EJ, Kuntz RE: Late loss in lumen diameter and binary restenosis for drug-eluting stent comparison. *Circulation* 111:3435–3442, 2005.
6. Pocock SJ, Lansky AJ, Mehran R, et al: Angiographic surrogate end points in drug-eluting stent trials: a systematic evaluation based on individual patient data from 11 randomized, controlled trials. *J Am Coll Cardiol* 51:23–32, 2008.
7. Byrne RA, Eberle S, Kastrati A, et al: Distribution of angiographic measures of restenosis after drug-eluting stent implantation. *Heart* 95:1572–1578, 2009.
8. Costa MA, Simon DI: Molecular basis of restenosis and drug-eluting stents. *Circulation* 111:2257–2273, 2005.
9. Byrne RA, Sarafoff N, Kastrati A, et al: Drug-eluting stents in percutaneous coronary intervention: a benefit-risk assessment. *Drug Saf* 32:749–770, 2009.
10. Nakazawa G, Otsuka F, Nakano M, et al: The pathology of neoatherosclerosis in human coronary implants bare-metal and drug-eluting stents. *J Am Coll Cardiol* 57:1314–1322, 2011.
11. Byrne RA, Joner M, Tada T, et al: Restenosis in bare metal and drug-eluting stents: distinct mechanistic insights from histopathology and optical intravascular imaging. *Minerva Cardioangiol* 60:473–489, 2012.
12. Nakano M, Otsuka F, Yahagi K, et al: Human autopsy study of drug-eluting stents restenosis: histomorphological predictors and neointimal characteristics. *Eur Heart J* 34:3304–3313, 2013.
13. Mehran R, Dangas G, Abizaid AS, et al: Angiographic patterns of in-stent restenosis: classification and implications for long-term outcome. *Circulation* 100:1872–1878, 1999.
14. Deleted in pages.
15. Mehilli J, Byrne RA, Tiroch K, et al: Randomized trial of paclitaxel- versus sirolimus-eluting stents for treatment of coronary restenosis in sirolimus-eluting stents: the ISAR-DESIRE 2 (intracoronary stenting and angiographic results: drug eluting stents for in-stent restenosis 2) study. *J Am Coll Cardiol* 55:2710–2716, 2010.
16. Teirstein PS, Massullo V, Jani S, et al: Catheter-based radiotherapy to inhibit restenosis after coronary stenting. *N Engl J Med* 336:1697–1703, 1997.
17. Waksman R, White RL, Chan RC, et al: Intracoronary gamma-radiation therapy after angioplasty inhibits recurrence in patients with in-stent restenosis. *Circulation* 101:2165–2171, 2000.
18. Leon MB, Teirstein PS, Moses JW, et al: Localized intracoronary gamma-radiation therapy to inhibit the recurrence of restenosis after stenting. *N Engl J Med* 344:250–256, 2001.
19. vom Dahl J, Dietz U, Haager PK, et al: Rotational atherectomy does not reduce recurrent in-stent restenosis: results of the angioplasty versus rotational atherectomy for treatment of diffuse in-stent restenosis trial (ARTIST). *Circulation* 105:583–588, 2002.
20. Albiero R, Silber S, Di Mario C, et al: Cutting balloon versus conventional balloon angioplasty for the treatment of in-stent restenosis: results of the restenosis cutting balloon evaluation trial (RESCUT). *J Am Coll Cardiol* 43:943–949, 2004.
21. Alfonso F, Zueco J, Cequier A, et al: A randomized comparison of repeat stenting with balloon angioplasty in patients with in-stent restenosis. *J Am Coll Cardiol* 42:796–805, 2003.
22. Waksman R, Cheneau E, Ajani AE, et al: Intracoronary radiation therapy improves the clinical and angiographic outcomes of diffuse in-stent restenotic lesions: results of the Washington radiation for in-stent restenosis trial for long lesions (long WRIST) studies. *Circulation* 107:1744–1749, 2003.
23. Ragosta M, Samady H, Gimple LW, et al: Percutaneous treatment of focal vs. diffuse in-stent restenosis: a prospective randomized comparison of conventional therapies. *Catheter Cardiovasc Interv* 61:344–349, 2004.
24. Sharma SK, Kini A, Mehran R, et al: Randomized trial of rotational atherectomy versus balloon angioplasty for diffuse in-stent restenosis (ROSTER). *Am Heart J* 147:16–22, 2004.
25. Kastrati A, Mehilli J, von Beckerath N, et al: Sirolimus-eluting stent or paclitaxel-eluting stent vs balloon angioplasty for prevention of recurrences in patients with coronary in-stent restenosis: a randomized controlled trial. *JAMA* 293:165–171, 2005.
26. Scheller B, Hehrlein C, Bocksch W, et al: Treatment of coronary in-stent restenosis with a paclitaxel-coated balloon catheter. *N Engl J Med* 355:2113–2124, 2006.
27. Alfonso F, Perez-Vizcayno MJ, Hernandez R, et al: A randomized comparison of sirolimus-eluting stent with balloon angioplasty in patients with in-stent restenosis: results of the restenosis intrastent: balloon angioplasty versus elective sirolimus-eluting stenting (RIBS-II) trial. *J Am Coll Cardiol* 47:2152–2160, 2006.
28. Holmes DR, Jr, Teirstein P, Satler L, et al: Sirolimus-eluting stents vs vascular brachytherapy for in-stent restenosis within bare-metal stents: the SISR randomized trial. *JAMA* 295:1264–1273, 2006.
29. Stone GW, Ellis SG, O'Shaughnessy CD, et al: Paclitaxel-eluting stents vs vascular brachytherapy for in-stent restenosis within bare-metal stents: the TAXUS V ISR randomized trial. *JAMA* 295:1253–1263, 2006.
30. Park SW, Lee SW, Koo BK, et al: Treatment of diffuse in-stent restenosis with drug-eluting stents vs. intracoronary beta-radiation therapy: INDEED Study. *Int J Cardiol* 131:70–77, 2008.
31. Unverdorben M, Vallbracht C, Cremers B, et al: Paclitaxel-coated balloon catheter versus paclitaxel-coated stent for the treatment of coronary in-stent restenosis. *Circulation* 119:2986–2994, 2009.

32. Habara S, Mitsudo K, Kadota K, et al: Effectiveness of paclitaxel-eluting balloon catheter in patients with sirolimus-eluting stent restenosis. *JACC Cardiovasc Interv* 4:149–154, 2011.
33. Wiemer M, Konig A, Rieber J, et al: Sirolimus-eluting stent implantation versus beta-irradiation for the treatment of in-stent restenotic lesions: clinical and ultrasound results from a randomised trial. *EuroIntervention* 6:687–694, 2011.
34. Rittger H, Brachmann J, Sinha AM, et al: A randomized, multicenter, single-blinded trial comparing paclitaxel-coated balloon angioplasty with plain balloon angioplasty in drug-eluting stent restenosis: the PEPCAD-DES study. *J Am Coll Cardiol* 59:1377–1382, 2012.
35. Song HG, Park DW, Kim YH, et al: Randomized trial of optimal treatment strategies for in-stent restenosis after drug-eluting stent implantation. *J Am Coll Cardiol* 59:1093–1100, 2012.
36. Chevalier B, Moulichon R, Teiger E, et al: One-year results of the CRISTAL trial, a randomized comparison of cypher sirolimus-eluting coronary stents versus balloon angioplasty for restenosis of drug-eluting stents. *J Interv Cardiol* 25:586–595, 2012.
37. Byrne RA, Neumann FJ, Mehilli J, et al: Paclitaxel-eluting balloons, paclitaxel-eluting stents, and balloon angioplasty in patients with restenosis after implantation of a drug-eluting stent (ISAR-DESIRE 3): a randomised, open-label trial. *Lancet* 381:461–467, 2013.
38. Habara S, Iwabuchi M, Inoue N, et al: A multicenter randomized comparison of paclitaxel-coated balloon catheter with conventional balloon angioplasty in patients with bare-metal stent restenosis and drug-eluting stent restenosis. *Am Heart J* 166:527–533 e2, 2013.
39. Alfonso F, Perez-Vizcayno MJ, Cardenas A, et al: A randomized comparison of drug-eluting balloon versus everolimus-eluting stent in patients with bare-metal stent-in-stent restenosis: the ribs v clinical trial (restenosis intra-stent of bare metal stents: paclitaxel-eluting balloon vs. everolimus-eluting stent). *J Am Coll Cardiol* 63:1378–1386, 2014.
40. Mehran R, Mintz GS, Popma JJ, et al: Mechanisms and results of balloon angioplasty for the treatment of in-stent restenosis. *Am J Cardiol* 78:618–622, 1996.
41. Macander PJ, Roubin GS, Agrawal SK, et al: Balloon angioplasty for treatment of in-stent restenosis: feasibility, safety, and efficacy. *Cathet Cardiovasc Diagn* 32:125–131, 1994.
42. Raja Y, Routledge HC, Doshi SN: A noncompliant, high pressure balloon to manage undilatable coronary lesions. *Catheter Cardiovasc Interv* 75:1067–1073, 2010.
43. Alfonso F, Perez-Vizcayno MJ, Gomez-Recio M, et al: Implications of the "watermelon seeding" phenomenon during coronary interventions for in-stent restenosis. *Catheter Cardiovasc Interv* 66:521–527, 2005.
44. Alfonso F, Garcia P, Fleites H, et al: Repeat stenting for the prevention of the early lumen loss phenomenon in patients with in-stent restenosis. Angiographic and intravascular ultrasound findings of a randomized study. *Am Heart J* 149:e1–e8, 2005.
45. Kobayashi Y, Teirstein P, Linnemeier T, et al: Rotational atherectomy (stentablation) in a lesion with stent underexpansion due to heavily calcified plaque. *Catheter Cardiovasc Interv* 52:208–211, 2001.
46. Vales L, Coppola J, Kwan T: Successful expansion of an underexpanded stent by rotational atherectomy. *Int J Angiol* 22:63–68, 2013.
47. Koster R, Hamm CW, Seabra-Gomes R, et al: Laser angioplasty of restenosed coronary stents: results of a multicenter surveillance trial. The Laser Angioplasty of Restenosed Stents (LARS) Investigators. *J Am Coll Cardiol* 34:25–32, 1999.
48. Mehran R, Mintz GS, Satler LF, et al: Treatment of in-stent restenosis with excimer laser coronary angioplasty: mechanisms and results compared with PTCA alone. *Circulation* 96:2183–2189, 1997.
49. Mehran R, Dangas G, Mintz GS, et al: Treatment of in-stent restenosis with excimer laser coronary angioplasty versus rotational atherectomy: comparative mechanisms and results. *Circulation* 101:2484–2489, 2000.
50. Mahdi NA, Pathan AZ, Harrell L, et al: Directional coronary atherectomy for the treatment of Palmaz-Schatz in-stent restenosis. *Am J Cardiol* 82:1345–1351, 1998.
51. Sanchez PL, Rodriguez-Alemparte M, Colon-Hernandez PJ, et al: Directional coronary atherectomy vs. rotational atherectomy for the treatment of in-stent restenosis of native coronary arteries. *Catheter Cardiovasc Interv* 58:155–161, 2003.
52. Adamian M, Colombo A, Briguori C, et al: Cutting balloon angioplasty for the treatment of in-stent restenosis: a matched comparison with rotational atherectomy, additional stent implantation and balloon angioplasty. *J Am Coll Cardiol* 38:672–679, 2001.
53. Kobayashi Y, Mehran R, Mintz GS, et al: Acute and long-term outcomes of cutting balloon angioplasty followed by gamma brachytherapy for in-stent restenosis. *Am J Cardiol* 92:1329–1331, 2003.
54. Fasseas P, Orford JL, Lennon R, et al: Cutting balloon angioplasty vs. conventional balloon angioplasty in patients receiving intracoronary brachytherapy for the treatment of in-stent restenosis. *Catheter Cardiovasc Interv* 63:152–157, 2004.
55. Takano M, Yamamoto M, Murakami D, et al: Optical coherence tomography after new scoring balloon angioplasty for in-stent restenosis and de novo coronary lesions. *Int J Cardiol* 141:e51–e53, 2010.
56. Cremers B, Schmitmeier S, Clever YP, et al: Inhibition of neo-intimal hyperplasia in porcine coronary arteries utilizing a novel paclitaxel-coated scoring balloon catheter. *Catheter Cardiovasc Interv* 2013.
57. Waksman R, Robinson KA, Crocker IR, et al: Intracoronary low-dose beta-irradiation inhibits neointima formation after coronary artery balloon injury in the swine restenosis model. *Circulation* 92:3025–3031, 1995.
58. Waksman R, Robinson KA, Crocker IR, et al: Endovascular low-dose irradiation inhibits neointima formation after coronary artery balloon injury in swine. A possible role for radiation therapy in restenosis prevention. *Circulation* 91:1533–1539, 1995.
59. Popma JJ, Suntharalingam M, Lansky AJ, et al: Randomized trial of 90Sr/90Y beta-radiation versus placebo control for treatment of in-stent restenosis. *Circulation* 106:1090–1096, 2002.
60. Waksman R, Raizner AE, Yeung AC, et al: Use of localised intracoronary beta radiation in treatment of in-stent restenosis: the INHIBIT randomised controlled trial. *Lancet* 359:551–557, 2002.
61. Waksman R, Ajani AE, Pinnow E, et al: Twelve versus six months of clopidogrel to reduce major cardiac events in patients undergoing gamma-radiation therapy for in-stent restenosis: Washington radiation for in-stent restenosis trial (WRIST) 12 versus WRIST PLUS. *Circulation* 106:776–778, 2002.
62. Sabate M, Costa MA, Kozuma K, et al: Geographic miss: a cause of treatment failure in radio-oncology applied to intracoronary radiation therapy. *Circulation* 101:2467–2471, 2000.
63. Costa MA, Sabate M, van der Giessen WJ, et al: Late coronary occlusion after intracoronary brachytherapy. *Circulation* 100:789–792, 1999.
64. Torguson R, Sabate M, Deible R, et al: Intravascular brachytherapy versus drug-eluting stents for the treatment of patients with drug-eluting stent restenosis. *Am J Cardiol* 98:1340–1344, 2006.
65. Moris C, Alfonso F, Lambert JL, et al: Stenting for coronary dissection after balloon dilation of in-stent restenosis: stenting a previously stented site. *Am Heart J* 131:834–836, 1996.
66. Alfonso F, Cequier A, Zueco J, et al: Stenting the stent: initial results and long-term clinical and angiographic outcome of coronary stenting for patients with in-stent restenosis. *Am J Cardiol* 85:327–332, 2000.
67. Elezi S, Kastrati A, Hadamitzky M, et al: Clinical and angiographic follow-up after balloon angioplasty with provisional stenting for coronary in-stent restenosis. *Catheter Cardiovasc Interv* 48:151–156, 1999.
68. Alfonso F, Melgares R, Mainar V, et al: Therapeutic implications of in-stent restenosis located at the stent edge. Insights from the restenosis intra-stent balloon angioplasty versus elective stenting (RIBS) randomized trial. *Eur Heart J* 25:1829–1835, 2004.
69. Morice MC, Serruys PW, Sousa JE, et al: A randomized comparison of a sirolimus-eluting stent with a standard stent for coronary revascularization. *N Engl J Med* 346:1773–1780, 2002.
70. Moses JW, Leon MB, Popma JJ, et al: Sirolimus-eluting stents versus standard stents in patients with stenosis in a native coronary artery. *N Engl J Med* 349:1315–1323, 2003.
71. Degertekin M, Regar E, Tanabe K, et al: Sirolimus-eluting stent for treatment of complex in-stent restenosis: the first clinical experience. *J Am Coll Cardiol* 41:184–189, 2003.
72. Singh IM, Filby SJ, El Sakr F, et al: Drug-eluting stents versus bare-metal stents for treatment of bare-metal in-stent restenosis. *Catheter Cardiovasc Interv* 76:257–262, 2010.
73. Alfonso F, Perez-Vizcayno MJ, Hernandez R, et al: Long-term clinical benefit of sirolimus-eluting stents in patients with in-stent restenosis results of the RIBS-II (restenosis intra-stent: balloon angioplasty vs. elective sirolimus-eluting stenting) study. *J Am Coll Cardiol* 52:1621–1627, 2008.
74. Dibra A, Kastrati A, Alfonso F, et al: Effectiveness of drug-eluting stents in patients with bare-metal in-stent restenosis: meta-analysis of randomized trials. *J Am Coll Cardiol* 49:616–623, 2007.
75. Lu YG, Chen YM, Li L, et al: Drug-eluting stents vs. intracoronary brachytherapy for in-stent restenosis: a meta-analysis. *Clin Cardiol* 34:344–351, 2011.
76. Steinberg DH, Gaglia MA, Jr, Pinto Slottow TL, et al: Outcome differences with the use of drug-eluting stents for the treatment of in-stent restenosis of bare-metal stents versus drug-eluting stents. *Am J Cardiol* 103:491–495, 2009.
77. Byrne RA, Cassese S, Windisch T, et al: Differential relative efficacy between drug-eluting stents in patients with bare metal and drug-eluting stent restenosis; evidence in support of drug resistance: insights from the ISAR-DESIRE and ISAR-DESIRE 2 trials. *EuroIntervention* 9:797–802, 2013.
78. Abizaid A, Costa JR, Jr, Banning A, et al: The sirolimus-eluting cypher select coronary stent for the treatment of bare-metal and drug-eluting stent restenosis: insights from the e-select 64-71 (multicenter post-market surveillance) registry. *JACC Cardiovasc Interv* 5:64–71, 2012.
79. Hehrlein C, Dietz U, Kubica J, et al: Twelve-month results of a paclitaxel releasing balloon in patients presenting with in-stent restenosis first-in-man (PEPPER) trial. *Cardiovasc Revasc Med* 13:260–264, 2012.
80. Lemos PA, van Mieghem CA, Arampatzis CA, et al: Post-sirolimus-eluting stent restenosis treated with repeat percutaneous intervention: late angiographic and clinical outcomes. *Circulation* 109:2500–2502, 2004.
81. Byrne R, Iijima R, Mehilli J, et al: [Treatment of paclitaxel-eluting stent restenosis with sirolimus-eluting stent implantation: angiographic and clinical outcomes]. *Rev Esp Cardiol* 61:1134–1139, 2008.
82. Cosgrave J, Melzi G, Biondi-Zoccai GG, et al: Drug-eluting stent restenosis the pattern predicts the outcome. *J Am Coll Cardiol* 47:2399–2404, 2006.
83. Song HG, Park DW, Kim YH, et al: Randomized trial of optimal treatment strategies for in-stent restenosis after drug-eluting stent implantation. *J Am Coll Cardiol* 59:1093–1100, 2012.
84. Cosgrave J, Melzi G, Corbett S, et al: Repeated drug-eluting stent implantation for drug-eluting stent restenosis: the same or a different stent. *Am Heart J* 153:354–359, 2007.
85. Garg S, Smith K, Torguson R, et al: Treatment of drug-eluting stent restenosis with the same versus different drug-eluting stent. *Catheter Cardiovasc Interv* 70:9–14, 2007.
86. Alfonso F, Perez-Vizcayno MJ, Dutary J, et al: Implantation of a drug-eluting stent with a different drug (switch strategy) in patients with drug-eluting stent restenosis. Results from a prospective multicenter study (RIBS III [restenosis intra-stent: balloon angioplasty versus drug-eluting stent]). *JACC Cardiovasc Interv* 5:728–737, 2012.
87. Li Y, Li L, Su Q, et al: Same versus different types of drug-eluting stents in the treatment of in-stent restenosis: a meta analysis. *Chinese Journal of Tissue Engineering Research* 17:565–570, 2013.
88. Abizaid A, Costa JR, Jr, Bartorelli AL, et al: The ABSORB EXTEND study: preliminary report of the twelve-month clinical outcomes in the first 512 patients enrolled. *EuroIntervention* pii:20130827-06, 2014.
89. Naganuma T, Costopoulos C, Latib A, et al: Feasibility and efficacy of bioresorbable vascular scaffolds use for the treatment of in-stent restenosis and a bifurcation lesion in a heavily calcified diffusely diseased vessel. *JACC Cardiovasc Interv* 7:e45–e46, 2014.
90. Ielasi A, Latib A, Naganuma T, et al: Early results following everolimus-eluting bioresorbable vascular scaffold implantation for the treatment of in-stent restenosis. *Int J Cardiol* 173:513–514, 2014.
91. Byrne RA, Joner M, Alfonso F, et al: Drug-coated balloon therapy in coronary and peripheral artery disease. *Nature Reviews Cardiology* 11:13–23, 2014.
92. Alfonso F, Perez-Vizcayno MJ: Drug-eluting balloons for restenosis after stent implantation. *Lancet* 381:431–433, 2013.
93. Scheller B, Clever YP, Kelsch B, et al: Long-term follow-up after treatment of coronary in-stent restenosis with a paclitaxel-coated balloon catheter. *JACC Cardiovasc Interv* 5:323–330, 2012.
94. Stone GW, Rizvi A, Newman W, et al: Everolimus-eluting versus paclitaxel-eluting stents in coronary artery disease. *N Engl J Med* 362:1663–1674, 2010.
95. Kedhi E, Joesoef KS, McFadden E, et al: Second-generation everolimus-eluting and paclitaxel-eluting stents in real-life practice (COMPARE): a randomised trial. *Lancet* 375:201–209, 2010.
96. Kwong JS, Yu CM: Drug-eluting balloons for coronary artery disease: an updated meta-analysis of randomized controlled trials. *Int J Cardiol* 168:2930–2932, 2013.
97. Indermuehle A, Bahl R, Lansky AJ, et al: Drug-eluting balloon angioplasty for in-stent restenosis: a systematic review and meta-analysis of randomised controlled trials. *Heart* 99:327–333, 2013.
98. Alfonso F, Garcia J, Perez-Vizcayno MJ, et al: New stent implantation for recurrences after stenting for in-stent restenosis: implications of a third metal layer in human coronary arteries. *J Am Coll Cardiol* 54:1036–1038, 2009.
99. Martin JL, Ellis SG, Colombo A, et al: Frequency of coronary artery bypass grafting following implantation of a paclitaxel-eluting or a bare-metal stent into a single coronary artery. *Am J Cardiol* 103:11–16, 2009.
100. Iqbal J, Onuma Y, Ormiston J, et al: Bioresorbable scaffolds: rationale, current status, challenges, and future. *Eur Heart J* 35:765–776, 2014.

14 Management of Thrombotic Lesions

Anthony A. Bavry

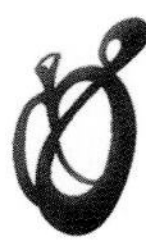

INTRODUCTION

Acute myocardial infarction is caused by thrombotic occlusion of a native coronary artery. While partial occlusion usually presents as a non ST-elevation myocardial infarction (NSTEMI), it is expected that complete occlusion will result in ST-elevation myocardial infarction (STEMI). Acute myocardial infarction can also occur as a result of thrombotic occlusion of a saphenous vein graft. Saphenous vein graft occlusion may be associated with larger thrombus burden than native coronary artery occlusion and therefore may require different strategies for management. Stent thrombosis is becoming increasingly recognized as a distinct cause of acute myocardial infarction.

Primary percutaneous coronary intervention (PCI) is effective at reperfusing or recanalizing the infarct related artery with a success rate that exceeds 90%.[1] Traditionally this has been accomplished by passing an uninflated coronary balloon "back and forth" across the thrombus, possibly coupled with serial balloon inflations at the site of occlusion. This established the term "door-to-balloon time" that is currently used as a quality metric for catheterization laboratories that offer primary PCI. Unfortunately, such disruption of thrombus likely results in macro- and micro-embolization into the downstream coronary bed. Impaired myocardial perfusion can be observed by failure of electrocardiographic ST-segments to return to baseline. This can also be observed during coronary angiography by assessment of myocardial blush grade, which represents flow in the microcirculation (0 = no blush, 1 = minimal blush, 2 = moderate blush, and 3 = normal blush). Despite successful epicardial coronary flow, impaired myocardial flow (blush grade 0 to 2) has been observed in over 70% of patients.[1] Impaired myocardial perfusion has been associated with poor prognosis. For example, after coronary flow is re-established in acute myocardial infarction, no ST-segment resolution is associated with 29% long-term mortality compared with 4% for complete resolution.[2] Similarly, poor myocardial blush (grade 0/1) is associated with 23% long-term mortality compared with 3% for normal blush (grade 3).[3]

Accordingly, different strategies have been developed to manage thrombus during primary PCI in order to mitigate the adverse effects associated with embolization. This review will principally center on the current pharmacological and mechanical approaches to manage thrombotic lesions.

STENT THROMBOSIS

An important etiology of acute myocardial infarction is stent thrombosis.[4] In fact, in a relatively large registry, the proportion of STEMI cases due to stent thrombosis increased from 6% in 2003 to 2004, to approximately 11% in 2009 to 2010.[5] This is important since primary PCI for stent thrombosis is less effective (76% to 80% successful reperfusion) than primary PCI for native artery occlusion.[6,7] STEMI due to stent thrombosis is also associated with an increased risk for long-term myocardial infarction (~23%) and repeat stent thrombosis (~15%) compared with STEMI due to native artery occlusion.[5]

With current generation drug-eluting stents (everolimus and zotarolimus-eluting), late and very late stent thrombosis is exceedingly rare; however, this complication is still seen during periods of inadequate antiplatelet therapy. Inadequate antiplatelet therapy might be the result of poor patient compliance, but is also seen among patients undergoing noncardiac surgical procedures who have been instructed to minimize or stop their antiplatelet therapy.[8]

PHARMACOLOGICAL STRATEGIES TO IMPROVE MYOCARDIAL PERFUSION

Facilitated PCI has been studied as a potential mechanism to improve outcomes during acute myocardial infarction. With this approach it was hoped that improvement in preprocedure coronary flow could reduce infarct size and improve survival. PCI can be facilitated by potent antiplatelet agents (i.e., glycoprotein IIb/IIIa inhibitors) or by thrombolytic agents. Dong et al. performed a metaanalysis on nearly 3000 STEMI patients who received upstream eptifibatide or tirofiban versus in-lab eptifibatide or tirofiban.[9] Although upstream glycoprotein inhibitor use was associated with improved preprocedure coronary flow, it did not reduce recurrent myocardial infarction or mortality. Glycoprotein IIb/IIIa inhibitors can also be administered intra-coronary, rather than intravenous; however, recent randomized trial data did not find a benefit in regard to survival or recurrent myocardial infarction from this approach.[10]

The Facilitated Intervention with Enhanced Reperfusion Speed to Stop Events (FINESSE) trial randomized nearly 2500 patients who presented within 6 hours of a STEMI to one of the following study drug strategies: upstream abciximab versus upstream abciximab with half-dose reteplase versus upstream placebo.[11] Efficacy was similar between all treatment arms; however, major bleeding was increased from a facilitated approach, especially with thrombolytic therapy. Major bleeding was 10.1% with upstream abciximab versus 14.5% with upstream abciximab with half-dose reteplase versus 6.9% with upstream placebo. Eitel et al. also conducted a metaanalysis to examine the association between facilitated PCI and mortality.[12] Compared with primary PCI, the odds ratio (OR) for mortality from glycoprotein IIb/IIIa inhibitor–facilitated PCI was 0.88, 95% confidence interval (CI), 0.59 to 1.33; for thrombolytic-facilitated PCI, OR = 1.47; 95% CI, 0.96 to 2.25; and for combination glycoprotein IIb/IIIa inhibitor/half-dose thrombolytic–facilitated PCI, OR = 1.22; 95% CI, 0.55 to 2.67.[12] Therefore, facilitated PCI does not appear to improve survival and, in the case of thrombolytics, may even be associated with harm.

MECHANICAL STRATEGIES TO IMPROVE MYOCARDIAL PERFUSION

Currently Approved Devices

The simplest way to retrieve coronary thrombus is with the use of a manual aspiration thrombectomy catheter. A variety of catheters are commercially available (**Table 14-1, Figure 14-1**). The catheter is attached to a stopcock and syringe that is prepped with negative pressure and advanced over a 0.014-inch wire proximal to the site of occlusion. When the stopcock is turned, the catheter aspirates blood/thrombotic debris from the catheter tip. The catheter is slowly advanced through the site of occlusion and returned to the guide catheter when the syringe is filled with blood and thus no longer aspirating. Normally one to two or more passes with the aspiration catheter are performed to restore epicardial blood flow. One can continue passes until there is no more debris noted in the aspirate when run through a mesh filter or gauze. Many catheters now come preloaded with a stylet that can facilitate deliverability of the device to the site of occlusion. There is no clear advantage of one device over another; however, most of the clinical trial data support the Export device. **Table 14-2** provides pearls to consider for optimal use.

TABLE 14-1 Commercially Available Aspiration Thrombectomy Catheters

MANUFACTURER	DEVICE	PRELOADED WITH STYLET	GUIDE CATHETER (Fr)
Medtronic	Export AP	No	6, 7
	Export Advance	Yes	6, 7
Terumo	PriorityOne	Yes	6, 7
Vascular solutions	Pronto V3	No	6
	Pronto V4	No	6, 7, 8
	Pronto LP	Yes	6
Maquet	ExpressWay	Yes	6
Spectranetics	QuickCat	No	6
Bayer	Fetch 2	No	6

Fr, French.
The Pronto V4 has an embedded wire for additional deliverability and kink resistance.
The Pronto LP is intended for small vessels (~1.5 mm).

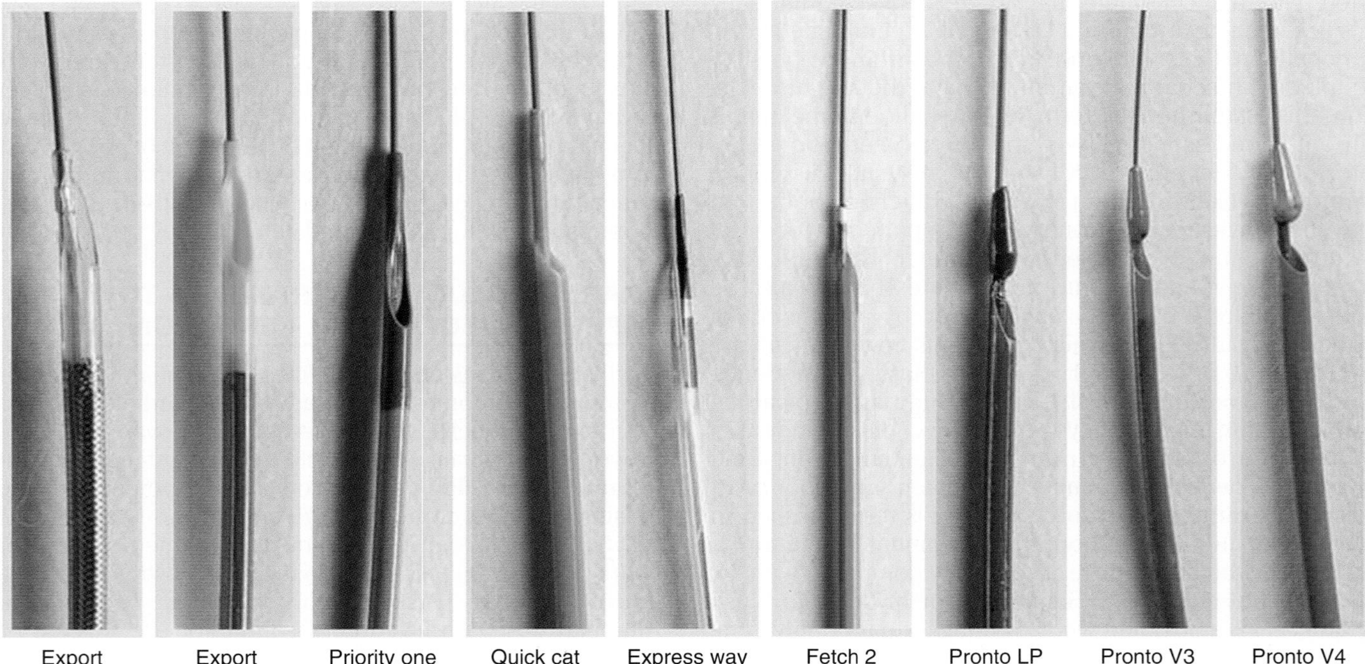

FIGURE 14-1 Composite of commercially available aspiration thrombectomy catheters.

TABLE 14-2 Pearls for Optimal Use of Aspiration Thrombectomy Catheters

PEARL	REASON/EXPLANATION
Activate suction proximal to lesion	Prevent systemic embolism of thrombus
Keep suction activated until device is completely removed from body	Firm thrombus might be trapped at catheter tip and prematurely stopping suction could liberate thrombus into guide catheter/systemic circulation
Once device is removed from body, back bleed from hemostatic valve	The device can entrain air. This is also to potentially discharge retained thrombus as above Caution if the guide catheter pressure is severely damped, since opening the hemostatic valve can entrain air rather than bleed back
Aspiration thrombectomy catheters can also be used to infuse medications into the myocardial bed	With poor coronary flow, intracoronary administration of medications through the guide catheter may end up in the systemic rather than coronary circulation
Aspiration thrombectomy catheter can be difficult to advance to the target. In this scenario, consider a catheter that comes loaded with a stylet or delivers through a guide extender	The sylet stiffens the catheter and enhances deliverability Similarly, a guide extender may provide enough support to allow the thrombectomy catheter to track into position
Despite being designed to be "kink-resistant," all catheters are relatively easy to kink	Slow down during advancement of catheter into the body

TABLE 14-3 Commercially Available Mechanical Thrombectomy Catheters

MANUFACTURER	DEVICE	RAPID EXCHANGE	GUIDE CATHETER (FR)
Bayer	Angiojet distaflex	No	6
	Angiojet spiroflex	Yes	6
	Angiojet spiroflex VG	Yes	7

Fr, French.
The Angiojet Distaflex is intended for small vessels (tip is 4 Fr and body of catheter is 5 Fr).

Alternatively, mechanical or rheolytic thrombectomy can be performed. This is represented by the AngioJet catheter (Bayer Healthcare; Warrendale, Pennsylvania) (**Table 14-3, Figure 14-2**). This device shares many similarities with aspiration thrombectomy. The catheters require a 6 French (Fr) guide catheter, except for the Spiroflex VG catheter that is intended for saphenous vein graft lesions and requires a 7 Fr guide catheter. High-pressure saline jets are directed retrograde within the catheter (**Figure 14-3**). This creates a low-pressure zone through which the thrombus can be withdrawn into the catheter through entry ports and externalized to a collection bag. Rheolytic thrombectomy catheters create −600 mm Hg at the catheter tip compared with −10 mm Hg for aspiration thrombectomy catheters. There is potential for blood loss with this device, especially with multiple and prolonged runs; however, it is likely similar to

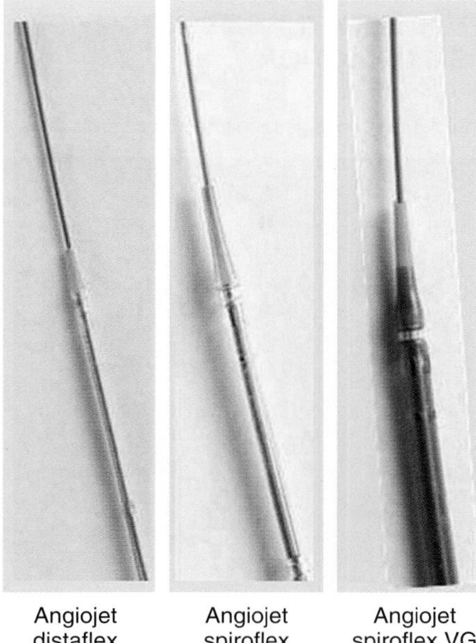

FIGURE 14-2 Composite of commercially available rheolytic thrombectomy catheters.

the degree of blood loss with aspiration thrombectomy catheters. Some patients will require a temporary pacemaker, especially when thrombectomy is performed in the right coronary artery. Some operators recommend theophylline infusion to prevent bradyarrhythmias, although there are few data to support this.

Case

Figure 14-3 and Videos 14-1 to 14-5 highlight the clinical application of aspiration and rheolytic thrombectomy devices within the same patient during an acute myocardial infarction. The patient was an 83-year-old man with prior coronary artery bypass grafting and percutaneous coronary intervention who presented to the hospital with an acute myocardial infarction. He was taken for cardiac catheterization and coronary angiogram revealed an occluded saphenous vein graft to the ramus intermedius that was presumed to be the culprit artery (**Figure 14-4,** Video 14-1). The site of occlusion was proximal to a previously placed stent. Aspiration thrombectomy was performed with an Export device; however, this only restored partial coronary flow (**Figure 14-5,** Videos 14-2 and 14-3). Next, rheolytic thrombectomy was performed with the Angiojet Spiroflex device (Video 14-4). Temporary pacing was not required. This was successful in restoring normal coronary flow (**Figure 14-6,** Video 14-5).

Potentially Useful Devices

An alternative approach is to trap the thrombus within the coronary artery rather than retrieve it. This strategy was studied in the Safety and Efficacy Study of the MGuard Stent After a Heart Attack (MASTER) trial.[13] In this feasibility trial, a polyethylene terephthalate micronet mesh-covered stent was compared with a commercially available bare-metal or drug-eluting stent during STEMI. The mesh-covered stent significantly improved postprocedure ST-segment resolution. Future studies will need to determine if this improves clinical outcomes.

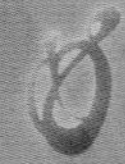

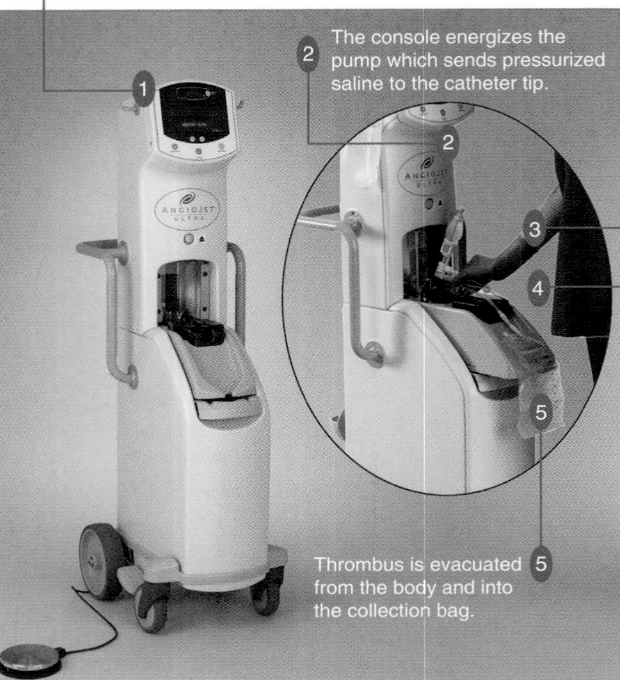

1 The angiojet ultra console monitors and controls the system.
2 The console energizes the pump which sends pressurized saline to the catheter tip.
Thrombus is evacuated from the body and into the collection bag. 5

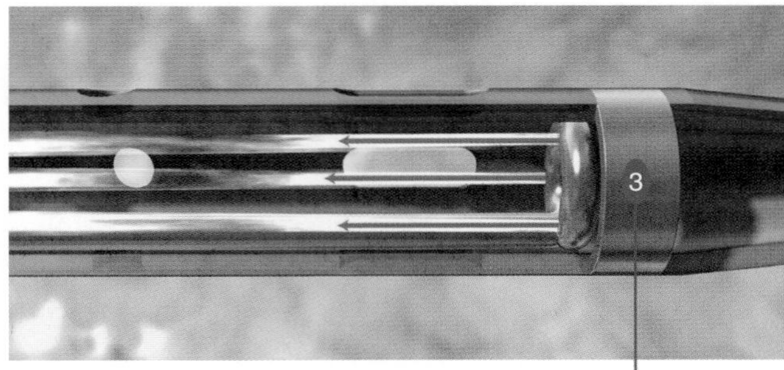

3
Saline jets travel backwards to create a low pressure zone causing a vacuum effect.

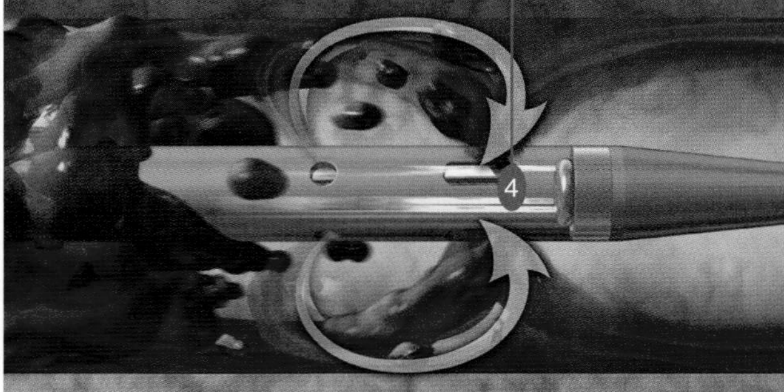

Thrombus is drawn into the in-flow windows and the jets push the thrombus back down the catheter.
4

FIGURE 14-3 Schematic of mechanism of action for rheolytic thrombectomy. *(Reprinted with permission from Bayer HealthCare LLC. The AngioJet is a registered trademark of Bayer.)*

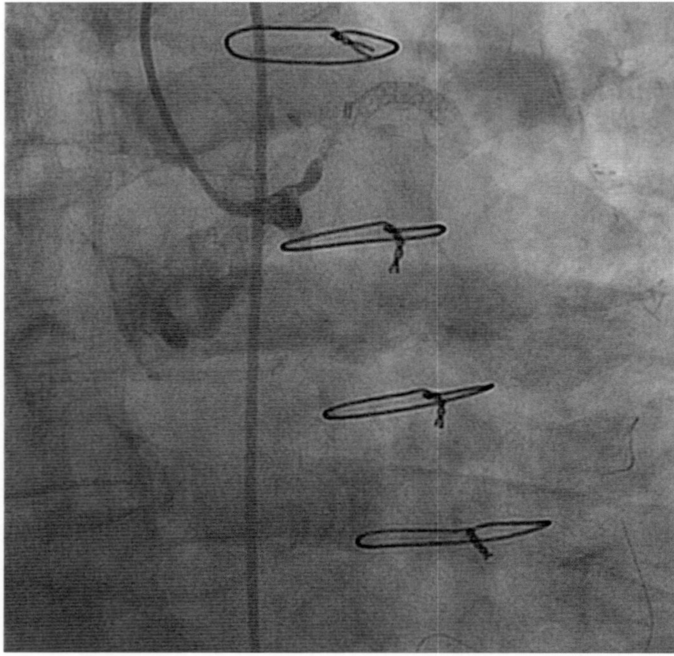

FIGURE 14-4 Saphenous vein graft occlusion. The site of occlusion is proximal to the previously placed stent.

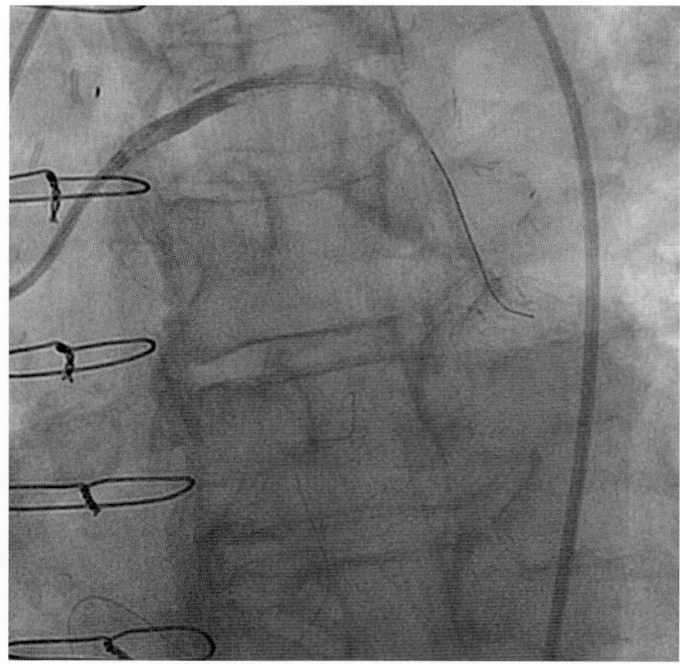

FIGURE 14-5 Improved but still poor flow after aspiration thrombectomy.

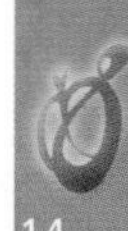

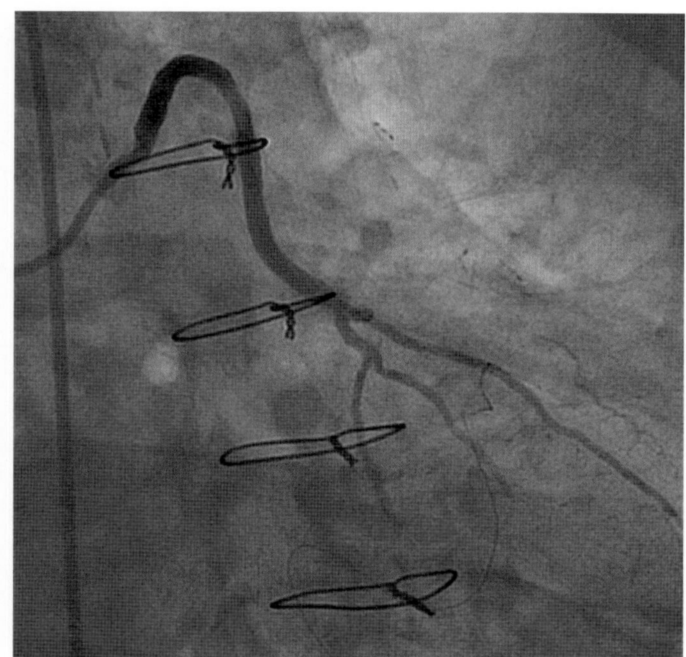

FIGURE 14-6 Successful reperfusion after rheolytic thrombectomy with the Angiojet Spiroflex device.

As mentioned previously, intracoronary administration of a glycoprotein IIb/IIIa inhibitor does not appear to be beneficial when compared with intravenous administration.[10] Part of the reason for the lack of efficacy from this strategy could be due to impaired coronary flow, thus resulting in much of the drug being dispersed systemically. The ClearWay catheter (Atrium Medical; Hudson, New Hampshire) is a device that was designed to infuse drug (e.g., glycoprotein IIb/IIIa inhibitors) locally rather than intracoronary.[14] This device is a 2.7 Fr rapid exchange catheter that has a "weeping" PTFE balloon that allows for local drug delivery.

Devices That Are Not Used

Embolic protection devices (i.e., a distal filter) are routinely used in saphenous vein graft lesions. The devices have been studied in native coronary artery occlusion; however, they are not used due to lack of efficacy.[15] Other devices that have been studied to some extent are the excimer laser and ultrasonic thrombectomy.[16,17]

CLINICAL TRIAL DATA

Aspiration Thrombectomy

The Thrombus Aspiration during Percutaneous Coronary Intervention in Acute Myocardial Infarction (TAPAS) trial randomized over 1000 participants to aspiration thrombectomy versus conventional PCI.[18] Aspiration was performed with the Export device (Medtronic; Minneapolis, Minnesota). This trial found that aspiration thrombectomy was associated with significantly improved myocardial blood flow (myocardial blush grade and ST-segment resolution). Although not powered for clinical endpoints, patients with good myocardial blood flow had improved clinical outcomes.

Metaanalyses have documented a reduction in major adverse cardiovascular events, including all-cause mortality from aspiration thrombectomy versus conventional PCI during acute myocardial infarction.[15,19] However, the mechanism for this benefit is not entirely clear since aspiration thrombectomy is only associated with a marginal improvement in recurrent myocardial infarction and target vessel revascularization, with no improvement in infarct size.[19]

The largest trial on the topic, Thrombus Aspiration during ST-Segment Elevation (TASTE) myocardial infarction, which included more than 7000 participants, was recently published. This trial was unable to document a mortality benefit from aspiration thrombectomy.[20] However, aspiration thrombectomy was associated with a marginal reduction in recurrent myocardial infarction ($p = 0.09$) and stent thrombosis at 30 days ($p = 0.06$). Additional randomized trial data on the topic are forthcoming, including from longer term follow-up of TASTE and from the ongoing randomized trial of routine aspiration ThrOmbecTomy with PCI versus PCI Alone (TOTAL) in patients with STEMI undergoing primary PCI.

Rheolytic Thrombectomy and Distal Embolic Protection

Data are not as robust or as supportive regarding the use of rheolytic thrombectomy.[15,19] One of the largest and most recent trials on the topic found the Angiojet device to be safe (i.e., no apparent increase in stroke).[21] Rheolytic thrombectomy might be especially useful for massive thrombus burden, acute myocardial infarction due to a saphenous vein graft lesion, or an inadequate result from aspiration thrombectomy.

A metaanalysis examined nine trials that randomized patients with acute myocardial infarction to distal embolic protection versus conventional PCI.[15] In summary, distal embolic protection was not associated with a reduction in major adverse clinical events.

Infusion Catheter

The ClearWay catheter was studied in the Intracoronary Abciximab Infusion and Aspiration Thrombectomy in Patients Undergoing Percutaneous Coronary Intervention for Anterior ST-Segment Elevation Myocardial Infarction (INFUSE-AMI) trial.[14] Patients were assigned to one of the following groups:

1. Aspiration thrombectomy followed by local delivery of abciximab
2. Aspiration thrombectomy with no abciximab
3. Local delivery of abciximab with no aspiration thrombectomy
4. No local delivery of abciximab and no aspiration thrombectomy

Aspiration thrombectomy did not reduce final infarct size at 30 days, although local delivery of abciximab was associated with a modest reduction in infarct size ($p = 0.03$).[14] At 1 year, compared with no active therapy, local delivery of abciximab was associated with a lower frequency of death (1.4% vs. 4.9%; $p = 0.04$), while aspiration thrombectomy was associated with a lower frequency of new-onset heart failure (0.9% vs. 4.5%; $p = 0.02$) and hospitalization for heart failure (0.9% vs. 5.49%; $p = 0.0008$).[22] Since this represents a potential paradigm shift, further study of this device, especially alongside of commercially available aspiration catheters, is warranted.

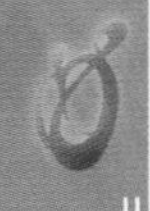

GUIDELINE RECOMMENDATIONS

The American College of Cardiology/American Heart Association 2013 practice guidelines, state that aspiration thrombectomy is reasonable among patients undergoing primary PCI (Class IIa recommendation; level of evidence [LOE] B).[23] In contrast, routine rheolytic thrombectomy is not given a recommendation due to lack of clinical benefit. The European Society of Cardiology 2012 guidelines also state that routine thrombus aspiration should be considered (Class IIa; LOE B).[24]

CONCLUSIONS

In summary, management of thrombus during acute coronary syndromes (NSTEMI and STEMI) is important to preserve myocardial function and improve clinical outcomes. Stent thrombosis is an important and increasing cause of acute myocardial infarction. Most of the facilitated pharmacological approaches, including intracoronary administration of glycoprotein IIb/IIIa inhibitors through the guiding catheter, have fallen out of favor. Local delivery of a glycoprotein IIb/IIIa inhibitor at the site of occlusion appears promising and deserves further study. The current standard of care for mechanical management of thrombus is manual aspiration thrombectomy; however, important questions remain with this strategy and further data will be forthcoming.

References

1. Stone GW, Peterson MA, Lansky AJ, et al: Impact of normalized myocardial perfusion after successful angioplasty in acute myocardial infarction. *J Am Coll Cardiol* 39:591–597, 2002.
2. van 't Hof AW, Liem A, de Boer MJ, et al: Clinical value of 12-lead electrocardiogram after successful reperfusion therapy for acute myocardial infarction. Zwolle Myocardial Infarction Study Group. *Lancet* 350:615–619, 1997.
3. van 't Hof AW, Liem A, Suryapranata H, et al: Angiographic assessment of myocardial reperfusion in patients treated with primary angioplasty for acute myocardial infarction: myocardial blush grade. Zwolle Myocardial Infarction Study Group. *Circulation* 97:2302–2306, 1998.
4. Bavry AA, Kumbhani DJ, Helton TJ, et al: Late thrombosis of drug-eluting stents: a meta-analysis of randomized clinical trials. *Am J Med* 119:1056–1061, 2006.
5. Brodie BR, Hansen C, Garberich RF, et al: ST-segment elevation myocardial infarction resulting from stent thrombosis: an enlarging subgroup of high-risk patients. *J Am Coll Cardiol* 60:1989–1991, 2012.
6. Chechi T, Vecchio S, Vittori G, et al: ST-segment elevation myocardial infarction due to early and late stent thrombosis a new group of high-risk patients. *J Am Coll Cardiol* 51:2396–2402, 2008.
7. Ergelen M, Gorgulu S, Uyarel H, et al: The outcome of primary percutaneous coronary intervention for stent thrombosis causing ST-elevation myocardial infarction. *Am Heart J* 159:672–676, 2010.
8. Bavry AA, Bhatt DL: Appropriate use of drug-eluting stents: balancing the reduction in restenosis with the concern of late thrombosis. *Lancet* 371:2134–2143, 2008.
9. Dong L, Zhang F, Shu X: Upstream vs deferred administration of small-molecule glycoprotein IIb/IIIa inhibitors in primary percutaneous coronary intervention for ST-segment elevation myocardial infarction: insights from randomized clinical trials. *Circ J* 74:1617–1624, 2010.
10. Thiele H, Wohrle J, Hambrecht R, et al: Intracoronary versus intravenous bolus abciximab during primary percutaneous coronary intervention in patients with acute ST-elevation myocardial infarction: a randomised trial. *Lancet* 379:923–931, 2012.
11. Ellis SG, Tendera M, de Belder MA, et al: Facilitated PCI in patients with ST-elevation myocardial infarction. *N Engl J Med* 358:2205–2217, 2008.
12. Eitel I, Franke A, Schuler G, et al: ST-segment resolution and prognosis after facilitated versus primary percutaneous coronary intervention in acute myocardial infarction: a meta-analysis. *Clin Res Cardiol* 99:1–11, 2010.
13. Stone GW, Abizaid A, Silber S, et al: Prospective, randomized, multicenter evaluation of a polyethylene terephthalate micronet mesh-covered stent (MGuard) in ST-segment elevation myocardial infarction: the MASTER trial. *J Am Coll Cardiol* 2012.
14. Stone GW, Maehara A, Witzenbichler B, et al: Intracoronary abciximab and aspiration thrombectomy in patients with large anterior myocardial infarction: the INFUSE-AMI randomized trial. *JAMA* 307:1817–1826, 2012.
15. Bavry AA, Kumbhani DJ, Bhatt DL: Role of adjunctive thrombectomy and embolic protection devices in acute myocardial infarction: a comprehensive meta-analysis of randomized trials. *Eur Heart J* 29:2989–3001, 2008.
16. Topaz O, Ebersole D, Das T, et al: Excimer laser angioplasty in acute myocardial infarction (the CARMEL multicenter trial). *Am J Cardiol* 93:694–701, 2004.
17. Brosh D, Bartorelli AL, Cribier A, et al: Percutaneous transluminal therapeutic ultrasound for high-risk thrombus-containing lesions in native coronary arteries. *Catheter Cardiovasc Interv* 55:43–49, 2002.
18. Svilaas T, Vlaar PJ, van der Horst IC, et al: Thrombus aspiration during primary percutaneous coronary intervention. *N Engl J Med* 358:557–567, 2008.
19. Kumbhani DJ, Bavry AA, Desai MY, et al: Role of aspiration and mechanical thrombectomy in patients with acute myocardial infarction undergoing primary angioplasty: an updated meta-analysis of randomized trials. *J Am Coll Cardiol* 62:1409–1418, 2013.
20. Frobert O, Lagerqvist B, Olivecrona GK, et al: Thrombus aspiration during ST-segment elevation myocardial infarction. *N Engl J Med* 369:1587–1597, 2013.
21. Migliorini A, Stabile A, Rodriguez AE, et al: Comparison of AngioJet rheolytic thrombectomy before direct infarct artery stenting with direct stenting alone in patients with acute myocardial infarction. The JETSTENT trial. *J Am Coll Cardiol* 56:1298–1306, 2010.
22. Stone GW, Witzenbichler B, Godlewski J, et al: Intralesional abciximab and thrombus aspiration in patients with large anterior myocardial infarction: one-year results from the INFUSE-AMI trial. *Circ Cardiovasc Interv* 6:527–534, 2013.
23. O'Gara PT, Kushner FG, Ascheim DD, et al: 2013 ACCF/AHA guideline for the management of ST-elevation myocardial infarction: executive summary: a report of the American College of Cardiology Foundation/American Heart Association Task Force on Practice Guidelines. *Circulation* 127:529–555, 2013.
24. Steg PG, James SK, Atar D, et al: ESC Guidelines for the management of acute myocardial infarction in patients presenting with ST-segment elevation. *Eur Heart J* 33:2569–2619, 2012.

15 Fractional Flow Reserve

Morton J. Kern

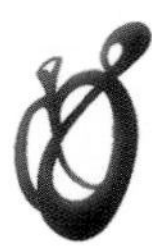

INTRODUCTION

Coronary blood flow and pressure measurements across a stenotic coronary artery provide information on the ischemic potential of a specific lesion at the time of catheterization. Physiologic assessment of coronary artery stenosis by fractional flow reserve (FFR) has become the gold standard for invasive assessment of myocardial ischemia. Its integration into the catheterization procedure as an adjunct to coronary angiography has made a significant impact on clinical decision making and outcomes for patients with a variety of angiographic presentations including intermediately severe single-vessel disease, multivessel disease, left main stenosis, diffuse disease, and bifurcation or ostial branch stenoses. The clinical outcome validation of FFR from several large randomized trials has led to favorable recommendations in guidelines for coronary revascularization, making it part of the standard of care for patients with coronary artery disease (CAD). This chapter reviews the concepts behind coronary physiology and FFR for clinical applications.

RATIONALE FOR IN-LAB CORONARY PHYSIOLOGIC MEASUREMENTS

The rationale for using coronary physiologic assessment arises from two sources: (1) that the coronary angiogram has significant limitations to demonstrating the clinical significance of lesions accurately, particularly in intermediately narrowed (between 30%-80% diameter stenosis), lesions and (2) that decisions for revascularization via percutaneous coronary intervention (PCI) or coronary artery bypass graft (CABG) surgery should be based on the presence of ischemia, information which may not be apparent from the angiogram or prior noninvasive testing.[1-3]

Coronary angiography produces a two-dimensional silhouette image of the three-dimensional vascular lumen. The interpretation of this image as representing an ischemia-producing lesion is both difficult and unreliable as evidenced from the poor correlation between noninvasive testing with angiographic percent diameter stenosis. Angiography does not provide vascular wall detail sufficient to characterize plaque size, length, or eccentricity. Viewed from different radiographic projections, the eccentric lesion produces an image with an unknown lumen dimension and is associated with at least six additional morphologic features known to contribute to the resistance to flow. Almost all of these features cannot be measured accurately from the angiogram (**Figures 15-1** and **15-2**). Other confounding artifacts of coronary angiography include contrast streaming, branch overlap, vessel foreshortening, calcifications, and ostial origins, which all contribute to uncertainty in gauging the ischemic potential of lesions.

The uncertainty of angiographic lesion assessment can be overcome with direct physiologic measurements in the catheterization laboratory (cath lab) using pressure and flow sensor guidewires.

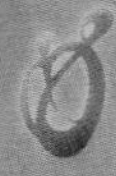

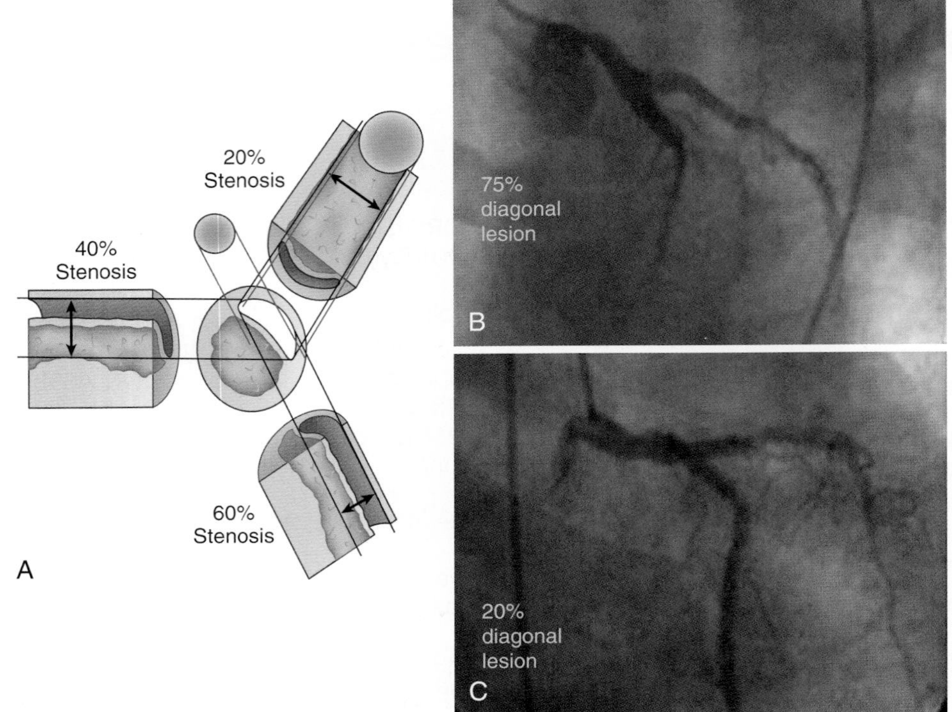

FIGURE 15-1 **A,** Viewed from different radiographic projections, the eccentric lumen produces an image with a high degree of uncertainty related to true lumen size and its impact on coronary blood flow **(C).** The same lesion may appear significant in one radiographic view **(B)** and nonsignificant in another **(C).**

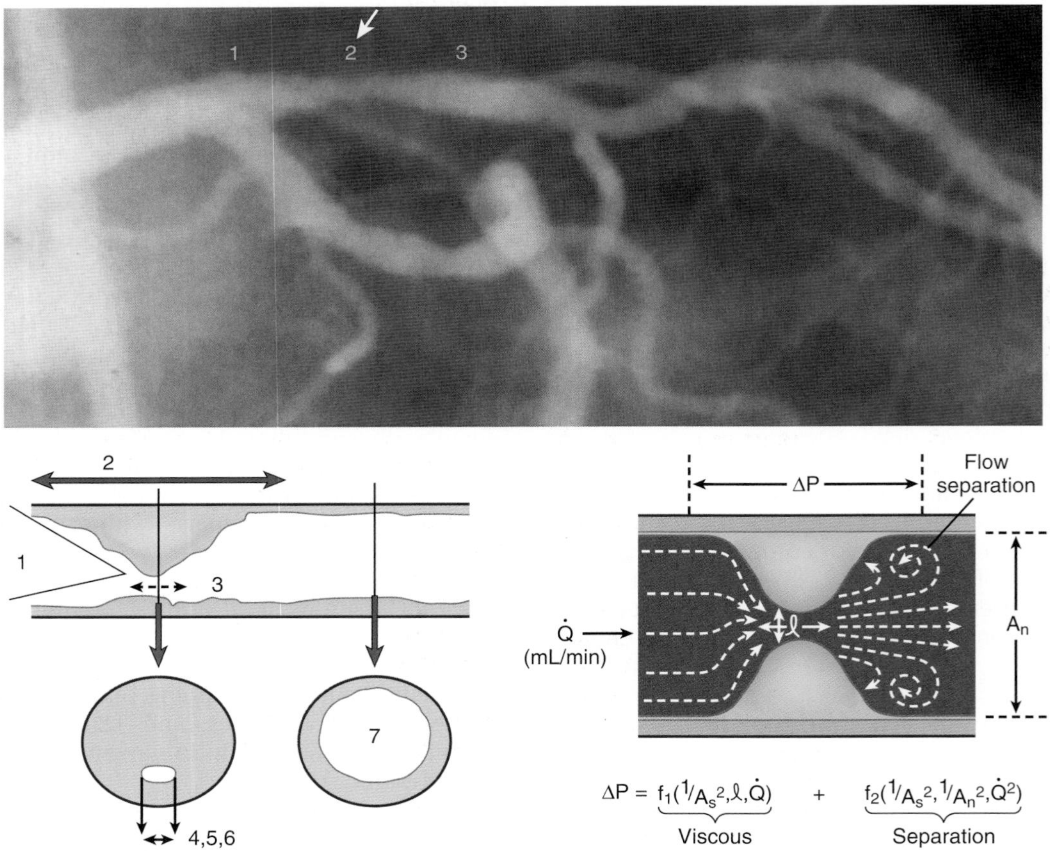

FIGURE 15-2 There are at least six morphological factors that produce pressure loss across a stenosis, most of which cannot be measured from the angiogram. *(1)* Entrance angle, *(2)* length of disease, *(3)* length of lesion, *(4, 5, 6)* type of lesion (eccentric, concentric, irregular), and *(7)* reference vessel size.

DERIVATION OF FRACTIONAL FLOW RESERVE FROM CORONARY PRESSURE MEASUREMENTS

Pijls and De Bruyne developed and validated an index for determining the physiologic impact of coronary stenoses, called the fractional flow reserve (FFR).[4-6] In the cath lab, FFR is measured as the ratio of mean distal coronary pressure divided by the mean proximal aortic pressure during maximal hyperemia. The coronary pressure beyond the stenosis is measured with a 0.014-inch guidewire with a high-fidelity pressure transducer mounted 1.5 cm from the tip of the wire, at the junction of the radio-opaque and radiolucent segments (**Figure 15-3**). The proximal coronary pressure is measured from the guide catheter and is equivalent to aortic pressure.

Using coronary pressure distal to a stenosis measured at constant and minimal myocardial resistances (i.e., maximal hyperemia), Pijls et al.[5] derived an estimate of the percentage of normal coronary blood flow expected to go through a stenotic artery. A simplified derivation for FFR is shown in **Figure 15-4.** FFR can be subdivided into three components describing the flow contributions by the coronary artery, the myocardium, and the collateral supply. FFR of the coronary artery (FFR_{cor}) is defined as the maximum coronary artery flow in the presence of a stenosis divided by the theoretic normal maximum flow of the same artery (i.e., the maximum flow in that artery if no stenosis were present). Similarly, FFR

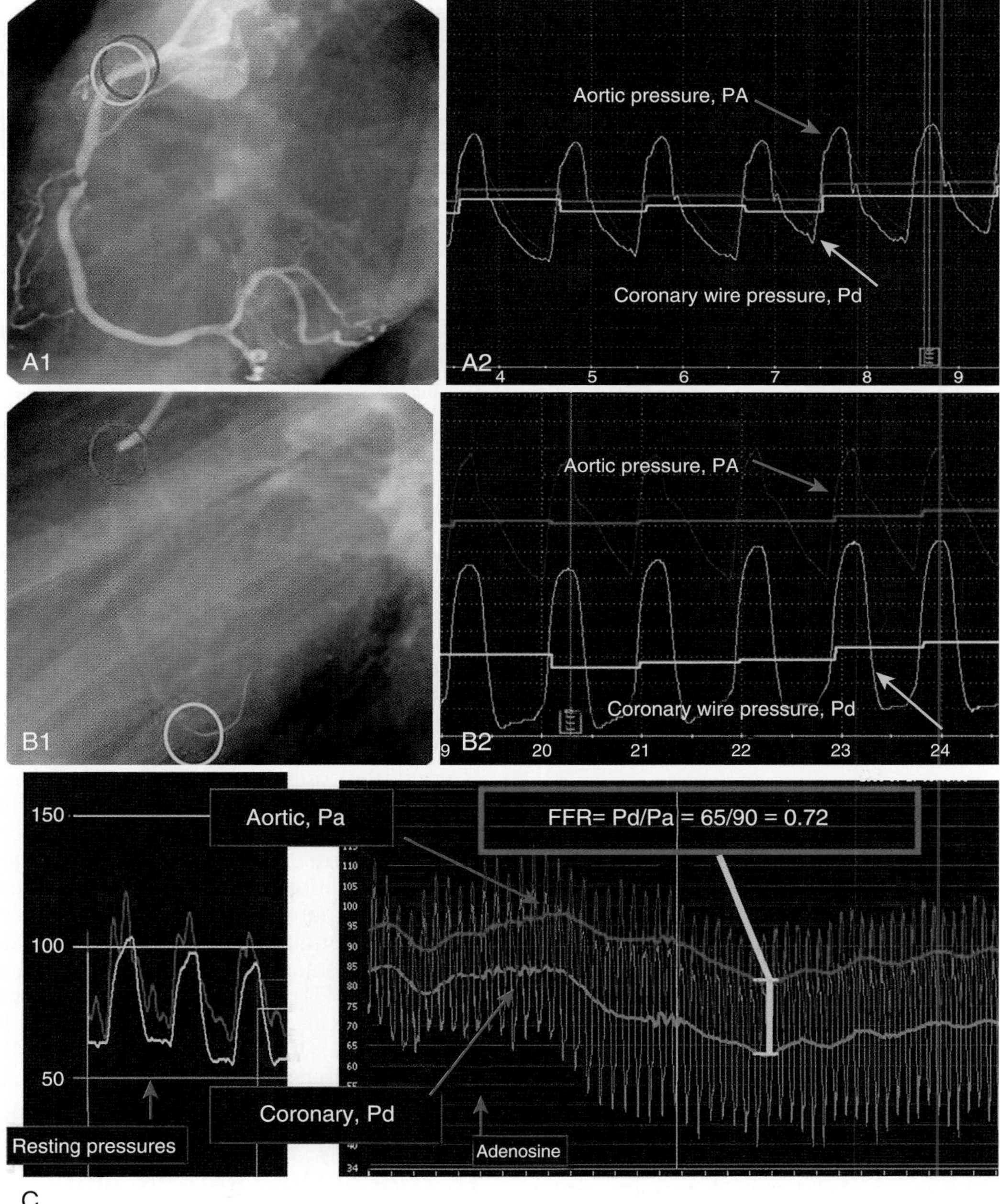

FIGURE 15-3 Method of fractional flow reserve (FFR) measurement. The first step is always to advance the pressure wire up to the tip of the catheter **(A1)** to be absolutely sure that the pressures are superimposed **(A2).** Then, the wire is advanced across the stenosis **(B1)** and obtains a corresponding FFR **(B2). C,** Left panel shows a mild resting gradient which becomes bigger with hyperemia (right panel). FFR is calculated as P_d/P_a at the nadir of distal pressure presumed to be the point of maximal hyperemia. In this example FFR = 0.72.

P_a P_d

Principles:

1. Aortic pressure, Pa, is the same along the length of the normal vessel
2. Resistance = P/Q
3. Flow, Q = P/R
4. FFR = $\frac{\text{Myocardial flow (Qs) across stenosis}}{\text{Myocardial flow (Qn) without stenosis}}$
5. Qs/Qn = $\frac{(Pd/Rs)}{(Pa/Rn)}$
6. If Rs = Rn, then Qs/Qn = Pd/Pa hence
7. FFR = Pd/Pa, at max hyperemia

FIGURE 15-4 Simplified derivation of fractional flow reserve (FFR). FFR is the ratio of maximal myocardial perfusion in the stenotic territory divided by maximal hyperemic flow in that same region in the hypothetical case the lesion was not present. FFR represents that fraction of hyperemic flow that persists despite the presence of the stenosis. This ratio of two flows is calculated solely from the ratio of mean coronary pressure (P_d) divided by mean aortic pressure (P_a) provided both pressures are recorded under conditions of maximal hyperemia. Aortic pressure, P_a, is the same along the length of the normal vessel. FFR is defined as myocardial flow (Q_s) across stenosis/myocardial flow (Q_n) without stenosis. To derive FFR, assume resistance = P/Q, then flow, Q = P/R, and that $Q_s/Q_n = (P_d/R_s)/(P_a/R_n)$, where R_s, R_n is resistance in stenotic and normal bed, which are identical at maximal hyperemia. If $R_s = R_n$, then $Q_s/Q_n = P_d/P_a$, which is FFR = $Q_s/Q_n = P_d/P_a$. *(Modified from Pijls NH, van Son JA, Kirkeeide RL, et al: Experimental basis of determining maximum coronary, myocardial, and collateral blood flow by pressure measurements for assessing functional stenosis severity before and after percutaneous transluminal coronary angioplasty. Circulation 87:1354–1367, 1993.)*

of the myocardium (FFR_{myo}) is defined as maximum myocardial (artery and bed) flow distal to an epicardial stenosis divided by its value if no epicardial stenosis were present. Stated another way, FFR represents that fraction of normal maximum flow that remains despite the presence of an epicardial lesion. Note that at maximal hyperemia FFR_{cor} is about equal to FFR_{myo} because myocardial bed resistance is minimal. The difference between FFR_{myo} and FFR_{cor} is FFR of the collateral flow.

The following equations are used to calculate the FFR of a coronary artery and its dependent myocardium:

$$FFR_{cor} = (P_d - P_w)/(P_a - P_w)$$

$$FFR_{myo} = (P_d - P_v)/(P_a - P_v)$$

$$FFR_{collateral} = FFR_{myo} - FFR_{cor}$$

(where P_a, P_d, P_v, and P_w are pressures of the aorta, distal artery, venous [or right atrial], and coronary wedge [during balloon occlusion] pressures, respectively; because FFR_{cor} uses P_w, it can be calculated only during coronary angioplasty).

In most clinical circumstances P_v is negligible relative to aortic pressure and omitted from the calculations. P_v may be included when right atrial pressure is >10 mm Hg and may influence FFR ± 0.02 units in patients with elevated right atrial pressure. FFR reflects both antegrade and collateral (or bypass graft) myocardial perfusion rather than merely trans-stenotic pressure loss (i.e., a stenosis pressure gradient). Because it is calculated only at peak hyperemia and excludes the microcirculatory resistance from the computation, FFR, unlike the coronary velocity reserve (CVR), is largely independent of basal flow, heart rate, systemic blood pressure, or status of the microcirculation.[6] **Table 15-1** lists the calculations for FFR. **Table 15-2** lists the thresholds for clinical applications of FFR.

TABLE 15-1 Calculations of FFR from Pressure Measurements

Myocardial fraction flow reserve (FFR_{myo}):
$FFR_{myo} = 1 - \Delta P/P_a - P_v$
$= P_d - P_v/P_a - P_v$
$\approx P_d/P_a$
Coronary fractional flow reserve (FFR_{cor}): $FFR_{cor} = 1 - \Delta P(P_a - P_w)$
Collateral fractional flow reserve (FFR_{coll}): $FFR_{coll} = FFR_{myo} - FFR_{cor}$

Modified from Pijls NH, van Son JA, Kirkeeide RL, et al: Experimental basis of determining maximum coronary, myocardial, and collateral blood flow by pressure measurements for assessing functional stenosis severity before and after percutaneous transluminal coronary angioplasty. Circulation 87:1354–1367, 1993.
Note: All measurements are made during hyperemia except P_w.
FRR, Fractional flow reserve; P_a, mean aortic pressure; P_d, distal coronary pressure; ΔP, mean translesional pressure gradient; P_v, mean right atrial pressure; P_w, mean coronary wedge pressure or distal coronary pressure during balloon inflation.

TABLE 15-2 Physiologic Thresholds Associated with Clinical Application of FFR

INDICATION	FFR
Ischemia detection	<0.75
Deferred PCI	>0.80
Endpoint of PCI*	>0.90

Modified from Kern MJ, et al: Physiological assessment of coronary artery disease in the cardiac catheterization laboratory: a scientific statement from the American Heart Association committee on diagnostic and interventional cardiac catheterization, council on clinical cardiology. Circulation 114:1321–1341, 2006.
FFR, Fractional flow reserve; *PCI,* percutaneous coronary intervention.
*Endpoint of stenting is anatomic apposition of stent struts best determined by IVUS. FFR can normalize despite malapposition of some stent struts.

Coronary Flow Reserve versus Fractional Flow Reserve

Coronary flow reserve (CFR) differs from FFR in several significant ways. CFR is defined as the ratio of peak hyperemic flow (or velocity) to basal flow (**Figure 15-5**).[7,8] CFR is altered by changing maximal and basal flow velocity values, which vary with heart rate, blood pressure, and contractility. FFR does not depend on basal flow levels since it is computed only at maximal flow and is unaffected by changing hemodynamics or the status of the microcirculation. CFR >2.0 represents a nonischemic value with an unknown normal value as CFR can change depending on existing conditions of the patient. In contrast, FFR has an absolute normal value of 1.0 for every artery, every patient, and every condition. FFR is specific for determining the ischemic potential of a specific epicardial coronary stenosis, whereas CFR provides the maximal flow across both the epicardial (R1) and microvascular (R2, R3) resistances (**Figure 15-6**). If either one or both is abnormal, CFR is abnormal, with no way to distinguish the contribution of the stenosis to impaired flow reserve. For these reasons FFR is preferred over CFR for in lab lesion assessment.

Fractional Flow Reserve and Myocardial Bed Size

An important concept to understanding the visual-functional mismatch of angiographic lesion severity and FFR is the relationship of myocardial bed size to epicardial flow. The

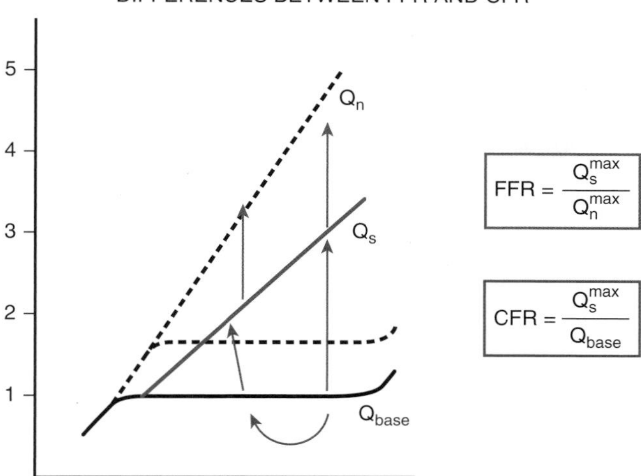

FIGURE 15-5 Fractional flow reserve (FFR) is defined as the ratio of myocardial flow (Q_{smax}) across stenosis to myocardial flow (Q_n) without stenosis. Coronary flow reserve (CFR) is defined as the ratio of peak hyperemic flow (Q_{smax}) to basal flow (Q_{base}). FFR is unaffected by changing baseline flow alterations in response to changing hemodynamics, contractility, or microvascular state, all factors that predictably alter CFR.

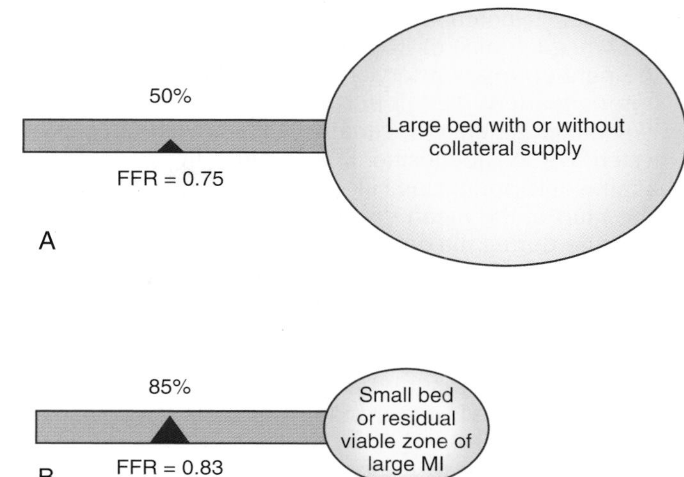

FIGURE 15-7 Influence of myocardial bed on fractional flow reserve (FFR). Myocardial bed (Mass) requires appropriate amount of blood flow and hence can affect FFR. A large bed **(A)** with a mild lesion (50%) can have a high flow and low FFR. The converse is true for a small myocardial **(B)** (such as may occur after myocardial infarction [MI]) and explains the common visual-functional mismatch between anatomic lesion severity and its physiologic impact.

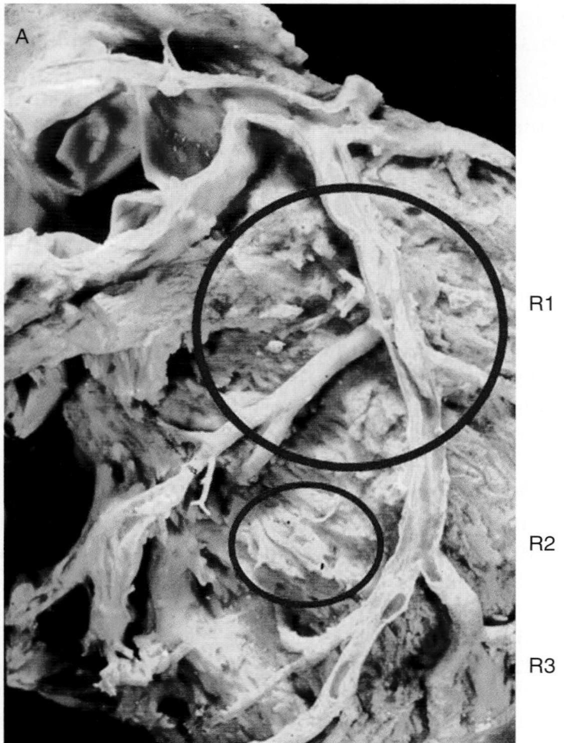

FIGURE 15-6 A, Pathological specimen demonstrating sources of myocardial perfusion: R1: Epicardial arteries, R2: Precapillary arterioles, R3: Microcirculation. Fractional flow reserve is specific for epicardial coronary stenosis (R1 resistance), whereas coronary flow reserve measures the sum of both the epicardial (R1) and microvascular (R2, R3) resistances.

larger the myocardial mass subtended by a vessel, the larger the hyperemic flow, and in turn, the larger the gradient and the lower the FFR for a given stenosis (**Figure 15-7**). This explains why a stenosis with a minimal cross-sectional area of 4 mm^2 has totally different hemodynamic significance in the proximal left anterior descending artery (LAD) versus a more distal location or region such as might be supplied by a second marginal branch in the lateral wall distribution. Proof of this concept was demonstrated by Iqbal et al.,[9] whereby an intermediately stenotic LAD supplying the anterior and inferior myocardial beds in a patient with an occluded right coronary artery (RCA) had an FFR of 0.72. After stenting and opening the RCA, reducing the LAD myocardial bed, the FFR across the LAD now rose to 0.84. In a similar manner the hemodynamic significance of a particular stenosis may change if the perfusion territory changes after myocardial infarction. It is for this reason that FFR in the ST-elevation myocardial infarction (STEMI) patient may not be valid until the dynamic changes of the acute injury are over. Regardless of the visual appearance, FFR accounts for the flow through the epicardial artery related to the bed supplied.

TECHNIQUES OF INTRACORONARY PRESSURE SENSOR WIRE MEASUREMENT

FFR can be easily measured using a 5 Fr or 6 Fr guide catheter and either of two available pressure wire systems (St. Jude Medical, Minneapolis, Minnesota, or Volcano Therapeutics, Rancho Cordova, California). After diagnostic angiography with a catheter seated in the coronary ostium, the steps to measure FFR are as follows:

1. Anticoagulation (intravenous [IV] heparin usually 40 U/kg or bivalirudin) and intracoronary (IC) nitroglycerin (100-200–mcg bolus) are administered before guidewire insertion.
2. The pressure wire is connected to the system's pressure analyzer and calibrated and zeroed to atmospheric pressure outside the body.
3. The wire is advanced through the guide to the coronary artery. The pressure wire and guide pressures are matched (i.e., equalized, also called normalized) before crossing the stenosis, usually at the tip of the guide.
4. The wire is then advanced across the stenosis about 2 centimeters distal to the coronary lesion.

5. Maximal hyperemia is induced with IV adenosine (140 mcg/kg/min) or IC bolus adenosine (20-30 mcg for the right coronary artery, 60 mcg or 100 mcg for the left coronary artery [LCA]). In some cases where borderline FFR values generate uncertainty, 180 mcg/kg/min can be tested. For IV adenosine, FFR is typically measured at 2 min. For IC adenosine, FFR is measured at 15-20 seconds.
6. The ratio of the mean distal pressure to mean proximal pressure during maximal hyperemia is calculated as the FFR. An FFR of ≤0.80 is correlated to abnormal ischemic testing and is useful as an indication to proceed with PCI.
7. PCI can be performed using the pressure wire as the working angioplasty guidewire. After the procedure, FFR can be remeasured to assess the adequacy of the intervention and any residual or new angiographic narrowings.
8. Finally, at the end of the procedure, the pressure wire is pulled back into the guide to confirm equal pressure readings, indicating signal stability.

Pitfalls and practice of measuring FFR are described in more detail elsewhere.[9]

PHARMACOLOGIC CORONARY HYPEREMIA

Stenosis severity should always be assessed using measurements obtained during maximal hyperemia. At maximal hyperemia, autoregulation is abolished and microvascular resistance fixed and minimal. Under these conditions, coronary blood flow is directly related to the driving pressure. Therefore, maximal hyperemic coronary blood flow is closely related to the coronary arterial pressure and is part of the derivation of pressure-derived FFR of the myocardium.

Hyperemia is most commonly achieved with IV or IC adenosine (**Table 15-3**). Alternative intravenous hyperemic agents include IV adenosine triphosphate (ATP) (140 mcg/kg/min), regadenoson 400 mcg IV bolus, and IV dopamine (10-40 mcg/min × 2 min increments). Less commonly used agents include IC ATP (50-100 mcg), and rarely used agents are IC papaverine (10-15 mg) and IC nitroprusside (50-100 mcg).[10]

Adenosine

IV adenosine is the preferred method of inducing hyperemia because it achieves a steady state and produces prolonged hyperemia and is weight based and operator independent. The onset of action of adenosine is rapid, its duration very brief with a half-life of <10 seconds. By providing prolonged hyperemia, IV adenosine infusion allows for a slow pullback of the pressure wire, useful to identify the exact location of the pressure drop-off for both simple and serial lesions or the presence of diffuse disease. IV adenosine also permits maximal coronary flow for assessment of aorto-ostial narrowings without guide catheter obstruction that may potentially occur with administration of IC adenosine.

While hyperemia of IC adenosine is equivalent to IV infusion in a large majority of patients, in a small percentage of cases, coronary hyperemia may be suboptimal with IC adenosine. Jeremias et al.[11] compared IC (15-20 mcg in the right and 18-24 mcg in the left coronary artery) to IV adenosine (140 mcg/kg/min) in 52 patients with 60 lesions. There was a strong linear relationship between IC and IV adenosine ($r = 0.978$ and $p < 0.001$). The mean measurement difference for FFR was 0.004 ± 0.03. In 8.3% of stenoses, FFR with IC adenosine differed by 0.05 or more compared with IV adenosine, suggesting an inadequate hyperemic response with IC adenosine. Subsequent studies have confirmed the correlation between IC and IV adenosine; however, it has been suggested that higher doses of IC adenosine (>60 mcg) may improve hyperemia and generate lower FFR values.[12]

The feasibility and efficacy of peripheral compared with central IV infusion of adenosine for FFR measurement were tested by Seo et al.[13] They measured FFR in 71 patients using IC bolus injection and continuous IV infusion (140 µg/min/kg) of adenosine via the femoral and the forearm vein (**Figure 15-8AB**). In 20 patients, hyperemic mean transit time and index of microcirculatory resistance were also measured. After bolus IC adenosine FFR (mean) was 0.81 ± 0.10; after femoral vein infusion (FFR, 0.80 ± 0.10); after forearm vein infusion of adenosine (FFR, 0.80 ± 0.11; p for noninferiority = 0.01). There was no difference in the number of functionally significant stenoses (FFR, <0.75; femoral vein vs. forearm vein, 17 (25.0%) vs. 17 (25.0%); p = 1.0) nor values of hyperemic mean transit time and index of microcirculatory resistance. This study suggests that continuous intravenous infusion of adenosine via the forearm vein is a convenient and effective way to induce steady-state hyperemia for FFR and other physiologic measurements.

Regadenoson

Adenosine activates several adenosine receptor subtypes, which may result in undesirable effects including nausea, flushing, shortness of breath, chest pain, and atrioventricular block.

To reduce the incidence of side effects without affecting hyperemia, selective adenosine A_{2A} receptor agonist agents

TABLE 15-3 Pharmacological Hyperemic Agents for FFR Measurements

	ADENOSINE	ADENOSINE	REGADENOSON	NTP	PAPAVERINE
Route	IV	IC	IV	IC	IC
Dosage	140 mcg/kg/min	60-100 mcg LCA 20-30 mcg RCA	0.4 mg	50-100 mcg	15 mg LCA 10 mg RCA
Half-life	1-2 min	30-60 sec	2-4 min (up to 30 min)	1-2 min	2 min
Time to max hyperemia	<1-2 min	5-10 sec	1-4 min	10-20 sec	20-60 sec
Advantage	Gold standard	Short action	IV bolus	Short action	Short action
Disadvantage	↓ BP, chest burning	AV Block, ↓ BP	↑ HR, long action, ?redose	↓ BP	Torsades, ↓ BP

AV, Atrioventricular; *BP,* blood pressure; *FFR,* fractional flow reserve; *HR,* heart rate; *IC,* intracoronary; *IV,* intravenous; *LCA,* left coronary artery; *RCA,* right coronary artery.

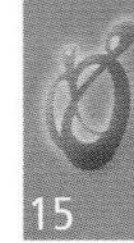

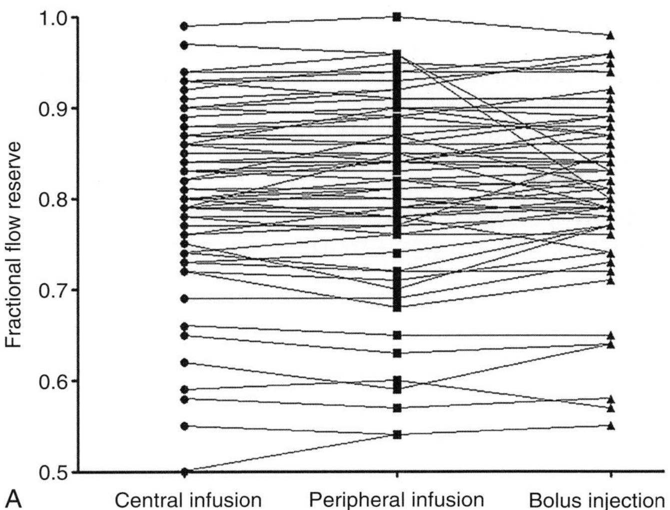

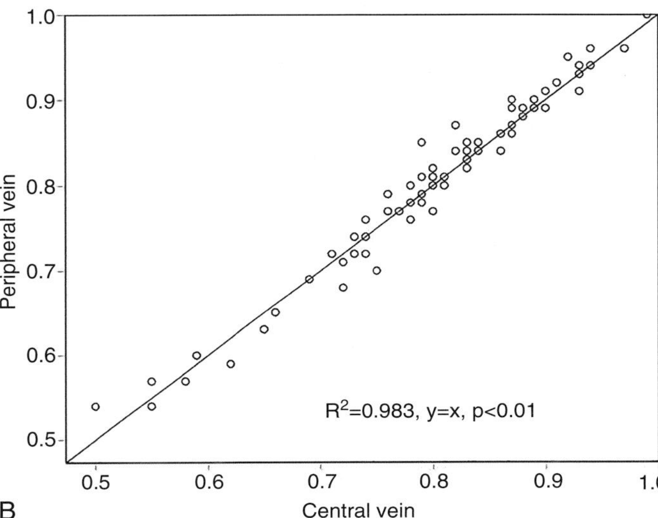

FIGURE 15-8 **A,** Individual values of fractional flow reserve with three different methods of adenosine administration. **B,** Correlation of fractional flow reserve between central and peripheral adenosine administration. *(From Seo MK, Koo BK, Kim JH, et al: Comparison of hyperemic efficacy between central and peripheral venous adenosine infusion for fractional flow reserve measurement. Circ Cardiovasc Interv 5(3):401–405, 2012.)*

such as regadenoson have been developed. Regadenoson is a low-affinity A_{2A} adenosine receptor agonist that induces coronary vasodilatation and increased myocardial blood flow in a manner reportedly equivalent to adenosine. By selectively targeting the A_{2A} receptor in coronary arteries, it has fewer adverse effects compared with adenosine. Regadenoson has a longer half-life of 2-3 minutes in the initial phase, 30 minutes in the intermediate phase, and 2 hours in the terminal phase and may prove to be easier to use than short-acting adenosine. With a single infusion bolus of regadenoson, coronary hyperemia may be achieved and maintained equivalent to that achieved with a constant infusion of adenosine. Because of these properties, regadenoson may be a promising coronary vasodilator for the measurement of FFR.[14,15]

Alternative Hyperemic Agents

Other agents that produce maximal coronary hyperemia include ATP, nitroprusside, and dobutamine. Coronary flow reserve was equivalent with ATP and papaverine[10] with IC ATP doses >15 µg. IV dobutamine (10 to 40 µg/kg per minute) has also been used to assess lesion severity with FFR. Compared with IV adenosine, peak dobutamine infusion produced similar distal coronary pressure and pressure ratios (Pd/Pa 60 ± 18 vs. 59 ± 18 mm Hg; FFR, 0.68 ± 0.18 and 0.68 ± 0.17, respectively; all p = NS). High-dose IV dobutamine did not modify the angiographic area of the epicardial stenosis, and much like adenosine, fully exhausted myocardial resistance regardless of inducible left ventricular dysfunction. Intracoronary nitroprusside (50, 100 mcg bolus) produces nearly identical results to IV and IC adenosine.[16]

The influence of caffeine (an adenosine receptor antagonist) on FFR remains controversial as it is unknown whether the concentration of caffeine after a cup of coffee prior to induction of hyperemia interferes with FFR measurement. A review of the literature[17] suggests that a serum caffeine level of 3 to 4 mg/L at the time of an adenosine-hyperemia study does not affect the diagnostic ability of myocardial perfusion imaging to detect coronary artery disease. While this likely holds true for patients undergoing intravenous adenosine-induced hyperemia, if there is any concern the operator can increase the adenosine dose administered to overcome any receptor inhibition.

TABLE 15-4 Factors Confounding the Interpretation of Fractional Flow Reserve

1. Equipment factors:
   - Erroneous zero
   - Incomplete pressure transmission (tubing/connector leaks)
   - Faulty electric wire connection
   - Pressure signal drift
   - Hemodynamic recorder miscalibration
2. Procedural factors
   - Guide catheter damping
   - Incorrect placement pressure sensor
   - Inadequate hyperemia
3. Physiological factors
   - Serial lesion
   - Reduced myocardial bed
   - Acute myocardial infarction

Theoretical conditions that might influence FFR
   - Severe left ventricular hypertrophy
   - Exuberant collateral supply
   - Adenosine insensitivity

Modified from Koolen JJ, Pijls NHJ: Coronary pressure never lies. Cathet Cardiovasc Intervent 72:248–256, 2008.
FFR, Fractional flow reserve.

PRECAUTIONS AND PITFALLS OF FRACTIONAL FLOW RESERVE

Consideration should be given to several possible reasons for a nonischemic FFR (>0.80) measurement despite apparently severe stenosis. Errors in the performance of FFR include hemodynamic artifacts and failure to induce maximal hyperemia.[18] **Table 15-4** lists factors that may lead to inaccurate FFR measurements.

Catheters with sideholes should not be used to measure FFR, as proximal pressure gradients may occur, complicating distal gradient evaluations. Moreover, sideholes may cause insufficient IC adenosine administration down the vessel. Larger guide catheters can partially occlude the coronary ostium as hyperemia is induced, impairing maximal flow.

Removing the guide catheter from the coronary ostium after giving the hyperemic agent will avoid this pitfall.

SAFETY OF INTRACORONARY SENSOR WIRE MEASUREMENTS

Qian et al.[19] examined the safety of intracoronary Doppler wire measurements in 906 patients. Severe transient bradycardia after intracoronary adenosine occurred in 14 patients undergoing RCA FFR and only one having LCA FFR (1.5%). Coronary spasm occurred in nine patients during passage of the Doppler guidewire. Ventricular fibrillation during the procedure occurred in two patients with asystole in one patient. Hypotension with bradycardia and ventricular asystole occurred in one patient. All complications could be managed medically. These data support the safety of using sensor wire measurements.

Validation and Threshold of Ischemia

FFR values <0.75 are associated with ischemic stress testing results in numerous comparative studies with high sensitivity (88%), specificity (100%), positive predicted value (100%), and overall accuracy (93%). FFR values >0.80 are associated with negative ischemic results with a predictive accuracy of 95%. Single stress testing comparisons with variations in testing methods and patient cohorts have produced a zone of FFR with overlapping positive and negative results (0.75-0.80). The interpretation of FFR values in this range requires clinical judgment. A metaanalysis of 31 studies[20] comparing the results of FFR to quantitative coronary angiography (QCA) and/or noninvasive imaging of the same lesions found QCA had a sensitivity of 78% and specificity of 51% against FFR (<0.75 cutoff). The receiver-operator characteristic estimates were similar for FFR compared with perfusion scintigraphy (sensitivity 75%, specificity 77%) and dobutamine stress echocardiography (sensitivity 82%, specificity 74%). Considering the limited accuracy and reproducibility of noninvasive tests in general, it is not surprising that this metaanalysis showed only modest concordance of FFR with noninvasive imaging tests. In contrast, the initial validation study[4] comparing FFR to a panel of three different stress tests in the same patients both before and after PCI remains the most rigorous study of an ischemic diagnostic test. Furthermore, because perfusion scintigraphy compares relative and not absolute myocardial flow in different coronary beds, scintigraphy has difficulty identifying the hemodynamic significance of individual lesions in patients with multivessel CAD.[21,22] Similarly, on stress echocardiography, severe ischemia in one region may mask the consequences of a less severe albeit hemodynamically significant lesion in another region. In contrast to noninvasive tests, FFR is a vessel- and lesion-specific index of ischemia.

USE OF FRACTIONAL FLOW RESERVE FOR SPECIFIC ANGIOGRAPHIC SUBSETS

The Intermediate Coronary Lesion

In the absence of prior objective evidence of ischemia, the operator faced with an intermediately severe angiographic stenosis (30%-70% narrowing) in the cath lab must deal with the uncertainty regarding the presence or absence of ischemia. Rather than presuming ischemia from imperfect angiographic views, or performing stress testing following angiography, FFR enables the operator to immediately treat or not treat coronary lesions based on ischemia. Several large studies have rendered favorable outcomes with the implementation of FFR as a guide to treat or not treat such lesions.[23-25] Ischemia test results and FFR have been compared extensively in single and multicenter trials (**Table 15-5**).

The deferral of percutaneous coronary intervention (DEFER) study[26] demonstrated that PCI can be safely deferred in patients with FFR-normal intermediate disease based on 5-year outcomes. The study randomized 325 patients scheduled for PCI into three groups: a deferral group (n = 91) with an FFR ≥0.75 and medical therapy was continued; or despite an FFR ≥0.75, the PCI performance group (n = 90), in which the lesions were treated with stents. The third group was the reference group (n = 144) who had an FFR <0.75 and stents were placed as planned. For the deferred and performed groups, the event-free survival was the same (80% and 73%, respectively, p = 0.52), and both were significantly better than in the reference group (63%, p = 0.03). The composite rate of cardiac death and acute myocardial infarction in the deferred, performed, and reference groups was 3%, 8%, and 16%, respectively (p = 0.21 for deferred vs. performed and p = 0.003 for reference vs. both of the deferred and performed groups) (**Figure 15-9**). The percentage of patients free from angina on follow-up was not different between the deferred and performed groups. The five-year risk of cardiac death or myocardial infarction in patients with a normal FFR was <1% per year and not

TABLE 15-5 Studies with FFR to Assess Intermediate Left Main Coronary Stenoses and Correlation with Stress Testing

AUTHOR	REF.	PATIENTS	NO.	TEST	THRESHOLD
De Bruyne	Circ 1995	1-VD	60	Bic ECG	0.72
Pijls	Circ 1995	1-VD (PCI)	60	Bic ECG	0.74
Pijls	NEJM 1996	1-VD	45	Bic ECG; Thallium; Dob ECHO	0.75
Bartunek	JACC 1996	1-VD	75	Dob ECHO	0.78
Chalmuleau	JACC 2000	MVD	127	MIBI	0.74
Abe	Circ 2000	1-VD	46	Thallium	0.75
De Bruyne	Circ 2001	Post MI	57	MIBI	0.75-0.80

From Lokhandwala J, Hodgson J: Assessing intermediate left main lesions with IVUS or FFR: how intravascular ultrasound and fractional flow reserve can be used in this challenging subset. Cardiac Interventions 2009.

Bic, Bicycle; *Dob ECHO,* dobutamine echo stress test; *FFR,* fractional flow reserve; *MI,* myocardial infarction; *MIBI,* radionuclide myocardial perfussion stress test; *PCI,* percutaneous coronary intervention; *VD,* vessel disease.

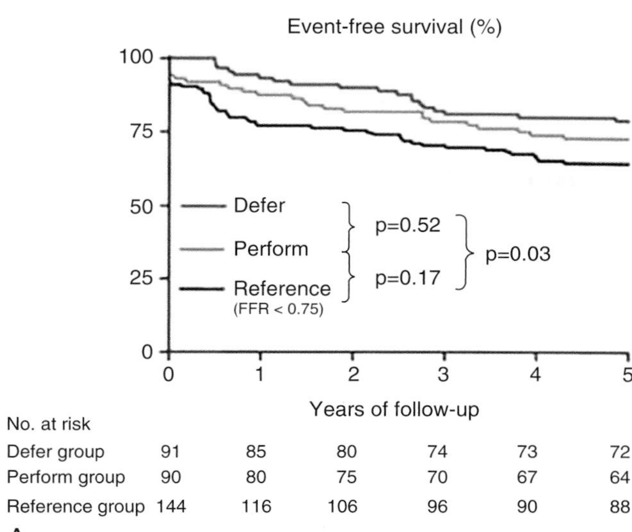

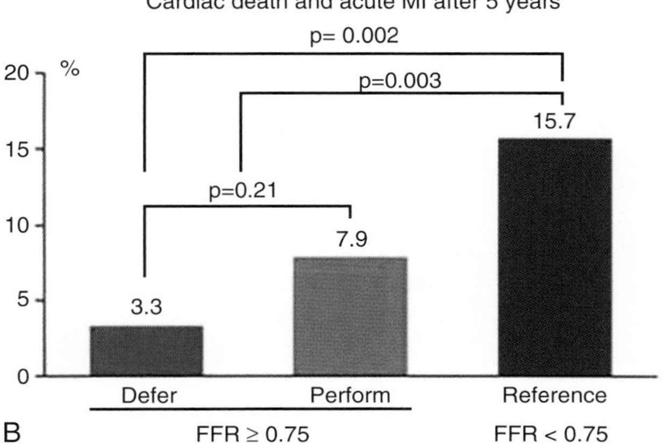

FIGURE 15-9 The DEFER study results. **A,** Kaplan-Meier survival curves from adverse cardiac events at 5-year follow-up. **B,** Cardiac death and acute myocardial infarction rate at 5-year follow-up. *FRR,* Fractional flow reserve; *MI,* myocardial infarction. *(Modified from Pijls NH, van Schaardenburgh P, Manoharan G, et al: Percutaneous coronary intervention of functionally non-significant stenoses: 5-year follow-up of the DEFER study. J Am Coll Cardiol 49(21):2105–2111, 2007.)*

decreased by stenting. Treating patients with intermediate lesions assisted by FFR is associated with a low event rate, comparable to event rates in patients with normal noninvasive testing. Similar outcomes for deferral of lesions with FFR >0.80 were also reported in patients in the FFR versus Angiography for Multivessel Evaluation (FAME) trial described below. **Table 15-6** presents patient outcomes after deferral of coronary intervention in intermediate coronary lesions.

Fractional Flow Reserve in Multivessel Disease

The FAME (FFR vs. Angiography for Multivessel Evaluation) trial by Tonino et al.[33] compared a physiologically guided PCI approach (FFR-PCI) to a conventional angiographic-guided PCI (Angio-PCI) in patients with multivessel CAD. One thousand five patients with multivessel CAD undergoing PCI with drug-eluting stents were enrolled. Operators identified all lesions by visual angiographic appearance (>50% diameter stenosis) to be treated in advance of randomization to a stenting strategy. For the FFR-PCI group (n = 496), all lesions had FFR measurements and only those with FFR <0.80 were stented. For the Angio-PCI group (n = 509), all lesions identified were stented. Clinical characteristics and angiographic findings were similar in both groups with average SYNTAX scores of 14.5 (indicating low to intermediate-risk patients).

Compared with the Angio-PCI group, the FFR-PCI group used fewer stents per patient (1.9 ± 1.3 vs. 2.7 ± 1.2; p < 0.001), less contrast (272 mL vs. 302 mL; p < 0.001), and had a lower procedure cost ($5332 vs. $6007, p < 0.001) and shorter hospital stay (3.4 vs. 3.7 days, p = 0.05). More importantly, the 2-year rates of mortality or myocardial infarction were 13% in the Angio-PCI group compared with 8% in the FFR-PCI group (p = 0.02) (**Figure 15-10**). Composite rates of death, nonfatal myocardial infarction, or revascularization were 22% and 18%, respectively (p = 0.08). For lesions deferred on the basis of FFR >0.80, the rate of myocardial infarction was only 0.2% and the rate of revascularization was 3.2% after 2 years.[34] A cost-effectiveness evaluation showed that FFR-guided PCI not

TABLE 15-6 Outcomes After Deferral of Coronary Intervention in Intermediate Coronary Lesions

INDEX	REFERENCE	REF	N	DEFERRAL RALVALUE	MACE	FOLLOW-UP (MO)
FFR	Bech	98	100	0.75	8%	18
	Bech	27	150	0.75	8%	24
	Hernandez Garcia	99	43	0.75	12%	11
	Bech	28	24	0.75	21%	29
	Rieber	29	47	0.75	13%	12
	Chamuleau	30	92	0.75	9%	12
	Rieber	31	24	0.75	8%	12
	Lessar†	100	34	0.75	9%	12
CFR	Kern	101	88	2.0	7%	9
	Ferrari	102	22	2.0	9%	15
	Chamuleau*	32	143	2.0	6%	12

Modified with permission from Kern MJ: Coronary physiology revisited: practical insights from the cardiac catheterization laboratory. Circulation 101:1344–1351, 2000. **http://content.onlinejacc.org/article.aspx?articleid=1140344**.

CFR, Coronary flow velocity reserve; *FFR,* fractional flow reserve; *MACE,* major adverse cardiac events principally rates of PCI, no significant rates of death/MI; *N,* number; *PCI,* percutaneous coronary intervention.

*Multivessel disease.

†Unstable angina pectoris.

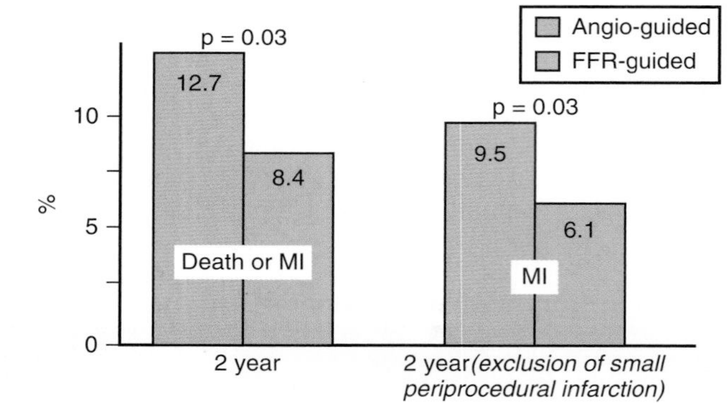

FIGURE 15-10 The FAME study results. Kaplan-Meier survival curves according to study group for 2-year outcomes. **A,** Major adverse cardiac events (MACE). **B,** Death. **C,** Death or myocardial infarction. **D,** Revascularization. **E,** FAME study: Death and MI after 2 years. *FFR,* Fractional flow reserve; *MACE,* major adverse cardiac events; *MI,* myocardial infarction; *PCI,* percutaneous coronary intervention. *(**A-D,** From Tonino PAL, et al: Fractional flow reserve versus angiography for guiding percutaneous coronary intervention. N Engl J Med 360:213–224, 2009. **E,** Data from Tonino PAL, et al: Fractional flow reserve versus angiography for guiding percutaneous coronary intervention. N Engl J Med 360:213–224, 2009; and Tonino PAL, et al: Fractional flow reserve versus angiography in multivessel evaluation. JACC, Vol. 55, 2010.)*

only improved outcomes in FAME, but did so at a significantly lower cost.[35]

In the subsequent FAME 2 trial,[36] the investigators identified 1220 patients with stable CAD who were scheduled for one-, two-, or three-vessel PCI. After FFR was performed, those with at least one stenosis with FFR $\leq$0.80 (n = 888) were enrolled in the randomized trial and those with stenoses with FFR >0.80 in all measured vessels were enrolled in a registry (n = 332). Patients enrolled in the trial were randomized to either optimal medical therapy or FFR-guided PCI plus optimal medical therapy. The primary endpoint was defined as death, myocardial infarction, or urgent revascularization at 2 years. However, the trial was stopped early because a highly significant difference was seen in this endpoint. At 12 months, those undergoing FFR-guided PCI and optimal medical therapy fared better than those with medical therapy alone (HR 0.32; CI, 0.19 to 0.53; $p < 0.001$). FFR-guided PCI also demonstrated a statistically significant relief in angina compared with medical therapy alone (**Figure 15-11**).

FAME 2 demonstrated that optimal medical therapy in addition to FFR-guided PCI in patients with stable coronary artery disease results in improved outcomes when compared with optimal medical therapy alone. Subsequently, the authors demonstrated that FFR-guided PCI is a cost-effective alternative to optimal medical management for stable angina.[35]

See Video 15-1 for a case example of a patient with 3V CAD and use of FFR.

Fractional Flow Reserve After Percutaneous Coronary Intervention

FFR after bare-metal stenting (BMS)[37,38] has been shown to predict adverse cardiac events at follow-up. Pijls et al. examined 750 patients with angiographically satisfactory PCI using postprocedural FFR. At 6 months, 76 patients (10%) suffered an adverse event. FFR immediately after stenting was the most significant independent variable related to all types of events. In 36% of patients, FFR normalized (>0.95) and patients had an event rate of only 5%. In 32% of patients with post-procedure FFR between 0.90 and 0.95, the event rate was 6%. In the remaining 32% with FFR <0.90, the event rate was 20%, and in those with FFR <0.80 the rate was 30%. Outcomes with FFR after drug-eluting stenting have not yet been reported.

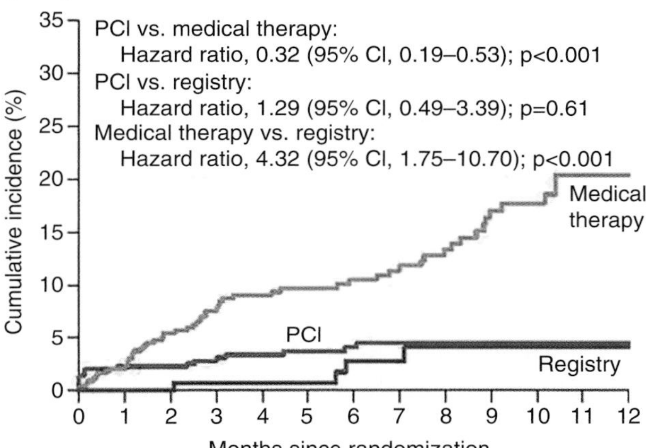

No. at risk													
Medical therapy	441	414	370	322	283	253	220	192	162	127	100	70	37
PCI	447	414	388	351	308	277	243	212	175	155	117	92	53
Registry	166	156	145	133	117	106	93	74	64	52	41	25	13

FIGURE 15-11 The FAME 2 study results. Kaplan-Meier curve for primary endpoint of death, myocardial infarction, or urgent revascularization at 12 months in the group assigned to PCI and optimal medical therapy vs. optimal medical therapy alone versus those who did not undergo revascularization. *PCI,* Percutaneous coronary intervention. *(Modified from De Bruyne B, Pijls NH, Kalesan B, et al: Fractional flow reserve-guided PCI versus medical therapy in stable coronary disease. N Engl J Med 367(11):991–1001, 2012.)*

Left Main Stenosis

Accurate assessment of the hemodynamic significance of left main (LM) coronary lesions is of critical importance when patients face possible CABG surgery. Because of the inherent limitations discussed above, angiography alone may not be reliable in intermediate LM stenoses, and FFR is useful for decision making.[39,40]

Numerous studies of FFR support its use in equivocal LM disease (**Table 15-7**). Most recently, Hamilos et al.[40] examined FFR and 5-year outcome in 213 patients with an angiographically equivocal LM coronary artery stenosis in a large multicenter prospective trial. When FFR was ≥0.80, patients were treated medically or another stenosis was treated by coronary angioplasty (nonsurgical group; n = 138). When FFR was <0.80, CABG surgery was performed (surgical group; n = 75). The 5-year survival estimates were 90% in the nonsurgical (FFR ≥0.80) group and 85% in the surgical (FFR <0.80) group (p = 0.48). The 5-year event-free survival estimates were 74% and 82% in the two groups, respectively (p = 0.50) (**Figure 15-12**). Of note, only 23% of patients with a diameter stenosis >50% had a hemodynamically significant LM by FFR.

See Video 15-2 for case example of a patient with left main stenosis assessed with FFR.

Complex Left Main Lesion Assessment (LM Plus Downstream Lesions) with Fractional Flow Reserve

One principal requirement of obtaining an accurate FFR is ensuring that maximal hyperemia is achieved across the target lesion. In the case of serial lesions (or LM plus downstream disease acting as serial lesions), each lesion blunts the maximal hyperemia of the other and thus neither can be relied on to produce an accurate FFR (unless we employ a coronary balloon catheter and use the occlusion wedge pressure and perform a complicated calculation; see later). In clinical practice, we measure the summed epicardial FFR

TABLE 15-7 Studies with FFR to Assess Intermediate Left Main Coronary Stenoses

			Medical Therapy			*Surgical Therapy*			
STUDY	**FFR THRESHOLD**	**N**	**N (%)**	**MACE**	**DEATH**	**N (%)**	**MACE**	**DEATH**	**FOLLOW-UP TIME (MO)**
Hamilos (2009)	0.8	213	136 (65%)	26%	9 (6.5%)	73 (35%)	17%	7 (9.6%)	35/25
Courtis (2009)	0.75 surg 0.8 med	142	82 (58%)	13%	3 (3.6%)	60 (42%)	7%	3 (5%)	14/11
Lindstraedt (2006)	0.75 surg 0.8 med	51	24 (47%)	31%	0	27 (53%)	34%	5 (19%)	29/16
Suemaru (2005)	0.75	15	8 (53%)	0	0	7 (47%)	29%	0	33/10
Legutko (2005)	0.75	38	20 (53%)	10%	0	18 (46%)	11%	2	24 mean
Jimenez-Navaro	0.75	27	20 (74%)	10%	0	7 (26%)	29%	2	12/12
Bech (2001)	0.75	54	24 (44%)	24%	0	30 (56%)	17%	1	29/15

Modified from Lokhandwala J, Hodgson J: Assessing intermediate left main lesions with IVUS or FFR: how intravascular ultrasound and fractional flow reserve can be used in this challenging subset. Cardiac Interventions, 2009.

FFR, Fractional flow reserve; *MACE,* major adverse cardiac events principally rates of PCI, no significant rates of death/MI; *N,* number; *PCI,* percutaneous coronary intervention.

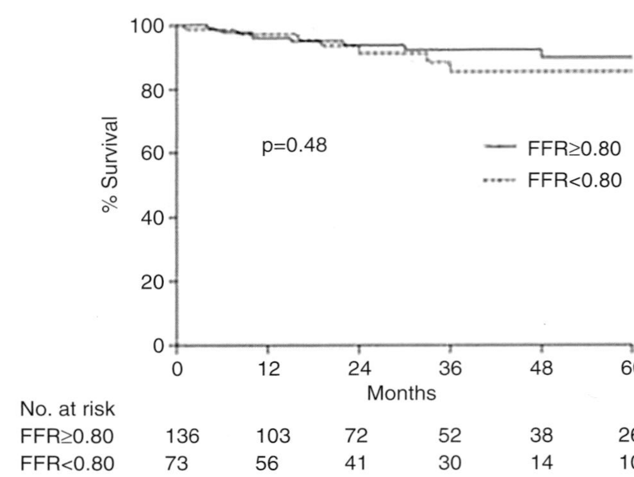

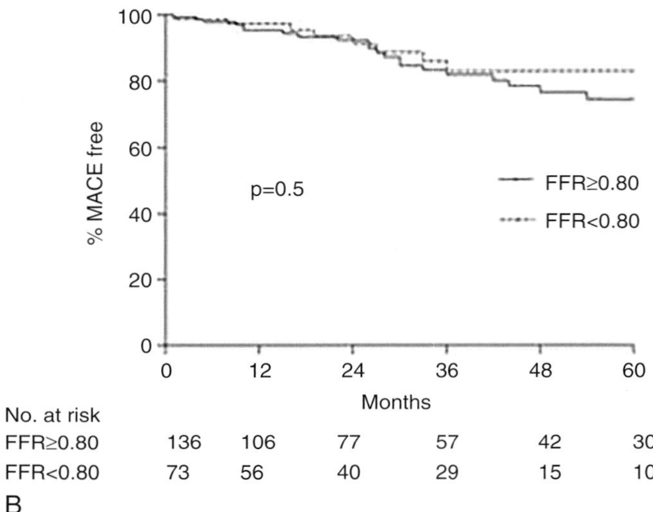

FIGURE 15-12 The left main fractional flow reserve (LM FFR) 5-year outcome study. **A,** Total survival and **(B)** Major adverse cardiac event-free survival by Kaplan-Meier mortality curves in the two study groups. The 5-year event-free survival estimates were 74% and 82% in the two groups, respectively (p = 0.50). *FFR,* Fractional flow reserve; *MACE,* major adverse cardiac events. *(From Hamilos M, Muller O, Cuisset T, et al: Long-term clinical outcome after fractional flow reserve–guided treatment in patients with angiographically equivocal left main coronary artery stenosis. Circulation 120:1505–1512, 2009.)*

across both lesions. If positive, we then record a pressure pullback during hyperemia, noting the largest pressure gradient (ΔP) as we pull back across each lesion individually. We then treat the largest gradient and repeat what now is a single lesion FFR. For the LM with downstream LAD/CFX disease, this combination of lesions potentially acts as lesions in series and so the FFR of the LM must be assessed in this manner.

Committing to PCI of a downstream lesion solely to measure the FFR of the LM may not be an option, however, as the patient may be best treated with CABG. Fortunately, the presence of concurrent downstream LAD lesion with an LM stenosis may or may not affect the FFR of the LM.[41] To illustrate the influence of a downstream LAD lesion, **Figure 15-13** depicts changes in the myocardial bed for the LM which is the summed territories of both the LAD and circumflex (CFX) arteries. The LM bed can be even larger if the RCA is occluded and collaterals supplied from the left coronary system. **Figure 15-13** illustrates various scenarios in which the FFR of the LM may be influenced by remote branch disease. Yong et al.[41] examined the effect of downstream LAD disease in six sheep. Balloon catheters were used to create variable stenoses in the LM and then in the LAD. Pressure guidewires were positioned in the LAD and LCX arteries so that the investigators were able to measure the difference between the true FFR in the LM alone (FFR_{true}) and the apparent (FFR_{app}) with an LAD stenosis. With increasing LAD occlusion severity, FFR was reduced by >0.02 to 0.03 units only when the epicardial (summed LM plus LAD) FFR was <0.50, meaning that for all practical purposes only a severe and proximal LAD stenosis is likely to influence the true LM FFR (**Figure 15-14**).

Fractional Flow Reserve and Small-Vessel Disease

Myocardial bed size contributes to the visual-functional mismatch of coronary stenoses as discussed previously. Small coronary vessels generally supply small myocardial territories and thus may have limited ischemic potential relative to their angiographic stenosis severity. FFR may thus be particularly helpful in small vessels. Puymirat et al.[42] assessed the clinical outcome of FFR-guided PCI in the treatment of small coronary vessel lesions as compared with an angio-guided PCI in a manner similar to the FAME trial. 717 patients were enrolled (495 angio-guided, 222 FFR-guided) from January 2004 to December 2008, and treated with PCI for stable or unstable angina in coronary vessels with reference diameters and stent sizes of <3 mm. Retrospective analyses of endpoints (death, nonfatal myocardial infarction (MI), combined death or nonfatal MI, target vessel revascularization (TVR), and procedure costs and major adverse cardiac events (MACE), defined as death, nonfatal MI, and TVR) were collected over 3.3 years (from 0.01-5 years). Using a propensity score-adjusted Cox analysis, patients treated with FFR-guided PCI had significantly lower rates of death or nonfatal MI (hazard ratio (HR), 0.413; $p = 0.004$), nonfatal MI (HR, 0.063; $p = 0.007$), TVR (HR, 0.517; $p = 0.006$), and MACE (HR, 0.458; $p < 0.001$). No difference was observed in mortality alone. Procedure costs were also reduced in the FFR-guided strategy (3253 ± 102 euros vs. 4714 ± 37 euros; $p < 0.0001$). These findings support the fact that FFR-guided PCI of small coronary arteries is safe and results in better clinical outcomes when compared with an angio-guided PCI.

Serial (Multiple) Lesions in a Single Vessel

As noted above, in order to obtain an accurate FFR, one must produce maximal (hyperemic) trans-stenotic flow. When there are two (or more) consecutive or serial stenoses, the first stenosis limits maximal flow across the downstream lesions, while all downstream stenoses limit the maximal flow across the more proximal lesion. Thus the interaction between the stenoses prevents us from using the simple FFR ratio (P_d/P_a) for each stenosis individually. Put another way, when there is more than one significant lesion in the same epicardial vessel, each lesion blunts maximal flow (i.e., produces submaximal flow) and therefore results in an inaccurate individual lesion FFR. The extent to which both stenoses influence each other is somewhat unpredictable. However, the simple FFR can assess the *summed* result of any group of stenoses.

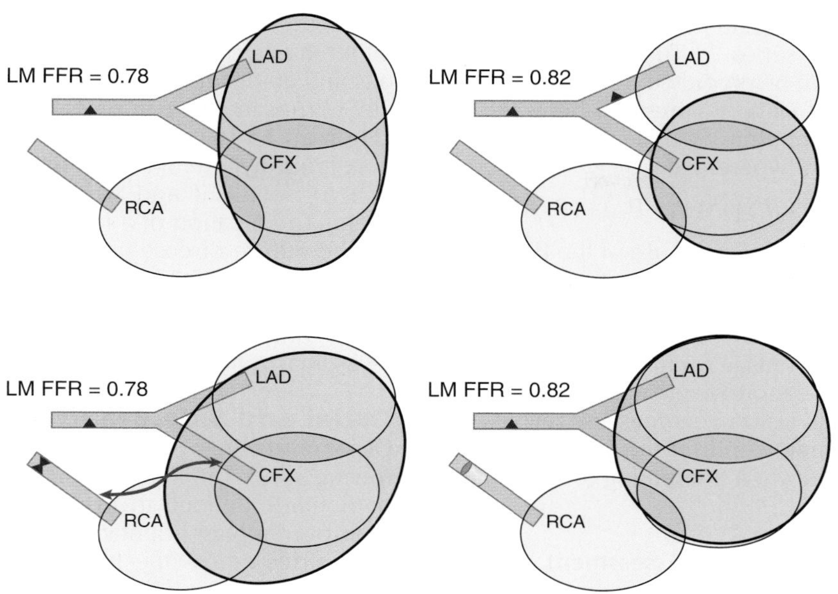

FIGURE 15-13 Diagram of hypothetical LM FFR and the potential change that might occur when the myocardial bed (yellow overlaid regions) is made smaller (right panels). Isolated LM narrowing, no LAD, CFX, RCA stenoses **(A).** For illustration the FFR is assigned 0.78. The FFR reflects the physiologic significance of just the LM narrowing. LM narrowing plus LAD stenosis **(B).** LM FFR rises to 0.82 because LM bed is decreased due to the LAD stenosis. The same scenario would apply when adding LCX narrowing. The LM FFR alone cannot be accurately measured when the myocardial bed flow is compromised. If the LAD and CFX are hemodynamically insignificant, the LM FFR will be accurate. LM narrowing plus totally occluded RCA with collaterals from LCA, no LAD/LCX disease **(C).** The LM FFR is again assigned 0.78. After RCA opening with resolution of collateral flow, LM FFR increases to 0.84 since LM myocardial bed size is reduced **(D)**. *CFX,* Circumflex artery; *FFR,* fractional flow reserve; *LAD,* left anterior descending artery; *LM FFR,* left main fractional flow; *RCA,* right coronary artery.

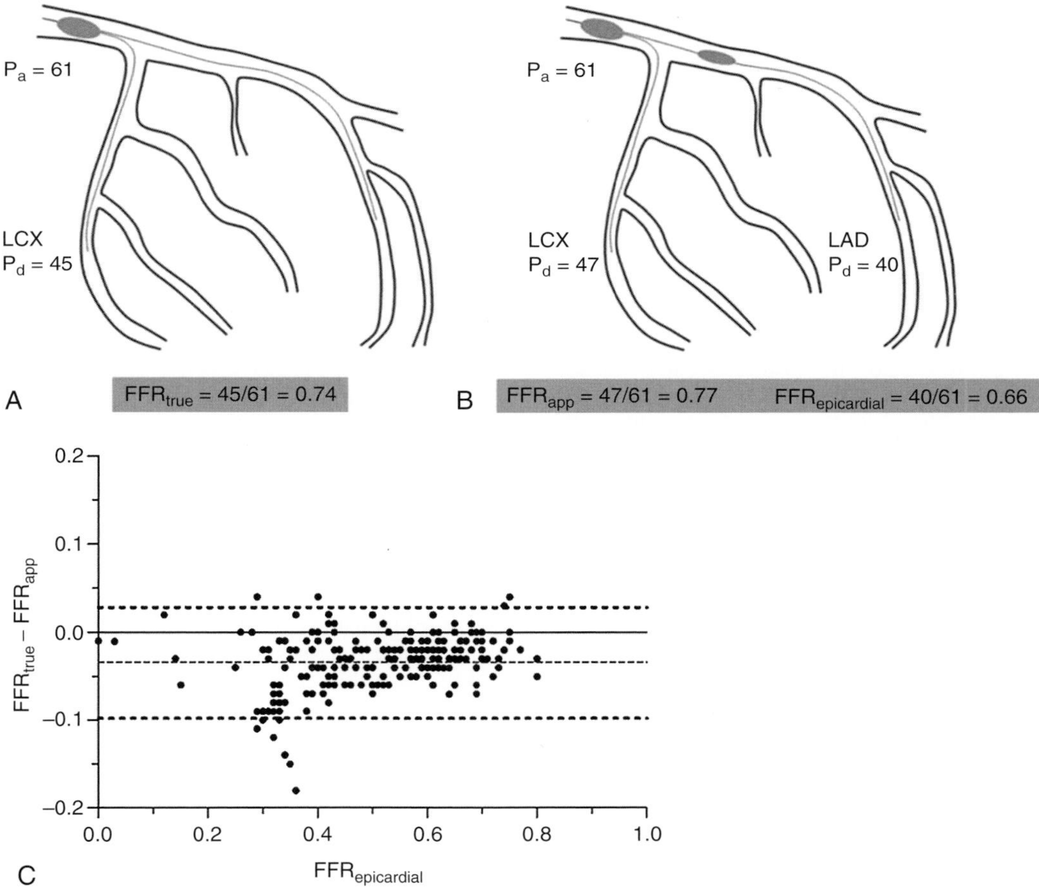

FIGURE 15-14 Animal model of LM +/– LAD stenosis. Example of physiological measurements. Schematic example of physiological measurements. **A,** True fractional flow reserve (FFR_{true}) of the left main coronary artery obtained during left main balloon inflation and no stenosis in the left anterior descending (LAD) artery (FFR_{true} = distal pressure [P_d]) in the left circumflex (LCX) artery divided by proximal arterial pressure (P_a). **B,** FFR_{app} obtained during balloon inflation in the LAD (FFR_{app} = LCX P_d/P_a during downstream balloon inflation). $FFR_{epicardial}$ represents FFR of left main plus LAD ($FFR_{epicardial}$ = LAD P_d/P_a during LAD balloon inflation). **C,** Impact of downstream LAD on left main fractional flow reserve (LM FFR). Plot of difference between true (FFR_{true}) and apparent (FFR_{app}) fractional flow reserve (FFR) versus composite FFR of left main and stenosed downstream vessel ($FFR_{epicardial}$). Dashed and dotted lines indicate bias and 95% confidence interval of the agreement, respectively. *FFR,* Fractional flow reserve; *LAD,* left anterior descending artery; *P_d,* distal pressure; *P_a,* aortic pressure. *(From Yong ASC, Daniels D, De Bruyne B, et al: Fractional flow reserve assessment of left main stenosis in the presence of downstream coronary stenoses. Circ Cardiovasc Interv 6:161–165, 2013.)*

Experimental studies demonstrate how to determine an individual lesion FFR in the series.[34,35] The individual FFR of each stenosis separately can be predicted by a different FFR equation from Pijls et al.[43] using P_a, pressure between the two stenoses (P_m), P_d, and coronary occlusion wedge pressure (P_w) during maximum hyperemia:

$$FFR_{predicted} = (P_d - [(P_m/P_a) * P_w])/((P_a - P_m) + (P_d - P_w))$$

This special calculation requires the use of the P_w during balloon inflation, a highly impractical way to make these measurements. Pijls et al.[43] and DeBruyne[44] demonstrate nicely the effect of increasing the severity of the distal lesion on the serial FFR measurements in an experimental model. As the distal lesion becomes more severe with a larger gradient, the FFR of the proximal lesion becomes less severe (i.e., FFR goes up). This experiment confirms the adverse interaction between serial lesions when attempting to use simple FFR alone.

Practical Technique of Serial Lesion Assessment

Serial lesion assessment involves the following five steps:

1. Pass the pressure wire beyond the last lesion. Measure the FFR (total) across all lesions with IV adenosine in standard fashion. For example, if the FFR = 0.84 then none of the lesions would need treatment and nothing further needs to be done.
2. If the summed FFR in step 1 is <0.80 then perform a pressure pullback during IV adenosine hyperemia.
3. Determine which of the lesions produces the biggest pressure gradient. Do NOT measure separate lesion FFR values; it is the pressure gradient (ΔP) that will be used to decide which lesion to treat first.
4. Stent the lesion with the largest ΔP.
5. After treating the first lesion, reassess the remaining lesion(s) repeating the standard FFR technique. If the FFR is <0.80, then stent the next lesion. (If more than two lesions, and FFR remains abnormal, then stent the lesion with the next largest ΔP). An example of serial lesion assessment and treatment is shown in **Figure 15-15**.

Kim[27] found that FFR-guided revascularization strategy using pullback pressure tracing in serial stenoses was safe and effective. A total of 131 patients (141 vessels and 298 lesions) with multiple intermediate stenoses within the same coronary artery were assessed with pullback pressure tracings. As expected, there was a weak negative correlation between FFR and angiographic percent diameter stenosis ($r = -0.282$; $p < 0.001$). In total, 116 stents were implanted and revascularization was deferred in 61.1% (182 of 298) of lesions. When the vessels with an initial FFR <0.8 were divided into two groups according to FFR after first stenting (FFR ≥0.8 vs. FFR <0.8), there were no differences in baseline angiographic and physiological parameters between the two groups. During the mean follow-up of 501 ± 311 days, there was only one target vessel revascularization due to in-stent restenosis. There were no events related to deferred lesions.

This strategy can reduce unnecessary intervention and maximize the benefit of percutaneous coronary intervention with drug-eluting stents in patients with multiple stenoses within 1 coronary artery.

Diffuse Coronary Disease

Using FFR during continuous pressure wire pullback from a distal to proximal location, the impact of diffuse atherosclerosis can be documented. Diffuse atherosclerosis, rather than a focal narrowing, is characterized by a continuous and gradual pressure recovery during pullback, without any abrupt increase in pressure related to a focal region[28] (**Figure 15-16**). The pressure pullback recording at maximum hyperemia will provide the necessary information to decide if and where stent implantation may be useful. The location of a focal pressure drop superimposed on the diffuse disease can be identified as an appropriate location for treatment. Diffuse CAD can produce an abnormal FFR in the absence of focal epicardial stenoses (**Figure 15-17**) and might be best treated medically or with surgical revascularization.

Ostial and Side Branch Lesions

Ostial narrowings of side branches or newly produced narrowing in side branches within stents ("jailed" branches) are particularly difficult to assess by angiography because of their overlapping orientation relative to the parent branch, stent struts across the branch, and image foreshortening. Koo et al.[29] compared FFR to angiography in 97 "jailed" side branch lesions (vessel size >2.0 mm, percent stenosis >50% by visual estimation) after stent implantation. No lesion with <75% stenosis had FFR < 0.75. Among 73 lesions with ≥75% stenosis, only 20 lesions (27%) were functionally significant. Of 91 patients, side branch intervention was performed in 26/28 patients with FFR < 0.75. In this subgroup, FFR increased to >0.75 despite residual stenosis of 69 ± 10%. At 9 months, functional restenosis was 8% (5/65) with no difference in events compared with 110 side branches treated by angiographic guidance alone (4.6% versus 3.7%, p = 0.7) (**Figure 15-18**). Measurement of FFR for ostial and side branch assessment thus identifies the minority of lesions that are functionally significant, reducing the need for complex, time-consuming, and potentially detrimental side branch interventions.[31,32] A case example is shown in **Figure 15-19**.

Video 15-3 shows a case example of a patient with ostial diagonal branch narrowing post PCI assessed by FFR.

Saphenous Vein Graft Lesions

When assessing a lesion in an SVG, recall that there are three potential sources of coronary blood flow to the myocardium: the epicardial artery, the bypass conduit, and collateral flow. The FFR is the summed responses of three competing flows (and pressures) from (1) the native vessel, (2) the CABG conduit, and (3) the collateral flow induced from long-standing native coronary occlusion.

After CABG surgery, the bypass conduit should act in a similar fashion to the native low-resistance epicardial vessel. However, the assessment of ischemia due to a stenosis in a CABG conduit is complicated by several features that include (1) the potential for competing flow (and pressure) from both the native and conduit vessels; (2) the presence of collaterals from long-standing native coronary occlusion; and (3) the potential for microvascular abnormalities due to ischemic fibrosis and scarring, preexisting or bypass surgery-related myocardial infarction, or chronic low flow ischemia. Despite these complicating features, the theory of FFR applies just as much to a lesion in a saphenous vein graft to the right coronary artery feeding a normal myocardial bed as a lesion in the native right coronary.

When measuring the FFR across an SVG lesion, the pressure sensor is positioned beyond the anastomosis into the

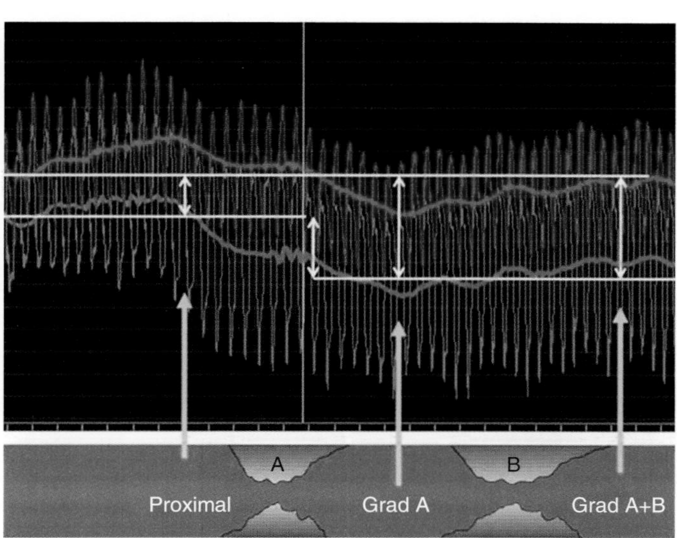

FIGURE 15-15 **A,** Serial (multiple) lesions in a single vessel. When more than one discrete stenosis is present in the same vessel, the hyperemic flow and pressure through the first lesion will be attenuated by the second and vice versa. The fractional flow reserve (FFR) value recorded reflects the value across both lesions. Individual lesion FFR cannot be determined without a coronary occlusion wedge pressure. In practice, identify the lesion with the largest translesional gradient. Proceed with treatment of this lesion and then reassess the remaining lesion with FFR. **B,** Two consecutive intermediate stenoses (labeled 1 and 2 with *arrows*) were observed in the left anterior descending artery. As the fractional flow reserve was 0.48, pullback pressure tracing was performed while simultaneously monitoring the intracoronary pressure *(green line),* aortic pressure *(red line),* and FFR *(yellow line).* Two step-ups of intracoronary pressure were observed during pullback pressure tracing under maximal hyperemia **(C).** Apparent FFR of lesions 1 and 2 were 0.67 (ratio of pressures across lesion 1 = 60/90) and 0.75 (ratio of pressures across lesion 2 = 45/60), respectively. As the larger pressure step-up was observed across lesion 1 (30 mm Hg) than lesion 2 (16 mm Hg), the proximal stenosis was regarded as the primary target lesion and stenting was performed. **D** and **E,** After stenting lesion 1 **(D),** pullback pressure tracings **(E)** were performed again. FFR was 0.59 and intracoronary pressure step-up across lesion 2 was 20 mm Hg. Therefore, stenting to the distal stenosis followed. True FFR of lesion 2 was 0.73 (55/75 mm Hg). **F** and **G,** After stenting both proximal and distal lesions, FFR was 0.85 and no significant pressure step-up was found across lesion 1 or lesion 2. *FFR,* Fractional flow reserve; P_d, distal pressure; P_a, aortic pressure. *(From Kim HL, Koo BK, Nam CW, et al: Comparison of hyperemic efficacy between central and peripheral venous adenosine infusion for fractional flow reserve measurement. J Am Coll Cardiol Intv 5(10):1013–1018, 2012.)*

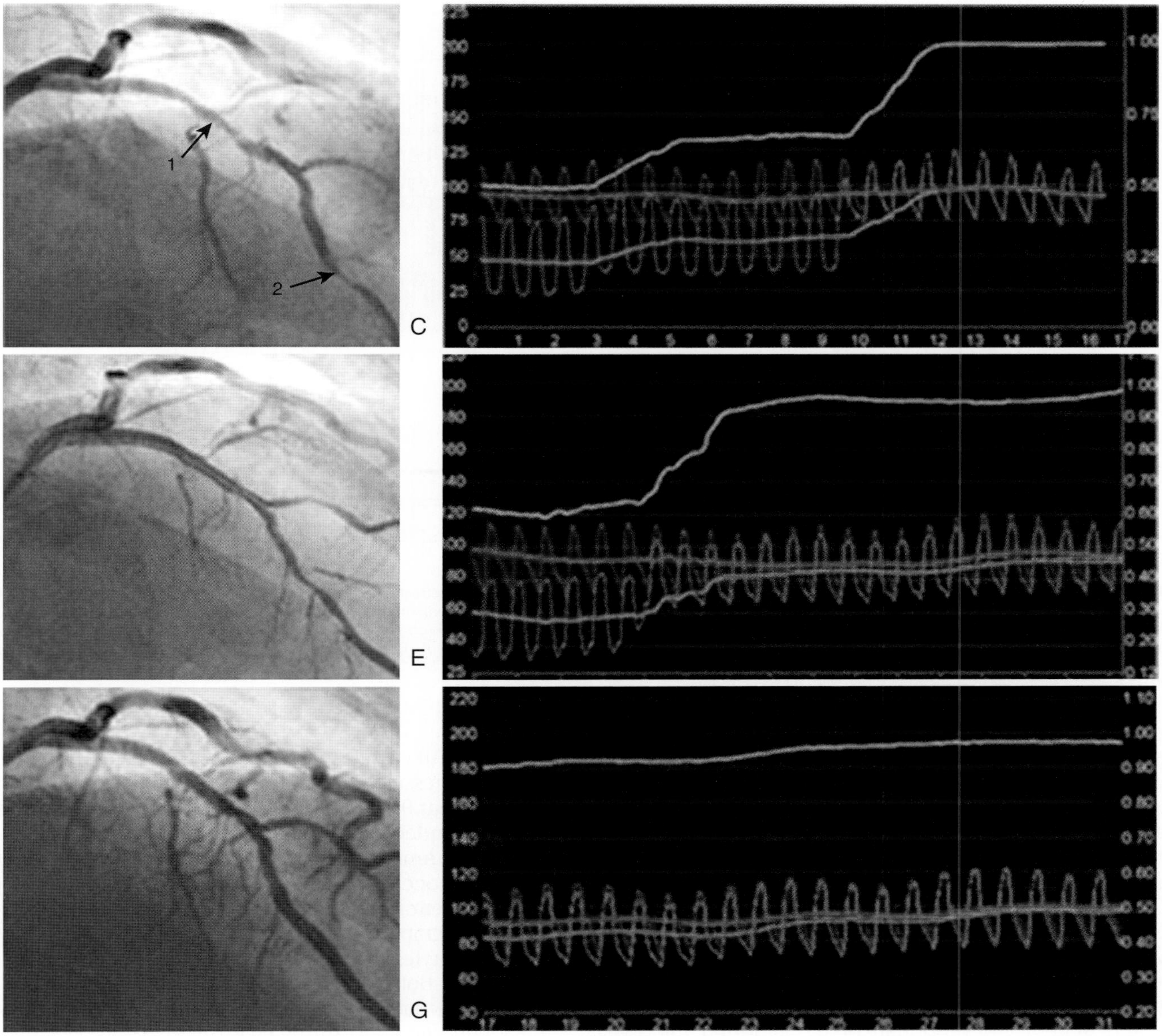

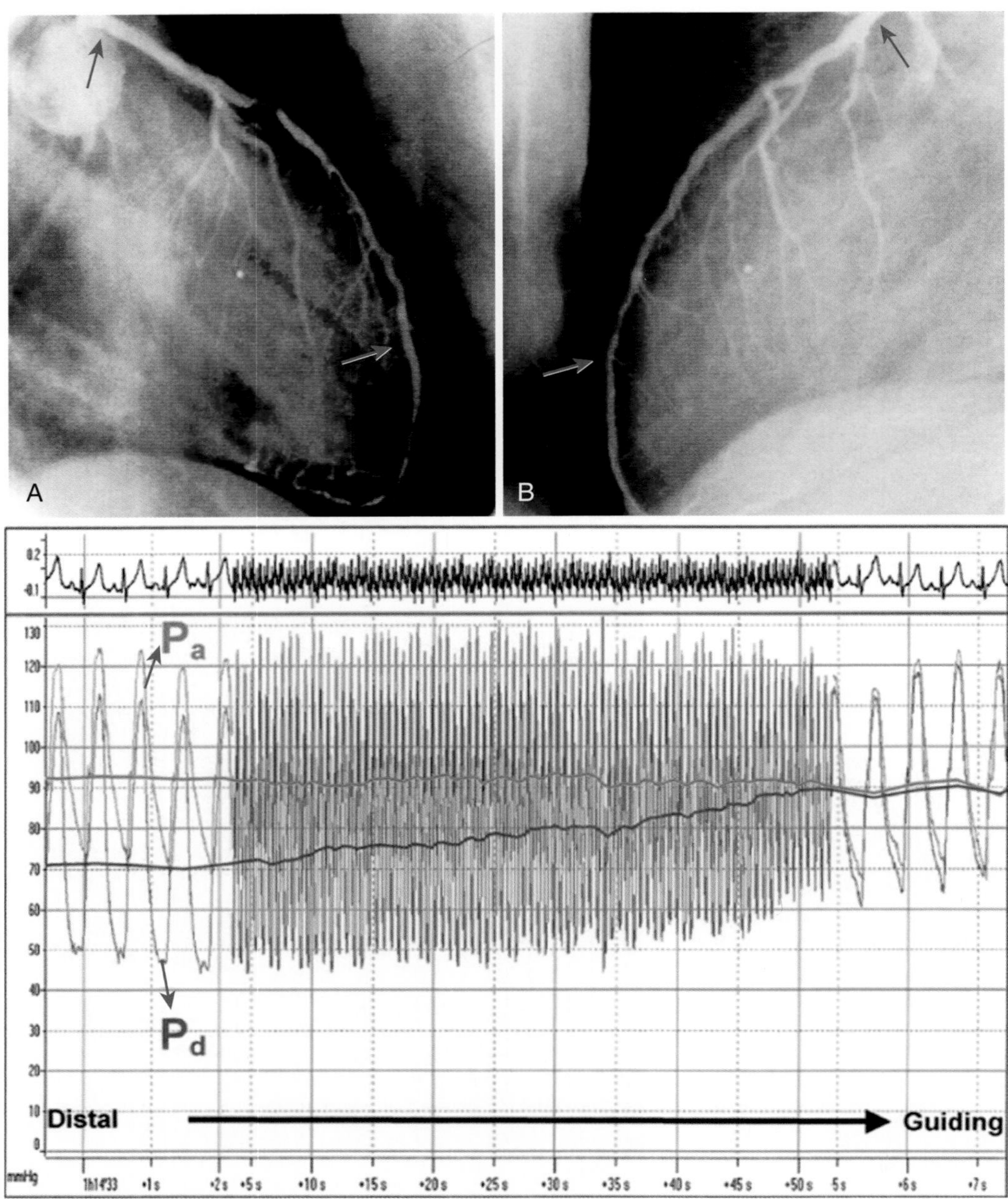

FIGURE 15-16 Fractional flow reserve (FFR) in diffuse disease. The tight stenosis in the mid-LAD was treated by angioplasty. The coronary angiogram of the LAD **(A** and **B)** did not show any focal stenosis, but luminal irregularities suggested diffuse atherosclerosis. Aortic *(red)* and distal coronary pressure *(blue)* recordings **(C)** show an FFR of 0.76. When the sensor is slowly pulled back, a graded, continuous increase in distal coronary pressure is observed, indicating diffuse atherosclerosis, not focal stenosis. The aortic and distal coronary pressure measurements are indicated by the red and blue arrows, respectively. P_d, Distal pressure; P_a, aortic pressure. *(Modified from De Bruyne B, Hersbach F, Pijls NH, et al: Abnormal epicardial coronary resistance in patients with diffuse atherosclerosis but "normal" coronary angiography. Circulation 104(20):2401–2406, 2001. Copyright © American Heart Association, Inc. All rights reserved.)*

native vessel. If the native vessel is occluded then the FFR reflects only the SVG lesion. If there is partial flow through the native vessel then the FFR reflects both the SVG and native vessel lesions. In this case, the SVG and native lesions act like lesions in series and a pressure pullback technique during hyperemia is needed to identify which lesion is producing the most gradient and responsible for the abnormal FFR. IV adenosine should be used when assessing FFR in SVG lesions.

FFR is related to the long-term outcome of SVG patency. Confirming the relevance of the physiologic stenosis severity and graft patency, Botman et al.[45] reported the 1-year follow-up of 164 patients undergoing coronary bypass grafts (n = 450). All vessels grafted had FFR measured beforehand with the pressure sensor angioplasty guidewire in the cath lab. At 1 year, 9% of grafts on functionally significant lesions were occluded while 21% of grafts on functionally nonsignificant lesions were occluded (**Figure 15-20**). A significant graft occlusion rate was observed for grafted vessels that had near normal physiology (FFR >0.80, normal = 1.0). The angiographic percent diameter narrowing displayed a similar but less precise correlation with graft failure. As shown by Botman's findings, competitive flow from nonobstructed native vessels causes early graft failure, which has been known to surgeons for many years. FFR provides objective data on the physiologic impact of intermediately severe stenosis, which has tremendous influence on the outcome of the grafts and the patient's future course.

Fractional Flow Reserve in Acute Coronary Syndrome

In acute coronary syndrome (ACS) settings and especially in acute myocardial infarction (AMI), the pathophysiology of the infarcted artery and its subtended microvascular bed is complex and dynamic. The predictive ability of FFR in ACS has several limitations: (1) The microvascular bed in the infarct zone may not have uniform, constant, or minimal resistance, (2) the severity of stenosis may evolve as thrombus and vasoconstriction abate, and (3) FFR measurements are not meaningful when normal perfusion has not been achieved. Thus, a negative (≥0.80) FFR has limited diagnostic utility in the infarct-related artery during the first 24-48 hours after ACS, while a positive (≤0.80) value still identifies a stenotic lesion. FFR also has demonstrated value in non-culprit remote lesion assessment and in target lesion assessment during the recovery phase of MI[30,46-50] (**Figure 15-21**).

DeBruyne et al.[46] compared single-photon emission computed tomography (SPECT) myocardial perfusion imaging and FFR (obtained before and after PCI) in 57 patients with an MI > 6 days (mean 20 days) prior to evaluation. Patients with positive SPECT before PCI had a significantly lower FFR than patients with negative SPECT (0.52 ± 0.18 vs. 0.67 ± 0.16; $p = 0.0079$). The best FFR cutoff found for determining peri-infarct ischemia was 0.78. In a similar study, Samady et al.[51] compared FFR to SPECT and myocardial contrast echo (MCE) in 48 patients 3.7 ± 1.3 days after infarction. To identify true reversibility, follow-up SPECT was performed 11 weeks after PCI. The sensitivity, specificity, and concordance of FFR ≤ 0.75 for detecting true reversibility on SPECT were 88%, 93%, and 91% (chi-square $p < 0.001$), and for detecting reversibility on MCE were 90%, 100%, and 93% (chi-square $p < 0.001$), respectively. The optimal FFR value for discriminating inducible ischemia on non-invasive imaging was also 0.78, similar to DeBruyne et al.[89] These studies suggest that within 3-6 days following AMI, FFR of the infarct-related artery correlates with non-invasive stress testing.

For patients with unstable angina or NSTEMI, FFR measurement at the time of angiography may be superior to a SPECT strategy. Leesar et al.[49] randomized 70 patients who received at least 48 hours of medical stabilization and had an intermediate single-vessel stenosis to one of two strategies: angiography followed by SPECT the next day or FFR-guided revascularization at the time of angiography. Compared with the SPECT strategy, the FFR-guided approach had a reduced hospital stay (11 ± 2 hours vs. 49 ± 5 hours, $p < 0.001$) and cost (1329 ± 44 US dollars vs. 2113 ± 120 US dollars, $p < 0.05$), with no increase in procedure time, radiation exposure time, or clinical event rates at 1-year follow-up.

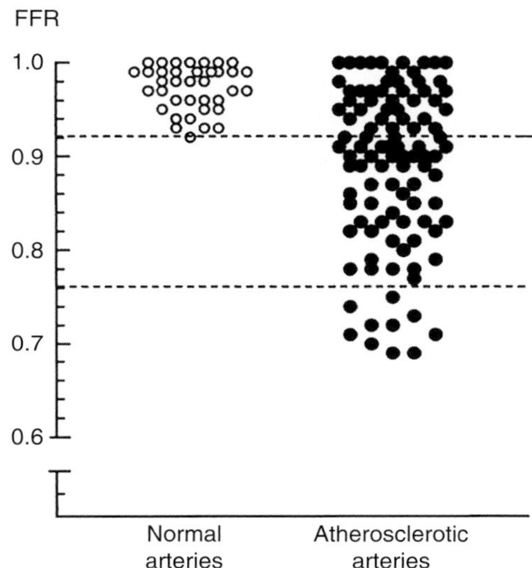

FIGURE 15-17 Fractional flow reserve (FFR) in diffuse coronary artery disease (CAD). Graphs of individual values of FFR in normal arteries and in atherosclerotic coronary arteries without focal stenosis on arteriogram. Diffuse CAD can produce an abnormal FFR in the absence of epicardial stenoses. The upper dotted line indicates the lowest value of FFR in normal coronary arteries. The lower dotted line indicates the 0.75 threshold level. *(Reused with permission from De Bruyne B, Hersbach F, Pijls NH, et al: Abnormal epicardial coronary resistance in patients with diffuse atherosclerosis but "normal" coronary angiography. Circulation 104:2401–2406, 2001.)*

INTRAVASCULAR ULTRASOUND AND FRACTIONAL FLOW RESERVE IN LESION ASSESSMENT

A normal FFR can be predicted reasonably well with IVUS dimensions, but accurate prediction of an abnormal FFR is

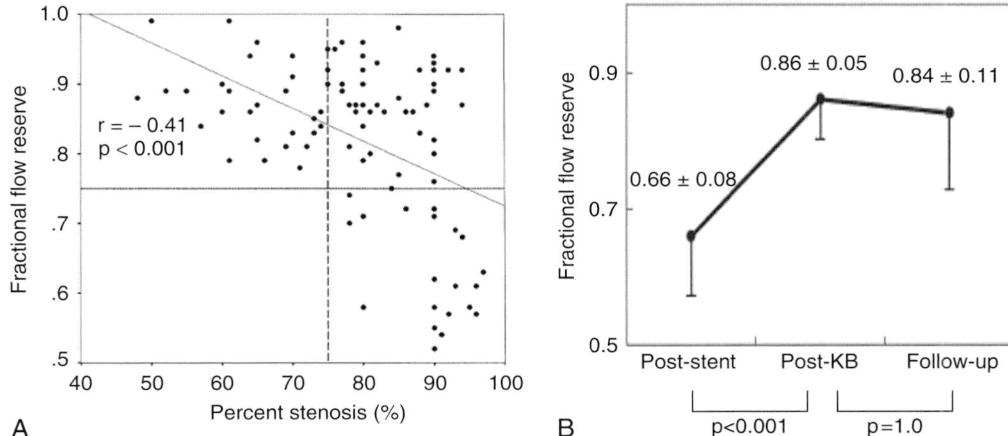

FIGURE 15-18 **A,** Side branch narrowing after stenting (percent diameter narrowing) compared with FFR. *FFR,* Fractional flow reserve; *KB,* kissing balloon. *(From Koo BK, Kang HJ, Youn TJ, et al: Physiologic assessment of jailed side branch lesions using fractional flow reserve. J Am Coll Cardiol 46;633–637, 2005.)* **B,** Long term outcome of FFR after kissing balloon treatment of jailed side branch. *(From Koo BK, Park KW, Kang HJ, et al: Physiological evaluation of the provisional side-branch intervention strategy for bifurcation lesions using fractional flow reserve. Eur Heart J 29(6):726–732, 2008.)*

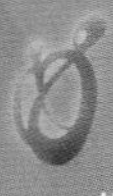

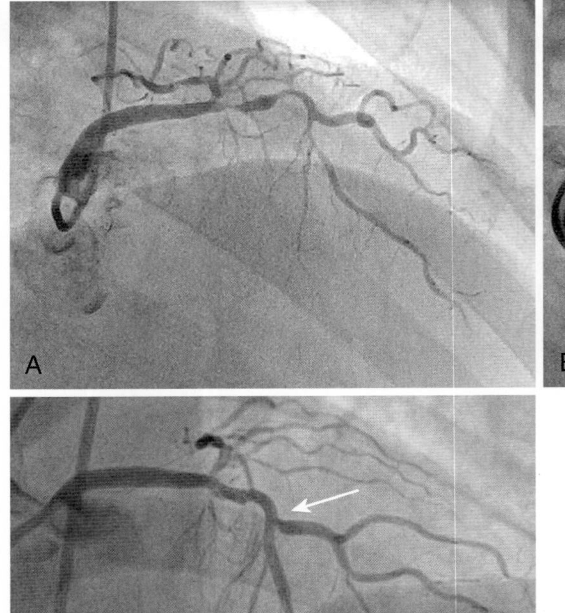

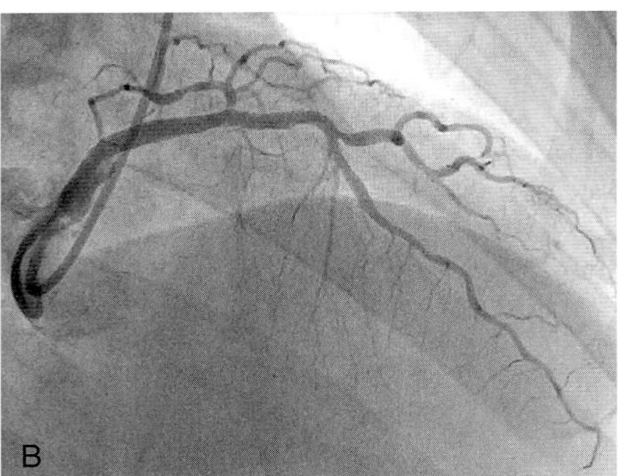

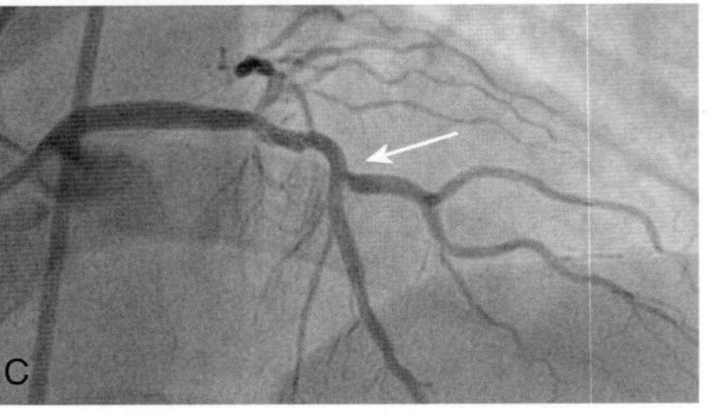

FIGURE 15-19 Cine angiogram frames before **(A)** and after stenting **(B)** ostial narrowing of the diagonal branch (*arrow,* **C**). FFR across side branch was 0.85. High pressure balloon of main branch was performed and the procedure terminated.

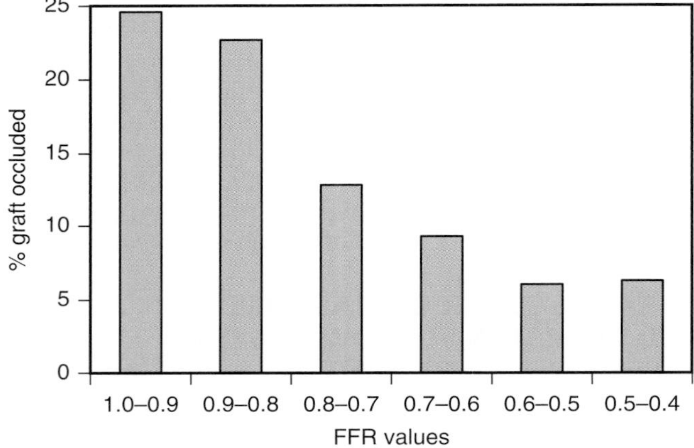

FIGURE 15-20 The fate of bypass grafts and FFR at time of surgery. High FFR is associated with high graft occlusion rates. *FFR,* Fractional flow reserve. *(From Botman CJ, Schonberger J, Koolen S, et al: Does stenosis severity of native vessels influence bypass graft patency? A prospective fractional flow reserve-guided study. Ann Thorac Surg 83:2093–2097, 2007.)*

a challenge with IVUS.[52,53] The primary limitation of IVUS MLA to predict hemodynamic significance is that the functional effects of a lesion are dependent on factors other than percent area stenosis. These include lesion length, eccentricity, entrance and exit angles and forces, reference vessel dimensions, and the amount of viable myocardium subtended by the lesion.[54]

There is better agreement between IVUS and FFR in assessing left main coronary artery (LMCA) than non-LMCA lesions; the better correlation being due to limited variability in LMCA length, size, and amount of supplied myocardium. Both techniques have theoretical and practical limitations. As noted above, proximal LAD and/or LCX disease may impact FFR of LMCA stenoses, so IVUS MLA may be simpler to measure for LMCA than FFR.

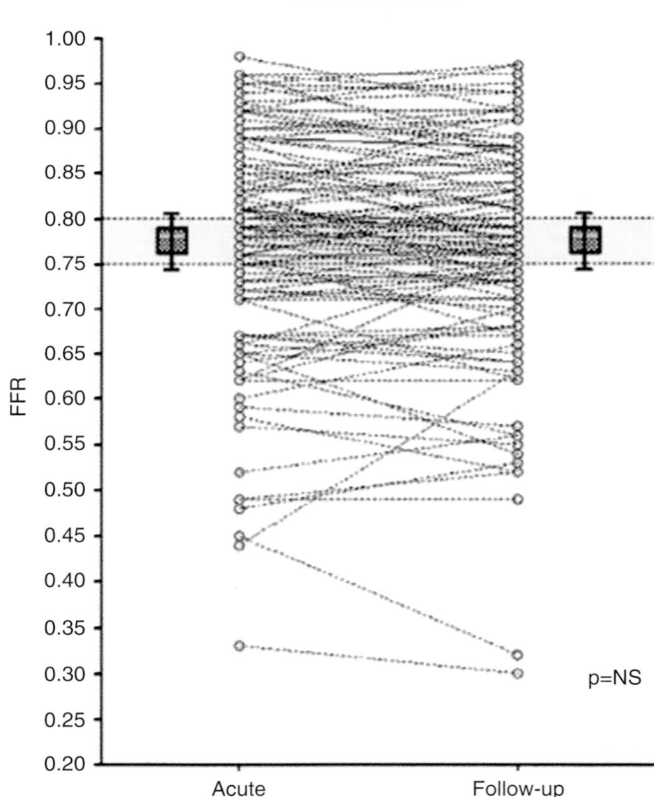

FIGURE 15-21 Fractional flow reserve (FFR) and acute coronary syndrome (ACS). FFR values are of nonculprit coronary artery stenoses during acute myocardial infarction and their FFR at follow-up. *FFR,* Fractional flow reserve; *ACS,* acute coronary syndrome. *(From Ntalianis A, Sels JW, Davidavicius G, et al: Fractional flow reserve for the assessment of nonculprit coronary artery stenoses in patients with acute myocardial infarction. J Am Coll Cardiol Intv 3:1274, 2010.)*

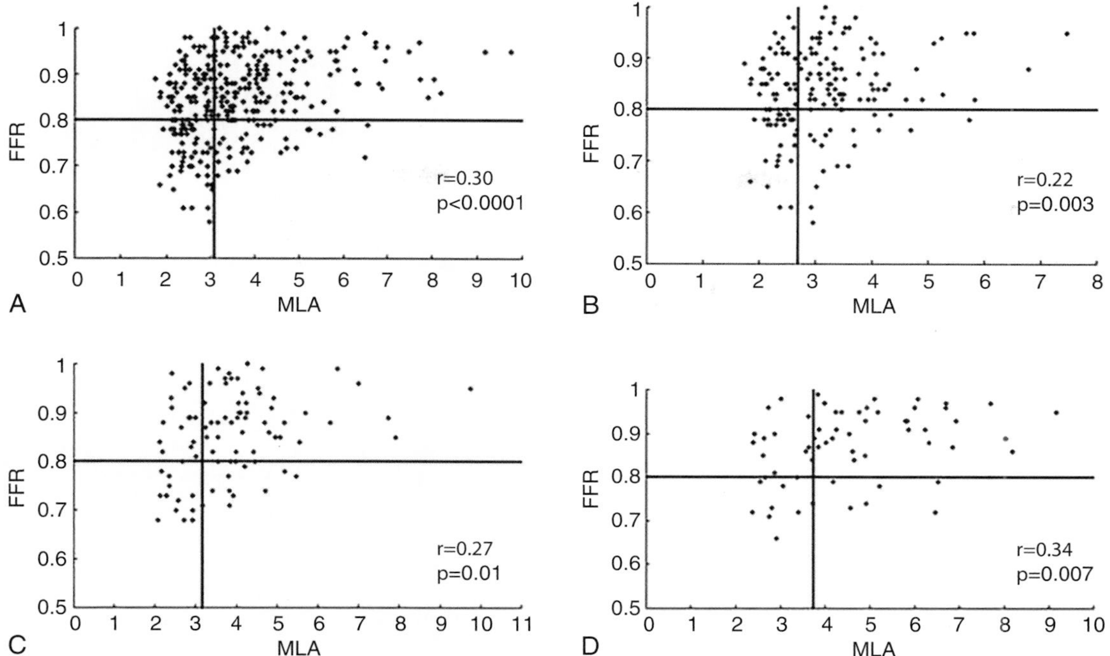

FIGURE 15-22 Left: Comparison of intravascular ultrasound (IVUS) and fractional flow reserve (FFR). **A,** Data for all reference vessel diameters (RVD) with FFR of 0.8 and minimum lumen area (MLA) cutoff of 3.07 mm². **B,** RVD < 3.0 mm with FFR of 0.8 and MLA of 2.68 mm². **C,** RVD of 3.0-3.5 mm with FFR of 0.8 and MLA of 3.16 mm². **D,** RVD >3.5 mm with FFR of 0.8 and MLA 3.74 mm². Right: Diagnostic sensitivity, specificity, positive predictive value (PPV), and negative predictive value (NPV) of IVUS MLA in the prediction of functionally significant stenosis overall based on RVD <3.0 mm, 3.0 to 3.5 mm, and >3.5 mm. *FFR,* Fractional flow reserve; *MLA,* minimum lumen area. *(From Waksman R, Legutko J, Singh J, et al: FIRST: fractional flow reserve and intravascular ultrasound relationship study. J Am Coll Cardiol 61(9):917–923, 2013.)*

Table 15-3 summarizes studies that correlated IVUS MLA in LMCA stenoses with FFR. Jasti et al.[55] showed good correlation between FFR and IVUS, with sensitivities and specificities >0.90. In a study of 55 intermediate LMCA lesions, an MLA < 5.9 mm² and an MLD < 2.8 mm² correlated well with FFR < 0.75.[55] The emerging consensus is that a cross-sectional area of <6.0 mm² is clinically significant, has fair correlation with FFR < 0.75, and may warrant intervention to improve 1-year mortality (44). In Asian populations, an MLA cutoff <4.8 mm² correlates well with reduced FFR < 0.8 and <4.1 mm² with FFR < 0.75.[56,57]

Fractional Flow Reserve and Intravascular Ultrasound Comparisons for Non–Left Main Coronary Artery Stenosis

In non-LMCA lesions there is only moderate correlation between anatomic dimensions by IVUS and ischemia by physiological assessment. IVUS and FFR correlation is best in demonstrating non-significant lesions[55]; the correlation in demonstrating significant stenoses is significantly weaker. Part of the reason for this deficiency is that attempting to determine a critical MLA without considering the reference vessel MLA leads to inaccuracy. An MLA of 3.0 mm² in a proximal versus distal arterial segment has entirely different effects on flow and subsequent clinical implications.

In the largest study to date, IVUS was compared with FFR in 544 lesions.[58] The optimal cutoff value to predict an FFR ≤ 0.80 was an MLA of 2.9 mm² by IVUS, but the overall accuracy was only 66%. Moreover, of the 240 lesions that had an MLA of <2.9 mm², only 47% were hemodynamically significant by FFR. Similarly concerning, 19% of lesions with an MLA of >2.9 mm² had an FFR of <0.80, limiting the utility of IVUS for hemodynamic lesion assessment.

Kang et al.[56] evaluated 236 angiographically intermediate coronary lesions in which both IVUS and FFR measurements were performed. An IVUS-measured MLA of 2.4 mm² had the maximal accuracy to predict an FFR < 0.80. However, the overall diagnostic accuracy was 68% with a confidence interval ranging from 1.8 to 2.6 mm².

FIRST was a multicenter prospective registry of patients who underwent elective coronary angiography and had intermediate coronary stenoses (40% to 80%).[59] An IVUS-measured MLA < 3.07 mm² had the best the best sensitivity and specificity (64% and 64.9%, respectively) for correlating with FFR < 0.80 (**Figure 15-22**). Even when IVUS MLA thresholds were adjusted for reference vessel diameter, the correlation with FFR was modest.

Therefore, FFR is the standard for assessing the hemodynamic significance of intermediate non-LMCA lesions for decisions regarding need for revascularization. An MLA ≥ 4.0 mm² reasonably accurately identifies non-significant lesions for which PCI can be safely deferred. However, an MLA < 4.0 mm² does not accurately predict a hemodynamically significant lesion and should not be used to justify revascularization. An MLA < 3.0 mm² most likely is a significant stenosis, but due to only modest sensitivity and specificity, physiologic testing is also desirable before proceeding with revascularization.

See Video 15-4 for a case example of a patient with ectatic and aneurysmal coronary artery, acute coronary syndrome managed with IVUS and FFR.

ASSESSING COLLATERAL FLOW

The pressure-derived fractional collateral flow is defined as the mean coronary wedge pressure (distal coronary pressure during balloon occlusion) divided by the mean aortic pressure (if the central venous pressure is abnormal, then it should be subtracted from both the wedge and aortic pressures). In general, a pressure-derived FFR of 0.25 or more suggests sufficient collaterals to prevent ischemia during PCI. Furthermore, these patients have a significantly lower adverse event rate during follow-up compared with those with insufficient collaterals at the time of PCI (pressure-derived collateral flow <0.25). Pressure-derived collateral flow has also been studied in patients with AMI and has been shown to be the major determinant of left ventricular recovery after primary PCI. Unfortunately, this technique for assessing collaterals is limited by the requirement for coronary artery occlusion.[60-62]

In order to quantify the presence and degree of collaterals, a Doppler collateral flow index (CFI) has been described. CFI is defined as the amount of flow via collaterals to a vascular region, divided by the amount of flow to the same region via the normally patent vessel. It is determined by summing the integral of systolic and diastolic flow velocities during balloon occlusion. In the case of temporally shifted bidirectional flow velocity signals, the antegrade and retrograde velocity integrals are added. The total velocity integral during balloon occlusion is then divided by the velocity integral after successful PCI, in order to calculate the CFI. A Doppler CFI >0.30 has been shown to accurately predict collateral circulation adequate to prevent myocardial ischemia during PCI. Moreover, the Doppler CFI is a more sensitive determinant of collateral flow than is angiographically visible collateral circulation. In another study, patients undergoing PCI who had a Doppler CFI of >0.25 had a fourfold decrease in the major adverse cardiac event rate at approximately 2 years compared with those with a CFI < 0.25. The obvious limitation of this technique is that it requires performance of PCI.[63]

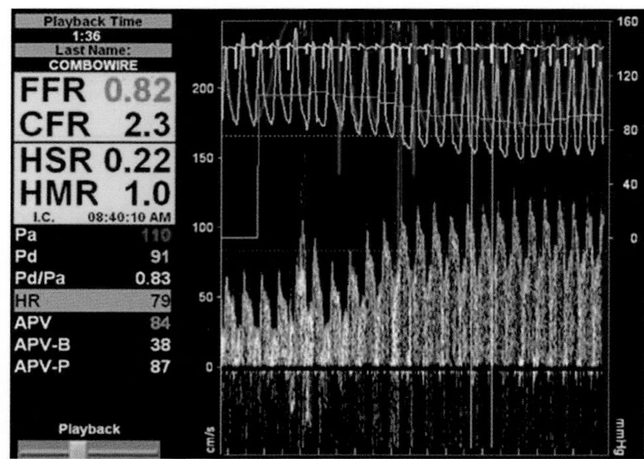

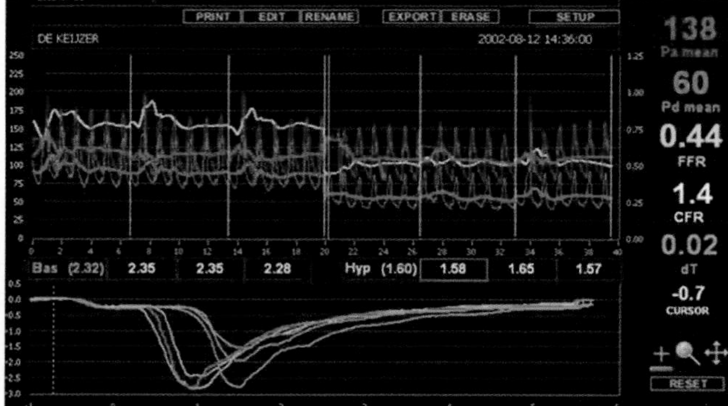

FIGURE 15-23 Characterizing the microcirculation. Pressure and Doppler flow measurements during adenosine-induced hyperemia. Hyperemic stenosis resistance index (HSRv) = Pa – Pv/APVhyper. IMR = Pa * Tmn [(Pd – Pw)/(Pa – Pw)]. *CFR,* Coronary flow velocity reserve; *FFR,* fractional flow reserve; *HSR,* Hyperemic stenosis resistance.

INDEX OF MICROCIRCULATORY RESISTANCE

Index of microcirculatory resistance (IMR) is defined as the ratio of distal coronary pressure to the inverse of the mean transit time during maximal hyperemia. It is a quantitative index that is unique to the microcirculation and independent of epicardial coronary artery disease.[64,65] While CFR has been studied in microvascular dysfunction, IMR is superior to CFR because it is not affected by resting hemodynamics, making it more reproducible, even after hemodynamic perturbations. When measured immediately after primary PCI for ST-elevation myocardial infarction, IMR predicts the amount of myocardial damage and left ventricular recovery better than other indices, such as CFR, ST-segment resolution, or TIMI myocardial perfusion grade and is an independent predictor of long-term clinical outcomes including death and rehospitalization for heart failure.[62] Examples of measurements characterizing the microcirculation are shown in **Figure 15-23**.

After primary angioplasty, Fearon et al.[65] found that patients with preserved IMR may have greater recovery of regional ventricular function after primary angioplasty for ST elevation myocardial infarction. In 253 patients, IMR was measured immediately after primary PCI using a pressure–temperature sensor wire. The prognostic value of IMR was compared with coronary flow reserve, TIMI myocardial perfusion grade, and clinical variables. The mean IMR was 40.3 ± 32.5. Patients with an IMR > 40 had a higher rate of death or rehospitalization at 1 year than those with an IMR ≤40 (17% vs. 7%; $p = 0.027$). During follow-up (2.8 years), 14% experienced the primary end point and 4% died. An IMR >40 was associated with an increased risk of death or rehospitalization for heart failure (hazard ratio (HR), 2.1; $p = 0.034$) and of death alone (HR, 3.95; $p = 0.028$). An IMR >40 was the only independent predictor of death alone (HR, 4.3; $p = 0.02$, **Figure 15-24**). Like a low reference vessel coronary flow velocity reserve (CFVR), an elevated IMR at the time of primary percutaneous coronary intervention predicts poor long-term outcomes. In addition to providing prognostic information in this important patient subset, IMR may potentially be used in selecting patients with relatively preserved post-infarct microvasculature that might most benefit from regional delivery of regenerative cell therapies.

ECONOMICS OF PHYSIOLOGIC GUIDED INTERVENTIONS

The economics of lesion assessment suggests that with disposable sensor-tipped guidewires that cost approximately $600, and initial capital expenses around $50,000, FFR has the ability to save overall health care costs. Measurements require <15 minutes of time with small amounts of heparin, nitroglycerin, and adenosine. Whether these costs are offset by elimination of non-invasive stress testing and the associated additional hospital time has been addressed. Studies have demonstrated a cost savings to the hospital by using

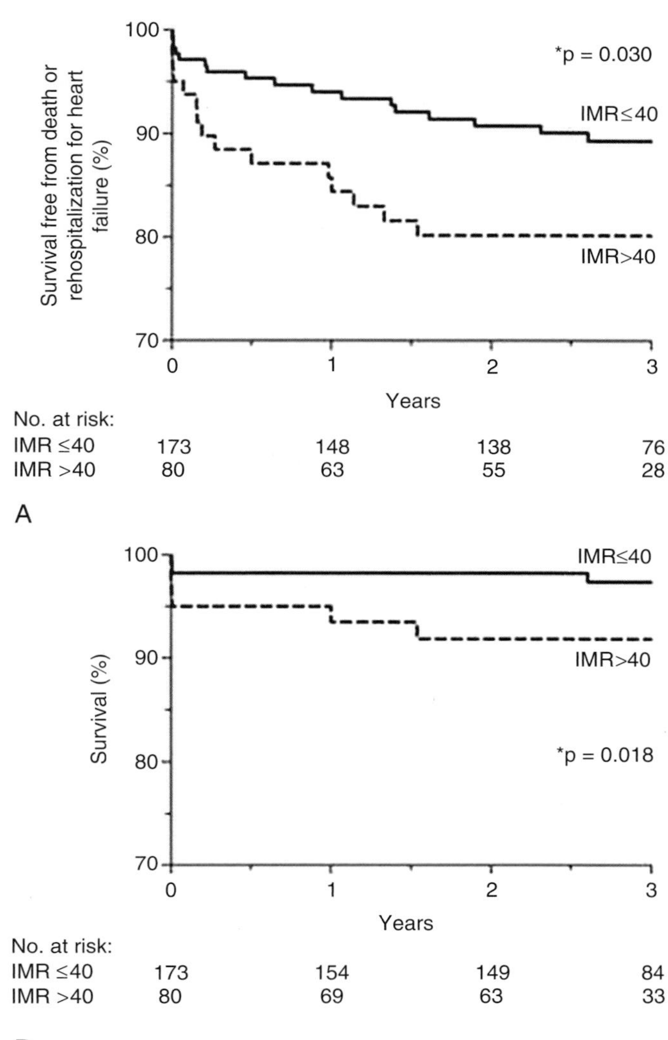

FIGURE 15-24 **A,** The Kaplan-Meier curves displaying the relationship between IMR >40 and survival free of death or rehospitalization for heart failure. **B,** The Kaplan-Meier curves displaying the relationship between IMR >40 and survival free of death. IMR indicates Index of Microcirculatory Resistance. *(From Fearon WF, Low AF, Yong AS, et al: Prognostic value of the index of microcirculatory resistance measured after primary percutaneous coronary intervention. Circulation 127:2436–2441, 2013.)*

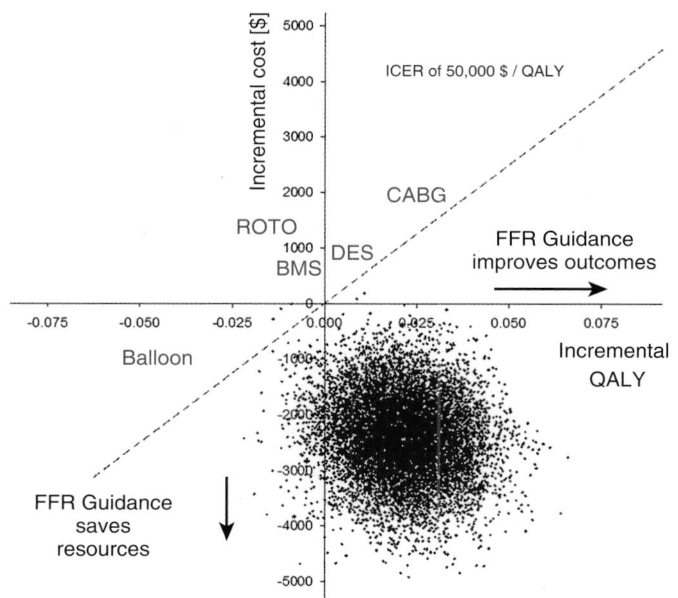

FIGURE 15-25 Bootstrap Cost Analysis of the FAME Study at 1 year. *BMS,* Bare-metal stent; *CABG,* coronary artery bypass graft surgery; *DES,* drug-eluting stent; *ROTO,* rotoblator. *(From Fearon W, Bornschein B, Tonino P, et al: Economic evaluation of fractional flow reserve–guided percutaneous coronary intervention in patients with multivessel disease / clinical perspective. Circulation 122(24):2545–2550, 2010.)*

in-lab lesion assessment. In one study,[66] a decision model was generated comparing the long-term costs and benefits of three strategies for treating patients with an intermediate coronary lesion and no prior functional study: (1) deferring the decision for percutaneous coronary intervention (PCI) to obtain a nuclear stress imaging study (NUC strategy), (2) measuring fractional flow reserve (FFR) at the time of angiography to help guide the decision for PCI (FFR strategy), and (3) stenting all intermediate lesions (STENT strategy). The investigators found that the FFR strategy saved $1795 per patient compared with the NUC strategy and $3830 compared with the STENT strategy. Quality-adjusted life expectancy was similar among the three strategies.

In another study,[67] 70 patients admitted with unstable angina/non-ST-segment elevation myocardial infarction and angiographically intermediate coronary lesions were randomized to either immediate measurement of FFR and interventional or medical treatment as dictated by the FFR value or to nuclear stress imaging with a return trip to the catheterization laboratory if abnormal. The investigators found that the FFR strategy significantly reduced the duration and cost of hospitalization. There were no significant differences or event rates at 1-year follow-up.

The FAME 1 study showed higher quality outcomes at lower cost with FFR compared with an angiographic guided strategy (**Figure 15-25**). The FAME 1 and 2[33,34] studies also demonstrated long-term cost savings when treating ischemic lesions directed by FFR rather than relying on angiography alone. Although the cost of the physiologic information translates into an operational expense for the catheterization laboratory, the data consistently show significant overall savings to the health care system and a substantial clinical benefit to the patient with FFR.

CONCLUSIONS

The integration of coronary physiology with angiography has proven to be invaluable in aiding the physician with decision making in equivocal stenosis and multivessel disease. Through physiological assessment of coronary artery stenosis, FFR identifies lesions with ischemic potential and essentially functions as a stress test in the cath lab. **Table 15-8** summarizes the derivations and unique features of intracoronary physiologic measurements. The remarkable improvement in patient outcomes with implementation of this strategy supports the ischemia-guided revascularization strategy and is prompting a shift in the existing coronary revascularization paradigm. **Table 15-9** provides applications of FFR in current clinical practice. Use of FFR is very likely to continue to increase in the coming years.

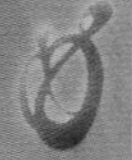

TABLE 15-8 Comparison and Derivations of Intracoronary Physiological Measurements

	DERIVATION	UNIQUE FEATURES
Fractional flow reserve	FFR = Q_{sten}/Q_{normal} at maximal hyperemia Q = flow, sten = stenotic artery, normal = theoretic same artery without stenosis $Q_{sten} = P_{sten}/Resistance_{sten}$, $Q_{normal} = P_{aorta}/Resistance_{sten}$, then $Q_{sten}/Q_{normal} = P_{sten}/P_{aorta}$ Hence FFR = $P_{distal\ to\ stenosis}/P_{aorta}$ (complete derivation includes venous pressure P_v as FFR = $P_{distal\ to\ stenosis} - P_v/P_{aorta} - P_v$, see reference 2)	• Nonischemic threshold range >0.75-0.80 • Normal value of 1.0 for every artery and every patient • Epicardial lesion specific • Linear relation with relative maximum blood flow • Independent of hemodynamic alterations • Value that accounts for total myocardial blood flow, including collaterals • Highly reproducible • High spatial resolution (pressure pullback recording)
Coronary flow velocity and reserve	CFVR = $Q_{hyperemia}/Q_{base}$ Q = Velocity if cross-sectional area unchanged during hyperemia	• Nonischemic threshold range of CFR >2.0 • Coronary flow reserve in non-obstructed vessels assesses microvascular integrity • Complements invasive coronary studies of endothelial function • Accurate estimation of volumetric flow when vessel cross-sectional area available • Valuable for blood flow research studies
Combined pressure and flow velocity measurements	HSR = $P_{aorta} - P_{distal\ to\ stenosis}/Q_{hyperemic}$ IMR = $P_{distal\ to\ stenosis}/(1/\text{mean transit time}_{hyperemic})$	• Separate assessment of stenosis and microvascular resistances • Allows construction of pressure-flow curves (assessment of compliant lesions, hemodynamic gain after PCI) Stenosis Resistance Index: • Normal value of 0 • Lesion specific • Highly reproducible, high sensitivity • Useful in cases of discordance between CFR and FFR

Modified From Kern MJ, Samady H: Current concepts of integrated coronary physiology in the cath lab. J Am Coll Cardiol 55:173–185, 2010.
CFR, Coronary flow velocity reserve; *FRR,* fractional flow reserve; *HSR,* hyperemic stenosis resistance; *IMR,* index of microcirculatory resistance.

TABLE 15-9 Applications of FFR in the Catheterization Laboratory

A. Applications Supported by PCI Guidelines
   1. 5.4.1 FFR: Recommendations*
   CLASS IIa
   1. FFR is reasonable to assess angiographic intermediate coronary lesions (50% to 70% diameter stenosis) and can be useful for guiding revascularization decisions in patients with SIHD. *(Level of Evidence: A)*
   2. Assessing the success of PCI in restoring flow reserve and to predict the risk of restenosis. (Class IIb, *Level of Evidence: C*)
   3. Evaluating patients with anginal symptoms without an apparent angiographic culprit lesion. (Class IIb, *Level of Evidence: C*)
   4. Routine assessment of the severity of angiographic disease in patients with a positive, unequivocal noninvasive functional study is not recommended. (Class III, *Level of Evidence: C*)

B. Clinical Applications of FFR
   1. Determination of one or more culprit stenoses (either serially or in separate vessels) in patients with multivessel disease
   2. Evaluation of ostial or distal left main and ostial right lesions, especially when these regions cannot be well visualized by angiography
   3. Guidance of treatment of serial stenoses in a coronary artery
   4. Determination of significance of focal treatable region in vessel with diffuse coronary artery disease
   5. Determination of prognosis after stent deployment
   6. Assessment of stenosis in patients with previous (non-acute, >6 days) myocardial infarction
   7. Assessment of lesions in patients with treated unstable angina pectoris
   8. Assessment of the collateral circulation

C. Clinical Applications of Combined Coronary Pressure and Doppler Flow Velocity under Study
   1. Assessment of intermediate stenosis
   2. Assessment of the microcirculation
   3. Identification of lesion compliance (change of pressure-velocity relationship)

*Levine GN, Bates ER, Blankenship JC, et al: 2011 ACCF/AHA/SCAI guideline for percutaneous coronary intervention: a report of the American College of Cardiology Foundation/American Heart Association Task Force on Practice Guidelines and the Society for Cardiovascular Angiography and Interventions. *Circulation* 124:e574–e651, 2011.
FFR, Fractional flow reserve; *PCI,* percutaneous coronary intervention.

References

1. Topol EJ, Nissen SE: Our preoccupation with coronary luminology. The dissociation between clinical and angiographic findings in ischemic heart disease. *Circulation* 92:2333–2342, 1995.
2. Meijboom WB, Van Mieghem CAG, van Pelt N, et al: Comprehensive assessment of coronary artery stenoses: computed tomography coronary angiography versus conventional coronary angiography and correlation with fractional flow reserve in patients with stable angina. *J Am Coll Cardiol* 52(8):636–643, 2008.
3. Ziaee A, Parham WA, Herrmann SC, et al: Lack of relation between imaging and physiology in ostial coronary artery narrowings. *Am J Cardiol* 93(11):1404–1407, 2004.
4. Pijls NH, De Bruyne B, Peels K, et al: Measurement of fractional flow reserve to assess the functional severity of coronary-artery stenoses. *N Engl J Med* 334:1703–1708, 1996.
5. Pijls NHJ, Van Gelder B, Van der Voort P, et al: Fractional flow reserve: a useful index to evaluate the influence of an epicardial coronary stenosis on myocardial blood flow. *Circulation* 92:318–319, 1995.
6. De Bruyne B, Bartunek J, Sys SU, et al: Simultaneous coronary pressure and flow velocity measurements in humans: feasibility, reproducibility and hemodynamic dependence of coronary flow velocity reserve, hyperemic flow versus pressure slope index and fractional flow reserve. *Circulation* 94:1842–1849, 1996.
7. Spaan JAE, Piek JJ, Hoofman JIE, et al: Physiological basis of clinically used coronary hemodynamic indices. *Circulation* 113:446–455, 2006.
8. Kern MJ, Lerman A, Bech JW, et al: Physiological assessment of coronary artery disease in the cardiac catheterization laboratory: a scientific statement from the American Heart Association committee on diagnostic and interventional cardiac catheterization. *Circulation* 114(12):1321–1341, 2006.
9. Iqbal MB, Shah N, Khan M, et al: Reduction in myocardial perfusion territory and its effect on the physiological severity of a coronary stenosis. *Circ Cardiovasc Interv* 3:89–90, 2010.
10. McGeoch RJ, Oldroyd KG: Pharmacological options for inducing maximal hyperaemia during studies of coronary physiology. *Catheter Cardiovasc Interv* 71(2):198–204, 2008.
11. Jeremias A, Whitbourn RJ, Filardo SD, et al: Adequacy of intracoronary versus IV adenosine-induced maximal coronary hyperemia for fractional flow reserve measurements. *Am Heart J* 140:651–657, 2000.
12. Casella G, Leibig M, Schiele TM, et al: Are high doses of intracoronary adenosine an alternative to standard intravenous adenosine for the assessment of fractional flow reserve? *Am Heart J* 148:590–595, 2004.
13. Seo MK, Koo BK, Kim JH, et al: Comparison of hyperemic efficacy between central and peripheral venous adenosine infusion for fractional flow reserve measurement. *Circ Cardiovasc Interv* 5(3):401–405, 2012.
14. Nair PK, Marroquin OC, Mulukutla SR, et al: Clinical utility of regadenoson for assessing fractional flow reserve. *JACC Cardiovasc Interv* 4(10):1085–1092, 2011.
15. Hodgson JM, Dib N, Kern MJ, et al: Coronary circulation responses to binodenoson, a selective adenosine A2A receptor agonist. *Am J Cardiol* 99:1507–1512, 2007.
16. Parham WA, Bouhasin A, Ciaramita JP, et al: Coronary hyperemic dose responses to intracoronary sodium nitroprusside. *Circulation* 109:1236–1243, 2004.
17. Salcedo J, Kern MJ: Effects of caffeine and theophylline on coronary hyperemia induced by adenosine or dipyridamole. *Cathet Cardiovasc Interv* 74:598–605, 2009.
18. Pijls NHJ, Kern MJ, Yock PG, et al. Practice and potential pitfalls of coronary pressure measurement. *Cath Cardiovasc Interv* 49:1–16, 2000.
19. Qian J, Ge J, Baumgart D, et al: Safety of intracoronary Doppler flow measurement. *Am Heart J* 140(3):502–510, 2000.
20. Christou MA, Siontis GC, Katritsis DG, et al: Meta-analysis of fractional flow reserve versus quantitative coronary angiography and noninvasive imaging for evaluation of myocardial ischemia. *Am J Cardiol* 99(4):450–456, 2007.
21. Potvin JM, Rodés-Cabau J, Bertrand OF, et al: Usefulness of fractional flow reserve measurements to defer revascularization in patients with stable or unstable angina pectoris, non-ST-elevation and ST-elevation acute myocardial infarction, or atypical chest pain. *Am J Cardiol* 98:289–297, 2006.

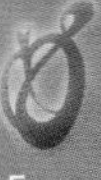

22. Ahn JM, Kang SJ, Mintz FS, et al: Validation of minimal luminal area measured by intravascular ultrasound for assessment of functionally significant coronary stenosis comparison with myocardial perfusion imaging. *J Am Coll Cardiol Intv* 4:665–671, 2011.
23. Kern MJ, Samady H: Current concepts of integrated coronary physiology in the cath lab. *J Am Coll Cardiol* 55(3):173–185, 2010.
24. Bech GJ, DeBruyne B, Pijls NH, et al: Fractional flow reserve to determine the appropriateness of angioplasty in moderate coronary stenosis: a randomized trial. *Circulation* 103(24):2928–2934, 2001.
25. Berger A, Botman KJ, MacCarthy PA, et al: Long-term clinical outcome after fractional flow reserve-guided percutaneous coronary intervention in patients with multivessel disease. *J Am Coll Cardiol* 46:438–442, 2005.
26. Pijls NHJ, Van Schaardenburgh P, Manoharan G, et al: Percutaneous coronary intervention of functionally non-significant stenoses: 5-year follow-up of the DEFER study. *J Am Coll Cardiol* 49:2105–2111, 2007.
27. Kim HL, Koo BK, Nam CW, et al: Clinical and physiological outcomes of fractional flow reserve-guided percutaneous coronary intervention in patients with serial stenoses within one coronary artery. *JACC Cardiovasc Interv* 5(10):1013–1018, 2012.
28. De Bruyne B, Hersbach F, Pijls NH, et al: Abnormal epicardial coronary resistance in patients with diffuse atherosclerosis but "normal" coronary angiography. *Circulation* 104(20):2401–2406, 2001.
29. Koo BK, Kang HJ, Youn TJ, et al: Physiologic assessment of jailed side branch lesions using fractional flow reserve. *J Am Coll Cardiol* 46(4):633–637, 2005.
30. Ntalianis A, Sels JW, Davidavicius G, et al: Fractional flow reserve for the assessment of nonculprit coronary artery stenoses in patients with acute myocardial infarction. *JACC Cardiovasc Interv* 3(12):1274–1281, 2010.
31. Koo BK, Park KW, Kang HJ, et al: Physiological evaluation of the provisional side-branch intervention strategy for bifurcation lesions using fractional flow reserve. *Eur Heart J* 29(6):726–732, 2008.
32. Koo BK, Waseda K, Kang HJ, et al: Anatomic and functional evaluation of bifurcation lesions undergoing percutaneous coronary intervention. *Circ Cardiovasc Interv* 3:113–119, 2010.
33. Tonino PAL, De Bruyne B, Pijls NHJ, et al: Fractional flow reserve versus angiography for guiding percutaneous coronary intervention. *N Engl J Med* 360:213–224, 2009.
34. Pijls NHJ, Fearon WF, Tonino PAL, et al: Fractional flow reserve versus angiography for guiding percutaneous coronary intervention in patients with multivessel coronary artery disease: 2-year follow-up of the FAME (fractional flow reserve versus angiography for multivessel evaluation) study. *J Am Coll Cardiol* 56:177–184, 2010.
35. Fearon WF, Bronschein B, Tonino PA, et al: Economic evaluation of fractional flow reserve-guided percutaneous coronary intervention in patients with multivessel disease. *Circulation* 122(24):2545–2550, 2010.
36. De Bruyne B, Pijls NH, Kalesan B, et al: Fractional flow reserve-guided PCI versus medical therapy in stable coronary disease. *N Engl J Med* 367(11):991–1001, 2012.
37. Pijls NH, Klauss V, Siebert U, et al: Fractional flow reserve (FFR) post-stent registry investigators. Coronary pressure measurement after stenting predicts adverse events at follow-up: a multicenter registry. *Circulation* 105:2950–2954, 2002.
38. Samady H, McDaniel M, Veledar E, et al: Baseline fractional flow reserve and stent diameter predict optimal post-stent fractional flow reserve and major adverse cardiac events after bare-metal stent deployment. *JACC Cardiovasc Interv* 2:357–363, 2009.
39. Bech GJ, Droste H, Pijls NH, et al: Value of fractional flow reserve in making decisions about bypass surgery for equivocal left main coronary artery disease. *Heart* 86(5):547–552, 2001.
40. Hamilos M, Muller O, Cuisset T, et al: Long-term clinical outcome after fractional flow reserve–guided treatment in patients with angiographically equivocal left main coronary artery stenosis. *Circulation* 120:1505–1512, 2009.
41. Yong ASC, Daniels D, De Bruyne B, et al: Fractional flow reserve assessment of left main stenosis in the presence of downstream coronary stenoses. *Circ Cardiovasc Interv* 6(2):161–165, 2013.
42. Puymirat E, Peace A, Mangiacapra F, et al: Long-term clinical outcome after fractional flow reserve–guided percutaneous coronary revascularization in patients with small-vessel disease. *Circ Cardiovasc Interven* 5:62–68, 2012.
43. Pijls NH, De Bruyne B, Bech GJ, et al: Coronary pressure measurement to assess the hemodynamic significance of serial stenoses within one coronary artery: validation in humans. *Circulation* 102:2371–2377, 2000.
44. De Bruyne B, Pijls NH, Heyndrickx GR, et al: Pressure-derived fractional flow reserve to assess serial epicardial stenoses: theoretical basis and animal validation. *Circulation* 101:1840–1847, 2000.
45. Botman CJ, Schonberger J, Koolen S, et al: Does stenosis severity of native vessels influence bypass graft patency? A prospective fractional flow reserve-guided study. *Ann Thorac Surg* 83:2093–2097, 2007.
46. De Bruyne B, Pijls NHJ, Bartunek J, et al: Fractional flow reserve in patients with prior myocardial infarction. *Circulation* 104:157–162, 2001.
47. Fischer JJ, Wang XQ, Samady H, et al: Outcome of patients with acute coronary syndromes and moderate lesions undergoing deferral of revascularization based on fractional flow reserve assessment. *Cath Cardiovasc Interv* 68:544–548, 2006.
48. Potvin JM, Rodés-Cabau J, Bertrand OF, et al: Usefulness of fractional flow reserve measurements to defer revascularization in patients with stable or unstable angina pectoris, non-ST-elevation and ST-elevation acute myocardial infarction, or atypical chest pain. *Am J Cardiol* 98:289–297, 2006.
49. Leesar MA, Abdul-Baki T, Akkus NI, et al: Use of fractional flow reserve versus stress perfusion scintigraphy after unstable angina. Effect on duration of hospitalization, cost, procedural characteristics, and clinical outcome. *J Am Coll Cardiol* 41:1115–1121, 2003.
50. McClish JC, Ragosta M, Powers ER, et al: Recent myocardial infarction does not limit the utility of fractional flow reserve for the physiologic assessment of lesion severity. *Am J Cardiol* 93(9):1102–1106, 2004.
51. Samady H, Lepper W, Powers ER, et al: Fractional flow reserve of infarct-related arteries identifies reversible defects on noninvasive myocardial perfusion imaging early after myocardial infarction. *J Am Coll Cardiol* 47:2187–2193, 2006.
52. Nishioka T, Amanullah AM, Luo H, et al: Clinical validation of intravascular ultrasound imaging for assessment of coronary stenosis severity: comparison with stress myocardial perfusion imaging. *J Am Coll Cardiol* 33(7):1870–1878, 1999.
53. Takagi A, Tsurumi Y, Ishii Y, et al: Clinical potential of intravascular ultrasound for physiological assessment of coronary stenosis: relationship between quantitative ultrasound tomography and pressure-derived fractional flow reserve. *Circulation* 100:250–255, 1999.
54. Kang SJ, Lee JY, Ahn JM, et al: Validation of intravascular ultrasound-derived parameters with fractional flow reserve for assessment of coronary stenosis severity. *Circ Cardiovasc Interv* 4:65–71, 2011.
55. Jasti V, Ivan E, Yalamanchii V, et al: Correlations between fractional flow reserve and intravascular ultrasound in patients with an ambiguous left main coronary artery stenosis. *Circulation* 110:2831–2836, 2004.
56. Kang SJ, Lee JY, Ahn JM, et al: Intravascular ultrasound-derived predictors for fractional flow reserve in intermediate left main disease. *JACC Cardiovasc Interv* 4:1168–1174, 2011.
57. de la Torre Hernandez JM, Hernández Hernandez F, Alfonso F, et al: Prospective application of pre-defined intravascular ultrasound criteria for assessment of intermediate left main coronary artery lesions: results from the multicenter LITRO study. *J Am Coll Cardiol* 58(4):351–358, 2011.
58. Stone G. VERDICT/FIRST: Prospective, Multicenter Study Examining the Correlation between IVUS and FFR Parameters in Intermediate Lesions. In press, 2012.
59. Waksman R, Legutko J, Singh J, et al: FIRST: fractional flow reserve and intravascular ultrasound relationship study. *J Am Coll Cardiol* 61(9):917–923, 2013.
60. Piek JJ, van Liebergen RA, Koch KT, et al: Clinical, angiographic and hemodynamic predictors of recruitable collateral flow assessed during balloon angioplasty coronary occlusion. *J Am Coll Cardiol* 29:275–282, 1997.
61. Pijls NH, Bech GJ, el Gamal MI, et al: Quantification of recruitable coronary collateral blood flow in conscious humans and its potential to predict future ischemic events. *J Am Coll Cardiol* 25:1522–1528, 1995.
62. Seiler C, Fleisch M, Billinger M, et al: Simultaneous intracoronary velocity- and pressure-derived assessment of adenosine-induced collateral hemodynamics in patients with one- to two-vessel coronary artery disease. *J Am Coll Cardiol* 34:1985–1994, 1999.
63. Billinger M, Kloos P, Eberli FR, et al: Physiologically assessed coronary collateral flow and adverse cardiac ischemic events: a follow-up study in 403 patients with coronary artery disease. *J Am Coll Cardiol* 40:1545–1550, 2002.
64. Fearon WF, Low AF, Yong AC, et al. Prognostic value of the index of microcirculatory resistance measured after primary percutaneous coronary intervention. *Circulation* 127(24):2436–2441, 2013.
65. Ng MK, Yeung AC, Fearon WF: Invasive assessment of the coronary microcirculation: superior reproducibility and less hemodynamic dependence of index of microcirculatory resistance as compared to coronary flow reserve. *Circulation* 113:2054–2061, 2006.
66. Potvin JM, Rodés-Cabau J, Bertrand OF, et al: Usefulness of fractional flow reserve measurements to defer revascularization in patients with stable or unstable angina pectoris, non-ST-elevation and ST-elevation acute myocardial infarction, or atypical chest pain. *Am J Cardiol* 98:289–297, 2006.
67. Leesar MA, Abdul-Baki T, Akkus NI, et al: Use of fractional flow reserve versus stress perfusion scintigraphy after unstable angina. Effect on duration of hospitalization, cost, procedural characteristics, and clinical outcome. *J Am Coll Cardiol* 41:1115–1121, 2003.

16 Intravascular Ultrasound Imaging

Khaled M. Ziada

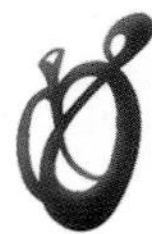

BACKGROUND AND LIMITATIONS OF ANGIOGRAPHY

Contrast angiography has been the gold standard of coronary artery imaging for over six decades. However, it is important to understand that angiograms only delineate the coronary lumen with no direct imaging or examination of the arterial wall. With the growing interest in vascular biology and understanding of the metabolically active atherosclerotic plaque, intravascular ultrasound (IVUS) imaging fills a gap in our understanding of coronary disease, as it allows in vivo examination of both the arterial wall and the lumen of the coronary arteries with high resolution. Although newer intravascular imaging modalities have evolved in the past decade, IVUS imaging remains the most mature adjunctive intravascular imaging modality and the one technique with a large body of literature to support its application.

Conceptually, it is easy to understand how angiography of the coronary arteries may not be the perfect imaging modality. The coronary arteries are constantly moving structures with complex, three-dimensional lumen shapes and atherosclerotic lesions of various distributions and compositions that need to be depicted on a two-dimensional display. Therefore, it is critically important for the angiographer to understand the limitations of the technique. This will allow a more realistic processing of the information, which is necessary when making diagnoses and in clinical decision making.[1,2] One of the most basic limitations is that fluoroscopy and cine angiography have limited resolution that is not adequate to delineate all the information needed from a coronary angiogram, even with near universal adoption of digital imaging and flat panel technology. Because of these complexities and limitations, interpretation of coronary angiograms has traditionally been marked by significant interobserver and intraobserver variability.[3,4]

As stated, and because angiograms are essentially contrast silhouettes of the lumen, it is not possible to directly discern whether the arterial wall is thickened (i.e., diseased). This is inferred by a reduction in the diameter of the luminogram in one segment compared to an adjacent one. Thus, the segmental construct in interpretation of angiograms is based on the assumption that narrower segments are the sites of disease, while adjacent larger segments represent the normal size of the artery or at least of its lumen. Yet autopsy studies have consistently demonstrated that atherosclerosis is diffuse, affecting almost all segments of an artery, albeit with varying severity.[5,6] Therefore, the "focal" lesions frequently described on angiography are the more diseased sites, but the "normal" or "mildly irregular" segments are almost always diseased as well. This leads to the angiographic underestimation of disease severity and degree of narrowing at the worst lesion sites (**Figure 16-1**).

Arterial remodeling, first described by Glagov et al., is another important phenomenon that can significantly affect angiographic interpretation.[7] Arterial remodeling describes the outward displacement of the arterial wall with increasing plaque size. This compensatory enlargement allows the artery to accommodate a certain amount of plaque volume without affecting the size of the lumen. Stenoses develop only when this mechanism is overwhelmed by increasing plaque size. Therefore, by definition, interpretation of contrast luminograms based on differences in lumen size from one segment to the other is not helpful in recognizing early, "well-compensated" stages of disease. Remodeled arterial segments with significant plaque burden can thus be described as "angiographically normal."

Another phenomenon, "negative remodeling," can also contribute to development of luminal narrowing in a reverse manner. In these cases, the reduction in the size of the artery itself contributes more to the reduction in lumen size than what the size of the plaque would indicate (**Figure 16-2A**).[8] The remodeling index is a metric relating the size of the artery at the lesion site to that at the proximal reference segment. An index exceeding 1.0 indicates compensatory enlargement at the lesion site and a value less than 1.0 indicates shrinkage or negative remodeling (**Figure 16-2B**). There is some evidence that positive remodeling is associated with acute presentations, while negative remodeling is more commonly seen in patients with stable angina.[9]

The complexity of coronary anatomy is another factor that limits the accuracy of angiographic depiction. The constantly moving tortuous arteries give off branches in different planes in a three-dimensional space. The lesions may be eccentric in distribution, at bifurcation points, ostial in

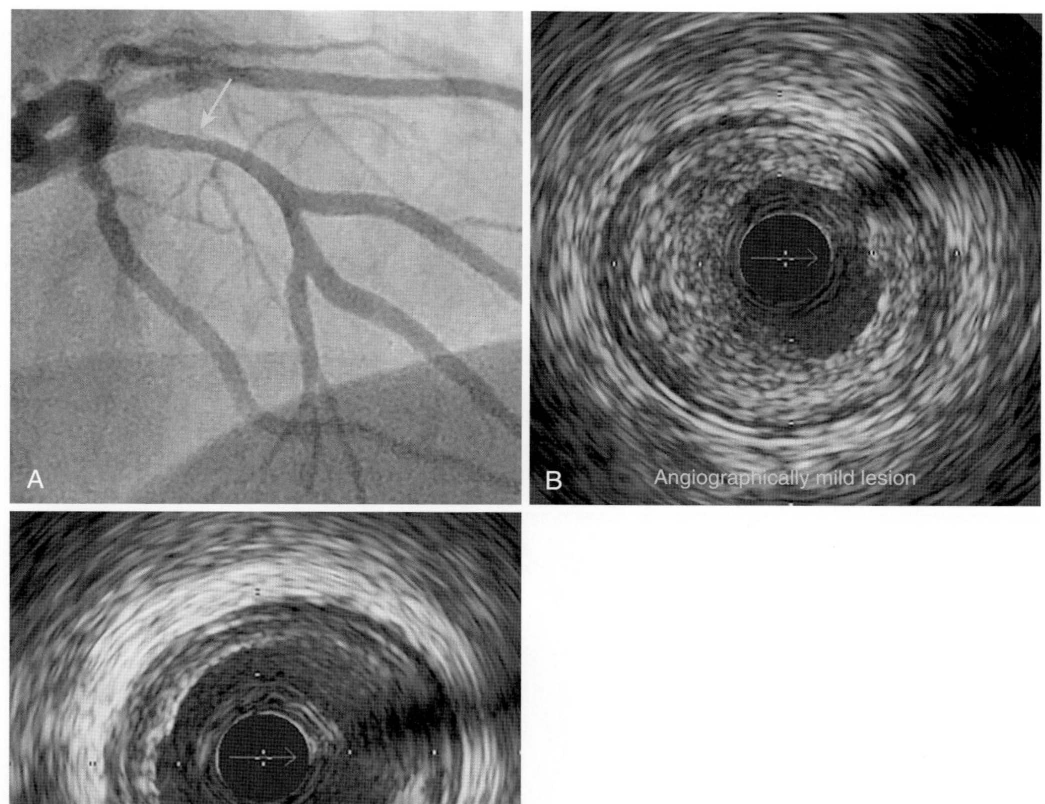

FIGURE 16-1 Angiographic underestimation of disease severity. **A,** A cranial angiographic projection of the left anterior descending artery. There is a proximal segment narrowing *(yellow arrow)* that appears mild to moderate in severity compared to the apparently "normal" proximal midsegment *(orange arrow)*. **B,** IVUS imaging reveals a severe stenosis at the site of the proximal stenosis, with a lumen area of <3.5 mm^2 and cross-sectional narrowing >70%. **C,** The angiographic underestimation is caused by the diffuse nature of disease involving the apparently "normal" segment distal to the lesion. Imaging of that segment reveals moderate stenosis and plaque burden with an eccentric distribution.

location, calcified, or have complex luminal topography. It takes a perfect orthogonal angiographic projection to delineate accurate information about one or more of those findings. Given that projections are frequently selected arbitrarily, it may be difficult for angiographers to visualize the lesion, define the percentage of stenosis, and proceed with a management decision (**Figures 16-3** and **16-4**).[1,2]

Contemporary, well-trained angiographers should be able to utilize adjunctive technologies that can resolve the clinical dilemmas caused by limitations of angiography and reach accurate conclusions. Currently, the most commonly utilized technologies in the cardiac catheterization laboratory are IVUS, optical coherence tomographic (OCT) imaging, and fractional flow reserve (FFR) measurement. While IVUS and OCT imaging address the limitations of angiography related to the resolution and complexities of severity and distribution of disease, FFR measurement addresses the discrepancy between the anatomical and functional significance of coronary lesions.

IVUS IMAGING, BASIC IMAGE, AND MEASUREMENTS

Imaging is performed using a miniaturized ultrasound transducer placed into the center of the vessel lumen on the tip of a catheter. Contemporary imaging catheters are 3 to 3.5 Fr in diameter and can be used within 5 or 6 Fr guiding catheters. Coronary imaging catheters are typically advanced over standard angioplasty guidewires, 0.014 inch in diameter. By emitting and receiving reflected ultrasound beams, sector images can then be generated. Two different technologic approaches are used to generate a circumferential tomographic image of the entire cross section of the vessel: (a) mechanical systems in which the transducer is composed of a single large piezoelectric crystal that is rotated at high speed to acquire images from all sectors of the circumference, and (b) phased array systems in which transducers are made of multiple small crystals that are sequentially activated to image adjacent sectors of the arterial cross section. The imaging frequency is 40 MHz to 45 MHz for the mechanical systems and 20 MHz for the phased array system. In both cases, the reflected ultrasound waveforms are processed into grayscale images and the sectors are reconstructed into the full tomographic cross section of the artery.

Definitions and methodology of acquiring IVUS images and measurements are outlined in the American College of Cardiology and the European Society of Cardiology expert consensus documents on the standards of IVUS imaging.[10-12] Tomographic images obtained by the IVUS transducer show

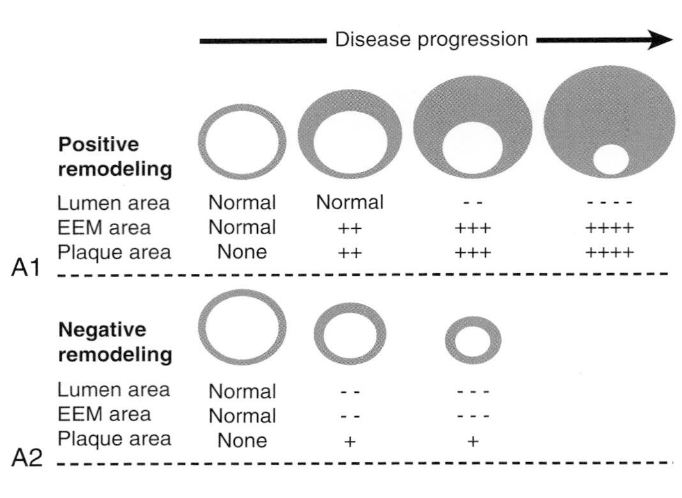

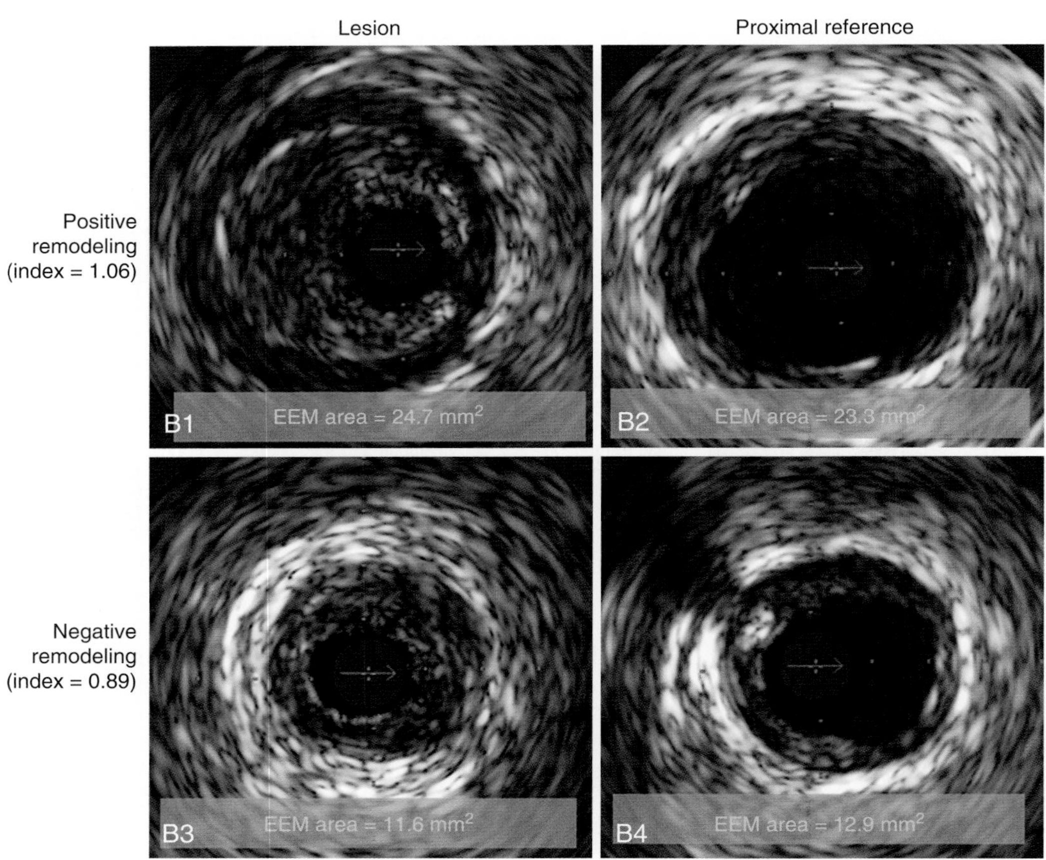

FIGURE 16-2 **A,** Arterial remodeling and disease progression. Schematic depiction of arterial remodeling in response to disease progression. In positive remodeling **(A1),** early plaque accumulation in the arterial wall is associated with compensatory enlargement of the vessel size. This allows plaque accumulation without compromise of lumen size. With disease progression, plaque deposition continues and can no longer be accommodated within the arterial wall, eventually leading to lumen compromise. In negative remodeling **(A2),** the driver of luminal narrowing is not accumulating plaque as much as "shrinkage" of the artery size. The origins of the negative remodeling process and whether it is related to positive remodeling remain unclear. *EEM,* External elastic membrane (outer boundary of the arterial wall). **B,** IVUS examples of coronary arterial remodeling. The remodeling index is calculated by dividing the EEM area at the lesion site by that of the proximal reference segment. **B1** and **B2,** ultrasound images from a patient with unstable clinical presentation obtained at the lesion and proximal reference sites. The lesion shows positive remodeling with a remodeling index of 1.06. **B3** and **B4,** ultrasound images from a patient with chronic stable angina. The lesion shows negative remodeling with an index of 0.89.

the reflection of the intima as an echodense layer, followed by the media as an echolucent stripe. The adventitia is the outer echodense layer that represents the outer boundary of the artery and the adherent connective tissue and gives the arterial wall a trilaminar appearance. Less commonly, and especially in very young individuals, the intima is so thin (<300 μm in thickness) that it leads to signal dropout and the traditional trilaminar appearance is replaced by a monolayer (**Figure 16-5**). Intimal thickening is the hallmark of arterial wall disease. When the intima thickens, it becomes more echodense and easier to visualize on display.

The basic IVUS measurements performed on a coronary artery image are shown in **Figure 16-6**. The echodense intimal leading edge defines the boundaries of the lumen, while the leading edge of the adventitia (the external elastic membrane [EEM]) defines the vessel area. The area between both tracings represents the plaque plus media or atheroma area. Lumen and vessel diameters can be measured as well.

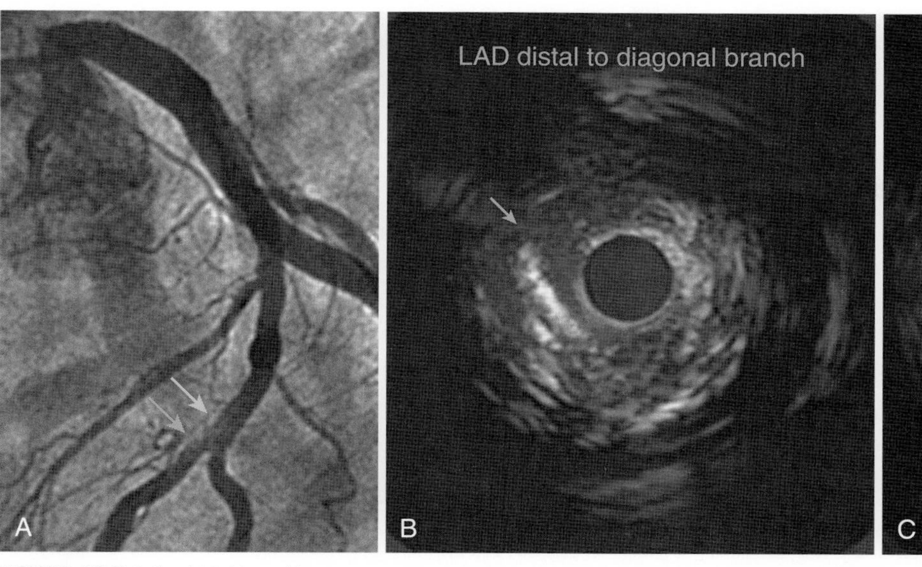

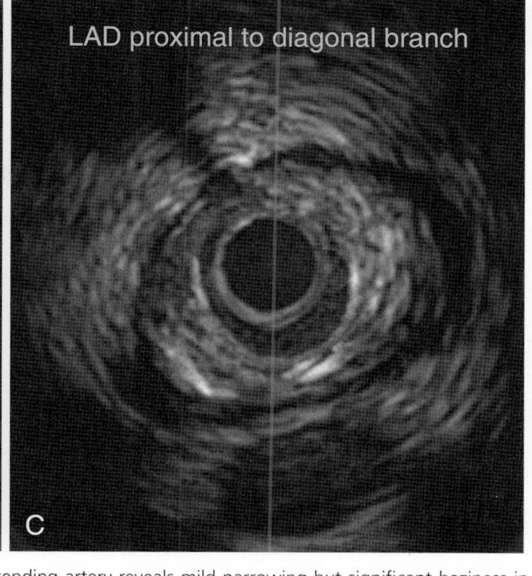

FIGURE 16-3 Role of IVUS in ambiguous coronary angiograms. **A,** An angiogram of the left anterior descending artery reveals mild narrowing but significant haziness in the midsegment opposite the origin of the main diagonal branch. IVUS imaging is performed in the mid-LAD with special attention to the haziness distal and proximal to the bifurcation (*orange* and *yellow arrows,* respectively). **B,** Distal to the diagonal branch, there is severe concentric disease with eccentric dense plaque and evidence of plaque disruption *(arrow).* **C,** Proximal to the diagonal branch, there is concentric plaque with severe luminal narrowing. The plaque disruption, the distribution of plaque, and the severity of disease around the bifurcation contribute to the haziness and result in angiographic underestimation of disease severity.

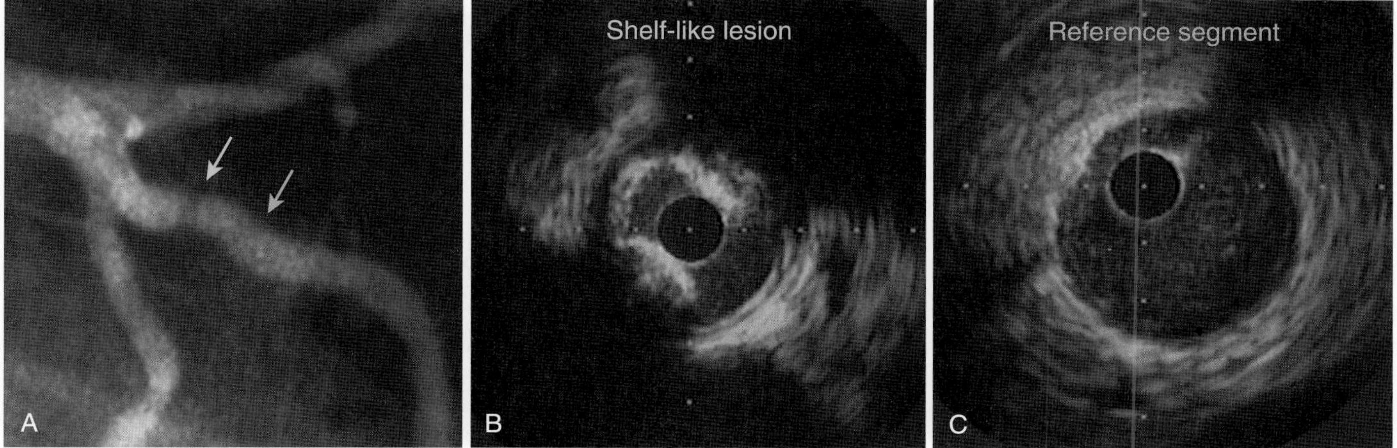

FIGURE 16-4 Role of IVUS in ambiguous coronary angiograms. **A,** The left coronary angiogram reveals a shelf-like lesion in a large, mildly tortuous marginal branch of the circumflex. Despite multiple projections, the lesion severity cannot be well defined. IVUS imaging at the lesion site *(yellow arrow)* reveals a severe, eccentric, heavily calcified plaque **(B)**. The lesion is very focal, such that the reference segment *(orange arrow)* is near normal on the IVUS pullback **(C)**. The calcification, eccentricity, tortuosity, and very short lesion length contributed to the indeterminate angiographic appearance.

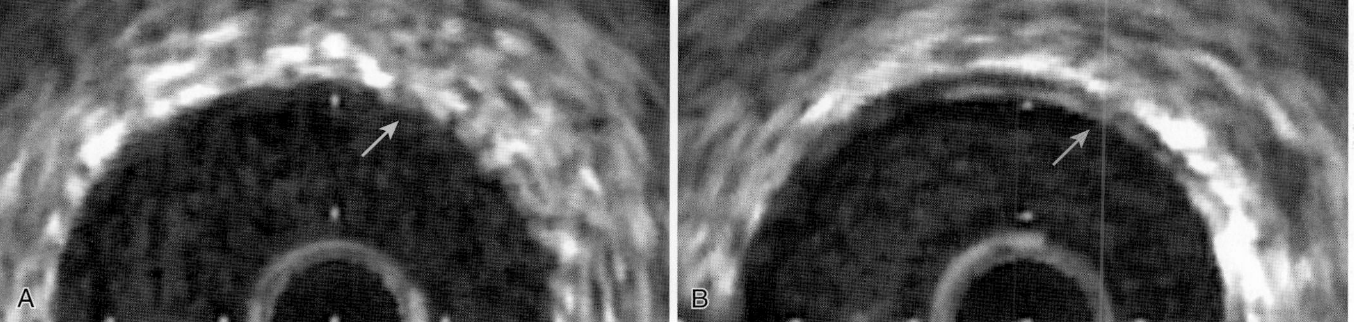

FIGURE 16-5 IVUS images of normal coronary arteries. **A,** The thickness of the normal intima is less than the resolution of the coronary IVUS catheter and thus it may not be visualized. In such a case, the only echodense layer is the adventitia, which leads to a monolayer appearance *(yellow arrow).* **B,** More frequently, the intima is mildly thickened so that it reflects ultrasound signals and can be seen as a leading echodense border *(orange arrow).* This gives the traditional trilaminar appearance of the normal or near-normal coronary arterial wall.

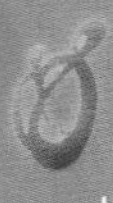

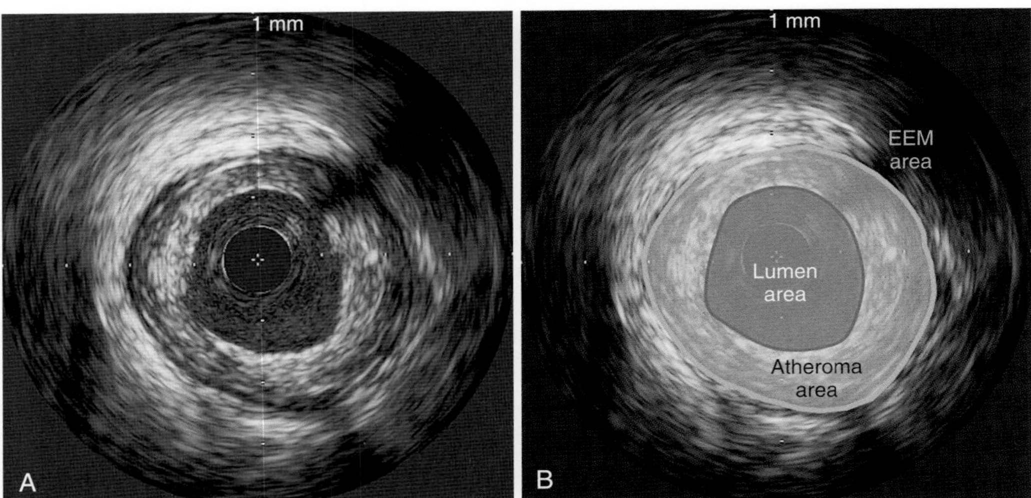

FIGURE 16-6 Basic IVUS measurements on still frames. A typical IVUS image from a patient with coronary artery disease reveals evidence of intimal thickening and some degree of luminal narrowing. A representative image is shown here. The same image is shown on panels **A** and **B,** with the electronic tracings of the intimal leading edge and the external elastic membrane (EEM) superimposed on panel **B.** The tracings form the boundaries of the lumen and vessel, respectively. Areas and diameters are often measured using automated software. The area between the lumen and EEM boundaries represents the atheroma or plaque area. Expressing the plaque area as a percentage of the EEM area is usually referred to as cross-sectional narrowing or plaque burden.

The plaque or atheroma area can be normalized to the size of the vessel by calculating a percentage of the cross-sectional narrowing or plaque burden (plaque area ÷ vessel area × 100).

The IVUS catheter can be mounted on an automatic pull-back device that moves it along the arterial segment at a known and constant velocity (0.5 or 1.0 mm/sec), thus allowing calculation of the length of the segment. Lumen and plaque areas, in addition to length, can then be used to calculate lumen and plaque volume. These are typically more accurate measures of disease burden and are commonly used in research studies, particularly those examining small degrees of progression or regression of plaque size. However, volumetric calculations are time consuming and of less value for everyday clinical applications of IVUS imaging.

Qualitatively, the echodensity of the plaque on grayscale displays is somewhat related to its tissue content. Using the adjacent adventitia as a visual reference, echodensity indicates a plaque is "bright" or "brighter" than adventitia (closer to the white end of the grayscale), while echolucency refers to plaques that appear "darker" than adventitia (closer to the black end of the grayscale). Most plaques are heterogeneous with varying densities, even on the same still frame image (**Figure 16-7**). Plaques rich in lipid are typically echolucent, whereas echodense ones are typically rich in fibrous tissue and calcification. Calcified lesions are usually very dense and have a back shadow due to the complete absorption of the ultrasound beam.[10] The association between echodensity and tissue content is not robust due to the overlap between various levels of grayscale and heterogeneous tissue content. As discussed later, advanced analysis of ultrasound backscatter (such as virtual histology technology) attempts to overcome the limitations of visual analysis of the reconstructed grayscale images.

GUIDELINES FOR USE AND APPROPRIATE INDICATIONS

Over the past two decades, numerous clinical studies have established a number of acceptable and appropriate applications of IVUS imaging in the cardiac catheterization laboratory. The updated clinical practice guideline for coronary interventions published by the ACC, AHA, and SCAI in 2010 outlines the recommendations for coronary IVUS imaging (**Table 16-1**).[11]

The following section reviews the current diagnostic and interventional applications outlined in the guideline statement. In addition, a few more advanced or highly specialized as well as research applications are discussed in detail.

Diagnostic Applications

Ambiguous Angiograms and Indeterminate Coronary Lesions

Vessel overlap, vessel tortuosity, eccentric lesions, ostial or bifurcation lesions, and severe calcification constitute the major reasons for suboptimal angiographic visualization of the lumen (see **Figures 16-3** and **16-4**).

This is particularly important when the lesions are of intermediate (40%-70%) severity in patients with mild or atypical symptoms. In these settings, IVUS imaging provides a tomographic perspective that is independent of the radiographic projection, which allows accurate quantification of lumen size, plaque burden, plaque distribution in relation to branch points, and distribution of calcified plaque.

When an angiographically intermediate lesion (50%-70% diameter stenosis) is encountered, interobserver and intraobserver variability is quite high. Further evaluation can be accomplished either by functional assessment (FFR measurement) or by a more accurate definition of the lumen size using IVUS or OCT imaging. Measurement of FFR accurately defines hemodynamically significant lesions.[13] Multiple prospective randomized trials have validated the use of FFR measurement in clinical decision making on the need for revascularization versus conservative management.[14-16]

IVUS measures that are used to define hemodynamically significant lesions have mostly been benchmarked against established FFR cutoff thresholds. In a small study of 51 lesions, a lesion was considered hemodynamically significant when FFR was <0.75. The IVUS measurements that identified such a lesion were minimum lumen area (MLA)

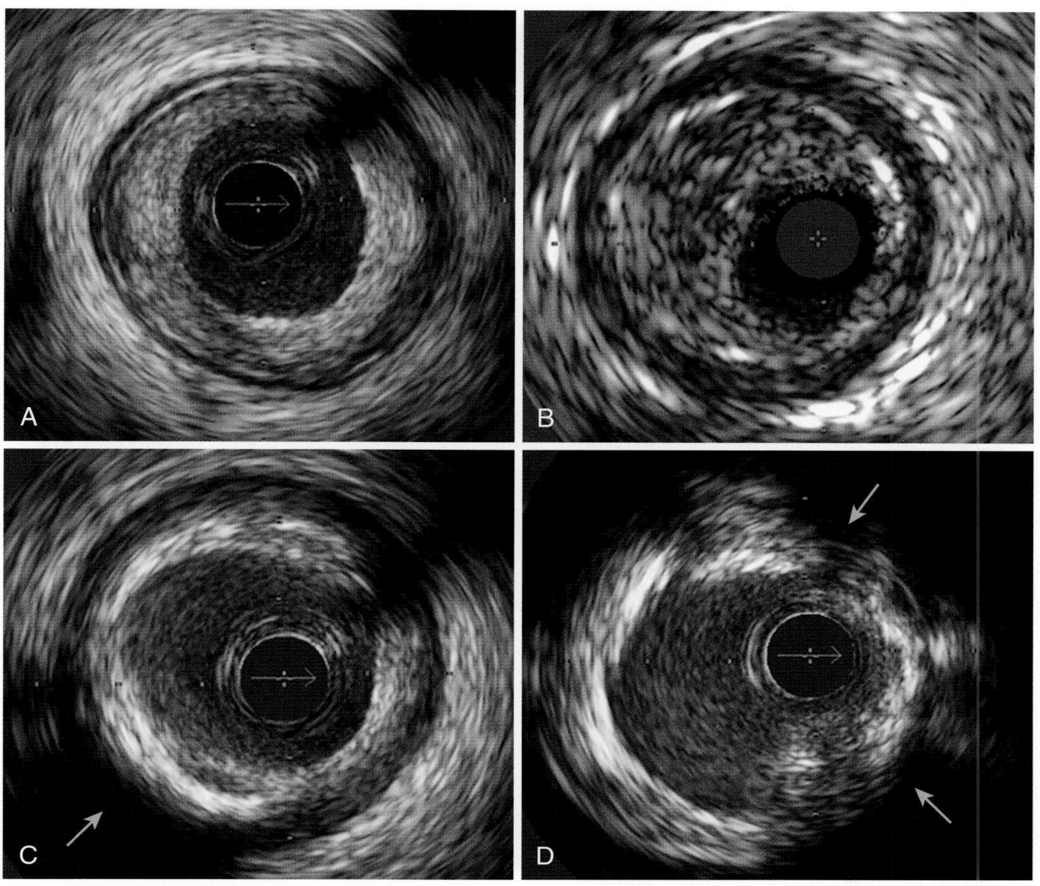

FIGURE 16-7 Typical IVUS plaque morphology and distribution. Atherosclerotic plaques are usually classified according to their echodensity on IVUS images. The density of the surrounding adventitia is used as a reference. Distribution can also be described according to the thickness of plaque on one wall versus the other. **A,** An example of a concentric echodense plaque with mild to moderate lumen compromise. **B,** An eccentric echolucent plaque with severe luminal narrowing. **C,** The plaque is concentric in distribution but heterogeneous in density. An arc of high echodensity and back shadow *(arrow)* is indicative of calcification. **D,** More extensive calcification and back shadow involving more than half the circumference of the artery *(arrows).*

TABLE 16-1 Indications of Coronary IVUS Imaging

Class I
• None
Class IIa
• Assessment of angiographically indeterminate left main CAD *(Level of Evidence: B)* • IVUS imaging and coronary angiography are reasonable 4-6 weeks and 1 year after cardiac transplantation to exclude donor CAD, detect rapidly progressive cardiac allograft vasculopathy, and provide prognostic information *(Level of Evidence: B)* • Determine the mechanism of stent restenosis *(Level of Evidence: C)*
Class IIb
• Assessment of non–left main coronary arteries with angiographically indeterminate coronary stenoses (50%-70% diameter stenosis) *(Level of Evidence: B)* • Guidance of coronary stent implantation, particularly in cases of left main coronary artery stenting *(Level of Evidence: B)* • Determination of the mechanism of stent thrombosis *(Level of Evidence: C)*
Class III
• Routine lesion assessment is not recommended when revascularization with PCI or CABG is not being contemplated *(Level of Evidence: C)*

From Levine GN, Bates ER, Blankenship JC, et al: 2011 ACCF/AHA/SCAI guideline for Percutaneous Coronary Intervention. A report of the American College of Cardiology Foundation/American Heart Association Task Force on practice guidelines and the Soceity for Cardiovascular Angiography and Interventions. J Am Coll Cardiol 58(24):e44–e122, 2011.

<3.0 mm^2 (sensitivity, 83.0%; specificity, 92.3%) and area stenosis >60% (sensitivity, 92.0%; specificity, 88.5%) (**Figure 16-8A**). The combination of both criteria (MLA <3.0 mm^2 and area stenosis <60%) had 100% sensitivity and specificity.[17] In another study of 53 lesions, a minimal luminal diameter (MLD) of <1.8 mm, MLA of ≤4 mm^2, and the cross-sectional area stenosis of >70% were the best indicators of hemodynamic significance, as determined by an FFR <0.75.[18] Methodological differences in the measurements of FFR (such as intracoronary vs. intravenous administration and use of adenosine vs. papaverine for generation of hyperemia) in these two studies may explain the discrepant cutoff values.

As the FFR threshold of <0.8 has been adopted more recently to define ischemia-producing lesions and to address discrepancies in reference vessel size, a larger retrospective analysis of 205 angiographically intermediate lesions was performed using both IVUS and FFR measurements. FFR was <0.8 in 26% of lesions. Overall, there was moderate correlation between FFR and IVUS measurements, including MLA ($r = 0.36$, $p < 0.001$), lesion length ($r = -0.43$, $p < 0.001$), and area stenosis ($r = 0.33$, $p = 0.01$). For the whole sample, an MLA >4.0 mm^2 had an excellent negative predictive value (>94%), and MLA <3.09 mm^2 was the best determinant of lesions with FFR <0.8 (sensitivity, 69.2%; specificity, 79.5%) (**Figure 16-8A**). The correlation between FFR and IVUS was better for large vessels

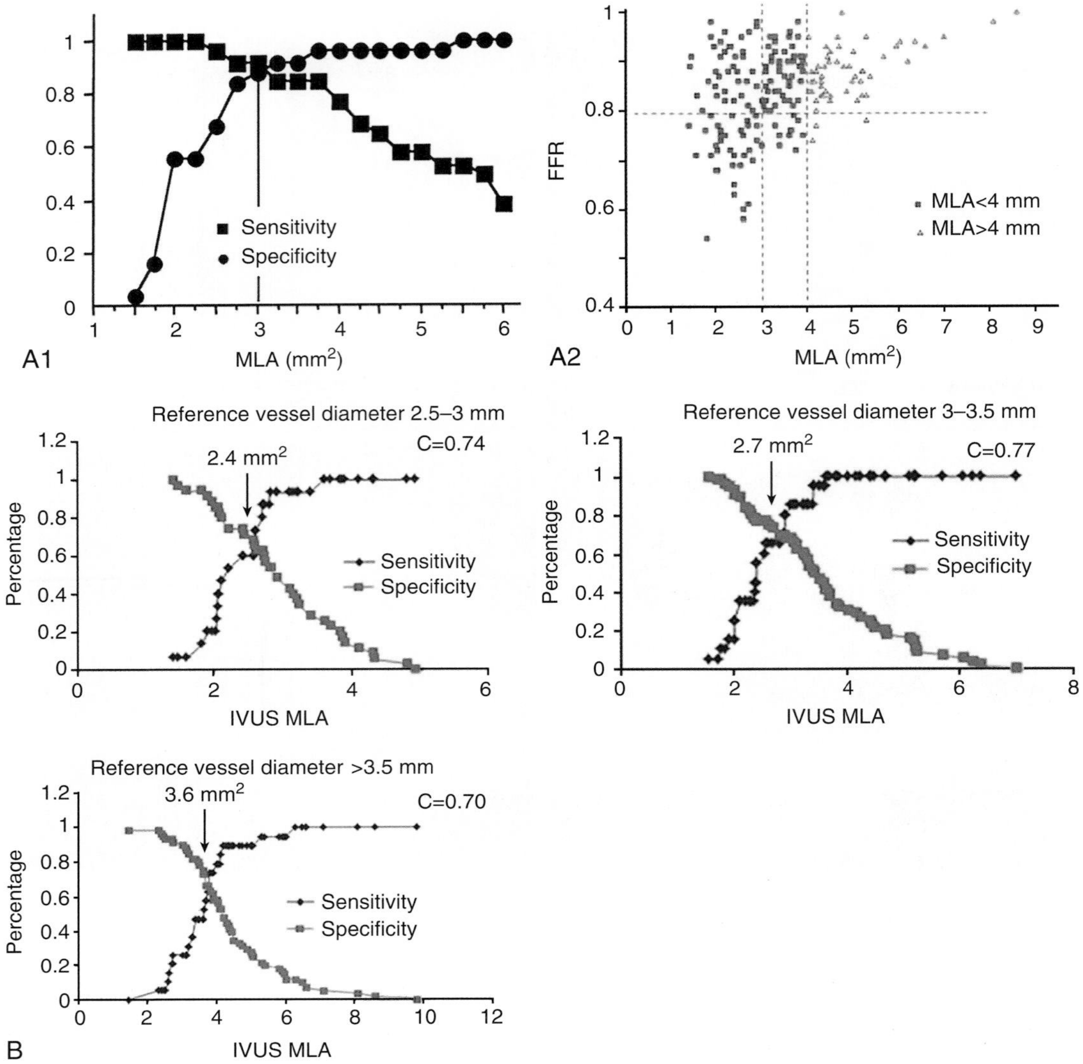

FIGURE 16-8 **A,** Role of IVUS imaging in defining the significance of angiographically intermediate lesions. A threshold of a minimal lumen area of 3.0 mm² provides the most reasonable compromise between sensitivity and specificity for defining hemodynamically significant lesions, based on FFR measurement as the gold standard. An MLA exceeding 4.0 mm² has a high negative predictive value as seen in the results of Ben-Dor I, Torguson R, Deksissa T, et al: Intravascular ultrasound lumen area parameters for assessment of physiological ischemia by fractional flow reserve in intermediate coronary artery stenosis. *Cardiovasc Revasc Med* 13(3):177–182, 2012. **A2,** Cross-sectional narrowing and lesion length are other measures that are predictive of hemodynamic significance (not shown). *(**A1,** From Takagi A, Tsurumi Y, Ishii Y, et al: Clinical potential of intravascular ultrasound for physiological assessment of coronary stenosis: relationship between quantitative ultrasound tomography and pressure-derived fractional flow reserve. Circulation 100:250–255, 1999. **A2,** From Ben-Dor I, Torguson R, Deksissa T, et al: Intravascular ultrasound lumen area parameters for assessment of physiological ischemia by fractional flow reserve in intermediate coronary artery stenosis. Cardiovasc Revasc Med 13(3):177–182, 2012.)* **B,** Role of IVUS imaging in defining significance of angiographically intermediate lesions. The minimal lumen area threshold used to correlate with hemodynamic significance as assessed by FFR varies according to the reference vessel size. *(From Ben-Dor I, Torguson R, Deksissa T, et al: Intravascular ultrasound lumen area parameters for assessment of physiological ischemia by fractional flow reserve in intermediate coronary artery stenosis. Cardiovasc Revasc Med 13(3):177–182, 2012.)*

compared to small vessels. Depending on the reference vessel diameter, threshold MLA values for ischemia-producing lesions (FFR <0.8) are as follows: MLA <2.4 mm² in small vessels, MLA <2.7 mm² in medium-sized vessels, and MLA <3.6 mm² in large vessels (**Figure 16-8B**).[19]

Evaluation of the Left Main Coronary Artery

Angiographic severity of left main coronary artery (LMCA) lesions is almost always difficult to quantify.[20] Visualizing the ostium and most proximal part of the vessel depends on the "reflux" of contrast into the aortic cusp. "Streaming" of contrast from the injection vortex can give a false impression of luminal narrowing near the tip of the injecting catheter. When the whole length of the LMCA is diseased, the absence of a near normal reference segment complicates the visual or automated quantification of stenosis severity. Furthermore, disease in the bifurcation or trifurcation into daughter branches is often complex in topography and is frequently concealed by the overlap of the branches in different projections (**Figure 16-9A**). Thus, reproducibility of quantitative angiography of the LMCA is worse than that of all other coronary arterial segments.[21] For these reasons, IVUS imaging is commonly used for better delineation of LMCA stenoses.

Similar to non–left main coronary lesions, a few studies were based on correlating cutoff values of IVUS measurements with FFR measures of hemodynamic significance of LMCA stenosis. In a study of 55 patients with angiographically ambiguous LMCA, both FFR and IVUS measurements were performed. The two IVUS measurements that

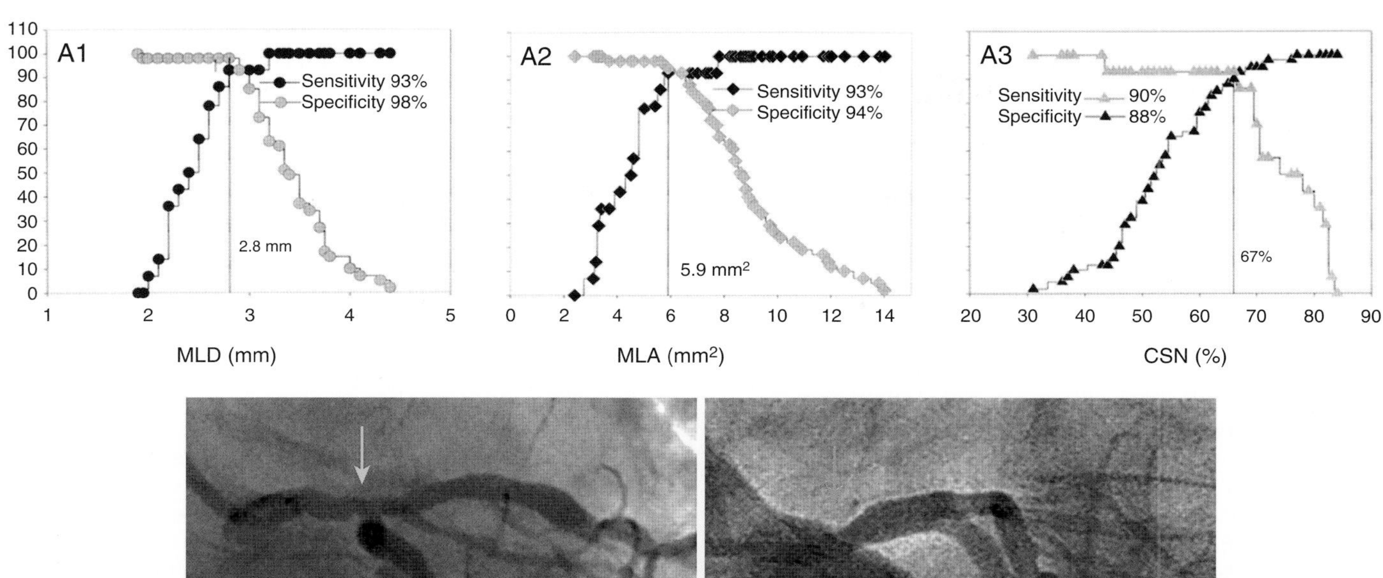

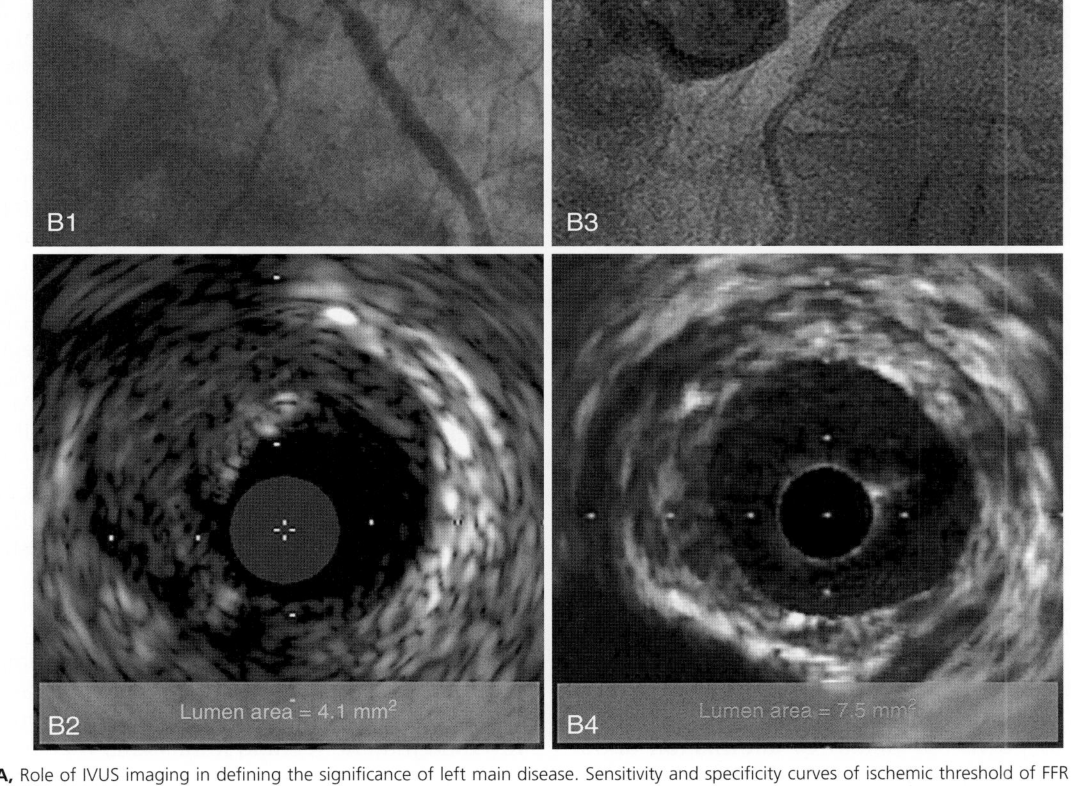

FIGURE 16-9 **A,** Role of IVUS imaging in defining the significance of left main disease. Sensitivity and specificity curves of ischemic threshold of FFR and IVUS parameters in cases of ambiguous left main coronary disease. The FFR cut point was 0.75. Best agreement was found when the minimum lumen diameter was ≤2.8 mm **(A1),** the minimum lumen area was ≤5.9 mm^2 **(A2),** and/or when the cross-sectional narrowing was ≥67% **(A3)**. *(From Jasti V, Ivan E, Yalamanchili V, et al: Correlations between fractional flow reserve and intravascular ultrasound in patients with an ambiguous left main coronary artery stenosis. Circulation 110:2831–2836, 2004.)* **B,** Examples of IVUS imaging of left main disease. **B1,** The caudal angiographic projection reveals a mild distal left main narrowing *(arrow)* in a patient with an early positive stress test. **B2,** IVUS imaging reveals a significant eccentric plaque with an MLA below the threshold of hemodynamic significance typically used (<5.9 mm^2). These findings prompted a referral to coronary bypass surgery. **B3,** an ostial left main lesion is seen on the angiogram without evidence of pressure dampening and in a patient with a marginally positive stress test. **B4,** IVUS imaging reveals an eccentric calcified plaque but a large uncompromised lumen. These findings led to deferral of any revascularization.

correlated best with hemodynamically significant lesions as determined by FFR were MLD <2.8 mm (sensitivity and specificity of 93% and 98%, respectively) and MLA <5.9 mm^2 (sensitivity, 93%; specificity, 95%) (**Figure 16-9B**).[22] In another series of 122 patients with intermediate LMCA stenosis, patients were followed for 1 year following a clinical decision to defer revascularization. Similar to the FFR-based studies, the MLD was the most important predictor of adverse cardiac events. A threshold MLD of 3 mm appeared to provide the best cutoff between those who developed clinical events and those who did not.[23] Other patient series demonstrated the safety of deferring revascularization in patients with LMCA stenosis when the minimum lumen area was >7.5 mm^2.[24]

Evaluation of Transplant Vasculopathy

Cardiac allograft vasculopathy (CAV) is a disease of unclear etiology that affects the coronary arteries of the transplanted heart and is characterized (at least in part) by progressive intimal proliferation of coronary arteries.[25] Due to its diffuse nature, the sensitivity of coronary angiography for detection of CAV is appreciably lower than its sensitivity in detection of the more segmental atherosclerotic lesions.[26,27] IVUS imaging provides a very useful and safe tool to study the early development and progression of CAV.[28-30] CAV is commonly defined as a site where the intimal thickness is ≥0.5 mm,[31,32] although a cutoff value of 0.3 mm is also used as a cutoff to diagnose earlier lesions.[33]

IVUS imaging of coronary arteries soon after transplantation has demonstrated that arteries that appear angiographically normal may contain evidence of early donor atherosclerosis. In one series with a mean donor age of 32 years, atherosclerotic lesions (maximal intimal thickness ≥0.5 mm) were detectable in >50% of patients. Donor atherosclerotic lesions are focal, noncircumferential, maybe calcified, and more commonly involve the proximal segments.[34] Presence of donor atherosclerosis does not seem to predispose to development of CAV.[35,36]

On serial IVUS studies with matched segments, CAV progression initially manifests as increasing intimal thickening associated with compensatory positive remodeling. Lumen compromise over a 5-year follow-up period can also be the result of a negative remodeling response.[37] Several studies have demonstrated an association between disease severity as assessed by IVUS and the clinical outcome in heart transplant recipients.[38,39] Serial studies allow the evaluation of disease progression, which is another important predictor of outcome. In a serial study of 143 patients followed for an average of 5.9 years, IVUS evidence of rapid progression of CAV (defined as ≥0.5-mm increase in intimal thickness in the first year after transplantation) was a powerful predictor of all-cause mortality and MI. Patients with rapidly progressive CAV had a higher mortality rate compared to those without (26% vs. 11%, $p = 0.03$). Death and nonfatal MI were also more frequent among those with rapid progression (51% vs. 16%, $p < 0.0001$).[40]

IVUS imaging has also been used in the evaluation of therapies directed toward control of CAV. The beneficial effects of pravastatin and everolimus in delaying the progression have been shown using IVUS imaging.[41,42]

Interventional Applications

In the 1990s, IVUS coronary imaging was rapidly adopted, as it was seen to provide a wealth of information about atherosclerotic disease patterns that overcame the limitations of angiography and favorably impacted interventional techniques. Hence, it was instrumental in better understanding the pathophysiologic mechanisms of action of various interventional devices and the arterial responses to interventions. This information resulted in improvement in device design and refinement of procedure techniques. Subsequently, the knowledge gained by operators from IVUS imaging became assimilated in the technical approaches. Widespread and routine use of IVUS imaging during interventional procedures tapered down to a more selective approach: situations when specific questions cannot be accurately answered on the basis of angiography alone.

With the predominance of coronary stenting, data supporting the use of IVUS imaging to aid in PCI device selection have become less relevant. In the selected cases where atherectomy is considered, IVUS evaluation may provide useful data about lesion characteristics that lead to the use of one particular device to "prepare" the lesion for stenting. In the following sections, the role of IVUS in guiding coronary stenting is discussed in more detail.

Vessel Sizing

The use of properly sized devices (such as balloons, stents, atherectomy burrs, etc.) is essential to achieve optimal procedural outcomes. The underestimation of reference vessel size and the use of undersized devices increase the risk of suboptimal outcomes such as early recoil, restenosis due to inadequate procedural lumen gain, or stent complications such as stent underexpansion and/or strut malapposition. On the other hand, an oversized device increases the risk of dissection or rupture.

As previously discussed, IVUS imaging frequently reveals significant disease burden in vessels that appear angiographically normal or mildly diseased; thus the true size of the reference vessel can be underestimated (see **Figures 16-1** and **16-3**). Certain clinical scenarios are associated with significant underestimation of angiographic reference vessel size. Examples include PCI in setting of acute myocardial infarction (higher degree of coronary vasomotor tone) and chronic total occlusion (distal segments are underfilled and diffusely diseased). In these situations, adequate coronary vasodilators and IVUS imaging can accurately delineate the reference vessel size, which is the most important determinant of device size selection. Often, after IVUS imaging and quick quantitative analysis, a larger balloon or stent size is accurately and safely selected for use.

It is important for operators to use IVUS imaging for vessel sizing judiciously. The reference vessel size is determined by the lumen diameter in the reference segments, that is, those segments that have no or minimal disease in the vicinity of the lesion to be treated. Using the EEM dimension at the reference or at the site of the lesion will result in overestimation of the vessel size, since EEM diameters reflect a degree of positive remodeling in most cases. This can result in device oversizing and should be avoided. The operator should focus on lumen size, with some adjustment depending on plaque burden.

IVUS Imaging in Coronary Stenting

Historically, IVUS imaging has been instrumental in optimizing the technique of coronary stenting as it is currently practiced. Initial IVUS observations in the early 1990s revealed that the technique of stents was frequently inadequately expanded and not fully opposed to the arterial wall despite satisfactory angiographic results.[43,44] These observations led to major refinements in the technique of stenting, most notably higher pressure postdilatations and the use of upsized balloons. Coupled with the introduction of dual antiplatelet therapy, these technical improvements resulted in a reduction in the incidence of stent thrombosis.[45]

A few terms commonly used in the discussion of IVUS imaging and stenting need to be defined. *Stent expansion* refers to the size of the stent lumen achieved after the stent is deployed and postdilated. That can be expressed in terms of minimum stent lumen diameter (MLD) or more frequently minimum lumen area (MLA). Expansion is also indexed to the size of the reference segments, where MLD

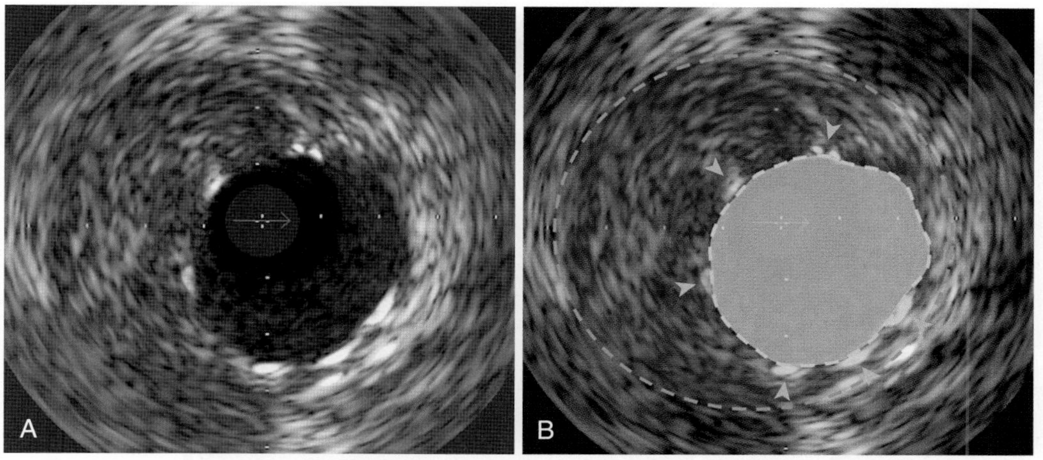

FIGURE 16-10 Stent expansion and strut malapposition. An IVUS image acquired after an undersized stent is deployed in the mid-right coronary artery. The same image is shown on both panels, with the electronic tracings of the stent lumen and the EEM superimposed on panel **B.** The dense metallic struts of the stent are seen in panel **A.** The small size of the stent lumen *(orange)* within the large EEM area *(blue)* represents stent underexpansion and is probably due to underestimation of vessel size. However, the stent struts *(arrowheads)* are all well opposed to the border of the plaque and thus there is no evidence of malapposition.

or MLA is divided by the mean diameter or area of the reference vessel to express a percentage of the reference. Stent MLA is an important predictor of restenosis, as is discussed later. *Stent* or *strut apposition* describes the contact between the stent struts and the underlying arterial wall. This is a qualitative metric of stenting that is detected with advanced imaging such as IVUS or OCT. It is related but not synonymous with stent expansion. It is common to see a well-opposed but underexpanded stent, for example, when the stent is slightly undersized or if a rigid lesion is not adequately predilated (**Figure 16-10**). *IVUS-guided stenting* refers to the strategy of using IVUS imaging to optimize all aspects of the stenting procedure, that is, using IVUS to assess vessel size, facilitate lesion preparation, assess adequate expansion and apposition, confirm results after post-dilation, and ensure the absence of complications in the reference segments (**Figure 16-11**).

Specific criteria to define optimal stent expansion were developed out of multiple observation studies that correlated final IVUS measurements with angiographic and/or clinical outcome.[46-50] The general consensus among those studies is that minimum in-stent lumen dimensions are the most important predictors of restenosis.[51]

Bare-Metal Stents

In bare-metal stents (BMS), minimum stent area <6 mm^2 was associated with the highest rates of restenosis and need for repeat revascularization (**Figure 16-12**).[50,52] The lumen area within the stented segment is primarily determined by the target vessel size, explaining the relatively higher rates of restenosis in smaller vessels despite the achievement of excellent procedural results in the majority of cases (**Figure 16-13**).

The strategy of IVUS-guided bare-metal stenting has been evaluated in several nonrandomized registries[52-56] and some randomized trials.[57-59] There is a general consensus that this did not alter the incidence of death and nonfatal MI, but it did consistently lead to a larger in-stent lumen dimension as a result of higher pressure and/or balloon upsizing. Whether that translates into a reduction in clinical restenosis and need for repeat revascularization remains controversial. Results have not been consistent and favorable results were observed more in the registries than in the randomized trials.

In the study by Schiele et al., 155 patients undergoing coronary stenting were randomized to IVUS guidance versus angiographic guidance.[57] Stent MLA was 20% larger in the IVUS-guided stenting arm, and at 6 months, there was a 22% relative reduction in angiographic binary restenosis in favor of the IVUS guidance arm (22.5% vs. 28.8%). However, this did not reach statistical significance ($p = 0.25$). This result was influenced by the small sample size and the overestimation of the expected benefit attributed to the use of IVUS guidance when the study was being designed. OPTICUS, the largest reported randomized trial on the comparison of IVUS-guided versus angiography-guided stenting, showed similar binary restenosis rates (24.5% and 22.8%, $p = 0.68$) and similar target vessel revascularization rates at follow-up, although acute gain was significantly higher in the IVUS-guided lesions.[58] OPTICUS specifically included patients with lesions ≤25 mm in length and vessels ≥2.5 mm in diameter. Another randomized study, the TULIP trial, investigated the possible role of IVUS in stenting long (≥20 mm) stenoses.[59] Binary restenosis and ischemia-driven target lesion revascularization were less common with IVUS guidance compared with angiography guidance (23% vs. 46%, $p = 0.008$, and 4% and 14%, $p = 0.037$, respectively). These studies do suggest that while IVUS imaging may not be needed to improve outcomes in every case, it may be of value in subsets of cases in which the risk of restenosis is elevated or carries a higher risk. In these cases, operators need to achieve a perfect or near perfect procedural result, which can only be accomplished by IVUS guidance.

Two recently published metaanalyses have also reached different conclusions. The first included seven randomized trials of IVUS versus angiographic guidance of bare-metal stenting in over 2000 patients. Overall, IVUS guidance results in improved procedural outcomes and significantly reduces the risk of repeat revascularization (13% vs. 18%, odds ratio 0.66, 95% CI, 0.48 to 0.91, $p = 0.004$).[60] Although this analysis does demonstrate an advantage of IVUS guidance, that conclusion was mostly driven by the results of two of the smaller studies that accounted for 25% of the weight of the analysis. Such a difference between IVUS and angiographic

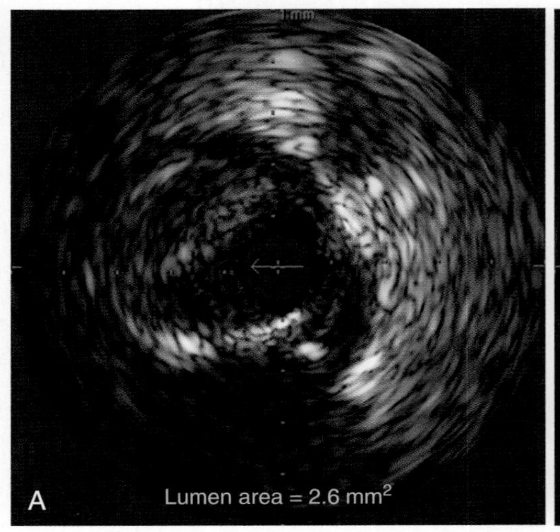

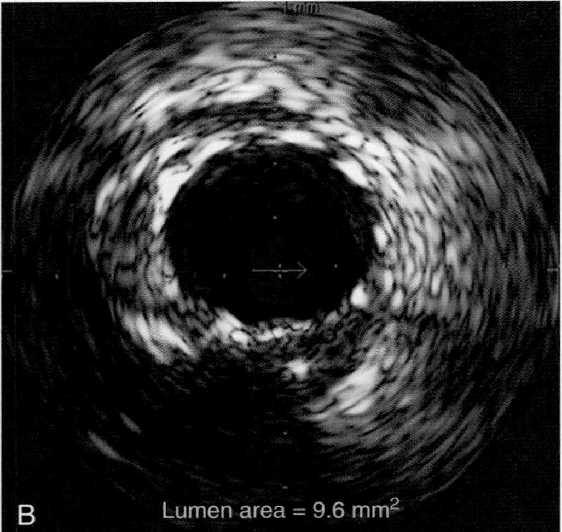

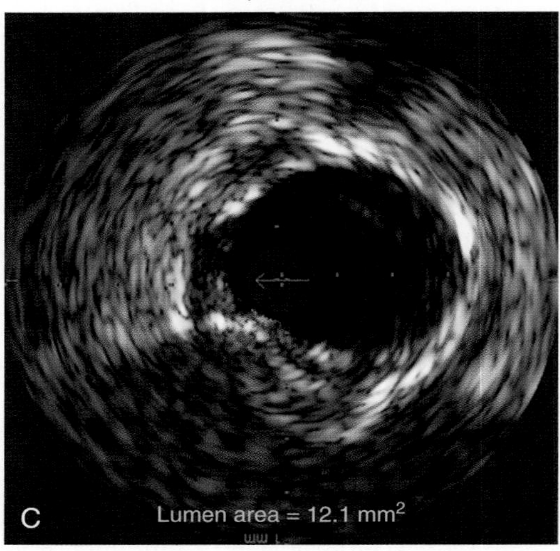

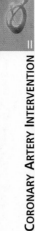

FIGURE 16-11 Example of IVUS-guided stenting. Preintervention IVUS **(A)** reveals a large plaque burden with mostly echolucent content but with eccentric calcification. Following balloon predilation and stent deployment at moderately high pressure **(B),** the struts are well opposed, but the stent lumen area appears small compared to the size of the vessel. Further postdilation using an appropriately sized noncompliant balloon improves the minimum stent lumen area (**C,** image rotated to facilitate comparison).

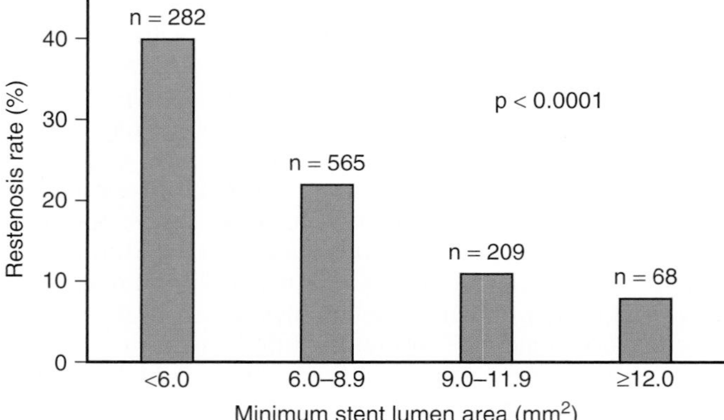

FIGURE 16-12 Impact of minimum stent lumen area on rate of restenosis after bare metal stenting. The relationship is what has traditionally been known as "bigger is better." The inverse correlation is continuous, but there is a near doubling of the restenosis rate when the area is <6 mm^2. *(From Kasaoka S, Tobis JM, Akiyama T, et al: Angiographic and intravascular ultrasound predictors of in-stent restenosis. J Am Coll Cardiol 32:1630–1635, 1998.)*

guidance could not be demonstrated in the larger included studies. Additionally, the included studies were not homogeneous in methodology or patient populations, which raises concerns about the generalizability of the conclusion. A second metaanalysis addressing the same topic included only five randomized controlled trials including 1754 patients.[61] The investigators were not able to demonstrate any improvement in clinical outcomes with IVUS guidance. This metaanalysis can also be criticized for the process of selection that may have left out studies fairly similar in methodology to ones that were included.

Drug-Eluting Stents

With more widespread use of DES and the lower rates of restenosis, the potential advantage of IVUS guidance to reduce restenosis has become less significant. Early in the DES era, several IVUS studies and substudies were performed to better understand the predictors and mechanisms of DES restenosis. Subsequently, there was significant interest in understanding mechanisms of stent thrombosis and the insights that IVUS can provide in these settings.

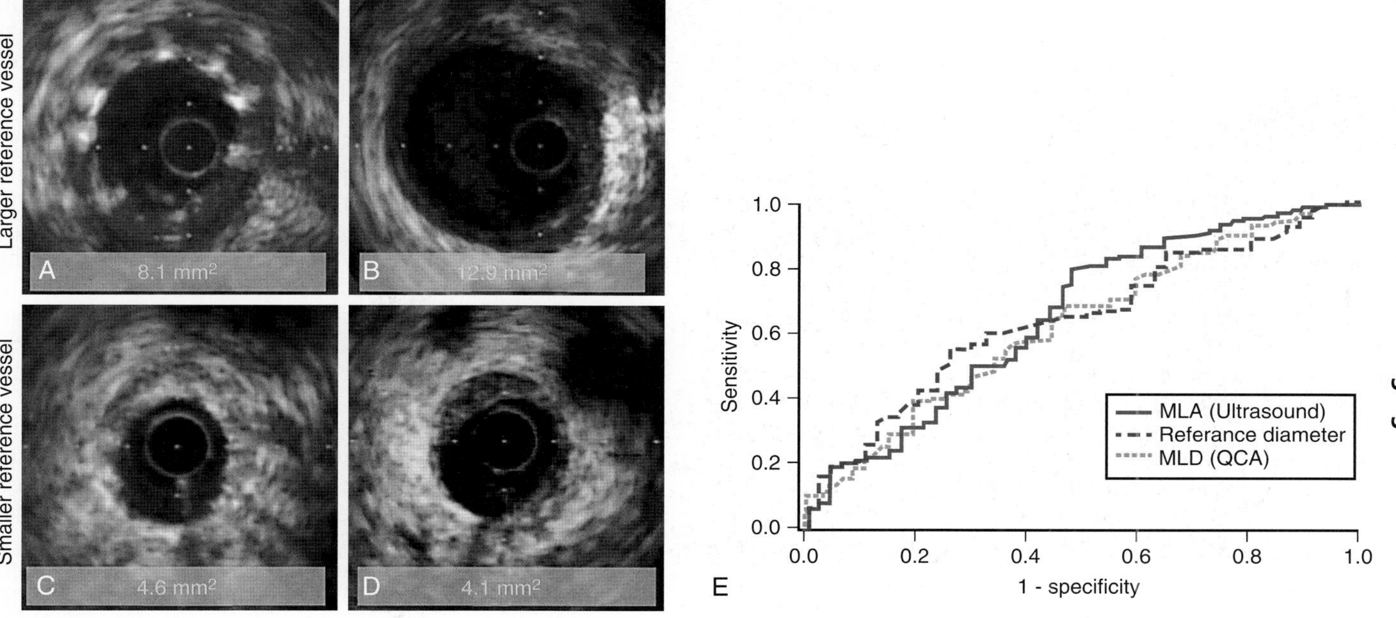

FIGURE 16-13 Impact of reference vessel size on outcome of stenting. The final stent lumen size is primarily determined by the reference vessel size. In larger vessels **(A, B)**, a larger stent MLA can be obtained even if there is a residual stenosis compared to the reference vessel. On the contrary, the stent lumen will be small even if there is no residual stenosis in a smaller reference vessel **(C, D)**. Receiver operator curves **(E)** demonstrate that the minimum stent lumen area is not a better predictor of target vessel revascularization than the reference vessel diameter, emphasizing the importance of vessel size in determining outcome. *(From Ziada KM, Kapadia SR, Belli G, et al: Prognostic value of absolute versus relative measures of the procedural result after successful coronary stenting: importance of vessel size in predicting long-term freedom from target vessel revascularization. Am Heart J 141:823–831, 2001.)*

IVUS imaging studies of the first generation sirolimus-eluting stents (SES) demonstrated that a postprocedural minimum stent area of <5 mm to 5.5 mm^2 was the most important predictor of angiographic binary restenosis at 6 to 9 months.[62,63] A larger analysis of a number of IVUS substudies performed within the TAXUS trial program examined the outcomes of the paclitaxel-eluting stents (PES).[64] This included 1580 PES and control group patients. Postprocedure, the stent MLA was similar in PES and BMS (6.6 mm ± 2.5 mm^2 vs. 6.7 mm ± 2.3 mm^2, $p = 0.92$). At 9 months, in-stent restenosis was significantly lower in the PES group (10% vs. 31%, $p < 0.0001$). Postintervention stent MLA by IVUS was the independent predictor of subsequent restenosis in both the PES and control BMS groups ($p = 0.0002$ for PES and $p = 0.0002$ for BMS). The optimal thresholds of postprocedure IVUS MLA that best predicted stent patency at 9 months were 5.7 mm^2 for PES and 6.4 mm^2 for BMS.

One of only two prospective randomized trials of IVUS-guided DES stenting included 284 patients and focused on complex lesions defined as bifurcations, long lesions, chronic total occlusions, or small vessels. The primary endpoint was the postprocedure MLD. This showed a statistically significant difference in favor of the IVUS group (2.70 mm ± 0.46 mm vs. 2.51 ± 0.46 mm, $p = 0.0002$). At 24 months, there was no difference in death or MI. Target vessel revascularization was nonsignificantly lowered in the IVUS-guided group compared to the angiography-guided arm (9.8% vs. 15.5%).[65] A similarly designed Korean randomized trial of 543 patients with long lesions treated with DES and randomized to IVUS guidance versus angiography guidance showed no difference in postprocedure stent length or MLD. The authors attributed that lack of improvement in the IVUS-guided arm to the high rate of crossover to IVUS utilization in the angiography-guided arm, which was allowed by protocol and occurred in 15% of patients.[66]

A specific high-risk group of patients in whom IVUS guidance has a valuable role are those undergoing unprotected LMCA stenting. In the MAIN-COMPARE registry, data from approximately 1000 stable patients undergoing unprotected left main stenting was compiled. IVUS guidance was used in 80% of cases. The 3-year outcomes were compared between the two groups using propensity-score matching in the entire population and separately in those receiving DES. In 201 matched pairs of the overall population, there was a trend toward reduced mortality with IVUS guidance compared with angiography guidance, but that did not reach statistical significance (6.0% vs. 13.6%, Cox-model $p = 0.061$). In the 145 matched pairs of patients receiving DES, mortality was lower with IVUS guidance (4.7% vs. 16.0%, log-rank $p = 0.048$; hazard ratio, 0.39; 95% CI, 0.15 to 1.02; Cox model $p = 0.055$). While the statistical significance of the benefit appears marginal and the underlying mechanism is unclear, it may be hypothesized that optimal expansion and apposition achieved by IVUS guidance may reduce the risk of late and very late stent thrombosis with DES.[67]

A large metaanalysis examined the role of IVUS guidance of DES procedures on clinical outcome. The metaanalysis included a very large number of patients (approximately 20,000), but it was weakened by the propensity of uncontrolled, nonrandomized patient registries (of the 20,000 patients included, there were only 105 randomized patients from one trial). That analysis demonstrated an improvement in death and rates of stent thrombosis with IVUS guidance compared to angiography alone but no difference in the need for repeat revascularization. While intriguing, these conclusions were primarily driven by results from two or three uncontrolled registries with unadjudicated outcomes and should be considered with caution.[68]

Recent data suggest much more significant advantages to IVUS guidance of DES procedures, with evidence of reduced risk of stent thrombosis, myocardial infarction, and major adverse events. This was generated from the ADAPT-DES trial, which was a prospective, multicenter registry of 8583 patients receiving DES, of whom 3349 (39%) were enrolled in a prespecified IVUS substudy. The study aimed to determine the frequency, timing, and correlates of early and late stent thrombosis. Patients in the IVUS imaging arm were more likely to have ACS. IVUS guidance led to a modification of the intended procedure in 74% of cases (larger stent, longer stent, additional stent, additional postdilation, and/or higher pressures). After 1 year of follow-up, definite/probable stent thrombosis occurred in 18 (0.6%) patients in the IVUS group versus 53 (1.0%) in the non-IVUS group (HR 0.4, 95% CI 0.20, 0.7, p = 0.003). Other adverse clinical outcomes were significantly reduced in the IVUS-guided arm (**Table 16-2**). After propensity matching, the use of IVUS remained an independent predictor of freedom from probable/definite stent thrombosis.[69]

Strut Malapposition

Due to the heightened awareness and concern about DES thrombosis events, the clinical impact of strut malapposition may be significant, and a lower threshold for IVUS examination may be justifiable after stenting (**Figure 16-14**) (Video 16-1). IVUS studies have demonstrated evidence of incomplete apposition of DES struts, more commonly seen at the distal stent edge than at the proximal or mid segments. Possible explanations include mismatch between the size of the lumen at the reference segment and the selected stent size. Lesion calcification is also another predictor of malapposition observed on IVUS studies.[70-72]

It is unclear whether minor strut malapposition is related to acute or subacute stent thrombosis with DES, although evidence for this appears circumstantial. In a small retrospective study of patients who returned with late DES thrombosis, the prevalence of strut malapposition was 77%, compared with 12% in a control group of DES patients whose stents were imaged at 8 months during routine follow-up and who did not have documented stent thrombosis. The highly statistically significant difference suggests that strut malapposition may have a role in precipitating this catastrophic complication.[73]

Importantly, other studies do not show that early strut malapposition may not be related to early thrombosis. In a small retrospective IVUS study, 15 patients with thrombosis and 45 control patients were examined. There was no difference in the prevalence of malapposition. However, stent MLA was significantly smaller in those who developed stent thrombosis (4.3 ± 1.6 mm^2 vs. 6.2 ± 1.9 mm^2, $p < 0.001$) compared to the matched controls. Additionally, severe reference segment disease was more common in the stent thrombosis group (67% vs. 9%, $p < 0.001$).[74] This highlights the importance of reference segment disease, which operators should consider carefully following stenting. Frequently, an additional stent to treat a severely diseased reference segment may avoid this concern, although no clear data exist to support this practice.

TABLE 16-2 ADAPT-DES Major Cardiac Adverse Outcomes within 1 Year of Follow-Up

	IVUS GROUP (N = 3343)	NON-IVUS GROUP (N = 5234)	HR (95% CI)	P VALUE
Probable/definite stent thrombosis	0.6%	1.0%	0.4 (0.2-0.7)	0.02
Myocardial infarction	2.5%	3.7%	0.7 (0.5-0.9)	0.002
Ischemic target vessel revascularization	2.4%	4.0%	0.6 (0.2-0.8)	0.0001
MACE (death/MI/stent thrombosis)	3.1%	4.7%	0.7 (0.6-0.9)	0.0006

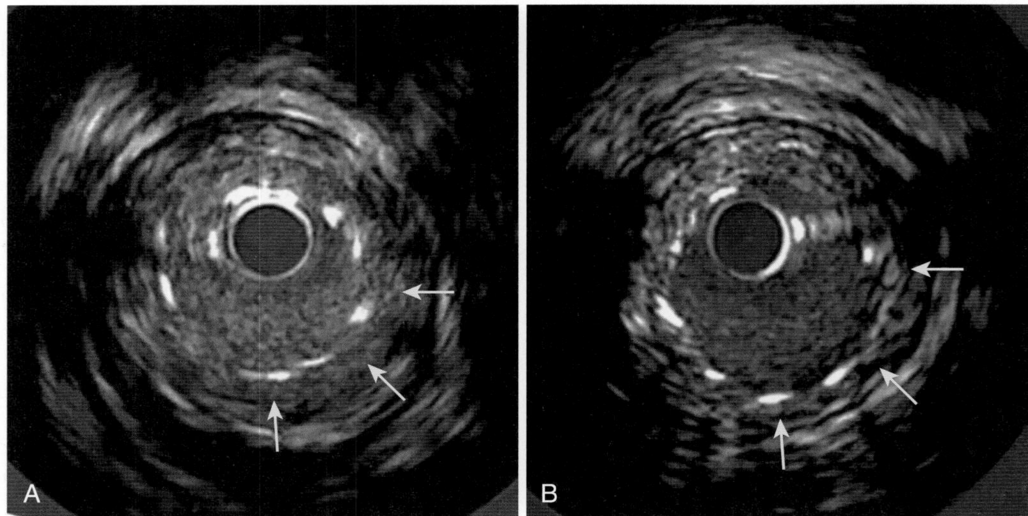

FIGURE 16-14 Strut malapposition. IVUS imaging after stenting reveals significant strut malapposition (**A,** *arrows*), probably due to an underestimation of the vessel size during stent selection. Subsequent postdilation using a larger noncompliant balloon results in complete apposition and a larger stent lumen area **(B)**.

Strut malapposition is not always a residual finding detected immediately after stent implantation. The phenomenon of late malapposition has also been described on follow-up IVUS imaging. That phenomenon has been estimated to occur in approximately 5% of BMS procedures but did not appear to have any clinical consequences.[75] Late malapposition has increased in prevalence with the use of DES. In a recent analysis of 705 lesions in 557 patients, the incidence was 12% in the overall population, with a higher prevalence in patients with longer stents, those who received DES in context of acute MI, or after chronic total occlusion.[76]

Yet, in this series, there was no evidence of increased clinical events in this subset of patients for a period of 10 months after the identification of late strut malapposition. These findings suggest that strut malapposition is of particular concern in situations in which there is difficulty in selecting an appropriate stent size, such as in long and diffusely diseased segments, MI angioplasty, and chronic total occlusions, or in case of a large vessel size mismatch between proximal and distal reference segments. While it is not definitive that this phenomenon is related to DES late thrombosis, it is prudent to optimize stent expansion and apposition with IVUS guidance in these situations.

Management of Stent Restenosis

IVUS imaging has provided an important perspective to study the mechanisms of restenosis following the use of various interventional devices including stents.[77-79] Unlike balloon angioplasty and stand-alone atherectomy, there is no significant recoil or negative remodeling associated with stent restenosis. True in-stent restenosis (ISR) is caused by neointimal hyperplastic response that is initiated at the time of arterial wall injury caused by stent implantation. Approximately 20% of stent "restenosis" results from initial underexpansion at the time of deployment, defined as a final in-stent MLA <80% of the average reference lumen area (**Figure 16-15**).[80] Additionally, the exact localization of the restenotic site is an important variable in deciding among treatment options. If restenosis is within the stent, higher pressure inflation can be effective. Conversely, this strategy may not be appropriate to treat edge restenosis or restenosis occurring primarily in the reference segments.

When stents are adequately expanded at the time of deployment, a more conventional restenosis is caused by intimal hyperplasia within the stent struts. In such cases, restenting with DES or brachytherapy are the available options for percutaneous therapy. Although the use of debulking devices (e.g., rotational atherectomy or laser ablation) makes theoretical sense in these cases, randomized trials have shown that these therapies are not superior to simple balloon angioplasty for treatment of ISR.[81,82] In cases in which the stent was never fully expanded at the time of deployment, treatment can be difficult. Further high-pressure and/or upsized balloon dilatations based on IVUS measurements can be performed, although the initial underexpansion is usually secondary to heavy calcification or dense fibrotic plaques, which may not yield to balloon dilation.

It is difficult to compare various strategies given the small absolute number of stent restenosis cases seen with widespread DES use. Late lumen loss, determined by IVUS, has been used as a surrogate endpoint to compare results of various strategies, including different DES and patient populations.[83]

Assessment of Complications After Intervention

Coronary dissection is the most common cause of acute arterial closure during PCI and can result in serious complications, including MI and emergency bypass surgery. IVUS is more sensitive in the detection of dissections as compared to angiography and can localize the extension of dissection in the arterial wall more accurately (**Figure 16-16**) (Video 16-2).

An IVUS classification of dissections is primarily based on the depth of the dissection (i.e., intimal, medial, or extending to the adventitia).[84] IVUS imaging is also helpful in identifying intramural hematoma that may accompany a dissection. However, the prognosis and treatment of an intramural hematoma after intervention remain largely unknown.[85] Although the axial and circumferential extent

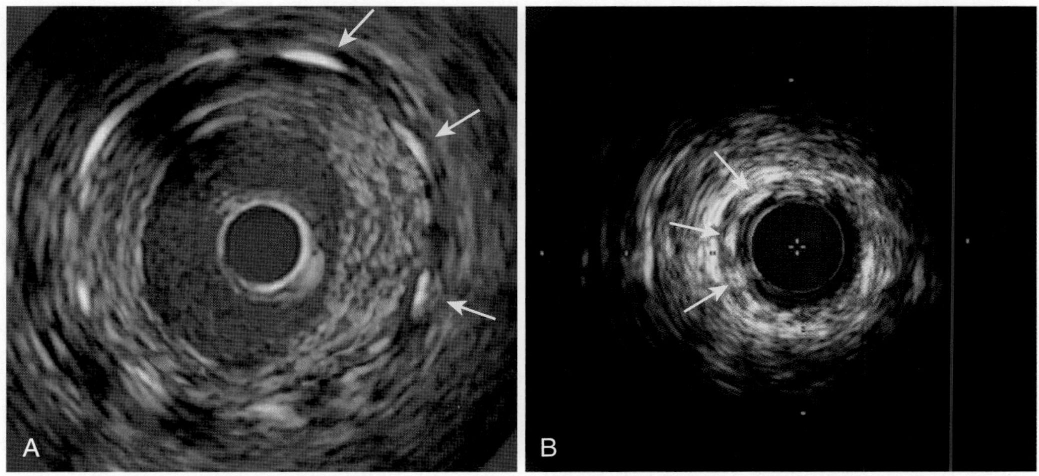

FIGURE 16-15 Mechanisms of stent restenosis. Stent lumen loss or true stent restenosis is caused by intimal hyperplasia within the boundaries of the stent struts **(A)**. The originally deployed stent appears to have been well expanded. In 20% of cases of restenotic stents, the mechanism is failure to expand at the time of deployment, frequently because of undersizing and/or dense or calcified plaque **(B)**. In these cases, neointima within the stent lumen is not the main mechanism of lumen loss; hence it can be considered "pseudo restenosis."

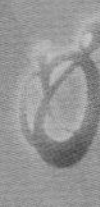

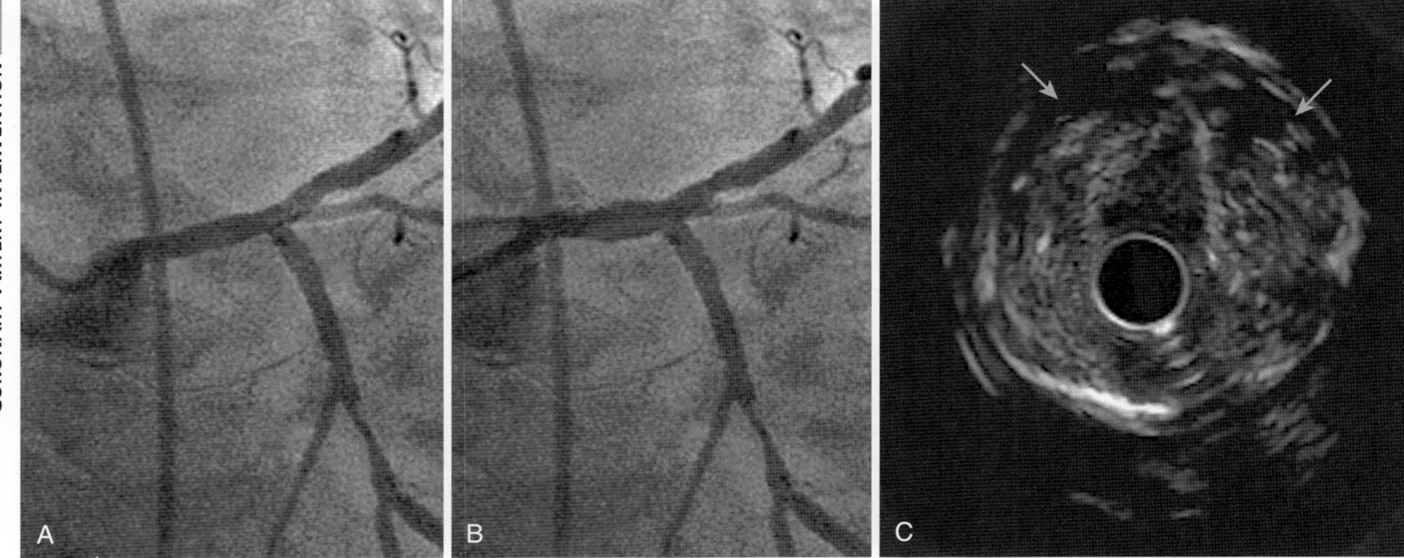

FIGURE 16-16 Role of IVUS imaging in delineating procedural complications. After obtaining diagnostic angiograms **(A)**, left circumflex intervention is planned. Minimal diffuse disease of the left main trunk and anterior descending artery is noted. Following guide catheter engagement **(B)**, the following angiograms reveal haziness and an "increase is size" of the left main trunk. IVUS imaging **(C)** delineates an extensive dissection, compromise of the lumen, and a developing intramural hematoma *(arrows)*.

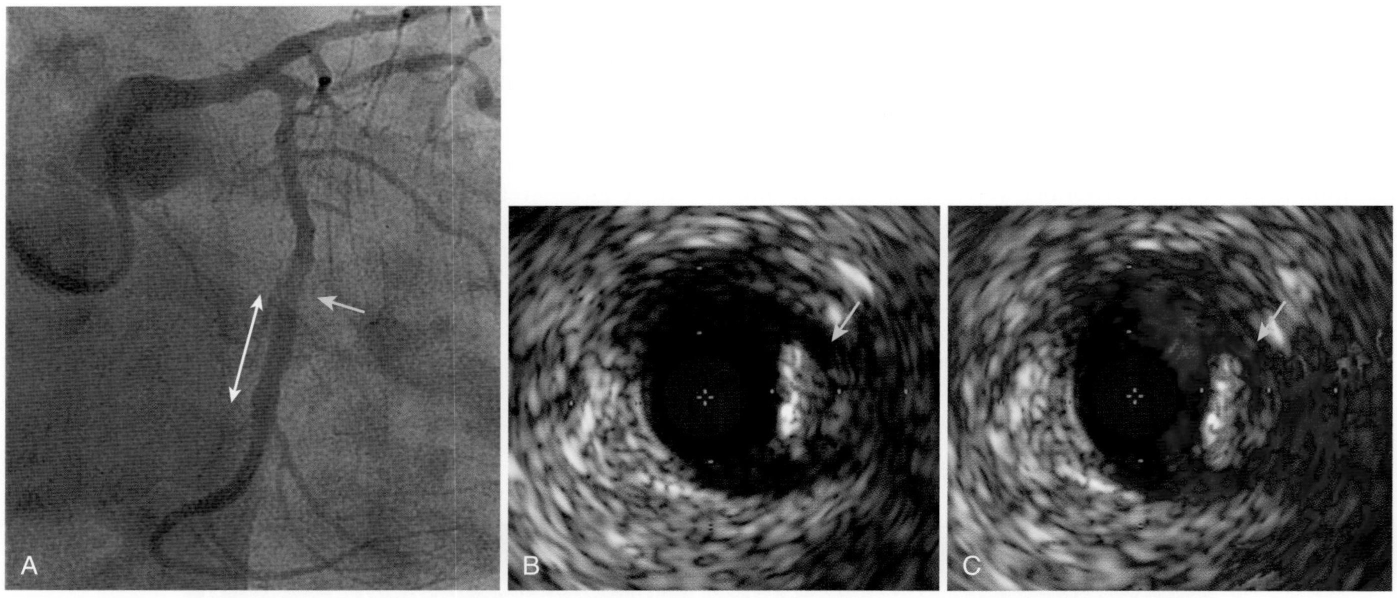

FIGURE 16-17 Peri-stent haziness. Following stent deployment in the mid circumflex artery (**A,** *white arrow*), an area of angiographic haziness was noted in the proximal reference segment *(yellow arrow)*. The stent appears slightly oversized. Grayscale IVUS imaging **(B)** demonstrates significant disease in the reference with a small lumen. In addition, intraluminal speckle appears to extend behind an intimal flap *(arrow)*, diagnostic of an edge dissection. Confirmation is obtained by ChromaFlo **(C),** where color flow is seen behind the intimal flap *(arrow)*. An additional stent was placed proximal to and overlapping with the first stent to cover the dissected segment.

of dissections can be better characterized on IVUS imaging, the prognostic value of IVUS findings remains unclear. Most non-flow-limiting dissections without high-risk features (i.e., persistence of contrast and spiral dissections) can be treated conservatively without additional mechanical interventions. Whenever stenting is indicated for an edge dissection, ultrasound imaging often reveals the involvement of a longer segment than can be appreciated angiographically. This is particularly relevant in cases of bailout stenting for threatened abrupt closure, where it is critical to cover the entire length of the dissected segment. In such cases, a residual dissection in the vicinity of the bailout stent(s) adds to the already higher risk of stent thrombosis.[86]

Angiographic "haziness" after stenting is used to describe the nonhomogeneous density or "ground glass" appearance that is seen in the stent reference segment. Frequently, haziness is subtle and angiography does not reveal a clear etiology. The incidence of peri-stent haziness without an obvious cause has been reported to be 15% with high-pressure stenting. The main causes usually revealed on IVUS imaging are edge dissections or a significant step-down of the luminal area from the edge of the stent to a moderately diseased reference segment (**Figures 16-17** and **16-18**).[87]

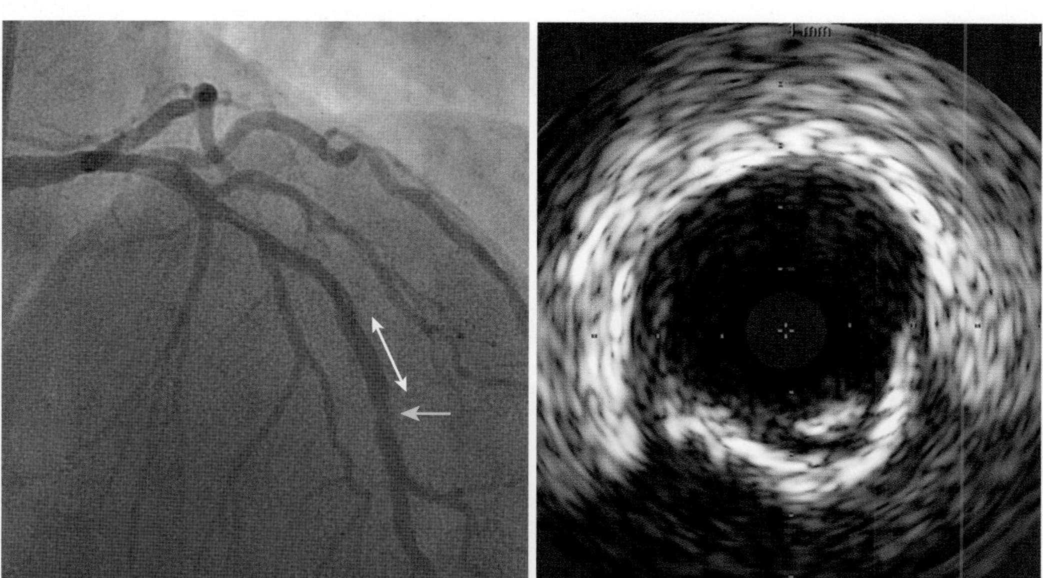

FIGURE 16-18 Peri-stent haziness. Following stent deployment in the mid anterior descending artery (**A,** *white arrow*), an area of angiographic haziness was noted in the distal reference segment *(yellow arrow)*. IVUS imaging **(B)** demonstrates significant and eccentric calcification in the reference vessel, but with adequate lumen size and no evidence of disruption. No further intervention was deemed necessary.

Ultrasound imaging is not particularly accurate in the delineation of intraluminal thrombus. These usually appear as echodense filling defects within the lumen. Mural thrombi cannot be distinguished from underlying plaque or tissue prolapse within the stent lumen because of suboptimal tissue characterization.

Advanced Applications of IVUS Imaging in Chronic Total Occlusion Angioplasty

Angioplasty for chronic total occlusion (CTO) cases has recently been gaining momentum, as newer techniques improved procedural success rates and DES reduced subsequent restenosis. IVUS imaging can facilitate certain steps of a usually long and complicated procedure. To date, there are no controlled data to support these advanced applications, but IVUS imaging during CTO PCI procedures is supported by reports from experienced operators performing relatively pioneering work.

One frequently used application of IVUS imaging in CTO cases is accurate vessel sizing. After crossing the occluded segment and due to diffuse disease and chronic underfilling, the distal vessel commonly appears smaller on angiography than its true size. IVUS imaging can delineate the burden of diffuse disease and allow the selection of a larger, more appropriately sized stent, which in turn can reduce the risk of restenosis.

Other applications of IVUS in CTO cases are more complex. For example, IVUS can be used to define the location of the occluded artery when the CTO is "stumpless" or has a vague stump on angiography.[88] This can be performed if the occlusion is in the proximity of a small branch or if the occlusion is at the ostium of a coronary artery. The IVUS catheter is advanced into the patent branch and a slow pullback is performed until the location of the occluded vessel is identified as a sector interruption of the wall, as typically seen at bifurcation points. The location is marked by filming the transducer on cine angiography. The IVUS transducer can be left in place to guide the passage of the wire into the occluded branch and can eventually help determine whether the wire is in the true lumen of the CTO by examining the wire location in the far field (**Figure 16-19**) (Video 16-3).

Another valuable application of IVUS imaging is to identify the true from false channels after a wire is passed through a CTO segment. If the catheter is advanced over the wire in the true lumen, the trilaminar appearance of the wall should be recognizable, and on pullback the orifices of side branches are seen. In a false channel, the wall is not trilaminar and the side branches may be seen arising from the lumen separated from the catheter by the linear echodensity of the dissection flap (**Figure 16-20**). Lower profile IVUS catheters have been used for this application in Asia and Europe. If the catheter is determined to be in a false channel, it can help guide the passage of a second wire into the true lumen, which can be seen in the far field.[89] This application can be performed via the retrograde and antegrade techniques and has proven valuable in salvaging procedures in which the true lumen could not be identified angiographically.[90]

IVUS Imaging in the Peripheral Arterial System

As with some other advanced applications, there are no guideline-based recommendations for use of IVUS imaging in the peripheral vasculature. The applications are driven by a need for additional information not accurately provided by angiography alone. Technically, imaging of larger arteries requires deeper penetration, which in turn means that imaging at a lower frequency, typically 10 MHz to 20 MHz. Peripheral imaging catheters are larger and can be advanced over 0.018-inch or 0.035-inch wires. Coronary imaging catheters can be used in the peripheral arteries that are 3 mm

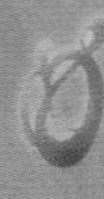

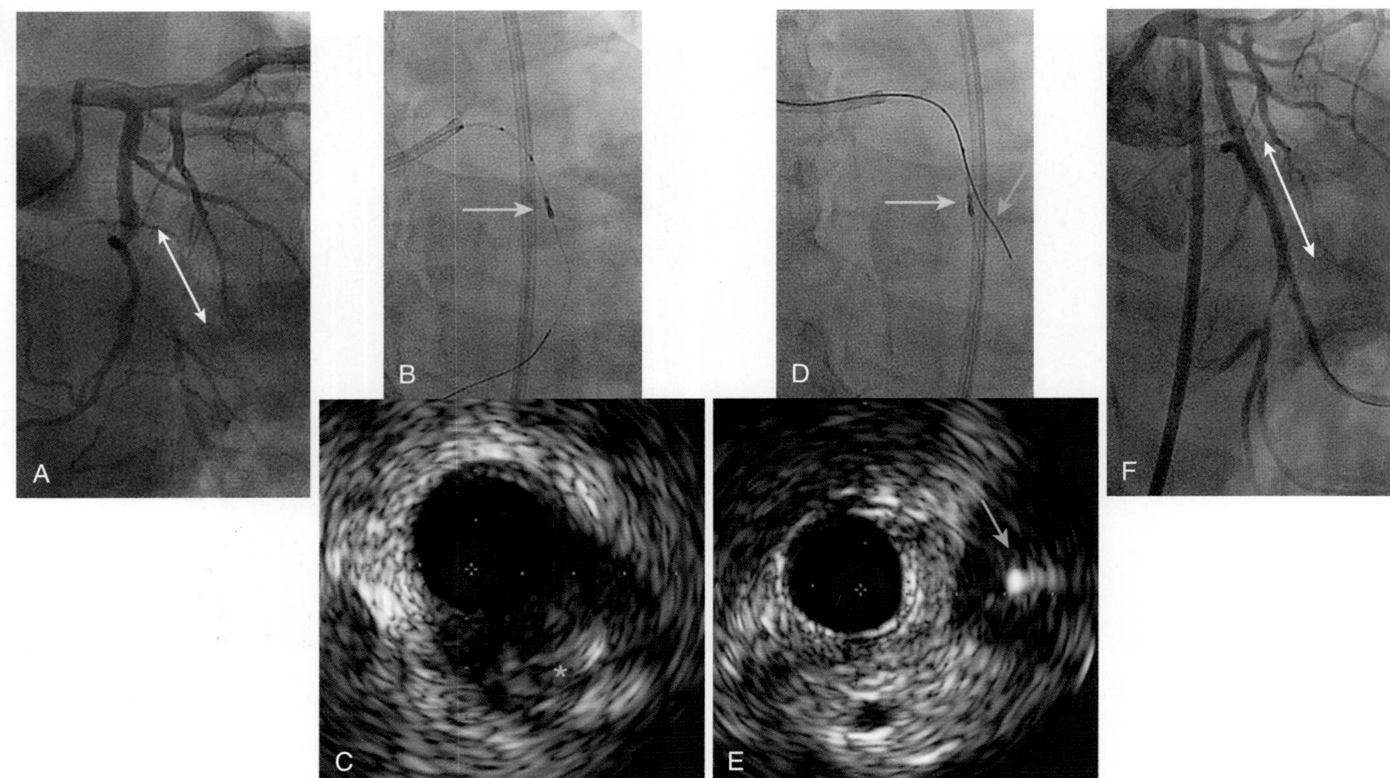

FIGURE 16-19 Use of IVUS imaging in locating an occluded ostium. **A,** Angiogram of a chronically occluded marginal branch of the circumflex artery with collateral filling of the distal segment. The proximal stump of the occluded artery cannot be visualized in multiple projections. **B,** The IVUS catheter *(yellow arrow)* is advanced into the AV continuation of the artery and pulled back until the bifurcation of the occluded marginal branch is visualized (*asterisk,* **C**). The location of the stump is marked on cine angiography and a stiff wire *(blue arrow)* is advanced through the proximal cap of the occlusion **(D)**. The entry of the wire into the marginal branch and confirmation of its intraluminal position is confirmed by keeping the IVUS probe in place and focusing on the wire artifact in the far field (*blue arrow,* **E**). After crossing, balloon angioplasty and stenting of the occluded segment are successfully performed (*white arrow,* **F**). *(Reused with permission from Wallace EL, Ziada KM: Intravascular ultrasound assisted localization and revascularization of an ostial chronic total occlusion: utility of near and far field imaging. Journal of Invasive Cardiology, 2015.)*

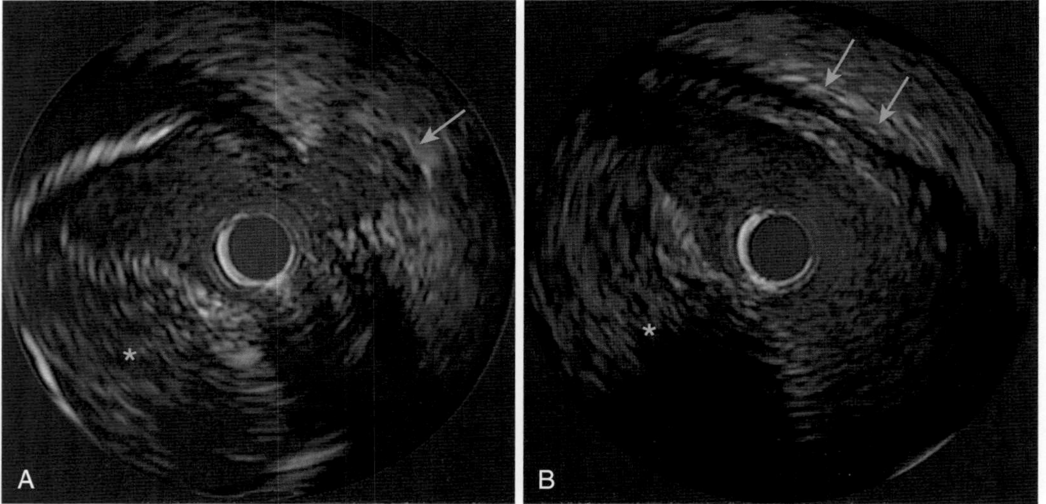

FIGURE 16-20 Distinguishing between true and false lumens. In complex interventions, particularly CTO PCI, it is crucial to define the true lumen before proceeding with angioplasty and stenting. Advancing an IVUS probe can provide two useful clues to distinguish between true and false lumens: branches always originate from true lumen (*arrow,* **A**), and the trilaminar appearance of the wall can only be present in a nondissected lumen (*arrows,* **B**). In this example, the IVUS catheter is in the true lumen and is separated from the false channel *(asterisk)* by a linear echodensity, which represents the dissection flap.

to 5 mm in diameter. IVUS imaging of peripheral arteries is not new. Some of the early validation studies were performed on femoral artery sections,[9] and much of the pioneering work in understanding remodeling in vivo was also done in peripheral arteries.[91,92] More recently, comparative studies demonstrated accuracy of IVUS in obtaining accurate lumen measurements and its superiority in defining plaque and calcification distribution in comparison to subtraction angiography.[93]

A simple application of IVUS in the peripheral arteries is accurate vessel sizing. This is important for device selection during atherectomy balloon angioplasty and/or for stent

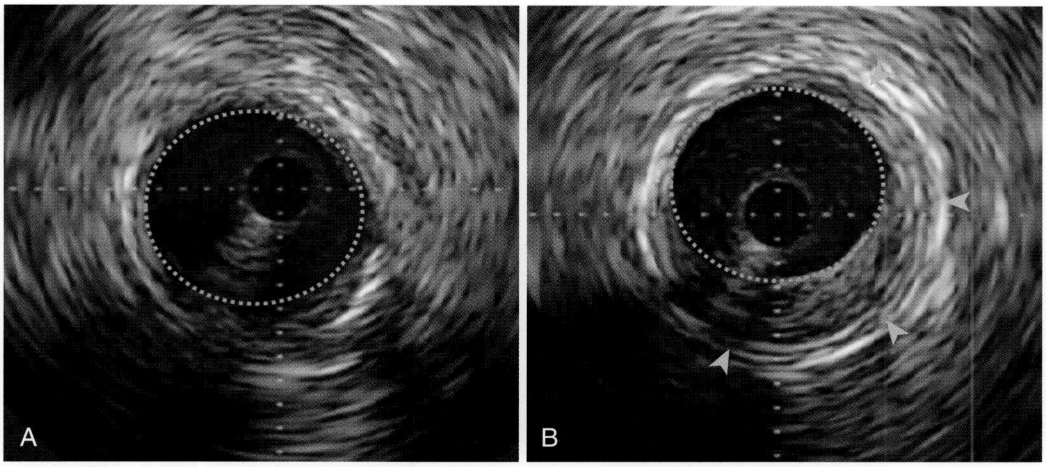

FIGURE 16-21 IVUS imaging of the iliac arteries. Peripheral IVUS imaging can provide accurate measurements of the iliac arteries and the aorta for interventional planning. To visualize the wall of the larger arteries from the center of the lumen, a lower frequency ultrasound is needed, typically 10 MHz to 20 MHz. This lowers the resolution, which can be seen as less definition of the arterial wall components. Additionally, the iliac arteries are less muscular than the coronaries, hence the media is thinner and harder to visualize. **A,** A near normal iliac artery with mild intimal thickening. **B,** A more distal segment with early disease seen as an eccentric plaque *(arrowheads).* This is an example of positive remodeling, as the lumen size (bound by the dotted gray border) remained unchanged with the development of atherosclerotic plaque in the distal vessel.

sizing. An important contemporary use of IVUS imaging is the sizing of the iliac artery prior to transfemoral transcutaneous aortic valve replacement. With the large size of the delivery system, it is critically important to define the size of the artery, the distribution of plaque burden, and the extent of calcification. Typically this is done using contrast CT imaging and/or angiography, but IVUS imaging can provide similar or more accurate information, without the use of contrast, which can be valuable in elderly patients with moderate degrees of renal insufficiency (**Figure 16-21**).[94]

IVUS imaging is also valuable to guide endovascular repair of abdominal aortic aneurysms (EVAR). Several measurements and morphologic information are important to delineate during such procedures. Diameter, length, branch vessels, and plaque distribution of the infrarenal neck of the aneurysm are important for accurate anchoring of the graft. Similar information can be obtained about the distal landing zone in the iliac artery. Imaging can also be used to define complications at the landing zones, if the angiograms are ambiguous. Importantly, this information can be obtained with minimal contrast and without excessive radiation exposure.[95] Some have advocated the use of IVUS imaging routinely in all EVAR cases.[96]

As previously described with CTO PCI, IVUS imaging from within the subintimal space can guide reentry into the true lumen and facilitate restoration of flow in cases in which antegrade access to the true lumen is not directly feasible. This technique is used in the femoral, popliteal, and iliac arteries as well. For this application, a dedicated 6 Fr dual-lumen IVUS catheter is equipped with a phased array transducer and a deployable needle at its tip. After gaining wire access into the subintimal space at the proximal cap, the dissection is extended along the length of the occluded segment. The catheter is then advanced over a wire placed in the subintimal space. When the transducer reaches the level of the distal cap, the true lumen can be identified in the far field. The IVUS catheter is rotated appropriately, such that the needle penetrates the intimal flap into the true lumen when deployed. Once that is achieved, an angioplasty wire can be advanced via the deployed needle to gain reentry into the true lumen (**Figure 16-22**) (Video 16-4). This technique facilitates difficult CTO cases with calcified caps and long occluded segments and saves contrast and radiation exposure as well as improves the success rate.[97]

RESEARCH APPLICATIONS—PROGRESSION/REGRESSION TRIALS

In addition to its value as a clinical tool to facilitate diagnosis and interventions in the catheterization laboratory, IVUS imaging has been a very valuable tool to gain insight into the atherosclerotic disease process. IVUS imaging was the first imaging modality used to demonstrate the process of arterial remodeling in vivo and its potential interaction with the propensity for plaque rupture and the development of clinical events.[8,98] It has also been used to study the impact of various therapeutic agents on progression and regression of atherosclerosis. The tested therapies included statins, antidiabetic agents, and renin-angiotensin system inhibitors. Such trials attempted to establish a new standard for the evaluation of drug therapy to limit the progression of atherosclerosis. To avoid variability in measured endpoints and to allow for comparison across trials, a consensus document outlined the most accepted methods of image acquisition, measurement, and endpoint reporting in studies of disease progression.[99] Serial and matched IVUS image that are essential for such studies require a high level of expertise during image acquisition and analysis. Volumetric quantification of the atheroma volumes is used to reduce variability. A number of endpoints are suggested in this document, although percent atheroma volume (PAV) has been the most commonly reported.

The trial of recombinant apolipoprotein A-I (apo A-I) Milano (a high-density lipoprotein mimetic) carried a lot of promise when it was first published. It demonstrated the potential of innovative therapies to impact atherosclerosis progression and the ability to utilize IVUS imaging to measure minimal morphometric changes in atheroma size. Coronary IVUS imaging was performed before and after 5 weeks of therapy. Analysis demonstrated a modest but statistically significant 4% reduction in PAV compared with

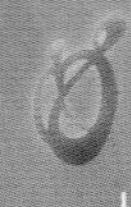

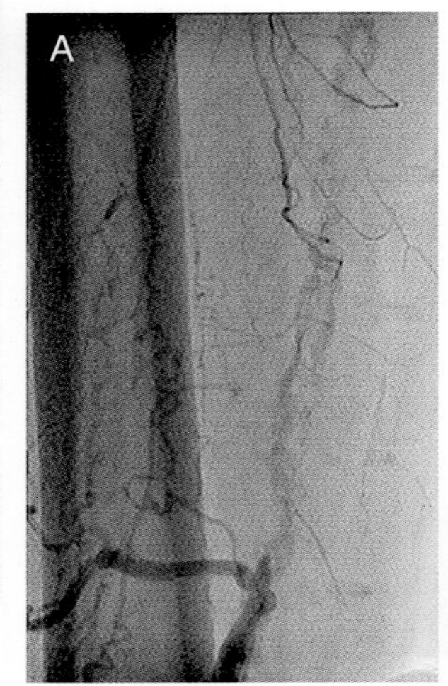

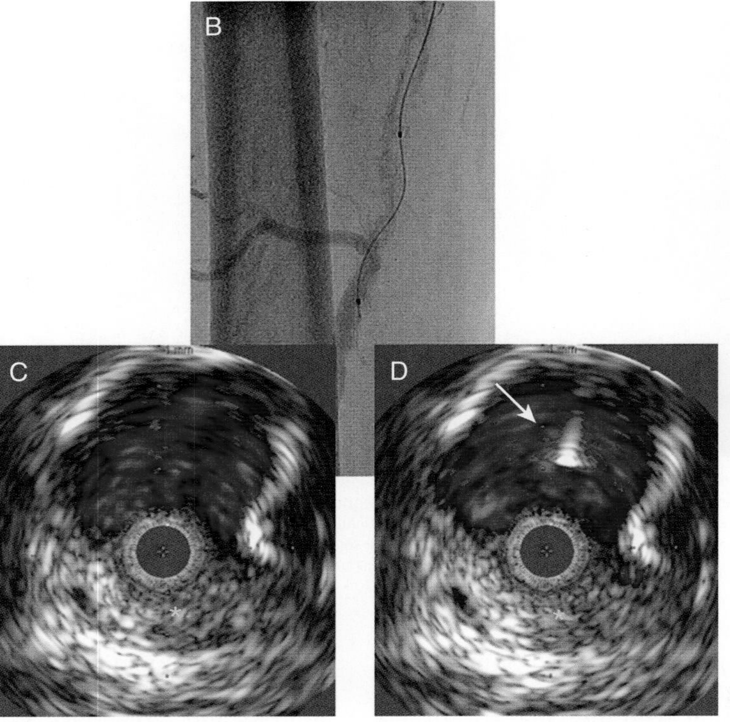

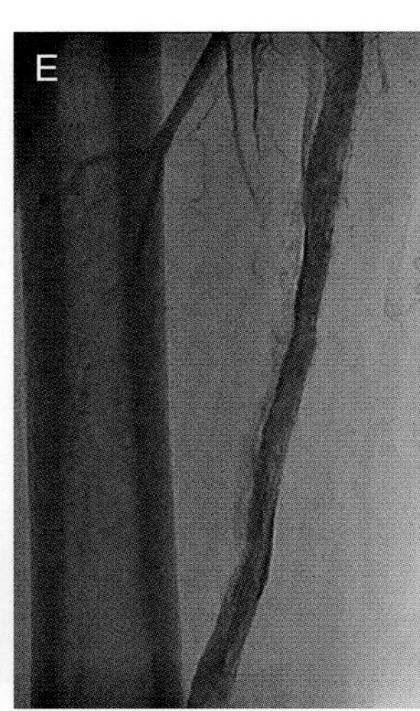

FIGURE 16-22 IVUS-facilitated reentry after subintimal tracking of an occluded femoral artery. **A,** An angiogram of a long and calcified superficial femoral artery occlusion *(arrows)* with reconstitution via collaterals from the profunda femoris artery. A stiff wire is used to penetrate the proximal cap and dissect the wall to create a subintimal track extending all the way to the distal stump **(B).** The dedicate reentry IVUS catheter is then delivered into the subintimal space (**C,** *asterisk*) until it reaches the level of the distal stump. The true channel is then visualized with the aid of ChromaFlo **(C).** After appropriate positioning, the needle is used for reentry and the angioplasty wire is advanced in the distal true lumen (*arrow,* **D**). Balloon angioplasty and a self-expanding stent follow to restore patency **(E).**

baseline in the apo A-I Milano group but a slight increase in the placebo group.[100]

A larger study of 654 patients sought to utilize serial IVUS imaging to examine the effect of intensive (atorvastatin 80 mg) versus standard (pravastatin 40 mg) lipid-lowering therapy on coronary atherosclerosis.[101] IVUS imaging was performed at baseline and after 18 months of therapy. As expected, LDL cholesterol was significantly lower in the high-dose statin arm, but the change in PAV was minimal compared with the baseline (–0.4%, p = 0.98 compared to baseline). In the pravastatin arm, there was significant progression in PAV (+2.7%, p = 0.001 compared with baseline). The difference between the groups was statistically significant in this primary endpoint as well as other secondary measures of disease progression. Subsequently, in a cohort treated with rosuvastatin to achieve more aggressive reduction of LDL cholesterol, and using a historic control group, rosuvastatin therapy was associated with a measurable regression in plaque size. With intense lipid lowering, the mean and median change in PAV for the entire vessel was –0.98% and –0.79%, respectively ($p < 0.001$ vs. baseline).[102]

While the absolute reduction in atheroma burden as measured by IVUS in each of these trials was small, its clinical significance remains unclear. Minimal progression may be a marker for arteries with more "active" disease and/or patients more susceptible to events. In an analysis of 4137 patients from six clinical trials that used serial IVUS to study plaque progression, there was a significant association between baseline disease burden and major adverse events, such that every standard deviation increase in PAV was associated with a 1.32-fold (95% CI: 1.22 to 1.42; $p < 0.001$) greater likelihood of experiencing an adverse event. Similarly, disease progression over the 2 years of follow-up was another predictor of adverse events: each standard deviation greater increase in PAV was associated with a 1.20-fold (95% CI: 1.10 to 1.31; $p < 0.001$) greater risk for adverse events.[103]

ADVANCING IVUS TECHNOLOGIES AND FUTURE DIRECTIONS

Over the past decade, there has been growing interest in better understanding of plaque composition and its role in defining plaque vulnerability. Using grayscale IVUS imaging for tissue characterization has modest accuracy and is not reliable clinically. In addition, resolution of IVUS is limited and may not allow detection of features considered essential to the diagnosis of plaque vulnerability. This led to the introduction of an advanced ultrasound-based tissue characterization technology, virtual histology (VH). IVUS tomography has also been combined with other tissue characterization techniques such as near infrared spectroscopy (NIRS). Going forward, other limitations of IVUS imaging may be overcome by technologic breakthroughs, some of which are on the horizon, such as high-definition catheters.

IVUS-Derived Virtual Histology

IVUS-derived VH is a more advanced imaging technique that depends on the analysis of the radio frequency backscatter of the ultrasound signal, using a larger number of parameters. Rather than just use the signal amplitude to define a shade of gray for each reflected line, this method utilizes a more complex mathematical autoregressive model to calculate the frequency spectrum from the region of interest (the coronary plaque).[104] The complex mathematical calculations do not lend themselves to quick interpretations by clinicians, hence the development of a simplified color-coded display that broadly distinguishes lipidic, fibrotic, necrotic, and calcific regions (**Figure 16-23**). This approach to analysis of the IVUS data can allow the identification of the thin-cap fibroatheroma (TCFA), considered by many pathologists to be the plaque most prone to rupture and cause acute clinical events.

TCFA is defined as a lipid-rich plaque (>10% confluent lipid core) with a very thin cap (<100 μm in thickness, not visible by VH) and with an area stenosis that is usually >40%. These plaques frequently contain speckles of calcification and are more prevalent in patients presenting with acute coronary syndromes, even in nonculprit segments (**Figure 16-24**). TCFA is most frequently located in proximal coronary arterial segments, which is consistent with the patterns of angiographic lesions underlying AMI.[105] It is important to note that in calcified plaques, the poor penetration of ultrasound signals through the calcium affects the accuracy of the backscatter interpretation. In such cases, the attenuation caused by the calcified plaque is interpreted as a necrotic core, thus artifactually overestimating its measured area by VH-IVUS.[106] Other plaque imaging modalities are more accurate in defining the size of the lipid core in calcified plaques (e.g., NIR).[107]

The PROSPECT trial (Providing Regional Observations to Study Predictors of Events in the Coronary Tree) is the largest study to date that provides insight into the natural history of various types of atherosclerotic plaques as defined by VH-IVUS.[108] In this study, 697 acute coronary syndrome patients entered into a registry with longitudinal follow-up. All underwent angiography and revascularization as clinically indicated. Three-vessel IVUS imaging and VH analysis were performed. Patients who developed events over the ensuing 3 years underwent repeat angiography and imaging. Adverse events were related to an originally nonculprit

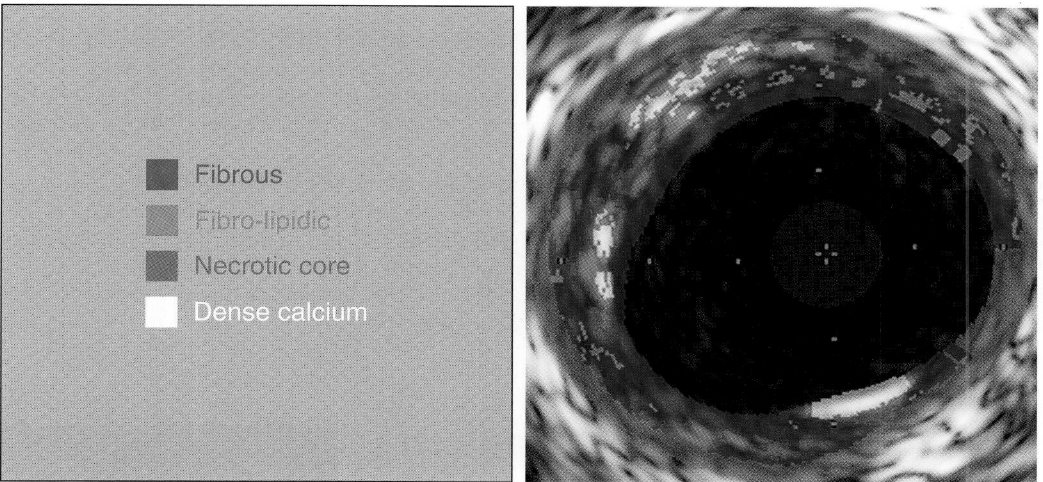

FIGURE 16-23 Virtual histology (VH) IVUS imaging. Using radiofrequency backscatter analysis, the variable components of the plaque (e.g., lipid, fibrous tissue, and calcium) can be identified. The display is then color-coded and an online evaluation of plaque structure can be available to the operator. *(From Nair A, Kuban BD, Tuzcu EM, et al: Coronary plaque classification with intravascular ultrasound radiofrequency data analysis. Circulation 106:2200–2206, 2002.)*

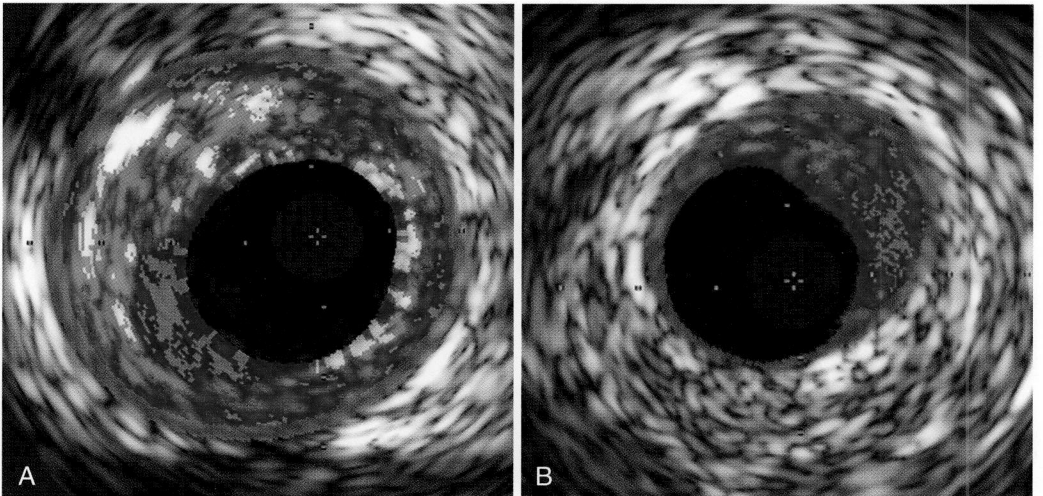

FIGURE 16-24 Examples of VH-IVUS imaging and plaque composition. **A,** A thin cap fibroatheroma (TCFA) as defined on VH-IVUS imaging: a lipid-rich plaque with a >10% confluent necrotic core, a very thin cap that is <100 μm in thickness (hence not visible by VH leading to direct proximity between the necrotic core and the lumen), and >40% cross-sectional area stenosis. These plaques are more likely seen in the context of acute coronary syndromes. **B,** A fibrous plaque with a minimal necrotic core and one that is more likely seen in patients with stable coronary disease.

lesion in 11.6% of patients. Lesion characteristics that predicted the development of future events included plaque burden ≥70%, MLA ≤4 mm², and TCFA on VH-IVUS. The presence of more than one feature increased the risk of future events (**Figure 16-25**).

In addition to the impact on progression, small-scale studies suggest that a VH-IVUS–defined lipid core may impact the remodeling process and outcome of PCI. Examining remodeling in 41 patients, there was a strong positive correlation between size of the necrotic core and the remodeling index, that is, plaques with large necrotic cores are more likely to be positively remodeled. Negatively remodeled plaques were predominantly fibrous.[109] In another study of patients undergoing PCI, the size of the necrotic core at the lesion site was associated with the development of peri-procedural MI, as defined by a rise in troponin I.[110]

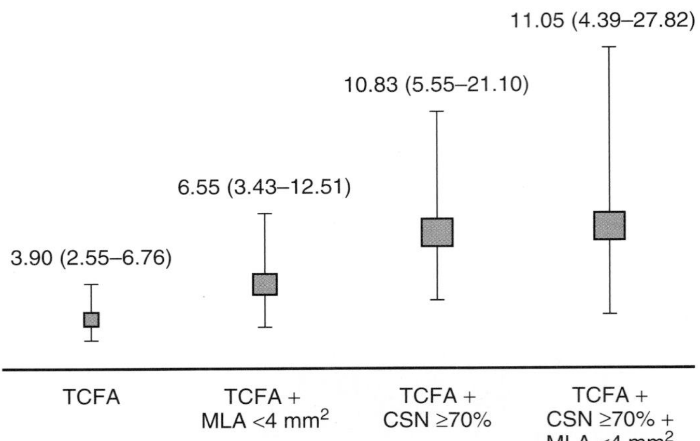

FIGURE 16-25 Hazard ratios of adverse events precipitated by nonculprit lesions based on VH and grayscale IVUS imaging. In the PROSPECT trial, the presence of TCFA increased the risk of future adverse events more than threefold. A lumen area ≤4 mm² and/or a cross-sectional narrowing ≥70% were also predictive of events. The combinations of VH-defined TCFA and grayscale quantitative metrics were stronger predictors of the risk of future adverse events. *(Data from Stone GW, Maehara A, Lansky AJ, et al: A prospective natural-history study of coronary atherosclerosis. N Engl J Med 364:226–235, 2011.)*

IVUS and Near Infrared Spectroscopy (NIRS)

Interest in identification of plaque vulnerability and recognition of the importance of the lipid core underlie the development of NIRS-equipped catheters. NIRS is a technology widely used to detect the chemical content of substances, and it can be used to detect lipid content with satisfactory accuracy.[111] A currently available combined NIRS-IVUS catheter provides simultaneous NIRS spectral data coregistered with traditional IVUS images in a single intracoronary pullback. This allows the recognition of lipid cores within the plaque and the morphometric features (such as area, volume, and distribution), both characteristics that can predict vulnerability.[112] This catheter is approved for use in the United States and around the world; clinical trials are ongoing to identify the best clinical and research applications for this intriguing technology (**Figure 16-26**).

IVUS and OCT Imaging

With the availability of catheter-based OCT imaging, the question of which intravascular imaging modality is more useful for the interventionalist is being considered. It is clear that both modalities provide additive insight over angiography alone in many diagnostic and interventional

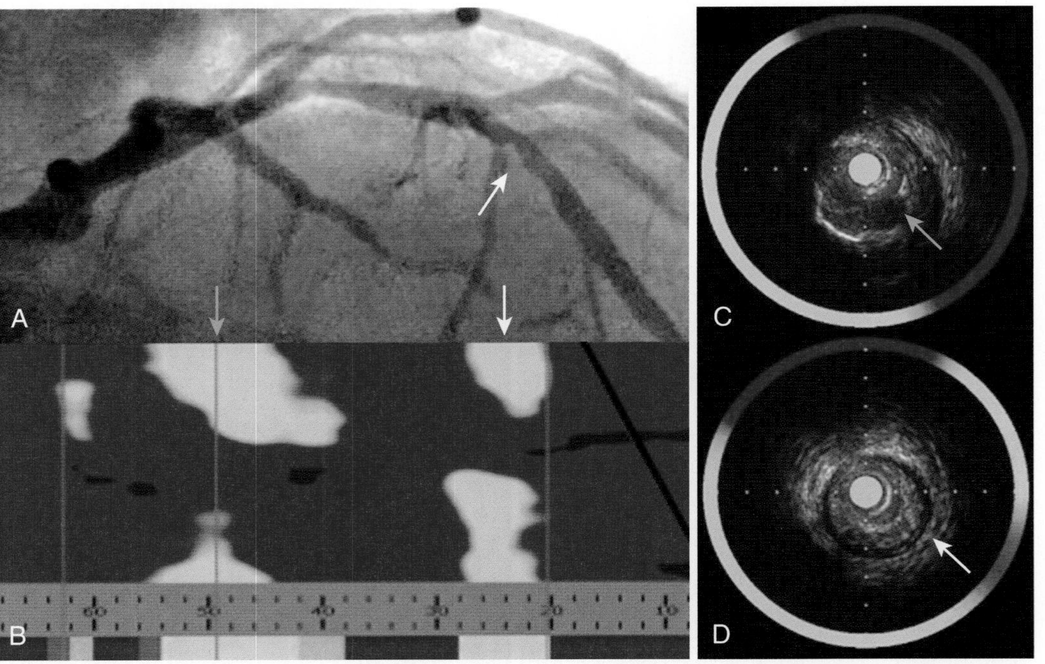

FIGURE 16-26 The combination of IVUS and near infrared spectroscopy (NIRS) in coronary imaging. An example of the value of multimodality imaging for the detection of plaque vulnerability/activity. **A,** An angiogram of the LAD reveals a proximal hazy lesion *(white arrow)* that is considered the culprit underlying the acute presentation. There is a midsegment lesion that appears mild in severity *(blue arrow)*. **B,** The chemogram generated by NIRS imaging reveals evidence of large lipid content in the proximal lesion *(white arrow)* but also in the midsegment lesion *(blue arrow)*. IVUS imaging confirms signs of plaque rupture and ulceration in the proximal lesion (**C,** *blue arrow*). The less severe lesion in the midsegment did show evidence of a large lipid core (*white arrow* on chemogram) and IVUS revealed a larger than expected plaque burden (**D,** *white arrow*). *(From Mader R, et al: Catheter Cardiovasc Interv 81:551–557, 2012.)*

applications. The judicious use of either modality is likely to answer a question or a concern that is not clearly resolved by angiographic examination. Nonetheless, each modality has its own advantages and disadvantages.[113,114]

There is little debate that the higher resolution of OCT provides significant advantages over IVUS imaging in certain categories, namely, (1) improved spatial resolution (20-40 μm) that allows better definition of TCFA and dissection flaps and (2) diagnosis of intraluminal thrombus. However, there are certain advantages to IVUS imaging that remain relevant despite its lower resolution. The use of light waves in OCT imaging does not allow penetration and imaging of the full thickness of the arterial wall, that is, OCT provides exquisite resolution but only of the luminal 1 mm to 2 mm of the wall. Thus deeper structures that can influence strategy and the results of an interventional procedure (such as deep calcification and/or dense fibrous plaques) may not be adequately visualized. Moreover, poor penetration does not allow the measurement of plaque thickness and volume, measures of plaque burden that have been shown to define future risk of clinical events in the PROSPECT trial. These measurements are also essential for the study of phenomena such as remodeling, disease progression, and/or response to therapeutic interventions.

In addition to the poor penetration, and due to its novelty, there are few data to support OCT use for guidance of interventional procedures. Compared to tens of thousands of patients undergoing IVUS-guided stenting, a number of observational and randomized trials, and multiple meta-analyses, only one study of 335 patients undergoing stenting with OCT guidance shed light on this subject.[115] While there is higher resolution that allows the detection of small dissection flaps or tissue prolapse after stenting, the clinical significance of such findings remains unclear. Concern remains that identifying such findings may lead to additional and possibly unnecessary interventions. There has been some debate about the accuracy of lumen measurements using frequency domain OCT compared to IVUS imaging,[116] although more recent studies support the accuracy of OCT measurements compared to IVUS and angiographic estimates.[117]

FUTURE DIRECTIONS

Although the pace of technologic progress of IVUS imaging seemed to stall for a decade or so, there have been more recent innovations in the past several years. These innovations address inadequate resolution, suboptimal tissue characterization, and the ability to predict plaque vulnerability. IVUS-VH and IVUS-NIRS combinations are examples of innovations that attempt to improve tissue characterization. More recently, a high-definition 60-MHz IVUS catheter system was developed to potentially bridge the image resolution gap between IVUS and OCT imaging. The challenge to develop a higher resolution transducer without affecting depth of penetration seems to have been overcome in this new device.[118] Preliminary data demonstrate significantly improved resolution compared to contemporary 40-MHz to 45-MHz transducers and image quality comparable to that acquired by OCT[119] (**Figure 16-27**). Forward-looking transducers are also being developed to allow guidance of interventions in occluded vessels. Using advanced imaging suites in which IVUS imaging pullbacks can be coregistered in three dimensions with biplane angiography will also allow the depiction of coronary trees that can be used in the

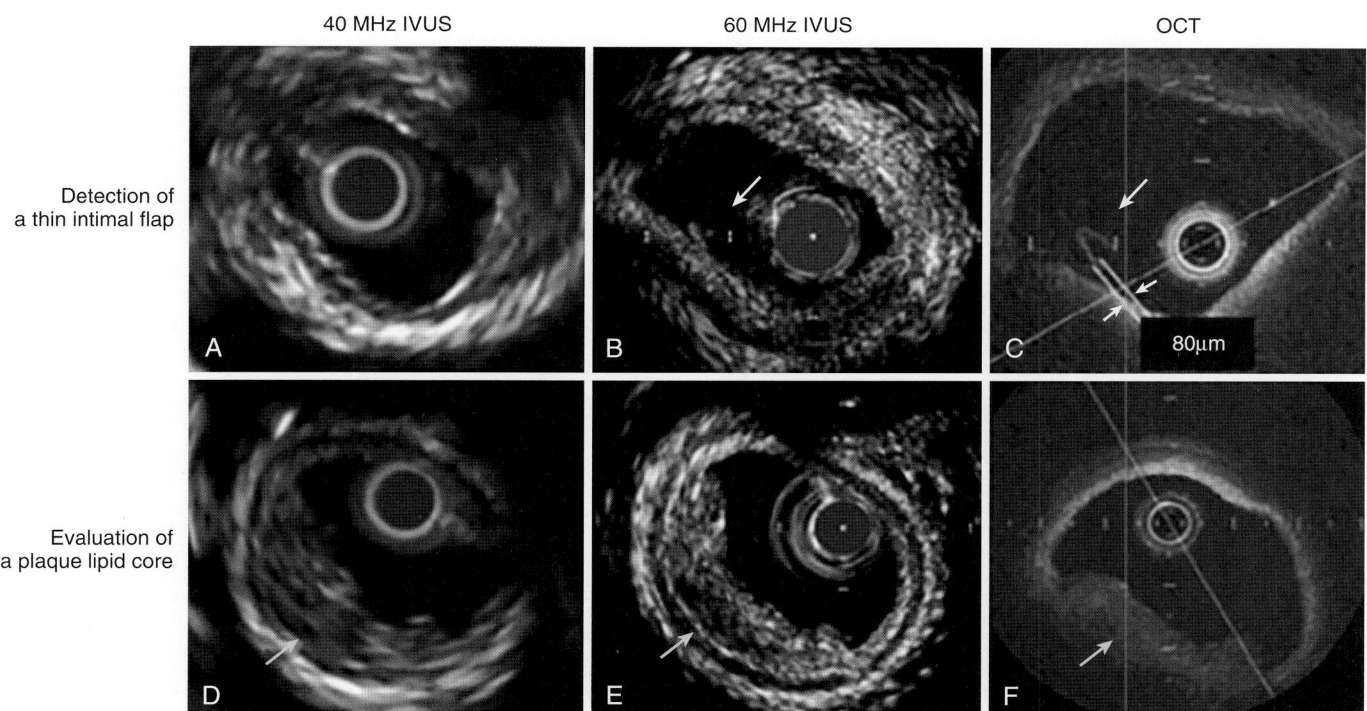

FIGURE 16-27 Improved resolution with high-definition IVUS imaging. With the development of 60-MHz high-definition IVUS probes, the difference in resolution between IVUS and OCT can be reduced significantly. In this experiment, all dissection flaps ≥80 μm were visualized on high-definition IVUS (*white arrow,* **B**). Similarly, the sensitivity of high-definition IVUS was identical to that of OCT in the detection of lipid core plaques (**D** through **F**, *yellow arrows*). The sensitivity of conventional 40-MHz IVUS imaging was inferior in both categories. *(From Tanka S, et al: J Am Coll Cardiol 61:E1878, 2013.)*

calculation of shear stress, another important predictor of cardiac events.

CONCLUSIONS

Due to inherent limitations of angiography, IVUS continues to play an important role in diagnostic and interventional procedures. For left main lesions and transplant vasculopathy, its role remains central. IVUS has provided great insight into the optimization of stent deployment and the understanding of mechanisms of stent failure. Applications in guiding CTO intervention are also valuable. The role of IVUS in peripheral arterial procedures is also expanding. With further evolution of the technology, IVUS will remain a useful tool, potentially being combined with other emerging imaging modalities to provide even more information to guide lesion- and patient-specific intervention.

ACKNOWLEDGMENT

The author would like to acknowledge Dr. Wael El Mallah for his invaluable assistance with preparation of the video illustrations accompanying this chapter.

References

1. Topol EJ, Nissen SE: Our preoccupation with coronary luminology. The dissociation between clinical and angiographic findings in ischemic heart disease. *Circulation* 92:2333–2342, 1995.
2. Ziada KM, Kapadia SR, Tuzcu EM, et al: The current status of intravascular ultrasound imaging. *Curr Probl Cardiol* 24:541–566, 1999.
3. Zir LM, Miller SW, Dinsmore RE, et al: Interobserver variability in coronary angiography. *Circulation* 53:627–632, 1976.
4. Galbraith JE, Murphy ML, de Soyza N: Coronary angiogram interpretation. Interobserver variability. *JAMA* 240:2053–2056, 1978.
5. Vlodaver Z, Frech R, Van Tassel RA, et al: Correlation of the antemortem coronary arteriogram and the postmortem specimen. *Circulation* 47:162–169, 1973.
6. Arnett EN, Isner JM, Redwood DR, et al: Coronary artery narrowing in coronary heart disease: comparison of cineangiographic and necropsy findings. *Ann Intern Med* 91:350–356, 1979.
7. Glagov S, Weisenberg E, Zarins CK, et al: Compensatory enlargement of human atherosclerotic coronary arteries. *N Engl J Med* 316:1371–1375, 1987.
8. Schoenhagen P, Ziada KM, Vince DG, et al: Arterial remodeling and coronary artery disease: the concept of "dilated" versus "obstructive" coronary atherosclerosis. *J Am Coll Cardiol* 38:297–306, 2001.
9. Schoenhagen P, Ziada KM, Kapadia SR, et al: Extent and direction of arterial remodeling in stable versus unstable coronary syndromes: an intravascular ultrasound study. *Circulation* 101(6):598–603, 2000.
10. Gussenhoven EJ, Essed CE, Lancee CT, et al: Arterial wall characteristics determined by intravascular ultrasound imaging: an in vitro study. *J Am Coll Cardiol* 14:947–952, 1989.
11. Levine GN, Bates ER, Blankenship JC, et al: 2011 ACCF/AHA/SCAI guideline for Percutaneous Coronary Intervention. A report of the American College of Cardiology Foundation/American Heart Association Task Force on practice guidelines and the Soceity for Cardiovascular Angiography and Interventions. *J Am Coll Cardiol* 58(24):e44–e122, 2011.
12. Di Mario C, Gorge G, Peters R, et al: Clinical application and image interpretation in intracoronary ultrasound. Study Group on Intracoronary Imaging of the Working Group of Coronary Circulation and of the Subgroup on Intravascular Ultrasound of the Working Group of Echocardiography of the European Society of Cardiology. *Eur Heart J* 19:207–229, 1998.
13. Pijls NH, De Bruyne B, Peels K, et al: Measurement of fractional flow reserve to assess the functional severity of coronary-artery stenoses. *N Engl J Med* 334:1703–1708, 1996.
14. Bech GJ, De Bruyne B, Pijls NH, et al: Fractional flow reserve to determine the appropriateness of angioplasty in moderate coronary stenosis: a randomized trial. *Circulation* 103:2928–2934, 2001.
15. Pijls NH, van Schaardenburgh P, Manoharan G, et al: Percutaneous coronary intervention of functionally nonsignificant stenosis: 5-year follow-up of the DEFER Study. *J Am Coll Cardiol* 49:2105–2111, 2007.
16. Tonino PA, De Bruyne B, Pijls NH, et al: Fractional flow reserve versus angiography for guiding percutaneous coronary intervention. *N Engl J Med* 360(3):213–224, 2009.
17. Takagi A, Tsurumi Y, Ishii Y, et al: Clinical potential of intravascular ultrasound for physiological assessment of coronary stenosis: relationship between quantitative ultrasound tomography and pressure-derived fractional flow reserve. *Circulation* 100:250–255, 1999.
18. Briguori C, Anzuini A, Airoldi F, et al: Intravascular ultrasound criteria for the assessment of the functional significance of intermediate coronary artery stenoses and comparison with fractional flow reserve. *Am J Cardiol* 87:136–141, 2001.
19. Ben-Dor I, Torguson R, Deksissa T, et al: Intravascular ultrasound lumen area parameters for assessment of physiological ischemia by fractional flow reserve in intermediate coronary artery stenosis. *Cardiovasc Revasc Med* 13(3):177–182, 2012.
20. Isner JM, Kishel J, Kent KM, et al: Accuracy of angiographic determination of left main coronary arterial narrowing. Angiographic–histologic correlative analysis in 28 patients. *Circulation* 63:1056–1064, 1981.
21. Fisher LD, Judkins MP, Lesperance J, et al: Reproducibility of coronary arteriographic reading in the coronary artery surgery study (CASS). *Cathet Cardiovasc Diagn* 8:565–575, 1982.
22. Jasti V, Ivan E, Yalamanchili V, et al: Correlations between fractional flow reserve and intravascular ultrasound in patients with an ambiguous left main coronary artery stenosis. *Circulation* 110:2831–2836, 2004.
23. Abizaid AS, Mintz GS, Abizaid A, et al: One-year follow-up after intravascular ultrasound assessment of moderate left main coronary artery disease in patients with ambiguous angiograms. *J Am Coll Cardiol* 34:707–715, 1999.
24. Fassa AA, Wagatsuma K, Higano ST, et al: Intravascular ultrasound-guided treatment for angiographically indeterminate left main coronary artery disease: a long-term follow-up study. *J Am Coll Cardiol* 45:204–211, 2005.
25. Mehra MR, Crespo-Leiro MG, Dipchand A, et al: International Society for Heart and Lung Transplantation working formulation of a standardized nomenclature for cardiac allograft vasculopathy—2010. *J Heart Lung Transplant* 29(7):717–727, 2010.
26. Uretsky BF, Murali S, Reddy PS, et al: Development of coronary artery disease in cardiac transplant patients receiving immunosuppressive therapy with cyclosporine and prednisone. *Circulation* 76:827–834, 1987.
27. Pascoe EA, Barnhart GR, Carter WH, Jr, et al: The prevalence of cardiac allograft arteriosclerosis. *Transplantation* 44:838–839, 1987.
28. Pflugfelder PW, Boughner DR, Rudas L, et al: Enhanced detection of cardiac allograft arterial disease with intracoronary ultrasonographic imaging. *Am Heart J* 125:1583–1591, 1993.
29. Pinto FJ, St Goar FG, Gao SZ, et al: Immediate and one-year safety of intracoronary ultrasonic imaging. Evaluation with serial quantitative angiography. *Circulation* 88:1709–1714, 1993.
30. Ramasubbu K, Schoenhagen P, Balghith MA, et al: Repeated intravascular ultrasound imaging in cardiac transplant recipients does not accelerate transplant coronary artery disease. *J Am Coll Cardiol* 41:1739–1743, 2003.
31. Tuzcu EM, De Franco AC, Hobbs R, et al: Prevalence and distribution of transplant coronary artery disease: insights from intravascular ultrasound imaging. *J Heart Lung Transplant* 14:S202–S207, 1995.
32. Escobar A, Ventura HO, Stapleton DD, et al: Cardiac allograft vasculopathy assessed by intravascular ultrasonography and nonimmunologic risk factors. *Am J Cardiol* 74:1042–1046, 1994.
33. St Goar FG, Pinto FJ, Alderman EL, et al: Intracoronary ultrasound in cardiac transplant recipients. In vivo evidence of "angiographically silent" intimal thickening. *Circulation* 85:979–987, 1992.
34. Kapadia SR, Nissen SE, Ziada KM, et al: Development of transplantation vasculopathy and progression of donor-transmitted atherosclerosis: comparison by serial intravascular ultrasound imaging. *Circulation* 98:2672–2678, 1998.
35. Gao HZ, Hunt SA, Alderman EL, et al: Relation of donor age and preexisting coronary artery disease on angiography and intracoronary ultrasound to later development of accelerated allograft coronary artery disease. *J Am Coll Cardiol* 29:623–629, 1997.
36. Botas J, Pinto FJ, Chenzbraun A, et al: Influence of preexistent donor coronary artery disease on the progression of transplant vasculopathy. An intravascular ultrasound study. *Circulation* 92:1126–1132, 1995.
37. Tsutsui H, Ziada KM, Schoenhagen P, et al: Lumen loss in transplant coronary artery disease is a biphasic process involving early intimal thickening and late constrictive remodeling: results from a 5-year serial intravascular ultrasound study. *Circulation* 104:653–657, 2001.
38. Mehra MR, Ventura HO, Stapleton DD, et al: Presence of severe intimal thickening by intravascular ultrasonography predicts cardiac events in cardiac allograft vasculopathy. *J Heart Lung Transplant* 14:632–639, 1995.
39. Rickenbacher PR, Pinto FJ, Lewis NP, et al: Prognostic importance of intimal thickness as measured by intracoronary ultrasound after cardiac transplantation. *Circulation* 92:3445–3452, 1995.
40. Tuzcu EM, Kapadia SR, Sachar R, et al: Intravascular ultrasound evidence of angiographically silent progression in coronary atherosclerosis predicts long-term morbidity and mortality after cardiac transplantation. *J Am Coll Cardiol* 45:1538–1542, 2005.
41. Kobashigawa JA, Katznelson S, Laks H, et al: Effect of pravastatin on outcomes after cardiac transplantation. *N Engl J Med* 333:621–627, 1995.
42. Eisen HJ, Tuzcu EM, Dorent R, et al: Everolimus for the prevention of allograft rejection and vasculopathy in cardiac-transplant recipients. *N Engl J Med* 349:847–858, 2003.
43. Nakamura S, Colombo A, Gaglione A, et al: Intracoronary ultrasound observations during stent implantation. *Circulation* 89:2026–2034, 1994.
44. Kiemeneij F, Laarman G, Slagboom T: Mode of deployment of coronary Palmaz-Schatz stents after implantation with the stent delivery system: an intravascular ultrasound study. *Am Heart J* 129:638–644, 1995.
45. Colombo A, Hall P, Nakamura S, et al: Intracoronary stenting without anticoagulation accomplished with intravascular ultrasound guidance. *Circulation* 91:1676–1688, 1995.
46. Kasaoka S, Tobis JM, Akiyama T, et al: Angiographic and intravascular ultrasound predictors of in-stent restenosis. *J Am Coll Cardiol* 32:1630–1635, 1998.
47. de Jaegere P, Mudra H, Figulla H, et al: Intravascular ultrasound-guided optimized stent deployment. Immediate and 6 months clinical and angiographic results from the Multicenter Ultrasound Stenting in Coronaries Study (MUSIC Study). *Eur Heart J* 19:1214–1223, 1998.
48. Hoffmann R, Mintz GS, Mehran R, et al: Intravascular ultrasound predictors of angiographic restenosis in lesions treated with Palmaz-Schatz stents. *J Am Coll Cardiol* 31:43–49, 1998.
49. Moussa I, Moses J, Di Mario C, et al: Does the specific intravascular ultrasound criterion used to optimize stent expansion have an impact on the probability of stent restenosis? *Am J Cardiol* 83:1012–1017, 1999.
50. Ziada KM, Kapadia SR, Belli G, et al: Prognostic value of absolute versus relative measures of the procedural result after successful coronary stenting: importance of vessel size in predicting long-term freedom from target vessel revascularization. *Am Heart J* 141:823–831, 2001.
51. de Feyter PJ, Kay P, Disco C, et al: Reference chart derived from post-stent implantation intravascular ultrasound predictors of 6 month expected restenosis on quantitative coronary angiography. *Circulation* 100:1777–1783, 1999.
52. Albiero R, Rau T, Schluter M, et al: Comparison of immediate and intermediate-term results of intravascular ultrasound versus angiography-guided Palmaz-Schatz stent implantation in matched lesions. *Circulation* 96:2997–3005, 1997.
53. Blasini R, Neumann FJ, Schmitt C, et al: Restenosis rate after intravascular ultrasound-guided coronary stent implantation. *Cathet Cardiovasc Diagn* 44:380–386, 1998.
54. Fitzgerald PJ, Oshima A, Hayase M, et al: Final results of the Can Routine Ultrasound Influence Stent Expansion (CRUISE) study. *Circulation* 102:523–530, 2000.
55. Choi JW, Goodreau LM, Davidson CJ: Resource utilization and clinical outcomes of coronary stenting: a comparison of intravascular ultrasound and angiographical guided stent implantation. *Am Heart J* 142:112–118, 2001.
56. Orford JL, Denktas AE, Williams BA, et al: Routine intravascular ultrasound scanning guidance of coronary stenting is not associated with improved clinical outcomes. *Am Heart J* 148:501–506, 2004.
57. Schiele F, Meneveau N, Vuillemenot A, et al: Impact of intravascular ultrasound guidance in stent deployment on 6-month restenosis rate: a multicenter, randomized study comparing two strategies–with and without intravascular ultrasound guidance. RESIST Study Group. REStenosis after IVUS guided STenting. *J Am Coll Cardiol* 32:320–328, 1998.
58. Mudra H, di Mario C, de Jaegere P, et al: Randomized comparison of coronary stent implantation under ultrasound or angiographic guidance to reduce stent restenosis (OPTICUS Study). *Circulation* 104:1343–1349, 2001.
59. Oemrawsingh PV, Mintz GS, Schalij MJ, et al: Intravascular ultrasound guidance improves angiographic and clinical outcome of stent implantation for long coronary artery stenoses: final results of a randomized comparison with angiographic guidance (TULIP Study). *Circulation* 107:62–67, 2003.
60. Parise H, Maehara A, Stone GW, et al: Meta-analysis of randomized studies comparing intravascular ultrasound versus angiographic guidance of percutaneous coronary intervention in pre-drug-eluting stent era. *Am J Cardiol* 107(3):374–382, 2011.

61. Lodi-Junqueira L, de Sousa MR, da Paixão LC, et al: Does intravascular ultrasound provide clinical benefits for percutaneous coronary intervention with bare-metal stent implantation? A meta-analysis of randomized controlled trials. *Syst Rev* 1:42, 2012.
62. Sonoda S, Morino Y, Ako J, et al: Impact of final stent dimensions on long-term results following sirolimus-eluting stent implantation: serial intravascular ultrasound analysis from the SIRIUS trial. *J Am Coll Cardiol* 43:1959–1963, 2004.
63. Hong MK, Mintz GS, Lee CW, et al: Intravascular ultrasound predictors of angiographic restenosis after sirolimus-eluting stent implantation. *Eur Heart J* 27:1305–1310, 2006.
64. Doi H, Maehara A, Mintz GS, et al: Impact of post-intervention minimal stent area on 9-month follow-up patency of paclitaxel-eluting stents: an integrated intravascular ultrasound analysis from the TAXUS IV, V, and VI and TAXUS ATLAS Workhorse, Long Lesion, and Direct Stent Trials. *JACC Cardiovasc Interv* 2(12):1269–1275, 2009.
65. Chieffo A, Latib A, Caussin C, et al: A prospective, randomized trial of intravascular-ultrasound guided compared to angiography guided stent implantation in complex coronary lesions: the AVIO trial. *Am Heart J* 165(1):65–72, 2013.
66. Kim JS, Kang TS, Mintz GS, et al: Randomized comparison of clinical outcomes between intravascular ultrasound and angiography-guided drug-eluting stent implantation for long coronary artery stenoses. *JACC Cardiovasc Interv* 6(4):369–376, 2013.
67. Park SJ, Kim YH, Park DW, et al: Impact of intravascular ultrasound guidance on long-term mortality in stenting for unprotected left main coronary artery stenosis. *Circ Cardiovasc Interv* 2:167–177, 2009.
68. Zhang Y, Farooq V, Garcia-Garcia HM, et al: Comparison of intravascular ultrasound versus angiography-guided drug-eluting stent implantation: a meta-analysis of one randomised trial and ten observational studies involving 19,619 patients. *EuroIntervention* 8(7):855–865, 2012.
69. Witzenbichler B, Maehara A, Weisz G, et al: Use of IVUS reduces stent thrombosis: results from the prospective, multicenter ADAPT-DES study. *Circulation* 129:463–470, 2014.
70. Serruys PW, Degertekin M, Tanabe K, et al: Intravascular ultrasound findings in the multicenter, randomized, double-blind RAVEL (RAndomized study with the sirolimus-eluting VElocity balloon-expandable stent in the treatment of patients with de novo native coronary artery Lesions) trial. *Circulation* 106:798–803, 2002.
71. Degertekin M, Serruys PW, Tanabe K, et al: Long-term follow-up of incomplete stent apposition in patients who received sirolimus-eluting stent for de novo coronary lesions: an intravascular ultrasound analysis. *Circulation* 108:2747–2750, 2003.
72. Kume T, Waseda K, Ako J, et al: Intravascular ultrasound assessment of postprocedural incomplete stent apposition. *J Invasive Cardiol* 24(1):13–16, 2012.
73. Cook S, Wenaweser P, Togni M, et al: Incomplete stent apposition and very late stent thrombosis after drug-eluting stent implantation. *Circulation* 115:2426–2434, 2007.
74. Fujii K, Carlier SG, Mintz GS, et al: Stent underexpansion and residual reference segment stenosis are related to stent thrombosis after sirolimus-eluting stent implantation: an intravascular ultrasound study. *J Am Coll Cardiol* 45(7):995–998, 2005.
75. Hong MK, Mintz GS, Lee CW, et al: Incidence, mechanism, predictors, and long-term prognosis of late stent malapposition after bare-metal stent implantation. *Circulation* 109:881–886, 2004.
76. Hong MK, Mintz GS, Lee CW, et al: Late stent malapposition after drug-eluting stent implantation: an intravascular ultrasound analysis with long-term follow-up. *Circulation* 113:414–419, 2006.
77. Painter JA, Mintz GS, Wong SC, et al: Serial intravascular ultrasound studies fail to show evidence of chronic Palmaz-Schatz stent recoil. *Am J Cardiol* 75:398–400, 1995.
78. Hoffmann R, Mintz GS, Dussaillant GR, et al: Patterns and mechanisms of in-stent restenosis. A serial intravascular ultrasound study. *Circulation* 94:1247–1254, 1996.
79. Lemos PA, Saia F, Ligthart JM, et al: Coronary restenosis after sirolimus-eluting stent implantation: morphological description and mechanistic analysis from a consecutive series of cases. *Circulation* 108:257–260, 2003.
80. Castagna MT, Mintz GS, Leiboff BO, et al: The contribution of "mechanical" problems to in-stent restenosis: an intravascular ultrasonographic analysis of 1090 consecutive in-stent restenosis lesions. *Am Heart J* 142:970–974, 2001.
81. Sharma SK, Kini A, Mehran R, et al: Randomized trial of Rotational Atherectomy Versus Balloon Angioplasty for Diffuse In-stent Restenosis (ROSTER). *Am Heart J* 147:16–22, 2004.
82. vom Dahl J, Dietz U, Haager PK, et al: Rotational atherectomy does not reduce recurrent in-stent restenosis: results of the angioplasty versus rotational atherectomy for treatment of diffuse in-stent restenosis trial (ARTIST). *Circulation* 105:583–588, 2002.
83. Abizaid A, Costa MA, Blanchard D, et al: Sirolimus-eluting stents inhibit neointimal hyperplasia in diabetic patients. Insights from the RAVEL Trial. *Eur Heart J* 25:107–112, 2004.
84. Mintz GS, Nissen SE, Anderson WD, et al: American College of Cardiology Clinical Expert Consensus Document on Standards for Acquisition, Measurement and Reporting of Intravascular Ultrasound Studies (IVUS). A report of the American College of Cardiology Task Force on Clinical Expert Consensus Documents. *J Am Coll Cardiol* 37:1478–1492, 2001.
85. Maehara A, Mintz GS, Bui AB, et al: Incidence, morphology, angiographic findings, and outcomes of intramural hematomas after percutaneous coronary interventions: an intravascular ultrasound study. *Circulation* 105:2037–2042, 2002.
86. Schuhlen H, Hadamitzky M, Walter H, et al: Major benefit from antiplatelet therapy for patients at high risk for adverse cardiac events after coronary Palmaz-Schatz stent placement: analysis of a prospective risk stratification protocol in the Intracoronary Stenting and Antithrombotic Regimen (ISAR) trial. *Circulation* 95:2015–2021, 1997.
87. Ziada KM, Tuzcu EM, De Franco AC, et al: Intravascular ultrasound assessment of the prevalence and causes of angiographic "haziness" following high-pressure coronary stenting. *Am J Cardiol* 80:116–121, 1997.
88. Park Y, Park HS, Jang GL, et al: Intravascular ultrasound guided recanalization of stumpless chronic total occlusion. *Int J Cardiol* 148(2):174–178, 2011.
89. Okamura A, Iwakura K, Date M, et al: Navifocus WR is the promising intravascular ultrasound for navigating the guidewire into true lumen during the coronary intervention for chronic total occlusion. *Cardiovasc Interv Ther* 2013. [Epub ahead of print].
90. Rathore S, Katoh O, Tuschikane E, et al: A novel modification of the retrograde approach for the recanalization of chronic total occlusion of the coronary arteries intravascular ultrasound-guided reverse controlled antegrade and retrograde tracking. *JACC Cardiovasc Interv* 3(2):155–164, 2010.
91. Losordo DW, Rosenfield K, Kaufman J, et al: Focal compensatory enlargement of human arteries in response to progressive atherosclerosis. In vivo documentation using intravascular ultrasound. *Circulation* 89:2570–2577, 1994.
92. Pasterkamp G, Wensing PJ, Post MJ, et al: Paradoxical arterial wall shrinkage may contribute to luminal narrowing in human atherosclerotic femoral arteries. *Circulation* 91:1444–1449, 1995.
93. Arthurs ZM, Bishop PD, Feiten LE, et al: Evaluation of peripheral atherosclerosis: a comparative analysis of angiography and intravascular ultrasound imaging. *J Vasc Surg* 51:933–938, 2010.
94. Toggweiler S, Leipsic J, Binder RK, et al: Management of vascular access in transcatheter aortic valve replacement: part 1: basic anatomy, imaging, sheaths, wires, and access routes. *JACC Cardiovasc Interv* 6(7):643–653, 2013.
95. Walker TG, Kalva SP, Yeddula K, et al: Clinical practice guidelines for endovascular abdominal aortic aneurysm repair: written by the Standards of Practice Committee for the Society of Interventional Radiology and endorsed by the Cardiovascular and Interventional Radiological Society of Europe and the Canadian Interventional Radiology Association. *J Vasc Interv Radiol* 21:1632–1655, 2010.
96. von Segesser LK, Marty B, Ruchat P, et al: Routine use of intravascular ultrasound for endovascular aneurysm repair: angiography is not necessary. *Eur J Vasc Endovasc Surg* 23:537–542, 2002.
97. Saket RR, Razavi MK, Padidar A, et al: Novel intravascular ultrasound-guided method to create transintimal arterial communications: initial experience in peripheral occlusive disease and aortic dissection. *J Endovasc Ther* 11(3):274–280, 2004.
98. Schoenhagen P, Ziada KM, Kapadia SR, et al: Extent and direction of arterial remodeling in stable versus unstable coronary syndromes: an intravascular ultrasound study. *Circulation* 101:598–603, 2000.
99. Mintz GS, Garcia-Garcia HM, Nicholls SJ, et al: Clinical expert consensus document on standards for acquisition, measurement and reporting of intravascular ultrasound regression/progression studies. *EuroIntervention* 6(9):1123–1130, 2011.
100. Nissen SE, Tsunoda T, Tuzcu EM, et al: Effect of recombinant ApoA-I Milano on coronary atherosclerosis in patients with acute coronary syndromes: a randomized controlled trial. *JAMA* 290:2292–2300, 2003.
101. Nissen SE, Tuzcu EM, Schoenhagen P, et al: Effect of intensive compared with moderate lipid-lowering therapy on progression of coronary atherosclerosis: a randomized controlled trial. *JAMA* 291:1071–1080, 2004.
102. Nissen SE, Nicholls SJ, Sipahi I, et al: Effect of very high-intensity statin therapy on regression of coronary atherosclerosis: the ASTEROID trial. *JAMA* 295(13):1556–1565, 2006.
103. Nicholls SJ, Hsu A, Wolski K, et al: Intravascular ultrasound-derived measures of coronary atherosclerotic plaque burden and clinical outcome. *J Am Coll Cardiol* 55(21):2399–2407, 2010.
104. Nair A, Kuban BD, Tuzcu EM, et al: Coronary plaque classification with intravascular ultrasound radiofrequency data analysis. *Circulation* 106:2200–2206, 2002.
105. Rodriguez-Granillo GA, Garcia-Garcia HM, Mc Fadden EP, et al: In vivo intravascular ultrasound-derived thin-cap fibroatheroma detection using ultrasound radiofrequency data analysis. *J Am Coll Cardiol* 46:2038–2042, 2005.
106. Sales FJ1, Falcão BA, Falcão JL, et al: Evaluation of plaque composition by intravascular ultrasound "virtual histology": the impact of dense calcium on the measurement of necrotic tissue. *EuroIntervention* 6(3):394–399, 2010.
107. Pu J, Mintz GS, Brilakis ES, et al: In vivo characterization of coronary plaques: novel findings from comparing greyscale and virtual histology intravascular ultrasound and near-infrared spectroscopy. *Eur Heart J* 33(3):372–383, 2012.
108. Stone GW, Maehara A, Lansky AJ, et al: A prospective natural-history study of coronary atherosclerosis. *N Engl J Med* 364:226–235, 2011.
109. Rodriguez-Granillo GA, Serruys PW, Garcia-Garcia HM, et al: Coronary artery remodeling is related to plaque composition. *Heart* 92:388–391, 2006.
110. Hong YJ, Mintz GS, Kim SW, et al: Impact of plaque composition on cardiac troponin elevation after percutaneous coronary intervention: an ultrasound analysis. *JACC Cardiovasc Imaging* 2(4):458–468, 2009.
111. Gardner CM, Tan H, Hull EL, et al: Detection of lipid core coronary plaques in autopsy specimens with a novel catheter-based near-infrared spectroscopy system. *JACC Cardiovasc Imaging* 1:638–648, 2008.
112. Madder RD, Steinberg DH, Anderson RD: Multimodality direct coronary imaging with combined near-Infrared spectroscopy and intravascular ultrasound: initial US experience. *Catheter Cardiovasc Interv* 81:551–557, 2013.
113. Waksman R, Kitabata H, Prati F, et al: Intravascular ultrasound versus optical coherence tomography guidance. *J Am Coll Cardiol* 62:S32–S40, 2013.
114. Maehara A, Mintz GS, Stone GW: OCT versus IVUS: accuracy versus clinical utility. *JACC Cardiovasc Imaging* 6:1105–1107, 2013.
115. Prati F, Di Vito L, Biondi-Zoccai G, et al: Angiography alone versus angiography plus optical coherence tomography o guide decision-making during percutaneous coronary intervention: the Centro per la Lotta contro l'Infarto-Optimisation of Percutaneous Coronary Intervention (CLI-OPCI) study. *EuroIntervention* 8:823–829, 2012.
116. Okamura T, Onuma Y, Garcia-Garcia HM, et al: First-in-man evaluation of intravascular optical frequency domain imaging (OFDI) of Terumo: a comparison with intravascular ultrasound and quantitative coronary angiography. *EuroIntervention* 6:1037–1045, 2011.
117. Kubo T, Akasaka T, Shite J, et al: OCT compared with IVUS in a coronary lesion assessment. The OPUS-CLASS study. *JACC Cardiovasc Imaging* 6:1095–1104, 2013.
118. Waters KR, Bautista R, Zelenka R, et al: Development of a high-definition intravascular ultrasound imaging system and catheter. *IEEE International Ultrasonic Symposium Proceedings* 1762–1765, 2011.
119. Tanaka S, Sakamoto K, Yamada R, et al: Plaque assessment with a novel high-definition 60-MHz IVUS imaging system: comparison with conventional 40 MHz IVUS and optical coherence tomography. *J Am Coll Cardiol* 61:E1878, 2013.

Optical Coherence Tomography

Farhad Abtahian and Ik-Kyung Jang

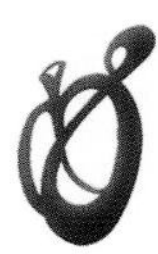

INTRODUCTION

Optical coherence tomography (OCT) is a tomographic imaging technology first described for use in ophthalmology[1] that has been adapted for real-time intravascular imaging. The resolution of OCT is significantly higher than other currently available intravascular imaging modalities, allowing for detailed characterization of the morphological features of coronary arteries, coronary plaques, and intracoronary stents. OCT is analogous to intravascular ultrasound (IVUS) with light as the energy source instead of sound.[1-3] Light is directed at a target, and the magnitude and echo time delay of the backscattered light signal is measured. Because it utilizes light, OCT has a resolution that is an order of magnitude greater than IVUS. Tissue-level properties can be assessed, allowing for differentiation of tissue types based on their optical characteristics. Higher resolution imaging also allows for more accurate assessment of vascular lumen size, vascular pathology, presence of thrombus, coronary stent strut apposition after percutaneous coronary intervention (PCI), and vascular response to previously placed coronary stents. Because of significant blood attenuation of light, OCT imaging requires a blood-free zone for imaging. First generation OCT imaging systems utilized an occlusive balloon with saline flush through a distal balloon lumen. Second generation OCT systems, utilizing a nonocclusive contrast flushing method to create a blood-free zone combined with faster catheter pullback, have significantly simplified image acquisition. These improvements allow for expansion of OCT use beyond research to more routine use to assess intravascular pathology and to guide PCI.

PHYSICS OF OPTICAL COHERENCE TOMOGRAPHY

OCT utilizes optical interference of near-infrared light to generate images.[1-3] Near-infrared light is emitted from a distal tip of an optical fiber located within the imaging catheter and directed at the target tissue (**Figure 17-1**). When light encounters a boundary between objects with varying optical impedances, a portion of the light is backscattered. The OCT catheter measures the magnitude and echo time delay of the backscattered light signal. To allow for recording of the reflected light, an interferometer is utilized to combine the reflected light from the sample with a reference beam reflected off of a reference mirror at a known distance. The summed beams from the sample and the reference mirror are then measured by the detector. The first generation time domain OCT (TD-OCT) systems utilized a broadband light source and determined tissue depth by changing the distance to the reference mirror.[4] Because of the need for mechanical sweep of the reference light source, the rate of image acquisition in TD-OCT is inherently limited. Maximum pullback speeds with TD-OCT systems are approximately 2-3 mm/second. In the context of need for a blood-free field, this limits the length of coronary artery that can be imaged during one pullback of the imaging catheter. In second generation Fourier-domain OCT (FD-OCT) systems, the light source is monochromatic and emits various wavelengths between 1250 nm and 1350 nm in a continuous sweep.[5] Fourier transformation of the interference signal generated allows for calculation of the reflections returning from different depths. As result, there is no

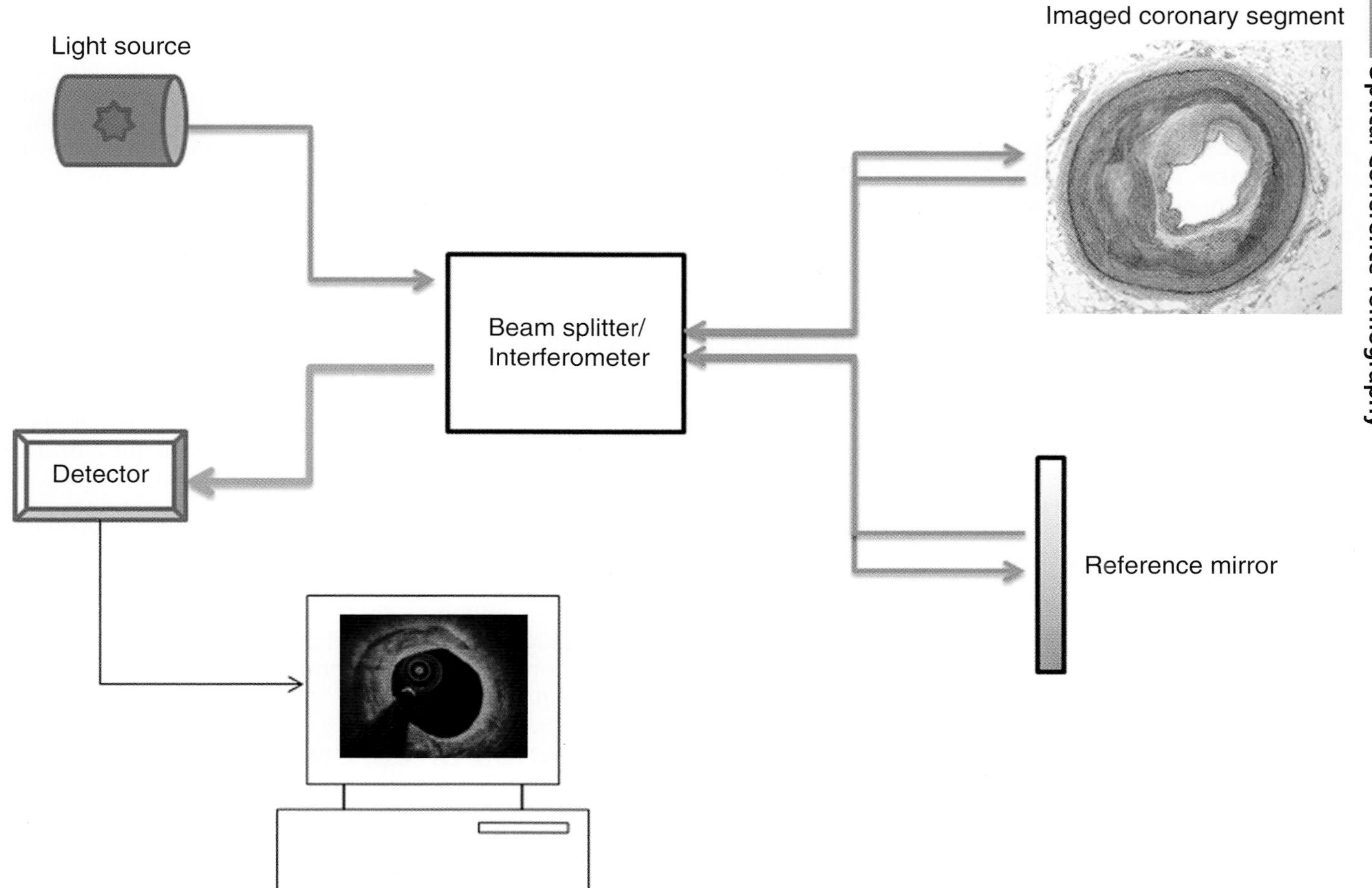

FIGURE 17-1 Near-infrared light is directed at a target and a reference mirror. Interference occurs when light from the sample and reference mirror arrive at the same time. The magnitude and echo time delay of the reflected light signal is measured. To allow for recording of the reflected light, an interferometer is utilized to combine the reflected light from the sample with a reference beam reflected off of a reference mirror at a known distance. The summed beams from the sample and the reference mirror are then measured by the detector. In a time domain (TD) optical coherence tomography (OCT) system, the reference mirror moves back and forth, allowing for measurement of depth. In a Fourier domain (FD) OCT system, the light sources sweeps across a frequency range. Because mechanical sweep of the reference mirror is not necessary, image acquisition is significantly faster with FD-OCT. *(From Abtahian F, Jang IK: Optical coherence tomography: basics, current application and future potential. Curr Opin Pharmacol 12:583–591, 2012.)*

need for mechanical adjustment of the reference light path. This allows all echo time delays to be measured simultaneously, leading to significantly faster image acquisition. FD-OCT systems allow pullback speeds of the imaging catheter of 20 mm/second.

Because light is the energy source, tissue can be imaged with an axial resolution of 10 μm and lateral resolution of 20 μm.[6] Tissue penetration is limited to a depth of 2 mm but varies significantly depending on the imaged tissue. Lipid, which is high attenuating, allows for significantly less tissue penetration than collagen or calcium, which are low attenuating. In comparison IVUS, which is currently the most commonly used intravascular imaging modality, provides a resolution of 150-250 μm to a depth of up to 10 mm.[7]

IMAGE ACQUISITION BY OPTICAL COHERENCE TOMOGRAPHY

Time Domain Optical Coherence Tomography

The first OCT used clinically was the M2 and M3 TD-OCT system manufactured by LightLab (Westford, Massachusetts, now part of St. Jude Medical). In the M2/M3 systems, a console contains the pullback device; the optical imaging components including the light source, beam splitter, reference arm, and detectors; and a computer for image creation. Images are recorded by a fiber-optic wire that rotates inside a protective sheath. The wire is attached to an automated pullback engine integrated with the console. An over-the-wire low-pressure occlusion balloon catheter with distal flush ports is used to occlude the imaged vessel at a low-pressure inflation (0.5 atm) and infuse saline or lactated Ringer's at approximately 0.5-1.0 mL/s to displace blood during imaging acquisition. Per manufacturer recommendations, the occlusion time should be limited to 30 seconds. Images are obtained during pullback at a rate of 0.5-2.0 mm/s. There are significant limitations from the occlusive technique for blood displacement, specifically transient ischemia, inability to image proximal segment of vessel due to balloon occlusion, and the complexity and time-consuming nature of the procedure. A nonocclusive technique for blood removal is also possible.[8] In this approach, blood is displaced by continuous injection of iso-osmolar contrast or mixture of dextran and lactated Ringer's through the guiding catheter by manual injection or automated injection. For automated injections, the volume of injection should be 50 mL at a rate of 1.5-3 mL/s depending on vessel size. Pullback is then performed at a speed of 2-3 mm/s during contrast injection. The nonocclusive technique for blood displacement has a safety profile similar to the occlusive technique.[9]

Frequency Domain Optical Coherence Tomography

The first commercially available OCT system in the United States was a frequency domain (FD)-OCT system, C7XR OCT manufactured by St. Jude Medical. In this second generation platform, the optical probe is integrated into a delivery catheter with a profile of 2.7 Fr and length of 140 cm. The catheter has a rapid exchange monorail tail compatible with standard 0.014 coronary wires and can be delivered via a 6 Fr guide catheter. Radio-opaque markers, identifying the distal tip, location of imaging lens, and 50 mm proximal to the lens allow for alignment of the catheter with the vessel segment of interest. During the pullback the optic fiber probe is pulled along the catheter sheath. As with the first generation TD-OCT systems, the FD-OCT systems contain a dedicated pullback device and a console that processes and stores the data. The C7 FD-OCT systems can acquire images at a pullback speed of 20 mm/s, allowing for imaging of a 50-mm vessel segment in less than 3 seconds. The newly available ILUMIEN OPTIS imaging system (St. Jude Medical, Minneapolis, Minnesota) allows for imaging of a 75-mm segment of vessel at a pullback speed of 40 mm/s. Because of the rapid pullback in these systems, adequate blood displacement can be achieved with a single bolus injection of contrast. Lactated Ringer's can also be used to minimize contrast load in patients with renal impairment. Guiding catheter should be positioned coaxially with vessel ostium to maximize delivery of contrast for blood clearance. The manufacture protocol recommends a 14-mL injection of contrast at a rate of 4 mL per second. The technique for image acquisition is significantly simplified and faster with the C7 and OPTIS system compared with the first generation M2/M3 systems.

Potential Risks and Complications

Overall, the technique appears to be safe[9,10] with 0.2% incidence of vessel dissection due to the imaging system and 1% incidence of ventricular fibrillation secondary to balloon occlusion, when the first generation TD-OCT system was used. Sinus bradycardia, tachycardia, and atrioventricular block have also been reported in the context of balloon occlusion but are rare. Blood clearance during OCT image acquisition can produce transient ischemia especially with the occlusive technique. This is of particular concern in patients with single-vessel myocardial blood supply. Chest pain and transient ST-segment elevation during vessel occlusion are common, occurring in about 50% of patients.[9] Risks of transient ischemia are significantly reduced with the second generation rapid pullback systems.[11] Coronary spasm and coronary dissection are potential complications whenever any device is introduced into a coronary artery and likewise can occur during OCT imaging. In order to reduce the risk of coronary spasm, intracoronary nitroglycerin should be administrated prior to image acquisition. The incidence appears to be less than 1% for either spasm or dissection. Similarly, there is a risk of air embolism and thrombus injection as would occur with any other intracoronary procedures. Complication rates with OCT are similar to those seen with IVUS in the PROSPECT study.[12] Fastidious attention to flush lines, contrast injection, and wire management is required as with any procedure. Anticoagulation prior to intracoronary introduction of OCT system is mandatory.

EVALUATION OF CORONARY PATHOLOGY

Normal Artery

By histology, the normal coronary artery has three tissue layers: intima, media, adventitia separated by an internal and external elastic lamina. All three layers can by visualized by OCT in a normal artery (**Figure 17-2**). The innermost adluminal intimal layer is seen by OCT as a signal-rich thin band.[13-15] The media is immediately below the intima and appears as an area of low signal intensity surrounded by the signal-rich adventitia. OCT assessment of intimal thickness is highly accurate,[14] allowing for detection of the earliest marker of atherosclerotic disease, intimal thickening secondary to deposition of lipids.[16] Coronary plaques are typically identified by the presence of focal thickening and loss

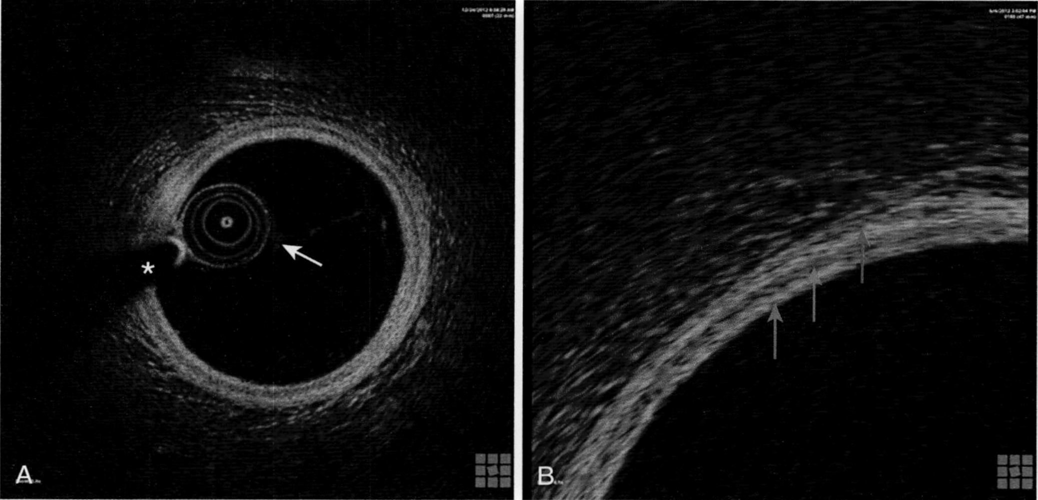

FIGURE 17-2 Optical coherence tomography (OCT) images from a normal coronary artery **(A)** with magnification **(B).** OCT catheter *(white arrow)* within a coronary artery reveals the normal three layers of the coronary artery: intima *(blue arrow)*, media *(red arrow)*, and adventitia *(green arrow)*. The guidewire causes a shadow artifact (*).

of the normal three-layered structure of the coronary artery. Mature coronary plaques are generally classified by histology as lipid-rich, fibrous, or fibrocalcific based on their tissue compositions,[17] each of which can be distinguished by its OCT appearance. In cadaveric studies of human arteries with histology as the gold standard, OCT has sensitivity for lipid plaque, fibrous plaque, and calcified plaque of 95%, 98%, and 100%, respectively. The specificity of OCT for the same three plaque tissue components was 98%, 94%, and 100%, respectively.[18] These results compare favorably to both integrated backscatter IVUS and conventional grayscale IVUS.

Lipid Plaque

Lipid plaque is defined by the presence of signal-poor areas with diffuse borders resulting from backscatter and rapid attenuation from the lipid-containing region located below a fibrous cap (**Figure 17-3A**). The fibrous cap is typically a homogeneous signal-rich band overlying the signal-poor lipid core. The minimal thickness of the fibrous cap is critical for identifying thin-cap fibroatheromas (TCFAs).[19]

Fibrous and Fibrocalcific Plaque

Fibrous plaques are visualized on OCT as homogeneous areas with high reflectivity and low attenuation (**Figure 17-3B**). Calcification within the coronary artery is demarcated by a signal-poor region with sharp edges and low attenuation (**Figure 17-3C**).[20] This is distinct from lipid pools that are signal-poor areas with diffuse borders and high attenuation. Because both calcium and lipid generate low backscatter, distinguishing calcified plaque from lipid-rich plaque can at times be difficult to untrained interpreters.[21]

Intraluminal and Intramural Pathology Seen by Optical Coherence Tomography

Macrophages

Increased inflammation and macrophage infiltration is a hallmark of vulnerable plaques. OCT can indirectly assess for macrophage density within vulnerable plaques on the basis of signal variance within the raw OCT data.[22,23] Fibrous caps containing macrophages have significant OCT signal variance, which when normalized for variations in OCT system settings to generate a normalized standard deviation (NSD) of the OCT signal, can be used to identify areas with significant macrophage infiltration. When the data are compressed to generate images, areas of macrophage infiltration show a granular pattern with heterogeneous back shadow (**Figure 17-3D**). Autopsy studies of lipid-rich plaques have shown that OCT can identify plaques with greater than 10% macrophage density within the fibrous cap (identified by CD68 positivity with immunohistochemistry) with near 100% sensitivity.[24] OCT studies of patients presenting with acute coronary syndrome (ACS) have shown significantly greater macrophage density within fibrous caps compared with patients with stable angina.[25] Sites of plaque rupture appear to have the highest density of macrophage infiltration. Although intriguing, the ability to identify macrophages

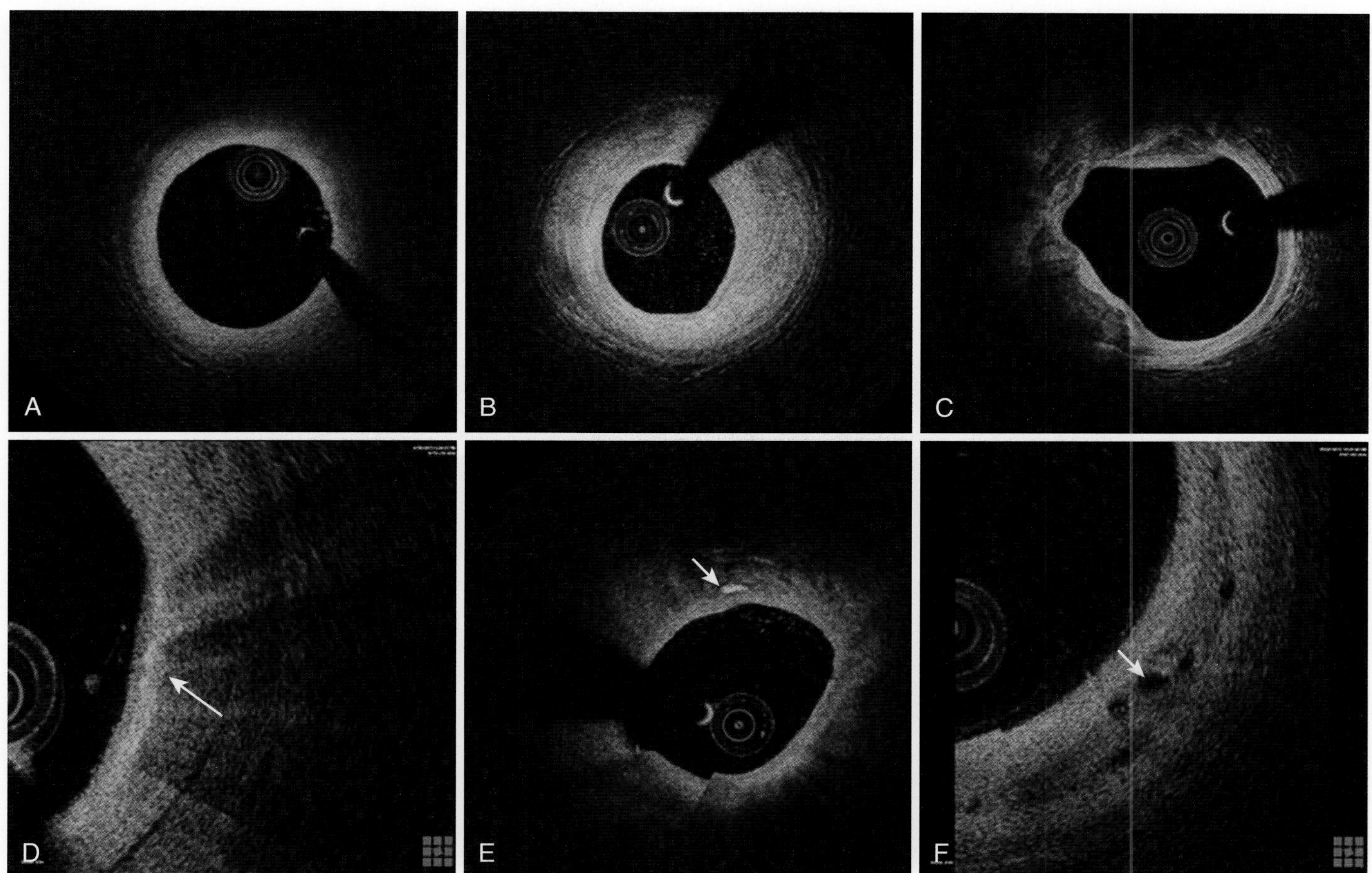

FIGURE 17-3 Optical coherence tomography (OCT) images of coronary pathology. **A,** Circumferential lipid-rich plaque. **B,** Fibrous plaque. **C,** Fibro-calcific plaque. **D,** Macrophages. **E,** Cholesterol crystal. **F,** Microchannels.

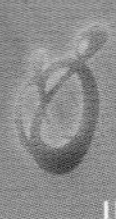

in vivo using signal variance has not been fully validated and further studies will be required to confirm.[22]

Cholesterol Crystal

Cholesterol crystals are identified by the presence of liner signal streaks typically in the context of a lipid-rich plaque (**Figure 17-3E**). The accuracy of OCT for the detection of cholesterol crystals has not been validated by histology.

Microchannels

OCT can detect within coronary plaque microchannels that appear as tubuloluminal structures with no signal inside (**Figure 17-3F**). These are believed to represent neovascularization and are found in higher abundance in thin capped lipid plaques and in patients presenting with plaque rupture. The presence of microchannels has also been associated with plaque progression.[23]

Thrombus

Thrombus is identified by the presence of an irregular mass either attached to the vessel wall (mural thrombus) or free within the vessel lumen. Platelet-rich white thrombus is a homogeneous signal-rich mass with low attenuation resulting in minimal shadowing, whereas red thrombus is a mass with rapid attenuation resulting in significant shadowing (**Figure 17-4A, B**).[26] The rate of signal attenuation, specifically a half attenuation width of 250 μm, can distinguish red and white thrombi with a sensitivity of 90% and specificity of 88%.[26]

Others

In addition to coronary plaques, acute coronary syndrome (ACS) can be caused by spontaneous coronary artery dissection and vasospasm. OCT is sensitive for detecting and characterizing coronary dissections and may be useful in guiding interventions to treat the dissection (**Figure 17-4C**).[27,28] The presence of double-lumen, dissection flap or intramural hematoma can be readily visualized by OCT even when angiographically not obvious. The morphological changes, specifically medial contraction and intimal gathering, that underlay coronary vasospasm have also been visualized by OCT.[29]

Thin-Cap Fibroatheroma

Coronary artery disease is the leading cause of death worldwide, most often by precipitating an ACS. ACS is an acute manifestation of the chronic process of atherosclerosis. As a result, there has been significant interest in understanding the mechanism by which coronary artery disease that is otherwise asymptomatic can lead to a sudden myocardial infarction. The term "vulnerable plaque" was initially coined in reference to coronary stenosis that did not appear to be significant by angiography but subsequently caused acute myocardial infarction.[30,31] Vulnerable plaques can be present in any location within the coronary arteries but are most commonly found in the proximal portion of the three main coronary vessels often at or near bifurcations.[32-35] ACS most frequently occurs when a vulnerable plaque ruptures, exposing the thrombogenic contents of the plaque to blood. Vulnerable plaques that are at high risk of precipitating an acute coronary event appear to have several histologic features that distinguish them from more stable coronary plaques. Autopsy studies have identified the presence of thin fibrous caps (<65 μm), large lipid cores (more than 40% of the overall plaque volume), and increased infiltration of macrophages into the plaque cap as the most common features of high-risk coronary plaques.[36] In addition, several other features have been linked to vulnerable plaques including positive remodeling of the affected vessel, increased vasa-vasorum neovascularization, and intraplaque hemorrhage. Because of a resolution capability of 10 μm, OCT is the only current modality that can readily identify and measure the thin fibrous caps of vulnerable plaques. Accurate and reproducible measurement of fibrous cap thickness is critical for the accurate identification of thin-cap fibroatheroma (TCFA). The typical method is averaging the measurement of cap width at several sites of minimal cap thickness based on visual estimation (**Figure 17-5**). Thickness is measured from the coronary artery lumen to inner border of the signal-poor region that identifies the lipid pool. In analyzing ruptured plaques, it can be challenging to identify the fibrous cap and accurately measure its thickness due to the presence of associated thrombus. Studies have either focused on the fibrous cap thickness at the preserved portions of the cap, which can overestimate cap thickness,[19] or measured the remnants of the cap at the rupture site.[37] A three-dimensional volumetric method has been proposed for more accurate measurement of fibrous cap area and thickness but has not been validated.[38] In a cadaveric study, OCT measurement of fibrous cap correlated well with histological measurements (r = 0.90).[39] Published

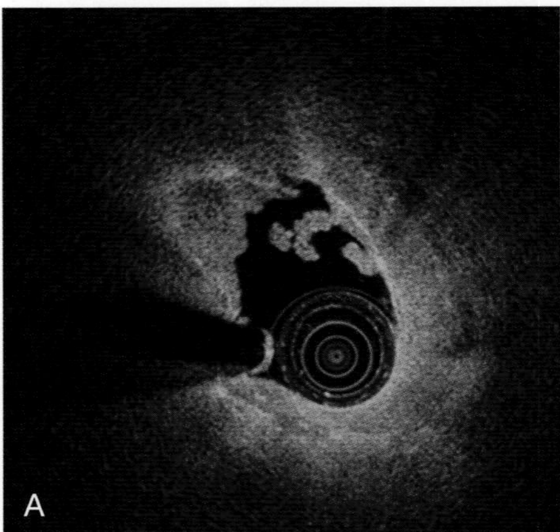

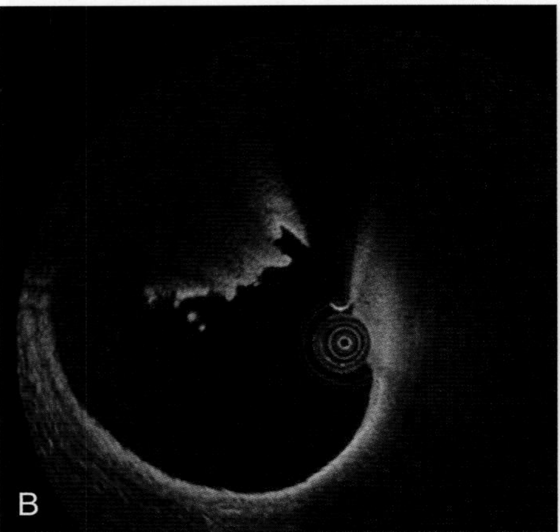

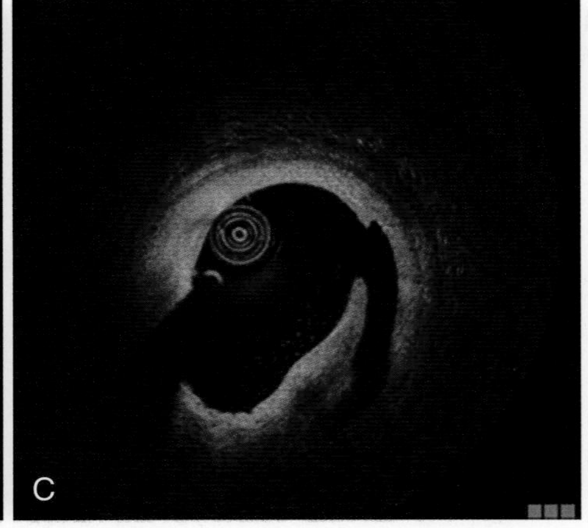

FIGURE 17-4 Optical coherence tomography (OCT) examples of intracoronary pathology. **A,** Platelet-rich white thrombus. **B,** Red blood cell-rich red thrombus. **C,** Dissection.

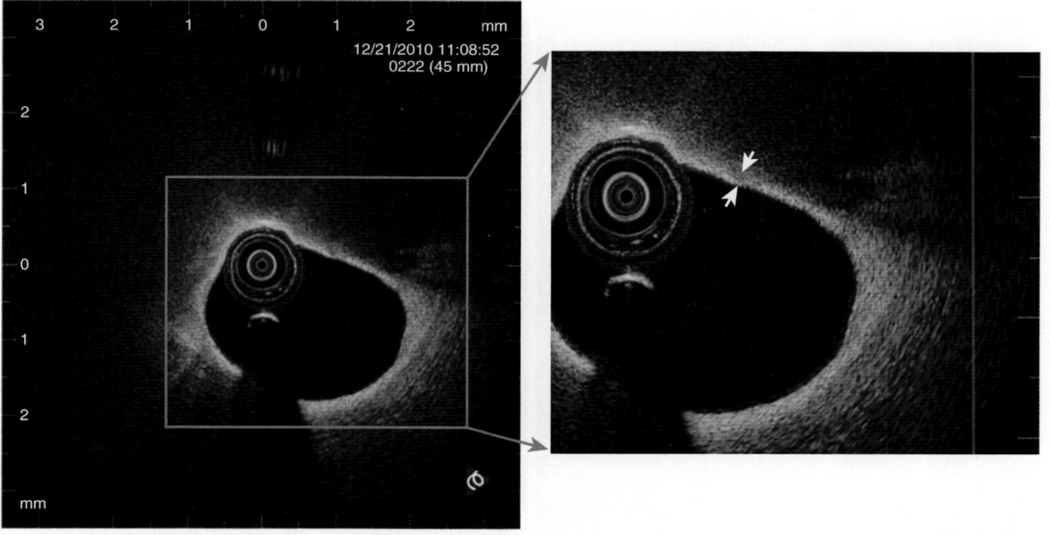

FIGURE 17-5 Example of thin-cap fibroatheroma (TCFA). The thinnest fibrous cap thickness of a lipid-rich plaque is measured. Lipid-rich plaques with a minimal cap thickness ≤65 μm are typically defined as TCFAs.

studies have varied in their definition of OCT defined TCFAs both in the cutoff for defining a cap as thin (65 μm vs. 70 μm vs. 80 μm) and the minimum lipid burden within the coronary plaque.[19,40,41]

PITFALLS OF IMAGE INTERPRETATION

Recognition of potential artifacts and limitations of OCT are crucial in proper interpretation of images. Incomplete clearance of blood is one of the most common causes of artifact during OCT imaging. Residual blood attenuates the light beam resulting in limited visualization of the vessel (**Figure 17-6A**). Significant blood attenuation can hamper accurate measurement of vessel size and can easily be confused for thrombus. With OCT, both lipid and calcium appear as signal-poor areas during OCT image acquisition. Lipid-rich plaques have indistinct borders while calcium-rich plaques have sharp borders surrounding the signal-poor areas. While these differences allow for distinguishing the two plaque types, there remains a significant overlap and potential to mischaracterize lipid-rich and calcium-rich plaques.[21] Because of the limited tissue penetration of OCT to 2-3 mm, determining the composition of thick plaques can become problematic with increasing signal drop-off. Attenuation of OCT signal deep within the artery wall can be confused for lipid pool and alternatively deep lipid can be misinterpreted as signal attenuation. Similarly, lack of tissue penetration prevents accurate measurement of total plaque burden and precludes assessing for vessel remodeling.

Optical Coherence Tomography Imaging Artifacts

- Shadowing is a result of signal drop-off distal to an object such as guidewire (**Figure 17-6B**), stent strut (**Figure 17-6C**), blood within the vessel or within the imaging catheter, macrophages, and thrombus. As result of signal loss, the underlying vessel structure cannot be visualized.
- Tangential signal dropout occurs when a catheter is nearly adjacent to a vessel wall, resulting in light being directed almost parallel with the vessel surface. As a result, the light source is significantly attenuated and there can be significant signal drop-off below the vessel lumen surface in the area immediately adjacent to the imaging catheter. It is important not to confuse this artifact with pathologic causes of signal-poor regions within vessel walls such as lipid-rich plaques.
- Nonuniform rotation distortion arises as a consequence of binding of the rotating optical components during image acquisition, typically due to a defective catheter or during imaging of tortuous or calcified vasculature or through a narrow stenosis. It appears as a smearing of the OCT image in the circumferential direction.
- Saturation artifact (**Figure 17-6D**) is caused by objects with highly reflective surface causing such high backscatter that they cannot be detected accurately. This results in linear streaks along an axial direction. Saturation artifact is typically caused by stent struts, guidewires, and occasionally by tissue surface.
- Motion artifact is caused by movement of the artery with respect to the imaging catheter (**Figure 17-6B**). It is a more significant problem with the TD-OCT systems that have a slower pullback speed and therefore acquire images over significantly more cardiac cycles. Seam lines, which are axial discontinuities, can arise when the imaging catheter moves relative to the vessel lumen during the acquisition of a single cross section. Movement of the artery can also disrupt the pullback, resulting in repeated images of the same anatomic area.
- Fold-over artifacts are specific to FD-OCT systems. They occur when the vessel lumen is larger than the imaging depth of the OCT system.
- Merry-go-round and sunflower effect are caused by eccentric wire positions that result in a light beam that is not perpendicular relative to the artery wall (**Figure 17-6C**).[42] Lateral resolution in the wall distal to the position of the wire is reduced ("merry-go-round effect") and the reflection of stent struts aligns toward the location of the wire, making it appear as if the stent struts are bending toward the wire ("sunflower effect").

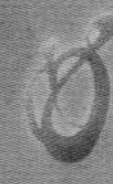

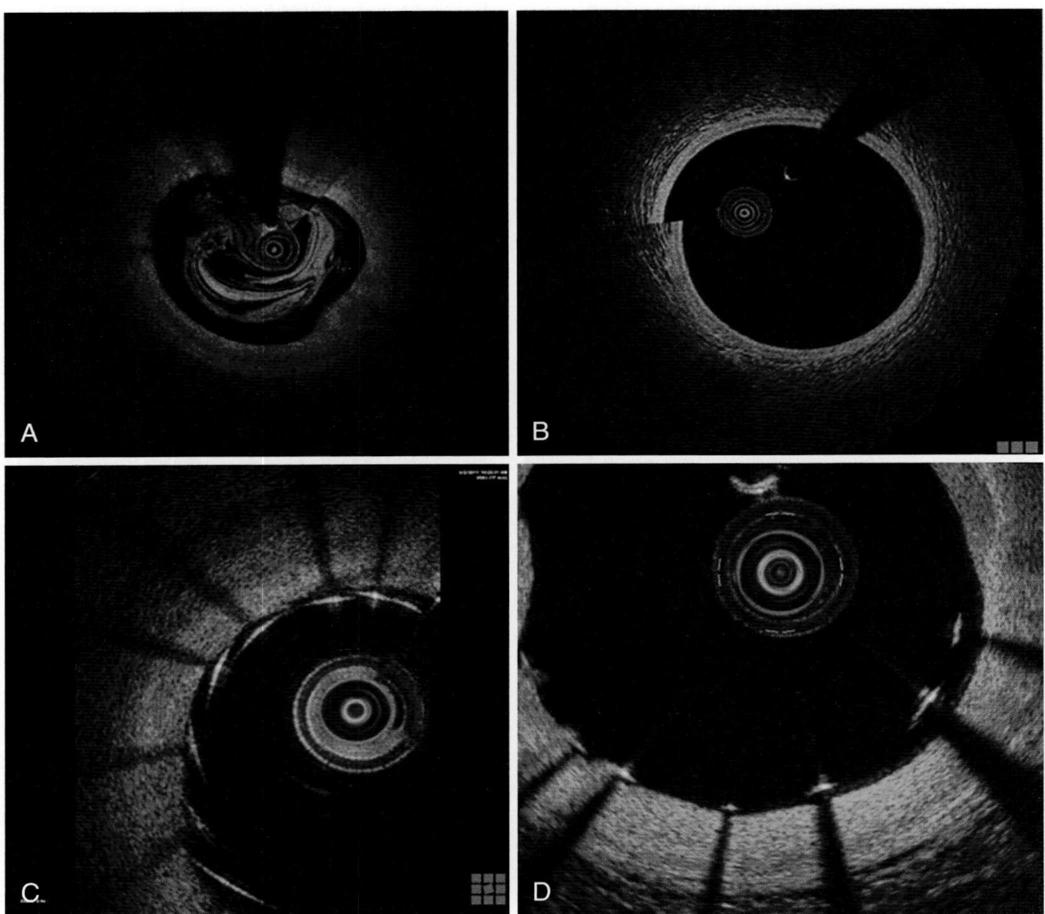

FIGURE 17-6 Examples of image artifact. **A**, Blood artifact. **B,** Motion artifact. **C,** Merry-go-round and sunflower. **D,** Saturation artifact.

ASSESSMENT OF CORONARY PLAQUE CHARACTERISTICS

Clinical Presentations and Plaque Morphology

The danger of TCFAs arises from their propensity to rupture and precipitate an acute coronary event. OCT identifies the presence of lipid-rich culprit plaques in 90% of patients presenting with ST-elevation myocardial infarction (STEMI) and 75% of patients presenting with non-ST-elevation myocardial infarction (NSTEMI). This compared to 60% of patients presenting with stable angina.[41] ACS patients also have thinner fibrous caps, large lipid burden, increased number of plaques with macrophages, and significantly more OCT-defined TCFAs (64.7% vs. 14.9%, $p < 0.001$).[43] Furthermore, patients with STEMI have a higher prevalence of OCT-defined TCFAs compared with patients with NSTEMI.[41] Ruptured plaques are seen more frequently in patients presenting with ACS compared with stable angina.[41,44]

One of the challenges of treating patients with coronary artery disease is recognizing plaques that are likely to progress with the goal of identifying patients who would benefit from either more aggressive pharmacological treatment or prophylactic intervention.[12] Studies involving small cohorts of patients with nonobstructive disease have identified TCFA and microchannels seen by OCT as potential predictors of plaque progression.[45] Specifically, plaques that had significant progression over a period of 7 months were significantly more likely to be TCFA or to have microchannels at baseline. Further prospective studies involving larger numbers of patients are needed to determine if these findings are significant enough to drive clinical decision making.

Etiology of Acute Coronary Syndrome

There are believed to be three principal mechanisms for acute coronary events leading to sudden cardiac death: rupture of thin-capped fibroatheromas, erosion of fibrous caps, and protruding calcific nodules (**Figure 17-7**).[21] Plaque rupture is defined by the presence of a fibrous cap discontinuity resulting in a cavity formation with communication between the cavity and the coronary artery lumen (Video 17-1).[46] By pathology, plaque erosions are identified by loss of the endothelial lining with overlying thrombus.[47] In a study comparing IVUS, angioscopy, and OCT, OCT was significantly better at detecting superficial plaque erosions.[44] With a resolution of 10-15 μm, OCT cannot visualize the endothelial lining of coronary arteries. Consequentially, surrogate markers must be utilized to identify plaque erosion by OCT. Erosions can potentially be identified by the presence of an intact fibrous cap with attached superficial thrombus or by the presence of an intact fibrous cap with irregular surface in the absence of superficial thrombus.[48] The presence of significant intracoronary thrombus, by limiting visualization of the underlying plaque and potentially hiding the presence of a fibrous cap discontinuity, significantly impairs the ability to distinguish plaque erosion from

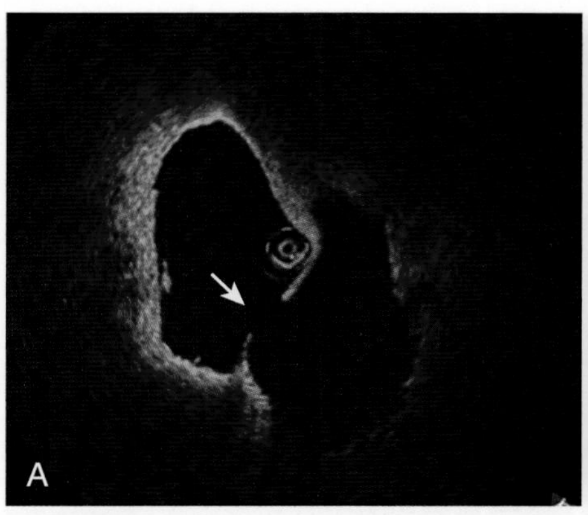

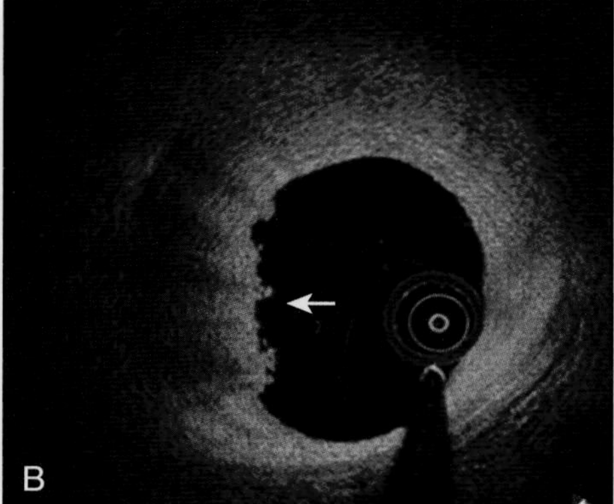

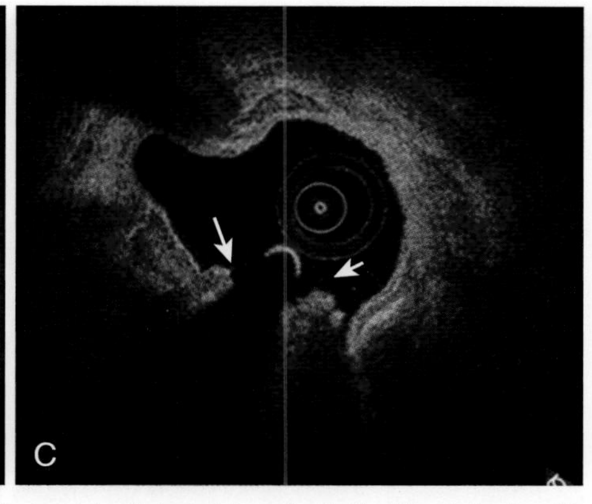

FIGURE 17-7 Etiology of acute coronary syndrome. **A,** Disrupted lipid-rich plaque. **B,** Plaque erosion. **C,** Calcified nodule. *(Adapted from Jia H, Abtahian F, Aguirre AD, et al: In vivo diagnosis of plaque erosion and calcified nodule in patients with acute coronary syndrome by intravascular optical coherence tomography. J Am Coll Cardiol 62:1748–1758, 2013.)*

plaque rupture.[49] Protruding calcific nodules have been defined by the presence of convex-shaped calcium that is covered by a thin fibrous cap or fully exposed to the lumen.[50] Fracture of calcific plate into the lumen frequently forms sharp angles which can be readily identified by OCT.

A study of patients presenting with ACS identified plaque erosions at the culprit lesion in 31.0% of cases, the majority in patients presenting with NSTEMI.[48] In contrast, plaque rupture was seen at the culprit site in 43.7% of patients, predominantly in patients with STEMI. Calcified nodules were causal in 7.9% of patients. Patients with plaque erosions are typically younger and appear to have higher levels of inflammatory markers compared with those with plaque rupture.[48,51] Vergallo et al. further showed that patients presenting with coronary plaque rupture at the culprit lesion were more likely to have ruptured plaques at nonculprit sites than patients presenting with ACS caused by erosion.[52] These results suggest that patients presenting with plaque rupture represent a subset of patients with increased pancoronary vulnerability. Distinguishing plaque erosion from plaque rupture may have therapeutic significance. Evaluation of patients' post-thrombolysis by OCT showed significantly more residual thrombus at sites of plaque rupture with a core of platelet-rich white thrombus surrounded by large amounts of red thrombus.[53] In contrast, sites of plaque erosion had significantly less thrombus that was predominantly platelet rich. Prati et al. analyzed 31 patients presenting with STEMI who were found to have an intact fibrous cap after aspiration thrombectomy.[54] Twelve patients with subcritical stenosis were treated with dual antiplatelet therapy and no stenting. At median 2 years' follow-up, all patients remained asymptomatic. This proof of concept study suggests an alternative treatment strategy forgoing stenting for patients with ACS and OCT verified nonobstructive plaque erosion may be possible.

Acute Myocardial Infarction at Rest versus with Exercise

The location of plaque rupture appears to correlate with the clinical scenario. Plaque rupture at the proximal portion of the plaque appears to occur more commonly with STEMI, while plaque rupture at the distal end of the plaque is seen more frequently with NSTEMI.[46] A study of culprit lesions in patients presenting with ACS revealed plaque rupture at the mid portion of the plaque correlates with the onset of coronary event at rest while plaque rupture at the plaque shoulder typically associates with coronary events occurring during activity.[55] The thickness of the ruptured fibrous cap in patients with ACS brought on by exertion was significantly higher than in patients with ACS at rest. Of note, in a significant minority of patients, the fibrous cap was thicker than the 65 μm used to define TCFAs.

ROLE OF OPTICAL COHERENCE TOMOGRAPHY IN PERCUTANEOUS CORONARY INTERVENTION

Pre-stent Deployment

The resolution of OCT makes it a potentially powerful tool to guide percutaneous coronary intervention (PCI). Accurate assessment of reference vessel size and lesion length are keys to appropriate stent sizing. Current OCT platforms contain software for semiautomatic vessel contour detection allowing for rapid, accurate, and reproducible measurements of reference vessel diameter and the minimal luminal diameter of the target lesion. The length of the lesion can also be measured rapidly in manual fashion. The potential exists for fully automated definition of luminal boundaries allowing for precise measurement of minimal lumen areas throughout the vessel segment analyzed.[56] The most recent OCT system (ILUMIEN OPTIS OCT, St. Jude Medical) catheter can acquire images over a longer segment of vessel (75 mm) at a faster pullback rate (40 mm/s). It is also reported to have a higher resolution then the previous generation system. The console allows for fully automated analysis of lumen contour in order to measure lesion length and reference vessel diameter. Using fractional flow reserve (FFR) as the gold standard, OCT is moderately accurate in determining lesion severity with similar accuracy to IVUS.[57] Minimal luminal areas of 1.91 mm^2 and percent lumen area stenosis >70% appear to be the best cutoff values to identify lesions with FFR <0.75.[58] Although OCT is sensitive for identifying severe lesions, the lack of specificity limits the positive predictive value of OCT-defined severe lesions.[57-59] Lesion characteristics such as fibrous, lipid, and calcium content, as defined by OCT, correlate with risk of post-procedure complications.[37,60-62] The presence of thrombus can also readily be identified prior to intervention. A recent randomized study evaluated the role of OCT in guiding in-stent thrombus removal for patients presenting with ACS and found

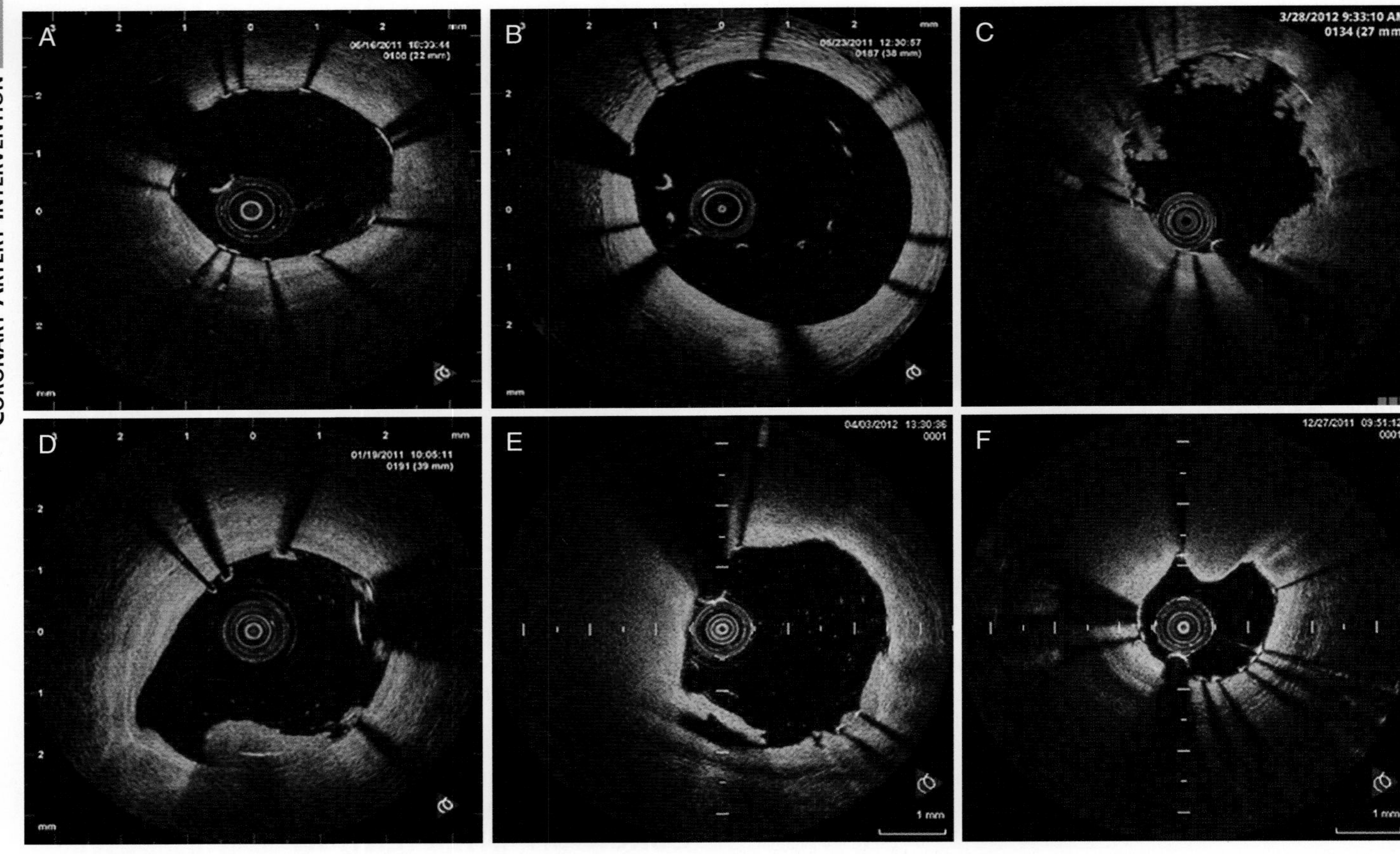

FIGURE 17-8 Optical coherence tomography (OCT) images immediately post-PCI. **A,** Well-apposed stent. **B,** Severely malapposed stent. **C,** Acute stent thrombosis. **D,** Mural thrombus. **E,** Edge dissection. **F,** Tissue prolapse.

significantly reduced thrombus volume in-stent and significantly larger stent area in the OCT-guided group.[63]

Immediate Post-stent Deployment

A key component of a successful intervention is adequate stent expansion resulting in a well-apposed stent (**Figure 17-8A** and Video 17-2). Metal stent struts are highly reflective and generate a strong signal with shadowing behind the stent strut ("blooming"). Bioabsorbable stents with polymeric struts, in contrast, do not cause shadowing.[64] Absorbable stents with metallic scaffolds appear similar to typical metal stents at implantation but overtime become less reflective and lose the blooming effect. Based on IVUS definitions for stent expansion,[65] adequate stent expansion is defined by OCT as a minimal in-stent lumen area that is >90% of the reference vessel lumen area. In the setting of significant artery tapering, adequate stent expansion is defined by a minimal in-stent area that is greater than 100% of the luminal area of the small distal reference segment.[66] Inadequate stent expansion leading to stent strut malapposition (**Figure 17-8B**) increases the risk of stent failure: either restenosis or in-stent thrombosis.

Because OCT can visualize individual stent struts and their distance from the vessel wall,[67] quantification of the degree of apposition or malapposition in simple and complex interventions are now possible.[68-70] Multiple methods for measuring stent strut apposition have been utilized in clinical studies. These include measuring from the center of the blooming artifact to the vessel wall or measuring from the outer surface of the blooming artifact to the vessel wall.[68,71,72] Accurate assessment of stent apposition requires measuring apposition at intervals of at maximum 1 mm and more typically 0.6 mm. Immediately post intervention, individual stent struts are either apposed or malapposed. Apposed stent struts are further classified as embedded or protruding. Struts buried in the vessel wall by more than half of the strut thickness are defined as embedded. Struts with the adluminal stent strut surface above the luminal surface of the vessel wall are defined as protruding.[68] There are two methods for defining malapposed stent struts. The distance from the stent strut to the vessel wall is measured and if this value is greater than the nominal stent strut thickness, the stent strut is classified as malapposed. For drug-eluting stents (DES) the distance includes the sum of the strut thickness and the thickness of the abluminal polymer. The extent of malapposition is determined by the number of cross sections containing malapposed struts. Alternatively, the maximum extent of malapposition at each stent strut can be measured to generate a total area of malapposition. Absolute cutoff distances have also been used based on studies associating these values with clinical outcomes. Gutierrez-Chico et al. found that stents with a maximal incomplete stent apposition of less than 270 μm uniformly showed complete stent strut neointimal coverage at follow-up whereas stents with maximal incomplete apposition greater than 850 μm invariably showed delayed strut coverage.[73]

In addition to inadequate stent expansion, OCT frequently identifies vessel dissection (a disruption in the vessel surface), intrastent thrombus, and tissue prolapse (protrusion of tissue between stent struts) post intervention (**Figure 17-8C-F**).[74-76] The sensitivity of OCT for the immediate effects of coronary stenting is significantly higher than IVUS.[77] The clinical significance of these findings is unclear as they appear to be very common. Tissue prolapse, defined as the projection of tissue into the lumen between stent struts, is seen in more than 90% of stented segments immediately post PCI. Dissections are defined by the presence of either an intimal flap without a fibrous cap disruption or a tear in the luminal surface that extends into the media or adventitia (**Figure 17-8E**).[78] Dissections can be located at the stent edge or within the stented segment. Gonzalo et al. evaluated 73 patients with OCT after stent implantation in 80 vessels and found tissue prolapse in 97.5% of stented segments, intra-stent dissection in 86.6%, and edge dissection in 25%.[74] A prospective study of 57 patients undergoing PCI on 63 lesions revealed an edge dissection in 21 lesions (20 patients), of which only two were angiographically visible.[79] At 1 year of follow-up, there was no associated stent thrombosis or target lesion revascularization and 20 of the dissections had healed on follow-up OCT imaging.

Bifurcation Intervention

PCI of bifurcating lesions may potentially be improved with OCT guidance. OCT imaging of patients undergoing provisional bifurcation stenting can identify a number of complications including stent under expansion and stent malapposition not noted on angiography. Malapposition is most commonly seen in the proximal section of the mother vessel.[80] Detection of malapposition can trigger more aggressive post-dilatation of the stent and improved stent apposition. Alegri-Barrero et al. utilized OCT to confirm re-crossing of a stent into a side branch via a distal cell. In a case control study, the authors found significantly improved stent apposition in the OCT-guided group.[81] Similarly, Viceconte et al. found significantly less malapposition in patients who had undergone OCT-guided bifurcation stenting compared with angiographic-guided.[82]

Clinical Benefit of Optical Coherence Tomography–Guided Percutaneous Coronary Intervention

A clear clinical benefit to OCT-guided PCI has not been established. Prati et al. evaluated angiography-guided PCI to OCT-guided PCI in a propensity matched case control study (n = 667 patients).[66] OCT identified complications requiring further intervention in 34.7% of patients. After multivariable analysis, OCT-guided PCI was associated with lower risk of cardiac death or myocardial infarction (MI) (odds ratio (OR)R 0.49; p = 0.037). Although intriguing, these results would need confirmation in a randomized controlled study to firmly establish a clinical benefit to OCT-guided PCI.

Late Stent Evaluation

In long-term follow-up of stents, stent strut apposition, tissue coverage, and extent of neointimal growth are key intermediate endpoints in comparing various stent platforms (**Figure 17-9**).[83] Stent strut coverage is of particular importance due to the association between an absence of neointimal stent coverage and late stent thrombosis (**Figure 17-10**).[84] Similar to immediately post intervention, stent struts at follow-up can be classified as embedded, protruding, or malapposed. Malapposition, or lack of contact between stents and intima, appears to correlate with PCI failure.[85,86] Different stent platforms appear to vary in their degree of malapposition at follow-up. For example, sirolimus-eluting stents appear to have higher rates of malapposition than zotarolimus stents.[87,88] Serial OCT studies have shown that inadequate stent deployment during the index PCI procedure is the most common cause of late stent malapposition.[89] Late-acquired stent malapposition in stents that were adequately apposed immediately post PCI is most frequently associated with significant plaque or thrombus prolapse immediately post intervention (**Figure 17-9C**).

Stent struts can be covered or uncovered by neointima (**Figure 17-9A, B**) Ideally, a coronary stent would allow for a thin layer of stent coverage without significant neointimal hyperplasia, which could proceed to in-stent restenosis. Stent coverage with neointima is probably protective against stent thrombosis as it separates the thrombogenic surface of the stent from blood. Bare-metal stents typically develop uniform neointimal coverage within several months of implantation that is visible by IVUS. In contrast, drug-eluting stents, by design, result in significantly less neointimal growth often below the level of detection of IVUS. OCT provides adequate resolution for the accurate and reproducible measurements of neonintima that correlate well with measurements obtained by histology.[90] The thickness of neointima is measured from the inner surface of the stent strut to the luminal surface of the neointima.[91] In order to quantify the degree of stent strut coverage, the number of uncovered struts is counted per frame analyzed (typically a frame every 1 mm of pullback) resulting in a total number of uncovered stent struts. Coverage of stent struts by endothelial cells is delayed in malapposed stents.[73] Fewer uncovered stents may correlate with decreased risk of stent thrombosis.[84] As might be expected, drug-eluting stents (DES) are found to have significantly more uncovered compared with bare-metal stents (BMS) even as far out as 2 years with significant heterogeneity in the extent of stent strut coverage.[87,92-98] The extent of stent strut coverage varies significantly between different stents likely as result of differing polymer coats and eluted drug[99-101] but not stent alloys.[102] For example, paclitaxel- and zotarolimus-eluting stents have been shown to have fewer uncovered stent struts at follow-up compared with sirolimus-eluting stents.[93]

Currently, the primary role of OCT in evaluating stent strut coverage is as an investigational tool to compare various stent platforms. Specifically, since stent thrombosis, the most feared complication post PCI, is relatively rare, it cannot reliably be utilized as study endpoint in the context of most randomized trials. OCT provides a potential surrogate endpoint, stent strut coverage, that makes feasible randomized studies comparing new stent designs and drug elutions.[99,103,104] As an example, recent studies have utilized OCT to evaluate bioresorbable vascular scaffolds[64,105-109] specifically looking at vascular response to stents and degree of bioabsorptions of the struts.

The inability to characterize the composition of the tissue covering stent struts, specifically distinguishing cellular coverage from fibrinous material, is an important limitation in the use of OCT to evaluate strut coverage. This is an important distinction as excess fibrin deposition has been linked to late stent thrombosis in autopsy studies.[110] In studies using animal models, the optical signal density of the coverage material could be used to differentiate fibrin from neointima, but these results have not been confirmed in humans.[111]

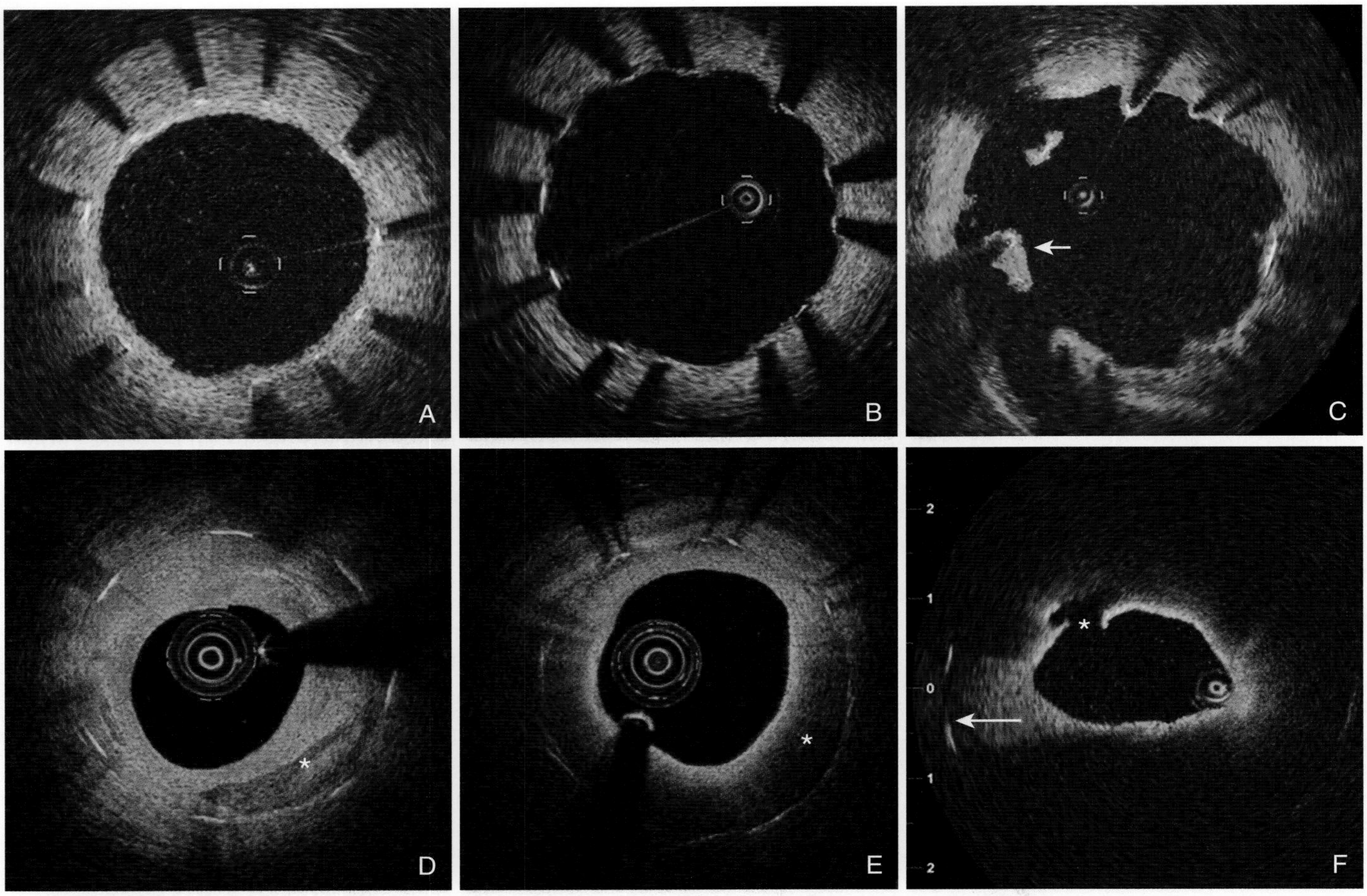

FIGURE 17-9 Optical coherence tomography (OCT) follow-up imaging of coronary stents. **A,** Well-opposed and covered stents. **B,** Well-opposed but uncovered stents. **C,** Malapposed sent struts with fibrin deposition *(arrow).* **D,** In-stent restenosis with area of calcification (*). **E,** In-stent restenosis with neoatherosclerosis and lipid-laden plaque (*). **F,** Ruptured neoatherosclerotic plaque (*) inside previously placed stent *(arrow).*

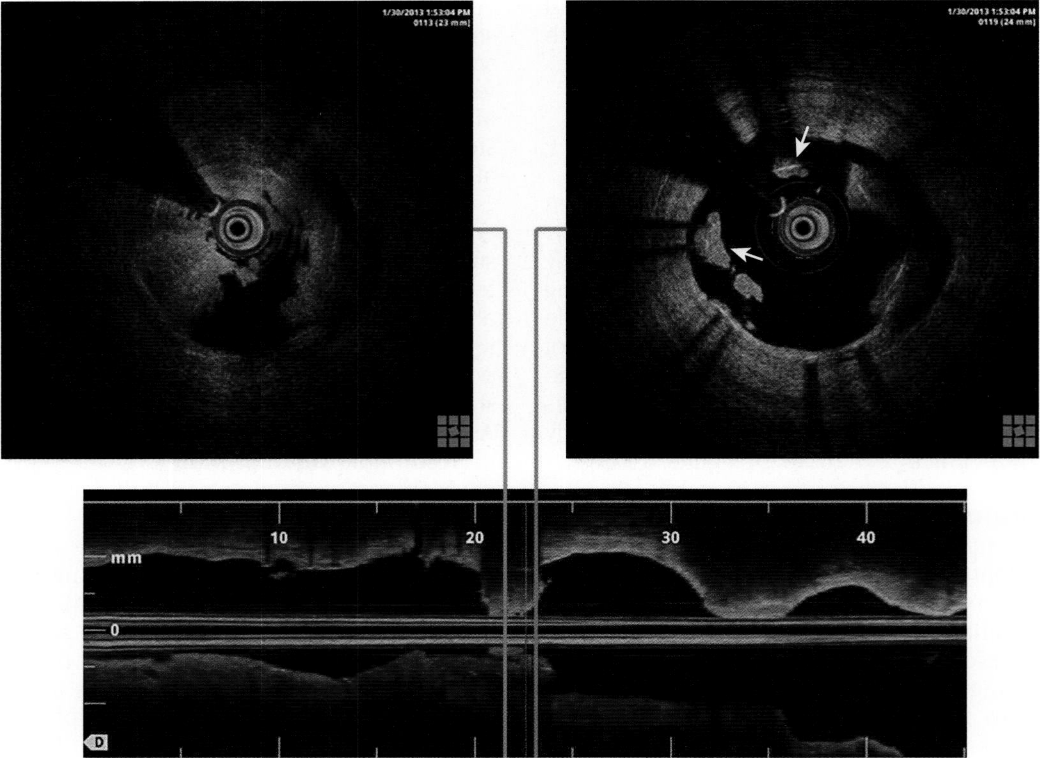

FIGURE 17-10 In-stent thrombosis due to malapposed stent. Cross-sectional images show significant burden of mixed thrombus *(blue line)* and an area immediately proximal *(red line)* with malapposed stent and attached white thrombus *(white arrows).*

Beyond describing the extent of tissue coverage, OCT can identify the tissue composition of the material causing in-stent restenosis (ISR) (**Figure 17-9D, E**). ISR secondary to smooth muscle cell proliferation has a homogeneous appearance and a smooth lumen contour when imaged with OCT.[112] Neoatherosclerosis is pathologically distinct from neointimal hyperplasia. Neoatherosclerosis within the stent is characterized by presence of calcification and lipid pools within the intima and formation of fibroatheromas.[113] Similar to coronary atherosclerosis, neoatherosclerosis can result in the formation of thin-cap fibroatheromas with lipid-rich neointima and a thin fibrous cap.[113] Macrophage infiltration and formation of microvessels have also been reported within neoatherosclerotic lesions.[114,115] Pathological studies have shown a distinct time course for the formation of neoatherosclerosis in bare-metal stents and drug-eluting stents. Within 6 months of bare-metal stent placement, smooth muscle cell proliferation results in the development of neointima visualized as a homogeneous OCT signal overlying the stent struts.[116] Neoatherosclerosis is not seen prior to 2 years after bare-metal stent implantation and typically not until 4 years after implantation.[113] In contrast, neoatherosclerosis is seen after 1 year of PCI with DES.[113] OCT studies have shown similarly distinct time course for neoatherosclerosis in BMS versus DES.[115,117,118] The degrees of neointimal hyperplasia, smoking history, chronic kidney disease, and use of drug-eluting stents appears to be associated with the formation of neoatherosclerosis.[114,119]

Disruption of TCFA present within the neointima can lead to acute coronary syndrome and may potentially explain a subset of cases with very late stent thrombosis (**Figure 17-9F**).[120] These finding have been corroborated by pathology and IVUS studies and may help identify a potential novel mechanism of late stent failure.[121,122]

ASSESSMENT OF NON–CORONARY ARTERY PATHOLOGY

Pulmonary Hypertension

OCT imaging of distal pulmonary artery in patients with pulmonary hypertension due to pulmonary arterial hypertension (PAH) and chronic thromboembolic disease (CTEPH) have been reported.[123,124] Intimal thickening in patients with PAH was readily visualized and measured by OCT. In contrast, patients with CTEPH displayed either a thrombotic occlusion or luminal flaps. A recent case series found OCT to be significantly more useful than IVUS in evaluating the pulmonary arteries of patients with CTEPH specifically to guide treatment with percutaneous transluminal pulmonary angioplasty.[125] At this time, evaluation of pulmonary vascular disease with OCT remains purely investigational.

Peripheral Vascular Disease

The experience with OCT in peripheral arterial disease is limited. The luminal diameter of peripheral arteries often exceeds the limits of OCT (6 mm). In an ex vivo study with arteries obtained from below knee amputations, OCT sensitivity and specificities for atherosclerotic plaque composition in peripheral arteries was comparable to findings for coronary arteries.[126] A similar pilot study showed OCT could accurately define the tissue features of carotid artery plaques.[127] In a feasibility study, Reimer et al. showed that OCT could be used safely to evaluate the results of carotid artery stenting.[128] Compared with IVUS, OCT appears to provide higher quality images of vascular wall structures and similar estimates of lumen and plaque size in an in vivo study of popliteal and infrapopliteal disease.[129] Renal artery fibromuscular dysplasia has been imaged by OCT in vivo revealing medial hyperplasia and fibrosis associated with areas of intimo-media dissection and aneurysm formation.[130] In a small study of 12 patients, OCT imaging of the renal arteries prior and post renal artery denervation revealed minimal morphological changes limited to three limited arterial dissections that required no intervention.[131] No clear clinical role has been established for OCT in peripheral intervention beyond case reports.[132]

Transplant Vasculopathy

Cardiac allograft vasculopathy is the primary cause of late graft failure in heart transplant recipients. It remains a diagnostic challenge as patients often lack signs and symptoms early in the disease process due to cardiac denervation. Angiography remains the standard screening diagnostic test but is limited at identifying graft vasculopathy due to the diffuse rather than focal nature of the disease. OCT has been found to be significantly more sensitive at identifying intimal hyperplasia, an early manifestation of allograft vasculopathy, than angiography or IVUS.[133] An OCT study of 53 patients enrolled after cardiac transplant found a progressive increase in the prevalence of atherosclerotic plaques, calcifications, TCFAs, and microchannels in patients further removed from their transplant. Importantly, this study showed that allograft vasculopathy includes the development of coronary lesions with characteristics of vulnerable plaques, placing these patients at risk of acute coronary events.[134]

FUTURE DIRECTIONS

Multimodality Systems

An integrated diagnostic system containing both a C7-XR OCT catheter and a pressure wire for FFR measurement is now available by St. Jude Medical, Inc. (St. Paul, Minnesota). The combined ILUMIEN system allows for assessment of both coronary lesion morphology by OCT and physiological significance by FFR using a single console.

Three-Dimensional Optical Coherence Tomography

Three-dimensional reconstruction of imaged coronary artery segments is possible using the data obtained during OCT image acquisition.[135] Currently, the technology is limited by the need for off-line reconstruction of images. Three-dimensional imaging could potentially allow for more accurate and global assessment of coronary plaque burden, presence of thin-cap fibroatheromas, intracoronary thrombus, stent deployment, or malapposition. The most recently approved OCT imaging system (ILUMIEN OPTIS OCT catheter, St. Jude Medical), allows for real-time three-dimensional reconstruction of the imaged vessel.

Micro-optical Optical Coherence Tomography

Current OCT systems with a resolution of approximately 10 μm cannot visualize cellular and sub-cellular structures. An OCT system with significantly higher resolution has recently been reported that may allow for resolution of single cells and potentially subcellular structures within coronary vasculature.[136] Imaging of cadaveric arteries readily identified endothelial cells, adherent leukocytes and macrophages, cholesterol crystals, and microcalcifications. The feasibility and utility of translating micro-optical OCT to clinical use are not known.

CONCLUSION

OCT is a real-time intravascular imaging technology that currently provides unmatched high-resolution images of superficial intracoronary structures including coronary plaques and stents. As a research tool, OCT has an established role in helping understand coronary pathology and vascular response to injury and stenting. With improving ease of use and the possibility of real-time three-dimensional imaging, the potential exists for the regular use of OCT in guiding PCI, especially during complex coronary intervention and after stent thrombosis.

References

1. Huang D, Swanson EA, Lin CP, et al: Optical coherence tomography. *Science* 254:1178–1181, 1991.
2. Takada K, Yokohama I, Chida K, et al: New measurement system for fault location in optical waveguide devices based on an interferometric technique. *Appl Opt* 26:1603–1606, 1987.
3. Youngquist RC, Carr S, Davies DE: Optical coherence-domain reflectometry: a new optical evaluation technique. *Opt Lett* 12:158–160, 1987.
4. Tearney GJ, Brezinski ME, Bouma BE, et al: In vivo endoscopic optical biopsy with optical coherence tomography. *Science* 276:2037–2039, 1997.
5. Bouma BE, Yun SH, Vakoc BJ, et al: Fourier-domain optical coherence tomography: recent advances toward clinical utility. *Curr Opin Biotechnol* 20:111–118, 2009.
6. Herrero-Garibi J, Cruz-Gonzalez I, Parejo-Diaz P, et al: Optical coherence tomography: its value in intravascular diagnosis today. *Rev Esp Cardiol* 63:951–962, 2010.
7. Suh WM, Seto AH, Margey RJ, et al: Intravascular detection of the vulnerable plaque. *Circ Cardiovasc Imaging* 4:169–178, 2011.
8. Prati F, Cera M, Ramazzotti V, et al: Safety and feasibility of a new non-occlusive technique for facilitated intracoronary optical coherence tomography (OCT) acquisition in various clinical and anatomical scenarios. *EuroIntervention* 3:365–370, 2007.
9. Barlis P, Gonzalo N, Di Mario C, et al: A multicentre evaluation of the safety of intracoronary optical coherence tomography. *EuroIntervention* 5:90–95, 2009.
10. Yamaguchi T, Terashima M, Akasaka T, et al: Safety and feasibility of an intravascular optical coherence tomography image wire system in the clinical setting. *Am J Cardiol* 101:562–567, 2008.
11. Imola F, Mallus MT, Ramazzotti V, et al: Safety and feasibility of frequency domain optical coherence tomography to guide decision making in percutaneous coronary intervention. *EuroIntervention* 6:575–581, 2010.
12. Stone GW, Maehara A, Lansky AJ, et al: A prospective natural-history study of coronary atherosclerosis. *N Engl J Med* 364:226–235, 2011.
13. Tearney GJ, Jang IK, Kang DH, et al: Porcine coronary imaging in vivo by optical coherence tomography. *Acta Cardiol* 55:233–237, 2000.
14. Kume T, Akasaka T, Kawamoto T, et al: Assessment of coronary intima—media thickness by optical coherence tomography: comparison with intravascular ultrasound. *Circ J* 69:903–907, 2005.
15. Jang IK, Bouma BE, Kang DH, et al: Visualization of coronary atherosclerotic plaques in patients using optical coherence tomography: comparison with intravascular ultrasound. *J Am Coll Cardiol* 39:604–609, 2002.
16. Uemura S, Ishigami KI, Soeda T, et al: Thin-cap fibroatheroma and microchannel findings in optical coherence tomography correlate with subsequent progression of coronary atheromatous plaques. *Eur Heart J* 33:78–85, 2011.
17. Yabushita H, Bouma BE, Houser SL, et al: Characterization of human atherosclerosis by optical coherence tomography. *Circulation* 106:1640–1645, 2002.
18. Kawasaki M, Bouma BE, Bressner J, et al: Diagnostic accuracy of optical coherence tomography and integrated backscatter intravascular ultrasound images for tissue characterization of human coronary plaques. *J Am Coll Cardiol* 48:81–88, 2006.
19. Yonetsu T, Kakuta T, Lee T, et al: In vivo critical fibrous cap thickness for rupture-prone coronary plaques assessed by optical coherence tomography. *Eur Heart J* 32:1251–1259, 2011.
20. Kume T, Akasaka T, Kawamoto T, et al: Assessment of coronary arterial plaque by optical coherence tomography. *Am J Cardiol* 97:1172–1175, 2006.
21. Manfrini O, Mont E, Leone O, et al: Sources of error and interpretation of plaque morphology by optical coherence tomography. *Am J Cardiol* 98:156–159, 2006.
22. Stamper D, Weissman NJ, Brezinski M: Plaque characterization with optical coherence tomography. *J Am Coll Cardiol* 47:C69–C79, 2006.
23. Sluimer JC, Kolodgie FD, Bijnens AP, et al: Thin-walled microvessels in human coronary atherosclerotic plaques show incomplete endothelial junctions relevance of compromised structural integrity for intraplaque microvascular leakage. *J Am Coll Cardiol* 53:1517–1527, 2009.
24. Tearney GJ, Yabushita H, Houser SL, et al: Quantification of macrophage content in atherosclerotic plaques by optical coherence tomography. *Circulation* 107:113–119, 2003.
25. MacNeill BD, Jang IK, Bouma BE, et al: Focal and multi-focal plaque macrophage distributions in patients with acute and stable presentations of coronary artery disease. *J Am Coll Cardiol* 44:972–979, 2004.
26. Kume T, Akasaka T, Kawamoto T, et al: Assessment of coronary arterial thrombus by optical coherence tomography. *Am J Cardiol* 97:1713–1717, 2006.
27. Alfonso F, Paulo M, Gonzalo N, et al: Diagnosis of spontaneous coronary artery dissection by optical coherence tomography. *J Am Coll Cardiol* 59:1073–1079, 2012.
28. Poon K, Bell B, Raffel OC, et al: Spontaneous coronary artery dissection: utility of intravascular ultrasound and optical coherence tomography during percutaneous coronary intervention. *Circ Cardiovasc Interv* 4:e5–e7, 2011.
29. Tanaka A, Shimada K, Tearney GJ, et al: Conformational change in coronary artery structure assessed by optical coherence tomography in patients with vasospastic angina. *J Am Coll Cardiol* 58:1608–1613, 2011.
30. Muller JE, Tofler GH, Stone PH: Circadian variation and triggers of onset of acute cardiovascular disease. *Circulation* 79:733–743, 1989.
31. Fuster V, Moreno PR, Fayad ZA, et al: Atherothrombosis and high-risk plaque: part I: evolving concepts. *J Am Coll Cardiol* 46:937–954, 2005.
32. Slager CJ, Wentzel JJ, Gijsen FJ, et al: The role of shear stress in the generation of rupture-prone vulnerable plaques. *Nat Clin Pract Cardiovasc Med* 2:401–407, 2005.
33. Slager CJ, Wentzel JJ, Gijsen FJ, et al: The role of shear stress in the destabilization of vulnerable plaques and related therapeutic implications. *Nat Clin Pract Cardiovasc Med* 2:456–464, 2005.
34. Naghavi M, Libby P, Falk E, et al: From vulnerable plaque to vulnerable patient: a call for new definitions and risk assessment strategies: part II. *Circulation* 108:1772–1778, 2003.
35. Wang JC, Normand SL, Mauri L, et al: Coronary artery spatial distribution of acute myocardial infarction occlusions. *Circulation* 110:278–284, 2004.
36. Burke AP, Farb A, Malcom GT, et al: Coronary risk factors and plaque morphology in men with coronary disease who died suddenly. *N Engl J Med* 336:1276–1282, 1997.
37. Yonetsu T, Kakuta T, Lee T, et al: Impact of plaque morphology on creatine kinase-MB elevation in patients with elective stent implantation. *Int J Cardiol* 146:80–85, 2011.
38. Bezerra HG, Attizzani GF, Costa MA: Three-dimensional imaging of fibrous cap by frequency-domain optical coherence tomography. *Catheter Cardiovasc Interv* 81:547–549, 2013.
39. Kume T, Akasaka T, Kawamoto T, et al: Measurement of the thickness of the fibrous cap by optical coherence tomography. *Am Heart J* 152(755):e1–e4, 2006.
40. Tanaka A, Imanishi T, Kitabata H, et al: Lipid-rich plaque and myocardial perfusion after successful stenting in patients with non-ST-segment elevation acute coronary syndrome: an optical coherence tomography study. *Eur Heart J* 30:1348–1355, 2009.
41. Jang IK, Tearney GJ, MacNeill B, et al: In vivo characterization of coronary atherosclerotic plaque by use of optical coherence tomography. *Circulation* 111:1551–1555, 2005.
42. Suzuki N, Guagliumi G, Bezerra HG, et al: The impact of an eccentric intravascular ImageWire during coronary optical coherence tomography imaging. *EuroIntervention* 6:963–969, 2011.
43. Kato K, Yonetsu T, Kim SJ, et al: Nonculprit plaques in patients with acute coronary syndromes have more vulnerable features compared with those with non-acute coronary syndromes: a 3-vessel optical coherence tomography study. *Circ Cardiovasc Imaging* 5:433–440, 2012.
44. Kubo T, Imanishi T, Takarada S, et al: Assessment of culprit lesion morphology in acute myocardial infarction: ability of optical coherence tomography compared with intravascular ultrasound and coronary angioscopy. *J Am Coll Cardiol* 50:933–939, 2007.
45. Uemura S, Ishigami K, Soeda T, et al: Thin-cap fibroatheroma and microchannel findings in optical coherence tomography correlate with subsequent progression of coronary atheromatous plaques. *Eur Heart J* 33:78–85, 2012.
46. Ino Y, Kubo T, Tanaka A, et al: Difference of culprit lesion morphologies between ST-segment elevation myocardial infarction and non-ST-segment elevation acute coronary syndrome: an optical coherence tomography study. *JACC Cardiovasc Interv* 4:76–82, 2011.
47. Farb A, Burke AP, Tang AL, et al: Coronary plaque erosion without rupture into a lipid core. A frequent cause of coronary thrombosis in sudden coronary death. *Circulation* 93:1354–1363, 1996.
48. Jia H, Abtahian F, Aguirre AD, et al: In vivo diagnosis of plaque erosion and calcified nodule in patients with acute coronary syndrome by intravascular optical coherence tomography. *J Am Coll Cardiol* 62:1748–1758, 2013.
49. Vergallo R, Yonetsu T, Kato K, et al: Evaluation of culprit lesions by optical coherence tomography in patients with ST-elevation myocardial infarction. *Int J Cardiol* 168:1592–1593, 2013.
50. Porto I, Di Vito L, Burzotta F, et al: Superficial calcified nodules and post-stenting microdissections imaged through 3-dimensional optical coherence tomography. *Int J Cardiol* 158:e62–e64, 2012.
51. Ferrante G, Nakano M, Prati F, et al: High levels of systemic myeloperoxidase are associated with coronary plaque erosion in patients with acute coronary syndromes: a clinicopathological study. *Circulation* 122:2505–2513, 2010.
52. Vergallo R, Ren X, Yonetsu T, et al: Pancoronary plaque vulnerability in patients with acute coronary syndrome and ruptured culprit plaque: a 3-vessel optical coherence tomography study. *Am Heart J* 167:59–67, 2014.
53. Hu S, Yonetsu T, Jia H, et al: Residual thrombus pattern in patients with ST-segment elevation myocardial infarction caused by plaque erosion versus plaque rupture following successful fibrinolysis: an optical coherence tomography study. *J Am Coll Cardiol* 63:1336–1338, 2013.
54. Prati F, Uemura S, Souteyrand G, et al: OCT-based diagnosis and management of STEMI associated with intact fibrous cap. *JACC Cardiovasc Imaging* 6:283–287, 2013.
55. Tanaka A, Imanishi T, Kitabata H, et al: Morphology of exertion-triggered plaque rupture in patients with acute coronary syndrome: an optical coherence tomography study. *Circulation* 118:2368–2373, 2008.
56. Sihan K, Botha C, Post F, et al: Fully automatic three-dimensional quantitative analysis of intracoronary optical coherence tomography: method and validation. *Catheter Cardiovasc Interv* 74:1058–1065, 2009.
57. Gonzalo N, Escaned J, Alfonso F, et al: Morphometric assessment of coronary stenosis relevance with optical coherence tomography: a comparison with fractional flow reserve and intravascular ultrasound. *J Am Coll Cardiol* 59:1080–1089, 2012.
58. Shiono Y, Kitabata H, Kubo T, et al: Optical coherence tomography-derived anatomical criteria for functionally significant coronary stenosis assessed by fractional flow reserve. *Circ J* 76:2218–2225, 2012.
59. Stefano GT, Bezerra HG, Attizzani G, et al: Utilization of frequency domain optical coherence tomography and fractional flow reserve to assess intermediate coronary artery stenoses: conciliating anatomic and physiologic information. *Int J Cardiovasc Imaging* 27:299–308, 2011.
60. Lee T, Kakuta T, Yonetsu T, et al: Assessment of echo-attenuated plaque by optical coherence tomography and its impact on post-procedural creatine kinase-myocardial band elevation in elective stent implantation. *JACC Cardiovasc Interv* 4:483–491, 2011.
61. Lee T, Yonetsu T, Koura K, et al: Impact of coronary plaque morphology assessed by optical coherence tomography on cardiac troponin elevation in patients with elective stent implantation. *Circ Cardiovasc Interv* 4:378–386, 2011.
62. Porto I, Di Vito L, Burzotta F, et al: Predictors of periprocedural (type IVa) myocardial infarction, as assessed by frequency-domain optical coherence tomography. *Circ Cardiovasc Interv* 5:89–96, S1–S6, 2012.
63. Di Giorgio A, Capodanno D, Ramazzotti V, et al: Optical coherence tomography guided in-stent thrombus removal in patients with acute coronary syndromes. *Int J Cardiovasc Imaging* 29:989–996, 2013.
64. Gomez-Lara J, Brugaletta S, Farooq V, et al: Head-to-head comparison of the neointimal response between metallic and bioresorbable everolimus-eluting scaffolds using optical coherence tomography. *JACC Cardiovasc Interv* 4:1271–1280, 2011.
65. de Jaegere P, Mudra H, Figulla H, et al: Intravascular ultrasound-guided optimized stent deployment. Immediate and 6 months clinical and angiographic results from the Multicenter Ultrasound Stenting in Coronaries Study (MUSIC Study). *Eur Heart J* 19:1214–1223, 1998.
66. Prati F, Di Vito L, Biondi-Zoccai G, et al: Angiography alone versus angiography plus optical coherence tomography to guide decision-making during percutaneous coronary intervention: the Centro per la Lotta contro l'Infarto-Optimisation of Percutaneous Coronary Intervention (CLI-OPCI) study. *EuroIntervention* 8:823–829, 2012.
67. Bouma BE, Tearney GJ, Yabushita H, et al: Evaluation of intracoronary stenting by intravascular optical coherence tomography. *Heart* 89:317–320, 2003.
68. Tanigawa J, Barlis P, Di Mario C: Intravascular optical coherence tomography: optimisation of image acquisition and quantitative assessment of stent strut apposition. *EuroIntervention* 3:128–136, 2007.

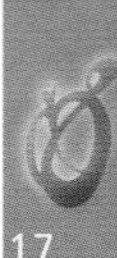

69. Tyczynski P, Ferrante G, Kukreja N, et al: Optical coherence tomography assessment of a new dedicated bifurcation stent. *EuroIntervention* 5:544–551, 2009.
70. Tyczynski P, Ferrante G, Moreno-Ambroj C, et al: Simple versus complex approaches to treating coronary bifurcation lesions: direct assessment of stent strut apposition by optical coherence tomography. *Rev Esp Cardiol* 63:904–914, 2010.
71. Miyoshi N, Shite J, Shinke T, et al: Comparison by optical coherence tomography of paclitaxel-eluting stents with sirolimus-eluting stents implanted in one coronary artery in one procedure.—6-month follow-up. *Circ J* 74:903–908, 2010.
72. Ishigami K, Uemura S, Morikawa Y, et al: Long-term follow-up of neointimal coverage of sirolimus-eluting stents—evaluation with optical coherence tomography. *Circ J* 73:2300–2307, 2009.
73. Gutierrez-Chico JL, Regar E, Nuesch E, et al: Delayed coverage in malapposed and side-branch struts with respect to well-apposed struts in drug-eluting stents: in vivo assessment with optical coherence tomography. *Circulation* 124:612–623, 2011.
74. Gonzalo N, Serruys PW, Okamura T, et al: Optical coherence tomography assessment of the acute effects of stent implantation on the vessel wall: a systematic quantitative approach. *Heart* 95:1913–1919, 2009.
75. Kawamori H, Shite J, Shinke T, et al: The ability of optical coherence tomography to monitor percutaneous coronary intervention: detailed comparison with intravascular ultrasound. *J Invasive Cardiol* 22:541–545, 2010.
76. Radu M, Jorgensen E, Kelbaek H, et al: Optical coherence tomography at follow-up after percutaneous coronary intervention: relationship between procedural dissections, stent strut malapposition and stent healing. *EuroIntervention* 7:353–361, 2011.
77. Kubo T, Imanishi T, Kitabata H, et al: Comparison of vascular response after sirolimus-eluting stent implantation between patients with unstable and stable angina pectoris: a serial optical coherence tomography study. *JACC Cardiovasc Imaging* 1:475–484, 2008.
78. Yonetsu T, Kakuta T, Lee T, et al: Assessment of acute injuries and chronic intimal thickening of the radial artery after transradial coronary intervention by optical coherence tomography. *Eur Heart J* 31:1608–1615, 2010.
79. Radu MD, Raber L, Heo J, et al: Natural history of optical coherence tomography-detected non-flow-limiting edge dissections following drug-eluting stent implantation. *EuroIntervention* 9:1085–1094, 2013.
80. Burzotta F, Talarico GP, Trani C, et al: Frequency-domain optical coherence tomography findings in patients with bifurcated lesions undergoing provisional stenting. *Eur Heart J Cardiovasc Imaging* 15:547–555, 2013.
81. Alegria-Barrero E, Foin N, Chan PH, et al: Optical coherence tomography for guidance of distal cell recrossing in bifurcation stenting: choosing the right cell matters. *EuroIntervention* 8:205–213, 2012.
82. Viceconte N, Tyczynski P, Ferrante G, et al: Immediate results of bifurcational stenting assessed with optical coherence tomography. *Catheter Cardiovasc Interv* 81:519–528, 2013.
83. Bezerra HG, Costa MA, Guagliumi G, et al: Intracoronary optical coherence tomography: a comprehensive review clinical and research applications. *JACC Cardiovasc Interv* 2:1035–1046, 2009.
84. Finn AV, Joner M, Nakazawa G, et al: Pathological correlates of late drug-eluting stent thrombosis: strut coverage as a marker of endothelialization. *Circulation* 115:2435–2441, 2007.
85. Cook S, Wenaweser P, Togni M, et al: Incomplete stent apposition and very late stent thrombosis after drug-eluting stent implantation. *Circulation* 115:2426–2434, 2007.
86. Sawada T, Shite J, Shinke T, et al: Very late thrombosis of sirolimus-eluting stent due to late malapposition: serial observations with optical coherence tomography. *J Cardiol* 52:290–295, 2008.
87. Kim JS, Jang IK, Kim TH, et al: Optical coherence tomography evaluation of zotarolimus-eluting stents at 9-month follow-up: comparison with sirolimus-eluting stents. *Heart* 95:1907–1912, 2009.
88. Kim JS, Shin DH, Kim BK, et al: Optical coherence tomographic comparison of neointimal coverage between sirolimus—and resolute zotarolimus-eluting stents at 9 months after stent implantation. *Int J Cardiovasc Imaging* 2011.
89. Ozaki Y, Okumura M, Ismail TF, et al: The fate of incomplete stent apposition with drug-eluting stents: an optical coherence tomography-based natural history study. *Eur Heart J* 31:1470–1476, 2010.
90. Murata A, Wallace-Bradley D, Tellez A, et al: Accuracy of optical coherence tomography in the evaluation of neointimal coverage after stent implantation. *JACC Cardiovasc Imaging* 3:76–84, 2010.
91. Yamamoto M, Takano M, Murakami D, et al: Optical coherence tomography analysis for restenosis of drug-eluting stents. *Int J Cardiol* 146:100–103, 2011.
92. Chen BX, Ma FY, Luo W, et al: Neointimal coverage of bare-metal and sirolimus-eluting stents evaluated with optical coherence tomography. *Heart* 94:566–570, 2008.
93. Kim JS, Kim TH, Fan C, et al: Comparison of neointimal coverage of sirolimus-eluting stents and paclitaxel-eluting stents using optical coherence tomography at 9 months after implantation. *Circ J* 74:320–326, 2010.
94. Xie Y, Takano M, Murakami D, et al: Comparison of neointimal coverage by optical coherence tomography of a sirolimus-eluting stent versus a bare-metal stent three months after implantation. *Am J Cardiol* 102:27–31, 2008.
95. Yao ZH, Matsubara T, Inada T, et al: Neointimal coverage of sirolimus-eluting stents 6 months and 12 months after implantation: evaluation by optical coherence tomography. *Chin Med J (Engl)* 121:503–507, 2008.
96. Guagliumi G, Sirbu V, Bezerra H, et al: Strut coverage and vessel wall response to zotarolimus-eluting and bare-metal stents implanted in patients with ST-segment elevation myocardial infarction: the OCTAMI (Optical Coherence Tomography in Acute Myocardial Infarction) study. *JACC Cardiovasc Interv* 3:680–687, 2010.
97. Tahara S, Bezerra HG, Sirbu V, et al: Angiographic, IVUS and OCT evaluation of the long-term impact of coronary disease severity at the site of overlapping drug-eluting and bare metal stents: a substudy of the ODESSA trial. *Heart* 96:1574–1578, 2010.
98. Katoh H, Shite J, Shinke T, et al: Delayed neointimalization on sirolimus-eluting stents: 6-month and 12-month follow up by optical coherence tomography. *Circ J* 73:1033–1037, 2009.
99. Guagliumi G, Musumeci G, Sirbu V, et al: Optical coherence tomography assessment of in vivo vascular response after implantation of overlapping bare-metal and drug-eluting stents. *JACC Cardiovasc Interv* 3:531–539, 2010.
100. Guagliumi G, Ikejima H, Sirbu V, et al: Impact of drug release kinetics on vascular response to different zotarolimus-eluting stents implanted in patients with long coronary stenoses: the LongOCT study (Optical Coherence Tomography in Long Lesions). *JACC Cardiovasc Interv* 4:778–785, 2011.
101. Guagliumi G, Capodanno D, Ikejima H, et al: Impact of different stent alloys on human vascular response to everolimus-eluting stent. An optical coherence tomography study. The OCTEVEREST. *Catheter Cardiovasc Interv* 2012.
102. Guagliumi G, Capodanno D, Ikejima H, et al: Impact of different stent alloys on human vascular response to everolimus-eluting stent: an optical coherence tomography study: the OCTEVEREST. *Catheter Cardiovasc Interv* 81:510–518, 2013.
103. Moore P, Barlis P, Spiro J, et al: A randomized optical coherence tomography study of coronary stent strut coverage and luminal protrusion with rapamycin-eluting stents. *JACC Cardiovasc Interv* 2:437–444, 2009.
104. Tearney GJ, Regar E, Akasaka T, et al: Consensus standards for acquisition, measurement, and reporting of intravascular optical coherence tomography studies: a report from the international working group for intravascular optical coherence tomography standardization and validation. *J Am Coll Cardiol* 59:1058–1072, 2012.
105. Onuma Y, Serruys PW, Ormiston JA, et al: Three-year results of clinical follow-up after a bioresorbable everolimus-eluting scaffold in patients with de novo coronary artery disease: the ABSORB trial. *EuroIntervention* 6:447–453, 2010.
106. Serruys PW, Ormiston JA, Onuma Y, et al: A bioabsorbable everolimus-eluting coronary stent system (ABSORB): 2-year outcomes and results from multiple imaging methods. *Lancet* 373:897–910, 2009.
107. Diletti R, Onuma Y, Farooq V, et al: 6-month clinical outcomes following implantation of the bioresorbable everolimus-eluting vascular scaffold in vessels smaller or larger than 2.5 mm. *J Am Coll Cardiol* 58:258–264, 2011.
108. Serruys PW, Onuma Y, Dudek D, et al: Evaluation of the second generation of a bioresorbable everolimus-eluting vascular scaffold for the treatment of de novo coronary artery stenosis: 12-month clinical and imaging outcomes. *J Am Coll Cardiol* 58:1578–1588, 2011.
109. Haude M, Erbel R, Erne P, et al: Safety and performance of the drug-eluting absorbable metal scaffold (DREAMS) in patients with de-novo coronary lesions: 12 month results of the prospective, multicentre, first-in-man BIOSOLVE-I trial. *Lancet* 381:836–844, 2013.
110. Nakazawa G, Finn AV, Vorpahl M, et al: Coronary responses and differential mechanisms of late stent thrombosis attributed to first-generation sirolimus—and paclitaxel-eluting stents. *J Am Coll Cardiol* 57:390–398, 2011.
111. Matsumoto D, Shinke T, Nakamura T, et al: Optical coherence tomography and histopathological assessment of delayed arterial healing after drug-eluting stent implant in a pig coronary model. *Int J Cardiol* 170:152–159, 2013.
112. Kwon SW, Kim BK, Kim TH, et al: Qualitative assessment of neointimal tissue after drug-eluting stent implantation: comparison between follow-up optical coherence tomography and intravascular ultrasound. *Am Heart J* 161:367–372, 2011.
113. Nakazawa G, Otsuka F, Nakano M, et al: The pathology of neoatherosclerosis in human coronary implants bare-metal and drug-eluting stents. *J Am Coll Cardiol* 57:1314–1322, 2011.
114. Yonetsu T, Kato K, Kim SJ, et al: Predictors for neoatherosclerosis: a retrospective observational study from the optical coherence tomography registry. *Circ Cardiovasc Imaging* 5:660–666, 2012.
115. Kang SJ, Mintz GS, Akasaka T, et al: Optical coherence tomographic analysis of in-stent neoatherosclerosis after drug-eluting stent implantation. *Circulation* 123:2954–2963, 2011.
116. Takarada S, Imanishi T, Ishibashi K, et al: The effect of lipid and inflammatory profiles on the morphological changes of lipid-rich plaques in patients with non-ST-segment elevated acute coronary syndrome: follow-up study by optical coherence tomography and intravascular ultrasound. *JACC Cardiovasc Interv* 3:766–772, 2010.
117. Yonetsu T, Kim JS, Kato K, et al: Comparison of incidence and time course of neoatherosclerosis between bare metal stents and drug-eluting stents using optical coherence tomography. *Am J Cardiol* 110:933–939, 2012.
118. Takano M, Yamamoto M, Inami S, et al: Appearance of lipid-laden intima and neovascularization after implantation of bare-metal stents extended late-phase observation by intracoronary optical coherence tomography. *J Am Coll Cardiol* 55:26–32, 2009.
119. Vergallo R, Yonetsu T, Uemura S, et al: Correlation between degree of neointimal hyperplasia and incidence and characteristics of neoatherosclerosis as assessed by optical coherence tomography. *Am J Cardiol* 112:1315–1321, 2013.
120. Hou J, Qi H, Zhang M, et al: Development of lipid-rich plaque inside bare metal stent: possible mechanism of late stent thrombosis? An optical coherence tomography study. *Heart* 96:1187–1190, 2010.
121. Higo T, Ueda Y, Oyabu J, et al: Atherosclerotic and thrombogenic neointima formed over sirolimus drug-eluting stent: an angioscopic study. *JACC Cardiovasc Imaging* 2:616–624, 2009.
122. Nakazawa G, Vorpahl M, Finn AV, et al: One step forward and two steps back with drug-eluting stents: from preventing restenosis to causing late thrombosis and nouveau atherosclerosis. *JACC Cardiovasc Imaging* 2:625–628, 2009.
123. Tatebe S, Fukumoto Y, Sugimura K, et al: Optical coherence tomography as a novel diagnostic tool for distal type chronic thromboembolic pulmonary hypertension. *Circ J* 74:1742–1744, 2010.
124. Hou J, Qi H, Zhang M, et al: Pulmonary vascular changes in pulmonary hypertension: optical coherence tomography findings. *Circ Cardiovasc Imaging* 3:344–345, 2010.
125. Tatebe S, Fukumoto Y, Sugimura K, et al: Optical coherence tomography is superior to intravascular ultrasound for diagnosis of distal-type chronic thromboembolic pulmonary hypertension. *Circ J* 77:1081–1083, 2013.
126. Meissner OA, Rieber J, Babaryka G, et al: Intravascular optical coherence tomography: comparison with histopathology in atherosclerotic peripheral artery specimens. *J Vasc Interv Radiol* 17:343–349, 2006.
127. Prabhudesai V, Phelan C, Yang Y, et al: The potential role of optical coherence tomography in the evaluation of vulnerable carotid atheromatous plaques: a pilot study. *Cardiovasc Intervent Radiol* 29:1039–1045, 2006.
128. Reimers B, Nikas D, Stabile E, et al: Preliminary experience with optical coherence tomography imaging to evaluate carotid artery stents: safety, feasibility and techniques. *EuroIntervention* 7:98–105, 2011.
129. Eberhardt KM, Treitl M, Boesenecker K, et al: Prospective evaluation of optical coherence tomography in lower limb arteries compared with intravascular ultrasound. *J Vasc Interv Radiol* 24:1499–1508, 2013.
130. Sanchez-Recalde A, Moreno R, Jimenez-Valero S: Renal artery fibromuscular dysplasia: in vivo optical coherence tomography insights. *Eur Heart J* 2013.
131. Stabile E, Ambrosini V, Squarcia R, et al: Percutaneous sympathectomy of the renal arteries: the OneShot Renal Denervation System is not associated with significant vessel wall injury. *EuroIntervention* 9:694–699, 2013.
132. Negi SI, Rosales O: The role of intravascular optical coherence tomography in peripheral percutaneous interventions. *J Invasive Cardiol* 25:E51–E53, 2013.
133. Hou J, Lv H, Jia H, et al: OCT assessment of allograft vasculopathy in heart transplant recipients. *JACC Cardiovasc Imaging* 5:662–663, 2012.
134. Cassar A, Matsuo Y, Herrmann J, et al: Coronary atherosclerosis with vulnerable plaque and complicated lesions in transplant recipients: new insight into cardiac allograft vasculopathy by optical coherence tomography. *Eur Heart J* 34:2610–2617, 2013.
135. Tearney GJ, Waxman S, Shishkov M, et al: Three-dimensional coronary artery microscopy by intracoronary optical frequency domain imaging. *JACC Cardiovasc Imaging* 1:752–761, 2008.
136. Liu L, Gardecki JA, Nadkarni SK, et al: Imaging the subcellular structure of human coronary atherosclerosis using micro-optical coherence tomography. *Nat Med* 17:1010–1014, 2011.

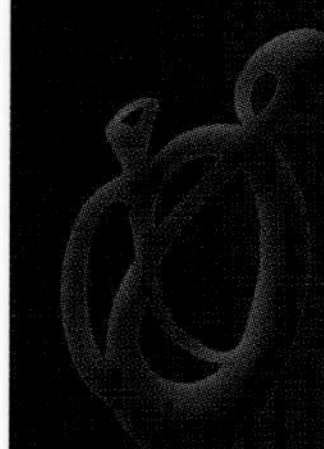

PART III

PERIPHERAL ARTERY INTERVENTION

18 Intervention for Lower Extremity Arterial Disease

Scott Kinlay

CLINICAL ASSESSMENT

Peripheral artery disease (PAD) is caused by a number of pathologies affecting the arteries of the lower extremities. The most common cause in industrialized countries is atherosclerosis, but the interventionalist needs to be aware of other pathologies that may be best treated by noninterventional approaches. The history and physical exam can distinguish most causes of peripheral artery disease and determine the need for further testing and urgency of interventional therapy.

Causes of Peripheral Artery Disease

Atherosclerosis is the most common cause of peripheral artery disease, principally related to the conventional risk factors of age, cigarette smoking, elevated cholesterol, hypertension, diabetes mellitus, and associated inactivity and obesity.[1,2] Other causes of large artery arterial disease include aneurysms, dissections, emboli, compression syndromes, and vasculitis.

About 50% to 90% of patients with atherosclerotic peripheral artery disease are asymptomatic.[3] The diagnosis is made by clinical exam or other tests that are clinically indicated or ordered for other reasons. Asymptomatic disease is a marker of elevated risk of cardiovascular events.[1,2] Thus, the interventionalist shares responsibility with the referring doctor in initiating risk factor modification by encouraging smoking cessation, initiating treatment for hyperlipidemia and hypertension, and promoting physical activity.

The symptoms of peripheral artery disease help distinguish acute from chronic presentations and often give an indication of the location of disease. The temporal relationship of disease onset is particularly important in determining the urgency of treatment.

Acute Limb Ischemia

Acute limb ischemia is a sudden decrease in perfusion (defined as within 14 days) that threatens the viability of the limb. Rapid assessment and treatment are needed to salvage the limb, although a high mortality often relates to coexisting comorbidities.[4] Acute limb ischemia is due to embolization most commonly from the heart, in situ thrombosis related to atherosclerosis (**Figure 18-1**), or increasingly, graft thrombosis or stent thrombosis.

Emboli may occur in patients without symptoms or signs of preceding peripheral artery disease. In situ thrombosis is often accompanied by signs of atherosclerosis in both limbs, but it can occur from impaired flow in a graft or stent (e.g., restenosis or graft hyperplasia), thrombosis of a popliteal aneurysm, hypercoagulable states, or dissection.

The classic symptoms and signs of acute limb ischemia are known as the *six P's*. These are pain, pallor, pulseless, poikilothermia (a cold limb), paresthesia, and paralysis. The order of these symptoms and signs also relates to the

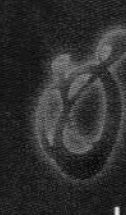

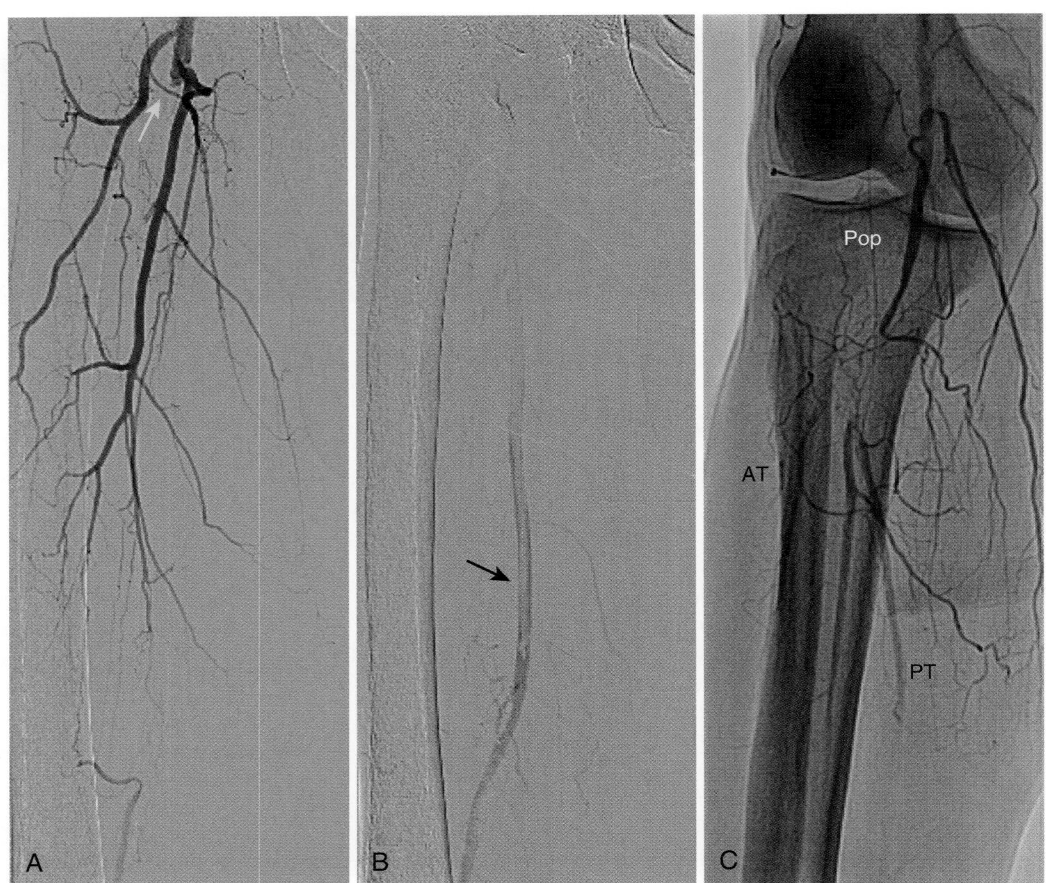

FIGURE 18-1 Angiography from a 73-year-old man with multiple comorbidities and acute limb ischemia. **A,** An occluded right superficial femoral artery *(arrow)* and patent profunda artery in the early phase of the angiogram. **B,** Late phase of the angiogram showing a long filling defect in the superficial femoral artery consistent with in situ thrombus *(arrow)*. **C,** Occlusion of the distal popliteal artery, peroneal tibial trunk, and proximal anterior tibial artery from embolized thrombus. *Pop,* Popliteal artery; *AT,* anterior tibial; *PT,* posterior tibial.

TABLE 18-1 Rutherford Classification of Acute Limb Ischemia

RUTHERFORD CLASS	PROGNOSIS	SENSORY EXAM	MOTOR EXAM	ARTERIAL DOPPLER SIGNAL	VENOUS DOPPLER SIGNAL	SKIN EXAM	INITIAL THERAPY	DEFINITIVE THERAPY
Class I Viable, Not Threatened	Not immediately threatened	Normal	Normal	Audible	Audible	Normal capillary return	Anti-coagulation	Imaging and revascularization
Class IIa: Marginally Threatened	Salvageable with prompt therapy	Minimal loss	Normal	Often inaudible	Audible	Decreased capillary return	Anti-coagulation	Imaging and revascularization
Class IIb: Immediately Threatened	Salvageable if treated immediately	Mild sensory loss and rest pain	Mildly to moderately abnormal	Usually inaudible	Audible	Pallor	Anti-coagulation	+/− Imaging and revascularization
Class III: Irreversible	Irreversible tissue and nerve damage	Profound loss	Paralysis and rigor	Inaudible	Inaudible	No capillary return and marbling	Anti-coagulation	Amputation

Adapted from Norgren L, Hiatt WR, Dormandy JA, et al: Inter-society consensus for the management of peripheral arterial disease (tasc ii). J Vasc Surg 45(Suppl S):S5–S67, 2007; and Rutherford RB, Baker JD, Ernst C, et al: Recommended standards for reports dealing with lower extremity ischemia: revised version. J Vasc Surg 26:517–538, 1997.

viability of the limb and whether revascularization will salvage it.[4] As sensory and motor function is lost progressively from the distal to proximal limb, a simple test of intact motor function is dorsiflexion of the big toe to resistance. **Table 18-1** shows the Rutherford classification[5] of acute limb ischemia and the management suggested by Inter-Society Consensus for the Management of Peripheral Arterial Disease.[2] Patients with Rutherford class I and IIa may be able to tolerate an overnight infusion of catheter-based thrombolysis. Patients with class IIb ischemia require more immediate revascularization by endovascular aspiration or mechanical thrombectomy in conjunction with thrombolysis[6,7] or classically by surgical embolectomy or bypass grafting. Typically, surgical treatment is employed if fasciotomy is required to prevent or treat a compartment syndrome associated with reperfusion injury and edema of the revascularized limb.

TABLE 18-2 Rutherford Categories and Fontaine Stages of Chronic Limb Ischemia in PAD[8]

PAD CLASSIFICATION	CLINICAL SYMPTOM	RUTHERFORD	FONTAINE
Asymptomatic	Asymptomatic	0	I
Intermittent claudication	Mild claudication	1	IIa
	Moderate claudication	2	IIb
	Severe claudication	3	IIb
Critical limb ischemia	Ischemic rest pain	4	III
	Minor tissue loss	5	IV
	Ulceration or gangrene	6	IV

Chronic Limb Ischemia

Chronic limb ischemia has an indolent presentation and is far more common than acute limb ischemia. The two classifications of chronic limb ischemia are the Rutherford scale commonly used in the United States and the Fontaine scale commonly used in Europe (**Table 18-2**).[1,2] Both scales distinguish the two main clinical presentations of intermittent claudication and critical limb ischemia.

Intermittent claudication is classically described as a cramping, aching discomfort or pain with exercise that is relieved by rest. Claudication results from muscle ischemia due to an inability to augment blood flow to a leg muscle related to a stenosis or occlusion of the large and/or small arteries. However, up to half of symptomatic patients describe atypical symptoms with exercise, including fatigue, slow walking speed, and gait disturbance.[3] Claudication has major effects on quality of life by impairing function and activity. It also relates to a high risk of cardiovascular events over the subsequent years. The risk of limb loss is usually low, so that it is perfectly safe and appropriate to attempt medical therapies (e.g., exercise programs and/or cilostazol) for several months before considering revascularization. In many cases, medical therapy resolves symptoms and improves quality of life and function to a level where revascularization is unlikely to offer extra benefits.

Critical limb ischemia occurs when blood flow at rest is inadequate to meet metabolic demands. Symptoms include pain at rest usually in the lower leg and often with a sensation of coldness or numbness in the limb. Symptoms are exacerbated by cold and leg elevation and relieved by leg dependency (e.g., hanging the leg over the edge of the bed) to improve blood flow to the foot by gravity. Ischemia can progress to infarction with gangrene and ulceration. Patients with critical limb ischemia are at high risk of major amputation (amputation above the ankle) and myocardial infarction and stroke.[1,2] Thus the goals of therapy are to improve blood flow through revascularization and ensure adequate treatment of risk factors for atherosclerosis.

Physical Exam

The exam should include a complete check of the skin, heart, lungs, abdomen, and upper and lower limbs to look for systemic disease and causes of lower limb ischemia.[9] Blood pressure should be measured in both arms, with a difference of more than 15 mm Hg to 20 mm Hg indicating significant unilateral upper extremity disease. All peripheral pulses are palpated and coded as absent (0), diminished (1), or normal (2). Expansile or hyperdynamic pulses may indicate aneurysms (e.g., of the abdominal aorta or popliteal artery). Ausculation of bruits indicates disturbed or turbulent flow and may indicate a stenosis. Shoes and socks should be removed to look for ulceration or gangrene, which may be missed by the patient with neuropathy. Arterial ulcers often have a dry base or an overlying eschar, in contrast to venous ulcers, which tend to be more beefy and moist. More severe forms of ischemia lead to pallor and coolness of the limb, particularly on elevation, and in critical limb ischemia, lowering the limb will reveal a dependent rubor due to hyperemia related to arteriolar and venule dilation and improved flow with gravity.

Physiological Tests

The ankle brachial index (ABI) is a simple office-based method to identify PAD. A handheld 5-MHz to 10-MHz Doppler device is used in conjunction with a conventional blood pressure cuff to measure the systolic pressure at both brachial arteries and the pedal arteries in both feet. Recent guidelines recommend recording the ABI for each limb as the highest pedal pressure in that limb over the highest brachial artery pressure.[10] A normal ABI is greater than 1.0 up to about 1.4. Higher ABIs often indicate calcification of the tibial arteries, in which case the ABI is unreliable for identifying obstructive disease. An ABI of 0.9 to 1.0 is borderline, and an ABI of less than 0.9 is abnormal and a sensitive and specific indicator of obstructive PAD as well as elevated risk of cardiovascular events.

Vascular laboratories are able to provide additional physiological data beyond the ABI.[9] These include segmental leg pressures that help to localize disease by using blood pressure cuffs at different locations to identify marked drops in systolic pressure between cuffs. Pulse volume recordings use blood pressure cuffs expanded to low pressure and identify the subtle expansion of the limb with each systole. These are particularly useful when calcified arteries prevent accurate measurements of ABI. Treadmill testing using standardized walking protocols can quantify the walking times or distances and identify a fall in ankle pressure with exercise in patients with PAD who have borderline results at rest.[8]

Arterial Imaging

Duplex ultrasound uses a combination of B-mode two-dimensional grayscale imaging with color-encoded Doppler imaging and pulsed-Doppler velocity analysis.[9] Grayscale imaging and color Doppler can identify the artery and direction of blood flow, but they are not reliable at grading the degree of stenosis. Stenoses are identified by turbulent flow with varying velocities and graded by pulsed-Doppler comparing velocities in the stenosed segment to a proximal

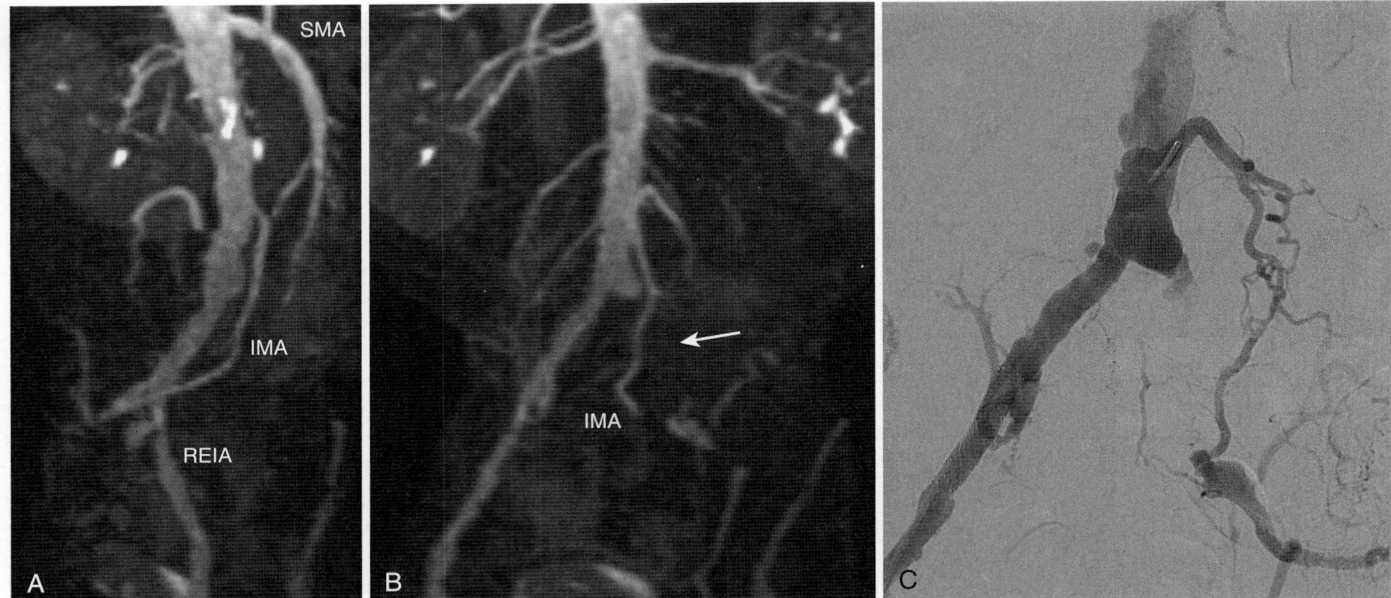

FIGURE 18-2 Comparison of magnetic resonance angiography and digital subtraction angiography (DSA). **A,** Lateral rotation of a maximum intensity image (MIP) of the lower aorta and iliac arteries. *SMA,* Superior mesenteric artery; *IMA,* inferior mesenteric artery; *REIA,* right external iliac artery. **B,** Anterior-posterior rotation from an MIP showing the left common iliac occlusion *(arrow)* and IMA supplying collaterals to the left external iliac artery. **C,** Corresponding image from conventional angiography with DSA. *(From Kinlay S, Bhatt DL: Treatment of noncoronary obstructive vascular disease. Braunwald heart disease, ed 10, Philadelphia, 2015, Elsevier, Figure 60-10, p 1353).*

reference segment. Greater stenosis relates to increasing peak and subsequently diastolic flow velocities.

Magnetic resonance angiography uses two techniques to identify arteries by coding blood flow white (**Figure 18-2**). These include time-of-flight techniques and contrast-enhanced imaging. Time-of-flight relies on laminar blood flow. It tends to overestimate stenosis severity compared to conventional angiography, particularly in regions of disturbed blood flow (e.g., at bifurcations) and regions with reversal of flow. Contrast-enhanced techniques use one of several contrast agents such as gadolinium. Contrast increases the accuracy of the imaging and is better able to define smaller distal arteries. Three-dimensional rendering can allow the reader to rotate the image to help identify eccentric stenoses. A disadvantage of gadolinium is the small risk of disabling nephrogenic systemic sclerosis, which is related to renal function and a particular concern in patients with end-stage renal disease on dialysis. For this reason, gadolinium is usually avoided in patients with severe renal dysfunction.

Computed tomographic angiography uses high-resolution x-ray scanners and iodinated contrast to image the arteries. Volume and three-dimensional rendering can strip surrounding tissue away from the artery images and provide images similar to conventional angiography or magnetic resonance imaging. High-resolution multidetector computed tomography is generally faster than magnetic resonance angiography, but it is sometimes difficult to assess stenosis severity in heavily calcified arteries due to the blooming effect around calcium. Most techniques require 100 mL or more of iodinated contrast, which limits its use in patients with renal dysfunction at risk of contrast nephropathy.

Invasive conventional angiography is still considered the gold standard for arterial imaging. Digital imaging equipment is now capable of conventional "cine" imaging as well as digital subtraction angiography, which removes nonarterial structures to better view the artery (**Figure 18-2**). Noninvasive angiography has largely superseded the need for conventional angiography in the diagnosis and location of disease, but invasive angiography can provide additional physiological assessment of specific lesions using pressure gradients at rest and with vasodilators. Generally a 10-mm Hg gradient at rest or a 15-mm Hg to 20-mm Hg gradient with vasodilators (e.g., nitroglycerin) is considered significant.[7] However, even a 4 Fr catheter placed through a lesion can falsely increase the gradient. Measuring gradients by pullback from proximal to distal or using 0.014-inch pressure wires helps avoid this error.

PERCUTANEOUS REVASCULARIZATION TOOLS

Approach and Access

The four major access sites for a lower limb artery are retrograde access from the contralateral femoral artery, antegrade access via the ipsilateral femoral artery, an upper extremity limb traversing the aorta, and retrograde access via an ipsilateral distal artery such as the popliteal or tibial arteries (**Figure 18-3**). Each access has its advantages and disadvantages.

Retrograde access of the contralateral femoral artery is familiar to many interventional cardiologists and sheath removal at the end of the case is facilitated by a number of closure devices (**Figure 18-4A-C**). Catheters and sheaths are directed over the aorto-iliac bifurcation into the contralateral leg. This provides easy access to the iliac, common femoral, and proximal superficial femoral arteries but is often used to treat more distal disease. The advantages of this approach are the ability to quickly balloon occlude the distal aorta or proximal contralateral iliac artery in the event of perforation of a more distal artery and the ability to treat the contralateral common femoral and proximal superficial femoral arteries. The disadvantages are that it may be difficult to negotiate a tortuous or calcified iliac artery system,

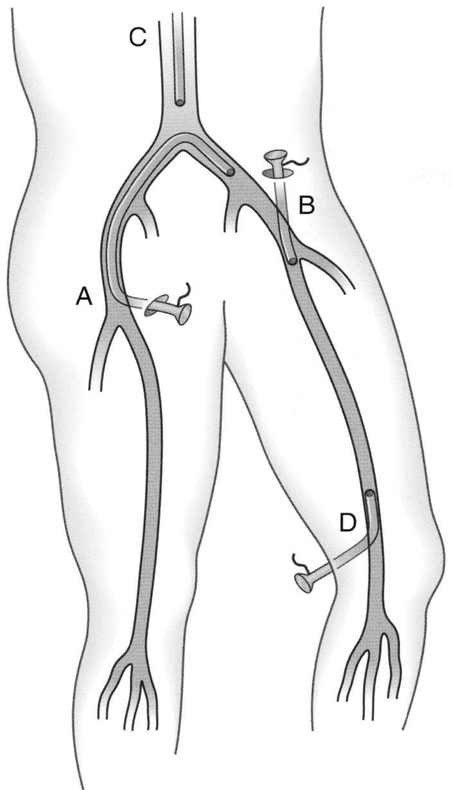

FIGURE 18-3 Potential access sites to treat peripheral artery disease. **A,** Contralateral common femoral access and up over the aortic bifurcation. **B,** Antegrade common femoral access. **C,** Brachial artery access with a guide or sheath in the lower aorta. **D,** Retrograde access from a more distal artery (e.g., popliteal or pedal artery).

and it may offer less support to push through extensive disease in the distal arteries (popliteal or tibial arteries).

An upper limb artery (typically the brachial artery) can provide access to the lower limbs, but due to distance, most equipment can only treat the distal aorta and iliac arteries (**Figure 18-5**). This technique is useful when a femoral artery approach is not possible due to disease or chronic occlusion of the iliac arteries. Although radial artery access is appealing, it is generally too far from the lower extremities for most interventional equipment.

Antegrade access of an ipsilateral femoral artery is useful for providing greater support for popliteal and tibial interventions (**Figure 18-4D**). It requires skin entry well above the common femoral artery and is therefore more difficult and often not feasible in overweight or obese patients. Since the subcutaneous path to the femoral artery is usually longer than with retrograde femoral artery access, closure devices are more difficult to use and tend to have a higher failure rate.

Retrograde access from a more distal artery is useful when antegrade access is unsuccessful (typically in crossing a chronic total occlusion) (**Figure 18-6**).[11-13] Manual compression is required to control hemostasis after the case, as the arteries are smaller. The key disadvantage of this approach is the potential to create an ischemic ulcer at the access site if revascularization is unsuccessful. Thus it is generally used as an approach of "last resort."

Guides and Sheaths

A variety of guides and sheaths are used for lower limb diagnostic cases and interventions. Both are measured in French size (1 French = 0.33 mm), but sheath French size

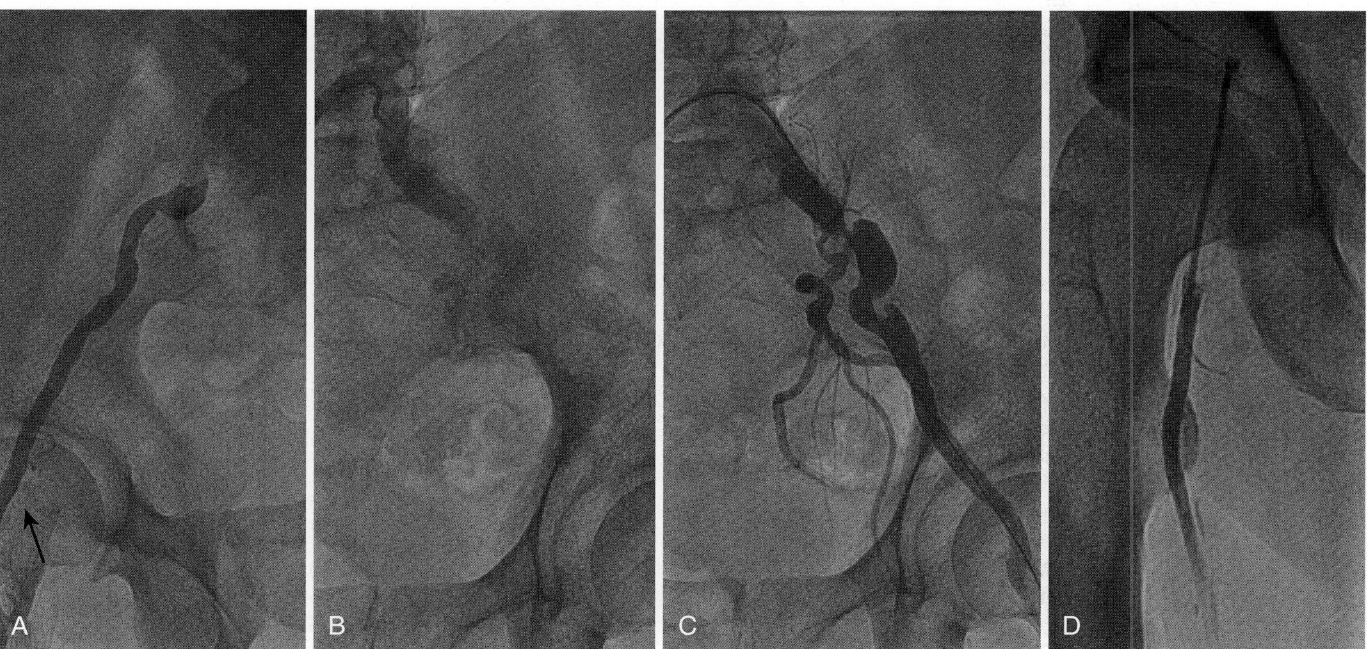

FIGURE 18-4 **A-C,** Access to a left iliac stenosis via the right common femoral artery. **A,** Access of the right femoral artery. Arrow indicates the tip of the femoral sheath. **B,** An Omniflush catheter is directed from the right iliac artery into the left iliac artery and a support wire is used to direct a sheath into the left iliac artery for the intervention. **D,** Antegrade access of the common femoral artery with the sheath tip directed into the superficial femoral artery. *(From Kinlay S, Bhatt DL: Treatment of noncoronary obstructive vascular disease. Braunwald heart disease, ed 10, Philadelphia, 2015, Elsevier, Figure 60-11, p 1354).*

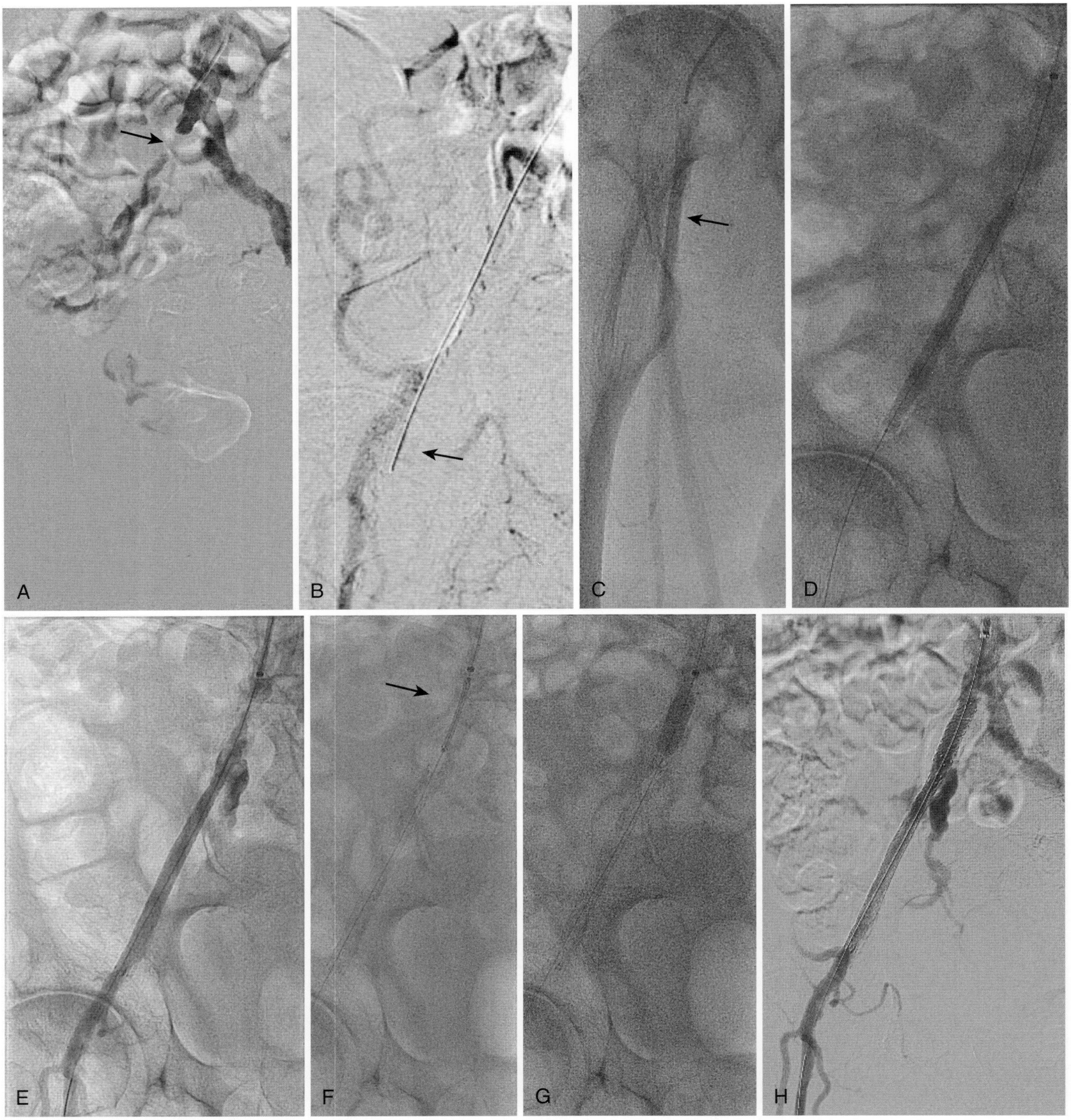

FIGURE 18-5 Brachial approach to a right common and external iliac occlusion. **A,** Angiogram from the brachial artery showing an occlusion at the right common iliac artery *(arrow)*. **B,** Wire tip in an extraluminal plane in the external iliac artery. **C,** After wire repositioning, injection distal to the occlusion shows the luminal location of the catheter. **D,** Balloon dilation of the external iliac artery. **E,** External iliac artery after a self-expanding stent used to dilate the artery (due to the close location to the common femoral artery). **F,** Deployment of a proximal balloon expandable stent at the origin of the right common iliac artery and avoiding the takeoff of the internal iliac artery. **G,** Postdilation of the proximal stent. **H,** Final result showing patent common, internal, and external iliac arteries.

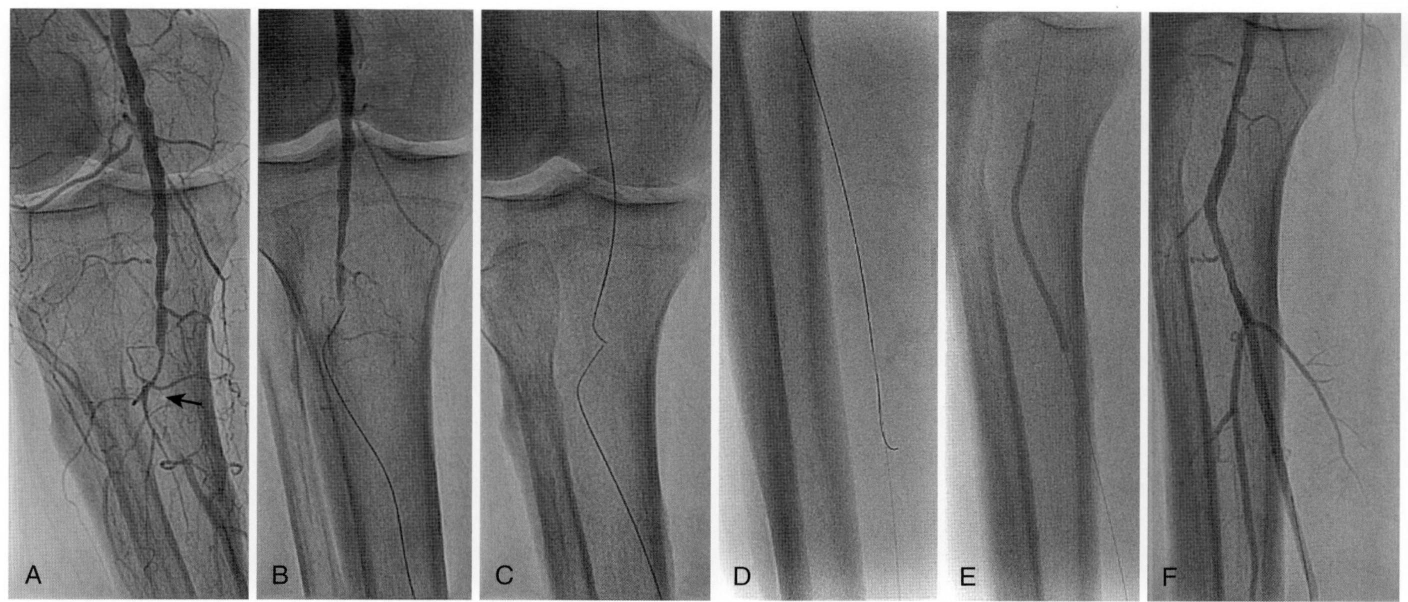

FIGURE 18-6 Antegrade and retrograde approach to an occluded below knee popliteal and posterior tibial artery. **A,** Occluded segment *(arrow)*. **B,** Retrograde wire from the posterior tibial artery accessed at the ankle. **C,** Antegrade and retrograde wires crossing the occlusion. **D,** The antegrade wire crossed the occlusion into the distal posterior tibial artery. **E,** Balloon angioplasty was followed by a short stent in the occluded segment. **F,** Final angiogram. *(From Kinlay S, Bhatt DL: Treatment of noncoronary obstructive vascular disease. Braunwald heart disease, ed 10, Philadelphia, 2015, Elsevier, Figure 60-13, p 1355).*

refers to the inner diameter and guide French size refers to the outer diameter. Thus sheaths have a larger external diameter than the same French guides.

Typical sheaths for the contralateral femoral artery access include the Balkin and Ansel sheaths, which have preformed curves but can be shaped further if required. Conventional short and long sheaths can be used for antegrade femoral artery access, including sheaths with radio-opaque tips that show where the tip of the sheath is in relation to the segment being treated.

If access is from the contralateral or ipsilateral femoral artery, a multipurpose guide can be directed into the distal superficial femoral or popliteal arteries for interventions below the knee (**Figure 18-7**) (Video 18-1). This can provide greater support than a femoral sheath and also reduce the amount of contrast required for an intervention. Conventional 0.014-inch coronary balloons or specific peripheral balloons can be used through a 5 Fr or 6 Fr multipurpose guide in this manner.

Wires

A multitude of wires are available to help navigate tortuous stenoses or long chronic total occlusions. These include 0.014-inch wires used for coronary artery interventions, which come in a range of tip stiffness and hydrophilic wires. Balloons designed for 0.018-inch wires usually have a low enough profile to be used with 0.014-inch wires, but 0.035-inch balloons have such a mismatch between the balloon nose and wire that they often do not track well on a 0.014-inch wire. Regular and hydrophilic 0.018-inch wires provide greater support than 0.014-inch wires but are often less torquable than the 0.014-inch wires.

Conventional and stiff 0.035-inch wires (e.g., Amplatz and Rosen wires) provide increased support for directing catheters and guides (e.g., from the contralateral femoral artery). The Wholey wire has a soft tip on a stiff shaft but is often less torquable than a hydrophilic wire. Angled hydrophilic wires can help select arteries for catheters and can be exchanged for stiffer J-wires to direct sheaths into position. Angled hydrophilic wires can be used to cross lesions but can perforate the artery quite easily, so confirmation of location by angiography from multiple views or other methods should be attempted prior to balloon angioplasty.

Anticoagulation

All interventions and often prolonged diagnostic cases require anticoagulation to prevent thrombus forming on wires and other equipment. Unfractionated heparin is often used at a lower activated clotting time (e.g., 220-250 seconds) compared to coronary interventions. Heparin is usually the anticoagulant of choice when treating long total occlusions due to the high incidence of wire perforation and the risk of larger perforations that may require immediate reversal of anticoagulation with protamine.

Perforation of the iliac arteries can be catastrophic due to the high volume of blood flow (approximately 200 mL/min at rest) and requires early identification and treatment. Although the recommended dose of protamine is approximately 10 mg per 1000 U of heparin used (and up to a maximum of 50 mg), often lower doses are successful in stopping bleeding, particularly when used with low-pressure balloon tamponade near the site of perforation. If unsuccessful, covered stents can be used to treat perforation (see below).

Newer anticoagulants such as bivalirudin and potent antiplatelet agents may offer better anticoagulation based on their experience in coronary interventions, but there are no direct comparisons of their safety and efficacy compared to heparin in lower extremity interventions.

Reentry Devices

Reentry devices are designed to locate the distal true lumen after dissecting through a chronic total occlusion.[6] All of these devices work on a principle that if a guidewire

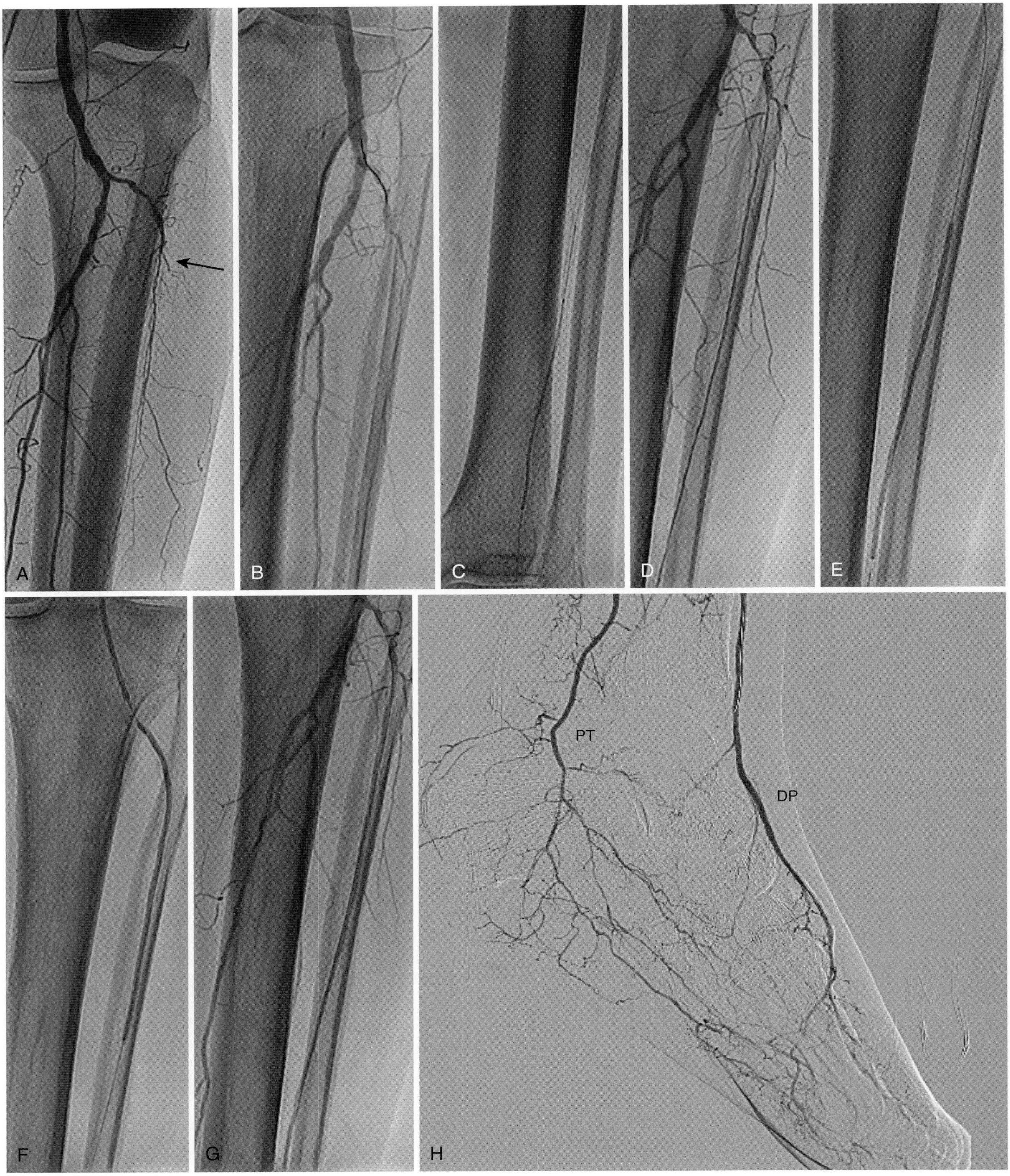

FIGURE 18-7 Antegrade access for balloon angioplasty to a totally occluded anterior tibial artery to treat a nonhealing ulcer of the antero-lateral foot using a multipurpose guide in the popliteal artery for support. **A,** Baseline angiogram showing occlusion of the anterior tibial artery *(arrow)*. **B,** 0.014-inch wire entering the occluded artery. **C,** Angioplasty of the distal anterior tibial artery with a 2.0 mm × 80 mm balloon. **D,** Angiogram after dilating the anterior tibial artery with a 2.0-mm balloon. **E,** Dilation of the distal artery with a 3.0-mm balloon. **F,** Dilation of the proximal anterior tibial artery with a 3.0-mm balloon. **G,** Final angiogram of the proximal anterior tibial artery. **H,** Final angiogram of the foot showing a patent dorsalis pedis artery (DP) and posterior tibial artery (PT) with a restored pedal arcade.

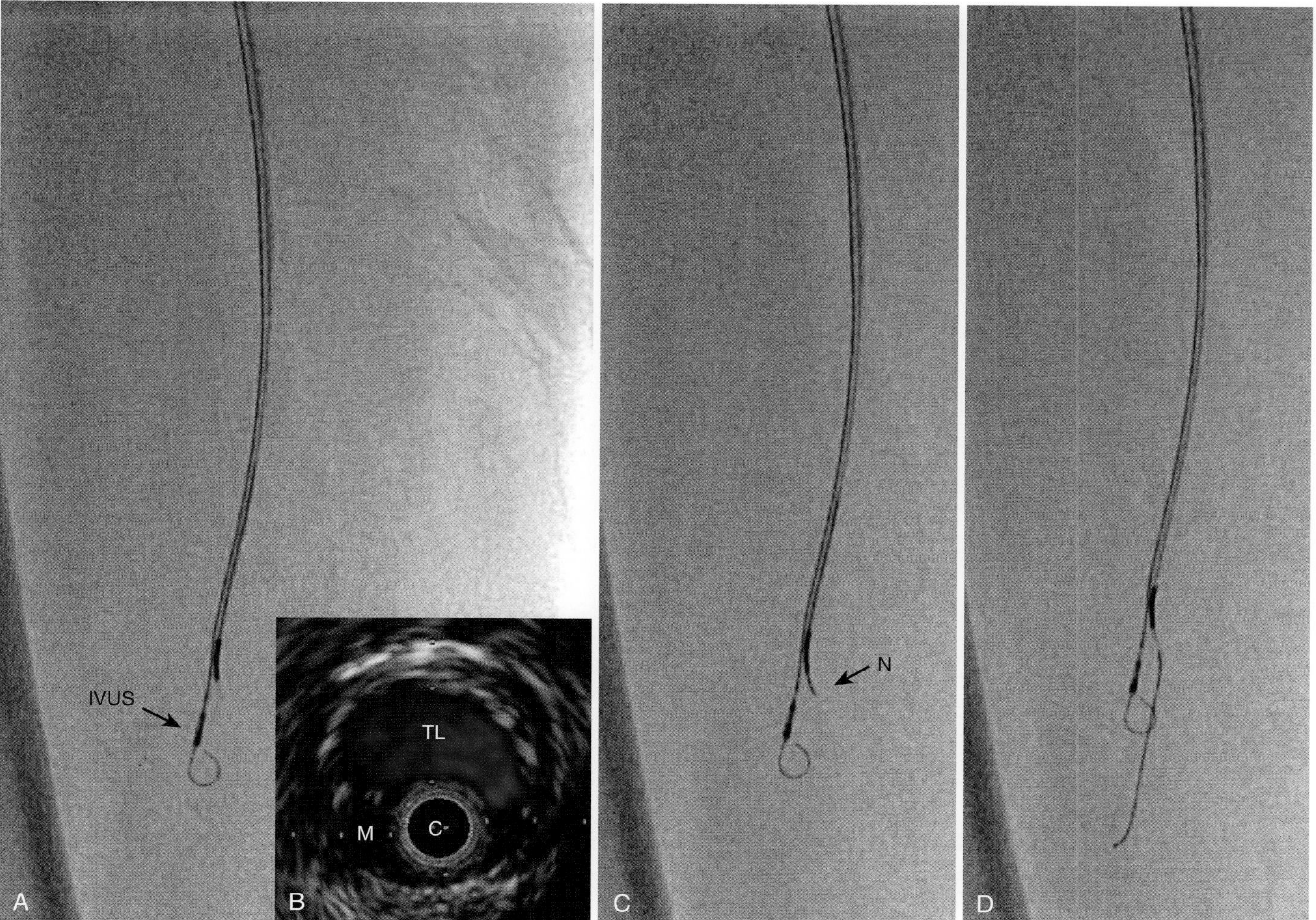

FIGURE 18-8 Pioneer catheter used to select the true lumen of a total occlusion of the superficial femoral artery. **A,** Pioneer catheter in a dissection plane just beyond the distal cap of the total occlusion. The intravascular ultrasound (IVUS) element of the catheter images the true lumen. **B,** IVUS image showing the catheter (C) in the media (M) of the artery imaging the true lumen (TL) with the aid of the chromoflo function showing moving blood in the lumen. **C,** The needle (N) is deployed into the true lumen. **D,** A 0.014-inch guidewire is advanced through the needle into the true lumen.

dissects down the side of a plaque into a plane beyond the distal cap, the reentry catheter will direct a guidewire into the true lumen. After accessing the distal artery lumen, the reentry device is removed and followed by conventional angioplasty and/or stenting. These devices await formal testing against standard interventional techniques to cross occlusions.

The Pioneer Plus catheter (Volcano Corp. San Diego, California) has a multiple array intravascular ultrasound at the end of the catheter. This is connected to a Volcano intravascular ultrasound system and used to image the true lumen. The catheter is rotated until the distal true lumen appears at the 12 o'clock position of the ultrasound image, which corresponds to the direction the curved needle at the tip of the device will deploy (**Figure 18-8**). Once the needle is in the true lumen, a 0.014-inch wire can be advanced through the needle into the true lumen.

The Outback LTD (Cordis, Miami Lakes, Florida) has an angled needle housed at the tip of a catheter with an L-shaped tip under fluoroscopy.[6] The catheter is advanced into a dissection plane adjacent to the distal true lumen and the catheter turned until the L-shaped marker is directed toward the lumen. In an orthogonal view, the tip should have a T-shape overlapping the distal true lumen. At this point a distal needle is deployed into the true lumen and an 0.014-inch wire advanced through the needle into the true lumen.

The OffRoad CTO (Boston Scientific, Natick, Massachusetts) uses a balloon advanced beyond the distal cap and inflated within the wall to point toward the lumen. A microcatheter lancet is advanced through the balloon to provide access for a wire to enter the distal lumen of the artery. The Enteer reentry system (Covidien, Mansfield, Massachusetts) uses a flat balloon with two side-exit ports. Fluoroscopy is used to avoid directing the wire to the port adjacent to the outer artery wall and instead chooses the exit port adjacent to the true lumen.

Other Chronic Total Occlusion (CTO) Devices

There are a number of devices designed to assist crossing total occlusions that often have tough entry and exit caps. Like the reentry devices above, case reports and series describe their use, but their value over conventional wire crossing techniques is untested. Reentry devices may be needed with CTO devices if the latter do not enter the distal lumen.

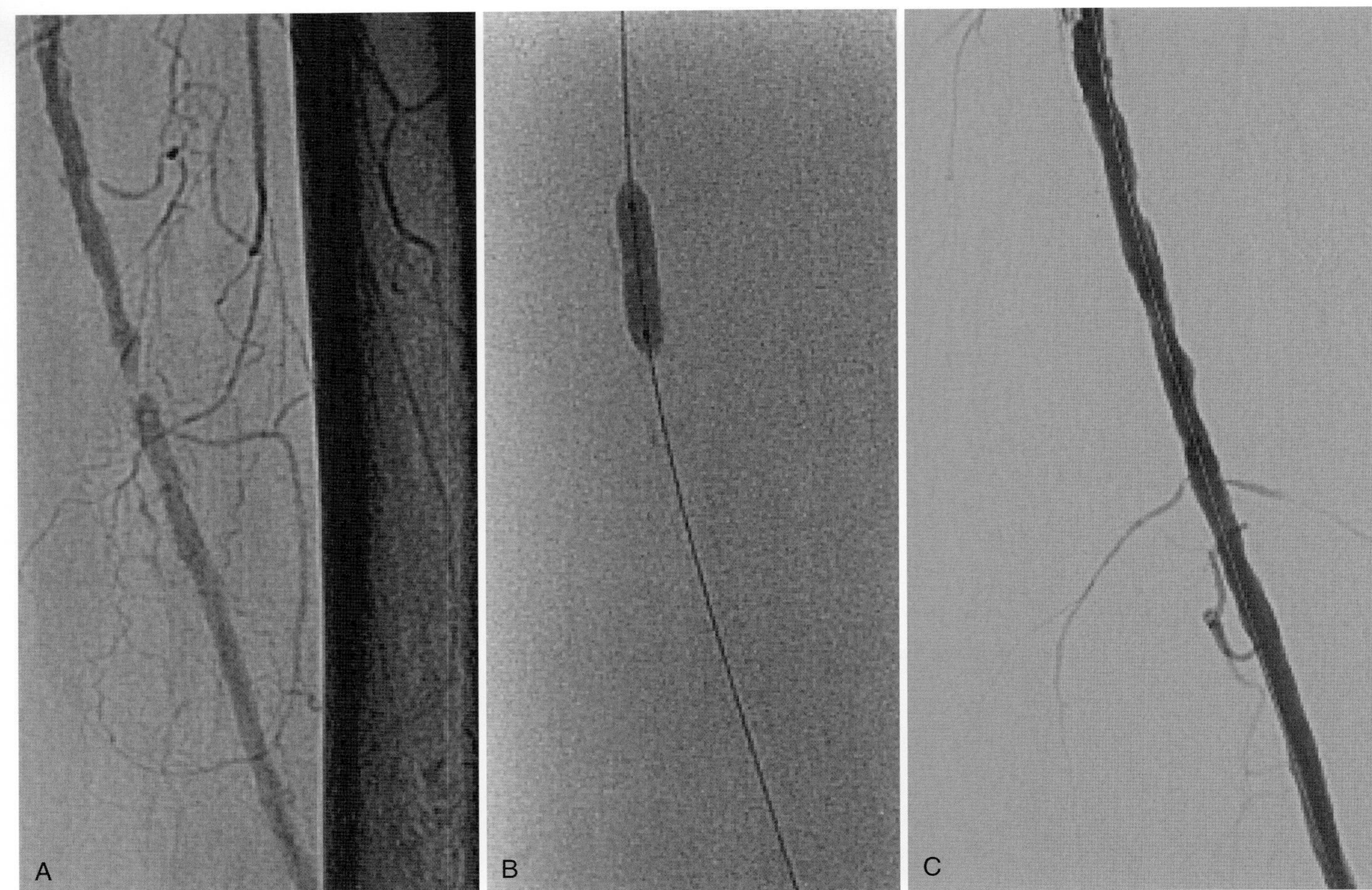

FIGURE 18-9 Treatment of a midsuperficial femoral artery stenosis **(A)**, with balloon angioplasty alone **(B)**, with an excellent final result **(C)**. *(From Kinlay S, Bhatt DL: Treatment of noncoronary obstructive vascular disease. Braunwald heart disease, ed 10, Philadelphia, 2015, Elsevier, Figure 60-2, p 1349).*

The Crosser CTO system (Bard, Murray Hill, New Jersey) uses a nitinol wire inserted into the proximal cap of an occlusion. The distal end of the wire is connected to an external transducer that generates high-frequency vibrations down the wire to the tip. The vibration assists the wire to traverse the occlusion. The Powerwire catheter (Baylis Medical Co., Montreal, Canada) uses radio frequency ablation to ablate plaque in a chronic total occlusion.

The TruePath CTO (Boston Scientific, Natick, Massachusetts) is an 0.018-inch wire with a diamond-encrusted tip that is connected to an external motor drive to burr through occlusions. The Viance catheter (Covidien, Mansfield, Massachusetts) uses a similar design with an atraumatic tip designed to blunt dissect down a plane in the artery media.

The Kittycat2 and Wildcat catheters (Avinger, Redwood City, California) have a rotating screw on the tip and are connected to an external motor drive to drill through an occlusion. A newer Ocelot catheter (Avinger, Redwood City, California) combines this design with a cross-sectional optical coherence tomography imaging system to avoid perforating the artery.

Balloon Angioplasty

Balloon angioplasty remains the standard revascularization technique for most interventions in the lower limbs (**Figure 18-9**), although it is often accompanied by stenting, particularly for long lesions. Although coronary 0.014-inch platform balloons can be used to cross lesions, they are generally too short for most lesions and less pushable than dedicated peripheral balloons.

Peripheral balloons are available in 0.014-inch, 0.018-inch, and 0.035-inch platforms. Most are compliant or semicompliant balloons and tend to grow with higher pressure inflations. Smaller diameter balloons are available in 0.014-inch and 0.018-inch platforms and are useful in the smaller tibial arteries (generally 2-4 mm diameter arteries) and to assist crossing long lesions in any artery. Larger diameter balloons are available in the 0.018-inch and 0.035-inch platforms, generally for treating iliac and femoral arteries.

Indeflator kits available for coronary interventions are suitable for inflating peripheral balloons. Since larger diameter balloons are used (compared to coronary interventions), the contrast used to dilate the balloons is usually more dilute (a 1:3 or 1:4 contrast:saline ratio). This allows faster inflation and deflation times and is usually an adequate density to visualize under fluoroscopy.

Angioplasty increases the arterial lumen through positive remodeling (acutely via expansion of the whole artery) and controlled dissections in the plaque and intima. Larger dissections that limit flow or have visible flaps greater than 50% of the lumen diameter increase the risk of abrupt closure in the proceeding 24 to 48 hours.[7] Over days to several months, angioplasty promotes a healing response associated with neointima produced largely by proteoglycan production from vascular smooth muscle cells. Restenosis over several months occurs by excessive neointima and negative remodeling of the whole artery. Over several years it is likely that neoatherosclerosis with lipid deposition and inflammatory cell recruitment can lead to renarrowing of the artery as it does in the coronary arteries.[14]

Drug-Eluting Balloons

Drug-coated balloons are recent innovations offering a lower rate of restenosis compared to noncoated balloons. These balloons are coated in drugs of the taxane class (e.g., paclitaxel), usually mixed with iodinated contrast or another molecule that acts as a detergent to promote release from the balloon and distribution into the injured arterial intima after balloon angioplasty. Results compared to conventional balloon angioplasty in the lower extremities show less restenosis and greater long-term patency of the femoral and tibial arteries when used as the initial intervention or as treatment for restenosis.[15-19]

They are used at the end of an intervention, as the drug is removed off the balloon with a single inflation. Thus multiple balloons may be required to treat long lesions.

Stents

The two stent designs for the lower extremity arteries are balloon expandable or self-expanding. Stent therapy requires aspirin and a thienopyridine (e.g., clopidogrel), although the evidence for dual antiplatelet therapy is derived largely from the coronary stent literature. Balloon expandable stents are made from stainless steel or alloys of steel and titanium or other metals (**Figure 18-10**). These provide a high degree of radial strength and are easier to deploy accurately (e.g., at ostial locations) compared to self-expandable stents, but they can be compressed by external force. For this reason, balloon expandable stents are often used for iliac artery lesions.

Originally, self-expanding stents were made from stainless steel, but they are now largely made from nitinol, which offers a lower rate of restenosis[7] (**Figure 18-11**). Their key advantage is their ability to recoil back to their baseline diameter after external compression and for this reason are used outside the torso and where there are greater torsion and compression forces on the artery (e.g., the superficial femoral artery). In lesions over 60 mm to 100 mm, self-expanding nitinol stents offer a lower restenosis rate and better functional results (as assessed by treadmill testing) compared to balloon angioplasty alone.[7]

Although newer designs are more durable and less prone to stent fracture,[7,20] they can be kinked or fractured with excessive flexion and torsion. This is particularly a concern over joints, for example, the popliteal artery. These stents tend to move on deployment and are therefore more difficult to use at ostial locations. Self-expanding stents that cover a large branch vessel (e.g., jail the profunda artery when treating a proximal superficial femoral lesion) are difficult to recover, as dilation through the stent struts is ineffective due to strut recoil. For these reasons, self-expanding stents are avoided where possible over the knee and hip joints and are used as a last resort in these locations (e.g., with critical limb ischemia and a poor angiographic result). Dissection per se does not define a poor angiographic result, as some dissection is present in all successful balloon angioplasty. A poor

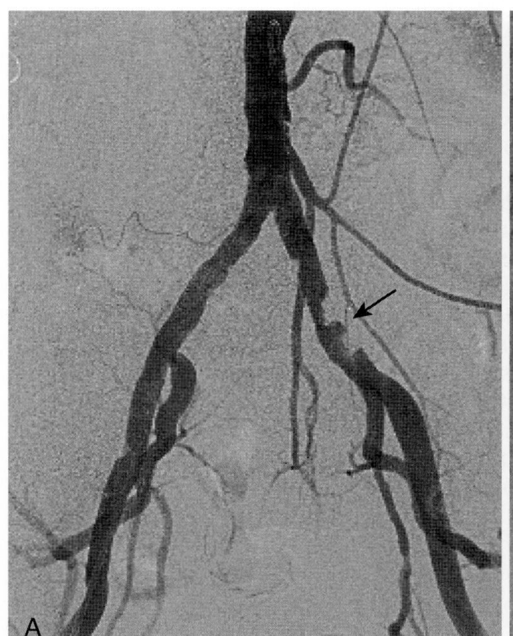

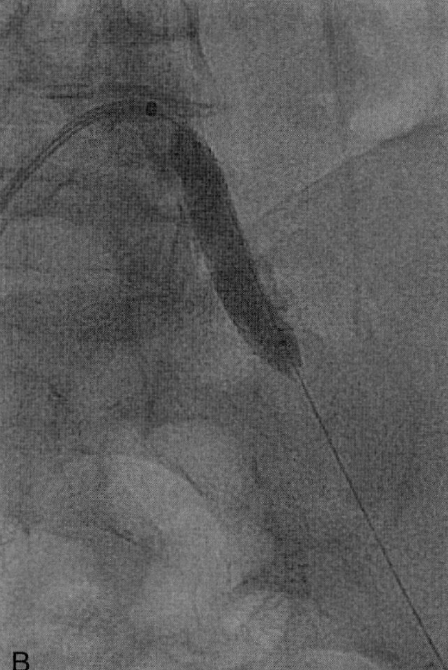

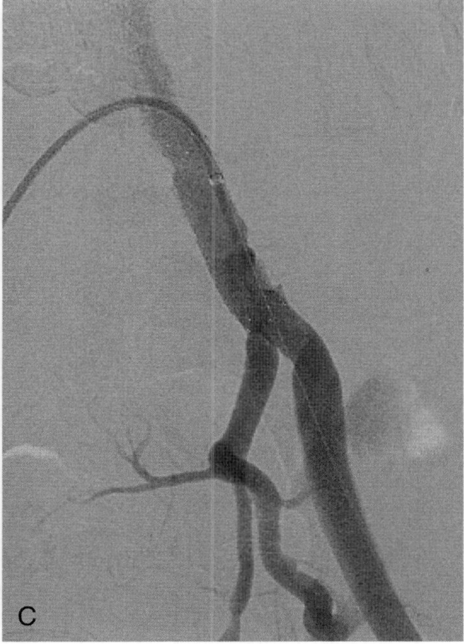

FIGURE 18-10 Treatment of left common iliac stenoses with a balloon expandable stent from the contralateral right femoral artery. **A,** Serial stenoses in the left common iliac artery *(arrow)*. **B,** Balloon expandable stent deployment. **C,** Final angiogram. *(From Kinlay S, Bhatt DL: Treatment of noncoronary obstructive vascular disease. Braunwald heart disease, ed 10, Philadelphia, 2015, Elsevier, Figure 60-3, p 1350).*

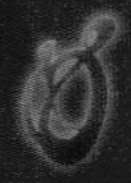

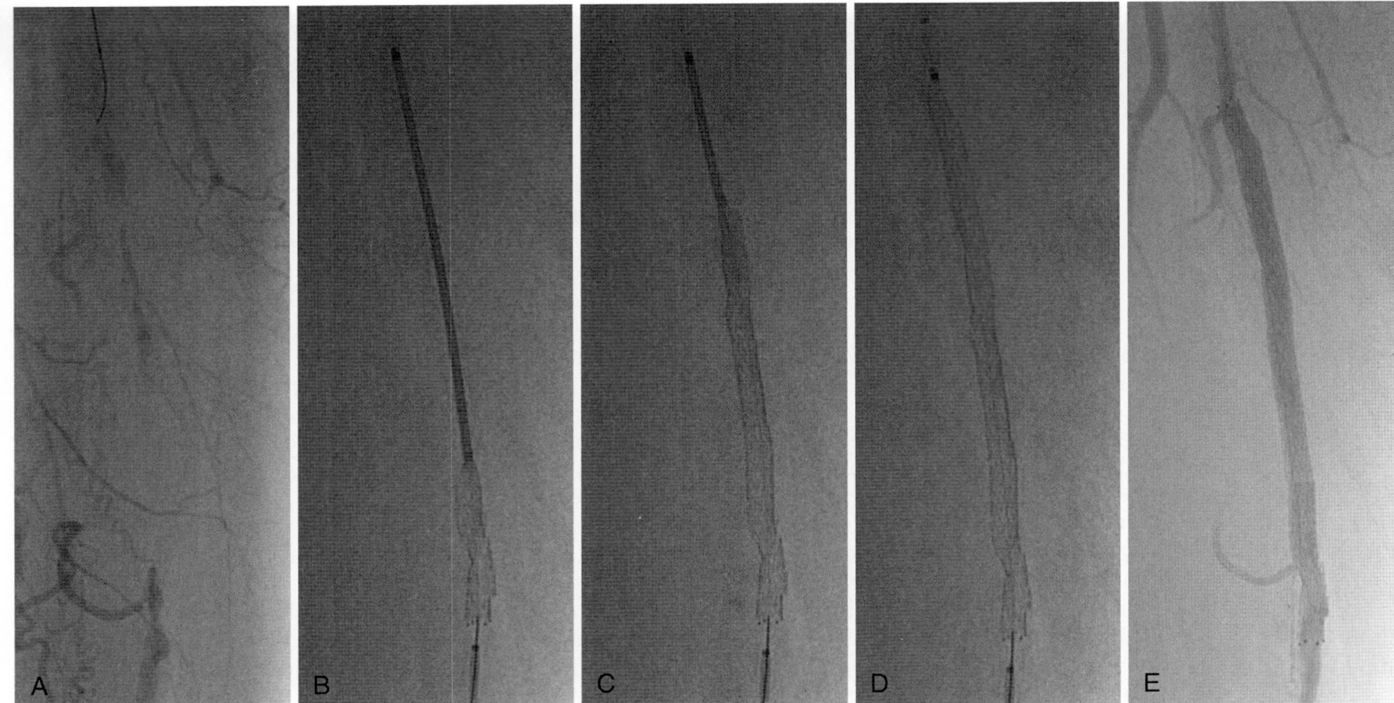

FIGURE 18-11 Treatment of a superficial femoral artery occlusion with a self-expandable nitinol stent. **A,** A wire approaches the occluded segment. **B-D,** The delivery catheter is pulled back to release the self-expanding stent. **E,** Final angiogram. *(From Kinlay S, Bhatt DL: Treatment of noncoronary obstructive vascular disease. Braunwald heart disease, ed 10, Philadelphia, 2015, Elsevier, Figure 60-4, p 1350).*

angiographic result is usually interpreted to mean dissection or recoil with poor flow (abnormally slow flow velocity) or a flap visibly extending beyond 50% of the lumen diameter.[7]

Covered Stents

Stents covered in a polytetrafluoroethylene (PTFE) jacket are available in both balloon expandable and self-expanding stent formats (**Figure 18-12**) (Video 18-2).[6,7] These are particularly useful in treating arterial perforations to prevent exsanguination or compartment syndromes. They are sometimes promoted as causing less restenosis (by excluding neointima), but the studies used to make this claim may be too short in duration to assess this outcome if restenosis is a longer process with covered stents.[21,22] In one study in iliac arteries, the difference in restenosis was due to an unusually high rate of restenosis in the uncovered stent arm.[21] Covered stents also risk covering important branch arteries or collaterals and predispose to acute limb ischemia in the case of stent occlusion (**Figure 18-13**, see part L). Stent thrombosis may also be higher with covered stents. It is uncertain if heparin-coated covered stents prevent stent thrombosis in longer term follow-up.

Drug-Eluting Stents

Drug-eluting balloon expandable stents developed for the coronary arteries can often be used for bailout situations after below knee balloon angioplasty (**Figure 18-6F**). In this situation, where angioplasty leads to flow-limiting dissections and where the lesion is focal (less than 30 mm), drug-eluting balloon expandable stents can reestablish flow and give acceptable patency up to 1 year.[23-25] However, they are subject to compressive forces and their use is generally reserved for revascularization with critical limb ischemia where major amputation is being prevented. The value of multiple overlapping drug-eluting stents is uncertain and likely to be related to a high incidence of stent occlusion by thrombosis or restenosis, particularly in more distal tibial arteries, which become more superficial.

More recent drug-eluting self-expanding stents offer the potential for less restenosis in the femoral artery, particularly for long lesions. These are created with drugs of the taxane class and in two studies reduced the risk of restenosis compared to bare-metal self-expanding stents.[26,27]

Atherectomy

Although various debulking and atherectomy devices may change the distensibility of arteries, there is little evidence that these devices provide better long-term patency over successful balloon angioplasty. Therefore, atherectomy is largely used as adjunctive therapy along with balloon angioplasty and/or stenting.[6,7] This strategy can be particularly useful for calcified lesions that may be difficult to expand by balloon or stent or in arteries over joints where atherectomy may reduce the risk of flow-limiting dissection with balloon angioplasty.

Rotational atherectomy uses a rotating burr to grind off particles of plaque that are either aspirated or small enough to go through capillaries and be removed by the reticular endothelial system. These include the Rotablater (Boston Scientific, Natick, Massachusetts), which was developed for coronary atherectomy but may be of use in the smaller distal arteries of the lower extremity (**Figure 18-14**), the Jetstream (Medrad, Warrendale, Pennsylvania), which

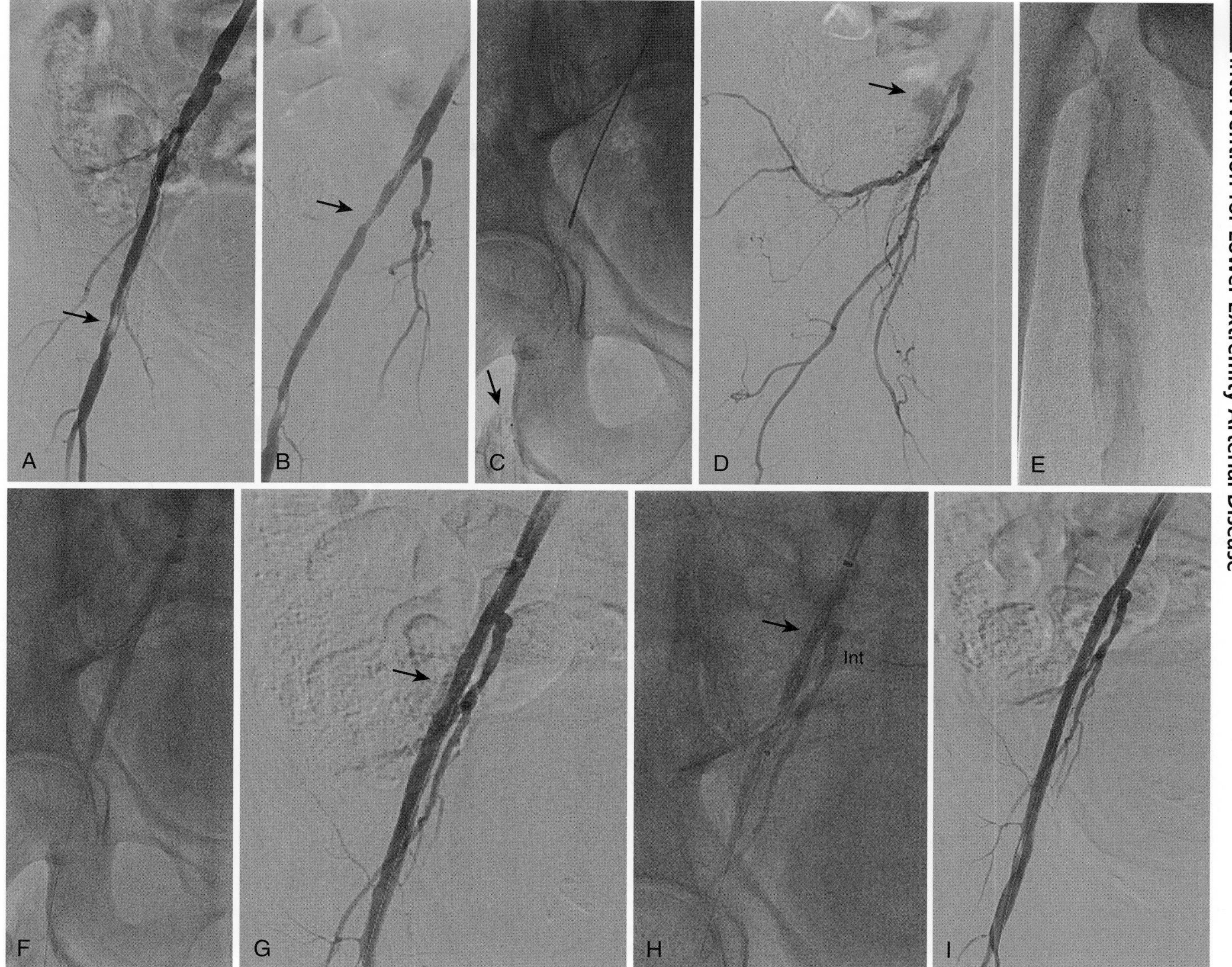

FIGURE 18-12 Treatment of sheath or guide perforation. **A,** The target lesion was a stenosis in the common femoral artery *(arrow)*. **B,** Oblique angiogram showing a more proximal stenosis in the external iliac artery *(arrow)*. **C,** Jetstream run of the common femoral lesion. Note the contrast extravasation, which was appreciated at the end of the Jetstream run *(arrow)*. **D,** Angiogram showing a perforation of the proximal external iliac artery, likely due to the sheath perforating the artery at the more proximal lesion. **E,** Contrast tracking in the extravascular tissues around the superficial femoral artery in the upper thigh. **F,** Balloon tamponade of the perforated external iliac lesion at low pressure with a 7.0 mm × 100 mm balloon. **G,** A smaller amount of extravasation of the dye at the perforation site *(arrow)*. **H,** Placing a 7.0 mm × 38 mm covered stent in the proximal external iliac using an oblique fluoroscopic image to position the proximal stent delivery marker *(arrow)* at the ostium of the external iliac artery so that it does not cover and exclude the internal iliac artery. *Int,* Internal iliac artery. **I,** Final angiogram showing no perforation and successful balloon angioplasty alone of the common femoral artery.

aspirates debris (**Figure 18-15**), and the Diamondback 360/Stealth 360/Predator 360 devices (Cardiovascular Systems Inc., St. Paul, Minnesota), which are wires with an eccentrically mounted diamond-encrusted burr to encourage a larger orbital cutting arc when the wire is rotated at high speed.

The directional atherectomy devices include the Turbohawk or Silverhawk (Covidien, Mansfield, Massachusetts), which has a cutting window that can be oriented to different directions prior to cutting and collecting plaque in the nose cone of the device (**Figure 18-16**).

All atherectomy devices have a tendency to embolize atheroma, even if they are designed to aspirate or collect atheroma. Long-segment atherectomy has greater risks of embolizing small material into the microcirculation, potentially leading to slow flow and critical limb ischemia. This can be prevented by deploying a distal filter embolic protection device to capture embolized debris, but this is only possible with the Jetstream and Silverhawk devices, as the other atherectomy devices run over their own proprietary wires.

In the event embolization occurs, large emboli can be removed by catheter aspiration or broken up by balloon angioplasty. Small-vessel embolization with slow flow may respond to bolus doses of microvascular dilators such as nitroprusside (100-300 micrograms).

Other Plaque-Modifying Technologies

Other technologies include cryoplasty, laser atherectomy, and cutting or scoring balloons. Cryoplasty (Polarcath,

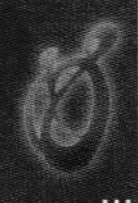

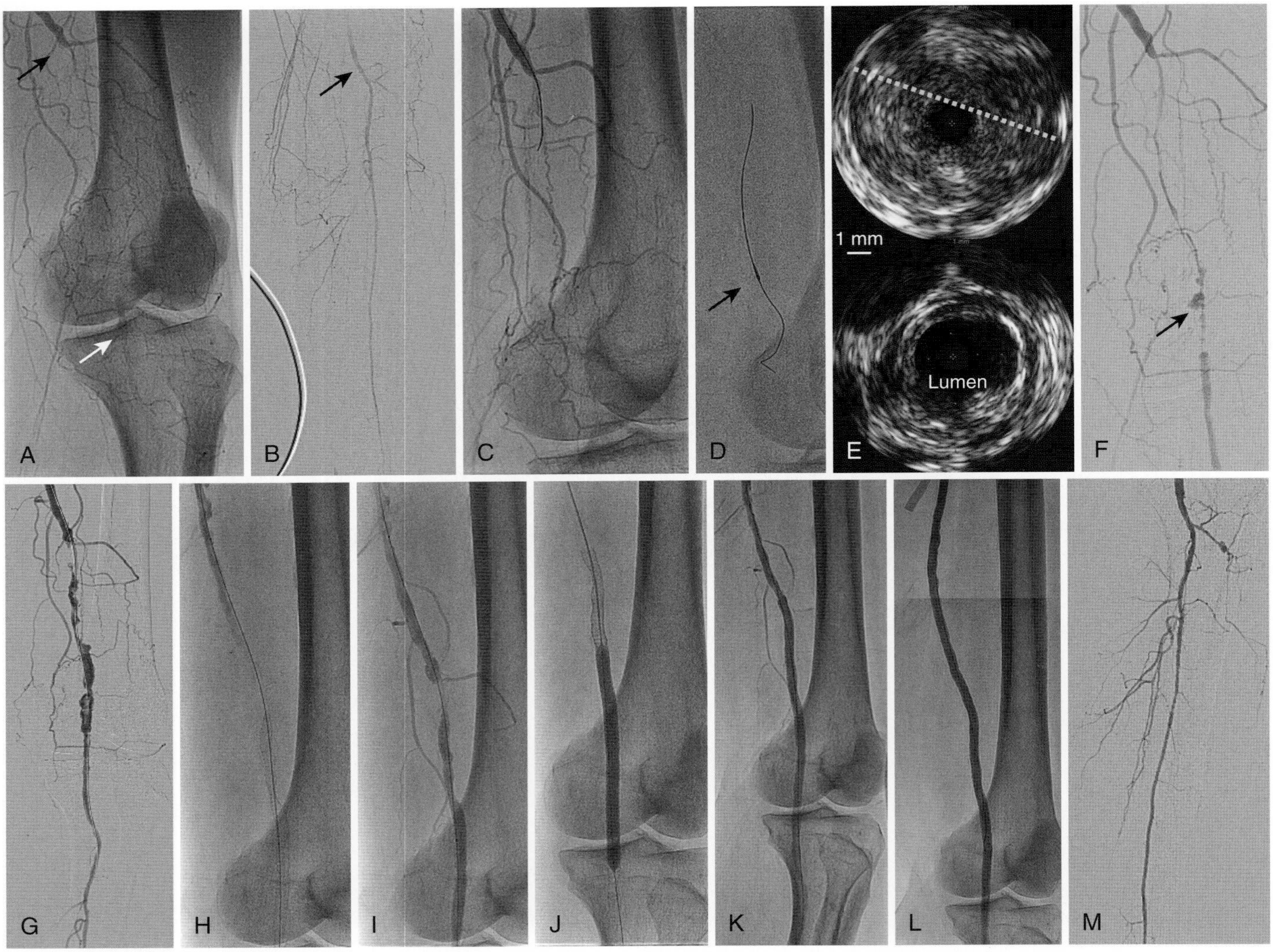

FIGURE 18-13 Endovascular treatment of a thrombosed popliteal aneurysm for a patient at high surgical risk. **A,** Occluded above knee popliteal artery *(black arrow),* with reconstitution of the below knee popliteal artery by collaterals *(white arrow).* **B,** Distal runoff into a peroneal artery *(arrow).* The anterior and posterior tibial arteries occluded. **C,** Wire in the proximal occlusion. **D,** IVUS catheter placed in occlusion to assess the popliteal artery. **E,** IVUS images. Upper image showing a thrombosed popliteal aneurysm (*yellow line* indicates a 9-mm vessel diameter). Lower image showing reentry into the distal lumen of the below knee popliteal artery. **F,** Thrombus in the popliteal artery *(arrow).* **G,** 24 hours after catheter directed thrombolysis. The angiogram shows extensive residual thrombus in an aneurysmal popliteal artery. **H,** Placement of a self-expanding covered stent in the mid to distal popliteal artery. **I,** Angiogram showing residual disease proximal to the stent. **J,** Postdilation after a second, more proximal covered self-expanding stent. **K,** Angiogram showing thrombus at the proximal margin of the stents. **L,** Final angiogram after a third proximal stent placed. Note the loss of collaterals. **M,** Final angiogram of the distal popliteal artery and peroneal artery below the knee.

Boston Scientific, Natick, Massachusetts) uses a proprietary technology to inflate a specially designed double balloon with nitrous oxide gas, which is delivered to the balloon for a 20-second inflation at −10 °C (**Figure 18-17**). In theory, this cooling is designed to induce apoptosis of vascular smooth muscle cells and prevent neointima formation and restenosis. In one single center study, restenosis after stenting was less common,[28] but the clinical effect seems relatively small. Laser atherectomy is designed to ablate tissue, but like other ablation technologies, it seems to offer no reduction in restenosis compared to balloon angioplasty alone. Cutting or scoring balloons use wires or cutting blades adjacent to a balloon. When the balloon is inflated at the lesion, the blades or wires are designed to cut the plaque to create a more controlled dissection. They may also concentrate force over the wires or blades to break resistant calcified or fibrous plaques. As such they have a niche role but of no proven benefit in clinical trials.

Brachytherapy

Brachytherapy in the lower limbs typically requires gamma radiation due to the larger distance between the delivery catheter and the wall of most lower extremity arteries (compared to coronary arteries). This technique is sometimes used to treat diffuse in-stent restenosis, but the extensive shielding and collaboration with radiation therapists make this technically difficult in most centers. The clinical effect of brachytherapy is not well studied, and the potential for drug-eluting balloons to be a much easier technology for this indication has decreased its popularity.

Catheter-Based Thrombolysis

Thrombosis of a major lower limb artery causing acute or critical limb ischemia can be treated successfully by catheter-based thrombolysis. All techniques require thrombolytic agents (e.g., recombinant tissue plasminogen activator—tPA) to be delivered into the thrombus, as

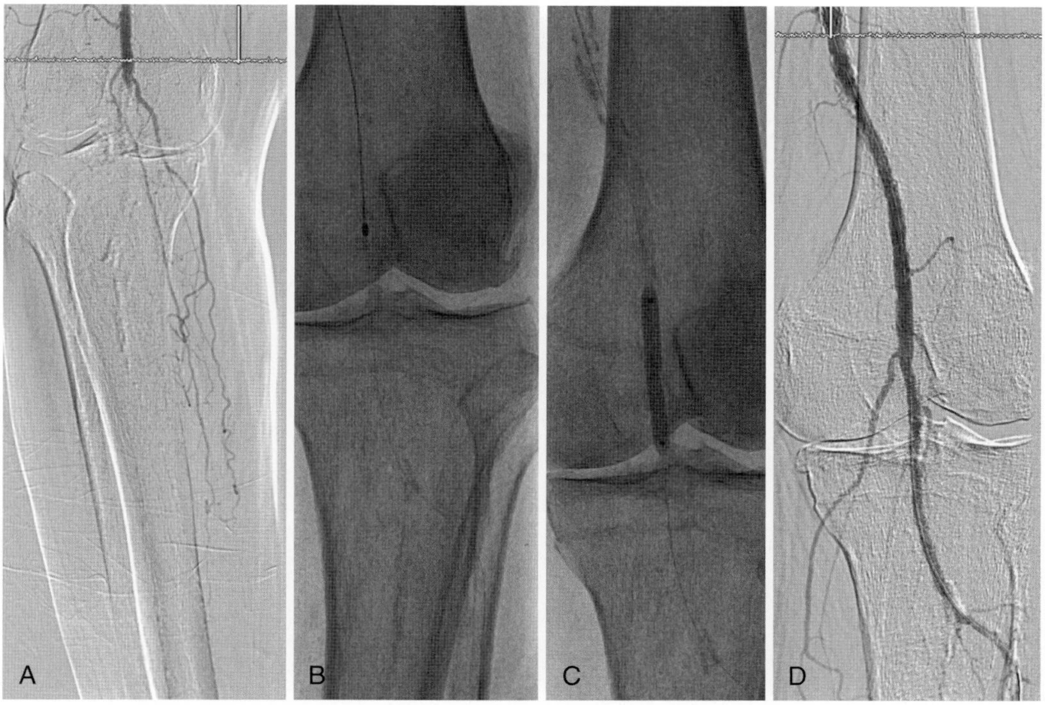

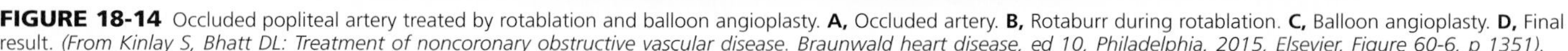

FIGURE 18-14 Occluded popliteal artery treated by rotablation and balloon angioplasty. **A,** Occluded artery. **B,** Rotaburr during rotablation. **C,** Balloon angioplasty. **D,** Final result. *(From Kinlay S, Bhatt DL: Treatment of noncoronary obstructive vascular disease. Braunwald heart disease, ed 10, Philadelphia, 2015, Elsevier, Figure 60-6, p 1351).*

intravenous therapy or infusing thrombolytic agents next to a thrombus is far less effective.[1,2]

Catheter-based infusion of thrombolytic drugs over 12 to 48 hours is best achieved after inserting a multiple hole infusion catheter (e.g., Cragg-McNamara catheter, Covidien, Mansfield, Massachusetts) over a wire into the thrombosed segment (**Figure 18-13**). The wire is removed and a valve at the tip closes to prevent the thrombolytic agent from exiting the end of the catheter. Instead, the thrombolytic agent infuses through multiple side holes over a 100-mm to 200-mm length of the catheter directly into the thrombus. An initial bolus of 10 mg to 20 mg tPA is given through the catheter and then a 1-mg to 2-mg per hour infusion over 12 to 48 hours. Usually 12 to 24 hours is adequate, with longer infusions increasing the risk of depleting fibrinogen and increasing bleeding from the access site or elsewhere.[29] Low-dose intravenous anticoagulation with heparin is often used concurrently. Systemic concentrations of fibrinogen levels of less than 100 mg/dL may indicate a higher risk of bleeding and the need to stop thrombolysis.[30]

In cases where a patient may not stay on bed rest, or where a lower dose of thrombolytic agent is preferred, or where the time required for catheter-based infusion may jeopardize the viability of a limb, two other endovascular techniques are available. These include the Angiojet (Possis Medical, Minneapolis, Minnesota), using the pulse spray option (**Figure 18-18**), and the Trellis catheter system (Covidien, Mansfield, Massachusetts). The Angiojet uses a Venturi effect to aspirate thrombus and debris from arteries.[6] However, in the pulse-spray mode, aspiration is blocked and the catheter sprays a solution of thrombolytic agent into the thrombosed artery (e.g., 10 mg tPA in 50 mL saline or 10-20 mg TNK in 50 mL saline). The solution is left for 20 minutes and then the Angiojet is converted to the usual aspiration setup and the solution and thrombus aspirated. The Trellis system contains a multihole infusion catheter with a balloon occluding the artery at the distal and proximal ends of the thrombus. The system uses a 6 Fr catheter (for balloon diameters up to 10 mm) or an 8 Fr system for balloon diameters up to 16 mm and two catheter lengths (80 or 120 cm). Depending on the catheter length, the system can treat segments of up to 15-cm or 30-cm lengths of thrombus. After the delivery of a thrombolytic agent, a moter oscillates a wire placed in the catheter lumen at 500 RPM to 3000 rpm to help mix the thrombolytic agent into the clot. After 10 minutes the lysed thrombus is aspirated.

Catheter-based thrombolysis can effectively restore perfusion to an ischemic limb. However, if there is substantial ischemia, reperfusion syndrome can occur, with tissue swelling leading to compartment syndrome. Compartment syndrome can cause tissue ischemia, infarction, and potentially limb loss that require specific fasciotomies to relieve the pressure. For this reason, thrombolysis in acute limb ischemia requires a collaborative approach, with surgeons who know how to assess compartment syndrome and perform an effective fasciotomy.

Intravascular Imaging

Intravascular imaging can help keep equipment within the artery wall when crossing an occlusion, measure the diameter of an artery for device sizing, and assess any angiographic features that could represent dissections or other structural abnormalities. The two key imaging techniques are intravascular ultrasound (IVUS) and optical coherence tomography (OCT). Although OCT has higher spatial resolution, its poor depth penetration compared to IVUS limits is usefulness in the large peripheral arteries.

IVUS is coupled with one reentry device to help locate the distal true lumen after dissecting through an occlusion (**Figure 18-8**). It can also show whether a wire is within the

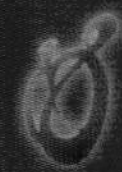

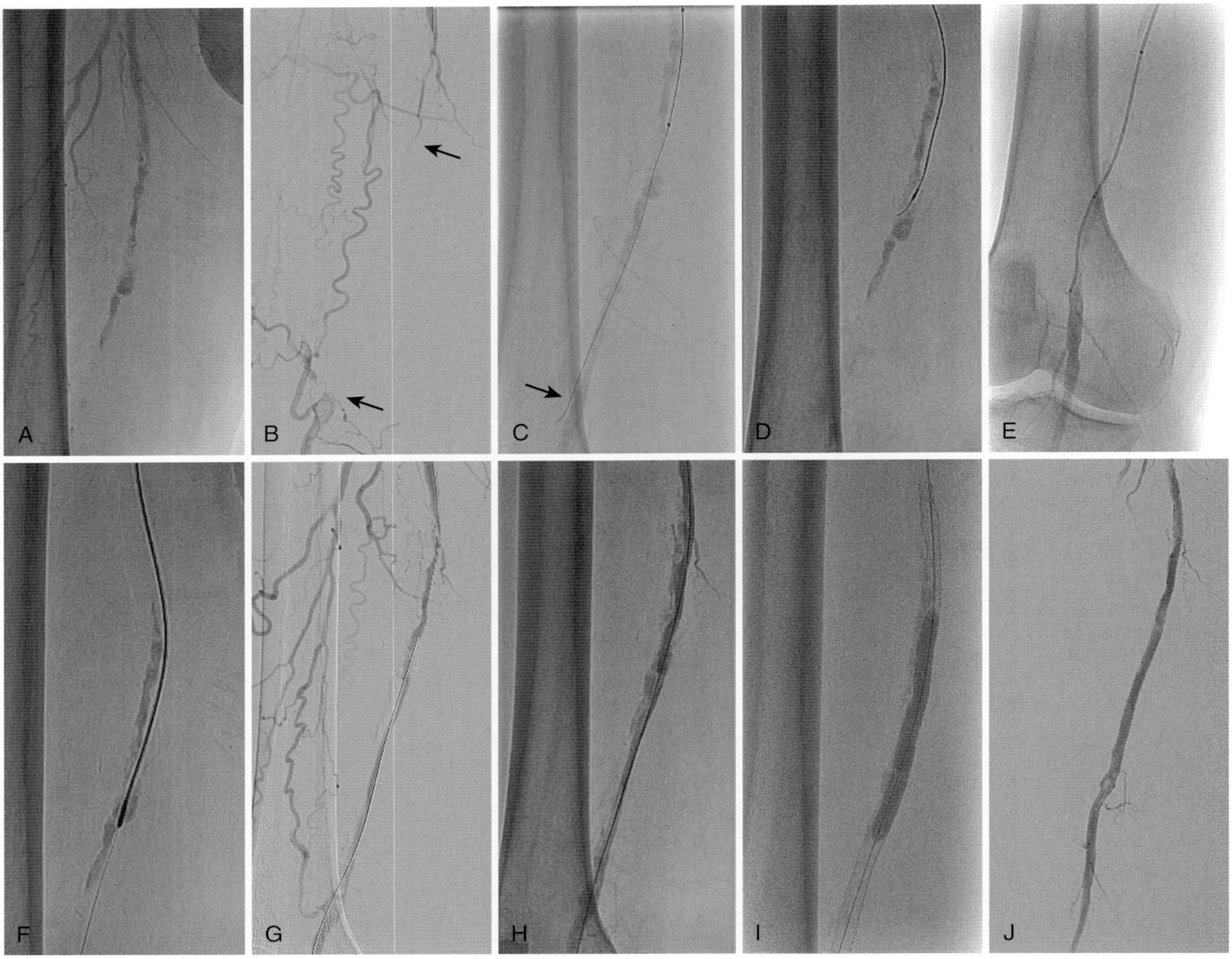

FIGURE 18-15 Rotational atherectomy in a heavily calcified total occlusion of the superficial femoral artery. **A,** Fluoroscopy without contrast shows heavy calcification. **B,** Digital subtraction showing a total occlusion between the two arrows and distal reconstitution by collaterals from the profunda femoral. **C,** Attempt to cross the lesion with a wire leads to the wire tip in an extraluminal plane *(arrow).* **D,** IVUS used to locate the most distal true lumen in the occlusion (see Figure 18-19). **E,** Injection through a support catheter demonstrating successful reentry into the true lumen in the above knee popliteal artery. **F,** Rotational atherectomy with a Jetstream device. **G,** Angiogram after atherectomy. **H,** Angiography after balloon angioplasty. **I,** Postdilating a self-expanding stent. **J,** Final result.

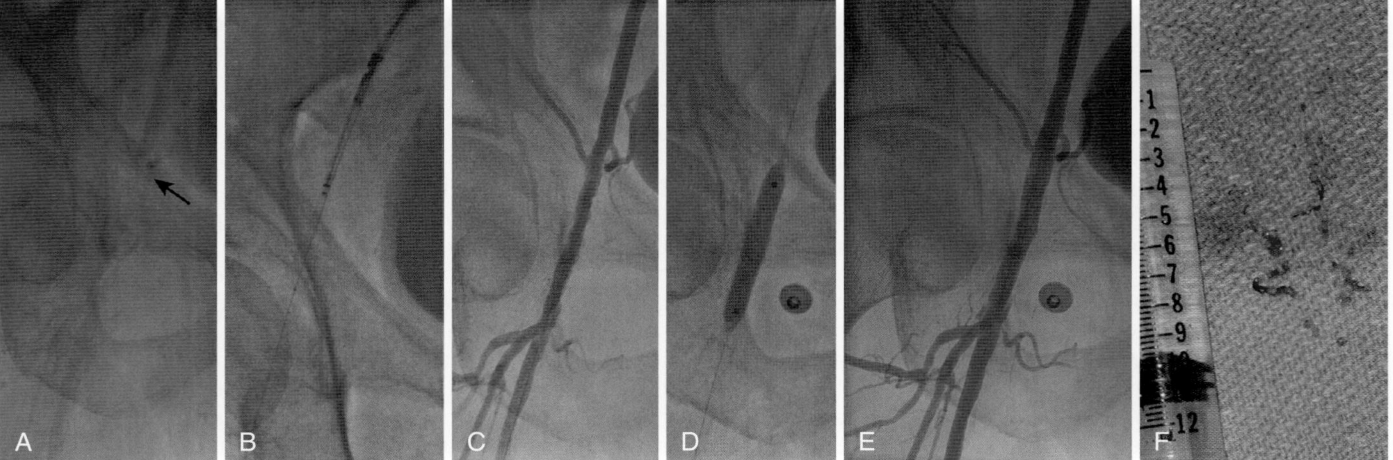

FIGURE 18-16 Common femoral artery occlusion treated with directional atherectomy. **A,** Occlusion in the right common femoral artery *(arrow).* **B,** Directional atherectomy catheter. **C,** After eight cutting runs. **D,** Adjunctive balloon angioplasty. **E,** Final angiogram. **F,** Atheromatous material removed by the atherectomy device. *(From Kinlay S, Bhatt DL: Treatment of noncoronary obstructive vascular disease. Braunwald heart disease, ed 10, Philadelphia, 2015, Elsevier, Figure 60-8, p 1352).*

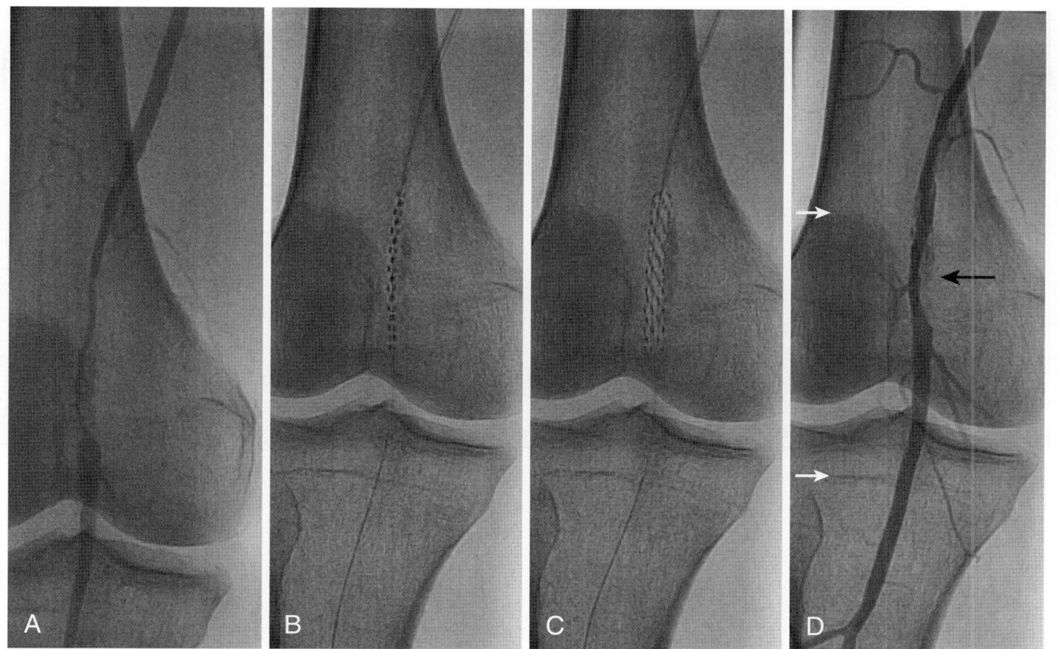

FIGURE 18-17 Cryoplasty of a popliteal artery stenosis. **A,** Popliteal artery stenosis. **B,** Cryoplasty balloon before inflation. **C,** Cryoplasty balloon during inflation. **D,** Final angiogram with some residual narrowing due to recoil adjacent to a heavily calcified segment of the popliteal artery *(black arrow)*. The popliteal artery between the top of the patella and tibial epiphyseal plate *(white arrows)* is exposed to extremes of flexion and torsion with physical activity and stents are generally avoided in this area. *(From Kinlay S, Bhatt DL: Treatment of noncoronary obstructive vascular disease. Braunwald heart disease, ed 10, Philadelphia, 2015, Elsevier, Figure 60-9, p 1353).*

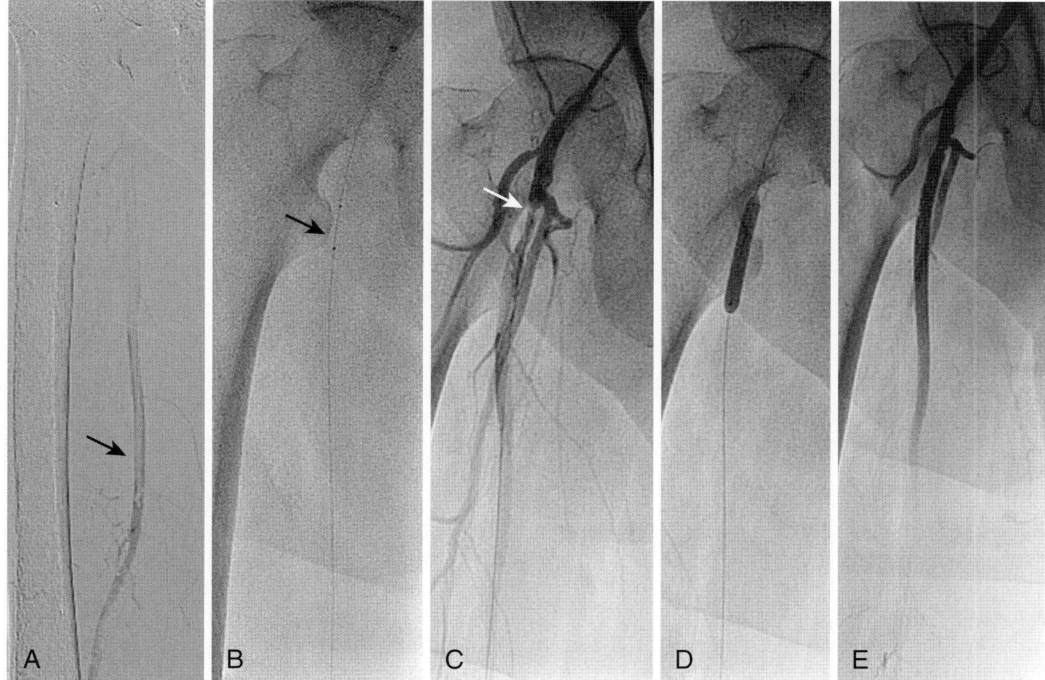

FIGURE 18-18 Thrombolysis using pulse-spray mechanical thrombolysis (same case as Figure 18-1). **A,** Late phase angiogram showing a long filling defect in the superficial femoral artery consistent with in situ thrombus *(arrow)*. **B,** Pulse-spray thrombolysis using a 4 Fr Angiojet catheter and 10 mg of recombinant tissue plasminogen activator over a 5.0-mm Spider X embolic protection device (*arrow* at tip of catheter). After 20 minutes, the catheter was switched to aspiration mode and the thrombus slurry removed with several aspiration runs. **C,** Residual stenosis at the origin of the superficial femoral artery *(arrow)*. **D,** Balloon angioplasty of the residual lesion. **E,** Final result.

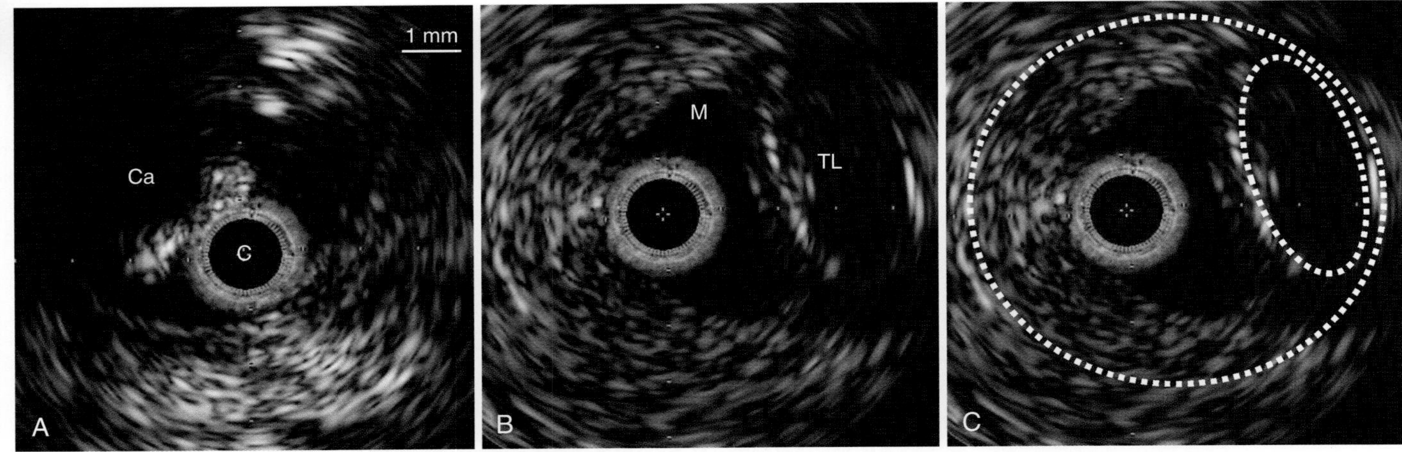

FIGURE 18-19 IVUS used to document the true lumen of a total superficial femoral artery (SFA) occlusion (see Figure 15D for corresponding angiogram). **A,** IVUS in the lumen of the proximal SFA showing a calcified plaque (Ca) at 9 to 12 o'clock adjacent to the catheter (C) in the artery lumen. **B,** IVUS in an intramedia location (M) with the true lumen appearing as an ellipse to the right of the catheter. **C,** Same image as B showing the true lumen (inner oval) and the total vessel area bounded by the adventia (outer circle).

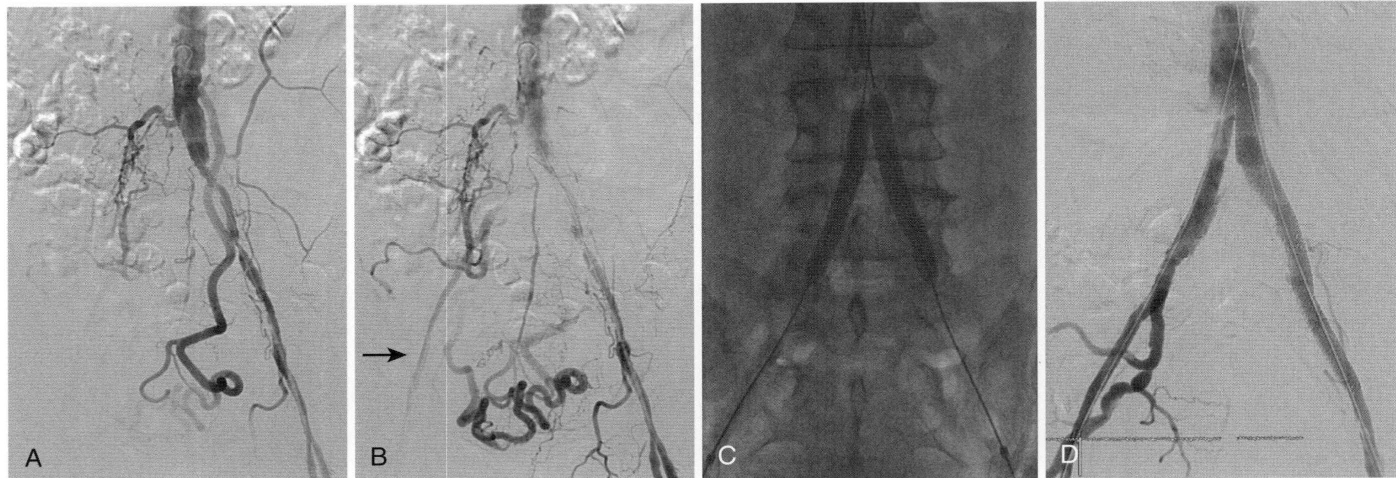

FIGURE 18-20 Aorto-iliac intervention for an occluded right common iliac and serial stenoses in the left iliac arteries. **A,** Early phase angiogram showing occlusion of the right common iliac artery. **B,** Late phase angiogram showing patent right external iliac artery *(arrow)*. **C,** Bilateral kissing balloon expandable stents in the common iliac arteries. **D,** Composite angiogram showing final result. *(From Kinlay S, Bhatt DL: Treatment of noncoronary obstructive vascular disease. Braunwald heart disease, ed 10, Philadelphia, 2015, Elsevier, Figure 60-14, p 1355).*

artery or exiting an occluded artery (**Figure 18-19**) and help show the underlying anatomical defect—for example, a popliteal aneurysm in an occluded popliteal artery (**Figure 18-13**).

INTERVENTIONS IN SPECIFIC ARTERIES

Aorto-iliac Interventions

Successful aortic or iliac interventions often make a great difference to function and quality of life in patients with symptoms due to peripheral artery disease. Although an ipsilateral common femoral access is often used, many operators will access the contralateral femoral artery, particularly when treating an iliac occlusion (**Figures 18-4A-C** and **18-10**). The external iliac artery dips into the pelvis from the common femoral artery and is the most common site of peripheral artery perforation by wires or balloon or stent expansion. Contralateral access allows the operator to rapidly deploy a proximal iliac or aortic occluding balloon if intervention from the ipsilateral side leads to perforation.

Ipsilateral retrograde access from the common femoral artery with a 6 Fr sheath offers good support for crossing an iliac lesion (**Figure 18-20**). Use of a sheath with a radio-opaque tip prevents inflating a balloon or stent within the tip of the sheath, particularly in lesions that are close to the sheath, such as the external iliac artery. The contralateral approach provides better visualization of the lesion and stent placement because contrast injected from the sheath moves distally toward the lesion. However, it is very difficult to treat an ostial or proximal common iliac lesion by this approach, as the sheath tip tends to migrate into the aorta and provides little support to advance balloons and stents.

Although balloon angioplasty has acceptable results in these large arteries, iliac stenting commonly uses stents due to better long-term patency and prevention of recoil after balloon deflation.[1,2] Balloon expandable stents are less likely to move on deployment and offer greater radial strength than self-expanding stents. They are therefore favored by many operators, except in the distal external iliac artery, as there may be some external compression as this artery ascends into the common femoral artery over the hip joint.

The origins of the common iliac arteries can be treated with "kissing stents" that create a higher carina. However, this technique makes it very hard to use a contralateral approach if this is needed in the future. Landing proximal common iliac stents at the ostia preserves this access for future interventions (**Figure 18-20**).

Durability of bare-metal iliac stents is excellent and similar to surgical revascularization, with over 80% patency at 5 years,[2,7] although it is slightly less in cigarette smokers. Covered stents are sometimes promoted as causing less restenosis; however, the evidence to support this is slim and there are concerns of higher risks of stent thrombosis and covering important branch vessels (e.g., the internal iliac artery or a contralateral common iliac artery). Covered stents have more clear indications for treating aneurysms or perforations.

Superficial Femoral Artery

The superficial femoral artery is the most common peripheral artery leading to symptomatic peripheral artery disease. The profunda femoral artery is rarely affected by obstructive atherosclerosis but usually provides an important source of collaterals when the superficial femoral artery is diseased. Thus endovascular interventions try to avoid the common femoral artery or jailing the profunda artery, as restenosis or occlusion of these arteries can lead to acute limb ischemia and limb loss.

The contralateral femoral access is the principal approach for disease involving the proximal superficial femoral artery, as there is not enough room to securely place a sheath from an ipsilateral antegrade common femoral approach (**Figures 18-15** and **18-18**). The contralateral iliac artery is engaged selectively with a mammary catheter or nonselectively with an Omniflush or pigtail catheter. These latter catheters are often used for diagnostic lower aorta and iliac angiograms prior to the intervention. An angled 0.035-inch hydrophilic wire is used to select the contralateral iliac system and deliver the catheter into the contralateral common femoral artery. The wire is exchanged for a stiff J-wire and the catheter and femoral sheath exchanged for a 45-cm to 55-cm sheath (e.g., Balkin or Ansel). The superficial femoral artery lesion is crossed with any type of wire. For stenosis, a highly torquable coronary 0.014-inch wire may be suitable initially and can be exchanged for an 0.018-inch or 0.035-inch wire for larger balloon angioplasty or stenting. Occlusions can be crossed with stiff 0.014-inch wires or hydrophilic 0.025-inch or 0.035-inch wires by leading with the wire tip or using a loop induced in the wire at the transition of the soft and stiff parts of the wire. This latter technique is sometimes called the "subintimal" technique, which is a misnomer, as an occlusion does not have an intima. In reality, this technique often dissects through the media and even close to the adventitia (**Figure 18-19**) and both techniques can lead to wire perforation of the artery. Successful crossing of an occlusion can be confirmed by angiography in one or two angulations or injection of contrast through a catheter or balloon delivered over the wire into the distal true lumen (**Figure 18-15E**).

Balloon angioplasty is the most common intervention using balloons with diameters of 5 mm to 6 mm for the superficial femoral artery and 4 mm to 5 mm for the above knee popliteal artery (**Figure 18-9**). Self-expanding stents are reserved for long lesions (greater than 100-150 mm) or flow limiting dissections, where there is evidence they lead to greater patency than balloon treatment alone (**Figure 18-11**).[7] Self-expanding stents are usually selected as a diameter 1 mm greater than the reference lumen of the artery to ensure they appose the artery wall. An undersized self-expanding stent cannot be made larger by bigger balloon inflation, as the nitinol memory leads it to recoil to the predetermined size. It is often difficult to place long self-expanding stents, as the most proximal end of the stent may shrink or extend longitudinally compared to the undeployed position. Often a short self-expanding stent is needed to treat the lesion back to the superficial femoral artery origin. In some cases it may be better to treat a short proximal length of the ostium of the superficial femoral artery by balloon angioplasty alone rather than risk jailing the profunda artery in an attempt to cover the ostium of the superficial femoral artery. This may be a more viable alternative with the advent of drug-eluting balloons.

Very long femoral artery stenting (>200 mm) is associated with fairly high rates of restenosis (up to 40-50% over 2.5 years[31]). However, it can be treated with repeat balloon angioplasty (**Figure 18-21**), improving the overall patency rates and justifying close outpatient surveillance in both claudication and critical limb ischemia.[31-33] Given the relatively high rates of restenosis with very long stented segments, drug-eluting self-expanding stents may be best used for very long lesions.[26] However, given the restricted lengths of the current stents (80 mm), multiple stents would be required for very long lesions, increasing the cost of this treatment. The routine use of drug-eluting balloons in conjunction with bare-metal self-expanding stents requires further evaluation.

Atherectomy may be used for lesions resistant to angioplasty (e.g., heavily calcified lesions) (**Figures 18-14** and **18-15**), but its value beyond balloon angioplasty for most lesions is uncertain, with increased risk of embolization and perforation. Embolic protection devices may be helpful in preventing distal embolization.

Retrograde access from the popliteal artery with a small 4 Fr or 5 Fr sheath can successfully cross a chronic total occlusion.[11,12] In this case a retrograde wire can be snared from a sheath placed contraterally in the common femoral artery and the wire tip externalized. This "dental floss" technique is also used in the iliac artery (**Figure 18-22**) (Video 18-3) and increases the support to deliver balloons across the occlusion for treatment. After successful intervention, the popliteal artery sheath is removed after anticoagulation has worn off and hemostasis achieved with manual compression. Although the popliteal approach is attractive, it is a smaller artery more prone to damage and potentially occlusion by dissection or manual compression on sheath removal. Also, an unsuccessful intervention can potentially lead to poor wound healing or an ischemic ulcer at the popliteal access site.

Popliteal Artery

The popliteal artery starts at Hunter's canal above the knee and ends at the junction of the anterior tibial and peroneal-tibial trunk arteries below the knee. This artery is subject to

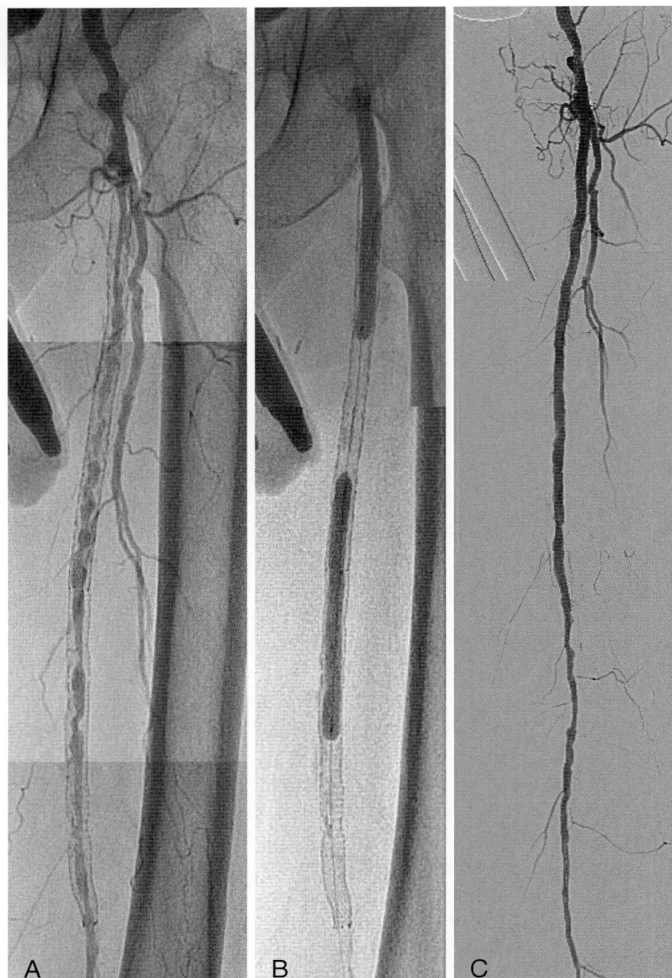

FIGURE 18-21 Balloon angioplasty of diffuse restenosis of a long superficial femoral artery stent. **A,** Diffuse in-stent restenosis. **B,** Collage of different angiograms showing balloon dilations with a 6.0 mm × 80 mm balloon along the length of the stents. **C,** Final angiogram showing a widely patent stent.

a great range of movement with walking and bending of the knee. Most of the flexion of the popliteal artery occurs below the upper margin of the patella to the lower margin of the tibial epiphyseal plate (**Figure 18-17D**). Therefore most operators try to avoid stenting this region unless they are treating critical limb ischemia and have a poor balloon angioplasty result (flow-limiting dissection). Occlusion of the popliteal artery can be treated with atherectomy and balloon angioplasty to avoid stenting (**Figure 18-14**), but it is important to recognize thrombosis of a popliteal aneurysm as a cause of occlusion (**Figure 18-13**). This latter condition is associated with catastrophic embolization and loss of the tibial arteries leading to major amputation and is best treated by surgical ligation and bypass. Although covered stents are used to treat popliteal aneurysms, their durability compared to surgery is uncertain. Covered stents can exclude important geniculate collaterals, and if they subsequently occlude, this can lead to an acute limb syndrome due to loss of the main artery and collaterals (**Figure 18-13L**).

Tibial Arteries

Disease of the tibial arteries rarely causes claudication, and most operators only intervene on these arteries for critical limb ischemia. Reperfusion syndrome (e.g., after revascularization of acute limb ischemia) or perforation of a tibial artery can also lead to catastrophic compartment syndrome with loss of muscle and need for amputation. An ipsilateral antegrade common femoral artery access allows insertion of balloons into the foot and provides greater support compared to a contralateral femoral approach (**Figures 18-4** and **18-7**). Since the tibial arteries are similar in size to coronary arteries, many of the coronary 0.014-inch wires, catheters, and balloons can be used to cross these lesions. Use of a multipurpose coronary intervention guide placed in the popliteal artery increases support and leads to better angiograms with reduced use of contrast.

Long 0.014-inch compatible peripheral balloons of 80-mm to 150-mm balloon lengths are often stiffer and prevent the need for multiple overlapping inflations with short coronary balloons. Although restenosis is more common after treating long, diffuse, and often calcified tibial arteries, increasing perfusion may allow wound and tissue healing prior to restenosis. In the event of poor wound healing due to restenosis, repeat angioplasty is often successful. Drug-eluting balloons are likely to have an important impact in preserving tibial artery patency and increasing wound healing rates in critical limb ischemia.[17]

In cases of critical limb ischemia where antegrade access to an occlusion is unsuccessful, retrograde access via a pedal artery can help cross a tibial occlusion (**Figure 18-6**). However, if this approach is unsuccessful, the pedal access site may become a nonhealing ulcer.

Venous and Prosthetic Graft Interventions

Bypass grafts can renarrow at the proximal and distal anastomoses with native arteries or in the body of the graft. Vein graft stenosis can be successfully treated with balloon angioplasty and stents used as bailout for flow-limiting dissections of recoil. If an anastomosis lesion occurs soon after the initial bypass graft, the surgeon may prefer surgical revision to endovascular treatment. Although short-term outcomes after endovascular intervention are similar to open surgical revision, the differences in long-term outcomes are uncertain. Prosthetic graft disease is more difficult to treat by endovascular methods, as positive remodeling of the prosthetic graft is not possible. Balloon angioplasty may remodel the plaque, displacing it longitudinally, but long-term results are unknown. Atherectomy could potentially remove plaque in prosthetic grafts, but the perforation is likely to lead to a rapid blood loss in part because there is no vasoconstriction reflex in prosthetic grafts (this is also likely in diseased vein grafts). Therefore covered stenting may be required in this case. Prosthetic graft disease is probably best treated by surgical revision. However, endovascular approaches may be required when a patient lacks vein conduit or the risks of repeat bypass are prohibitively high due to comorbidities or extensive fibrosis in the surgical field.

Catheter-based thrombolysis can successfully treat a thrombosed prosthetic graft (**Figure 18-23**) (Video 18-4). Long-term patency is higher if a correctable causal lesion is treated (e.g., a graft anastomosis stenosis).[29]

CONCLUSIONS

Advances in percutaneous intervention techniques and equipment have increased the options and success of treating occlusive disease of arteries, veins, and bypass grafts of

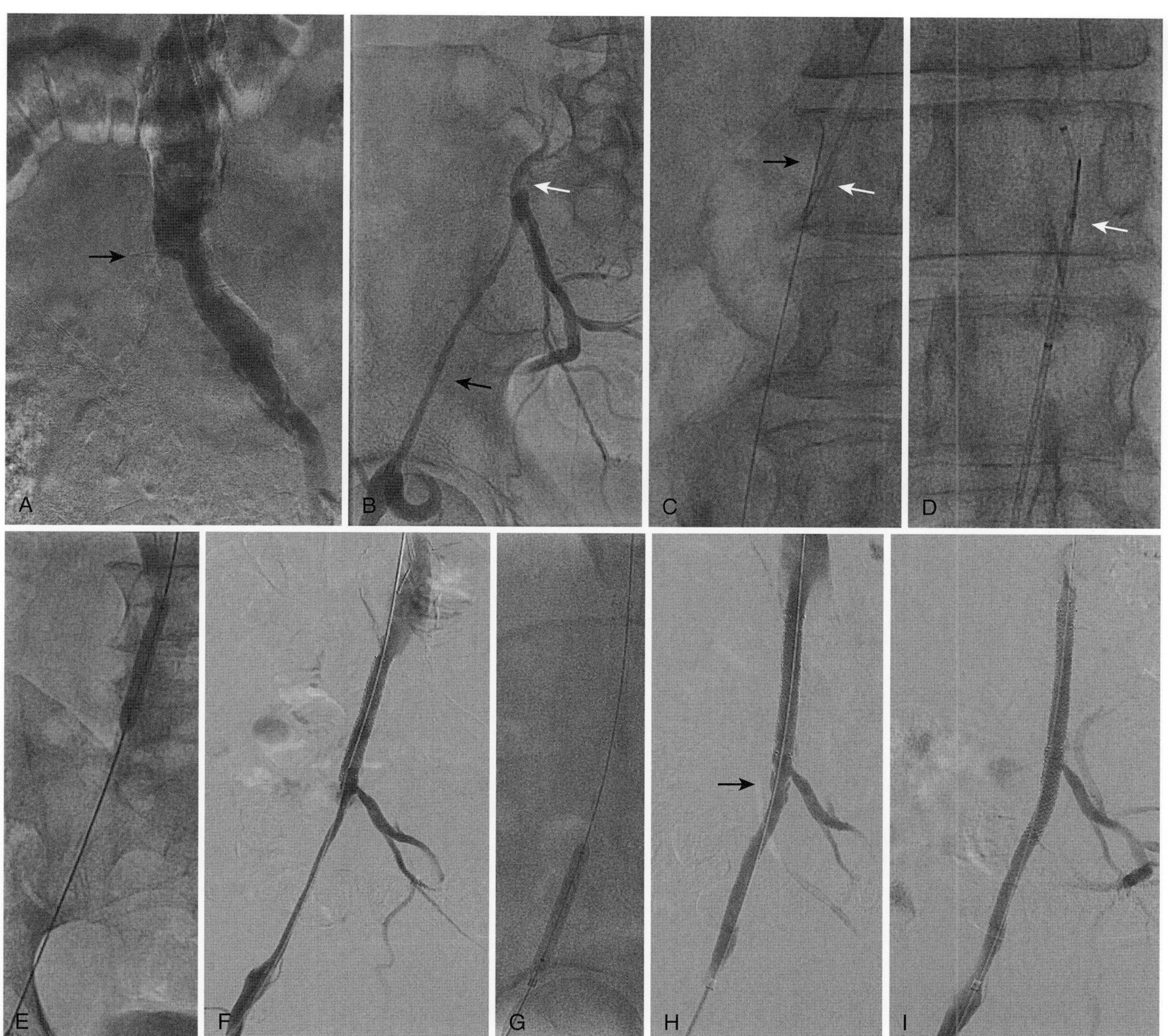

FIGURE 18-22 Antegrade and retrograde approach to an occluded right common iliac artery. **A,** Angiogram using a multipurpose catheter from the right brachial artery and positioned at the aortic bifurcation and shows an occluded right iliac artery *(arrow).* **B,** Angiogram from a sheath placed in the right common femoral artery showing a long stenosis of the right external iliac artery *(black arrow),* a patent internal iliac artery, and the distal occlusion cap of the common iliac artery *(white arrow).* **C,** A 0.025-inch hydrophilic wire is advanced retrograde through the occluded common iliac artery *(black arrow)* and adjacent to the multipurpose catheter *(white arrow).* **D,** The wire and a 0.035-inch support catheter are snared from above and pulled through the occlusion. **E,** The common iliac artery is dilated and stented from below using an 8.0 mm × 60 mm balloon expandable stent. **F,** Angiogram showing a patent right common iliac artery and stenosis in the external iliac artery. **G,** Several dilations of the external iliac artery and common femoral artery made with low-medium pressure dilations of a 7.0-mm balloon. **H,** Dissection of the ostium of the external iliac artery *(arrow).* **I,** After stenting, the proximal external iliac artery showing a patent right common iliac, internal iliac, external iliac, and common femoral arteries.

the lower extremities. Although de novo atherosclerosis and neointimal hyperplasia after percutaneous or surgical revascularization are the most common causes of obstructive disease in industrialized countries, the interventionalist needs to recognize other causes (e.g., inflammation or entrapment) or irreversible tissue damage (e.g., acute limb ischemia), which will determine the suitability or timing of percutaneous revascularization. Atherosclerosis risk factor modification and surveillance for new or recurrent disease are essential parts of the approach to managing peripheral artery disease. When percutaneous revascularization is appropriate, planning the procedure to optimize success includes considering vascular access, the use of specialized equipment, and ingenuity to tackle complex lesions, such as chronic total occlusions. Backup plans, knowing when to stop a procedure, and an adequate inventory (e.g., covered stents for perforation) are part of forward planning to avoid or treat complications.

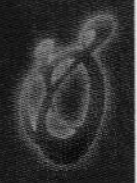

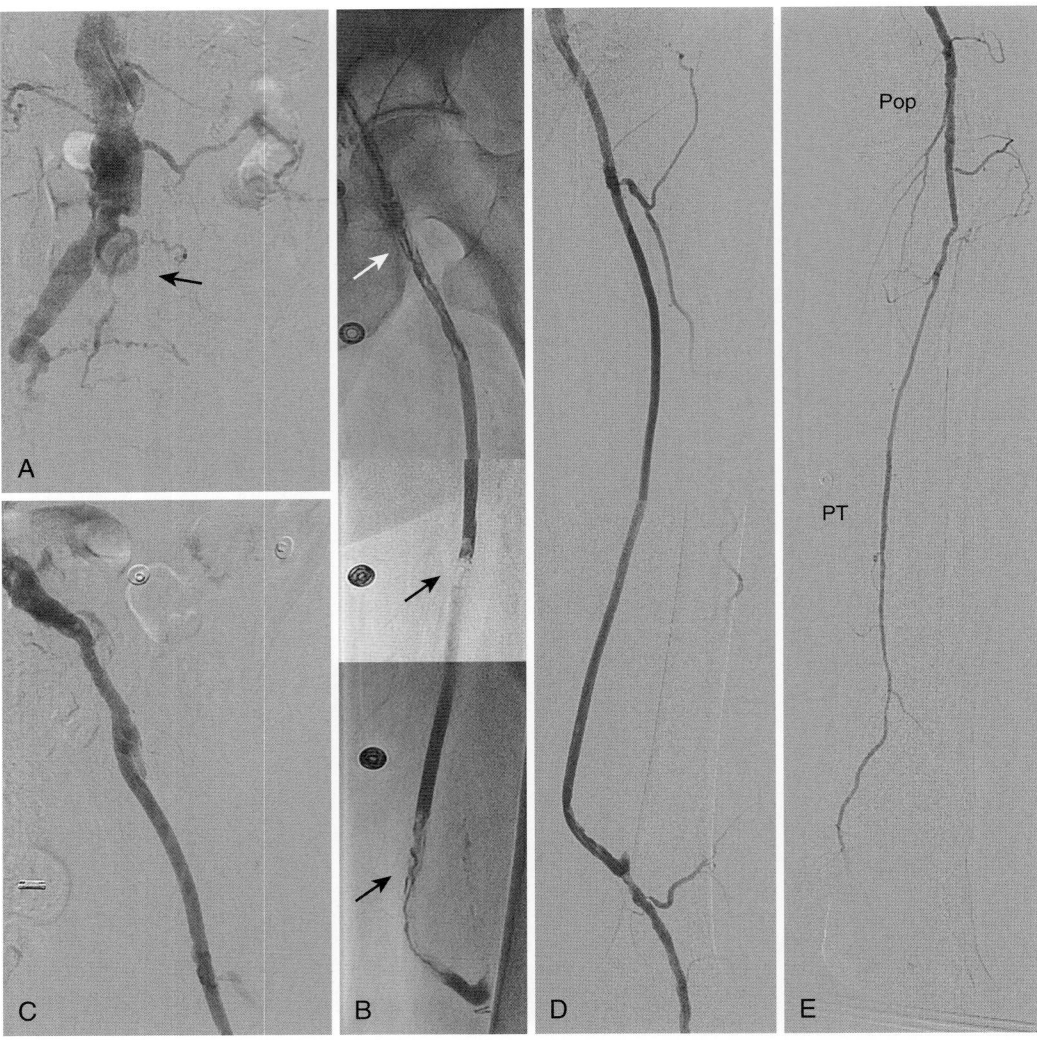

FIGURE 18-23 Thrombolysis of a thrombosed femoral to popliteal prosthetic graft. **A,** The proximal left common iliac artery is occluded with thrombus *(arrow)*. **B,** The thrombus extends through a left external iliac stent with filling defects in the proximal mid and distal graft *(arrows)* and no distal outflow from the graft. **C,** 24 hours after catheter-based thrombolysis, the left common and external iliac arteries are patent. **D,** Similarly, graft patency is restored and there is distal ouflow into the native popliteal artery. **E,** Distal runoff below the knee through the distal popliteal artery and posterior tibial artery. *Pop,* Popliteal artery; *PT,* posterior tibial artery.

References

1. 2011 Writing Group Members, 2005 Writing Committee Members, ACCF/AHA Task Force Members: 2011 ACCF/AHA focused update of the guideline for the management of patients with peripheral artery disease (updating the 2005 guideline): a report of the American College of Cardiology Foundation/American Heart Association task force on practice guidelines. *Circulation* 124:2020–2045, 2011.
2. Norgren L, Hiatt WR, Dormandy JA, et al: Inter-society consensus for the management of peripheral arterial disease (tasc ii). *J Vasc Surg* 45(Suppl S):S5–S67, 2007.
3. McDermott MM, Greenland P, Liu K, et al: Leg symptoms in peripheral arterial disease: associated clinical characteristics and functional impairment. *JAMA* 286:1599–1606, 2001.
4. Creager MA, Kaufman JA, Conte MS: Clinical practice. acute limb ischemia. *N Engl J Med* 366:2198–2206, 2012.
5. Rutherford RB, Baker JD, Ernst C, et al: Recommended standards for reports dealing with lower extremity ischemia: revised version. *J Vasc Surg* 26:517–538, 1997.
6. Rogers JH, Laird JR: Overview of new technologies for lower extremity revascularization. *Circulation* 116:2072–2085, 2007.
7. Schillinger M, Minar E: Percutaneous treatment of peripheral artery disease: novel techniques. *Circulation* 126:2433–2440, 2012.
8. Kinlay S: Outcomes for clinical studies assessing drug and revascularization therapies for claudication and critical limb ischemia in peripheral artery disease. *Circulation* 127:1241–1250, 2013.
9. Wennberg PW: Approach to the patient with peripheral arterial disease. *Circulation* 128:2241–2250, 2013.
10. Aboyans V, Criqui MH, Abraham P, et al: Measurement and interpretation of the ankle-brachial index: a scientific statement from the American Heart Association. *Circulation* 126:2890–2909, 2012.
11. Montero-Baker M, Schmidt A, Braunlich S, et al: Retrograde approach for complex popliteal and tibioperoneal occlusions. *J Endovasc Ther* 15:594–604, 2008.
12. Noory E, Rastan A, Schwarzwalder U, et al: Retrograde transpopliteal recanalization of chronic superficial femoral artery occlusion after failed re-entry during antegrade subintimal angioplasty. *J Endovasc Ther* 16:619–623, 2009.
13. Rogers RK, Dattilo PB, Garcia JA, et al: Retrograde approach to recanalization of complex tibial disease. *Catheter Cardiovasc Interv* 77:915–925, 2011.
14. Otsuka F, Vorpahl M, Nakano M, et al: Pathology of second-generation everolimus-eluting stents versus first-generation sirolimus- and paclitaxel-eluting stents in humans. *Circulation* 129:211–223, 2014.
15. Cassese S, Byrne RA, Ott I, et al: Paclitaxel-coated versus uncoated balloon angioplasty reduces target lesion revascularization in patients with femoropopliteal arterial disease: a meta-analysis of randomized trials. *Circ Cardiovasc Interv* 5:582–589, 2012.
16. Micari A, Cioppa A, Vadala G, et al: Clinical evaluation of a paclitaxel-eluting balloon for treatment of femoropopliteal arterial disease: 12-month results from a multicenter Italian registry. *JACC Cardiovasc Interv* 5:331–338, 2012.
17. Schmidt A, Piorkowski M, Werner M, et al: First experience with drug-eluting balloons in infrapopliteal arteries: restenosis rate and clinical outcome. *J Am Coll Cardiol* 58:1105–1109, 2011.
18. Tepe G, Zeller T, Albrecht T, et al: Local delivery of paclitaxel to inhibit restenosis during angioplasty of the leg. *N Engl J Med* 358:689–699, 2008.
19. Werk M, Langner S, Reinkensmeier B, et al: Inhibition of restenosis in femoropopliteal arteries: paclitaxel-coated versus uncoated balloon: femoral paclitaxel randomized pilot trial. *Circulation* 118:1358–1365, 2008.
20. Laird JR, Katzen BT, Scheinert D, et al: Nitinol stent implantation versus balloon angioplasty for lesions in the superficial femoral artery and proximal popliteal artery: twelve-month results from the resilient randomized trial. *Circ Cardiovasc Interv* 3:267–276, 2010.
21. Mwipatayi BP, Thomas S, Wong J, et al: A comparison of covered vs bare expandable stents for the treatment of aortoiliac occlusive disease. *J Vasc Surg* 54:1561–1570, 2011.
22. Saxon RR, Dake MD, Volgelzang RL, et al: Randomized, multicenter study comparing expanded polytetrafluoroethylene-covered endoprosthesis placement with percutaneous transluminal angioplasty in the treatment of superficial femoral artery occlusive disease. *J Vasc Interv Radiol* 19:823–832, 2008.
23. Fusaro M, Cassese S, Ndrepepa G, et al: Drug-eluting stents for revascularization of infrapopliteal arteries: updated meta-analysis of randomized trials. *JACC Cardiovasc Interv* 6:1284–1293, 2013.
24. Rastan A, Noory E, Zeller T: Drug-eluting stents for treatment of focal infrapopliteal lesions. *VASA Zeitschrift fur Gefasskrankheiten* 41:90–95, 2012.
25. Scheinert D, Katsanos K, Zeller T, et al: A prospective randomized multicenter comparison of balloon angioplasty and infrapopliteal stenting with the sirolimus-eluting stent in patients with ischemic peripheral arterial disease: 1-year results from the Achilles trial. *J Am Coll Cardiol* 60:2290–2295, 2012.

26. Dake MD, Ansel GM, Jaff MR, et al: Paclitaxel-eluting stents show superiority to balloon angioplasty and bare metal stents in femoropopliteal disease: 12-month zilver ptx randomized study results. *Circ Cardiovasc Interv* 4:495–504, 2011.
27. Lammer J, Bosiers M, Zeller T, et al: First clinical trial of nitinol self-expanding everolimus-eluting stent implantation for peripheral arterial occlusive disease. *J Vasc Surg* 54:394–401, 2011.
28. Banerjee S, Das TS, Abu-Fadel MS, et al: Pilot trial of cryoplasty or conventional balloon post-dilation of nitinol stents for revascularization of peripheral arterial segments: the cobra trial. *J Am Coll Cardiol* 60:1352–1359, 2012.
29. van den Berg JC: Thrombolysis for acute arterial occlusion. *J Vasc Surg* 52:512–515, 2010.
30. Piazza G, Goldhaber SZ: Fibrinolysis for acute pulmonary embolism. *Vasc Med* 15:419–428, 2010.
31. Connors G, Todoran TM, Engelson BA, et al: Percutaneous revascularization of long femoral artery lesions for claudication: patency over 2.5 years and impact of systematic surveillance. *Catheter Cardiovasc Interv* 77:1055–1062, 2011.
32. Sobieszczyk P, Eisenhauer A: Management of patients after endovascular interventions for peripheral artery disease. *Circulation* 128:749–757, 2013.
33. Todoran TM, Connors G, Engelson BA, et al: Femoral artery percutaneous revascularization for patients with critical limb ischemia: outcomes compared to patients with claudication over 2.5 years. *Vasc Med* 17:138–144, 2012.

19 Upper Extremity Intervention

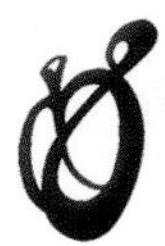

Amjad T. AlMahameed

INTRODUCTION

Atherosclerotic upper extremity obstructive disease is predominantly secondary to subclavian or innominate artery stenosis (SAS or IAS). The diagnosis is usually suspected when a significant (often ≥15 mm Hg) systolic brachial blood pressure discrepancy (SBBP) is detected between the two arms.[1,2] Applying this threshold, the prevalence of SAS in the general population is estimated at approximately 2% and increases with advancing age. In a high-risk population with known or suspected vascular disease, including individuals referred for coronary artery bypass surgery, the prevalence is estimated at about 7%.[1,2] Involvement of the left subclavian artery (L-SCA) is three to four times more common than the right brachiocephalic and subclavian arteries.[3-5] This may be explained by increased flow turbulence in the L-SCA due to its acute angle of origin. Moreover, one third of the stenotic lesions on the right side are found in the innominate trunk, proximal to the subclavian origin.[6,7]

The presence of SAS correlates well with known atherosclerotic risk factors and is a strong indicator of the presence of PAD, defined as ABI ≤0.90.[2,8] The incidence is much higher in patients with symptomatic PAD. In one study of 48 subjects with PAD who underwent aortic arch angiography, 19% had more than 50% stenosis of at least one brachiocephalic artery.[9] Furthermore, SAS predicts total and cardiovascular mortality (independent of both risk factors and existent cardiac disease at baseline) and all-cause mortality.[8,10] On the other hand, SAS is present in 11.5% of patients with known PAD. Therefore, we routinely recommend bilateral blood pressure measurements in high-risk patients.[2,11]

Nonatherosclerotic conditions that can result in SBPD and SAS include Takayasu's arteritis,[12] giant cell arteritis,[13] coarctation of the aorta,[14] thoracic outlet syndrome causing compression from an overlying rib,[15] radiation-induced vascular disease,[16] and, rarely, fibromuscular dysplasia (FMD),[17] arterial thrombosis (**Figure 19-1**), and neurofibromatosis.[18] Therefore, routine evaluation for these disorders is not warranted. FMD is more likely to affect small and medium size arteries, notably the brachial artery, and can occasionally lead to upper extremity ischemia and bilateral pulse discrepancy. Importantly, the presence of a BBPD with associated acute chest pain should alert the clinician for the possibility of aortic dissection.

DIAGNOSIS AND CLINICAL SYNDROMES

Isolated SAS rarely leads to symptoms, perhaps due to the lower muscular mass it supplies (compared to that supplied by the lower extremity inflow arteries) and the high degree of collaterals that develop. Symptoms related to vertebrobasilar insufficiency (also referred to as vertebral subclavian steal syndrome, or vSSS) remain uncommon with isolated SAS and most likely occur when multiple craniocervical arteries are stenotic or occluded.[19] The clinical manifestations of SAS are listed in **Table 19-1**.

Lord et al. showed that the discontinuity of the circle of Willis due to the vertebral-vertebral shunt (from the patent vertebral artery [VA] to the occluded one, across the circle of Willis) is responsible for symptoms experienced during repetitive use of the affected upper extremity.[19] Occasionally, the blood is routed from the anterior circulation through the descending cervical branches of the ipsilateral external carotid artery, providing collateral pathways to the occluded subclavian artery. In these case, symptoms of anterior circulation ischemia, such as transient hemiparesis paresis, speech disturbances, and sensory loss, may be reported.[20] On the other hand, ischemic syndromes attributable to the anterior circulation are common in symptomatic patients presenting with occlusive lesions of the right innominate trunk. Fifty percent of such patients express anterior ischemia, while 40% present with posterior symptoms, and up to 10% manifest global (anterior and posterior) symptoms.[21]

Javid test is a highly reliable clinical maneuver in demonstrating flow reversal via the circle of Willis. In this test, the examiner compresses the ipsilateral carotid artery, thereby decreasing intracranial pressure and flow and abolishing retrograde flow into the arm. This leads to an abrupt change in the quality of the ipsilateral radial pulse.[22]

Acute symptoms of arm or cerebral ischemia usually result from acute injury to the subclavian artery, as seen with sharp and blunt trauma, inadvertent misplacement of a large venous catheter into an SCA,[23-26] and coverage by a stent graft during TEVAR.[27]

Most cases of SAS are asymptomatic and diagnosed either incidentally on imaging studies or during routine physical exam. In addition to BBPD ≥15 mm Hg, careful physical examination can yield absent or markedly diminished distal pulses and a systolic supraclavicular bruit. The bruit is best auscultated by lightly applying the stethoscope

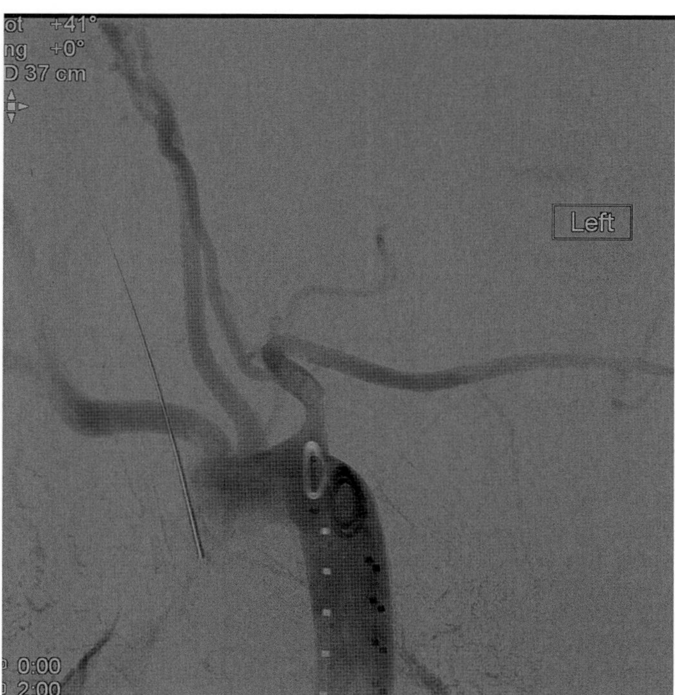

FIGURE 19-1 Thrombus noted in the proximal L-SCA. This patient presented with left hand ischemia.

TABLE 19-1 Clinical Manifestations of Subclavian Artery Stenosis

Arm ischemia	Arm claudication, muscle fatigue, hand or finger pain, paresthesias, coldness in the arm, Raynaud's phenomenon, distal embolization, and its sequelae of tissue loss and necrosis.
Vertebral subclavian steal syndrome (vSSS)	Symptoms of vertebrobasilar insufficiency: paroxysmal vertigo, drop attacks, ataxia, diplopia, motor dysphagia, dysarthria, and facial motor deficits. Typically seen with concurrent vertebral and carotid disease.
Coronary subclavian steal syndrome (cSSS)	Angina pectoris, refractory unstable angina, myocardial infarction, heart failure in patients with LIMA (or, rarely, RIMA) graft.
CVA or paralysis after TEVAR with coverage of the L-SCA[20]	Risk estimated at 4.7% vs. 2.7% in patients without LSA coverage. Preemptive revascularization offers no protection against CVA when coverage is applied.
Lower extremity claudication following AXF bypass	
Arm ischemia	Arm claudication, muscle fatigue, hand or finger pain, paresthesias, Raynaud's phenomenon, distal embolization, tissue loss, and necrosis.
Vertebral subclavian steal syndrome (vSSS)	Symptoms of vertebrobasilar insufficiency: vertigo, syncope, ataxia, diplopia, motor dysphagia, dysarthria, and facial motor deficits. Typically seen with concurrent vertebral and carotid disease.
Carotid subclavian steal syndrome	Rare, except in proximal innominate artery stenosis.

bell in each supraclavicular fossa while the patient sits looking forward with the shoulders relaxed and hands resting on the lap. Once detected, firm compression of the patient's ipsilateral radial artery decreases the SCA outflow and should shorten or obliterate the bruit. Arm exercises that can be carefully performed in the office (with the patient in a supine position to avoid provoking syncope) will induce peripheral vasodilation, thus augmenting the SCA outflow, which increases the turbulence across the stenotic lesion, rendering the bruit louder and longer.

Duplex ultrasound (DUS) with color flow is the diagnostic first test of choice. This modality provides excellent information of the lesion, identifies disease in the rest of the aortic arch vessels, and adequately assesses flow direction in the vertebral artery. Once the diagnosis is made and the symptoms are considered significant enough to warrant intervention, we routinely obtain a CTA or MRA to confirm the diagnosis, exclude proximal VA stenosis or occlusion (difficult to visualize by DUS and when present can manifest as retrograde vertebral flow, mimicking vSSS), and clearly define the anatomic relationships between the SCA lesion, the aortic arch (since ostial lesions represent an extension of atherosclerosis arising in the aortic arch), and the origins of the ipsilateral vertebral and internal mammary arteries. This information can be very useful in planning the treatment modality. Angiography is reserved for patients who were determined to undergo endovascular therapy.

We advise all patients referred to CABG with BBPD ≥15 mm Hg or history of a nonatherosclerotic condition that is known to be associated with SAS (see above) and those with known vascular disease to undergo screening for SAS prior to their open heart surgery. This can be done in the outpatient setting by DUS or angiography during the index cardiac catheterization procedure.

TREATMENT

Asymptomatic SAS is treated medically by applying global cardiovascular risk reduction strategies, including smoking cessation, antiplatelet therapy, and achieving target blood pressure, glucose, and cholesterol. The goal of therapy in asymptomatic patients is to stabilize the systemic atherosclerotic process and prevent progressive disease. Currently the evidence for revascularization of asymptomatic patients with hemodynamically significant SAS is lacking.[28] The exception to this rule is patients who are undergoing CABG with plans to utilize the LIMA, those who need an arteriovenous fistula for hemodialysis purposes and, rarely, when an axillo-femoral graft is considered.

Currently, more than 90% of patients undergoing subclavian artery revascularization are symptomatic.[29] Indications for revascularization procedures include the presence of one or more of the clinical syndromes outlined in **Table 19-1**.

Surgical Revascularization

Although surgical revascularization procedures were employed since the 1950s, endovascular therapy is now considered the modality of choice in contemporary practice.

Early surgical procedures employed a direct revascularization via transthoracic approach and were associated with significant morbidity and mortality.[29-33] Anatomic revascularization procedures include endarterectomy and bypass grafts. These are technically demanding and associated with relatively high peri-procedural complications. The evolution of extraanatomic cervical repair techniques improved surgical outcomes significantly.[32] Therefore, extraanatomic revascularization procedures have been employed and include carotid-subclavian transposition, carotid-subclavian bypass, axillo-axillary bypass, subclavian-subclavian bypass, and carotid-contralateral subclavian bypass (**Figure 19-2**).[32,33] Hybrid procedures are generally reserved for aneurysmal disease when the stent graft (TEVAR) is extended to cover the subclavian artery. An open extraanatomical bypass is performed prior to deploying the graft. Of note, while this strategy may reduce the risk of spinal cord ischemia, it offers no protection against it, as demonstrated by Cooper et al.[34]

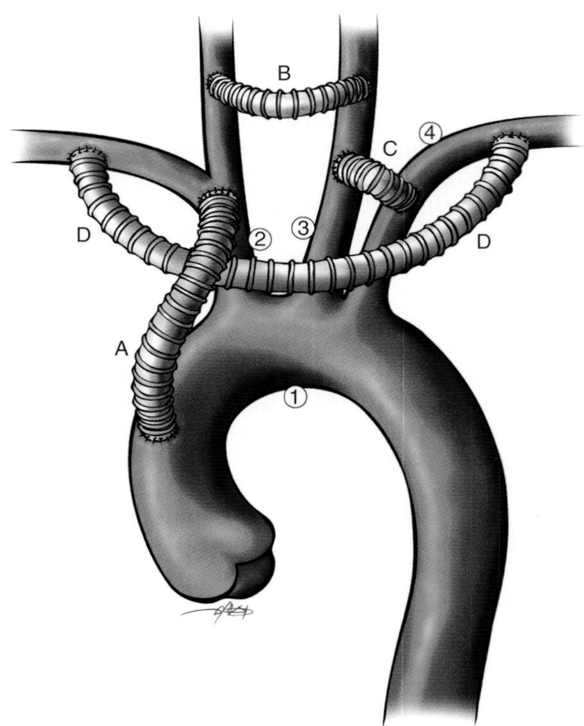

FIGURE 19-2 Illustration of brachiocephalic arteries and treatment strategies for revascularization. *(1)* Aortic arch; *(2)* innominate artery; *(3)* left common carotid artery; *(4)* left subclavian artery; *(A)* aortoinnominate bypass; *(B)* carotid-carotid bypass; *(C)* left subclavian-carotid bypass; *(D)* subclavian-subclavian/axillo-axillary bypass. *(From Aziz F, Gravett MH, Comerota AJ: Endovascular and Open Surgical Treatment of Brachiocephalic Arteries. Ann Vasc Surg 25:569–581, 2011.)*

A recent report by Aziz and Comerota elegantly reviewed the English literature and reported the outcomes of the different endovascular and open surgical treatment modalities of the brachiocephalic arteries (**Table 19-2**).[33] Their findings verified the remarkable improvement in surgical outcomes compared to the 22% mortality rate described in early experiences 50 years ago.[30,31,34,35] Subclavian-to-carotid artery transposition appears to have the greatest long-term patency for proximal subclavian artery occlusive disease (100% at 10 years), whereas axillo-axillary artery bypass surgery has the lowest patency rates, ranging from 88% to 89%.[36,37]

Endovascular Therapy

The combination of recent advancements in endovascular techniques, along with the technical challenges of surgical procedures and their associated serious complications (such as phrenic, vagus, and recurrent laryngeal nerve palsies, thoracic duct injuries, Horner's syndrome, and cerebral ischemia imposed by the need for proximal and distal cross clamping), made surgical revascularization progressively less popular.[38] Since its introduction in 1980 by Bachman and Kim, percutaneous transluminal angioplasty became the treatment of choice for SAS and IAS.[39] Endovascular therapy of completely occluded subclavian and innominate arteries was first reported in 1993 by Mathias et al.[40]

Interventional Technique

Once the decision to proceed with endovascular revascularization is made, a careful review of noninvasive studies (CTA or MRA) is critical for procedure planning. The anatomical relationships among the diseased segment, aortic arch, and other craniocervical arteries (carotid, VA, and IMA in the case of IAS and the VA and IMA when the L-SCA is being treated), as well as flow hemodynamics and collateral patterns, are reviewed. Special attention is given to the lesion characteristics, such as length, involvement of the ostium,

TABLE 19-2 Endovascular and Open Surgical Treatment of Brachiocephalic Arteries[33]

PROCEDURE	NO. OF STUDIES	NO. OF PATIENTS	MEAN FU	SURGICAL MORTALITY (%)	CVA (%)	10-YEAR SURVIVAL (%)	PATENCY RATE (%)	TECHNICAL SUCCESS
Anatomic revascularization of the brachiocephalic arteries[26]	22	1650	58 months	7.8	3.8%	NA		
Carotid-subclavian transposition	8	381		0.4	1	83% (one study)	100% (one study)	
Carotid-subclavian bypass	18	1041	53.8 months	1.5	1.3	89% (four studies)	91% (five studies)	
Axillo-axillary bypass	16	426	51 months	0.5	1.1	90% (one study)	87% at 10 years (one study)	
Hybrid	9	173		7.9	6.9		100% at 1 year	
Endovascular	26	1305 (1379 lesions)	31 months					94% (stenosis) 64% (occlusion)

presence of thrombus, atheromatous material or heavy calcification, proximal artery angulation, as well as the aortic arch type, orientation, and calcifications. Since peripheral vascular disease is common in these patients, access options are also evaluated. The innominate artery is short (2-5 cm) and large in diameter. It gives rise to the right carotid and vertebral subdivisions. It is also usually highly calcified and can be tortuous with a difficult takeoff depending on the aortic arch pattern. Therefore it is more challenging to treat endovascularly compared to the L-SCA.

Patients are started on ASA 325 mg daily and clopidogrel 75 mg daily 5 days prior to the procedure. We carefully perform a complete preprocedure and postprocedure neurologic and ipsilateral upper extremity examination to assess for possible periprocedure complications. The procedure is performed generally under conscious sedation and we apply the same protocols employed in cardiac catheterization procedures.

The common femoral artery (CFA) is the preferred primary route in most cases, when possible. A long (24 cm) 6 Fr sheath is placed for better catheter stability, particularly when iliac tortuousity is noted. Once access is obtained, unfractionated heparin boluses are given to maintain ACT ≥250 seconds. A complete aortic arch angiogram is then performed (utilizing DSA technique) to confirm the exact location, length, and severity of the stenotic lesion and collateral pathways. Late phase angiography allows for documentation of retrograde flow in the VA (or via branches of the carotid system).

Given the considerable movement of the ascending portion of the left SCA during respiration, which can occasionally cause kinking of the proximal segment during expiration, we perform angiography during breath hold immediately after expiration. The quality of the image depends on the patient's ability to comply.

Identifying fluoroscopic landmarks can facilitate engagement of the destination vessel. The left SCA extends from the aorta (along the left side of the mediastinum) to the outer edge of the first rib while the right brachiocephalic trunk arises on a level with the upper border of the second right costal cartilage and ascends obliquely upward, over the trachea. It divides at the level of the upper border of the right sternoclavicular articulation.

We approach the lesion with a 6 Fr guiding catheter and an exchange-length hydrophilic 0.035 inch wire is utilized to traverse the stenosis in antegrade fashion. The wire tip is positioned in the axillary artery, within the fluoroscopic field of view, to provide stability to the system. Balloon angioplasty is then carried out with a properly sized balloon (for the reconstituted SCA). Tight calcific lesions and an unstable guiding catheter system may not allow passage of the intended balloon. Therefore, preliminary dilatation with a smaller (2 or 4 mm) balloon may facilitate delivery of the larger balloon. We typically dilate the balloon slowly to complete expansion. We then deploy a balloon expandable stent (BES), as these allow for precise placement, particularly when the SCA ostium is involved. We routinely allow the proximal edge of the BES to protrude into the aortic arch by about 1 mm to ensure coverage of the plaque extension into the aortic arch wall.[41] We usually oversize the stent by 1 mm while the postdilatation balloon matches the vessel size and tolerate a mild waist, avoiding aggressive postdilatation, which can trigger the release of atheromatous debris.

Self-expanding stents (SES) have greater radial strength compared to BES. Therefore we utilized them in lesions distal to the VA, as these sites are subject to movement that may incur significant stress on the stent and cause fractures. SES are utilized for lesions distal to the vertebral artery and those involving the axillary and brachial arteries, as well as for lesions longer than 40 millimeters. Covered stents are reserved to repair direct injuries to the SCA, axillary, or brachial arteries.

We always avoid jailing the VA, when possible, to prevent VA closure (by plaque shift) or embolization. In cases of associated VA origin stenosis, however, we employ the "kissing balloon" technique and routinely advocate the use of distal embolus protection (DEP) devices when accessing the VA. Once the DEP device is deployed in the midcervical VA, we advance a coronary balloon over a 0.014 inch wire into the VA lesion and inflate both balloons simultaneously. The VA is accessed via the ipsilateral radial or brachial artery, after placement of a 6 Fr sheath. If the VA PTA result is unsatisfactory, it can be stented with a coronary drug-eluting stent.[42,43] The "double balloon" technique can also be used. Here, the balloon is kept inflated while the SCA is accessed via the transfemoral route and treated with angioplasty and stenting.[44]

When engagement of the SCA ostium with the guiding catheter is unsuccessful, we use a longer 4 Fr diagnostic catheter (curved or straight) through the 6 Fr guide or shuttle sheath. We then try to engage the ostium of the SCA with the 4 Fr catheter to support wire passage. When wire crossing is unsuccessful despite several careful attempts, which is usually the case in complete occlusion or when severe tortuousity is present, we combine the transfemoral antegrade with a transbrachial (or transradial) retrograde approach. We occasionally resort to this approach when the transfemoral catheter and guiding wire assembly stability remain unsatisfactory or in cases where severe ostial SCA stenosis (string sign, **Figure 19-3**) is noted. In a large series of 170 patients treated between 1993 and 2006,

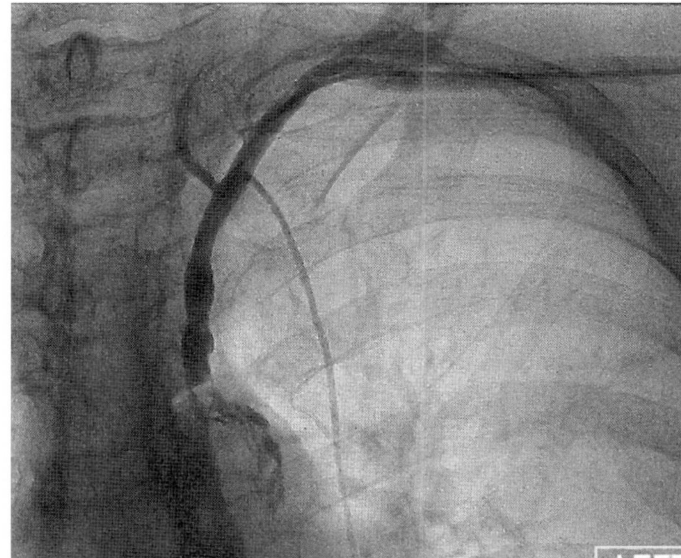

FIGURE 19-3 String sign indicative of very severe stenosis in the L-SCA.

revascularization was attempted on 177 subclavian or innominate arteries (98% and 6%, respectively). The retrograde approach, mainly via the brachial artery, was used in 13 out of 21 (62%) total occlusion cases.[45]

Given the diminished brachial (and radial) pulses imposed by the proximal occlusion, when accessing the ipsilateral brachial (or radial) artery, we always employ ultrasonographic guidance. An adequate length sheath is advanced over the wire and positioned proximal to the VA origin. Simultaneous angiography (via the transfemoral guiding catheter and the transbrachial sheath) is performed to delineate the length of the occlusion and its anatomic characteristics. Using these images, we carefully advance the transfemoral sheath and reattempt to cross the lesion antegradely. If this is unsuccessful, we then proceed to cross the lesion retrogradely. The brachial sheath is advanced carefully to engage the distal cap of the occlusion and the stiff guidewire is pushed through the occlusion into the descending aorta. We frequently evaluate the course of the wire during its passage by switching between AP to angulated views to ensure continued intraluminal position. Once in the descending aorta, the wire is snared and externalized through the transfemoral sheath. The wire is reversed and the soft tip is placed alongside the brachial sheath.

When treating a primarily atheromatous or thrombotic lesion, we introduce EPD through the brachial (or radial) sheath and deploy it into the midcervical VA, as long as the VA diameter is greater than 3.5 mm. In cases of innominate artery occlusion, both femoral arteries will need to be accessed so that an additional EPD is deployed into the right internal carotid artery.[46] Once EPD is deployed, angioplasty and stenting are carried out as described. Upon achieving satisfactory results, the EPDs are retrieved in the usual fashion. We do not recommend using EPD in the VA through the transfemoral approach, as removal may be difficult due to device entrapment by the subclavian or innominate stent once deployed.[47] Attention should be made to recognize and immediately treat potential EPD complications, such as vasospasm or vertebral or carotid artery dissection.[47]

The argument against using DEP in SCA and IA intervention relies largely on the early report of Ringelstein and Zeumer, which suggested that reversal of retrograde VA flow following SCA recanalization occurs gradually within 20 seconds to several minutes. A reasonable counterargument can be made that the protection provided by this brief delay is suboptimal and unreliable, particularly when thrombus is present, the lesion is mostly erythematous, and when intervention is performed at the right innominate artery where the right carotid artery is at risk.[48] This counterargument is further supported by the observation that almost a quarter of the patients in Ringelstein and Zeumer's study (two of nine) had immediate restoration of antegrade vertebral flow as assessed by continuous US monitoring of the vertebral artery. Nonetheless, routine use of EPD is not mandatory in all lesions.[47]

Generally, fibrotic lesions encountered in patients with fibromuscular dysplasia respond well to PTA alone. However, when angioplasty alone is used to treat subclavian and innominate artery lesions, adequate time (Dabus et al. advocated waiting 1 hour in their series) should be given to document persistent patency and absence of vessel recoil or closure prior to terminating the procedure.[43] In atherosclerotic lesions, where calcifications are common, stenting reduces acute closure, improves patency rates, facilitates recanalization of restenotic lesions, and reduces the risk of distal embolization by trapping debris between stent struts and the arterial wall during stent expansion. Based on the latter benefit, some authors went as far as advocating direct stenting.[29]

Technical success is usually defined as ≤30% residual stenosis (**Figure 19-4A-C**) and lowering the BBPD (≤10 mm Hg) and the pressure gradient (≤5 mm Hg). Clinical success is defined as improvement or resolution of the symptoms that justified the revascularization procedure.[49] In a single center study that evaluated trends and outcomes of subclavian revascularization in 114 patients who underwent 137 procedures, Palchick reported that the endoluminal approach became the predominant method since 2004 and that most procedures in recent years were performed for either arm ischemia or cardiac indication.[38]

The initial procedural success rates with endovascular therapy of subclavian and innominate artery stenosis is around 93% to 100%,[45,50-56] averaging 94%,[33] and 83% to 94% for occlusions.* A recent large series published by Patel et al. showed an intermediate (3-year) patency rate of 83%.[45] Other series confirmed long-term (5 to 10 years) patency rates between 80% to 90%, with better results achieved with stenting compared to angioplasty alone.[38,44,52,53]

Overall complication rates of endovascular interventions are significantly lower compared to open surgical procedures and range between 0 and 10%.† Potential complications of endovascular intervention include major and minor stroke, TIA, access site hematoma, pseudoaneurysm or AV fistula, radial, brachial, or axillary artery thrombosis, dissection or perforation, and digital ischemia.

Rarely, stent fractures (**Figure 19-5**) and distal embolization were reported.[66] These events are likely related to compression forces exerted by the clavicle and first rib on the stented lateral segment of the subclavian vessels as it traverses between them. The phenomenon was described in stented subclavian arteries and veins and it was reported with all types of stents, including BES, SES, and covered stents.[66,67] Nonetheless, we agree that the SES memory makes it more likely to resume its configuration following deformation and continue to recommend using SES for the distal segment of the SCA.[66]

CONCLUSIONS

In summary, atherosclerosis is the most common cause of upper extremity occlusive disease and revascularization procedures are an integral part of contemporary practice. Symptomatic individuals presenting with upper extremity ischemia, neurological symptoms, or coronary insufficiency due to compromised flow to a LIMA graft should be considered for treatment. Endovascular therapy is the treatment of choice in most cases and excellent results can be achieved with careful patient selection, thoughtful procedure planning, and when experienced operators follow best practices, including the retrograde approach and the use of EPD when appropriate.

*References 4, 33, 39, 40, 45, 57.
†References 38, 45, 50, 56, 58-65.

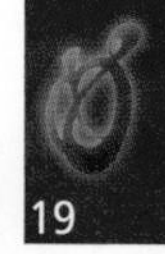

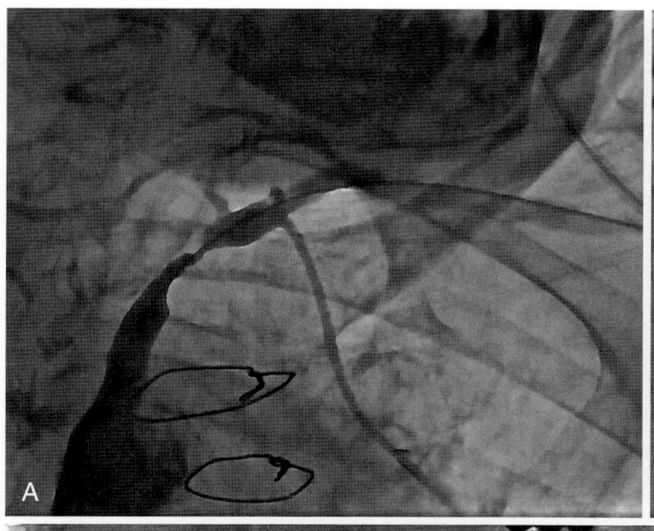

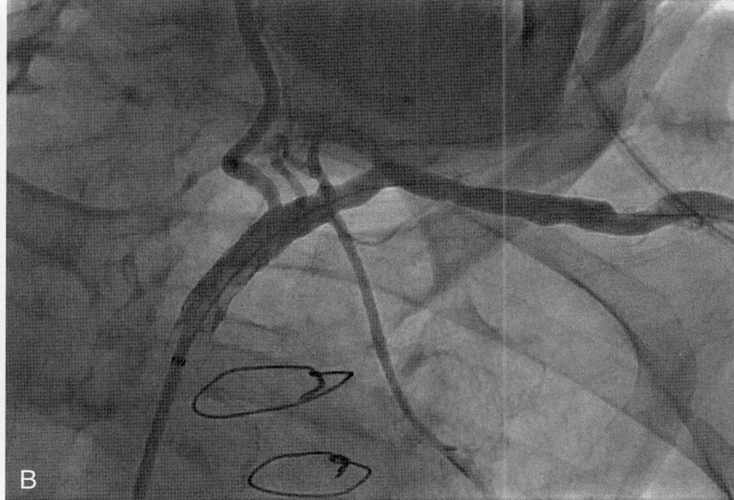

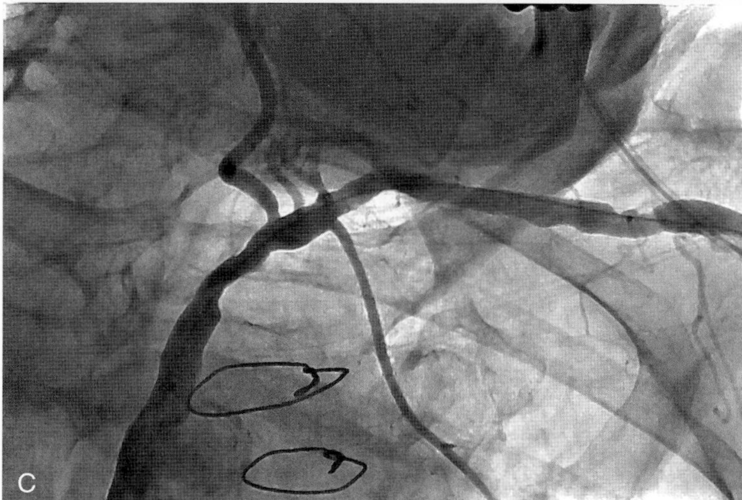

FIGURE 19-4 **A,** The L-SCA lesion is seen proximal to the vertebral artery. Note competitive flow in VA indicative of a retrograde pattern. **B,** RAO of the L-SCA poststenting with excellent results. **C,** RAO for LSC post-PTA alone. Good results are achieved. Note restoration of antegrade arterial flow.

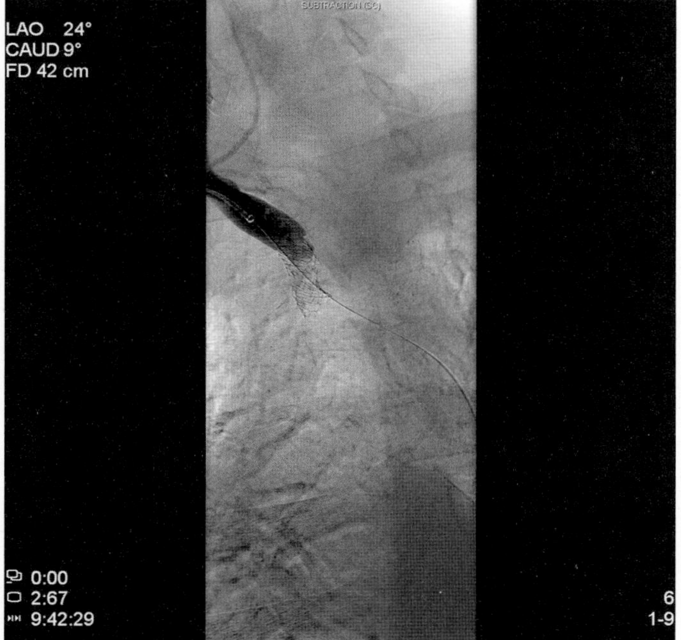

FIGURE 19-5 Stent fracture presented as restenosis. The aortic-right brachial gradient was 60 mm Hg.

References

1. Osborn LA, Vernon SM, Reynolds B, et al: Screening for subclavian stenosis in patients who are candidates for coronary bypass surgery. *Cathet Cardiovasc Intervent* 56:162–165, 2002.
2. Shadman R, Criqui MH, Bundens WP, et al: Subclavian stenosis: the prevalence, risk factors and association with other cardiovascular diseases. *J Am Coll Cardiol* 44:618–623, 2004.
3. Schillinger M, Haumer M, Schillinger S, et al: Outcome of conservative versus interventional treatment of subclavian artery stenosis. *J Endovasc Ther* 9:139–146, 2002.
4. Ochoa VM, Yeghiazarians Y: Subclavian artery stenosis: a review for the vascular medicine practitioner. *Vasc Med* 16:29–34, 2011.
5. Labropoulos N, Nandivada P, Bekelis K: Prevalence and Impact of the subclavian steal syndrome. *Ann Surg* 252:166–170, 2010.
6. Wylie EJ, Effeney DJ: Surgery of the aortic arch branches and vertebral arteries. *Surg Clin North Am* 59:669–680, 1979.
7. Hass WK, Fields WS, North RR, et al: Joint study of extracranial arterial occlusion. II. Arteriography, techniques, sites, and complications. *JAMA* 203:961–968, 1968.
8. Aboyans V, Criqui MH, McDermott MM, et al: The vital prognosis of subclavian stenosis. *J Am Coll Cardiol* 49:1540–1545, 2007.
9. Gutierrez GR, Mahrer P, Aharonian V, et al: Prevalence of subclavian artery stenosis in patients with peripheral vascular disease. *Angiology* 52(3):189–194, 2001.
10. Clark CE, Taylor RS, Shore AC, et al: Association of a difference in systolic blood pressure between arms with vascular disease and mortality: a systematic review and meta-analysis. *Lancet* 379:905–914, 2012.
11. English JA, Carell ES, Guidera SA, et al: Angiographic prevalence and clinical predictors of left subclavian stenosis in patients undergoing diagnostic cardiac catheterization. *Cathet Cardiovasc Intervent* 54:8–11, 2001.
12. Sharma BK, Jain S, Suri S, et al: Diagnostic criteria for Takayasu arteritis. *Int J Cardiol* 54(Suppl):S141–S147, 1996.
13. Nuenninghoff DM, Hunder GG, Christianson TJ, et al: Incidence and predictors of large-artery complication (aortic aneurysm, aortic dissection, and/or large-artery stenosis) in patients with giant cell arteritis: a population-based study over 50 years. *Arthritis Rheum* 48:3522–3531, 2003.
14. Backer CL, Mavroudis C: Coarctation of the aorta and interrupted aortic arch. In Baue AE, Geha AS, Hammond GI, et al, editors: *Glenn's thoracic and cardiovascular surgery*, Stamford, CT, 1996, Appleton and Lange, pp 1244–1247.
15. Durham JR, Yao JST, Pearce WH, et al: Arterial injuries in the thoracic outlet syndrome. *J Vasc Surg* 21:57–70, 1995.
16. Rubin DI, Scomberg PJ, Shepherd RF, et al: Arteritis and brachial plexus neuropathy as delayed complications of radiation therapy. *Mayo Clin Proc* 76:849–852, 2001.
17. Rice RD, Armstrong PJ: Brachial artery fibromuscular dysplasia. *Ann Vasc Surg* 24:255e1–e4, 2010.

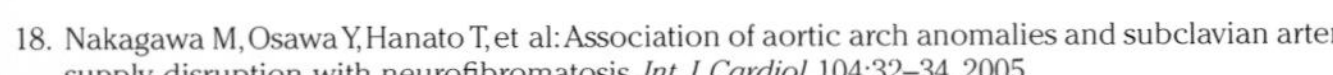

18. Nakagawa M, Osawa Y, Hanato T, et al: Association of aortic arch anomalies and subclavian artery supply disruption with neurofibromatosis. *Int J Cardiol* 104:32–34, 2005.
19. Lord RSA, Adar R, Stein RL: Contribution of the circle of Willis to the subclavian steal syndrome. *Circ* 40:871–878, 1969.
20. Goldenberg E, Arlazoroff Ar, Pajewski M, et al: Unusual clinical signs in left subclavian artery occlusion: clinical and angiographic correlation. *Stroke* 14(3), 396–398, 1983.
21. Cherry KJ, Jr, McCullough JL, Hallett JW, Jr, et al: Technical principles of direct innominate artery revascularization: a comparison of endarterectomy and bypass grafts. *J Vasc Surg* 9(5):718–723, 1989.
22. Javid H, Julian OC, Dye WS, et al: Management of cerebral arterial insufficiency caused by reversal of flow. *Arch Surg* 90:634–643, 1965.
23. Guilbert MC, Elkouri S, Bracco D, et al: Arterial trauma during central venous catheter insertion: case series, review and proposed algorithm. *J Vasc Surg* 48:918–925, 2008.
24. Cayne NS, Berland TL, Rockman CB, et al: Experience and technique for the endovascular management of iatrogenic subclavian injury. *Ann Vasc Surg* 24:44–47, 2010.
25. Park H, Kim HJ, Chan MJ, et al: A case of cerebellar infarction caused by acute subclavian thrombus following minor trauma. *Yonsei Med J* 54(6):1538–1541, 2013.
26. Klocker J, Falkensammer J, Pellegrini L, et al: Repair of arterial injury after blunt trauma in the upper extremity—immediate and long-term outcome. *Eur J Vasc Endovasc Surg* 39:160–164, 2010.
27. Cooper DG, Walsh SR, Sadat U, et al: Neurological complications after left subclavian artery coverage during thoracic endovascular aortic repair: a systematic review and meta-analysis. *J Vasc Surg* 49:1594–1601, 2009.
28. Schillinger M, Haumer M, Schillinger S, et al: Outcome of conservative versus interventional treatment of subclavian artery stenosis. *J Endovasc Ther* 9:139–146, 2002.
29. Sixt S, Rastan A, Schwarzwälder U, et al: Long term outcome after balloon angioplasty and stenting of subclavian artery obstruction: a single centre experience. *Vasa* 37:174–182, 2008.
30. De Bakey ME, Crawford ES, Fields WS: Surgical treatment of patients with cerebral arterial insufficiency associated with extracranial arterial occlusive lesions. *Neurology* 11:145–149, 1961.
31. Crawford ES, DeBakey ME, Morris GC, et al: Surgical treatment of occlusion of the innominate, common carotid, and subclavian arteries: a 10-year experience. *Surgery* 65:17–31, 1969.
32. Berguer R, Morasch MD, Kline RA, et al: Cervical reconstruction of the supra aortic trunks: a 16-year experience. *J Vasc Surg* 29:239–248, 1999.
33. Aziz F, Gravett MH, Comerota AJ: Endovascular and open surgical treatment of brachiocephalic arteries. *Ann Vasc Surg* 25:569–581, 2011.
34. Cooper DG, Walsh SR, Sadat U, et al: Neurological complications after left subclavian artery coverage during thoracic endovascular aortic repair: a systematic review and meta-analysis. *J Vasc Surg* 49:1594–1601, 2009.
35. De Bakey ME, Crawford ES, Cooley DA, et al: Surgical considerations of occlusive disease of innominate, carotid, subclavian, and vertebral arteries. *Ann Surg* 149:690–710, 1959.
36. Chang JB, Stein TA, Liu JP, et al: Long-term results with axillo-axillary bypass grafts for symptomatic subclavian artery insufficiency. *J Vasc Surg* 25:173–178, 1997.
37. Cina CS, Hussein SA, Lagana A, et al: Subclavian carotid transposition and bypass grafting: consecutive cohort study and systematic review. *J Vasc Surg* 35:422–429, 2002.
38. Palchik E, Bakken AM, Wolford HY, et al: Subclavian artery revascularization: an outcome analysis based on mode of therapy and presenting symptoms. *Ann Vasc Surg* 22:70–78, 2008.
39. Bachman DM, Kim RM: Transluminal dilatation for subclavian steal syndrome. *AJR Am J Roentgenol* 135:995–996, 1980.
40. Mathias KD, Luth I, Haarmann P: Percutaneous transluminal angioplasty of proximal subclavian artery occlusions. *Cardiovasc Intervent Radiol* 16:214–218, 1993.
41. Brountzos EN, Malagari K, Kelekis DA: Endovascular treatment of occlusive lesions of the subclavian and innominate arteries. *Cardiovasc Intervent Radiol* 29(4):503–510, 2006.
42. Henry M, Henry I, Klonaris C, et al: Percutaneous transluminal angioplasty and stenting of extracranial VA stenosis. In Henry M, Ohki T, Polydorou A, editors: *Angioplasty and stenting of the carotid and supra-aortic trunks*, ed 1, London (UK), 2003, Taylor and Francis Medicine, pp 673–682.
43. Dabus G, Moran CJ, Derdeyn CP, et al: Endovascular treatment of vertebral artery-origin and innominate/subclavian disease: indications and technique. *Neuroimaging Clin N Am* 17:381–392, ix, 2007.
44. Staikov IN, Do DD, Remonda L, et al: The site of atheromatosis in the subclavian and vertebral arteries and its implication for angioplasty. *Neuroradiology* 41(7):537–542, 1999.
45. Patel SN, White CJ, Collins TJ, et al: Catheter-based treatment of the subclavian and innominate arteries. *Catheter Cardiovasc Interv* 71:963–968, 2008.
46. Albuquerque FC, Ahmed A, Stiefel M, et al: Endovascular recanalization of the chronically occluded brachiocephalic and subclavian arteries: technical considerations and an argument for embolic protection. *World Neurosurg* 6:e327–e336, 2013.
47. Dumont1 TM, Eller JL, Hopkins LN: Embolic protection for great vessel revascularization: is this best practice? *World Neurosurg* 80(6):e199–e200, 2013.
48. Ringelstein EB, Zeumer H: Delayed reversal of vertebral artery blood flow following percutaneous transluminal angioplasty for subclavian steal syndrome. *Neuroradiology* 26:189–198, 1984.
49. Aiello F, Morrissey NJ: Open and endovascular management of subclavian and innominate arterial pathology. *Semin Vasc Surg* 24:31–35, 2011.
50. Rodriguez-Lopez JA, Werner A, Martinez R, et al: Stenting for artherosclerotic occlusive disease of the subclavian artery. *Ann Vasc Surg* 13:254–260, 1999.
51. Westerband A, Rodriguez JA, Ramaiah VG, et al: Endovascular therapy in prevention and management of coronary-subclavian steal. *J Vasc Surg* 38:699–704, 2003.
52. Berger L, Bouziane Z, Felisaz A, et al: Long-term results of 81 prevertebral subclavian artery angioplasties: a 26-year experience. *Ann Vasc Surg* 25:1043–1049, 2011.
53. deVries JP, Jager LC, van den Berg JC, et al: Durability of percutaneous transluminal angioplasty for obstructive lesions of proximal subclavian artery: long-term results. *J Vasc Surg* 41:19–23, 2005.
54. Miyakoshi A, Hatano T, Tsukahara T, et al: Percutaneous transluminal angioplasty for atherosclerotic stenosis of the subclavian or innominate artery: angiographic and clinical outcomes in 36 patients. *Neurosurg Rev* 35:121–126, 2012.
55. Huttl K, Nemes B, Simonffy A, et al: Angioplasty of the innominate artery in 89 patients: experience over 19 years. *Cardiovasc Intervent Radiol* 25(2):109–114, 2002.
56. Brountzos EN, Petersen B, Binkert C, et al: Primary stenting of subclavian and innominate artery occlusive disease: a single center's experience. *Cardiovasc Intervent Radiol* 27(6):616–623, 2004.
57. Martinez R, Rodriguez-Lopez J, Torruella L, et al: Stenting for occlusion of the subclavian arteries. *Tex Heart Inst J* 24:23–27, 1997.
58. Amor M, Eid-Lidt G, Chati Z, et al: Endovascular treatment of the subclavian artery: stent implantation with or without predilatation. *Catheter Cardiovasc Interv* 63(3):364–370, 2004.
59. Brountzos EN, Malagari K, Kelekis DA: Endovascular treatment of occlusive lesions of the subclavian and innominate arteries. *Cardiovasc Intervent Radiol* 29(4):503–510, 2006.
60. Bates MC, Broce M, Lavigne PS, et al: Subclavian artery stenting: factors influencing long-term outcome. *Catheter Cardiovasc Interv* 61(1):5–11, 2004.
61. Przewlocki T, Kablak-Ziembicka A, Pieniazek P, et al: Determinants of immediate and long-term results of subclavian and innominate artery angioplasty. *Cathet Cardiovasc Intervent* 67:519–526, 2006.
62. Sixt S, Rastan A, Schwarzwalder U, et al: Results after balloon angioplasty or stenting of atherosclerotic subclavian artery obstruction. *Cathet Cardiovasc Interv* 73:395–403, 2009.
63. AbuRahma AF, Bates MC, Stone PA, et al: Angioplasty and stenting versus carotid-subclavian bypass for the treatment of isolated subclavian artery disease. *J Endovasc Ther* 14:698–704, 2007.
64. Henry M, Amor M, Henry I, et al: Percutaneoous transluminal angioplasty of the subclavian arteries. *J Endovasc Surg* 6:33–41, 1991.
65. Gonzalez A, Gil-Peralta A, Gonzalez-Marcos JR, et al: Angioplasty and stenting for total symptomatic atherosclerotic occlusion of the subclavian or innominate arteries. *Cerebrovasc Dis* 13:107–113, 2002.
66. Phipp LH, Scott DJ, Kessel D, et al: Subclavian stents and stent-grafts: cause for concern? *J Endovasc Surg* 6:223–226, 1999.
67. Hinke DH, Zandt-Stastny D, Goodman LR: Pinch-off syndrome: a complication of implantable subclavian venous access devices. *Radiology* 177:353–356, 1990.

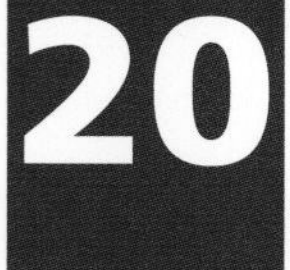

Renal Artery Intervention: Catheter-Based Therapy for Renal Artery Stenosis

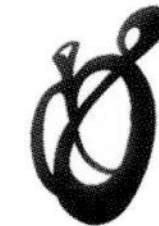

Christopher J. White

INTRODUCTION

A key principle governing renal artery stenting (RAS) is that clinical benefit will result from relieving a significant renal artery stenosis causing renal hypoperfusion. Published meta-analyses suggest that a very high RAS technical success rate (>95%) is accompanied by a surprisingly modest and inconsistent clinical improvement (**Figure 20-1**).[1-8] The discordance between the high technical success rate for RAS and the inconsistent clinical response suggests the following:

1. Successful RAS procedures were performed on nonobstructive RAS (stenoses not causing symptomatic renal hypoperfusion).
2. That the clinical syndrome being treated (hypertension or renal insufficiency) was not caused by renal hypoperfusion.

We must improve our ability to discriminate between ischemia-producing and nonischemia-producing renal artery stenoses, if we hope to obtain concordance between the very high technical success and a high expectation of clinical response.

DIAGNOSIS

Screening for Renal Artery Stenosis

Screening for renal artery stenosis is appropriate in patients at increased risk for this disease (**Table 20-1**). Whenever possible, screening tests for renal artery stenosis should be performed noninvasively using direct imaging tests such as Doppler ultrasound, computed tomographic angiography (CTA), or magnetic resonance angiography (MRA). Noninvasive imaging has become so sophisticated and accurate that it is seldom necessary to perform catheter-based angiography for the diagnosis of renal artery disease.

The appropriateness of screening angiography for RAS at the time of cardiac or peripheral vascular angiography of other vascular beds has been addressed by recommendations and guidelines endorsed by an expert consensus panel of the American College of Cardiology (ACC) and the American Heart Association (AHA).[9,10] For patients with risk factors as outlined in **Table 20-1** or clinical syndromes suggestive of RAS, aortography is given a Class I indication for screening at the time of angiography performed for other clinical indications. There is published evidence that nonselective, diagnostic, screening renal angiography is safe and is not associated with any incremental risk when performed at the time of cardiac catheterization.[11]

Duplex Ultrasonography

Duplex ultrasonography (DUS) is an excellent test to detect renal artery stenosis but is highly dependent upon the skills of the technician performing the test. It is the least expensive of the imaging modalities and provides useful information about the degree of stenosis, the kidney size and other associated disease processes such as obstruction. The location and degree of stenosis can accurately be determined by duplex ultrasound of the renal artery.

Overall, when compared with angiography, DUS has a sensitivity and specificity of 84% to 98% and 62% to 99%, respectively, when used to diagnose renal artery stenosis.[12,13] Renal artery duplex is an excellent test for the follow-up of RAS after revascularization. Following endovascular therapy a renal artery duplex should be obtained within the first few weeks to establish a baseline, at 6 months, 12 months, and yearly thereafter.[14,15]

One drawback of DUS is that the sensitivity is lower for identifying accessory renal arteries (67%) compared with main renal arteries (98%).[12] Therefore, if the patient has hypertension that cannot be adequately controlled with a

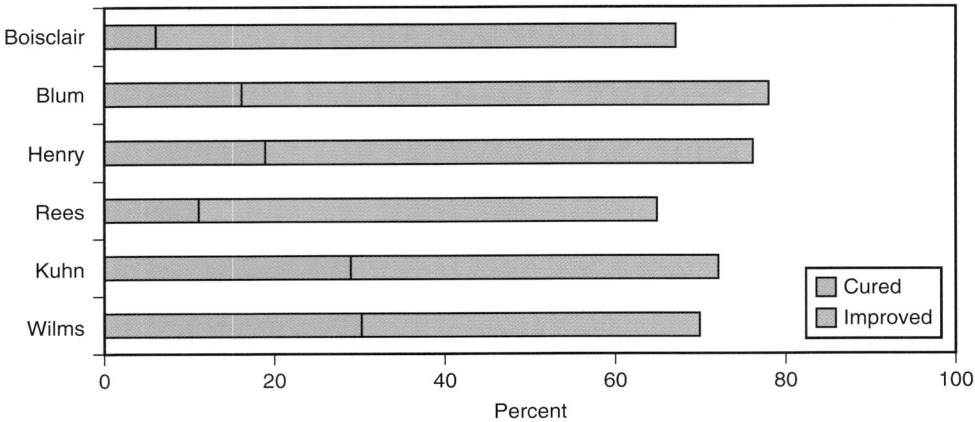

FIGURE 20-1 Hypertension response to renal intervention. Graphic representation of the cure and improvement rate after renal artery stenting (RAS). *(From Boisclair C, Therasse E, Oliva VL, et al: Treatment of renal angioplasty failure by percutaneous renal artery stenting with Palmaz stents: midterm technical and clinical results. AJR Am J Roentgenol 168:245–251, 1997; Blum U, Krumme B, Flugel P, et al: Treatment of ostial renal-artery stenoses with vascular endoprostheses after unsuccessful balloon angioplasty [see comments]. N Engl J Med 336:459–465, 1997; Henry M, Amor M, Henry I, et al: Stent placement in the renal artery: three-year experience with the Palmaz stent. J Vasc Interv Radiol 7:343–350, 1996; Rees CR, Palmaz JC, Becker GJ, et al: Palmaz stent in atherosclerotic stenoses involving the ostia of the renal arteries: preliminary report of a multicenter study. Radiology 181:507–514, 1991; Kuhn FP, Kutkuhn B, Torsello G, et al: Renal artery stenosis: preliminary results of treatment with the Strecker stent. Radiology 180:367–372, 1991; Wilms GE, Peene PT, Baert AL, et al: Renal artery stent placement with use of the Wallstent endoprosthesis. Radiology 179:457–462, 1991.)*

TABLE 20-1 Increased Prevalence of Renal Artery Stenosis

- Onset of hypertension ≤30 years or ≥55 years
- Malignant, accelerated, or resistant hypertension
- Unexplained renal dysfunction
- Development of azotemia with an angiotensin converting enzyme inhibitor or angiotensin II receptor blocker medication
- Unexplained pole to pole diameter discrepancy of ≥1.5 cm between kidneys
- Cardiac disturbance syndrome (flash pulmonary edema)
- Peripheral arterial disease (abdominal aortic aneurysm or ankle-brachial index <0.9)
- Multivessel (≥2) coronary artery disease

good regimen, and the DUS fails to demonstrate RAS, another imaging modality may be considered to identify stenosis of an accessory renal artery.

Detecting renal artery in-stent restenosis (ISR) is a potential problem when native vessel parameters are used for diagnosis. Recently a cohort of 132 patients with renal artery stents had angiographic correlation with DUS findings.[16] There was no single peak systolic velocity (PSV) cutoff that would accurately discriminate 60% to 99% from 0% to 59% restenosis in all patients. A PSV <241 cm/s was useful in excluding ISR (negative predictive value 96%): 78 of 81 renal arteries with PSV <241 cm/s had 0% to 59% restenosis. A PSV ≥296 cm/s was accurate in predicting ISR (positive predictive value 94%): 33 of 35 renal arteries with a PSV ≥296 cm/s had ISR by angiography. A PSV between 241 and 295 cm/s represented an indeterminate zone in which renal artery restenosis could not be diagnosed or excluded on the basis of DUS alone.

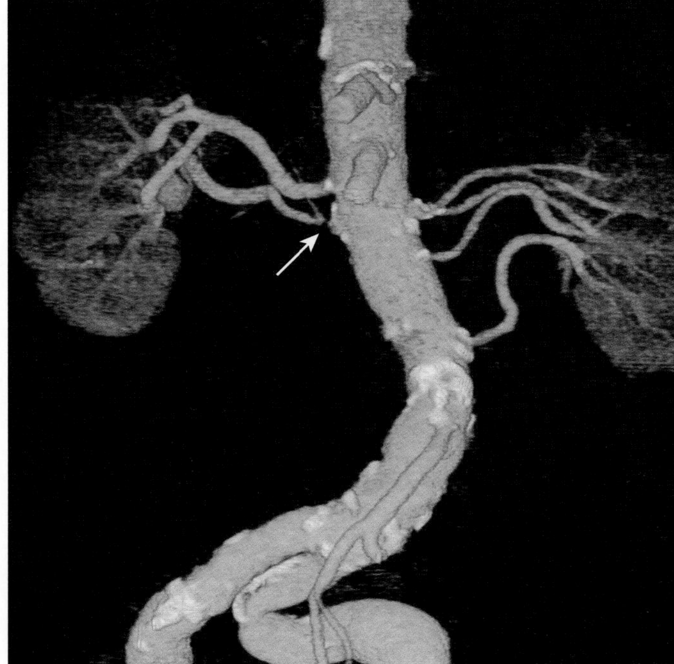

FIGURE 20-2 Computed tomographic angiography (CTA) of the abdominal aorta showing bilateral renal arteries (n = 5). Note the stenosis of the right renal accessory artery *(white arrow)*, that could be missed by duplex ultrasonography (DUS).

Resistive Index

The resistive index (RI) is obtained by measuring the peak systolic velocity (PSV) and the end diastolic velocity within the renal parenchyma at the level of the cortical blood vessels. It is an indication of the amount of small vessel arterial disease (i.e., nephrosclerosis) within the renal parenchyma. The renal artery RI has inappropriately been suggested as a method to stratify patients likely to respond to renal intervention.[17] However, a prospective study of renal stent placement by Zeller et al.[18] demonstrated that an elevated RI predicted a favorable blood pressure response and renal functional improvement at 1 year after renal arterial intervention. If there are good clinical reasons to revascularize a kidney, then it should be performed independently of the RI.

Noninvasive Angiography

Computed tomographic angiography (CTA) uses ionizing radiation and iodinated contrast to produce excellent images of the abdominal vasculature (**Figure 20-2**). CTA has a sensitivity and specificity for detecting RAS of 89% to 100% and specificity of 82% to 100%.[19-21] Excellent three-dimensional image quality with enhanced resolution can be obtained with multidetector-row CTA technology.[14] The advantages of CTA over magnetic resonance angiography (MRA) includes higher spatial resolution, absence of flow-related phenomena that may overestimate the degree of stenosis, and the capability to visualize calcification and metallic implants such as endovascular stents and stent grafts. CTA is generally well tolerated with an open gantry and thus claustrophobia is not as limiting a factor as it is for MRA. The disadvantages of CTA compared with MRA are exposure to ionizing radiation and the need to administer potentially nephrotoxic iodinated contrast agents.

MRA also provides excellent imaging of the abdominal vasculature and associated anatomical structures. When compared with angiography, MRA has demonstrated a sensitivity of 91% to 100% and a specificity of 71% to 100%.[22-25] Contrast-enhanced MRA using gadolinium improves image quality when compared with noncontrast studies and shortens imaging time, thereby eliminating some of the artifact created by gross patient movement.[26] However, MRA does not have the same sensitivity and specificity in patients with fibromuscular dysplasia (FMD) and is generally not a good screening test if FMD is suspected.[27]

MRA should not be used in patients with a glomerular filtration rate less than 30 mL/min/1.73 m^2 because of the increased likelihood of developing nephrogenic systemic sclerosis.[28] MRA may not be used in patients with metallic (ferromagnetic) implants such as some mechanical heart valves, cerebral aneurysm clips, and electrically activated implants (pacemakers, spinal cord stimulators). At the present time, MRA is not useful in following patients after stent implantation due to artifact produced by the metallic stent.

Invasive Angiography

The "Achilles' heel" of renal stenting is the inaccuracy of the angiographic determination of the severity of renal stenoses. The traditional "gold" standard for determining the severity of renal artery stenosis has been invasive angiography. Even with quantitative measurement, angiography may be unable to discriminate between nonobstructive stenoses and clinically significant ones (**Figure 20-3**).[29] Most would agree that interventionalists are able to identify "critical" stenoses in renal arteries, but for mild to moderately severe lesions, physiological confirmation is necessary.[30]

Translesional Pressure Gradients

Confirmation of the correlation with hemodynamic evidence of significant renal artery stenosis and renin release has been documented by De Bruyne and colleagues.[31] Other investigators have now established that hemodynamic parameters of significant renal artery stenosis (peak systolic gradient >21 mm Hg,[32] renal fractional flow reserve of ≤0.8,[33] and a dopamine-induced mean translesional gradient ≥20 mm Hg)[34] are associated with clinical improvement after renal stenting in patients with mild to moderate renal artery stenoses.

TIMI Frame Count

Angiographic measurements of renal blood flow by using renal frame counts (RFC) and renal blush grades (RBG) for microvascular flow can differentiate normal patients from patients with FMD.[35] Hypertensive patients with renal artery stenoses have also been shown to have decreased renal perfusion as measured by RFC.[36] Clinical responders tended to have higher baseline RFCs than nonresponders and had greater improvement in their RFC values following RAS. Three-quarters of the hypertensive patients who responded to RAS had a baseline RFC ≥25, and if the RFC improved by >4, then 79% were responders to RAS.

RENAL ARTERY INTERVENTION

The pathophysiology of renovascular hypertension has been well understood since the experiments of Goldblatt and others.[37] Modern confirmation of this cause and effect relationship was demonstrated by DeBruyne and colleagues, who performed an in vivo experiment that showed a threshold gradient (Pd/Pa ≤0.9) for the release of renin following graded renal artery obstruction.[31] Much confusion was brought to the field by the early introduction of percutaneous balloon angioplasty as a very successful treatment for renal artery FMD,[38] but it suffered a moderately high failure rate for atherosclerotic renal artery stenosis.[39] The over-estimation of the success rate for atherosclerotic lesions led to underpowered clinical trials, making it very difficult to demonstrate successful treatment outcomes.[40-42] Balloon angioplasty was subsequently shown

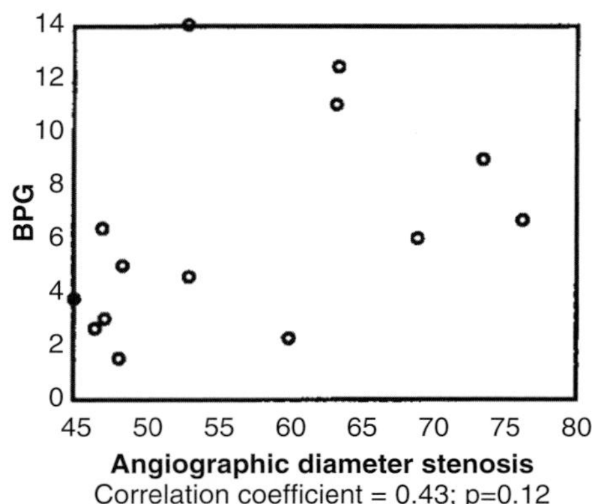

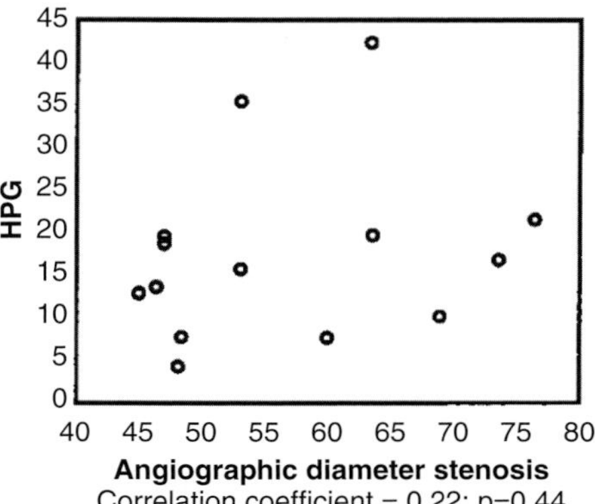

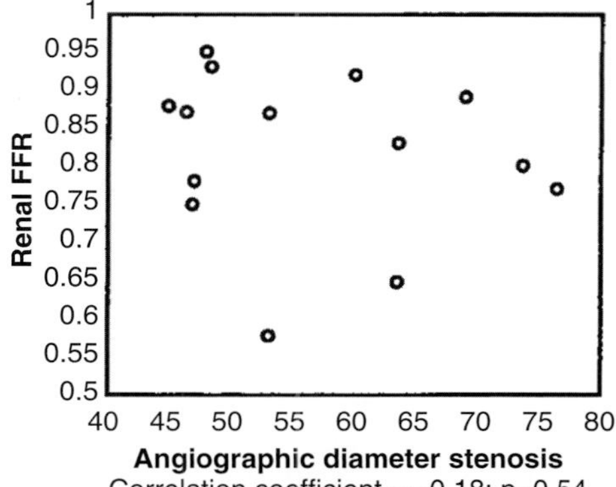

FIGURE 20-3 Lack of correlation between visual estimated renal artery stenosis and an objective measure of the hemodynamic gradient across the stenosis. *(Reproduced with permission from Subramanian R, White CJ, Rosenfield K, et al: Renal fractional flow reserve: a hemodynamic evaluation of moderate renal artery stenoses. Catheter Cardiovasc Interv 64:480–486, 2005, Figure 4.)*

TABLE 20-2 Renal Stent Patency at 12 Months

AUTHOR	ARTERIES TREATED (n)	RESTENOSIS RATE (%)
Blum et al.[4]	74	11.0
Tuttle et al.[46]	148	14.0
Henry et al.[47]	209	11.4
Van de Ven et al.[43]	43	14.0
Rocha-Singh et al.[48]	180	12.0

to be inferior to renal stenting in atherosclerotic renal artery stenosis.[43]

Renal artery restenosis after stent placement is related to both acute gain and late loss, similar to coronary artery restenosis. Quantitative angiography on a series of 100 consecutive patients was carried out and found that patients with patent renal arteries had significantly larger renal stent minimal lumen diameters (MLD) (4.3 ± 0.7 mm vs. 4.9 ± 0.9 mm; $p = 0.025$), and had significantly less late loss (1.3 ± 0.9 mm vs. 3.0 ± 1.4 mm; $p < 0.001$).[44] In the largest single series of renal stent implantation, a larger reference vessel diameter (RVD), and larger acute gain (i.e., poststent MLD) after stent deployment were strongly associated with a lower incidence of restenosis. For example, restenosis in a vessel with an RVD of <4.5 mm was 36% compared with only 6.5% for an artery with an RVD of >6.0 mm in diameter.[45] Renal stenting has been shown to be a durable treatment with 1-year patency rates ≥85% (**Table 20-2**)[4,43,46-48] and 5-year primary patency approaching 80%.[4,47]

Percutaneous catheter-based therapy with primary stent placement has replaced open surgery as the treatment of choice for atherosclerotic renal artery stenosis (Videos 20-1 and 20-2).[10] However, despite a technical success rate exceeding 95% for renal artery stent placement, there remains wide variation in the reported success rates in improving hypertension. While at least some of the variability in outcomes is attributable to a lack of standard reporting criteria,[49] the dominant factor appears to be poor patient and lesion selection for treatment.[31-33] Variability in the angiographic assessment of the hemodynamic severity of renal artery stenoses has undermined the predictability of a treatment response with success stenting. While the majority of hypertensive patients with atherosclerotic renal artery stenosis and hypertension will experience improved blood pressure control and/or the need for fewer medications, very few patients will be cured of hypertension (see **Figure 20-1**).[1-8]

Technique for Renal Artery Intervention

Aspirin is started at least one day prior to the procedure, while the use of dual antiplatelet therapy is at the discretion of the operator, but not supported by any evidence base. Retrograde femoral access is most commonly chosen, although radial artery access is rapidly gaining acceptance (see further on). For retrograde common femoral artery access, a 6 Fr or 7 Fr sheath is placed and 3000 to 5000 U of unfractionated heparin are given to achieve a target activated clotting time (ACT) of approximately 250 seconds. A 4 Fr diagnostic catheter (internal mammary or Judkins right coronary shape) is placed through a 6 Fr "short" (50-60 cm) angled (hockey-stick or renal shaped) guiding catheter, to engage the ostium of the renal artery. A 0.014-inch coronary angioplasty guidewire is advanced across the lesion, and the guide catheter is then telescoped (advanced) over the 4 Fr diagnostic catheter, allowing the larger catheter to atraumatically engage the renal artery ostium.

A second technique for safely engaging the atherosclerotic renal ostium is the "no touch" technique.[50] A 0.035-inch J-guidewire is advanced into the descending thoracic aorta above the renal arteries. The renal guide catheter is advanced over the J-wire until it is near the renal ostium. By gently manipulating (advancing and/or withdrawing) the 0.035-inch J-wire in the aorta, the tip of the guide catheter can be steered nearer to the renal artery ostium. When the guide is near the renal artery ostium, a 0.014-inch steerable guidewire is advanced through the guide catheter (alongside the 0.035-inch wire) and exiting the guide catheter near the ostium to enter into the renal artery and cross the stenosis into the distal portion of the renal artery. As the 0.035-inch guidewire is withdrawn, the guide catheter will atraumatically engage the renal ostium over the 0.014-inch wire.

A balloon sized 1:1 with the reference vessel diameter is inflated using the lowest pressure that will fully expand the balloon. This ensures that the calcified renal artery stenosis is dilatable, and also helps to choose the stent size. If the patient experiences discomfort during balloon inflation, the inflation should be terminated and the patient, lesion, and sizing reassessed. Pain may be due to stretching of the adventitial layers of the vessel and may be a precursor to arterial rupture or dissection. Balloon expandable stents, long enough to cover the lesion and sized 1:1 with the reference diameter, are used to scaffold the lesion and maximize the angiographic result.

Renal Artery Atherosclerotic Lesions

Atherosclerotic renal artery stenosis usually involves the ostial and very proximal portion of the main renal artery. These lesions are morphologically complex and can be difficult to visualize with two-dimensional angiography. The errors made with angiography are increased when interventionalists rely on "visual estimation" as the only means to determine lesion severity.[30] Under the best of circumstances, visual estimation of angiographic stenoses lacks reproducibility and precision. Confirmation of the hemodynamic significance of the renal artery stenosis is encouraged. Balloon angioplasty is associated with a lower success rate for atherosclerotic lesions, with a restenosis rate of approximately 50% over 6 months.[43] Aorto-ostial renal artery lesions are particularly difficult to effectively treat with balloon dilation alone. They are especially prone to restenosis due to vascular recoil caused by confluent plaque from the wall of the aorta extending into the ostium of the renal artery and are considered by many experts as unsuitable lesions for balloon angioplasty alone.

A strategy of primary renal artery stent placement has replaced provisional (bail-out) stent placement. A randomized controlled trial clearly demonstrated superiority of renal stents over balloons alone in atherosclerotic renal artery stenoses for procedure success, late patency, and cost-effectiveness.[43]

Atheroemboli are a concern with atherosclerotic lesions. Henry and coworkers placed renal stents in 65 renal arteries in 56 patients using emboli protection devices (EPDs).[51] They noted debris retrieval following renal stent deployment in 100% of the patients with distal balloon occlusion (Percusurge (n = 38), Medtronic, Minnesota), and in 80% of the filter cases (FilterWire (n = 26), BSC, Natick, Massachusetts) and (Angioguard (n = 1), Cordis, Miami, Florida). Interestingly, there was no difference in the size or number of particles regardless of whether balloon predilation was performed or not. With the reported frequency of visible atherosclerotic debris recovered with EPDs well above 50%, it is not surprising that 25% of successfully revascularized kidneys show a decline in renal function.[51-59]

Fibromuscular Dysplasia

Fibromuscular dysplasia (FMD) is commonly found in young adults, especially women, but the condition can persist into later life. The angiographic appearance of a corrugated vessel is diagnostic of FMD. In a patient with FMD who is hypertensive despite maximal medical therapy, balloon angioplasty alone is indicated and the patient will usually respond to balloon angioplasty without the need for stenting. Balloon angioplasty is the treatment of choice for renal artery stenoses caused by FMD. If the patient fails to respond to balloon angioplasty alone, or restenosis occurs, then renal stenting is a reasonable option.

Procedural Complications

Complications associated with catheter-based renal intervention are related to vascular access, catheter trauma, or systemic complications related to contrast reactions or renal toxicity. Vascular access complications are the most common complication in renal artery intervention. They include access site bleeding and hematoma (1.5% to 5%), access site vessel injury (1% to 2%), retroperitoneal hematoma (<1%), pseudoaneurysm (0.5% to 1%), arteriovenous fistula, and nerve injury (<1%).[1,2,44] Major complications of peripheral vascular angiography range from 1.9% to 2.9% (**Table 20-3**).[60]

Catheter-related renal artery complications include atheroembolism, vessel dissection, or arterial perforation, which are rare (<1%) but often devastating events. Anaphylactoid contrast reactions occur in fewer than 3% of cases, and less than 1% require hospitalization.[65] The risk of contrast-induced nephropathy (CIN) is increased in patients with baseline chronic renal insufficiency, diabetes mellitus, multiple myeloma, and those who are receiving other nephrotoxic drugs such as aminoglycosides. Prevention of CIN requires vigorous hydration and the use of as little iso-osmolar contrast as possible.[66]

Embolus Protection Devices

Embolus protection devices (EPDs) have been developed for clinical use in saphenous vein coronary bypass grafts and for cerebral protection during carotid stent placement. EPDs are percutaneous devices that can be divided into three categories as follows:

- filters
- dista locclusion balloons with aspiration of debris
- proximal occlusion balloons with reversal of flow

The aorto-ostial nature of most renal artery stenoses makes proximal occlusion devices unsuitable, which is why distal occlusion balloons and filters are the most common devices used in an off-label manner for renal protection.

In a single small randomized study of 100 patients that compared four arms, these were:

- control
- EPD
- IIb/IIIa antagonist
- EPD + IIb/IIIa inhibitor[67]

The control group, EPD group, and IIb/IIIa antagonist group demonstrated a decline in glomerular filtration rate ($p < 0.05$), but group 4 (combination therapy with EPD + IIb/IIIa antagonist), did not decline and was superior to the other groups ($p < 0.01$). The main effects of treatment demonstrated no overall improvement in glomerular filtration rate; although abciximab was superior to placebo ($0 \pm 27\%$ vs. $-10 \pm 20\%$; $p < 0.05$), embolic protection was not ($-1 \pm 28\%$ vs. $-10 \pm 20\%$; $p < 0.08$). An interaction was observed between abciximab and embolic protection ($p < 0.05$), favoring combination treatment. Abciximab reduced the occurrence of platelet-rich emboli in the filters from 42% to 7% ($p < 0.01$).

Radial Artery Access

Vascular access complications account for the majority of clinical complications of renal stenting. One way to minimize access site bleeding is to use the radial artery. The coronary interventional literature has demonstrated a marked reduction in vascular access complications with radial artery access compared with both brachial and femoral artery access.[68] Low profile radial sheaths and the ability to use a "sheathless" technique with 6 Fr guiding catheters make the radial artery approach a viable option (**Figure 20-4**).[69] In addition to minimizing vascular access complications, the radial artery approach has other advantages including increased patient acceptance and improved guiding catheter engagement due to the downward or caudal orientation of most renal arteries. The radial approach requires 125-cm guide catheters with 150-cm shaft length balloons and stents and there is a minor learning curve. The undeniable benefit of the radial access approach, however, is a major reduction in the vascular access related complications with same day discharge and increased patient satisfaction.[70]

TABLE 20-3 Complications of Renal Stent Placement

AUTHOR	PATIENTS (n)	DEATH (%)	DIALYSIS (%)	MAJOR COMPLICATIONS (%)
Tuttle et al.[61]	148	0	0	4.1
Rocha-Singh et al.[62]	180	0.6	0	2.6
Burket et al.[63]	171	0	0.7	0.7
White et al.[44]	133	0	0	0.75
Dorros et al.[64]	163	0.6	0	1.8
TOTAL/MEAN	795	<1.0	<1.0	2.0

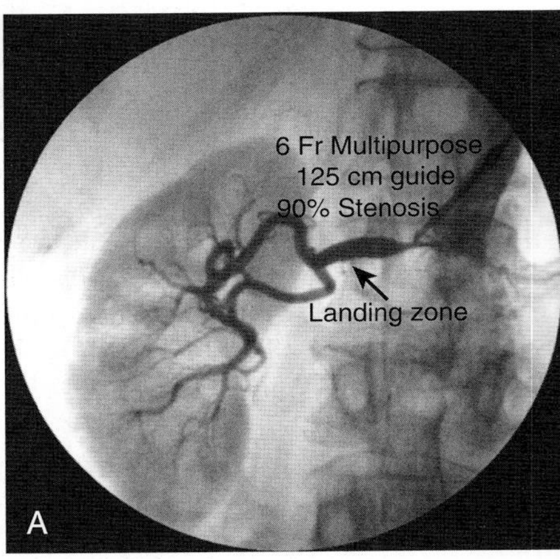

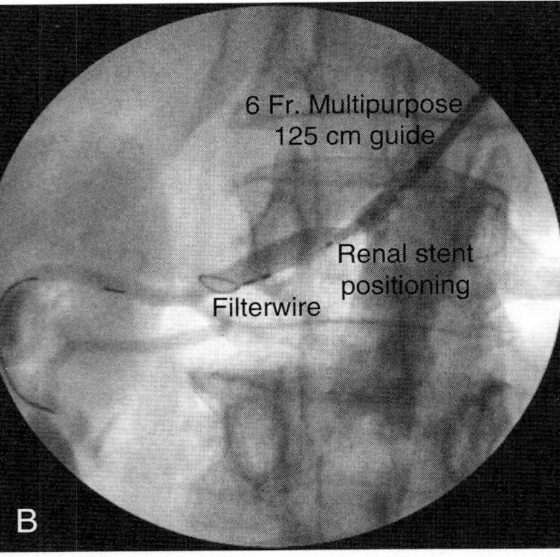

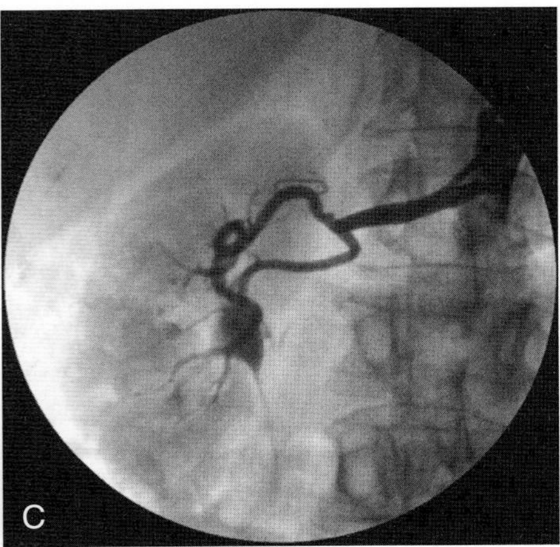

FIGURE 20-4 **A,** Baseline angiography using right radial artery access of a 90% stenosis of right renal artery using a 6 Fr multipurpose (125 cm) guide catheter. Note the landing zone prior to the bifurcation, suitable for a filter device (off-label use). **B,** The filter device has been deployed and the undeployed stent is being positioned across the lesion. **C,** Final angiography following stent deployment and filter retrieval.

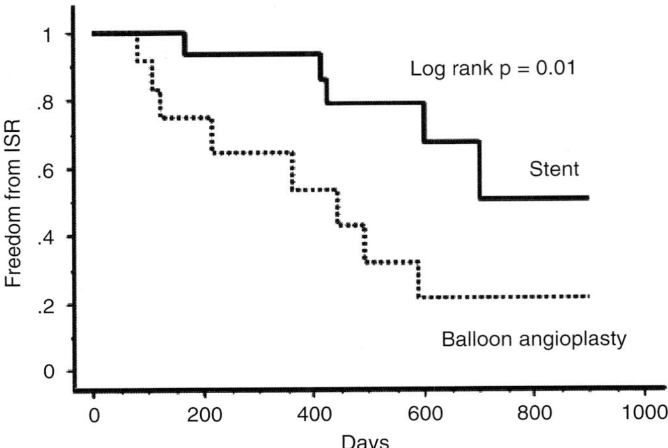

FIGURE 20-5 Kaplan-Meier curve comparing freedom from in-stent restenosis (ISR) for restenosis patients treated with a stent or balloon angioplasty.

Renal Artery In-Stent Restenosis

The optimal treatment of renal artery in-stent restenosis (ISR) is uncertain. Primary renal artery stent placement versus successful balloon angioplasty of ISR lesions demonstrated improved patency compared with balloon angioplasty alone with a 58% reduction in recurrent ISR (29.4% vs. 71.4%; p = 0.02) and a 30% reduction in follow-up diameter stenosis (41% vs. 58.2%; p = 0.03) (**Figure 20-5**).[71] The repeat stent group also had better secondary patency (p = 0.05) and a greater freedom from repeat ISR (p = 0.01) when compared with balloon angioplasty alone. Other methodologies such as coronary drug-eluting stents, covered stents, cutting balloons, and brachytherapy have been reported, but no systemic studies or any comparative data are available to support any strategy other than repeat bare-metal stenting.[72-74]

ASYMPTOMATIC RENAL ARTERY STENOSIS

There is no evidence to support beneficial outcomes for revascularization of an asymptomatic renal artery stenosis, regardless of the severity of the stenosis. The current ACC/AHA guidelines make renal intervention for unilateral asymptomatic, bilateral asymptomatic, or solitary asymptomatic RAS a Class IIb, level of evidence (LOE) C recommendation that suggests there is an uncertain risk to benefit ratio for this treatment. Patients with compelling anatomic lesions, threatening global renal function, may be considered for treatment on a case-by-case basis.[10]

RENOVASCULAR HYPERTENSION

Clinical Characteristics

It has been shown that patients with the highest systolic blood pressures have the greatest decrease in systolic pressure,[75] but there is no correlation between blood pressure improvement after renal stent placement and the variables of age, sex, race, severity of stenosis, number of vessels treated, baseline diastolic pressure, or baseline serum creatinine.[63] Two variables, bilateral renal artery stenosis (odds ratio [OR] = 4.6; p = 0.009), and mean arterial pressure >110 mm Hg (OR = 2.9; p = 0.003), are associated with improved blood pressure response following renal artery stent placement.[48] Studies comparing the results in elderly (≥75 years) versus younger (<75 years) patients, or in females versus males have failed to show any difference in response to renal stent placement.[76,77]

Prevalence

The prevalence of atherosclerotic renal artery stenosis depends upon the population examined. In an outpatient Medicare population (mean age of 77 years), screening renal ultrasound duplex studies demonstrated greater than 60% stenosis in 6.8%.[78] There were almost twice as many males (9.1%) as females (5.5%, p = 0.053) and there were no racial differences (Caucasian = 6.9% and African-American = 6.7%) in the prevalence of renal artery stenosis. Among the general hypertensive population, renal artery stenosis is the most common (2% to 5%) secondary cause of hypertension.[79] An autopsy series of patients aged older than 50 years found renal artery stenosis in 27%, rising to 53% if there was a history of diastolic hypertension.[80] Among patients entering dialysis treatment 10% to 15% have renal artery stenosis as the cause of their end-stage renal disease.[81-83] Approximately 25% of elderly patients with

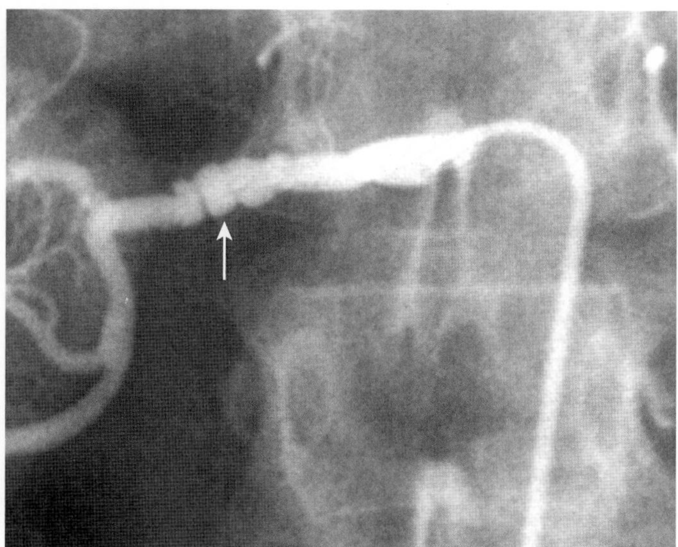

FIGURE 20-6 Angiography of the classic string of pearls sign for renal fibromuscular dysplasia.

unexplained chronic kidney disease (CKD) have unsuspected renal artery stenosis.[84-86]

Epidemiology

Renal artery stenosis is predominantly due to atherosclerosis in the adult population, with FMD (**Figure 20-6**) being more common in younger females.[38] RAS is more common in patients who have atherosclerosis involving any other vascular bed.[87] In patients undergoing cardiac catheterization for suspected coronary artery disease, the prevalence of RAS ranges from 25% to 30%[11,88-91] while peripheral arterial disease or abdominal aortic aneurysm is associated with renal artery stenosis in 30% to 40%.[92,93]

Evidence-Based Treatment

Recently data from 527 patients enrolled in five modern prospective, multicenter (117 centers), industry-sponsored, U.S. Food and Drug Administration investigational device exemption (IDE) approved studies, were combined into a database and a pooled analysis was performed. Following renal stenting systolic blood pressure (SBP) and diastolic blood pressure (DBP) were significantly decreased at 9 months. An SBP reduction >10 mm Hg occurred in 61% of patients. A baseline SBP >150 mm Hg was strongly associated with blood pressure (BP) response, but other clinical characteristics were not. In hypertensive patients in whom renal artery stenosis is identified, the only reliable predictor of benefit is SBP >150 mm Hg before the procedure.

The current ACC/AHA guideline indications for RAS in hypertensive patients with hemodynamically significant RAS and a viable kidney (linear length >7 cm) includes the following:

- accelerated hypertension
- refractory hypertension (failure of three appropriate drugs, one of which should be a diuretic[94])
- hypertension with a small kidney
- hypertension with intolerance to medications (Class IIa, LOE B)[95]

By convention, a hemodynamically significant lesion requires demonstration of a ≥70% RAS by visual estimation, ≥70% RAS by intravascular ultrasound measurement, or a 50% to 70% RAS with a systolic gradient of ≥20 mm Hg or a mean translesional gradient of ≥10 mm Hg.[95]

The findings of the recently published Cardiovascular Outcomes in Renal Atherosclerotic Lesions (CORAL) trial that compared the initial treatment strategy for renovascular hypertension patients between multifactorial medical therapy (e.g., an angiotensin receptor blocking agent, a thiazide-type diuretic, amlodipine, atorvastatin, antiplatelet therapy, and diabetes managed according to clinical practice guidelines) with medical therapy plus renal stenting are consistent with the guidelines.[96] The CORAL study found that the primary composite endpoint (death from cardiovascular or renal causes, myocardial infarction, stroke, hospitalization for congestive failure, progressive renal insufficiency, or the need for renal replacement therapy) in patients with renal artery stenosis (>60% diameter stenosis) and poorly controlled hypertension, on at least two or more medications, did not differ between groups. The number of blood pressure medications did not differ between the groups (medical 3.5 ± 1.4 vs. stent 3.3 ± 1.5) at the completion of the trial and both groups had a similar fall in systolic blood pressure, 15.6 mm Hg ± 25.8 mm Hg in the medical therapy group and 16.6 mm Hg ± 21.2 mm Hg in the stent group. The CORAL recommendations for an initial trial of multifactorial medical therapy is consistent with the current ACC/AHA guidelines, which require that patients fail medical therapy for renovascular hypertension prior to revascularization.

ISCHEMIC NEPHROPATHY

Prevalence

Ischemic nephropathy, its incidence and its reversibility, continues to be a source of debate among experts.[97,98] The number of patients with atherosclerotic RAS requiring dialysis therapy is increasing.[99] Opponents of aggressive revascularization of RAS patients with renal insufficiency contend that the kidney is supplied with an excess of nutrient blood flow and therefore few kidneys will benefit from revascularization.[98]

Evidence-Based Treatment

The literature is replete with patient series in which RAS improves renal function[86,100-103] as well as counterbalancing reports of worsening of renal failure after successful RAS.[1,104,105] However, there are no large randomized studies demonstrating benefit of revascularization over medical therapy alone for improving renal function.

Unfortunately, there are several poorly done studies such as the recently completed STAR (STent placement and blood pressure and lipid-lowering for the prevention of progression of renal dysfunction caused by Atherosclerotic ostial stenosis of the Renal artery) trial[106] and the Angioplasty and Stenting for Renal Artery Lesions (ASTRAL) trial, comparing RAS plus medical therapy to medical therapy alone.[107] Unfortunately, methodological problems, such as enrolling study patients with mild (<50%) or nonobstructive RAS, weakened these "intention to treat" trials. The sweeping negative statements regarding the efficacy of RAS were not supported by the evidence presented.

Dramatic benefit for RAS versus medical therapy in the patients with the most severe renal disease was demonstrated in a large cohort study.[108] One center offered patients (n =182) medical therapy only and the other center offered RAS plus medical therapy (n = 348). Patients were matched

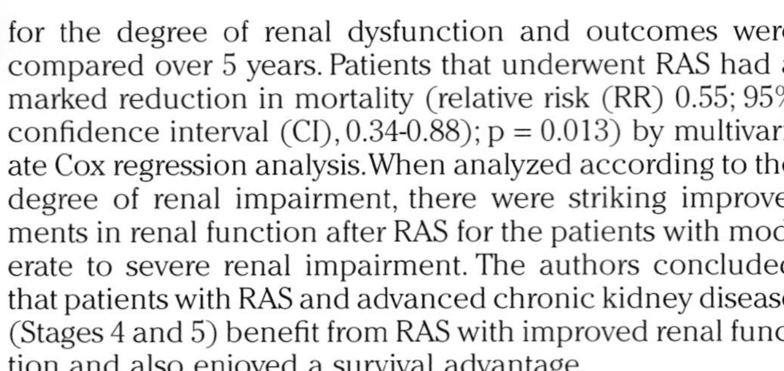

for the degree of renal dysfunction and outcomes were compared over 5 years. Patients that underwent RAS had a marked reduction in mortality (relative risk (RR) 0.55; 95% confidence interval (CI), 0.34-0.88); p = 0.013) by multivariate Cox regression analysis. When analyzed according to the degree of renal impairment, there were striking improvements in renal function after RAS for the patients with moderate to severe renal impairment. The authors concluded that patients with RAS and advanced chronic kidney disease (Stages 4 and 5) benefit from RAS with improved renal function and also enjoyed a survival advantage.

Currently, there are several parameters that suggest that a patient is likely to improve renal function after revascularization. First, there must be an obstructive renal artery stenosis lesion causing hypoperfusion of the kidney. The more renal tissue at risk, the more likely there will be a response or improvement with RAS. Patients with bilateral renal stenosis and solitary kidney stenosis are traditionally thought to be most likely to improve. Last, patients with small kidneys (<7 cm) and those with significant proteinuria are less likely to benefit.[109]

Patients with rapidly declining renal function, as opposed to those with stable renal failure, have the most to gain from revascularization.[102,110] The rate of decline in renal function, determined as the slope of the regression line of serum creatinine over time, is a very strong predictor of benefit with RAS.[102] A multivariate analysis demonstrated the only significant predictor of benefit following RAS was the rate of decline of renal function that preceded the procedure. Baseline creatinine, the presence of proteinuria, renal size, and diabetes were not significant predictors of improvement in this study.

The current ACC/AHA guideline recommendation[10] for catheter-based therapy to preserve renal function concludes that RAS is reasonable for patients with significant renal artery stenosis and progressive chronic kidney disease with bilateral renal artery stenosis or a solitary functioning kidney with stenosis (Class IIa, LOE B) RAS may also be considered on an individual basis for patients with hemodynamically significant stenosis and chronic renal insufficiency with unilateral RAS (Class IIb, LOE C).

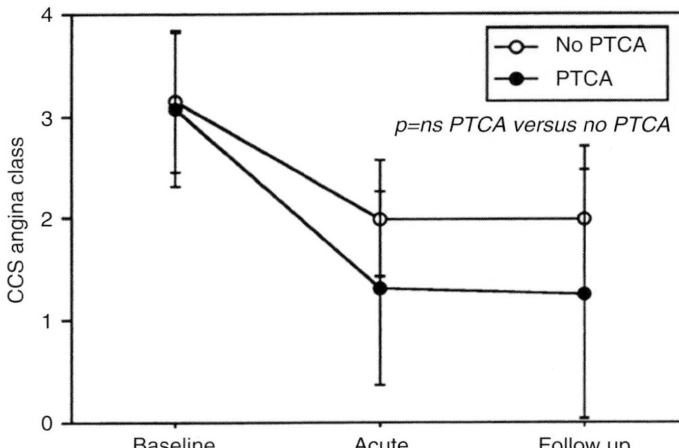

FIGURE 20-7 Effect of renal artery stent implantation with percutaneous transluminal coronary angioplasty (PTCA) (group I, n = 13) and without PTCA (group II, n = 7) on Canadian Cardiovascular Society (CCS) angina Class in patients presenting with unstable angina. *(Reprinted with permission from Khosla S, White CJ, Collins TJ, et al: Effects of renal artery stent implantation in patients with renovascular hypertension presenting with unstable angina or congestive heart failure. Am J Cardiol 80(3):363–366, 1997, Figure 3.)*

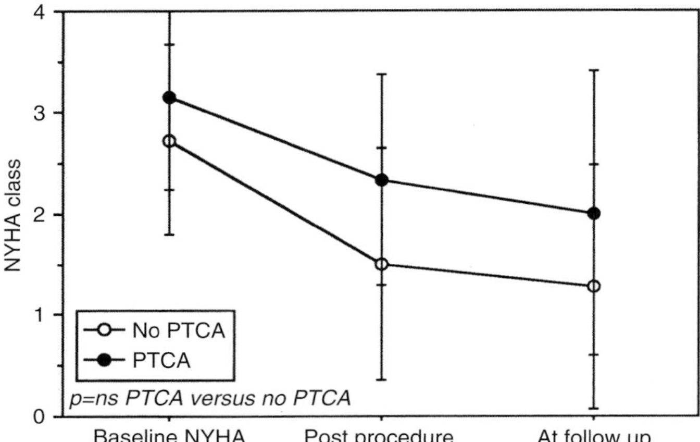

FIGURE 20-8 Effect of renal artery stent implantation with percutaneous transluminal coronary angioplasty (PTCA) (group III, n = 28) or without PTCA (group IV, n = 6) on New York Heart Association (NYHA) functional class of patients presenting with congestive heart failure (CHF). *(Reprinted with permission from Khosla S, White CJ, Collins TJ, et al: Effects of renal artery stent implantation in patients with renovascular hypertension presenting with unstable angina or congestive heart failure. Am J Cardiol 80(3):363–366, 1997, Figure 4.)*

CARDIAC DESTABILIZATION SYNDROMES

Cardiac destabilization syndromes attributable to renal artery stenosis include exacerbations of coronary ischemia and congestive heart failure (CHF) due to peripheral arterial vasoconstriction and/or volume overload.[111] Renovascular disease may also complicate the management of heart failure patients by preventing administration of an angiotensin converting enzyme inhibitor (ACEI) or angiotensin II receptor blocker (ARB).

The importance of renal artery stent placement in the treatment of cardiac disturbance has been described in a series of patients presenting with either CHF or an acute coronary syndrome.[112] Successful renal stent placement resulted in a significant decrease in blood pressure and control of symptoms in 88% (42 of 48) of all patients. Assessment of the treatment effects acutely and at 8 months using the Canadian Cardiovascular Society (CCS) angina classification (**Figure 20-7**) and the New York Heart Association (NYHA) functional classification (**Figure 20-8**) were not different between the combined coronary and renal revascularization group compared with those who had only renal stent placement, suggesting that renal revascularization was the most significant intervention.[112]

Gray and colleagues reported a case series of 39 patients treated with renal artery stent implantation for control of CHF.[113] Eighteen (46%) patients had bilateral RAS and 21 (54%) patients had stenosis to a solitary functioning kidney. Renal artery stent implantation was technically successful in all 39 patients. Blood pressure improved in 72% of patients. Renal function improved in 51% and was stable in 26% of patients. The mean number of hospitalizations for CHF prior to stenting was 2.37 + 1.42 (range 1-6) and after renal stenting was 0.30 + 0.065 (range 0-3) ($p < 0.001$). Seventy-seven percent of patients had no further hospitalizations after RAS over a mean follow-up period of 21.3 months.

Percutaneous therapy can relieve the RAS and result in marked improvement in both heart failure and angina symptoms.[112] The ACC/AHA guidelines make percutaneous revascularization for hemodynamically significant RAS and recurrent, unexplained congestive heart failure, or sudden unexplained pulmonary edema a Class I, LOE B indication. RAS for renal artery stenosis and refractory unstable angina earned a Class IIa, LOE B indication.[10]

CONCLUSIONS

Patients with presumed atherosclerotic renovascular hypertension should initially be given a trial of multifactorial medical therapy to treat their blood pressure as suggested by the results of CORAL. For patients whose blood pressure is not controlled with medical therapy, one should follow the recommendation of the ACC/AHA guidelines document, which states that it is reasonable to offer renal artery stenting to patients with an atherosclerotic severe renal artery stenosis (>70% angiographic diameter renal artery stenosis, or 50% to 70% stenosis with hemodynamic confirmation of lesion severity) associated with resistant hypertension and failure of three drugs, one of which is a diuretic, or in patients with hypertension, and intolerance to medication.[10]

Catheter-based therapy for symptomatic (hypertension, ischemic nephropathy, or cardiac destabilization syndromes), hemodynamically significant, atherosclerotic RAS is the preferred method of revascularization. The discordance between the high (>95%) procedural success and the moderate (60% to 70%) clinical response is most likely due to three major factors: poor patient selection, poor discrimination of lesion severity by angiography, and the presence of severe parenchymal renal disease. There is encouraging data that suggest that the use of physiologic lesion assessment can enhance selection for revascularization and improve clinical response rates.[31-33] In addition to maximizing the clinical benefit by better patient and lesion selection for RAS, the broader use of radial artery access for RAS will decrease vascular access complications, improve patient satisfaction, and enable same day discharge in a subset of the patients.

References

1. Isles CG, Robertson S, Hill D: Management of renovascular disease: a review of renal artery stenting in ten studies. *QJM* 92:159–167, 1999.
2. Leertouwer TC, Gussenhoven EJ, Bosch JL, et al: Stent placement for renal arterial stenosis: where do we stand? A meta-analysis. *Radiology* 216:78–85, 2000.
3. Boisclair C, Therasse E, Oliva VL, et al: Treatment of renal angioplasty failure by percutaneous renal artery stenting with Palmaz stents: midterm technical and clinical results. *AJR Am J Roentgenol* 168:245–251, 1997.
4. Blum U, Krumme B, Flugel P, et al: Treatment of ostial renal-artery stenoses with vascular endoprostheses after unsuccessful balloon angioplasty [see comments]. *N Engl J Med* 336:459–465, 1997.
5. Henry M, Amor M, Henry I, et al: Stent placement in the renal artery: three-year experience with the Palmaz stent. *J Vasc Interv Radiol* 7:343–350, 1996.
6. Rees CR, Palmaz JC, Becker GJ, et al: Palmaz stent in atherosclerotic stenoses involving the ostia of the renal arteries: preliminary report of a multicenter study. *Radiology* 181:507–514, 1991.
7. Kuhn FP, Kutkuhn B, Torsello G, et al: Renal artery stenosis: preliminary results of treatment with the Strecker stent. *Radiology* 180:367–372, 1991.
8. Wilms GE, Peene PT, Baert AL, et al: Renal artery stent placement with use of the Wallstent endoprosthesis. *Radiology* 179:457–462, 1991.
9. White CJ, Jaff MR, Haskal ZJ, et al: Indications for renal arteriography at the time of coronary arteriography: a science advisory from the American Heart Association Committee on Diagnostic and Interventional Cardiac Catheterization, Council on Clinical Cardiology, and the Councils on Cardiovascular Radiology and Intervention and on Kidney in Cardiovascular Disease. *Circulation* 114:1892–1895, 2006.
10. Hirsch AT, Haskal ZJ, Hertzer NR, et al: ACC/AHA 2005 guidelines for the management of patients with peripheral arterial disease (lower extremity, renal, mesenteric, and abdominal aortic): executive summary a collaborative report from the American Association for Vascular Surgery/Society for Vascular Surgery, Society for Cardiovascular Angiography and Interventions, Society for Vascular Medicine and Biology, Society of Interventional Radiology, and the ACC/AHA Task Force on Practice Guidelines (Writing Committee to Develop Guidelines for the Management of Patients With Peripheral Arterial Disease) endorsed by the American Association of Cardiovascular and Pulmonary Rehabilitation; National Heart, Lung, and Blood Institute; Society for Vascular Nursing; TransAtlantic Inter-Society Consensus; and Vascular Disease Foundation. *J Am Coll Cardiol* 47:1239–1312, 2006.
11. Rihal CS, Textor SC, Breen JF, et al: Incidental renal artery stenosis among a prospective cohort of hypertensive patients undergoing coronary angiography. *Mayo Clin Proc* 77:309–316, 2002.
12. Hansen KJ, Tribble RW, Reavis SW, et al: Renal duplex sonography: evaluation of clinical utility. *J Vasc Surg* 12:227–236, 1990.
13. Hoffmann U, Edwards JM, Carter S, et al: Role of duplex scanning for the detection of atherosclerotic renal artery disease. *Kidney Int* 39:1232–1239, 1991.
14. Olin JW, Kaufman JA, Bluemke DA, et al: Atherosclerotic Vascular Disease Conference: Writing Group IV: imaging. *Circulation* 109:2626–2633, 2004.
15. Morvay Z, Nagy E, Bagi R, et al: Sonographic follow-up after visceral artery stenting. *J Ultrasound Med* 23:1057–1064, 2004.
16. Del Conde I, Galin ID, Trost B, et al: Renal artery duplex ultrasound criteria for the detection of significant in-stent restenosis. *Catheter Cardiovasc Interv* 2013.
17. Radermacher J, Chavan A, Bleck J, et al: Use of Doppler ultrasonography to predict the outcome of therapy for renal-artery stenosis. *N Engl J Med* 344:410–417, 2001.
18. Zeller T, Frank U, Muller C, et al: Predictors of improved renal function after percutaneous stent-supported angioplasty of severe atherosclerotic ostial renal artery stenosis. *Circulation* 108:2244–2249, 2003.
19. Urban BA, Ratner LE, Fishman EK: Three-dimensional volume-rendered CT angiography of the renal arteries and veins: normal anatomy, variants, and clinical applications. *Radiographics* 21:373–386, questionnaire 549–555, 2001.
20. Willmann JK, Wildermuth S, Pfammatter T, et al: Aortoiliac and renal arteries: prospective intraindividual comparison of contrast-enhanced three-dimensional MR angiography and multi-detector row CT angiography. *Radiology* 226:798–811, 2003.
21. Kawashima A, Sandler CM, Ernst RD, et al: CT evaluation of renovascular disease. *Radiographics* 20:1321–1340, 2000.
22. De Cobelli F, Venturini M, Vanzulli A, et al: Renal arterial stenosis: prospective comparison of color Doppler US and breath-hold, three-dimensional, dynamic, gadolinium-enhanced MR angiography. *Radiology* 214:373–380, 2000.
23. Schoenberg SO, Rieger J, Johannson LO, et al: Diagnosis of renal artery stenosis with magnetic resonance angiography: update 2003. *Nephrol Dial Transplant* 18:1252–1256, 2003.
24. Fain SB, King BF, Breen JF, et al: High-spatial-resolution contrast-enhanced MR angiography of the renal arteries: a prospective comparison with digital subtraction angiography. *Radiology* 218:481–490, 2001.
25. Tan KT, van Beek EJ, Brown PW, et al: Magnetic resonance angiography for the diagnosis of renal artery stenosis: a meta-analysis. *Clin Radiol* 57:617–624, 2002.
26. Saloner D: Determinants of image appearance in contrast-enhanced magnetic resonance angiography. A review. *Invest Radiol* 33:488–495, 1998.
27. Vasbinder GB, Nelemans PJ, Kessels AG, et al: Accuracy of computed tomographic angiography and magnetic resonance angiography for diagnosing renal artery stenosis. *Ann Intern Med* 141:674–682, discussion 682, 2004.
28. Prchal D, Holmes DT, Levin A: Nephrogenic systemic fibrosis: the story unfolds. *Kidney Int* 73:1335–1337, 2008.
29. Subramanian R, White CJ, Rosenfield K, et al: Renal fractional flow reserve: a hemodynamic evaluation of moderate renal artery stenoses. *Catheter Cardiovasc Interv* 64:480–486, 2005.
30. Topol EJ, Nissen SE: Our preoccupation with coronary luminology: the dissociation between clinical and angiographic findings in ischemic heart disease. *Circulation* 92:2333–2342, 1995.
31. De Bruyne B, Manoharan G, Pijls NH, et al: Assessment of renal artery stenosis severity by pressure gradient measurements. *J Am Coll Cardiol* 48:1851–1855, 2006.
32. Leesar MA, Varma J, Shapira A, et al: Prediction of hypertension improvement after stenting of renal artery stenosis: comparative accuracy of translesional pressure gradients, intravascular ultrasound, and angiography. *J Am Coll Cardiol* 53:2363–2371, 2009.
33. Mitchell J, Subramanian R, White C, et al: Predicting blood pressure improvement in hypertensive patients after renal artery stent placement. *Catheter Cardiovasc Interv* 69:685–689, 2007.
34. Mangiacapra F, Trana C, Sarno G, et al: Translesional pressure gradients to predict blood pressure response after renal artery stenting in patients with renovascular hypertension. *Circ Cardiovasc Interv* 2010.
35. Mulumudi MS, White CJ: Renal frame count: a quantitative angiographic assessment of renal perfusion. *Catheter Cardiovasc Interv* 65:183–186, 2005.
36. Mahmud E, Smith TW, Palakodeti V, et al: Renal frame count and renal blush grade: quantitative measures that predict the success of renal stenting in hypertensive patients with renal artery stenosis. *JACC Cardiovasc Interv* 1:286–292, 2008.
37. Goldblatt H, Lynch J, Hanzal RF, et al: Studies on experimental hypertension I, the production of persistent elevation of systolic blood pressure by means of renal ischemia. *J Exp Med* 59:347–379, 1934.
38. Slovut DP, Olin JW: Fibromuscular dysplasia. *N Engl J Med* 350:1862–1871, 2004.
39. Sos TA, Pickering TG, Sniderman K, et al: Percutaneous transluminal renal angioplasty in renovascular hypertension due to atheroma or fibromuscular dysplasia. *N Engl J Med* 309:274–279, 1983.
40. van Jaarsveld BC, Krijnen P, Pieterman H, et al: The effect of balloon angioplasty on hypertension in atherosclerotic renal-artery stenosis. Dutch Renal Artery Stenosis Intervention Cooperative Study Group. *N Engl J Med* 342:1007–1014, 2000.
41. Webster J, Marshall F, Abdalla M, et al: Randomised comparison of percutaneous angioplasty vs continued medical therapy for hypertensive patients with atheromatous renal artery stenosis. Scottish and Newcastle Renal Artery Stenosis Collaborative Group. *J Hum Hypertens* 12:329–335, 1998.
42. Plouin PF, Chatellier G, Darne B, et al: Blood pressure outcome of angioplasty in atherosclerotic renal artery stenosis: a randomized trial. Essai Multicentrique Medicaments vs Angioplastie (EMMA) Study Group. *Hypertension* 31:823–829, 1998.
43. van de Ven PJ, Kaatee R, Beutler JJ, et al: Arterial stenting and balloon angioplasty in ostial atherosclerotic renovascular disease: a randomised trial. *Lancet* 353:282–286, 1999.
44. White CJ, Ramee SR, Collins TJ, et al: Renal artery stent placement: utility in lesions difficult to treat with balloon angioplasty. *J Am Coll Cardiol* 30:1445–1450, 1997.
45. Lederman R, Mendelsohn F, Santos R, et al: Primary renal artery stenting: characteristics and outcomes after 363 procedure. *Am Heart J* 142:314–323, 2001.
46. Tuttle KR, Chouinard RF, Webber JT, et al: Treatment of atherosclerotic ostial renal artery stenosis with the intravascular stent. *Am J Kidney Dis* 32:611–622, 1998.
47. Henry M, Amor M, Henry I, et al: Stents in the treatment of renal artery stenosis: long-term follow-up. *J Endovasc Surg* 6:42–51, 1999.
48. Rocha-Singh KJ, Mishkel GJ, Katholi RE, et al: Clinical predictors of improved long-term blood pressure control after successful stenting of hypertensive patients with obstructive renal artery atherosclerosis. *Catheter Cardiovasc Interv* 47:167–172, 1999.
49. Rundback JH, Sacks D, Kent KC, et al: Guidelines for the reporting of renal artery revascularization in clinical trials. American Heart Association. *Circulation* 106:1572–1585, 2002.
50. Feldman RL, Wargovich TJ, Bittl JA: No-touch technique for reducing aortic wall trauma during renal artery stenting. *Catheter Cardiovasc Interv* 46:245–248, 1999.
51. Henry M, Henry I, Klonaris C, et al: Renal angioplasty and stenting under protection: the way for the future? *Catheter Cardiovasc Interv* 60:299–312, 2003.
52. Henry M, Klonaris C, Henry I, et al: Protected renal stenting with the PercuSurge GuardWire device: a pilot study. *J Endovasc Ther* 8:227–237, 2001.
53. Holden A, Hill A: Renal angioplasty and stenting with distal protection of the main renal artery in ischemic nephropathy: early experience. *J Vasc Surg* 38:962–968, 2003.
54. Henry M, Henry I, Polydorou A, et al: Renal angioplasty and stenting: long-term results and the potential role of protection devices. *Expert Rev Cardiovasc Ther* 3:321–334, 2005.
55. Hagspiel KD, Stone JR, Leung DA: Renal angioplasty and stent placement with distal protection: preliminary experience with the FilterWire EX. *J Vasc Interv Radiol* 16:125–131, 2005.

56. Edwards MS, Craven BL, Stafford J, et al: Distal embolic protection during renal artery angioplasty and stenting. *J Vasc Surg* 44:128–135, 2006.
57. Holden A, Hill A, Jaff MR, et al: Renal artery stent revascularization with embolic protection in patients with ischemic nephropathy. *Kidney Int* 70:948–955, 2006.
58. Edwards MS, Corriere MA, Craven TE, et al: Atheroembolism during percutaneous renal artery revascularization. *J Vasc Surg* 46:55–61, 2007.
59. Henry M, Henry I, Polydorou A, et al: Embolic protection for renal artery stenting. *J Cardiovasc Surg (Torino)* 49:571–589, 2008.
60. Balduf LM, Langsfeld M, Marek JM, et al: Complication rates of diagnostic angiography performed by vascular surgeons. *Vasc Endovascular Surg* 36:439–445, 2002.
61. Tuttle KR, Puhlman ME, Cooney SK, et al: Urinary albumin and insulin as predictors of coronary artery disease: an angiographic study. *Am J Kidney Dis* 34:918–925, 1999.
62. Rocha-Singh K, Jaff MR, Rosenfield K, et al: Evaluation of the safety and effectiveness of renal artery stenting after unsuccessful balloon angioplasty: the ASPIRE-2 study. *J Am Coll Cardiol* 46:776–783, 2005.
63. Burket M, Cooper C, Kennedy D, et al: Renal artery angioplasty and stent placement: predictors of a favorable outcome. *Am Heart J* 139:64–71, 2000.
64. Dorros G, Jaff MR, Mathiak L, et al: Stent revascularization for atherosclerotic renal artery stenosis. 1-year clinical follow-up. *Tex Heart Inst J* 25:40–43, 1998.
65. Bettmann MA, Heeren T, Greenfield A, et al: Adverse events with radiographic contrast agents: results of the SCVIR contrast agent registry. *Radiology* 203:611–620, 1997.
66. Barrett BJ, Parfrey PS: Clinical practice. Preventing nephropathy induced by contrast medium. *N Engl J Med* 354:379–386, 2006.
67. Cooper C, Haller S, Colyer W, et al: Embolic protection and platelet inhibition during renal artery stenting. *Circulation* 117:2752–2760, 2008.
68. Kiemeneij F, Laarman GJ, Odekerken D, et al: A randomized comparison of percutaneous transluminal coronary angioplasty by the radial, brachial and femoral approaches: the access study. *J Am Coll Cardiol* 29:1269–1275, 1997.
69. Kessel DO, Robertson I, Taylor EJ, et al: Renal stenting from the radial artery: a novel approach. *Cardiovasc Intervent Radiol* 26:146–149, 2003.
70. Trani C, Tommasino A, Burzotta F: Transradial renal stenting: why and how. *Catheter Cardiovasc Interv* 74:951–956, 2009.
71. N'Dandu ZM, Badawi RA, White CJ, et al: Optimal treatment of renal artery in-stent restenosis: repeat stent placement versus angioplasty alone. *Catheter Cardiovasc Interv* 71:701–705, 2008.
72. Munneke GJ, Engelke C, Morgan RA, et al: Cutting balloon angioplasty for resistant renal artery in-stent restenosis. *J Vasc Interv Radiol* 13:327–331, 2002.
73. Spratt JC, Leslie SJ, Verin V: A case of renal artery brachytherapy for in-stent restenosis: four-year follow-up. *J Invasive Cardiol* 16:287–288, 2004.
74. Ellis K, Murtagh B, Loghin C, et al: The use of brachytherapy to treat renal artery in-stent restenosis. *J Interv Cardiol* 18:49–54, 2005.
75. Weinberg I, Keyes MJ, Giri J, et al: Blood pressure response to renal artery stenting in 901 patients from five prospective multicenter FDA-approved trials. *Catheter Cardiovasc Interv* 83:603–609, 2014.
76. Bloch MJ, Trost DA, Whitmer J, et al: Ostial renal artery stent placement in patients 75 years of age or older. *Am J Hypertens* 14:983–988, 2001.
77. Harjai K, Khosla S, Shaw D, et al: Effect of gender on outcomes following renal artery stent placement for renovascular hypertension. *Cathet Cardiovasc Diagn* 42:381–386, 1997.
78. Hansen KJ, Edwards MS, Craven TE, et al: Prevalence of renovascular disease in the elderly: a population-based study. *J Vasc Surg* 36:443–451, 2002.
79. Simon N, Franklin S, Bleifer K, et al: Clinical characteristics of renovascular hypertension. *JAMA* 220:1209–1218, 1972.
80. Holley KE, Hunt JC, Brown AL, Jr, et al: Renal artery stenosis. A clinical-pathologic study in normotensive and hypertensive patients. *Am J Med* 37:14–22, 1964.
81. Guo H, Kalra PA, Gilbertson DT, et al: Atherosclerotic renovascular disease in older US patients starting dialysis, 1996 to 2001. *Circulation* 115:50–58, 2007.
82. Mailloux LU, Napolitano B, Bellucci AG, et al: Renal vascular disease causing end-stage renal disease, incidence, clinical correlates, and outcomes: a 20-year clinical experience. *Am J Kidney Dis* 24:622–629, 1994.
83. Cairns HS: Atherosclerotic renal artery stenosis (Letter). *Lancet* 340:298–299, 1992.
84. O'Neil EA, Hansen K, Canzanello V, et al: Prevalence of ischemic nephropathy in patients with renal insufficiency. *Am Surg* 58:485–490, 1992.
85. Uzu T, Inoue T, Fujii T, et al: Prevalence and predictors of renal artery stenosis in patients with myocardial infarction. *Am J Kidney Dis* 29:733–738, 1997.
86. Rimmer JM, Gennari FJ: Atherosclerotic renovascular disease and progressive renal failure. *Ann Intern Med* 118:712–719, 1993.
87. Scoble J: The epidemiology and clinical manifestations of atherosclerotic renal disease. In Novick AC, Scoble JE, Hamilton G, editors: *Renal vascular disease*, London, 1996, W. B. Saunders, pp 303–314.
88. Jean WJ, Al-Bitar I, Zwicke DL, et al: High incidence of renal artery stenosis in patients with coronary artery disease. *Cathet Cardiovasc Diagn* 32:8–10, 1994.
89. Weber-Mzell D, Kotanko P, Schumacher M, et al: Coronary anatomy predicts presence or absence of renal artery stenosis. A prospective study in patients undergoing cardiac catheterization for suspected coronary artery disease. *Eur Heart J* 23:1684–1691, 2002.
90. Harding MB, Smith LR, Himmelstein SI, et al: Renal artery stenosis: prevalence and associated risk factors in patients undergoing routine cardiac catheterization. *J Am Soc Nephrol* 2:1608–1616, 1992.
91. Vetrovec GW, Landwehr DM, Edwards VI: Incidence of renal artery stenosis in hypertensive patients undergoing coronary angiography. *J Interven Cardiol* 2:69–76, 1989.
92. Valentine R, Myers S, Miller G, et al: Detection of unsuspected renal artery stenoses in patients with abdominal aortic aneurysms: refined indicatns for preoperative aortography. *Ann Vasc Surg* 7:220–224, 1993.
93. Olin J, Melia M, Young J, et al: Prevalence of atherosclerosis renal artery stenosis in patients with atherosclerosis elsewhere. *Am J Med* 88:46N–51N, 1990.
94. Chobanian AV, Bakris GL, Black HR, et al: Seventh report of the Joint National Committee on Prevention, Detection, Evaluation, and Treatment of High Blood Pressure. *Hypertension* 42:1206–1252, 2003.
95. Hirsch AT, Haskal ZJ, Hertzer NR, et al: ACC/AHA 2005 Practice Guidelines for the management of patients with peripheral arterial disease (lower extremity, renal, mesenteric, and abdominal aortic): a collaborative report from the American Association for Vascular Surgery/Society for Vascular Surgery, Society for Cardiovascular Angiography and Interventions, Society for Vascular Medicine and Biology, Society of Interventional Radiology, and the ACC/AHA Task Force on Practice Guidelines (Writing Committee to Develop Guidelines for the Management of Patients With Peripheral Arterial Disease): endorsed by the American Association of Cardiovascular and Pulmonary Rehabilitation; National Heart, Lung, and Blood Institute; Society for Vascular Nursing; TransAtlantic Inter-Society Consensus; and Vascular Disease Foundation. *Circulation* 113:e463–e654, 2006.
96. Cooper CJ, Murphy TP, Cutlip DE, et al: Stenting and medical therapy for atherosclerotic renal-artery stenosis. *N Engl J Med* 2013.
97. Safian RD, Textor SC: Renal-artery stenosis. *N Engl J Med* 344:431–442, 2001.
98. Textor SC, Lerman L, McKusick M: The uncertain value of renal artery interventions: where are we now? *JACC Cardiovasc Interv* 2:175–182, 2009.
99. Foley RN, Collins AJ: End-stage renal disease in the United States: an update from the United States Renal Data System. *J Am Soc Nephrol* 18:2644–2648, 2007.
100. Harden P, MacLeod M, Rodger R, et al: Effect of renal artery stenting on progression of renovascular renal failure. *Lancet* 349:1133–1136, 1997.
101. Watson P, Hadjipetrou P, Cox S, et al: Effect of renal artery stenting on renal function and size in patients with atherosclerotic renovascular disease. *Circulation* 102:1671–1677, 2000.
102. Muray S, Martin M, Amoedo M, et al: Rapid decline in renal function reflects reversibility and predicts the outcome after angioplasty in renal artery stenosis. *Am J Kidney Dis* 39:60–66, 2002.
103. Beutler JJ, Van Ampting JM, Van De Ven PJ, et al: Long-term effects of arterial stenting on kidney function for patients with ostial atherosclerotic renal artery stenosis and renal insufficiency. *J Am Soc Nephrol* 12:1475–1481, 2001.
104. Dejani H, Eisen TD, Finkelstein FO: Revascularization of renal artery stenosis in patients with renal insufficiency. *Am J Kidney Dis* 36:752–758, 2000.
105. Textor SC: Ischemic nephropathy: where are we now? *J Am Soc Nephrol* 15:1974–1982, 2004.
106. Bax L, Algra A, Mali WP, et al: Renal function as a risk indicator for cardiovascular events in 3216 patients with manifest arterial disease. *Atherosclerosis* 200:184–190, 2008.
107. Wheatley K, Ives N, Gray R, et al: Revascularization versus medical therapy for renal-artery stenosis. *N Engl J Med* 361:1953–1962, 2009.
108. Kalra PA, Chrysochou C, Green D, et al: The benefit of renal artery stenting in patients with atheromatous renovascular disease and advanced chronic kidney disease. *Catheter Cardiovasc Interv* 75:1–10, 2010.
109. Chrysochou C, Cheung CM, Durow M, et al: Proteinuria as a predictor of renal functional outcome after revascularization in atherosclerotic renovascular disease (ARVD). *QJM* 102:283–288, 2009.
110. Rivolta R, Bazzi C, Stradiotti P, et al: Stenting of renal artery stenosis: is it beneficial in chronic renal failure? *J Nephrol* 18:749–754, 2005.
111. Messerli FH, Bangalore S, Makani H, et al: Flash pulmonary oedema and bilateral renal artery stenosis: the Pickering syndrome. *Eur Heart J* 2011.
112. Khosla S, White CJ, Collins TJ, et al: Effects of renal artery stent implantation in patients with renovascular hypertension presenting with unstable angina or congestive heart failure. *Am J Cardiol* 80:363–366, 1997.
113. Gray BH, Olin JW, Childs MB, et al: Clinical benefit of renal artery angioplasty with stenting for the control of recurrent and refractory congestive heart failure. *Vasc Med* 7:275–279, 2002.

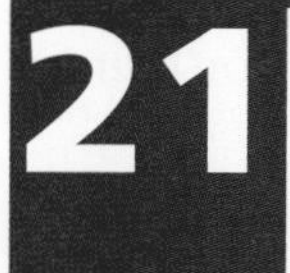

Mesenteric Artery Intervention: Catheter-Based Therapy for Chronic Mesenteric Ischemia

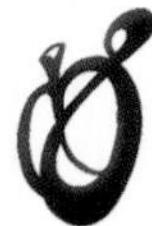

Christopher J. White

INTRODUCTION

Prevalence

The prevalence of mesenteric arterial stenoses is much more common than is the clinical manifestation of chronic mesenteric ischemia (CMI), likely due to the rich vascular communication among the three mesenteric vessels. CMI is twice as common in women than men. Asymptomatic mesenteric stenosis was documented angiographically in 40% of patients with an abdominal aortic aneurysm, 29% with aortoiliac obstructive disease, and in 25% of patients with peripheral arterial disease of the lower extremities.[1] In a healthy group of elderly individuals (>65 years) ultrasound imaging found a 17.5% prevalence of asymptomatic (>70%) stenosis of at least one mesenteric artery.[2] Symptomatic CMI is uncommon, accounting for less than 2% of all atheromatous revascularization procedures,[3] and it is usually the consequence of atherosclerotic disease involving aorto-ostial stenosis of the celiac, superior mesenteric, and/or inferior mesenteric arteries often in the context of concomitant atherosclerotic disease of the aorta.

Etiology

Classical teaching suggests that CMI occurs when only one of three mesenteric arteries (celiac, superior mesenteric, and inferior mesenteric) remains patent due to the rich collateral supply and the most commonly intervened on vessel is the superior mesenteric artery. Causes of CMI include vascular conditions such as fibromuscular dysplasia, Takayasu disease, Buerger disease, radiation and autoimmune arteritis, and aortic dissection, but atherosclerosis is the predominant (>95%) cause of clinical mesenteric arterial stenosis.[4] The median arcuate syndrome, also called the celiac axis compression syndrome, can occur if the origin of the celiac trunk arising from the aorta is extrinsically compressed by the arcuate ligament of the diaphragm. This can cause significant, sometimes critical, stenosis of this vessel.[5]

Natural History

The natural history of asymptomatic mesenteric artery stenosis is that clinical symptoms do not develop in the majority of patients.[6] Abdominal angiography was performed in 980 patients, demonstrating >50% stenosis of at least one mesenteric artery in 82 patients. After 2.6 years of follow-up, CMI developed in only 4 (4.9%) of the 82 patients, and these individuals all had involvement of all three mesenteric arteries.[7]

The natural history of patients with symptomatic CMI is that between 20% and 50% of patients will progress to develop acute mesenteric ischemia.[8] The remaining patients continue to suffer chronic postprandial abdominal pain, weight loss, and emaciation.

DIAGNOSIS

Clinical Presentation

The classical symptoms of CMI include abdominal pain triggered by food ingestion and accompanied by significant unexplained weight loss (**Table 21-1**). The abdominal pain is often periumbilical and described as dull aching or sometimes as "crampy" and begins within 1 hour after food ingestion and subsides 1 to 2 hours later. Many patients develop a "fear of food" and decrease their caloric intake, resulting in unintended weight loss. It is not unusual for patients with classic CMI to present with a 20- to 40-pound weight loss. Significant weight loss often helps to differentiate patients with functional bowel symptoms from those with CMI.

Ischemic gastropathy, ischemic colitis, and malabsorption are less common manifestations of CMI. Ischemic gastropathy usually manifests as nausea, vomiting, fullness, right upper quadrant discomfort, abdominal pain, and weight loss. Ischemic colitis presents with abdominal pain, gastrointestinal bleeding, and/or hematochezia.[9] The diagnosis may be delayed as patients may be referred for a malignancy evaluation for weight loss. However, evidence of significant stenosis of two or more mesenteric vessels in conjunction with endoscopic findings of bowel ischemia should prompt the diagnosis.[10] CMI may occur in single mesenteric artery disease particularly after surgery if mesenteric collaterals have been disrupted.

CMI often masquerades as a severe functional bowel syndrome. In a series of 59 patients with CMI from the Ochsner Clinic a typical presentation was found in 78%, with

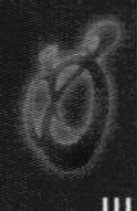

the remainder presenting with ischemic gastropathy or ischemic colitis in the remaining 22% of patients.[11] The diagnosis of CMI is based upon symptoms of bowel ischemia in the presence of hemodynamically significant stenoses in more than one mesenteric artery. Due to the difficulty in making this diagnosis, a multidisciplinary team approach is encouraged. On physical examination patients with CMI may have an abdominal bruit localized in the epigastrium, and they may have other signs of peripheral vascular disease.

Imaging

Duplex ultrasonography, as well as cross-sectional imaging with computed tomographic angiography (CTA), and magnetic resonance angiography (MRA), are adequate to establish the presence of mesenteric arterial stenosis.[12-17]

Invasive angiography remains the gold standard for visualizing the mesenteric arterial tree. Visualization of the mesenteric vessels requires a lateral aortogram (**Figure 21-1**). The anterior-posterior aortogram may reveal the arc of Riolan, an engorged collateral connecting the inferior mesenteric artery (IMA) to the superior mesenteric artery (SMA) and indicative of proximal mesenteric artery disease. Invasive angiography is used less frequently for screening, but is recommended for patients with an inconclusive noninvasive imaging study or in whom revascularization therapy is being considered.

TABLE 21-1 Most Frequent Symptoms of Chronic Mesenteric Ischemia

Typical symptoms	78%
Post-prandial abdominal pain	
Fear of food	
Weight loss (>20 pounds)	
Ischemic gastropathy	14%
Nausea, vomiting	
Fullness	
Abdominal pain	
Right upper quadrant discomfort	
Weight loss	
Ischemic colitis	8%
Abdominal pain	
Gastrointestinal bleeding	
Hematochezia	

MANAGEMENT OF CHRONIC MESENTERIC ISCHEMIA

Medical Therapy

Patients with asymptomatic CMI should be treated as other patients with atherosclerotic vascular disease with aggressive multimodality therapy to treat risk factors including lipid-lowering therapy with a statin drug, smoking cessation, blood pressure control, diabetes control, and treated with aspirin antiplatelet therapy. In addition, treatment with digoxin should be avoided due to the detrimental actions of digoxin in the splanchnic circulation causing vasoconstriction and ischemia.[18]

Current guideline recommendations are that patients with symptomatic CMI should be evaluated for revascularization.[19] Without revascularization they will have progression of their disease and risk the development of acute myocardial infarction (AMI), inanition, and death.

Catheter-Based Endovascular Therapy

Catheter-based endovascular revascularization techniques are preferred to open surgery due to their lower procedural morbidity (**Figure 21-2**). Endovascular therapies may be repeated if necessary, generally without increased patient risk compared with the first procedure, and prior angioplasty does not preclude surgery if required at a later date.

The aorto-ostial location of the stenoses, as is the case for renal artery stenoses, is the most common cause of CMI, and is difficult to treat with balloon angioplasty alone due to elastic recoil. Scaffolding the lesion with a stent defeats this recoil resulting in a larger lumen diameter and higher procedural success rate than for balloon dilation alone (**Figure 21-3**) (Videos 21-1 and 21-2).[11,21-24] The results of primary stent placement for CMI in 59 patients (79 vessels) yielded a procedural success rate of 96%, with symptom relief in 88%.[11] At a mean follow-up of 38 ± 15 months, 17% had a recurrence of symptoms but none developed acute

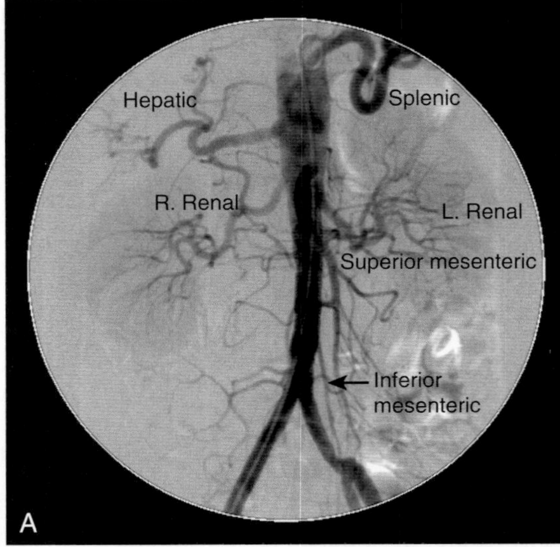

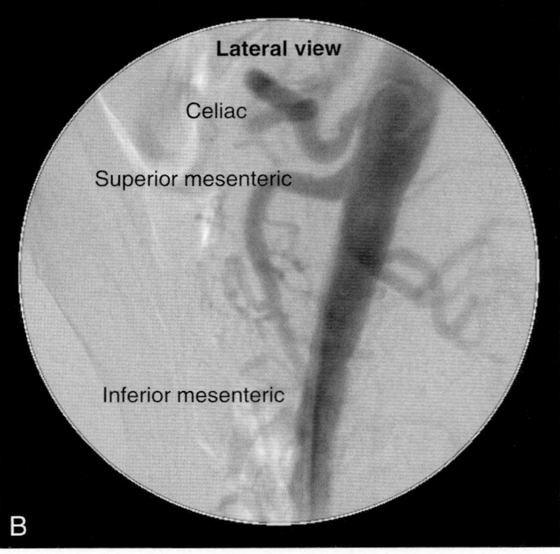

FIGURE 21-1 **A,** Antero-posterior abdominal aortic angiogram showing branches. **B,** Lateral abdominal aortic angiogram showing mesenteric branches.

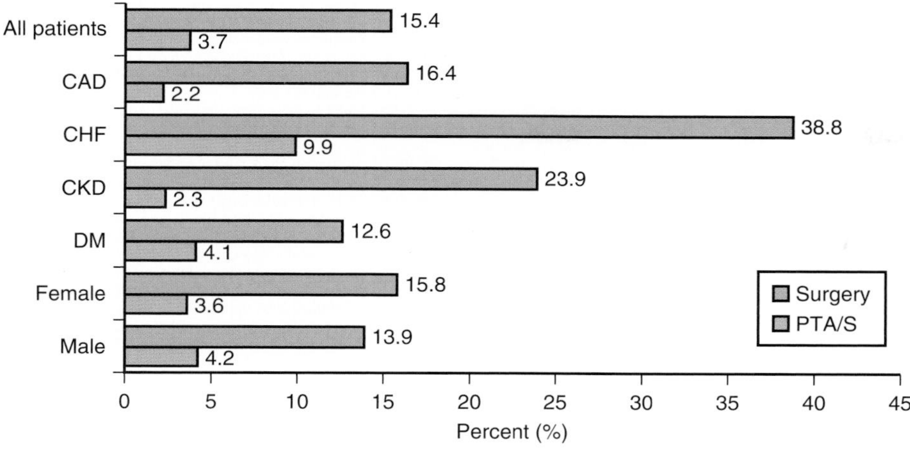

FIGURE 21-2 Bar graph of mortality rates for surgery and endovascular treatment of CMI. *(From the National Inpatient Sample database. Schermerhorn ML, Giles KA, Hamdan AD, et al: Mesenteric revascularization: management and outcomes in the United States, 1988–2006. J Vasc Surg 50:341–348.e1, 2009.[20])*

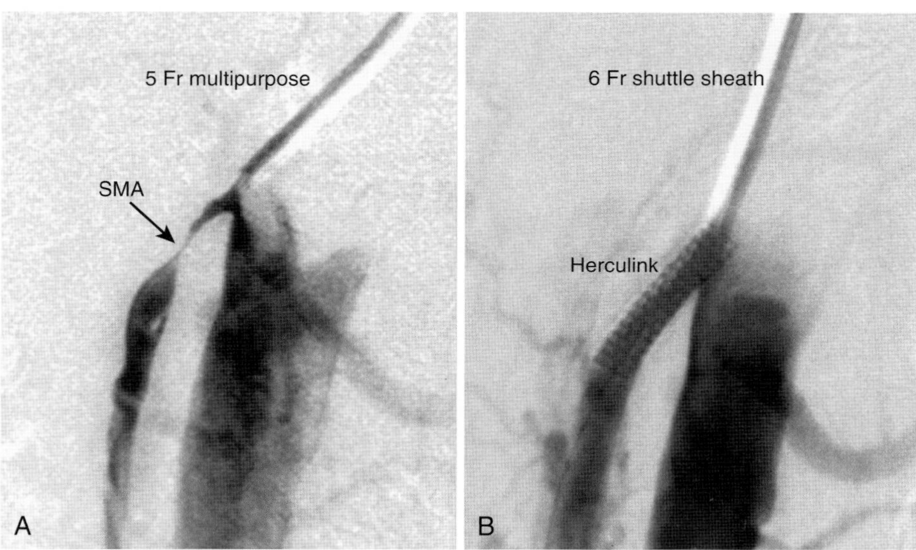

FIGURE 21-3 **A,** Baseline lateral angiogram of tight superior mesenteric artery (SMA) stenosis. **B,** Angiogram following successful balloon expandable stent placement.

mesenteric ischemia and all underwent successful repeat revascularization without complication. Many of the same techniques in terms of guide catheter selection and manipulation for renal artery stenting are applicable to mesenteric artery intervention.

There are no clinical trials directly comparing surgical versus catheter-based revascularization strategies for CMI. Because patients with CMI have systemic atherosclerosis and are malnourished, they frequently have increased risk for surgical complications. It is not surprising that surgical revascularization carries high periprocedural morbidity (~45%) and mortality rates (~15%).[25] Whether patients who survive surgery have higher patency rates and symptom-free survival than patients treated with stent revascularization is controversial.[25,26]

The results of percutaneous revascularization have prompted several investigators to advocate the use of this strategy as the treatment of choice for patients with CMI, or as a bridging procedure for further surgical revascularization in patients who develop recurrence of symptoms after percutaneous treatment once the surgical risk has been decreased.[27] The complications of endovascular therapy are usually related to vascular access and they include hematomas, pseudoaneurysms, abrupt occlusion, and retroperitoneal bleeding.

Surgical Therapy

A variety of surgical techniques for mesenteric revascularization have reported early success rates of 91% to 96% and late success rates between 80% and 90%. In **Figure 21-1**, the mortality outcomes of surgical studies are summarized, showing a periprocedural mortality rate as high as 29%.[28]

Post-procedure Management and Follow-up

Follow-up evaluation at 1, 3, 6, and 12 months with mesenteric artery duplex ultrasound is advisable to evaluate continued patency. Any recurrence of symptoms should prompt investigation for recurrent stenosis. Restenosis by duplex does not always correlate with recurrence of symptoms.[29] Doppler ultrasound (duplex) is the standard modality used by most centers,[3] but the advent of CTA and MRA may provide alternative modalities for follow-up in the future.[16]

CONCLUSIONS

The infrequent occurrence of CMI has made randomized control trials comparing treatment outcomes very difficult to perform. Case series have shown that percutaneous therapy with stent placement offers the lowest morbidity and roughly equivalent long-term outcomes when compared with surgery. The current treatment recommendation is that patients who are candidates for either surgery or percutaneous therapy should receive percutaneous therapy with primary stent placement, analogous to ostial renal artery stenting.

References

1. Valentine RJ, Martin JD, Myers SI, et al: Asymptomatic celiac and superior mesenteric artery stenoses are more prevalent among patients with unsuspected renal artery stenoses. *J Vasc Surg* 14:195–199, 1991.
2. Hansen KJ, Wilson DB, Craven TE, et al: Mesenteric artery disease in the elderly. *J Vasc Surg* 40:45–52, 2004.
3. Kougias P, Kappa JR, Sewell DH, et al: Simultaneous carotid endarterectomy and coronary artery bypass grafting: results in specific patient groups. *Ann Vasc Surg* 21:408–414, 2007.
4. Harris MT, Lewis BS: Systemic diseases affecting the mesenteric circulation. *Surg Clin North Am* 72:245–259, 1992.
5. Bech FR: Celiac artery compression syndromes. *Surg Clin North Am* 77:409–424, 1997.
6. van Bockel JH, Geelkerken RH, Wasser MN: Chronic splanchnic ischaemia. *Best Pract Res Clin Gastroenterol* 15:99–119, 2001.
7. Thomas JH, Blake K, Pierce GE, et al: The clinical course of asymptomatic mesenteric arterial stenosis. *J Vasc Surg* 27:840–844, 1998.
8. Stoney RJ, Cunningham CG: Acute mesenteric ischemia. *Surgery* 114:489–490, 1993.
9. Cappell MS: Intestinal (mesenteric) vasculopathy. II. Ischemic colitis and chronic mesenteric ischemia. *Gastroenterol Clin North Am* 27:827–860, vi, 1998.
10. Matsumoto AH, Tegtmeyer CJ, Fitzcharles EK, et al: Percutaneous transluminal angioplasty of visceral arterial stenoses: results and long-term clinical follow-up. *J Vasc Interv Radiol* 6:165–174, 1995.
11. Silva JA, White CJ, Collins TJ, et al: Endovascular therapy for chronic mesenteric ischemia. *J Am Coll Cardiol* 47:944–950, 2006.
12. Bowersox JC, Zwolak RM, Walsh DB, et al: Duplex ultrasonography in the diagnosis of celiac and mesenteric artery occlusive disease. *J Vasc Surg* 14:780–786, discussion 786–788, 1991.
13. Zwolak RM, Fillinger MF, Walsh DB, et al: Mesenteric and celiac duplex scanning: a validation study. *J Vasc Surg* 27:1078–1087, discussion 1088, 1998.
14. Chow LC, Chan FP, Li KC: A comprehensive approach to MR imaging of mesenteric ischemia. *Abdom Imaging* 27:507–516, 2002.
15. Geelkerken RH, van Bockel JH: Duplex ultrasound examination of splanchnic vessels in the assessment of splanchnic ischaemic symptoms. *Eur J Vasc Endovasc Surg* 18:371–374, 1999.
16. Shih MC, Hagspiel KD: CTA and MRA in mesenteric ischemia: part 1, role in diagnosis and differential diagnosis. *AJR Am J Roentgenol* 188:452–461, 2007.
17. Shih MC, Angle JF, Leung DA, et al: CTA and MRA in mesenteric ischemia: part 2, normal findings and complications after surgical and endovascular treatment. *AJR Am J Roentgenol* 188:462–471, 2007.
18. Kim EH, Gewertz BL: Chronic digitalis administration alters mesenteric vascular reactivity. *J Vasc Surg* 5:382–389, 1987.
19. Hirsch AT, Haskal ZJ, Hertzer NR, et al: ACC/AHA 2005 guidelines for the management of patients with peripheral arterial disease (lower extremity, renal, mesenteric, and abdominal aortic): executive summary a collaborative report from the American Association for Vascular Surgery/Society for Vascular Surgery, Society for Cardiovascular Angiography and Interventions, Society for Vascular Medicine and Biology, Society of Interventional Radiology, and the ACC/AHA Task Force on Practice Guidelines (Writing Committee to Develop Guidelines for the Management of Patients With Peripheral Arterial Disease) endorsed by the American Association of Cardiovascular and Pulmonary Rehabilitation; National Heart, Lung, and Blood Institute; Society for Vascular Nursing; TransAtlantic Inter-Society Consensus; and Vascular Disease Foundation. *J Am Coll Cardiol* 47:1239–1312, 2006.
20. Schermerhorn ML, Giles KA, Hamdan AD, et al: Mesenteric revascularization: management and outcomes in the United States, 1988-2006. *J Vasc Surg* 50:341–348.e1, 2009.
21. Sheeran SR, Murphy TP, Khwaja A, et al: Stent placement for treatment of mesenteric artery stenoses or occlusions. *J Vasc Interv Radiol* 10:861–867, 1999.
22. Sharafuddin MJ, Olson CH, Sun S, et al: Endovascular treatment of celiac and mesenteric arteries stenoses: applications and results. *J Vasc Surg* 38:692–698, 2003.
23. AbuRahma AF, Stone PA, Bates MC, et al: Angioplasty/stenting of the superior mesenteric artery and celiac trunk: early and late outcomes. *J Endovasc Ther* 10:1046–1053, 2003.
24. Resch T, Lindh M, Dias N, et al: Endovascular recanalisation in occlusive mesenteric ischemia–feasibility and early results. *Eur J Vasc Endovasc Surg* 29:199–203, 2005.
25. Kasirajan K, O'Hara PJ, Gray BH, et al: Chronic mesenteric ischemia: open surgery versus percutaneous angioplasty and stenting. *J Vasc Surg* 33:63–71, 2001.
26. Sivamurthy N, Rhodes JM, Lee D, et al: Endovascular versus open mesenteric revascularization: immediate benefits do not equate with short-term functional outcomes. *J Am Coll Surg* 202:859–867, 2006.
27. Brown DJ, Schermerhorn ML, Powell RJ, et al: Mesenteric stenting for chronic mesenteric ischemia. *J Vasc Surg* 42:268–274, 2005.
28. Derrow AE, Seeger JM, Dame DA, et al: The outcome in the United States after thoracoabdominal aortic aneurysm repair, renal artery bypass, and mesenteric revascularization. *J Vasc Surg* 34:54–61, 2001.
29. Fenwick JL, Wright IA, Buckenham TM: Endovascular repair of chronic mesenteric occlusive disease: the role of duplex surveillance. *ANZ J Surg* 77:60–63, 2007.

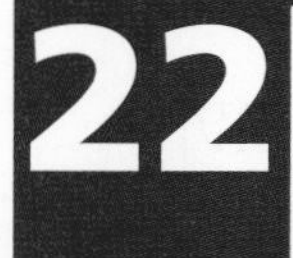

Renal Denervation

Stefan C. Bertog, Laura Vaskelyte, Todd Drexel, Ilona Hofmann, Dani Id, Sameer Gafoor, Markus Reinartz, and Horst Sievert

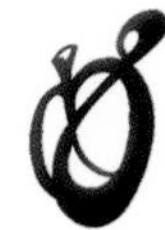

INTRODUCTION

Hypertension is a leading cause of death worldwide, with 13% of all deaths attributed to it in 2004 (World Health Organization, 2009). A prevalence of 29% (1.56 billion) has been predicted for 2025.[1] In the United States, approximately 65 million individuals have hypertension.[2] It is associated with cardiovascular and cerebrovascular morbidity and mortality with a direct relationship of blood pressure and event risk.[3] Antihypertensive therapy has been shown to reduce strokes, heart attacks, and cardiovascular deaths.[4,5] However, some patients' blood pressures remain in a suboptimal range despite multi-drug antihypertensive therapy. If the blood pressure remains below target despite ≥3 antihypertensive medications of different classes, one of which optimally should be a diuretic, or requires ≥4 antihypertensive medications for adequate control, it is generally considered to be "resistant."[6] The reported prevalence of resistant hypertension varies widely depending on definitions used and populations studied. In some nonpopulation-based tertiary referral studies[7] and clinical trials,[8-10] the prevalence ranges between 12% and 34%. In population-based studies, the reported prevalence is lower. For example, in the National Health and Nutrition Examination Surveys (NHANES) it was 9%[11] and, in a population study from northern California and Colorado, 2%.[12] Risk factors for developing resistant hypertension include male gender, age, diabetes, obesity, chronic kidney disease, and Framingham 10-year coronary risk >20%.[12,13] Importantly, patients with resistant hypertension have a higher risk for cardiovascular events.[12] The sympathetic nervous system plays a substantial role in development and maintenance of resistant hypertension and has recently been the target of catheter-based intervention. In this context, the physiology of the renal sympathetic nervous system, the role in hypertension, and the effects and techniques of interrupting the renal sympathetic nervous system are discussed.

ROLE OF THE KIDNEY IN HYPERTENSION

Before reviewing the specifics of the renal sympathetic nervous system in blood pressure regulation, an important concept should be mentioned first: Kidneys have a dominant role in blood pressure control.[14] This has been shown by kidney cross-transplantation. When kidneys from hypertensive rats are removed and implanted into normotensive rats and vice versa, normotensive rats become hypertensive and hypertensive rats normotensive.[15] It is, therefore, the kidney and not the host that primarily determines blood pressure. The kidneys' ability to regulate blood pressure can take place (regardless of external influences) by the principle of pressure natriuresis. It is the ability to conserve or excrete sodium and water to an extent that maintains blood pressure at an intrinsic goal unique to the kidney. In support of this concept, when kidneys are isolated from external influences by denervation, bilateral adrenalectomy, and continuous infusion of high doses of catecholamines and glucocorticoids, cross clamping the aorta (thereby increasing perfusion pressure of the kidneys) causes pronounced natriuresis and diuresis.[16,17] Hence, the kidneys largely determine blood pressure by maintaining an intrinsic blood pressure goal by pressure natriuresis. Though this can be achieved in the absence of external influences, external signals can change the intrinsic blood pressure goal. One such signal comes from the renal sympathetic nervous system.

ANATOMY AND PHYSIOLOGY OF THE RENAL SYMPATHETIC NERVOUS SYSTEM

Every component of the kidney is supplied by *efferent* sympathetic nerve fibers.[18-21] Equally important, the kidneys send signals to the central nervous system via *afferent* sympathetic fibers.

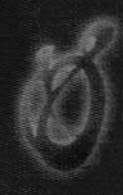

FIGURE 22-1 Illustration of the anatomy of the efferent renal sympathetic nervous system (for description, see text). *JGA,* Juxtaglomerular apparatus; *NTS,* solitary tract nucleus; *RVLM,* rostroventrolateral medulla; *VLN,* ventrolateral nucleus of the hypothalamus.

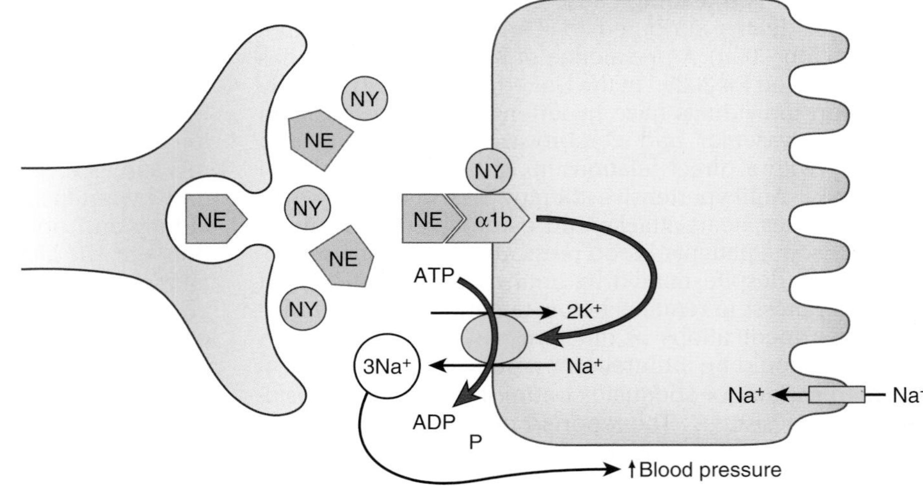

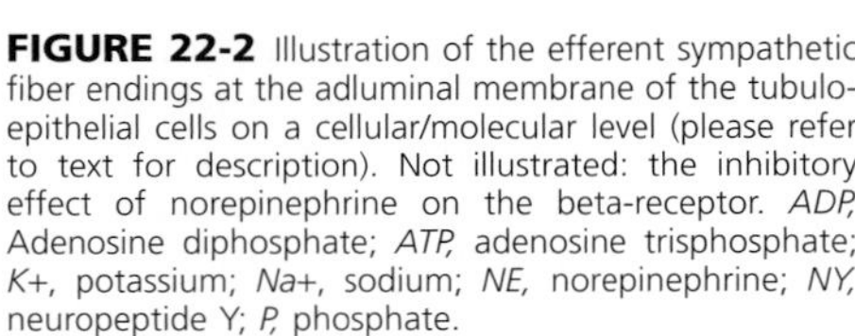

FIGURE 22-2 Illustration of the efferent sympathetic fiber endings at the adluminal membrane of the tubulo-epithelial cells on a cellular/molecular level (please refer to text for description). Not illustrated: the inhibitory effect of norepinephrine on the beta-receptor. *ADP,* Adenosine diphosphate; *ATP,* adenosine trisphosphate; *K+,* potassium; *Na+,* sodium; *NE,* norepinephrine; *NY,* neuropeptide Y; *P,* phosphate.

Efferent Fibers (Figure 22-1)

Signals from the central nervous system (amygdala, ventrolateral nucleus of the hypothalamus, cortex, pons) and chemo- and baroreceptors are integrated in the medulla oblongata (solitary tract nucleus and rostral ventral medulla oblongata) from where sympathetic nerve fibers course within the spinal cord to the intermediolateral nucleus (Th10-L2).[22] In the intermediolateral nucleus, signals are relayed to presynaptic fibers that exit the spinal cord and terminate at postsynaptic fibers in the celiac, superior, and inferior mesenteric ganglion. Postsynaptic fibers (located predominantly within the adventitia of the renal arteries) supply the tubuloepithelial cells, granular cells of the juxtaglomerular apparatus, and arteriolar smooth muscle cells. Norepinephrine and neuropeptide Y are released (**Figure 22-2**). Norepinephrine binds to both alpha-1b receptors and beta-receptors (located in the adluminal membrane of the tubuloepithelial cells[23,24]) causing stimulation[25] and inhibition[26] of the sodium/potassium ATPase, respectively, with an overall neutral effect. However, neuropeptide Y enhances the stimulatory effect of norepinephrine.[26] The net effect is a stimulation of the sodium/potassium ATPase causing sodium and water retention and a blood pressure increase. At the granular cells of the juxtaglomerular apparatus, norepinephrine binds to beta-1 receptors, causing G-protein-coupled activation of adenyl cyclase, generating cyclic AMP that stimulates renin release (**Figure 22-3**).[27] Renin causes activation of the renin angiotensin system,

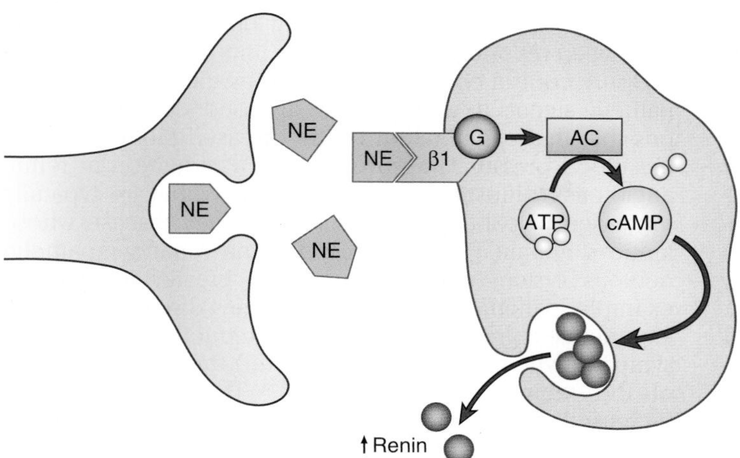

FIGURE 22-3 Illustration of the efferent sympathetic nerve fiber endings at the juxtaglomerular apparatus on a cellular/molecular level (please refer to text for description). *AC,* Adenylcyclase; *ATP,* adenosine trisphosphate; *cAMP,* cyclic adenosine monophosphate; *G,* G-protein; *NE,* norepinephrine.

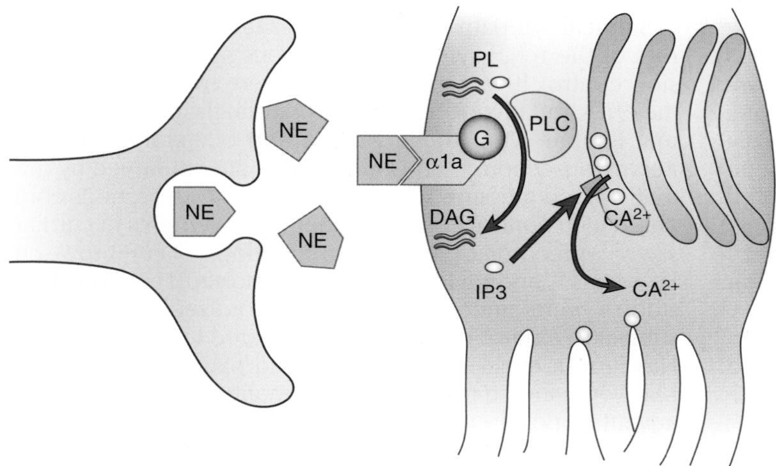

FIGURE 22-4 Illustration of the efferent sympathetic nerve fiber ending at the renal arterioles on a cellular/molecular level (see text for description). *Ca^{2+},* Calcium; *DAG,* diacylglycerol; *G,* G-protein; *IP3,* inositol trisphosphate; *NE,* norepinephrine; *PL,* phospholipid; *PLC,* phospholipase C.

generating angiotensin II and aldosterone and causing vasoconstriction and sodium and water retention, respectively, with subsequent blood pressure increase.[28] Hormones of the angiotensin-aldosterone system also cause vascular remodeling[28,29] and changes in cardiac architecture such as left ventricular hypertrophy and fibrosis.[30] At arteriolar smooth muscle cells, norepinephrine binds to alpha-1a receptors and (via G-protein-coupled mechanism) activates phospholipase C, releasing inositol trisphosphate and diacylglycerol (**Figure 22-4**).[31] Inositol trisphosphate stimulates calcium release from the sarcoplasmic reticulum that binds to the contractile apparatus, triggering smooth muscle contraction and vasoconstriction.[32]

Afferent Fibers

Renal afferent nerve fiber endings are most abundant within the renal pelvis. Mechano- and chemoreceptors stimulate the renal afferent nervous system.[33] Mechanoreceptors provide feedback on hydrostatic pressure within the renal pelvis, arteries, and veins. Chemoreceptors are a gauge for the renal interstitial milieu and are activated by mediators released during renal parenchymal ischemia. Signals are relayed from the kidney via afferent sympathetic fibers with nuclei located in the dorsal root ganglia to the ipsilateral posterior gray column (lamina I-III). The neurotransmitters are substance P– and calcitonin gene–related peptide. Signals are then further transmitted from the spinal cord to central nervous system autonomic centers (paraventricular nucleus of the hypothalamus and solitary tract nucleus in the brainstem) and to the contralateral kidney.[34,35] Autonomic center stimulation, in turn, increases the overall sympathetic tone causing vasoconstriction, fluid retention, and, consequently, blood pressure increase. Stimulation of the contralateral kidney alters the sodium and water balance (renorenal reflex). The impact of renal afferent sympathetic nervous stimulation on blood pressure has been shown in animal studies that target activation or inhibition of afferent fibers. Renal injury in rats by toxin injection or ischemia results in activation of the afferent sympathetic fibers causing an increase in overall sympathetic nervous system activity and blood pressure that can be attenuated or prevented by prior dorsal rhizotomy (transection of the dorsal roots—the equivalent to interruption of the afferent sympathetic pathway).[36-38] Likewise, a blood pressure reduction has been shown in renal insufficiency rat models after dorsal rhizotomy. In this model, the hypertensive response after near total nephrectomy is less pronounced if these animals have first undergone dorsal (Th10-L2) rhizotomy.[39]

ANIMAL AND HUMAN DATA SUPPORTING A LINK BETWEEN THE RENAL SYMPATHETIC NERVOUS SYSTEM AND HYPERTENSION

Several pivotal animal experiments, in addition to those previously described, warrant mention. Direct stimulation of the splanchnic nerve in a dog model causes a blood pressure increase,[40] whereas interruption of the renal sympathetic fibers (by removal and re-implantation of the kidneys) causes diuresis and blood pressure reduction. Similarly, splanchnic nerve transection causes natriuresis and diuresis.[41] An increase in blood pressure seen in the Goldblatt model of a single kidney supplied by a stenotic artery or in the Goldblatt two kidneys, one clip model (only one of the renal arteries has a stenosis in this model), can be attenuated by denervation of the clipped renal artery.[37] Hypertension in a rat model caused by renal injury, for example, by intrarenal phenol injection, can be attenuated by renal sympathetic denervation.[36] Comparison of genetically spontaneous hypertensive rats with genetically normotensive rats identified increased renal sympathetic nerve activity in the hypertensive rats.[42] Renal denervation in spontaneous hypertensive rats was shown to delay the onset of hypertension and to mitigate the hypertensive response.[43] It is noteworthy that hypertension returned to spontaneously hypertensive because of re-innervation of renal sympathetic nerves but was again attenuated by repeat denervation.[44] Renal denervation in other animal hypertensive models, including other rats, dogs, pigs, and rabbits, has also been shown to prevent or delay the development of hypertension and diminish the severity of hypertension.[45]

In humans, the sympathetic nervous system has been shown to play an important role in the pathogenesis and maintenance of hypertension. Increased plasma catecholamine levels have been shown in borderline hypertension[46] and in young patients with hypertension.[47] However, the plasma catecholamine concentrations are not universally elevated. Particularly in older hypertensive patients, levels similar to normotensive individuals have been reported.[48] Plasma catecholamine concentrations depend not only on its release at the nerve terminals but also on metabolism and reuptake. In addition, differences in sympathetic nerve activity between end organs have been demonstrated[49,50]; therefore, it may not consistently reflect overall and regional sympathetic nervous system activity. Instead, muscle sympathetic nervous system activity and norepinephrine spillover measurements are more reliable indicators of overall and regional sympathetic tone. In this context, compared with normotensive individuals, higher muscle sympathetic nerve activity and reduced norepinephrine reuptake have been described in hypertensive patients.[48,50-52] Increased sympathetic nerve activity has also been identified in individuals with secondary hypertension related to renal artery stenosis, obesity, and obstructive sleep apnea.[53-55]

The consequences of interrupting the renal sympathetic nervous system on blood pressure have also been demonstrated in humans. The increased sympathetic tone in patients with chronic kidney disease requiring dialysis normalizes following bilateral nephrectomy.[56] The increased sympathetic activity persists following kidney transplant if the native kidneys remain.[57] Blood pressure reductions following nephrectomy in patients with kidney disease including those with unilateral disease and single nephrectomy (e.g., for pyelonephritis or congenital hypoplasia)[58-60] and in patients with bilateral disease and bilateral nephrectomy have been reported.[61,62] Though the improvements in blood pressure control could be explained by elimination of sympathetic signals to and from the diseased kidneys, it is also possible that explantation of the diseased kidneys causes the blood pressure improvement by a reduction in renin-angiotensin-aldosterone system activity that is typically increased in patients with chronic kidney disease whose kidneys remain in place. However, the renal sympathetic nervous system appears to have a greater impact. For example, patients with chronic kidney disease generally experience a greater blood pressure reduction with central sympatholytic therapy (e.g., clonidine) than with blockade of the renin-angiotensin system.[63] The mechanism for increased renal sympathetic activity is unclear but could be related to renal ischemia as sympathetic nervous system activity decreases following angioplasty in patients with renal artery stenosis.[64] Blood pressure has also been shown to improve following unilateral nephrectomy in patients with renal artery stenosis.[65]

Surgical sympathectomy provides further insight into the role of the renal sympathetic nervous system in hypertension control. It was used to treat severe hypertension until the1970s and involved resection of distal thoracic and proximal lumbar sympathetic ganglia and bilateral splanchnic nerve transection.[66,67] The surgery was accompanied by dramatic blood pressure[67-70] and mortality[67,71-73] reductions compared with control groups. Further, improvements in cardiac size,[74,75] precordial pain,[76] renal function,[74-76] cerebrovascular events,[76] and headaches[76] were reported. However, these studies were uncontrolled, nonrandomized comparisons subject to a number of limitations related to placebo effect, Hawthorne effect, selection bias, and patient and operator bias. Operative morbidity and mortality together with the advent of novel antihypertensive agents led to the discontinuation of surgical sympathectomy for the treatment of hypertension in the 1970s. Nonetheless, the results further support the importance of the renal sympathetic nervous system in the pathogenesis of hypertension and potential benefits after sympathectomy.

Percutaneous Renal Sympathetic Denervation

The aforementioned physiological and clinical observations underlining the importance of the renal sympathetic nervous system in blood pressure control and the convenient location of the sympathetic nerve fibers (predominantly in the renal artery adventitia and perivascular space) led to the concept and evaluation of catheter-based renal sympathetic denervation by radiofrequency application. The efficacy and safety were first assessed in pigs. Renal denervation using the Symplicity Flex Renal Denervation System (Medtronic Inc., Minneapolis, Minnesota) (**Figure 22-5**) was accompanied by histological evidence of neuronal injury in the perivascular space of the renal artery, as well as a reduction in sympathetic axons in the renal cortex (by tyrosine hydroxylase staining) and a 90% reduction in renal norepinephrine concentration (unpublished report by Medtronic). Optical coherence tomography (OCT) examination of the renal artery after renal denervation in a pig demonstrated endothelial denudation, transmural tissue coagulation followed by tissue fibrosis, and re-endothelialization and renal nerve necrosis 10 days after ablation.[77] Six months after ablation, histology demonstrated

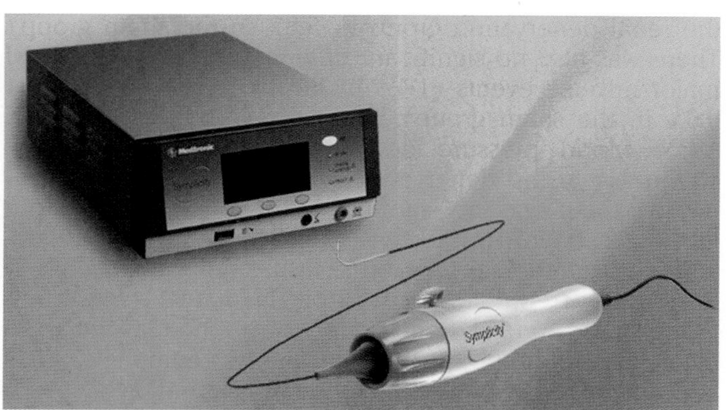

FIGURE 22-5 Image illustrating the Symplicity Flex Renal Denervation System (Medtronic Inc., St. Paul, Minn.). The generator and the Symplicity catheter are shown.

necrotic nerve fibers and fibrosis involving 10% to 25% of the media and adventitia without stenosis.[78]

In Symplicity-1, 45 patients with severe resistant hypertension underwent radiofrequency renal sympathetic denervation.[79] A significant 27/17 mm Hg 1-year office blood pressure reduction was observed. An increase in antihypertensive therapy occurred in four patients; however, a significant and pronounced blood pressure reduction remained after excluding these patients from analysis. In addition, blood pressure medications were reduced in nine patients due to improved blood pressure control. Thirteen percent of patients were considered nonresponders (defined as systolic blood pressure reduction of <10 mm Hg). Ambulatory blood pressure reductions were less pronounced (11 mm Hg systolic) than office blood pressures, a common theme in all subsequent studies examining renal denervation.

Renal and total body norepinephrine spillover decreased after renal denervation (n = 10), supporting the notion that renal denervation reduces renal and overall sympathetic nervous system activity. A reduction in overall sympathetic tone assessed by muscle sympathetic nerve activity has been demonstrated in one patient from Symplicity HTN-1[80] and subsequently in a separate study.[81] One guide catheter–induced renal artery dissection requiring stenting and one femoral artery pseudoaneurysm were reported.

In a registry including Symplicity HTN-1 patients and others, office blood pressure reductions were durable, 33/14 mm Hg at 24 months[82] and 32/14 mm Hg at 36 months (n = 87), regardless of age, diabetic status, or baseline renal function.[83] Furthermore, the responder rate increased over time from 70% at 1 month to 93% at 36 months.[83] One de novo renal artery stenosis possibly related to renal denervation requiring stenting, one renal artery stenosis at a site remote from the treatment site (with some degree of preexistent stenosis) requiring stenting, and two hemodynamically insignificant mild renal artery stenoses were reported throughout the 36-month follow-up.

In Symplicity HTN-2 (n = 106), patients with severe resistant hypertension were randomized to renal sympathetic denervation (in addition to conventional medical therapy) or conventional medical therapy alone.[84] There was a significant 32/12 mm Hg office blood pressure reduction in the denervation group versus none in the control group at 6 months with a responder rate of 84% (vs. 35% in the control group). The ambulatory pressure (11/7 mm Hg) was, once again, less pronounced than the office blood pressure reduction after renal denervation; however, it remained significant (vs. no change in the control group). There were no major adverse events. No changes in renal function or urine albumin to creatinine ratios were seen in either group. Forty-six patients from the control group crossed over to renal denervation and experienced a significant 24/8 mm Hg blood pressure reduction 6 months after cross-over.[85] In addition, a lasting 33/14 mm Hg reduction in office blood pressure has been demonstrated in those 40 patients of the initial group who underwent 36-month follow-up.[85]

Renal denervation has more recently been studied in a small number (n = 20) of patients with milder forms of resistant hypertension (systolic office blood pressure 140 to 160 mm Hg) with significant 13/5 mm Hg office and 11/4 mm Hg ambulatory blood pressure reductions at 6 months.[86] Similar findings were reported subsequently in 54 patients with mild resistant hypertension with 13/7 mm Hg and 14/7 mm Hg office and ambulatory blood pressure reductions at 6 months.[87] Therefore, it appears that hypertension severity predicts the magnitude of response.

Limitations

All limitations that accompany unblinded studies without a control group including selection and observer bias, placebo effect, and Hawthorne effect apply to Symplicity HTN-1, and the same limitations, with the exception of selection bias, apply to Symplicity HTN-2. In addition, given inclusion of patients into the study based on systolic office blood pressure and comparison of follow-up blood pressure with the blood pressure used for inclusion, regression to the mean may lead to overestimation of the treatment effect. Though it does not eliminate regression to the mean, comparison of ambulatory blood pressures before and after treatment attenuates (but does not completely eliminate) the consequences of this statistical phenomenon. It is, therefore, not surprising that ambulatory blood pressure effects are invariably lower than office blood pressure effects unless measures are taken to prevent regression to the mean.

Any injury to the renal artery as it occurs with radiofrequency or ultrasound energy application may, in addition to the intraprocedural risk of renal artery dissection or thrombus formation with or without embolization, lead to renal artery stenosis. In this context, pulmonary vein stenosis has been reported after radiofrequency application for the purpose of pulmonary vein isolation in patients with atrial fibrillation.[88] However, the radiofrequency energy used for renal denervation (e.g., 8 W with the Symplicity Renal Denervation System) is lower than for pulmonary vein isolation (up to 30 W). In studies with imaging follow-up, renal artery stenosis has been a rare event. For example, at the 36-month follow-up of Symplicity HTN-1 and registry patients, only one of 153 patients was found to have a renal artery stenosis potentially related to renal denervation requiring stenting.[83] Nevertheless, renal artery stenoses have been reported not only with radiofrequency[89,90] but also with ultrasound energy application.[91] It is noteworthy that imaging follow-up in many studies is limited and the exact incidence of renal artery stenoses at long-term follow-up remains to be determined.

Renal denervation has not led to meaningful blood pressure responses in approximately 15% of patients, for unclear reasons. Possibilities include incomplete denervation due to technical limitations, procedural shortcomings, or the presence of hypertension not driven by sympathetic overactivity. In this context, it would be desirable to measure renal and/or overall sympathetic nerve activity routinely prior to, during, and after renal denervation; however, this is cumbersome and not without risks (norepinephrine spillover measurements require invasive measurements). Moreover, it is also not clear whether such measurements would help predict clinical success. Discrepant regional sympathetic activity may further complicate matters. For example in some hypertensive patients, renal norepinephrine spillover is normal whereas muscle sympathetic nerve activity is increased.[50] To date, the only known independent predictors of response are baseline blood pressure (more pronounced response in patients with higher baseline blood pressures[82,84,86,92]) and baseline baroreceptor sensitivity (more pronounced blood pressure reduction the lower the baseline baroreceptor activity).[93] In an effort to establish methods to gauge sympathetic nerve activity during denervation, Chinushi et al. have studied blood pressure, heart rate, heart rate variability, and plasma catecholamines during transcatheter electrical nerve stimulation in dogs. Autonomic nerve stimulation of the nondenervated renal artery was accompanied by a pronounced increase in heart rate, blood pressure, and catecholamine levels, whereas these parameters increased only minimally after stimulation of the denervated artery.[94] Similar techniques and methods, provided they can safely be performed, may have merit by providing feedback regarding procedural and, perhaps, clinical success.

The possibility of renal sympathetic re-innervation has been raised as it occurs in some animal models.[44] Moreover, sympathetic cardiac re-innervation has been described in humans after heart transplantation.[95] In this context, histologic examination of transplanted kidneys suggests re-innervation[96]; however, it does not appear to be of functional relevance.[97] The durability of blood pressure reductions in HTN-1 and -2 (described above) does not suggest relevant sympathetic re-innervation, at least up to 36 months.

Symplicity HTN-3

The above-mentioned potential shortcomings of Symplicity 1 and 2 and of a number of other uncontrolled studies demonstrating a blood pressure reduction have led to the performance of the Symplicity HTN-3.[98] In this trial, maximum efforts were made to minimize the possibility that a blood pressure difference between the treatment and control group might be driven by placebo and Hawthorne effect by randomly assigning patients with resistant hypertension to renal denervation or a sham procedure (renal angiography without denervation) in a 2:1 fashion with blinding of investigators and patients at follow-up. The design also eliminated a potential operator and patient bias. A total of 535 patients were enrolled. Renal denervation with the Symplicity Flex Renal Denervation System (Medtronic Inc.) was performed in those assigned to renal denervation (in 364 patients) and renal artery angiography in the control group. Endpoints were safety (composite of death from any cause, end-stage renal disease, embolic event resulting in end-organ damage, vascular complications, hypertensive crisis within 30 days, or renal artery stenosis within 6 months) and efficacy (change in systolic office blood pressure at 6 months with a superiority margin of 5 mm Hg). The study demonstrated an excellent safety profile. There was no significant difference in the composite safety endpoint at 6 months (4% in the renal denervation group vs. 5.8% in the sham group). There was also no significant difference in the number of major adverse events (1.4% in the denervation group vs. 0.6% in the sham group). However, although the systolic office blood pressure decreased in both groups (by 14 mm Hg in the denervation group vs. 11.7 in the sham group), there was no significant difference between the groups (2.39 mm Hg). Likewise, there was no significant difference in ambulatory blood pressure reduction between the groups (reduction of 6.8 mm Hg in the denervation group vs. 4.8 mm Hg in the sham group). The reason for the discrepant findings between the first two Symplicity trials and a number of other studies demonstrating a favorable blood pressure response and Symplicity HTN-3 remains unclear. It is possible that effects of previous trials were artificial and driven by above described limitations, particularly regression to the mean, also referred to as "big day bias" (by which the blood pressure that was used to enter the trial was also used as the baseline), placebo/Hawthorne effect, and observer bias. However, several aspects deserve consideration.

First, there is sound physiological evidence supporting a reduction in renal and overall sympathetic nervous system activity after renal denervation both from animal and human experience, described in detail previously. This suggests the possibility of technical limitations in the trial. It is, for example, conceivable that the procedural technique did not lead to the desired interruption of the renal sympathetic nervous fibers. In this context, it has been pointed out that the mean number of ablations (3.9 per artery) was smaller than is common practice. However, the number of ablations was no different in Symplicity HTN-1 (4 per artery) and it has yet to be shown that the number of ablations corresponds to efficacy. Furthermore, operator experience was limited as reflected by the number of procedures per operator. Only one denervation was performed by 31% of operators and all procedures (364) were performed by 111 operators (average number of procedures: 3.3). It is, therefore, possible that limited experience may have affected the efficacy. Yet there was no difference in efficacy between those operators who performed ≥5 and those who performed <5 procedures. Further, there was no difference in efficacy when results after first were compared with later denervations.

Second, patient selection may have influenced the results. It is possible that patient characteristics differed between patients enrolled in Symplicity HTN-3 and prior studies. To this effect, subgroup analyses have been performed and demonstrated a more pronounced office blood pressure reduction with a significant difference compared with the sham group in patients who were not of African-American descent, patients younger than 65 years, and those with a GFR ≥60 mL/min/173 m^2. In this context, in the population in which renal denervation was studied and taking a smaller treatment effect than predicted into account, Symplicity HTN-3 may have been underpowered to demonstrate a significant difference in blood pressure reductions between the treatment and control groups. It should be noted, however, that the ambulatory blood pressure monitoring did not confirm a significant effect in the above subgroups.[99]

Until further data are available, aforementioned aspects remain speculations.

PRACTICAL ASPECTS: PATIENT SELECTION AND PERFORMANCE OF THE PROCEDURE

Case Selection

For the first few cases, for those who do not have prior experience with renal artery intervention, definition of the anatomy may be helpful for appropriate case selection. It may be prudent to select cases with no or only mild abdominal aortic tortuosity and/or atherosclerosis. Prior computed tomographic (CT) or magnetic resonance angiography (MRA) outline the abdominal aortic anatomy and illustrate potential challenges due to tortuosity or pronounced atherosclerosis. Some imaging software programs may allow determination of the optimal fluoroscopy angle to visualize the ostium and takeoff of the renal artery. Of note, MRA using gadolinium is contraindicated in patients with a glomerular filtration rate of <30 mL/min. However, the use of special imaging techniques may allow adequate visualization of the aorta and renal arteries without the use of contrast.[100-103] Nevertheless, noninvasive imaging does not replace an abdominal aortography, as all current methods, Duplex ultrasound, and CT or MRI may not adequately identify accessory renal arteries. Hence, generally, abdominal aortography should be part of most renal denervation procedures.

Patient Selection

Patient selection can be performed with a simple algorithm (**Figure 22-6**). The first question that must be answered is: Does the patient have severe resistant hypertension? In pivotal trials, *severe* resistant hypertension was defined as a blood pressure of ≥160 mm Hg (or ≥150 mm Hg in the presence of diabetes mellitus).[79,84] Milder forms of resistant hypertension appear to benefit from renal denervation but the magnitude of blood pressure reduction is generally lower.[86,87] Key elements of accurate office blood pressure measurement have been well described in the attached reference.[104] If it is measured accurately and the patient meets these criteria, the next step is to rule out white coat hypertension (normal blood pressures except when the patient is in a medical environment). This can be done with ambulatory blood pressure measurement or, if unavailable, by periodic home blood pressure measurements, provided the patient's device is well calibrated. To eliminate the possibility of medical noncompliance, one might consider administration of all antihypertensive medications under the physician's or nurse's supervision prior to ambulatory blood pressure device hook-up to assure at least compliance with morning medications. If there are serious doubts, one could ask the patient to return for supervised evening medication administration (though this may pose logistical challenges) while the patient is wearing the monitor. Other techniques to enhance surveillance of medical compliance may be pill counts or measurement of antihypertensive medication blood levels but this has proven unreliable or costly in our experience. The next question is: Are there medications or illicit drugs that may cause a blood pressure increase, and, if so, can these be replaced by alternative medications? **Table 22-1** provides a list of the more common medications and illicit drugs that one needs to consider. When it is determined by ambulatory blood pressure measurement that the patient indeed has resistant hypertension, and after all medications or illicit drugs that may cause a high blood pressure are eliminated, the next step is an assessment for secondary hypertension. A list of the most common causes is outlined in **Table 22-2**. Many can be eliminated by history, physical exam (including measurement of blood

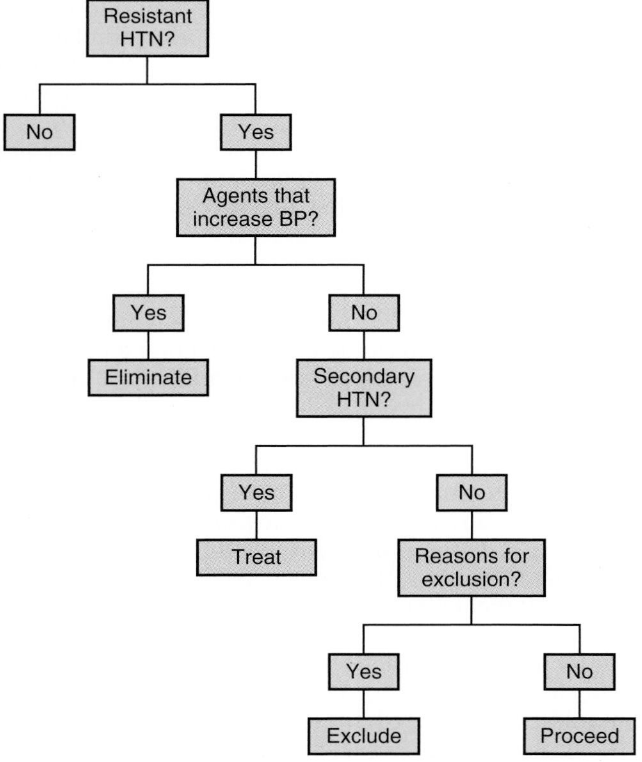

FIGURE 22-6 Patient selection.

TABLE 22-1 Common Substances That May Increase Blood Pressure

Alcohol
Caffeine
Selective and nonselective COX inhibitors/NSAIDs
Exogenous steroids (e.g., prednisone or oral contraceptives)
Cocaine and amphetamines
Appetite suppressants
Nasal congestants
Licorice (including chewing tobacco)
Antidepressants
Ketoconazole
Cyclosporine
Antiemetics (e.g., metoclopramide)
Erythropoietin

TABLE 22-2 Causes for Secondary Hypertension

Renal artery stenosis
Hyperaldosteronism
Glucocorticoid excess
Pheochromocytoma
Hyperthyroidism
Hypothyroidism
Hyperparathyroidism
Coarctation of the aorta
Chronic renal insufficiency

pressure in both upper and lower extremities to rule out aortic coarctation and subclavian artery stenosis), and standard laboratory tests that would be recommended in any patient with hypertension (including serum electrolytes [calcium included], creatinine, uric acid, complete blood count, urinalysis including check for microalbuminuria, and analysis of the urinary sediment). Screening for endocrine causes of secondary hypertension requires a set of laboratory tests that can easily be performed in most practices. A comprehensive discussion of endocrine hypertension is beyond the scope of this chapter, but a practical approach (and that pursued in our practice) may be the following: The patient is instructed to take 1 mg of dexamethasone orally at 11 PM and to come to the office the following morning when plasma renin, aldosterone, cortisol, and thyroid-stimulating hormone (TSH) levels are measured (at 8 AM). In addition, 24-hour collection for urinary catecholamines and metanephrines is started. If urinary metanephrines pose a logistical challenge, alternatively, plasma metanephrines can be measured, recognizing a higher rate of false positive results than with urinary metanephrines. The upper limit of normal for renin/aldosterone ratio is 20 to 30 and the aldosterone level is typically above >15 ng/dL with an undetectable renin concentration in primary hyperaldosteronism.[105] The above ratio takes into account that plasma renin activity is measured in ng/mL/hr and plasma aldosterone concentration in measured in ng/dL. However, the upper normal ratio may vary if other units or assays are used as outlined in the attached reference.[105] In healthy individuals, the 8 AM cortisol level should be less than 1.8 mcg/dL.[106] This cutoff provides a sensitivity of >95% and a specificity of 80%.[107] The urinary catecholamines should be less than twice the upper limit of normal.[108] In the presence of a pheochromocytoma, typically the urinary metanephrine levels are significantly elevated (several-fold higher than the upper reference limit).[108] There are a few important aspects when considering endocrine secondary hypertension:

1. **Hyperaldosteronism.** The estimated prevalence of primary hyperaldosteronism in patients with hypertension and resistant hypertension is 5% to 12% and 23% to 26%, respectively.[109-113] This estimate was lower (0.05% to 2%) when hypokalemia was considered to be an essential component of hyperaldosteronism.[114] It is now recognized that most patients with primary hyperaldosteronism are, in fact, normokalemic.[115] Nevertheless, lab clues may include hypokalemia and a slightly increased sodium concentration. Plasma renin and aldosterone levels are measured while the patient has been sitting for at least 5 minutes, in the morning, and after at least 2 hours of upright posture (standing, walking, or sitting).[105] Postural maneuvers are not necessary. It is essential that the patient is normokalemic at the time of measurement because hypokalemia suppresses aldosterone secretion (potentially leading to false negative results) and, under optimal circumstances, liberal salt intake should be encouraged.[105] Though a number of medications may interfere with test accuracy, for practical purposes, all antihypertensive medications may be continued with the exception of aldosterone inhibitors (spironolactone or eplerenone) and direct renin inhibitors (e.g., aliskiren). Aldosterone inhibitors should be discontinued 6 weeks prior to measurement. Further, chewing tobacco and licorice may affect test accuracy and must be discontinued before testing. It is best to keep in mind that most commonly used antihypertensive agents (including angiotensin conversion enzyme inhibitors, angiotensin receptor blockers, diuretics, and dihydropyridine calcium channel blockers) have a tendency to cause false negative results by virtue of primarily increasing the renin level. Therefore, if these agents are continued, a markedly positive test result and/or a renin level above the upper limit of detection are accompanied by a high likelihood of primary aldosteronism. Treatment with beta-blockers or central alpha-2 agonists (e.g., clonidine and methyldopa) may lower the plasma renin activity but it also lowers plasma aldosterone concentrations typically leaving the renin:aldosterone ratio unchanged;[116] however, false positive test results have been reported (related to a more pronounced reduction in renin levels compared with aldosterone concentration).[117] Depending on whether renin activity or concentration is measured, false positive and false negative results, respectively, have been reported. Hence with regard to the aforementioned antihypertensives, if test results are not diagnostic, discontinuation of these medications and temporary replacement with alternative antihypertensive medications that do not interfere with testing (e.g., verapamil, hydralazine, prazosin, doxazosin, terazosin)[105] followed by test repetition can be considered. When an abnormal renin:aldosterone level is encountered, collaboration with an endocrinologist for the purpose of confirmatory tests (oral or intravenous salt loading[105,118] or fludrocortisone stimulation[105] test) will facilitate further management. When screening and confirmatory tests are positive, most would proceed with imaging (CT with protocol focusing on the adrenal gland) and adrenal vein sampling, with adrenal gland removal in case of lateralization (particularly if this corresponds with an adrenal mass). An argument can also be made to proceed with unilateral removal of the adrenal gland in young patients (<40 years) who are found to have an unequivocal adrenal mass without prior adrenal vein sampling as an incidental adrenal mass (incidentaloma) is uncommon in this age category.[119] However, it is important to keep in mind that CT scanning alone to localize an adrenal adenoma can be misleading as misidentification is not uncommon. Adrenal vein sampling can be technically challenging but the success rate has been reported as high as 74% to 96%.[118,120-124] The sensitivity of adrenal vein sampling for the detection of a unilateral adrenal adenoma is 95% and 100%, respectively, and superior to CT imaging.[120,121] Adrenal vein sampling is important because it helps to determine whether a patient has "surgical disease" (adrenal adenoma [35%] or unilateral primary adrenal hyperplasia [2%])[125] with a potential cure after unilateral adrenalectomy or idiopathic hyperaldosteronism (60%)[125] or glucocorticoid remediable hyperaldosteronism (<3%),[125] both of which are treated medically. Adrenal aldosterone-producing carcinomas (<1%) and ectopic aldosterone-producing carcinomas (<0.1%) are so rare[125] that they will not be discussed here.

What if the patient has hypertension and hypokalemia and very low renin and aldosterone concentrations? Under these circumstances, conditions that mimic hyperaldosteronism but do not cause aldosterone excess should be considered. These include exogenous administration of substances such glucocorticoids or licorice ingestion, conditions that lead to an excess of substances with mineralocorticoid activity other than aldosterone

(11-beta hydroxylase deficiency, deoxycorticosterone-producing tumors, glucocorticoid-producing tumors, congenital adrenal hyperplasia), or Liddle syndrome, caused by a sodium channel defect in the tubuloepithelial cells leading to sodium retention and potassium wasting.

2. **Glucocorticoid excess.** Though the most convenient screening test, especially in patients with a low clinical suspicion, is the overnight dexamethasone suppression test, alternative tests (midnight salivary cortisol [should be measured twice] and urinary free cortisol [should be measured twice]), particularly in patients with a higher degree of suspicion, are reasonable.[106] Potential pitfalls are medications that interact with the cytochrome P450 enzyme thereby interfering with cortisol metabolism causing false positive or negative results. If feasible, these should be discontinued prior to testing. In patients with renal failure, dexamethasone suppression test should be preferred over urinary free cortisol.[106] In patients with suspected cyclic Cushing syndrome, urinary free cortisol or midnight salivary cortisol are preferred over dexamethasone suppression test.[106] In those without renal insufficiency, if urinary free cortisol is chosen as the screening test, high performance liquid chromatography has a better performance than immunoassays and the upper normal is 40 to 50 mcg/24 hours with a greater than four times upper limit of normal highly suggestive of Cushing syndrome.[126] If the screening test is abnormal it is best to collaborate with an endocrinologist for confirmatory testing and determination if the underlying problem is a pituitary adenoma (68%) or ectopic ACTH syndrome (usually the consequence of small cell lung cancer [12%], adrenal adenoma [10%], or adrenal carcinoma [8%]).[126] Other tumors (ectopic corticotropin-releasing hormone [CRH] secreting tumors or micronodular hyperplasia) are rare, <2%.[126] Under most circumstances the next steps would be brain MRI, CRH stimulation test, ACTH level determination, and high-dose 48-hour dexamethasone suppression test.
3. **Pheochromocytoma.** Though pheochromocytomas are rare even in patients with resistant hypertension, screening in resistant hypertension is recommended, as the consequences of a missed tumor are serious and appropriate treatment may offer a potential cure. The use of plasma metanephrines for screening is more convenient than urinary collection; however, it is important to recognize that the specificity is limited with a false positive rate of 15% to 25% depending on age.[127,128] Therefore, given the rarity of this tumor, the chance that an elevated plasma metanephrine result is, in fact, related to a pheochromocytoma in a patient with a low clinical suspicion is very low. Hence, urine metanephrine collection (specificity >90%[127]) may be a better screening test in patients with low clinical suspicion. Importantly, provided high power liquid chromatography or mass spectrometry methods are used, most medications, including antihypertensives, can be continued[129] with the exception of tricyclic antidepressants and flexeril. Measurement during major stress (e.g., critical illness, postsurgery, during drug withdrawal) is not recommended, due to a high false positive rate. It probably does not matter whether the patient is supine or upright when the blood sample is obtained.
4. **Hyperparathyroidism, hyperthyroidism.** These conditions can easily be ruled out by including a TSH level and calcium level in the routine laboratory investigations.

Procedure

Antiplatelet Therapy and Anticoagulation

There is no universally accepted, standard protocol for renal denervation. However, endothelial injury (denudation with or without thrombus formation) and/or thrombus/char formation at the catheter tip is to be expected[77,130] with the use of most current denervation technology. Therefore, though not proven, antiplatelet therapy prior to the procedure (e.g., 81-325 mg aspirin, or 600 mg of clopidogrel in those who are intolerant to aspirin), followed by 2 to 4 weeks of therapy (81-100 mg of aspirin or 75 mg of clopidogrel daily) to cover the presumed duration for re-endothelialization and healing,[77] seems to be justified (longer in the presence of other indications for antiplatelet therapy). In addition, prior to insertion of any equipment into the renal arteries, intravenous anticoagulation with heparin (goal ACT >250 seconds) or bivalirudin should be performed to avoid thrombus adherent to wires or ablation equipment used for the procedure.

For most interventional cardiologists, nephrologists, or interventional radiologists, the routine performance of the procedure is not technically challenging. When challenges do occur, they are usually related to aortic and/or iliac tortuosity.

Access

With rare exceptions, femoral arterial access is used. An alternative access site is the brachial artery. However, given the length of the currently available Symplicity Flex denervation catheter (90 cm), several procedural aspects for brachial approach denervation need to be considered (see later discussion). Standard femoral access using the Seldinger technique is performed with insertion of a sheath, the size of which depends on the denervation system used (6 Fr for the Symplicity Renal Denervation System). In case of severe iliac tortuosity, the use of a long (e.g., 40-45 cm) sheath can be considered to reduce friction and facilitate torque transmission to the guide catheter by straightening the iliac vasculature. Device manufacturers are developing newer generation devices that will allow performance of renal denervation from the radial approach. However, more pronounced respiratory and cardiac motion via the brachial or radial approach can cause significant catheter instability and may compromise consistent wall contact.

Angiography

A pigtail or Omni Flush catheter (AngioDynamics Inc., Queensbury, New York) is advanced into the abdominal aorta over a 0.035-inch guidewire with the tip position between L1 and L2. The wire is removed and contrast injected (15-20 cc if digital subtraction angiography is used, 20-30 cc if conventional angiography is used). Another option preferred by the authors is to place the renal guide catheter to be used for angiography and denervation into the abdominal aorta with the tip between L1 and L2 over a 0.035-inch guidewire with injection through the guide catheter while the wire remains in the distal thoracic aorta well ahead of the guide catheter tip (this requires the use of a Y-connector prior to angiography) (Video 22-1). The guide catheter may then be used to perform selective angiography. A shallow (10-20 degrees) left anterior oblique (LAO) projection given the typically slightly more anterior takeoff of the right compared with the left renal artery is used for abdominal aortic angiography. Size, takeoff, course, tortuosity, and bifurcation pattern of the renal arteries are examined and attention is directed to presence and size of accessory renal arteries and any significant atherosclerosis. The guide catheter is selected according to anatomy. In the overwhelming majority of cases, the renal artery takeoff is slightly inferiorly oriented and the shape of an internal mammary (IM) catheter is most suitable for selective engagement. When the takeoff is horizontal, a renal double curve (RDC) guide catheter or a Judkins right (JR-4) may be well suited. For a superior takeoff, a multipurpose (MP) catheter may be preferred. The guide catheter may be engaged into the renal arteries directly after guidewire removal. However, we prefer the use of the "no touch technique" by which the guide catheter, with the wire still in place several centimeters ahead of the catheter tip (in the thoracic aorta), is oriented toward the renal artery ostium (small contrast injections during maneuvering can confirm optimal position) (Video 22-2). A second, smaller coronary (0.014-inch, e.g., Iron Man) or peripheral (0.018-inch, e.g., Spartacore) guidewire may be advanced into the renal artery to further facilitate engagement. Subsequently, the 0.035-inch guidewire is removed, allowing the guide catheter to "fall into" or passively engage the renal artery. This may lower the risk of plaque disruption and embolization in a hostile aorta or dissection of the renal artery at engagement. When engagement proves difficult, consideration may be given to advancing a glide wire into the renal artery as a rail for the guide catheter. For most renal denervation devices, catheter positioning 3 to 4 mm into the renal artery facilitates denervation catheter entry into the renal artery as most devices will, once they reach the catheter tip, straighten it out, causing it to point upward roofing the renal artery, impeding further advancement. When deeper guide catheter positioning is difficult, a glide wire can first be advanced into the renal artery, and, if necessary, a smaller (e.g., 4 Fr) diagnostic catheter (e.g., JR-4) advanced through the guide catheter into the renal artery in a telescoping fashion as a rail for the guide catheter to allow deeper engagement. Selective angiography is performed (2-3 cc are typically sufficient for this purpose) with extended cineangiographic imaging for visualization of the contrast nephrogram. Rarely more than 10 cc are necessary for selective angiography of both renal arteries. In case of renal insufficiency, consideration may be given not to perform abdominal aortography and selective angiography during denervation may be performed with carbon dioxide. The imaging quality is inferior to conventional angiography but sufficient to provide guidance for catheter positioning.[131]

Denervation

Some operators routinely use a vasodilator (e.g., 200-400 mcg of intra-arterial nitroglycerine, 200 mcg of nicardipine, 100 mcg of verapamil, or 100 mcg of nitroprusside) to prevent or minimize vasospasm prior to denervation; however, the value of this approach is questionable. The following discussion focuses on the use of the Symplicity catheter, as it is currently the most frequently used. After guide catheter engagement, the Symplicity catheter is advanced into the renal artery in a neutral configuration to a distal position (Video 22-3). Sometimes, particularly in the presence of tortuosity, resistance can be encountered. In this case, slight withdrawal followed by tip flexion (see later) and re-advancement may facilitate negotiation of tortuosity. Once in the distal most desired location, the tip is flexed to provide wall contact with the renal artery. Tip flexion is achieved by pulling a lever on the catheter handle backward and tip straightening occurs by pushing the handle forward (Video 22-4). A foot pedal is pushed to initiate radiofrequency energy delivery by a preset algorithm. The generator will provide feedback by illustrating the impedance, impedance drop, temperature, and duration of denervation (Video 22-5). The desired impedance and drop range is between 220 and 250 ohm and >10%, respectively. Very high impedance is typically related to catheter position in a small side branch and low impedance or significant (>10-20 ohm) variability to inadequate wall contact. In this case, catheter repositioning will improve wall contact. If an error signal is encountered during ablation, radiofrequency application is interrupted. Reasons for an error signal are invariably too little wall contact or too high temperature recorded related to side branch positioning or renal artery spasm requiring catheter repositioning. After successful ablation, the catheter tip is straightened into the neutral position (by pulling the lever on the handle) and the catheter slightly (5 mm) pulled back, flexed, and turned either by torque on the catheter itself or by turning a rotator on the handle. The advantage of using the handle rotator is tactile feedback by a "click" every 45 degrees and visual reference on the handle. The aforementioned steps are repeated with an aim of eight ablations per artery in a stepwise circumferential spiral manner if the anatomy allows. Contrast injection may be performed after every ablation to assess the renal artery and confirm position; however, consideration may be given to forgo angiography or use carbon dioxide injections in patients with renal insufficiency.

Luminal irregularities and reduction in renal artery caliber at the site of ablation are frequently encountered. The histological correlate appears to be vessel wall edema, endothelial denudation, and adherent thrombotic material.[77,130] Spasm may contribute; however, administration of vasodilators frequently does not lead to angiographic improvements. It is important not to succumb to the temptation to treat such angiographic findings with balloon angioplasty or stenting because the angiographic changes will invariably resolve (with the rare exception of renal artery stenosis[89,90]).

In the Symplicity trials, patients with renal arteries <4 mm in diameter and/or accessory renal arteries were excluded.[80,84] However, some operators including ourselves perform (off-label) denervation in arteries with diameters ≥3.5 mm, including all suitable accessory renal arteries. Some data suggest that accessory renal artery denervation can be safely performed and is accompanied by blood pressure reductions albeit perhaps less pronounced than in patients with bilateral single renal arteries.[132] When early renal artery bifurcation is encountered, both branches should be denervated if they are of adequate size.

Tortuosity of the renal artery can complicate advancement of the denervation catheter. To provide more stability and support, consideration may be given to position a 0.014-inch or 0.018-inch buddy wire into the renal artery during advancement of the denervation catheter, reminding oneself to remove it prior to energy application as this may interfere with the ablation or cause adverse effects due to heat transmitted to the renal artery wall.

In cases of severe iliac tortuosity, acute angle inferior renal artery takeoff, or distal aortic, iliac, or femoral occlusions, consideration may be given to renal denervation from the brachial approach. Under these circumstances, it is important to remember that most conventional guide catheters are too long (100 cm) to accommodate the Symplicity catheter or too short to reach the renal artery. Under these circumstances the use of a 90-cm sheath may allow engagement of the renal arteries. To minimize the risk of renal artery trauma by the sheath, a diagnostic catheter (e.g., multipurpose) can be used to engage the renal artery first using it as a rail for the guide sheath. Once it is engaged, the diagnostic catheter is removed and the ablation catheter advanced into the renal artery. A potential disadvantage using a brachial access route is respiratory and cardiac motion translated to the catheter particularly using the right brachial approach. This motion causes unstable catheter position with the Symplicity catheter. However, some other denervation technologies fix the catheter tip in the renal artery thereby counteracting respiratory variations.

Occasionally, patients have undergone prior renal artery stenting. Though patients with renal artery stents have been excluded from participation in most trials, denervation distal to the stent is feasible and may be accompanied by blood pressure reductions.[133] Application of radiofrequency energy within the stent cannot be recommended given the unpredictable safety (e.g., heat injury) and efficacy.

When atherosclerotic renal artery stenoses are encountered at angiography prior to deneration, a possible approach is to proceed with renal artery balloon angioplasty first followed by denervation at a later date if the desired blood pressure goal cannot be reached.

Sedation, Analgesia, and Other Necessary Medications

Routine administration of benzodiazepines (e.g., midazolam) and opioid analgesics (e.g., fentanyl or morphine) prior to radiofrequency or ultrasound energy application is recommended because severe visceral (abdominal, lower back, and pelvic) pain is almost always encountered with radiofrequency or ultrasound energy application. The location of pain fibers has not been well studied; however, some evidence points to the media.[134] In this context, lesser degrees or absence of pain with ablation techniques sparing the media (e.g., chemical neurolysis) have been reported (personal communication: Tim Fischell, Borgess Heart Institute, Kalamazoo, Michigan). Antiemetics (e.g., 1-mg intravenous granisetron or 4-8 mg intravenous ondansetron) are not prophylactically used but should be readily available for opioid- or pain-induced nausea. In addition, intravenous atropin (1 mg) should be available in case of a vagal reaction and flumazenil and naloxone should be available to reverse respiratory depression caused by benzodiazepines and opioids.

Equipment

All the usual tools for angiography and medications that have been mentioned above should be available. In addition, bailout equipment is important. This should include stents of 4- to 7-mm diameter (the typical diameter of renal arteries) and 10- to 20-mm length as well as 0.014-inch or 0.018-inch guidewires (e.g., Iron Man or Spartacore [Abbott, Abbott Park, Illinois]) and balloon expandable covered stents (e.g., Atrium iCast covered stent [Atrium, Hudson, New Hampshire]) in case of renal artery perforation (no such report published to date). Necessary equipment for emergent airway management (including for endotracheal intubation) in case of excessive sedation with respiratory compromise must be in the catheterization laboratory and personnel trained in emergent airway management must be readily available.

EFFECT OF RENAL DENERVATION ON CONDITIONS OF SYMPATHETIC OVERACTIVITY OTHER THAN HYPERTENSION

In patients with diabetes mellitus, improved fasting glucose, insulin levels, C-peptide levels, glucose levels after oral glucose tolerance test, and homeostasis assessment model-insulin resistance (HOMA-IR) have been reported in a small cohort, supporting improvements in glucose control and insulin sensitivity after denervation.[135-137] The physiological basis for these observations is not certain. Enhanced skeletal muscle blood flow is conceivable.[138] Decreases in sympathetic nervous system activity and the corresponding reduction in adrenergic alpha-1 receptor mediated vasoconstriction may improve skeletal muscle blood flow and capillary density thereby promoting glucose transport into insulin sensitive skeletal muscle.[139]

Early studies have excluded patients with more than mild renal insufficiency. Hence, the safety and efficacy of renal denervation in patients with advanced renal failure is not clear. Moreover, concerns have been raised that the change in renal hemodynamics after renal denervation may accelerate renal injury. However, on theoretical grounds, renal denervation would be expected to have a favorable effect on blood pressure given the observed increase in renal and overall sympathetic nervous system activity and blood pressure demonstrated in animal models of renal injury (attenuated by prior renal denervation)[36,39] and pronounced increase in muscle sympathetic nerve activity, a surrogate for sympathetic nervous system activity, seen in a number of studies of patients with renal injury including dialysis patients,[56] patients with advanced renal insufficiency,[63] polycystic kidney disease,[140] and kidney transplantation[57] with a direct relationship between severity of renal insufficiency and muscle sympathetic nerve activity.[141] In neither of the Symplicity trials, including hypertensive patients with normal or mildly reduced renal function at baseline, did an adverse effect on renal function occur.[98,142] Moreover, small studies suggest safety and efficacy of renal denervation in patients with renal insufficiency and end-stage renal disease. In one study of 15 patients with stage 3 to 4 chronic kidney disease, office blood pressure reductions after renal denervation were similar to those reported in Symplicity HTN-1 and 2 with a more favorable dipping profile related to nocturnal blood pressure reductions but no significant change in average ambulatory blood pressures.[143] In this study there was no deterioration of renal function up to 12 months based on serum creatinine and cystatine C and no difference in proteinuria. Further, in a small (n = 12) study of patients with end-stage renal failure on dialysis, renal denervation could be performed without complications in nine.[144] Three patients' renal arteries were atrophic and of too small caliber for denervation. There were no complications suggesting that renal denervation can safely be performed in patients with end-stage renal failure.

Limited data suggest a reduction in atrial fibrillation recurrence after pulmonary vein isolation.[145] In addition, reductions in ventricular arrhythmias in patients with incessant ventricular arrhythmias have been reported.[146] Furthermore, an improvement in apnea/hypopnea indices has been reported in hypertensive patients with obstructive sleep apnea after renal sympathetic denervation.[137]

Finally, beneficial effects of renal denervation in patients with heart failure may be expected. Sympathetic overactivity is common in heart failure patients[147] and associated with increased mortality.[148] A mortality reduction with beta adrenoreceptor and renin-angiotensin system inhibition has been shown in large clinical trials.[149,150] Given the favorable effects on sympathetic tone, similar beneficial effects would be expected after renal denervation. In this context, decreased left ventricular filling pressures and improved left ventricular systolic function have been demonstrated following renal denervation in an animal model.[151] The feasibility and safety of renal denervation was recently explored in a small (n = 7) pilot study. No adverse effects occurred and functional class improved.[152] Ongoing studies may further clarify the role of renal denervation in this patient population.

NEW CONCEPTS AND DEVICES

The sound physiological data underlying the concept of renal denervation and the encouraging results of Symplicity HTN-1 and 2 led to the design of a number of new concepts and technologies for renal denervation.

The review of all devices is beyond the scope of this chapter. Therefore, the following device description is not all-inclusive. New concepts have focused on facilitating denervation by reducing procedural times (e.g., by using multi-electrode catheters) and attempt to allow more reliable circumferential energy delivery and minimize collateral renal artery injury (e.g., by cooling or avoiding wall contact).

Medtronic has designed a spiral radiofrequency catheter, SPYRAL System (**Figure 22-7**), with multiple electrodes thereby minimizing catheter manipulations and procedural time and possibly offering more reliable circumferential ablation results. This catheter has undergone a first-in-man study with preliminary results in 40 patients demonstrating a systolic office blood pressure reduction of 16/7 mm Hg at one-month follow-up.[153] A similar spiral radiofrequency catheter (**Figure 22-7**) that provides irrigation during ablation is manufactured by Johnson & Johnson (New Brunswick, New Jersey) and undergoing an early clinical safety and efficacy trial (RENABLATE) with an estimated enrollment of 35 patients. There are two balloon-mounted radiofrequency systems, the Covidien One Shot (Covidien Ltd., Dublin, Ireland) and Vessix Renal Denervation System (Boston Scientific, Natick, Massachusetts), that have multiple radiofrequency electrodes mounted on balloon catheters delivered into the renal artery over a 0.014-inch guidewire (**Figure 22-7**). The balloon is inflated and radiofrequency energy applied. The Covidien One Shot system (monopolar electrodes, 7-8 Fr guide catheter system) has an integrated irrigation system for cooling during the procedure. In a first-in-man (RHAS trial, n = 9)[154] and subsequent study (RAPID, n = 47),[155,156] office blood pressure reductions were 34/13 mm Hg and 20/8 mm Hg respectively at 6 months with a less pronounced ambulatory blood pressure reduction of 11/6 mm Hg. No major acute complications occurred, and in those 41 patients who underwent renal artery imaging, no renal artery stenosis was seen. Covidien has since aborted its clinical denervation program. The Vessix Renal Denervation System (bipolar electrodes) (demonstrated in Videos 22-6 to 22-10) has been studied in a first-in-man and post market study (REDUCE-HTN). Together, 6-month follow-up data were available at the writing of this chapter on 107 patients with a significant 25/10 mm Hg office blood pressure reduction.[157] One renal artery stenosis progression was reported and no other major adverse events. A potential advantage of the system is the applicability in renal arteries with a diameter of 3.5 mm. During the aforementioned study, patients with accessory renal arteries were included

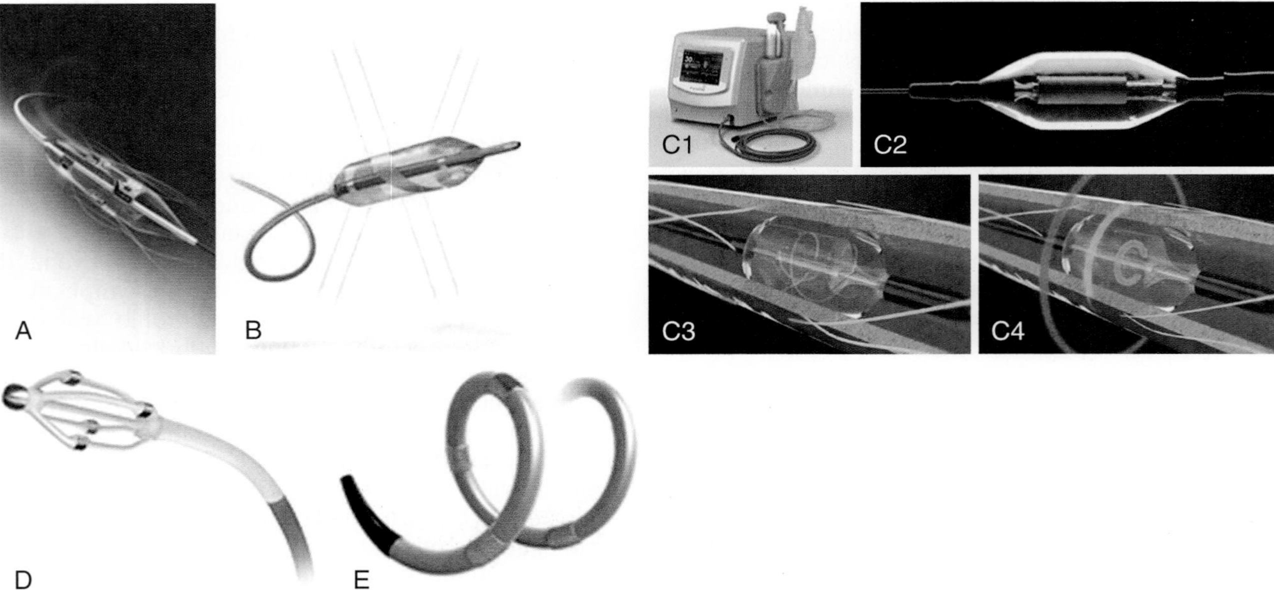

FIGURE 22-7 Renal denervation systems: **A,** Vessix Renal Denervation System (Boston Scientific, Natick, Mass.). **B,** Covidien OneShot (Covidien Ltd., Dublin, Ireland). **C,** Paradise System: *C1,* Paradise generator. *C2,* Cylindrical transducer within a cooling balloon. *C3,* Illustration of catheter within the artery demonstrating endothelial and medial cooling and centering of the transducer within the artery. *C4,* Illustration of circumferential heating with concomitant balloon cooling (Recor Medical, Ronkonkoma, NY). **D,** EnligHTN catheter (St. Jude Medical, St. Paul, Minn.). **E,** SPYRAL denervation catheter (Medtronic Inc., Minneapolis, Minn.).

and experienced a significant but slightly less pronounced office blood pressure reduction of 20/10 mm Hg.[157] The EnligHTN™ Renal Denervation System (St. Jude Medical, St. Paul, Minnesota) is a basket-shaped multi-electrode ablation catheter delivered through an 8 Fr system (**Figure 22-7**). After the basket unfolds, allowing contact of the electrodes with the renal artery wall, radiofrequency energy is applied simultaneously to all electrodes. In a first safety and efficacy trial including denervation of 46 patients, an office blood pressure reduction of 25/10 mm Hg was achieved at 6 months with a lasting effect demonstrated up to 18 months and no significant changes in renal function.[158]

The Paradise Ultrasound Denervation System (ReCor Medical, Palo Alto, California) is a catheter based system (6 Fr) featuring a cylindrical nonfocused ultrasound transducer centered within a balloon that circulates cooling fluid and that outputs a uniform circumferential energy pattern designed to ablate tissues located 1 to 6 mm from the arterial wall and protect tissues within 1 mm (**Figure 22-7**). The technology has been evaluated in over 135 patients, in 3 clinical studies, and through commercial use in Europe. Preliminary results from the REDUCE first-in-human study conducted in South Africa (n = 15) demonstrated a mean office blood pressure reduction of 28/13 mm Hg at 3-month follow-up.[91] One guidewire associated renal artery dissection occurred and two renal artery stenosis were reported. These were attributed to a low cooling flow rate. Design modifications were implemented including an increased cooling flow rate prior to initiation of two post-market approval studies. Preliminary results from REALISE, a post-market study in moderate resistant hypertensive patients in France (n = 20) demonstrated a mean reduction in office systolic blood pressure of −18 mm Hg and a mean reduction in ambulatory systolic blood pressure of −14 mm Hg at 12 months. Preliminary results from ACHIEVE, a post-market study in resistant hypertensive patients in Europe (n = 100) demonstrated a mean reduction in office systolic blood pressure of −17 mm Hg and a mean reduction in ambulatory systolic blood pressure of −5 mm Hg at 6 months. There have been no reports of new onset renal artery stenosis in either of these studies.[91] A similar concept using a cooling balloon catheter but microwave energy is designed by Denervx LLC (Maple Grove, Minnesota). It is currently undergoing animal studies. Ultrasound energy can also be applied by an external source focusing on the perirenal arterial tissue guided by ultrasound imaging (Surround Sound Ablative Field, Kona Medical Inc., Bellevue, Washington). This concept has been examined in a first-in-man (WAVE-I) study of 24 patients with a 6-month office blood pressure reduction of 29/12 mm Hg and no major adverse events.[159] Similar results (office blood pressure reduction of 26/9 mm Hg, n = 17) were demonstrated in a second study (WAVE-II) at 3 months.[159]

Finally, renal nerve disruption can be achieved without energy but by injection of neurotoxic substances such as alcohol into the perivascular space. In this context, Ablative Solutions (Menlo Park, California) has designed a catheter that delivers ethanol into the renal artery adventitia via ultrafine needles. This concept may minimize intimal and media injury and perhaps the potential for renal artery stenosis while allowing denervation of sympathetic nerves in deeper tissue layers. In addition, by sparing injury to the media (where pain fibers are presumably located) it may reduce the amount of procedural pain.

Radiofrequency application has recently been explored for the treatment of primary pulmonary hypertension resistant to conventional medications with a dramatic reduction in mean pulmonary artery pressure from 55 mm Hg to 36 mm Hg and pulmonary vascular resistance from 1800 dynes to 760 dynes in a small cohort of patients. This is one of the most pronounced improvements in pulmonary artery pressure reported to date.[160]

CONCLUSIONS

Renal and overall sympathetic nervous system activity plays an important role in development and maintenance of hypertension. A number of animal experiments and human observations support a potential role for renal denervation in hypertension and, perhaps, other conditions associated with sympathetic overactivity. In addition, early experience with the Symplicity catheter and other novel approaches support a blood pressure-lowering effect. Enthusiasm for the concept of renal denervation has recently been dampened by the results of the only sham-controlled blinded trial available to date, Symplicity HTN-3, and the procedure remains investigational in the United States, though it is widely available in other parts of the world. Though it is conceivable that, contrary to our current physiological concepts, renal denervation does not cause the desired blood pressure reduction, it would be premature to make this conclusion. Completion of the Symplicity HTN-3 data analysis and ongoing trials will hopefully enhance our understanding of the renal sympathetic nervous system and provide answers as to whether, how well, and for what patient renal denervation works. In the meantime, very careful patient selection limiting renal denervation to those with severe resistant hypertension with no other treatment options or to controlled clinical trials is called for.

Most frequently, hypertension is asymptomatic. The treatment rationale is cardiovascular risk reduction. Therefore, ideally, establishment of any (medical or device) treatment modality in our armamentarium should be based on demonstration of a reduction in major adverse cardiovascular and cerebrovascular events; an outcome trial of renal artery denervation has been planned, but it remains to be seen if such a large and long-term study will in fact be carried out.

References

1. Kearney PM, Whelton M, Reynolds K, et al: Global burden of hypertension: analysis of worldwide data. *Lancet* 365:217–223, 2005.
2. Egan BM, Zhao Y, Axon RN: US trends in prevalence, awareness, treatment, and control of hypertension, 1988-2008. *JAMA* 303:2043–2050, 2010.
3. Lewington S, Clarke R, Qizilbash N, et al: Age-specific relevance of usual blood pressure to vascular mortality: a meta-analysis of individual data for one million adults in 61 prospective studies. *Lancet* 360:1903–1913, 2002.
4. Psaty BM, Lumley T, Furberg CD, et al: Health outcomes associated with various antihypertensive therapies used as first-line agents: a network meta-analysis. *JAMA* 289:2534–2544, 2003.
5. Psaty BM, Smith NL, Siscovick DS, et al: Health outcomes associated with antihypertensive therapies used as first-line agents. A systematic review and meta-analysis. *JAMA* 277:739–745, 1997.
6. Calhoun DA, Jones D, Textor S, et al: Resistant hypertension: diagnosis, evaluation, and treatment: a scientific statement from the American Heart Association Professional Education Committee of the Council for High Blood Pressure Research. *Circulation* 117:e510–e526, 2008.
7. Garg JP, Elliott WJ, Folker A, et al: Resistant hypertension revisited: a comparison of two university-based cohorts. *Am J Hypertens* 18:619–626, 2005.
8. Cushman WC, Ford CE, Cutler JA, et al: Success and predictors of blood pressure control in diverse North American settings: the antihypertensive and lipid-lowering treatment to prevent heart attack trial (ALLHAT). *J Clin Hypertens (Greenwich)* 4:393–404, 2002.
9. Jamerson K, Weber MA, Bakris GL, et al: Benazepril plus amlodipine or hydrochlorothiazide for hypertension in high-risk patients. *N Engl J Med* 359:2417–2428, 2008.
10. Gupta AK, Nasothimiou EG, Chang CL, et al: Baseline predictors of resistant hypertension in the Anglo-Scandinavian Cardiac Outcome Trial (ASCOT): a risk score to identify those at high-risk. *J Hypertens* 29:2004–2013, 2011.
11. Persell SD: Prevalence of resistant hypertension in the United States, 2003-2008. *Hypertension* 57:1076–1080, 2011.
12. Daugherty SL, Powers JD, Magid DJ, et al: Incidence and prognosis of resistant hypertension in hypertensive patients. *Circulation* 125:1635–1642, 2012.

13. Egan BM, Zhao Y, Axon RN, et al: Uncontrolled and apparent treatment resistant hypertension in the United States, 1988 to 2008. *Circulation* 124:1046–1058, 2011.
14. Bertog SC, Sobotka PA, Sievert H: Renal denervation for hypertension. *JACC Cardiovasc Interv* 5:249–258, 2012.
15. Rettig R: Does the kidney play a role in the aetiology of primary hypertension? Evidence from renal transplantation studies in rats and humans. *J Hum Hypertens* 7:177–180, 1993.
16. Roman RJ, Cowley AW, Jr: Characterization of a new model for the study of pressure-natriuresis in the rat. *Am J Physiol* 248:F190–F198, 1985.
17. Cowley AW, Jr: Long-term control of arterial blood pressure. *Physiol Rev* 72:231–300, 1992.
18. Barajas L: The innervation of the juxtaglomerular apparatus. An electron microscopic study of the innervation of the glomerular arterioles. *Lab Invest* 13:916–929, 1964.
19. Ljungqvist A, Wagermark J: The adrenergic innervation of intrarenal glomerular and extra-glomerular circulatory routes. *Nephron* 7:218–229, 1970.
20. Muller J, Barajas L: Electron microscopic and histochemical evidence for a tubular innervation in the renal cortex of the monkey. *J Ultrastruct Res* 41:533–549, 1972.
21. Barajas L, Wang P: Localization of tritiated norepinephrine in the renal arteriolar nerves. *Anat Rec* 195:525–534, 1979.
22. Drexel T, Bertog SC, Vaskelyte L, et al: Renal denervation. *Anadolu Kardiyol Derg* 14:186–191, 2014.
23. Insel PA, Snavely MD, Healy DP, et al: Radioligand binding and functional assays demonstrate postsynaptic alpha 2-receptors on proximal tubules of rat and rabbit kidney. *J Cardiovasc Pharmacol* 7(Suppl 8):S9–S17, 1985.
24. Meister B, Dagerlind A, Nicholas AP, et al: Patterns of messenger RNA expression for adrenergic receptor subtypes in the rat kidney. *J Pharmacol Exp Ther* 268:1605–1611, 1994.
25. Ibarra F, Aperia A, Svensson LB, et al: Bidirectional regulation of Na+,K(+)-ATPase activity by dopamine and an alpha-adrenergic agonist. *Proc Natl Acad Sci U S A* 90:21–24, 1993.
26. Holtback U, Ohtomo Y, Forberg P, et al: Neuropeptide Y shifts equilibrium between alpha- and beta-adrenergic tonus in proximal tubule cells. *Am J Physiol* 275:F1–F7, 1998.
27. Aldehni F, Tang T, Madsen K, et al: Stimulation of renin secretion by catecholamines is dependent on adenylyl cyclases 5 and 6. *Hypertension* 57:460–468, 2011.
28. Tomaschitz A, Pilz S, Ritz E, et al: Aldosterone and arterial hypertension. *Nat Rev Endocrinol* 6:83–93, 2010.
29. Duprez DA: Role of the renin-angiotensin-aldosterone system in vascular remodeling and inflammation: a clinical review. *J Hypertens* 24:983–991, 2006.
30. Schiffrin EL: Effects of aldosterone on the vasculature. *Hypertension* 47:312–318, 2006.
31. Hwang KC, Gray CD, Sweet WE, et al: Alpha 1-adrenergic receptor coupling with Gh in the failing human heart. *Circulation* 94:718–726, 1996.
32. Berridge MJ: Inositol trisphosphate and diacylglycerol as second messengers. *Biochem J* 220:345–360, 1984.
33. Ciriello J, de Oliveira CV: Renal afferents and hypertension. *Curr Hypertens Rep* 4:136–142, 2002.
34. Ciriello J, Calaresu FR: Central projections of afferent renal fibers in the rat: an anterograde transport study of horseradish peroxidase. *J Auton Nerv Syst* 8:273–285, 1983.
35. Rosas-Arellano MP, Solano-Flores LP, Ciriello J: c-Fos induction in spinal cord neurons after renal arterial or venous occlusion. *Am J Physiol* 276:R120–R127, 1999.
36. Ye S, Zhong H, Yanamadala V, et al: Renal injury caused by intrarenal injection of phenol increases afferent and efferent renal sympathetic nerve activity. *Am J Hypertens* 15:717–724, 2002.
37. Katholi RE, Whitlow PL, Winternitz SR, et al: Importance of the renal nerves in established two-kidney, one clip Goldblatt hypertension. *Hypertension* 4:166–174, 1982.
38. Katholi RE, Winternitz SR, Oparil S: Decrease in peripheral sympathetic nervous system activity following renal denervation or unclipping in the one-kidney one-clip Goldblatt hypertensive rat. *J Clin Invest* 69:55–62, 1982.
39. Campese VM, Kogosov E: Renal afferent denervation prevents hypertension in rats with chronic renal failure. *Hypertension* 25:878–882, 1995.
40. Kottke FJ, Kubicek WG, Visscher MB: The production of arterial hypertension by chronic renal artery-nerve stimulation. *Am J Physiol* 145:38–47, 1945.
41. Bernard C: Lecons sur les Proprietes et les Alterations Pathologiques des Liquides de l'Organisme. *Paris: Bailliers et Fils* 2:170–171, 1859.
42. Thoren P: Efferent renal nerve traffic in the spontaneously hypertensive rat. *Clin Exp Hypertens A* 9(Suppl 1):259–279, 1987.
43. Abramczyk P, Zwolinska A, Oficjalski P, et al: Kidney denervation combined with elimination of adrenal-renal portal circulation prevents the development of hypertension in spontaneously hypertensive rats. *Clin Exp Pharmacol Physiol* 26:32–34, 1999.
44. Norman RA, Jr, Dzielak DJ: Role of renal nerves in onset and maintenance of spontaneous hypertension. *Am J Physiol* 243:H284–H288, 1982.
45. DiBona GF, Esler M: Translational medicine: the antihypertensive effect of renal denervation. *Am J Physiol Regul Integr Comp Physiol* 298:R245–R253, 2010.
46. Anderson EA, Sinkey CA, Lawton WJ, et al: Elevated sympathetic nerve activity in borderline hypertensive humans. Evidence from direct intraneural recordings. *Hypertension* 14:177–183, 1989.
47. Esler M, Jennings G, Biviano B, et al: Mechanism of elevated plasma noradrenaline in the course of essential hypertension. *J Cardiovasc Pharmacol* 8(Suppl 5):S39–S43, 1986.
48. Goldstein DS: Plasma catecholamines and essential hypertension. An analytical review. *Hypertension* 5:86–99, 1983.
49. Esler M, Jennings G, Lambert G, et al: Overflow of catecholamine neurotransmitters to the circulation: source, fate, and functions. *Physiol Rev* 70:963–985, 1990.
50. Esler M, Lambert G, Jennings G: Regional norepinephrine turnover in human hypertension. *Clin Exp Hypertens A* 11(Suppl 1):75–89, 1989.
51. Schlaich MP, Lambert E, Kaye DM, et al: Sympathetic augmentation in hypertension: role of nerve firing, norepinephrine reuptake, and angiotensin neuromodulation. *Hypertension* 43:169–175, 2004.
52. Smith PA, Graham LN, Mackintosh AF, et al: Relationship between central sympathetic activity and stages of human hypertension. *Am J Hypertens* 17:217–222, 2004.
53. Grassi G, Seravalle G, Colombo M, et al: Body weight reduction, sympathetic nerve traffic, and arterial baroreflex in obese normotensive humans. *Circulation* 97:2037–2042, 1998.
54. Narkiewicz K, Pesek CA, Kato M, et al: Baroreflex control of sympathetic nerve activity and heart rate in obstructive sleep apnea. *Hypertension* 32:1039–1043, 1998.
55. Zoccali C, Mallamaci F, Parlongo S, et al: Plasma norepinephrine predicts survival and incident cardiovascular events in patients with end-stage renal disease. *Circulation* 105:1354–1359, 2002.
56. Converse RL, Jr, Jacobsen TN, Toto RD, et al: Sympathetic overactivity in patients with chronic renal failure. *N Engl J Med* 327:1912–1918, 1992.
57. Hausberg M, Kosch M, Harmelink P, et al: Sympathetic nerve activity in end-stage renal disease. *Circulation* 106:1974–1979, 2002.
58. Ask-Upmark: Ueber juvenile maligne Nephrosclerose und ihr Verhael- tnis zu Stoerungen in der Nierenentwicklung [Juvenille malignant nephrosclerosis and its role in disorders in kidney development]. *Acta Pathol Microbiol Scand* 6:383–442, 1929.
59. Butler AM: Chronic pyelonephritis and arterial hypertension. *J Clin Invest* 16:889–897, 1937.
60. Smith HW: Hypertension and urologic disease. *Am J Med* 4:724–743, 1948.
61. Cohen SL: Hypertension in renal transplant recipients: role of bilateral nephrectomy. *Br Med J* 3:78–81, 1973.
62. McHugh MI, Tanboga H, Marcen R, et al: Hypertension following renal transplantation: the role of the host's kidney. *Q J Med* 49:395–403, 1980.
63. Ligtenberg G, Blankestijn PJ, Oey PL, et al: Reduction of sympathetic hyperactivity by enalapril in patients with chronic renal failure. *N Engl J Med* 340:1321–1328, 1999.
64. Miyajima E, Yamada Y, Yoshida Y, et al: Muscle sympathetic nerve activity in renovascular hypertension and primary aldosteronism. *Hypertension* 17:1057–1062, 1991.
65. Perry CB: Malignant hypertension cured by unilateral nephrectomy. *Br Heart J* 7:139–142, 1945.
66. Allen EV: Sympathectomy for essential hypertension. *Circulation* 6:131–140, 1952.
67. Smithwick RH, Thompson JE: Splanchnicectomy for essential hypertension; results in 1,266 cases. *J Am Med Assoc* 152:1501–1504, 1953.
68. Newcombe CP, Shucksmith HS, Suffern WS: Sympathectomy for hypertension; follow-up of 212 patients. *Br Med J* 1:142–144, 1959.
69. Grimson KS, Orgain ES, Anderson B, et al: Total thoracic and partial to total lumbar sympathectomy, splanchnicectomy and celiac ganglionectomy for hypertension. *Ann Surg* 138:532–547, 1953.
70. Peet MM, Isberg EM: The surgical treatment of essential hypertension. *J Am Med Assoc* 130:467–473, 1946.
71. Hinton JW: End results of thoracolumbar sympathectomy for advanced essential hypertension. *Bull N Y Acad Med* 24:239–252, 1948.
72. Evelyn KA, Alexander F, Cooper SR: Effect of sympathectomy on blood pressure in hypertension; a review of 13 years' experience of the Massachusetts General Hospital. *J Am Med Assoc* 140:592–602, 1949.
73. Hammarstrom S, Bechgaard P: Prognosis in arterial hypertension; comparison between 251 patients after sympathectomy and selected series of 435 non-operated patients. *Am J Med* 8:53–56, 1950.
74. Peet M, Woods P, Braden S: The surgical treatment of hypertension: results in 350 consecutive cases treated by bilateral supradiaphragmatic splanchnicectomy and lower dorsal sympathetic gangliectomy. Clinical lecture at the New York Session. *JAMA* 115:1875–1885, 1940.
75. Smithwick RH: Surgery in hypertension. *Lancet* 2:65, 1948.
76. Grimson KS, Orgain ES, Anderson B, et al: Results of treatment of patients with hypertension by total thoracic and partial to total lumbar sympathectomy, splanchnicectomy and celiac ganglionectomy. *Ann Surg* 129:850–871, 1949.
77. Steigerwald K, Titova A, Malle C, et al: Morphological assessment of renal arteries after radiofrequency catheter-based sympathetic denervation in a porcine model. *J Hypertens* 30:2230–2239, 2012.
78. Rippy MK, Zarins D, Barman NC, et al: Catheter-based renal sympathetic denervation: chronic preclinical evidence for renal artery safety. *Clin Res Cardiol* 100:1095–1101, 2011.
79. Krum H, Schlaich M, Whitbourn R, et al: Catheter-based renal sympathetic denervation for resistant hypertension: a multicentre safety and proof-of-principle cohort study. *Lancet* 373:1275–1281, 2009.
80. Schlaich MP, Sobotka PA, Krum H, et al: Renal sympathetic-nerve ablation for uncontrolled hypertension. *N Engl J Med* 361:932–934, 2009.
81. Hering D, Lambert EA, Marusic P, et al: Substantial reduction in single sympathetic nerve firing after renal denervation in patients with resistant hypertension. *Hypertension* 61:457–464, 2013.
82. Symplicity HTN-1 Investigators: Catheter-based renal sympathetic denervation for resistant hypertension: durability of blood pressure reduction out to 24 months. *Hypertension* 57:911–917, 2011.
83. Krum H, Schlaich MP, Sobotka PA, et al: Percutaneous renal denervation in patients with treatment-resistant hypertension: final 3-year report of the Symplicity HTN-1 study. *Lancet* 383:622–629, 2014.
84. Symplicity HTNI, Esler MD, Krum H, et al: Renal sympathetic denervation in patients with treatment-resistant hypertension (The Symplicity HTN-2 Trial): a randomised controlled trial. *Lancet* 376:1903–1909, 2010.
85. Whitbourn R: Persistent and Safe Blood Pressure Lowering Effects of Renal Artery Denervation: Three Year Follow-up From the Symplicity HTN-2 Randomized Controlled Trial. Transcatheter Therapeutics (TCT), San Francisco, 2013.
86. Kaltenbach B, Franke J, Bertog SC, et al: Renal sympathetic denervation as second-line therapy in mild resistant hypertension: a pilot study. *Catheter Cardiovasc Interv* 81:335–339, 2013.
87. Ott C, Mahfoud F, Schmid A, et al: Renal denervation in moderate treatment-resistant hypertension. *J Am Coll Cardiol* 62:1880–1886, 2013.
88. Robbins IM, Colvin EV, Doyle TP, et al: Pulmonary vein stenosis after catheter ablation of atrial fibrillation. *Circulation* 98:1769–1775, 1998.
89. Kaltenbach B, Id D, Franke JC, et al: Renal artery stenosis after renal sympathetic denervation. *J Am Coll Cardiol* 60:2694–2695, 2012.
90. Vonend O, Antoch G, Rump LC, et al: Secondary rise in blood pressure after renal denervation. *Lancet* 380:778, 2012.
91. Zeller T: Percutaneous Renal Denervation System. The new ultrasound solution for the management of hypertension. Transcatheter Therapeutics (TCT), San Francisco, 2013.
92. Mahfoud F, Cremers B, Janker J, et al: Renal hemodynamics and renal function after catheter-based renal sympathetic denervation in patients with resistant hypertension. *Hypertension* 60:419–424, 2012.
93. Zuern CS, Eick C, Rizas KD, et al: Impaired cardiac baroreflex sensitivity predicts response to renal sympathetic denervation in patients with resistant hypertension. *J Am Coll Cardiol* 62:2124–2130, 2013.
94. Chinushi M, Izumi D, Iijima K, et al: Blood pressure and autonomic responses to electrical stimulation of the renal arterial nerves before and after ablation of the renal artery. *Hypertension* 61:450–456, 2013.
95. Kaye DM, Esler M, Kingwell B, et al: Functional and neurochemical evidence for partial cardiac sympathetic reinnervation after cardiac transplantation in humans. *Circulation* 88:1110–1118, 1993.
96. Gazdar AF, Dammin GJ: Neural degeneration and regeneration in human renal transplants. *N Engl J Med* 283:222–224, 1970.
97. Hansen JM, Abildgaard U, Fogh-Andersen N, et al: The transplanted human kidney does not achieve functional reinnervation. *Clin Sci* 87:13–20, 1994.
98. Bhatt DL, Kandzari DE, O'Neill WW, et al: A controlled trial of renal denervation for resistant hypertension. *N Engl J Med* 370:1393–1401, 2014.
99. Bakris GL, Townsend RR, Liu M, et al: Impact of renal denervation on 24-hour ambulatory blood pressure: results from symplicity HTN-3. *J Am Coll Cardiol* 2014, [Epub ahead of print].
100. Saranathan M, Bayram E, Worters PW, et al: A 3D balanced-SSFP Dixon technique with group-encoded k-space segmentation for breath-held non-contrast-enhanced MR angiography. *Magn Reson Imaging* 30:158–164, 2012.
101. Khoo MM, Deeab D, Gedroyc WM, et al: Renal artery stenosis: comparative assessment by unenhanced renal artery MRA versus contrast-enhanced MRA. *Eur Radiol* 21:1470–1476, 2011.
102. Shonai T, Takahashi T, Ikeguchi H, et al: Improved arterial visibility using short-tau inversion-recovery (STIR) fat suppression in non-contrast-enhanced time-spatial labeling inversion pulse (Time-SLIP) renal MR angiography (MRA). *J Magn Reson Imaging* 29:1471–1477, 2009.
103. Wilson GJ, Maki JH: Non-contrast-enhanced MR imaging of renal artery stenosis at 1.5 tesla. *Magn Reson Imaging Clin N Am* 17:13–27, 2009.

104. Pickering TG, Hall JE, Appel LJ, et al: Recommendations for blood pressure measurement in humans: an AHA scientific statement from the Council on High Blood Pressure Research Professional and Public Education Subcommittee. *J Clin Hypertens (Greenwich)* 7:102–109, 2005.
105. Funder JW, Carey RM, Fardella C, et al: Case detection, diagnosis, and treatment of patients with primary aldosteronism: an endocrine society clinical practice guideline. *J Clin Endocrinol Metab* 93:3266–3281, 2008.
106. Nieman LK, Biller BM, Findling JW, et al: The diagnosis of Cushing's syndrome: an Endocrine Society Clinical Practice Guideline. *J Clin Endocrinol Metab* 93:1526–1540, 2008.
107. Wood PJ, Barth JH, Freedman DB, et al: Evidence for the low dose dexamethasone suppression test to screen for Cushing's syndrome–recommendations for a protocol for biochemistry laboratories. *Ann Clin Biochem* 34(Pt 3):222–229, 1997.
108. Kudva YC, Sawka AM, Young WF, Jr: Clinical review 164: the laboratory diagnosis of adrenal pheochromocytoma: the Mayo Clinic experience. *J Clin Endocrinol Metab* 88:4533–4539, 2003.
109. Gordon RD, Stowasser M, Tunny TJ, et al: High incidence of primary aldosteronism in 199 patients referred with hypertension. *Clin Exp Pharmacol Physiol* 21:315–318, 1994.
110. Loh KC, Koay ES, Khaw MC, et al: Prevalence of primary aldosteronism among Asian hypertensive patients in Singapore. *J Clin Endocrinol Metab* 85:2854–2859, 2000.
111. Young WF, Jr: Primary aldosteronism: a common and curable form of hypertension. *Cardiol Rev* 7:207–214, 1999.
112. Stowasser M: Primary aldosteronism: rare bird or common cause of secondary hypertension? *Curr Hypertens Rep* 3:230–239, 2001.
113. Calhoun DA, Nishizaka MK, Zaman MA, et al: Hyperaldosteronism among black and white subjects with resistant hypertension. *Hypertension* 40:892–896, 2002.
114. Young WF, Jr: Endocrine hypertension: then and now. *Endocr Pract* 16:888–902, 2010.
115. Mulatero P, Stowasser M, Loh KC, et al: Increased diagnosis of primary aldosteronism, including surgically correctable forms, in centers from five continents. *J Clin Endocrinol Metab* 89:1045–1050, 2004.
116. Ahmed AH, Gordon RD, Taylor P, et al: Effect of atenolol on aldosterone/renin ratio calculated by both plasma renin activity and direct renin concentration in healthy male volunteers. *J Clin Endocrinol Metab* 95:3201–3206, 2010.
117. Seifarth C, Trenkel S, Schobel H, et al: Influence of antihypertensive medication on aldosterone and renin concentration in the differential diagnosis of essential hypertension and primary aldosteronism. *Clin Endocrinol (Oxf)* 57:457–465, 2002.
118. Young WF, Jr, Klee GG: Primary aldosteronism. Diagnostic evaluation. *Endocrinol Metab Clin North Am* 17:367–395, 1988.
119. Young WF, Jr, Hogan MJ: Renin-independent hypermineralocorticoidism. *Trends Endocrinol Metab* 5:97–106, 1994.
120. Young WF, Stanson AW, Thompson GB, et al: Role for adrenal venous sampling in primary aldosteronism. *Surgery* 136:1227–1235, 2004.
121. Nwariaku FE, Miller BS, Auchus R, et al: Primary hyperaldosteronism: effect of adrenal vein sampling on surgical outcome. *Arch Surg* 141:497–502, discussion –3, 2006.
122. Daunt N: Adrenal vein sampling: how to make it quick, easy, and successful. *Radiographics* 25(Suppl 1):S143–S158, 2005.
123. Stowasser M, Gordon RD: Familial hyperaldosteronism. *J Steroid Biochem Mol Biol* 78:215–229, 2001.
124. Doppman JL, Gill JR, Jr: Hyperaldosteronism: sampling the adrenal veins. *Radiology* 198:309–312, 1996.
125. Young WF: Primary aldosteronism: renaissance of a syndrome. *Clin Endocrinol (Oxf)* 66:607–618, 2007.
126. Findling JW, Raff H: Cushing's Syndrome: important issues in diagnosis and management. *J Clin Endocrinol Metab* 91:3746–3753, 2006.
127. Young WF, Jr: Adrenal causes of hypertension: pheochromocytoma and primary aldosteronism. *Rev Endocr Metab Disord* 8:309–320, 2007.
128. Singh RJ: Advances in metanephrine testing for the diagnosis of pheochromocytoma. *Clin Lab Med* 24:85–103, 2004.
129. Perry CG, Sawka AM, Singh R, et al: The diagnostic efficacy of urinary fractionated metanephrines measured by tandem mass spectrometry in detection of pheochromocytoma. *Clin Endocrinol (Oxf)* 66:703–708, 2007.
130. Taylor GW, Kay GN, Zheng X, et al: Pathological effects of extensive radiofrequency energy applications in the pulmonary veins in dogs. *Circulation* 101:1736–1742, 2000.
131. Bertog SC, Blessing E, Vaskelyte L, et al: Renal denervation: tips and tricks to perform a technically successful procedure. *EuroIntervention* 9(Suppl R):R83–R88, 2013.
132. Id D, Kaltenbach B, Bertog S, et al: Does the presence of accessory renal arteries affect the efficacy of renal denervation? American College of Cardiology annual scientific meeting, San Francisco, 2013.
133. Ziegler AK, Franke J, Bertog SC: Renal denervation in a patient with prior renal artery stenting. *Catheter Cardiovasc Interv* 81:342–345, 2013.
134. Schenk EA, el-Badawi A: Dual innervation of arteries and arterioles. A histochemical study. *Z Zellforsch Mikrosk Anat* 91:170–177, 1968.
135. Mahfoud F, Schlaich M, Kindermann I, et al: Effect of renal sympathetic denervation on glucose metabolism in patients with resistant hypertension: a pilot study. *Circulation* 123:1940–1946, 2011.
136. Schlaich MP, Straznicky N, Grima M, et al: Renal denervation: a potential new treatment modality for polycystic ovary syndrome? *J Hypertens* 29:991–996, 2011.
137. Witkowski A, Prejbisz A, Florczak E, et al: Effects of renal sympathetic denervation on blood pressure, sleep apnea course, and glycemic control in patients with resistant hypertension and sleep apnea. *Hypertension* 58:559–565, 2011.
138. Mancia G, Bousquet P, Elghozi JL, et al: The sympathetic nervous system and the metabolic syndrome. *J Hypertens* 25:909–920, 2007.
139. Koistinen HA, Zierath JR: Regulation of glucose transport in human skeletal muscle. *Ann Med* 34:410–418, 2002.
140. Klein IH, Ligtenberg G, Oey PL, et al: Sympathetic activity is increased in polycystic kidney disease and is associated with hypertension. *J Am Soc Nephrol* 12:2427–2433, 2001.
141. Grassi G, Quarti-Trevano F, Seravalle G, et al: Early sympathetic activation in the initial clinical stages of chronic renal failure. *Hypertension* 57:846–851, 2011.
142. Esler MD, Krum H, Sobotka PA, et al: Renal sympathetic denervation in patients with treatment-resistant hypertension (The Symplicity HTN-2 Trial): a randomised controlled trial. *Lancet* 376:1903–1909, 2010.
143. Hering D, Mahfoud F, Walton AS, et al: Renal denervation in moderate to severe CKD. *J Am Soc Nephrol* 23:1250–1257, 2012.
144. Schlaich MP, Bart B, Hering D, et al: Feasibility of catheter-based renal nerve ablation and effects on sympathetic nerve activity and blood pressure in patients with end-stage renal disease. *Int J Cardiol* 168:2214–2220, 2013.
145. Pokushalov E, Romanov A, Katritsis DG, et al: Renal denervation for improving outcomes of catheter ablation in patients with atrial fibrillation and hypertension: early experience. *Heart Rhythm* 11:1131–1138, 2014.
146. Remo BF, Preminger M, Bradfield J, et al: Safety and efficacy of renal denervation as a novel treatment of ventricular tachycardia storm in patients with cardiomyopathy. *Heart Rhythm* 11:541–546, 2014.
147. Hasking GJ, Esler MD, Jennings GL, et al: Norepinephrine spillover to plasma in patients with congestive heart failure: evidence of increased overall and cardiorenal sympathetic nervous activity. *Circulation* 73:615–621, 1986.
148. Cohn JN, Levine TB, Olivari MT, et al: Plasma norepinephrine as a guide to prognosis in patients with chronic congestive heart failure. *N Engl J Med* 311:819–823, 1984.
149. Packer M, Coats AJ, Fowler MB, et al: Effect of carvedilol on survival in severe chronic heart failure. *N Engl J Med* 344:1651–1658, 2001.
150. Effects of enalapril on mortality in severe congestive heart failure. Results of the Cooperative North Scandinavian Enalapril Survival Study (CONSENSUS). The CONSENSUS Trial Study Group. *N Engl J Med* 316:1429–1435, 1987.
151. Nozawa T, Igawa A, Fujii N, et al: Effects of long-term renal sympathetic denervation on heart failure after myocardial infarction in rats. *Heart Vessels* 16:51–56, 2002.
152. Davies JE, Manisty CH, Petraco R, et al: First-in-man safety evaluation of renal denervation for chronic systolic heart failure: primary outcome from REACH-Pilot study. *Int J Cardiol* 162:189–192, 2013.
153. Kandzari DE: Symplicity HTN Program: Expanding Therapeutic Options for HTN and New Indications. Transcatheter Therapeutics (TCT), San Francisco, 2013.
154. Ormiston JA, Watson T, van Pelt N, et al: First-in-human use of the OneShot renal denervation system from Covidien. *EuroIntervention* 8:1090–1094, 2013.
155. Verheye S: Preliminary results of the Rapid Renal Sympathetic Denervation for Resistant Hypertension Using the Maya Medical OneShot Ablation System (RAPID) Study. *JACC* 62, 2013.
156. Verheye S: Rapid renal sympathetic denervation for Resistant Hypertension Using the OneShot Ablation System (RAPID) Study: primary endpoint 6-month results. Transcatheter Therapeutics (TCT), San Francisco, 2013.
157. Kirtane A: Device and clinical trial update: the BSC vessix renal denervation system. Transcatheter Therapeutics (TCT), San Francisco, 2013.
158. Worthley SG: Longer-term safety and efficacy of sympathetic renal artery denervation using a multi-electrode renal artery denervation catheter in patients with drug-resistant hypertension: eighteen month results of a First-in Human, Multicenter Study. Transcatheter Therapeutics (TCT), San Francisco, 2013.
159. Brinton T: Extra-vascular focused ultrasonic denervation. Transcatheter Therapeutics (TCT), San Francisco, 2013.
160. Chen SL, Zhang FF, Xu J, et al: Pulmonary artery denervation to treat pulmonary arterial hypertension: the single-center, prospective, first-in-man PADN-1 study (first-in-man pulmonary artery denervation for treatment of pulmonary artery hypertension). *J Am Coll Cardiol* 62:1092–1100, 2013.

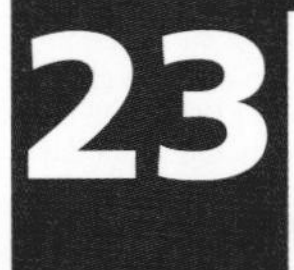

Endovascular Management of Aortic and Thoracic Aneurysms

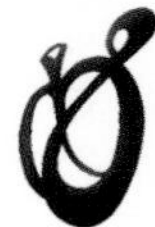

Aravinda Nanjundappa

A. Abdominal Aortic Aneurysm

INTRODUCTION

Abdominal aortic aneurysm (AAA) is defined as a 50% increase in the diameter of the aorta when compared with a normal segment.[1] The average infrarenal aortic diameters for men and women are 1.5 cm and 1.7 cm, respectively. The universal standard for an infrarenal aneurysmal aorta is greater than 3.0 cm.[2]

Natural History

An AAA is usually asymptomatic and is most commonly discovered as an incidental finding on a radiological examination. The prevalence of AAA increases with age, and the incidence in patients 45 to 54 years is 2.6% in men and 0.5% in women. In the older population (age 75 to 84 years), the incidence of AAA is 19.8% in men and 5.2% in women. The overall prevalence of AAA varies from 5% to 7% in patients over 65 years of age,[3] and men are affected 4 to 6 times more often than women.[3] A variety of cardiovascular and noncardiovascular co-morbidities, such as hypertension, coronary artery disease, cerebrovascular disease, and malignancy, co-exist with AAA. In patients with AAA, coronary artery disease and cerebrovascular disease are noted in 40% and 25%, respectively. Hypertension is present in more than half (55%) of patients with AAA; while malignancy is noted in 23% and claudication in 28%.[4] Approximately two thirds (66%) of AAA patients die from cardiovascular etiologies.[5]

Most aortic aneurysms increase at a rate of 0.2 to 0.3 cm/yr when the size is less than 5.5 cm. However, once the aneurysm reaches 5 to 6 cm, there is a rapid increase of up to 3 cm/yr.[6] A rapid growth in an AAA is usually seen in smokers and females. The devastating sequela of an enlarging AAA is catastrophic rupture and death. Ruptured AAA accounts for 1% of all deaths and it is the tenth leading cause of death in patients over 50 years in age.[7] Another clinical manifestation of AAA is distal embolization, resulting in acute limb ischemia, gangrene, blue toe syndrome, and limb loss.

Risk Factors

The risk factors for AAA are similar to those for atherosclerosis: male gender, age over 65 years, a history of ever smoking (>100 cigarettes in a person's lifetime), hypertension, hypercholesterolemia, and genetic predisposition.[8-10]

One of the potential risk factors is a family history of AAA and surgical interventions for AAA in a family member.[11-13] Five percent of patients with AAA have associated thoracic aneurysms, and approximately 15% have associated femoral or popliteal aneurysms.[14]

Inflammatory aneurysms are a unique subset (5%) of AAA and usually present with vague flank pain, abdominal discomfort, and fever. A computerized tomography (CT) scan or magnetic resonance imaging (MRI) usually demonstrate concentric thickening around the abdominal wall. The inflammatory process in the retroperitonium is extensive and often involves the inferior vena cava, ureters, renal vein, and duodenum. When such an AAA reaches 5.5 cm, the endovascular approach may be optimal.[15]

A minority of AAAs are associated with a nonatherosclerotic degenerative connective tissue disease, such as Ehlers-Danlos syndrome, Marfan syndrome, and Loeys-Dietz syndrome.[16,17] Mycotic aneurysms are rare, but can cause pseudoaneurysms; and the most common etiologies are *Salmonella* and *Staphylococcal aureus*. Surgical options include resection and extra-anatomic bypass or aorta bi-femoral bypass using the deep femoral veins. Patients with mycotic aneurysms commonly have co-morbidities and, therefore, the surgical approach may be prohibitive. Endovascular aneurysm repair (EVAR) for treatment of abdominal mycotic aneurysms may be a short-term solution to avoid catastrophic rupture.[18,19] A rare complication of AAA is aortoenteric fistula and case reports have successfully excluded these using an endograft.[20]

Laplace Law

Laplace law indicates that wall tension of a symmetric shape is directly proportional to the intraluminal pressure and inversely proportional to the wall thickness. However, in reality, AAAs are not symmetrical in shape and have variations in wall thickness and strength.

Predictors of Rupture

The maximum AAA diameter is the most extensively accepted single parameter that predicts the risk of rupture.[21,22] The risk of rupture increases when the AAA size is greater than 5.5 cm in men and women. The expansion rate is also an important determinant of risk of rupture.[23,24] Rapidly enlarging AAAs, defined as a growth of 0.5 cm every 6 months, are also considered to be at high risk for rupture.[25] Continued smoking and lifting heavy weights can cause a rupture in patients with aneurysms.[26]

DIAGNOSIS

Physical Exam

Despite the novelty and importance of a physical exam, the only reliable finding is a widened palpable or pulsatile aorta above the umbilicus. Only 30% of these asymptomatic AAAs are detected on routine physical examination as a pulsatile abdominal mass.[27] Auscultation of the aneurysm is useful, as the presence of a bruit may indicate associated aortic or mesenteric artery occlusive disease. Occasionally, a machinery murmur over the aneurysm may indicate an aortocaval fistula. The physical examination is dependent on the clinician's experience and the patient's body habitus. A large aneurysm in a thin individual is detected easily, while accuracy of physical examination is reduced by an obese body habitus. The overall sensitivity is approximately 29%, but can reach 96% in patients with an aneurysm ≥5.0 cm.[28,29] The absence of a widened or palpable aorta does not exclude the presence of an AAA. Concomitant aneurysms, such as femoral and popliteal aneurysms, can be more easily diagnosed, yet continue to be under diagnosed. Other physical exam findings can be distal arterial embolization, blue toe syndrome, or livedo reticularis, and diminished distal pulses.

Abdominal Ultrasound

This is a safe, cost-effective, and simple test of choice for screening patients with AAA. The sensitivity and specificity of ultrasound, when performed by trained personnel, is close to 96% and 100%, respectively, for detection of infrarenal AAA.[30] Ultrasound can serve as an excellent tool for the diagnosis and follow-up of AAA. Poor imaging quality, due to patient body habitus and variations in interpretations, are a few of the notable limitations.

Magnetic Resonance Angiography

Magnetic resonance angiography (MRA) is a noninvasive nonradiation test used to diagnose and evaluate the size of the AAA; however, MRA cannot usually be performed on patients with metallic implants, such as pacemakers.[31]

Computerized Tomography

Computerized tomography (CT) scans can not only confirm the precise size, they can also delineate thrombus, occlusion, or stenosis.[32] CT scanning plays a pivotal role in planning EVAR versus open repair and follow-up for shrinkage of size and endoleaks. The details of utilization of CT scan in preplanning an EVAR will be described later in this chapter.

INDICATIONS FOR REVASCULARIZATION

Symptomatic Patients

When an AAA becomes symptomatic it can be categorized into the following:

1. Impending rupture
2. Embolic or thrombotic complications
3. Mass effect

Symptomatic AAA patients usually present with abdominal pain, low back pain, and flank pain. A sudden onset of back pain or abdominal pain, hypotension, and a palpable abdominal mass are the classic triad of symptoms for a ruptured AAA. However, a clinical diagnosis for ruptured AAA requires a high index of suspicion and misdiagnosis that includes renal colic, perforated viscus, abdominal wall hernia, diverticulitis, and ischemic bowel.[33,34]

Thromboembolic symptoms from AAA can cause acute limb ischemia, gangrene, and limb loss. Baxter et al. identified 15 patients, among a review of 302 patients undergoing open AAA repair, to have distal embolization as the first manifestation. Among these patients, only two had an AAA size greater than 5 cm, which is suggestive of the potentially dangerous nature of small AAAs that are more likely to present with thromboembolic symptoms (**Figure 23-1**).[35] Large AAAs may cause vague symptoms, such as back pain, early satiety, ureteral compression, and venous thrombosis due to iliocaval compression.

Asymptomatic Aneurysms

AAA patients are generally asymptomatic and are found during incidental radiological tests, such as x-ray, ultrasound,

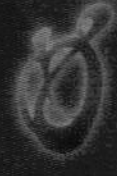

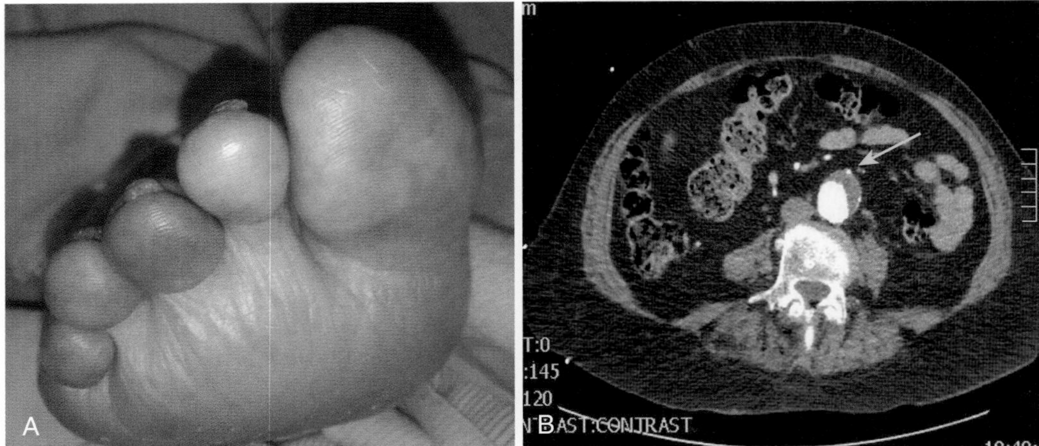

FIGURE 23-1 76-year-old patient with **(A)** blue toe syndrome from a **(B)** 3.5-cm abdominal aortic aneurysm (AAA).

CT scan, MRI, and positron emission tomography (PET) scan. The maximum diameter of the AAA is the best indicator of rupture.[36] The generally accepted indications are that men and women with an AAA greater than 5.0 to 5.5 cm require revascularization due to an increased risk of rupture.[37] Rapidly growing aneurysms, defined by a growth rate greater than 0.5 cm in 6 months or 1.0 cm in 1 year, also need revascularization.[38] Factors which should be considered include estimated risk of rupture under observation, the operative risk involved, life expectancy of the patient, and the patient's personal preferences.

CLINICAL DATA

The first EVAR was performed by Drs. Parody, Palmaz, and Barone on September 7, 1990; by 1991 five more patients were treated with EVAR.[39] A Dacron tube prosthesis was inserted via the transfemoral approach and the fixation was by balloon expandable stents. Subsequently, the nonstented bifurcated or straight devices were described by White et al.[40] White and colleagues published the data in 25 patients with the use of a novel graft attachment device (GAD). Successful EVAR was achieved with low morbidity and mortality in those patients who met the selection criteria.

Ivancev et al. performed an endoluminal exclusion of AAA using an aortomonoiliac stent graft.[41] A total of 45 patients underwent exclusion of AAA using the uni-limb device, which was deployed with the "Lancey-Mamosystem." Open surgical conversion was performed in six patients due to the short length of the endograft device. Several complications were noted, such as two patients with inadvertent renal artery occlusions, six patients with iliac artery dissections, seven patients with kinked grafts, and three patients had perioccluder leaks. A total of five patients died in the perioperative period and five more patients had significant migrations. The study proved the feasibility of graft use, but complications from a learning curve were clearly noted. This study also demonstrated the need for adherence to a strict inclusion protocol to improve mortality and reduce complications.

By 1997, six endovascular grafts were commercially available. The individual treatment strategies for each device and specific inclusion criteria were described.[42] The initial treatment of ruptured AAA with EVAR was reported by Dr. Yusuf et al.[43]

Initial Comparisons of Open Surgical Repair Versus Endovascular AAA Repair

The widespread use of EVAR to treat AAA followed the Food and Drug Administration (FDA) approval of second generation abdominal aortic endograft in 1999. The early EVAR outcomes noted in nonrandomized trials, registries, and single-center trials demonstrated lower rates of mortality and morbidity. A comparison of endoluminal versus open repair in the treatment of AAAs was analyzed in 303 patients.[44] Open repair was performed in 195 patients and endovascular repair in 108 patients. The perioperative mortality rates were 5.6% each in the open repair group and the endovascular group. The advantages of endovascular repair were lower blood loss, shorter intensive care unit (ICU) stay, and reduced neurological complications. However, the Achilles heel for EVAR continued to be late complications such as endoleak and migration.

After 15 years of initial EVAR, by 2006 in the United States 21,725 endovascular exclusion of AAA procedures were performed, and thus EVAR numbers exceeded the number of open surgical AAA revascularization.[45,46] The recent developments in catheter-based, endovascular techniques led to a substantial increase in the proportion of AAAs managed electively with EVAR. As of 2012, more than 70% of all infrarenal AAA was being treated with EVAR in the United States.[47]

Randomized Controlled Trials of EVAR Versus Open Surgical Repair

The landmark trials that demonstrated the safety, efficacy, and long-term results of EVAR versus open surgical repair for AAA were the Dutch randomized endovascular aneurysm management (DREAM) trial, EVAR I, EVAR 2, and OVER trial (**Table 23-1**).

DREAM

The DREAM trial was first published in 2004 and subsequently the long-term results in 2010.[48] DREAM was a randomized, controlled, multicenter trial (24 centers in Netherlands and 4 centers in Belgium) comparing EVAR with open repair in 351 patients with greater than 5 cm AAA who were suitable for both techniques. The primary endpoint was mortality from any cause and intervention. A total of 173 patients were randomly assigned to EVAR and 178 patients to open repair. There was no statistically significant

TABLE 23-1 Summary of Randomized Control Trials Comparing Outcomes of Open Versus Endovascular Repair for AAA

	DREAM		EVAR1		OVER	
OUTCOMES	OPEN REPAIR	ENDO REPAIR	OPEN REPAIR	ENDO REPAIR	OPEN REPAIR	ENDO REPAIR
30-day mortality %	4.6	1.2	4.3	1.8	3	0.5
Long-term mortality	30.1% at 6 yr	31.1% at 6 yr	22.3% at 4 yr	23.1% at 4 yr	9.8% at 2 yr	7.0% at 2 yr

difference found in the primary endpoint at 30 days between the surgical group and EVAR (9.8% vs. 4.7%; p = 0.10). At 6 years the cumulative survival rates were 68.9% for endovascular repair and 69.9% for surgical repair (95% confidence interval [CI], −8.8 to 10.8; p = 0.97). The rate of secondary intervention at 6 years in the EVAR group was 29.6% and open repair 18.1% (p = 0.03). The EVAR did have a lower procedural blood loss, systemic complications, need for mechanical ventilations, and shorter ICU and hospital stay.

EVAR 1

In this trial, 1252 patients from 37 hospitals in the United Kingdom between 1999 and 2004 were enrolled.[49] All patients had AAA greater than 5.5 cm and were considered to be acceptable candidates for either open repair or EVAR. A total of 626 patients were enrolled into each group and they were followed until 2009 for mortality rates, complications from graft, reinterventions, and resource use. The 30-day mortality for endovascular group was 1.8% versus 4.3% in the open repair group (p = 0.02). Despite the early benefit with aneurysm-related mortality in the EVAR group, by the end of the study there was no difference in mortality from any cause between the two groups (p = 0.73). Similar to the DREAM trial, EVAR 1 also showed higher rates of graft-related complications and re-interventions with EVAR and higher costs.

EVAR 2

The EVAR 1 investigators randomized 338 patients with AAA greater than 5.5 cm unfit for open repair to endovascular repair (n = 166) versus no intervention (n = 177).[50] The 30-day operative mortality in the endovascular group was 9%. The rupture rate in the no intervention group was 9 per 100 person years. At 4 years follow-up there was no difference in all-cause mortality (p = 0.25). The aneurysm-related mortality was lower in the EVAR group (adjusted ratio [AR] 0.53; p = 0.02). However, EVAR was associated with higher hospital costs and no benefit in terms of patient quality of life compared with the noninterventional group. The complication rates were higher in the endovascular group—48% versus 18% in the noninterventional group (p = <0.0001)

The OVER Trial

The open versus endovascular repair (OVER) trial was conducted at 42 veteran affairs medical centers in the United States.[51] OVER was a multicenter, randomized trial that enrolled a total 881 AAA patients who were eligible for open surgical repair or EVAR. The enrolled patients had an AAA maximum diameter of >5.0 cm, iliac artery aneurysm of >3.0 cm, or AAA >4.5 cm, and who had rapid AAA enlargement (>0.5 cm in 6 months) or secular aneurysms. A total of 437 patients were randomized to open repair and 444 patients to EVAR. The primary outcomes measured were procedure failure, secondary procedures, and length of stay, quality of life, erectile dysfunction, mortality, and major morbidity. The 30-day perioperative mortality was lower for EVAR compared with open repair (0.5% vs. 3.0%; p = 0.04). However, this early EVAR benefit was lost at 2 years; the perioperative mortality rates for open and EVAR were 9.8% versus 7.0% (p = 0.13). The EVAR group had reduced procedure time, transfusion requirement, blood loss, and hospital and intensive care stay. There were no differences in procedural failure, secondary procedures, quality of life, and erectile dysfunction incidence between the two groups.

ENDOVASCULAR REPAIR

Preoperative Imaging

Multiple modalities such as CT angiogram, MRA, intravascular ultrasound (IVUS), and angiogram are available to image AAA. A contrasted CT scan using the thin slices (0.9 to 3 mm) is the imaging modality of choice for preoperative evaluation of AAA prior to EVAR. In patients with significant renal insufficiency CT scan without contrast and MRA without gadolinium may be used. Such alternative techniques may miss important anatomical information such as: laminated thrombus, patent inferior mesenteric artery (IMA), and severe iliofemoral occlusive disease.[52] Besides the axial cuts, a review of sagittal, coronal, and three-dimensional (3D) reconstructions is necessary to fully understand the aneurysm anatomy, including its angulation (**Table 23-2**). IVUS can be used to size the aortic and iliac artery seal zones, and evaluate potential eccentric thrombus in the aortic neck and the external iliac artery for occlusive disease (**Figures 23-2 and 23-3**).

Anesthesia

All patients scheduled for elective EVAR should undergo appropriate preoperative risk stratification according to American College of Cardiology (ACC)/American Heart Association (AHA) guidelines. Patients who are considered inoperable for open surgical repair of AAA carry a risk of 18% to 43% perioperative cardiovascular events if primary conversion of EVAR to surgical open repair becomes necessary.[53] Initially, the majority of patients received general anesthesia for EVAR. The smaller sheath size and closure devices have enabled patients to undergo EVAR with monitored anesthesia care (MAC).[54,55] EVAR operators should coordinate and plan the procedure with the anesthesia for procedure safety and reduce complications.

Strategic Planning and Multispecialty Team

A careful and well thought out strategic plan of EVAR is essential for optimal outcomes. The planning should include a physical examination and detailed history and a thorough explanation of natural history of AAA to the patient and family. The multispecialty (vascular surgeon, cardiologist, and/or radiologist) discussion should include all treatment

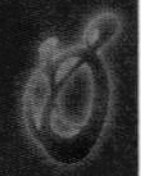

TABLE 23-2 Various Characteristics That Should Be Evaluated on the Preoperative CT Angiogram of an AAA

LOCATION	PARAMETER	MEASUREMENTS	DEVICE INSTRUCTIONS FOR USE
Aortic neck	Diameter	Measure at the level of lowest renal artery and 15 mm caudal a. 10 mm for Medtronic Endurant device b. 7 mm for Trivascular Ovation device	Should be 16-32 mm
	Length	Distance from lowest renal artery to the origin of aneurysm	>15 mm for most devices a. 10 mm for Medtronic Endurant device b. 7 mm for Ovation Trivascular device
	Angulation	Between the central line of aorta and aneurysm	Less than 60° a. Less than 90° for Lombard Aorfix device
	Thrombus	Should be <25% of vessel circumference	
	Calcification	Extensive/circumferential predicts problems with good seal	
	Taper	Look for reverse taper (>4 mm diameter increase over 10 mm aortic length)	Increase chances of proximal Type I endoleak
Distal aortic bifurcation		Look for narrowing that may preclude the accommodation of two limbs of the graft except for Endologix Powerlink device	
External iliac artery		Should be able to accommodate 14 Fr to 20 Fr sheath depending on the type of device A minimum of 6 mm EIA is recommended for the low-profile device	
Hypogastric artery		For patency, length between CIA and hypogastric origin and aneurysms	
Femoral arteries		For anterior versus posterior calcium, plaque, patency, and aneurysmal dilatation	

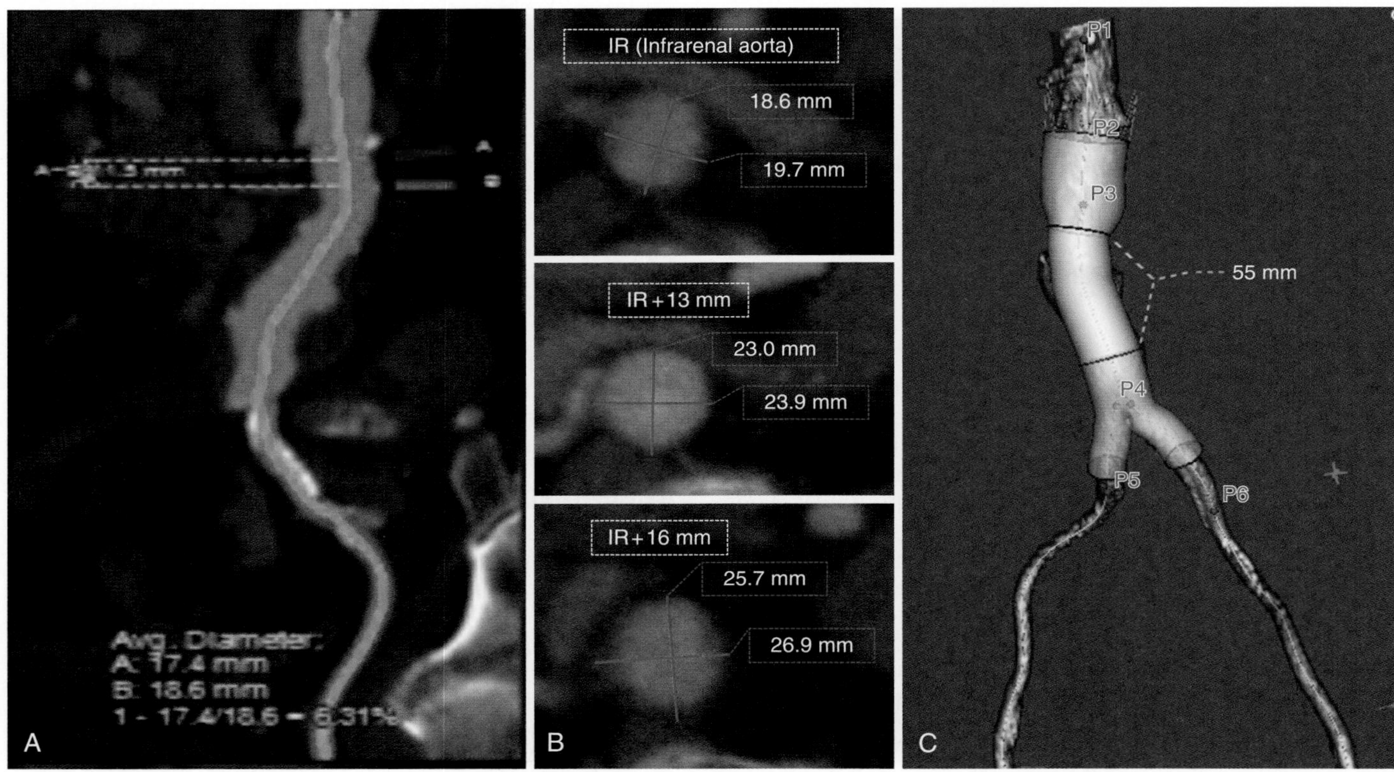

FIGURE 23-2 Computed tomography (CT) scan for pre-EVAR planning: **A,** center line measurements for infrarenal neck length and diameter. **B,** Infrarenal neck measured at 1 mm, 13 mm, and 16 mm below the lowest renal artery. **C,** 3D image reconstruction of EVAR graft superimposed on the abdominal aortic aneurysm (AAA).

options for AAA revascularization, and risk benefit and alternatives of EVAR. Each EVAR case should be preferably planned with a vascular surgeon and anesthesiologist in a team-based approach. Recent advances in CT software technology include availability of 3D measurements to assist in intraoperative navigation techniques.[56] All high-risk patients should have risk factor reduction by appropriate treatment with aspirin, beta blockers, ACE inhibitors, and statins prior to EVAR. Baseline pulmonary functions test and lab works such as blood urea nitrogen (BUN), creatinine, hemoglobin levels, and prothrombin time should be known prior to surgery. Anticoagulants such as warfarin or newer ones should be held in advance and, if needed, bridged with heparin. A type and screen of blood type rather than type and cross can reduce the number of transfusions.[57] All the devices and auxiliary equipment such as snares, covered

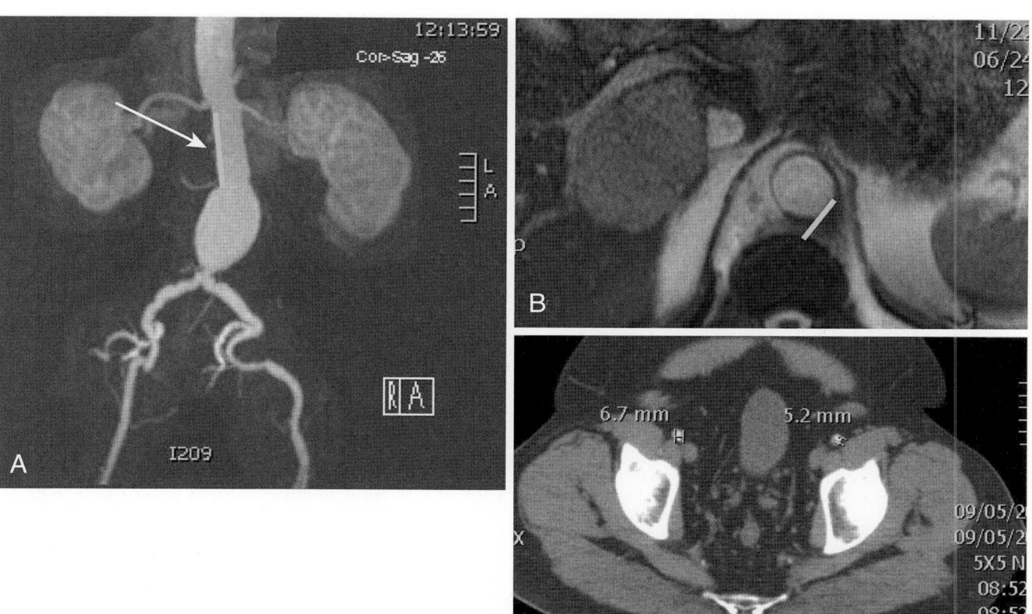

FIGURE 23-3 Shows magnetic resonance angiography (MRA) for pre-EVAR planning. **A,** Neck length. **B,** Diameter. **C,** External iliac diameter.

stents, and a Palmaz stent (Cordis corp., Miami Lakes, Florida) should be available before the start of the case.

EVAR is performed by various specialists who have proficiency in the procedure and follow-up. The multispecialty team usually should include vascular surgery, cardiology or radiology, and anesthesia. Despite the ability of a nonvascular surgery physician to perform EVAR, it is highly recommended to have a team approach with vascular surgery. Such a team approach plays a vital role in endovascular management of ruptured AAA.[58] Acute complications such as vessel rupture, distal embolization, requirement for a surgical cut down for vessel access and repair, or emergent conversion to open repair will need vascular surgery expertise.[59]

Anatomic Considerations

Anatomical considerations that are important for AAA suitability for EVAR are as follows:

- Proximal and distal attachment site
- Diameter and characteristics of access vessels
- Percutaneous access for EVAR
- Aorto iliac artery side branches with potential for exclusion during EVAR: hypogastric artery, accessory or anomalous origin of renal artery, and patent inferior mesenteric artery

Proximal and Distal Attachment Sites

One of the most important anatomical factors that predicts the suitability for EVAR is the character of aortic neck. Important measurements and characteristics include length, diameter, angulations, presence of thrombus, reverse taper, and calcification. The majority of the endovascular grafts have prespecified instructions for use (IFU)—the infrarenal neck length should be at least 10 mm in length and less than 32 mm in diameter with infrarenal angulations less than 90° (**Figures 23-4 and 23-5**).[60,61]

Aortic Neck: Diameter, Length, Angulation, Taper, Reverse Taper, and Thrombus

Aortic neck diameters that can be treated can range from 18 to 32 mm. Most measurements are based on the CT scan outer wall to outer wall except for Gore (W.L. Gore and associates, Inc., Flagstaff, Arizona), which measures inner to inner wall. The two important dimensions of the infrarenal neck of the AAA are measured as D1 and D2. D1 is the first image of the infrarenal aorta measured outer to outer wall in the short axis. D2 is the diameter below D1 at 10 mm or 15 mm distal based the graft. The length of the aortic neck is determined by counting the number of images from lower renal artery to the start of the aneurysm based on the CT scan slices at the time of imaging (0.9 to 5 mm).

The distal attachment site is equally important to ensure adequate seal and prevent endoleak (discussed later). The distal landing zone is preferable in the common iliac artery and allows perfusion of the hypogastric artery. In patients with common iliac artery (CIA) aneurysms, the endovascular approach can be performed with low morbidity, blood loss, hospital stay, and short-term mortality.[62] The mid-term durability and survival from endovascular approach offers the advantage of first-line treatment option for patients with iliac artery aneurysms (**Figure 23-6**).[63,64] The diameter of the CIA and morphology such as calcification, thrombus, and stenosis should be evaluated. CIA diameters up to 25 mm can be treated with endograft using a flared 28-mm limb available with Endurant stent graft system[65] (Medtronic Inc., Santa Rosa, California).

The two main issues of obliteration of hypogastric arteries are pelvic ischemia and Type II endoleak (explained later). A large series of EVAR patients who underwent hypogastric embolization had persistent buttock claudication in 12% of unilateral and 11% of bilateral hypogastric artery interruptions. Erectile dysfunction occurred in 9% of unilateral and 13% of bilateral hypogastric occlusions.[66] The dreaded

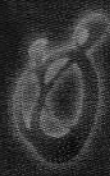

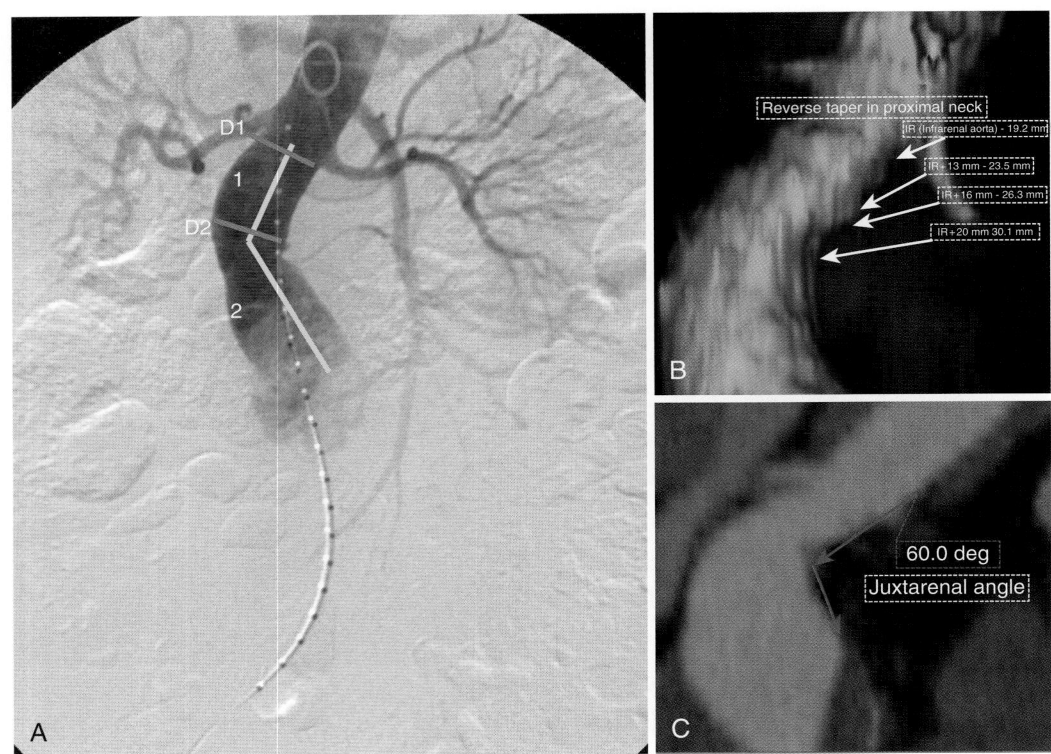

FIGURE 23-4 Case example of aortic neck characteristics that are ideal for EVAR. **A,** *1,* Length of the aneurysmal neck; *D1,* Diameter of the proximal neck; *D2,* Diameter of the distal neck; *2,* Angulation of the neck. **B** and **C,** Reverse taper of the aortic neck.

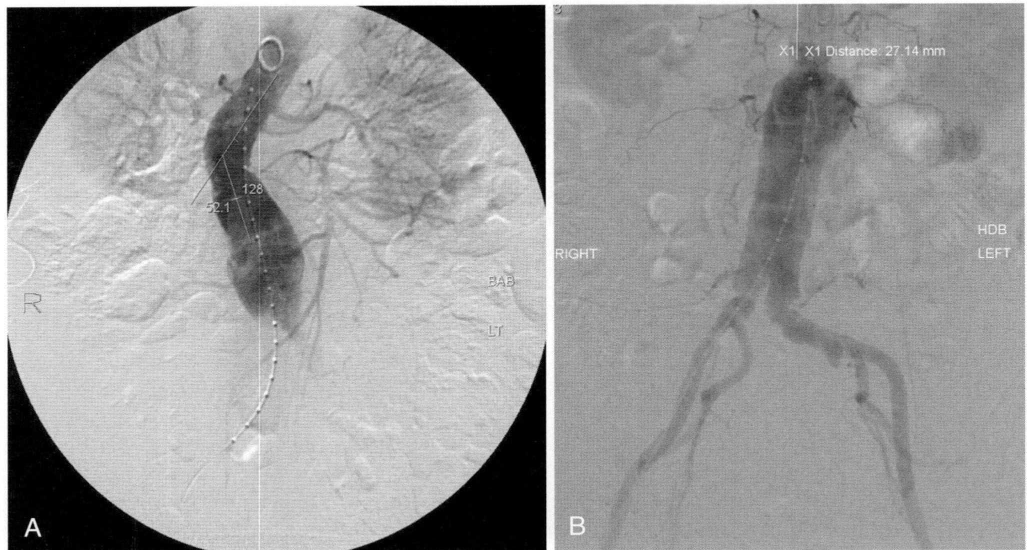

FIGURE 23-5 Angiographic confirmation of aortic neck measurements. **A,** Infrarenal neck angulation. **B,** Infrarenal neck length.

complication of ischemic colitis develops in less than 2% of EVAR cases.[67] The risk for colon necrosis increases in EVAR patients who have an occlusive disease of all three mesenteric vessels, or if previous colon surgery has interrupted the mesenteric collateral pathways. Colon ischemia is more likely to result from atheroembolism to the pelvic circulation rather than hypogastric artery occlusion.[68]

The characteristics of the common iliac artery can determine the following options that are available to manage the distal landing zone during EVAR (**Figure 23-7**).

1. If the internal iliac artery is not aneurysmal, coil embolization of the internal iliac artery is performed at its origin to reduce the postprocedure rates of buttock claudication.[69] The patency of branches of internal iliac artery may help in reducing the buttock postprocedure. The limb can be further extended across the embolized hypogastric artery into the external iliac artery (EIA) to obtain adequate seal.
2. If flow to the internal iliac artery has to be preserved then a surgical bypass from internal iliac artery to the external iliac artery can be performed. This hybrid technique has

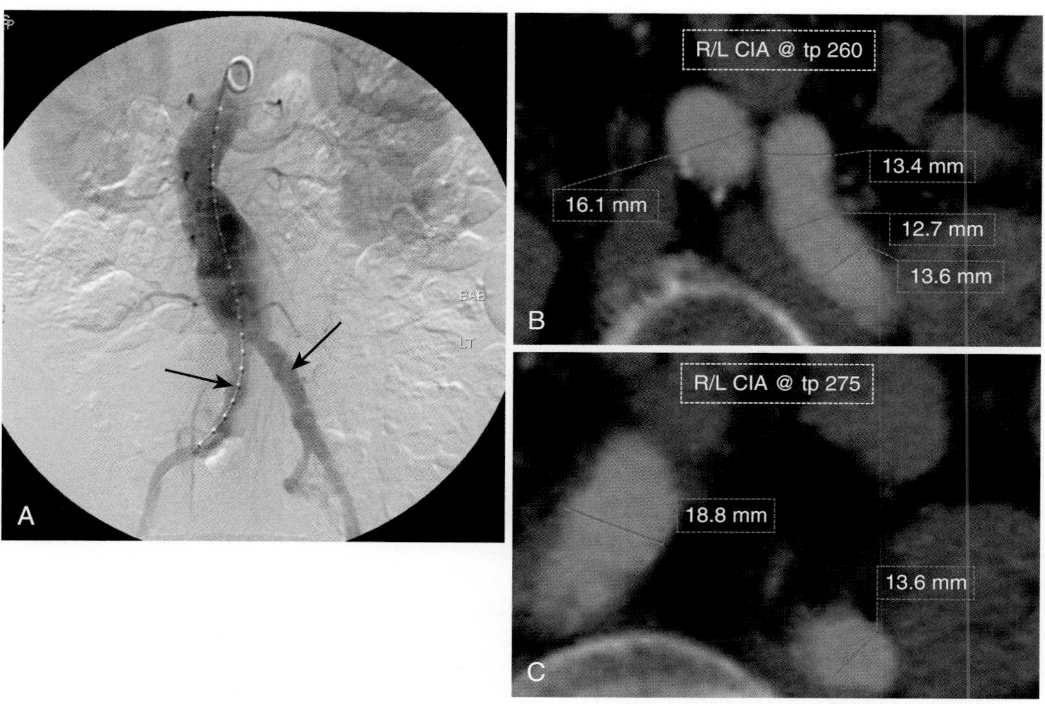

FIGURE 23-6 Common iliac artery with a good landing zone in a patient evaluated for EVAR. **A,** Angiography. **B** and **C,** Computed tomography (CT) scan.

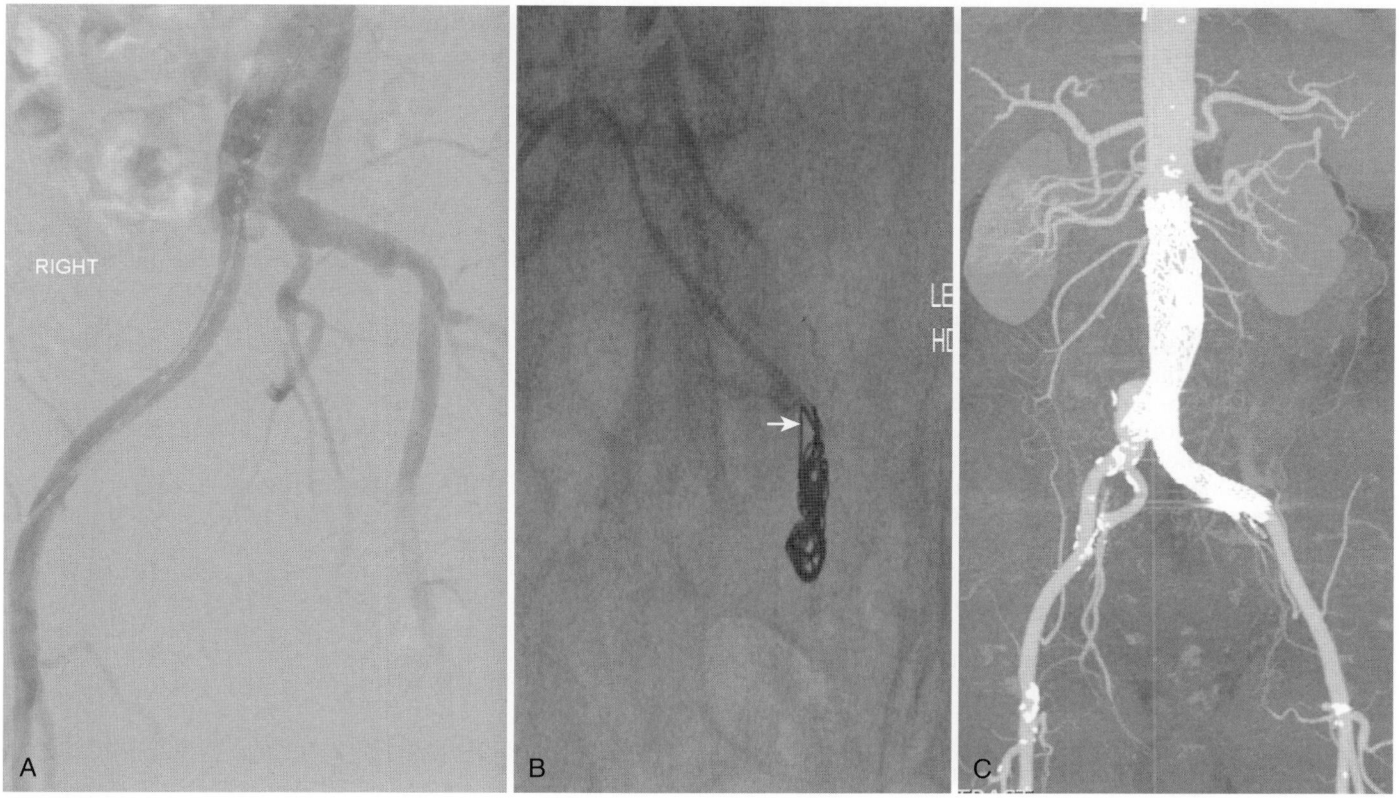

FIGURE 23-7 **A,** Pre-EVAR angiogram to treat CIA aneurysm of 3.2 cm and abdominal aortic aneurysm (AAA). **B,** The internal iliac artery is occluded at the origin by coil embolization. **C,** Computed tomography (CT) follow-up shows limb of the EVAR graft extended into the external iliac artery.

demonstrated good mid- and long-term patency.[70] However, the operative times, length of hospital stay, and blood loss are increased.[71]

3. If the hypogastric artery needs to be preserved, a double-barrel stenting can preserve the flow to the internal iliac artery and obtain adequate seal at the common iliac artery.[72,73] In this technique one covered stent is placed from the CIA into the hypogastric artery and a simultaneous limb of the EVAR graft will extend from CIA to the EIA (**Figure 23-8**).

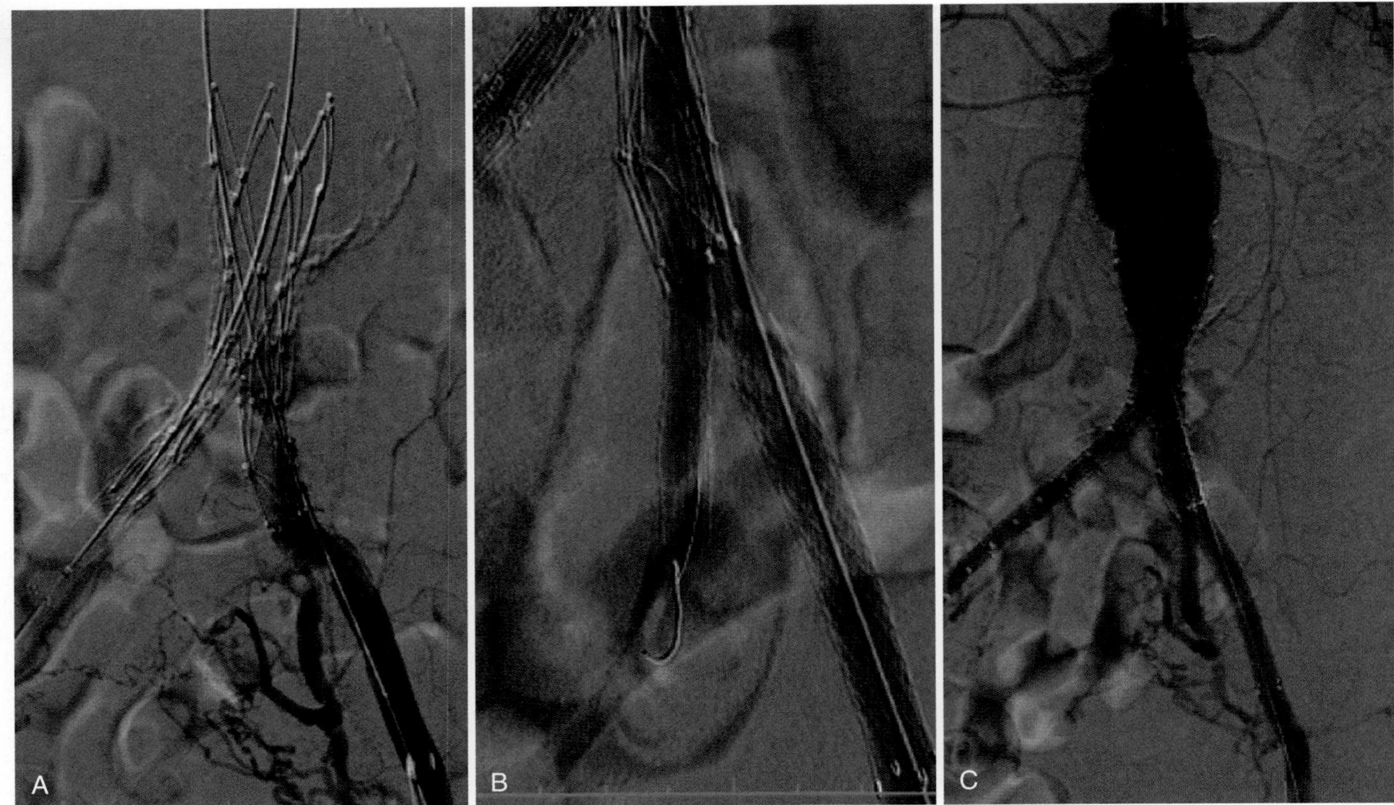

FIGURE 23-8 A case of sandwich technique during EVAR to maintain hypogastric artery patency. **A,** The left hypogastric artery shows severe ostial stenosis. **B,** Simultaneous stenting of left hypogastric artery and left external iliac artery (EIA). **C,** Final angiogram to show preservation of the left hypogastric artery and the left external iliac artery (EIA).

4. If the common iliac artery is occluded then a uni-aortic limb placement with femoral-femoral bypass is performed. A contralateral placement of flexible covered stent from external iliac artery to internal iliac artery will allow retrograde perfusion.[74,75]

Access Arteries

The bilateral common femoral artery (CFA) is the most common access site for insertion of the delivery sheath or the device. The majority of the devices need a prespecified sheath through which the device can be inserted. The access vessels are evaluated for atherosclerosis, stenosis, calcification, and vessel diameters (**Figure 23-9**). The CFA should be accessed for vessel length, depth of the artery from skin surface, and diameter. The calcification of the CFA is a critical determinant of the technical success and outcomes of EVAR.[76-78]

Calcification, atherosclerosis, and stenosis of the common femoral artery can be dealt with CFA cutdown by vascular surgery. The cutdown procedure, despite increasing the success rate of EVAR, carries a low degree of complications such as seroma/lymphocele, hematoma, bleeding, blood transfusion, vessel dissection, femoral nerve injury, infection, delay in wound healing, and scar tissue.[79,80] The diameter of the EIA plays an important role in device insertion and removal. A rupture of EIA can result in a catastrophic event requiring covered stent placement, transfusion, emergency vessel repair, and/or death. EIA rupture is associated with higher mortality and length of stay.[81]

One of the limitations for EVAR can be related to access due to small caliber arteries, calcification, and stenosis. These limitations can cause significant complications such as vessel dissection, perforation, rupture, and sudden occlusion. Emergent management of these complications in an urgent setting of EVAR can result in significant mortality and morbidity. CIA conduit can be a creative and very useful access modality for large-bore sheath management during EVAR.[82] However, a CIA conduit needs retroperitoneal incision, blood transfusion, general anesthesia, and prolonged stay in the hospital. A CIA conduit can be placed using a Dacron patch 8 mm to 10 mm sutured to the CFA (**Figure 23-10**).

Percutaneous Endovascular Aneurysm Repair

The advent of arterial access closure devices has enabled percutaneous endovascular aneurysm repair (PEVAR). PEVAR has demonstrated the low incidence of early and late access site complications.[83,84] The "preclose" technique for percutaneous access and closure uses Perclose ProGlide Suture Mediated Closure System (ProGlide SMC) (Abbott Vascular Inc., Redwood City, California) and is as follows (**Figure 23-11**).

Step-by-step approach to the "preclose" technique for PEVAR (Video 23-1):

1. Select the common femoral artery that is free of calcium, plaque, and stenosis based on CT scan imaging in cross-sectional and sagittal views.
2. Use micro-puncture needle for access and obtain a sheath angiogram to ensure mid-common femoral access at the start of the case.
3. The first ProGlide is advanced over a 0.035-inch guidewire until bleeding is noted from the side port and then the guidewire is removed.

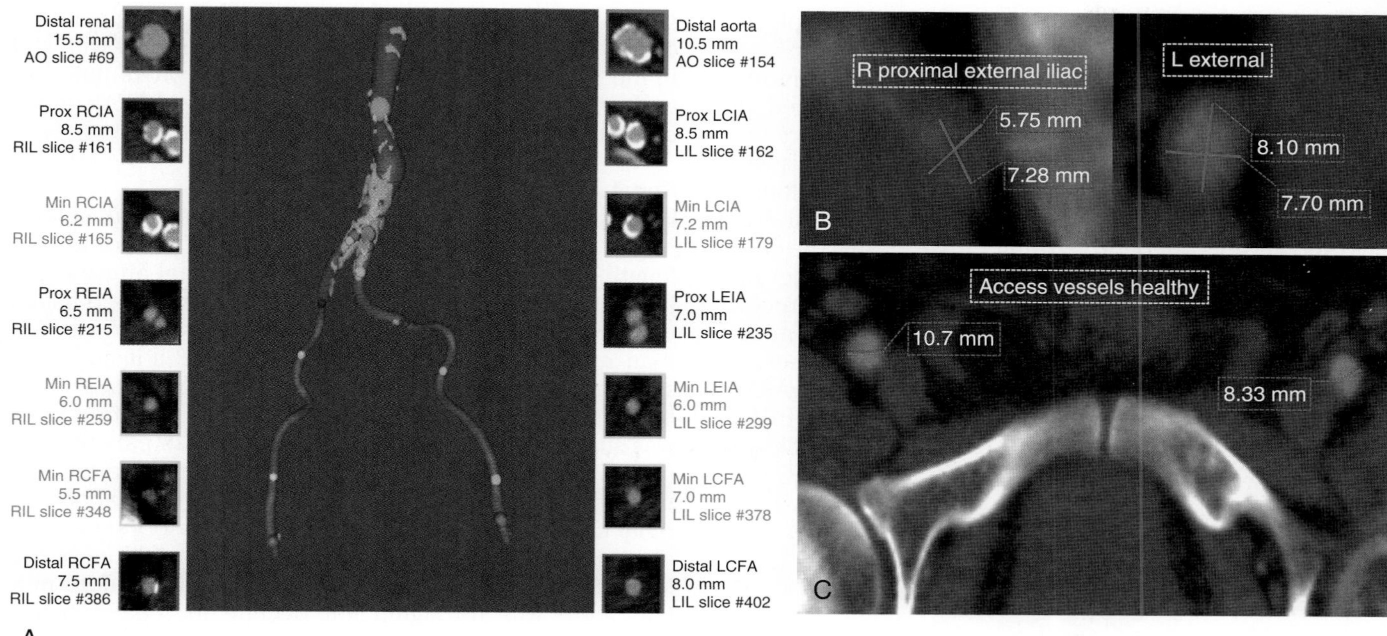

FIGURE 23-9 Computed tomography (CT) angiography measurements of the access vessels. **A,** Measurements using M2S software. **B,** Individual external iliac artery (EIA) measurements. **C,** CFA measurements.

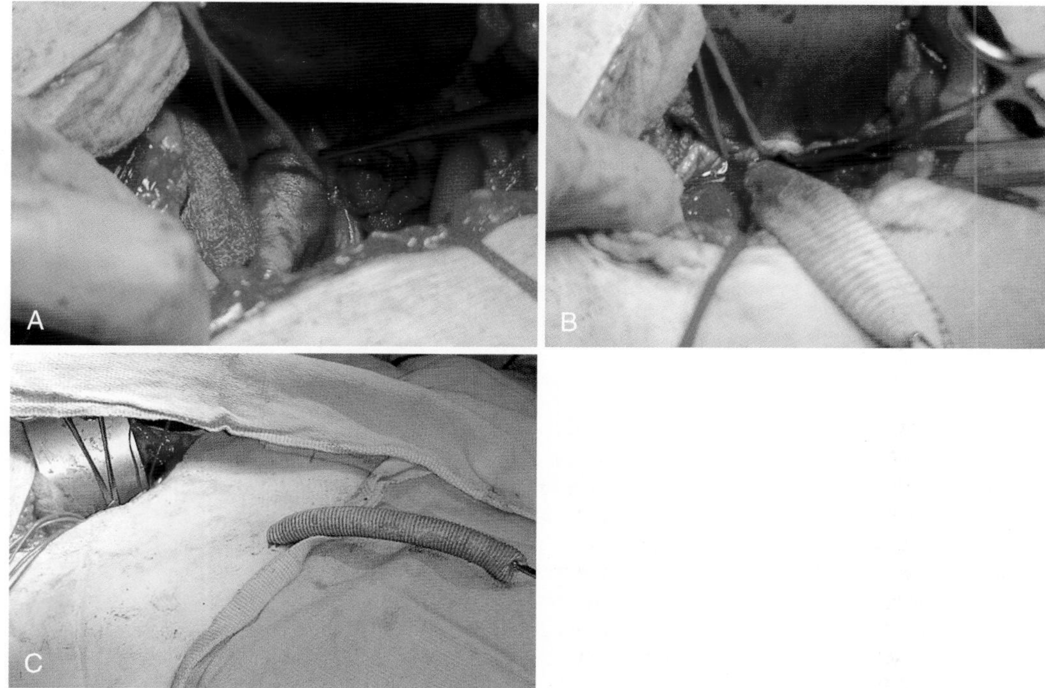

FIGURE 23-10 Access management for EVAR with an iliac artery conduit. **A,** Retroperitoneal incision to demonstrate the common iliac artery exposure. **B,** Dacron graft sutured to common iliac artery. **C,** Dacron graft tunneled to the skin surface for access.

4. Rotate the closure device to 30° medially and deploy the suture. Carefully retrieve the monofilament sutures and secure them with a rubber hemostasis.
5. Replace the guidewire into the ProGlide device via the wire port and remove the device, maintaining the wire access.
6. Deploy a second ProGlide rotating the device 30° laterally over the same guidewire.
7. Insert an 8 Fr to 10 Fr sheath for hemostasis and secure.
9. If large-bore access is needed on the contralateral side, the same steps are repeated to secure the Preclose ProGlide sutures.
10. At the end of the EVAR procedure carefully guide the knot pusher over the top of the arterial puncture and tighten the knot and then lock the suture.

11. If suture breaks, maintain wire access and deploy a second device.
12. The guidewires are removed when reasonable hemostasis is achieved and the sutures are cut, followed by manual pressure for 5 minutes if needed.

Anterior wall calcification of the access artery and severe fibrosis have been shown to be predictors of vessel failure while the sheath size and obesity have not.[85] Mousa et al. have shown that operator learning curve for the pre-close technique, vessel calcification, age, and female gender are predictors of failure of PEVAR and the need for open conversion.[86] The PEVAR trial was a multicenter, randomized prospective trial that compared percutaneous "pre-close" technique to surgical femoral cutdown for EVAR (SEVAR).[87] A total of 192 patients were enrolled, including 41 in the roll-in phase, and 151 patients were randomized to PEVAR or SEVAR. The 30-day ipsilateral access site vascular complication rate was 6% in the PEVAR group compared with 10% in the SEVAR group (p = 0.0048). The total procedure time and time to hemostasis was shorter in the PEVAR group compared with SEVAR.

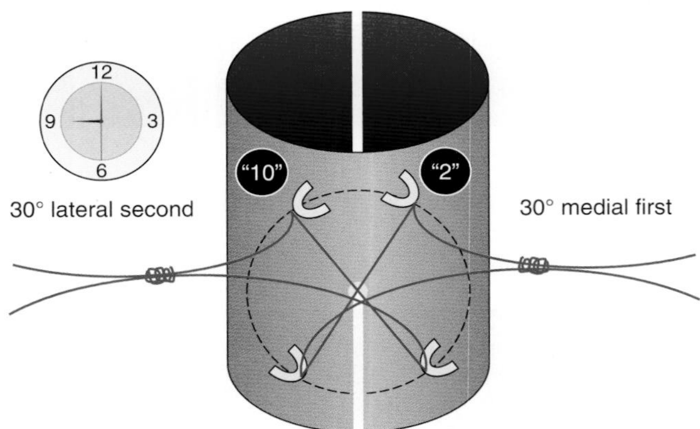

FIGURE 23-11 Demonstrates a cartoon concept of "preclose" using a ProGlide SMC for percutaneous access and closure. The two Preclose ProGlide sutures are deployed 30° medial first and 30° lateral second. *(Redrawn, courtesy Dr. Z. Kracjer, Texas Heart Institute.)*

Renal Artery Anomalies

Horseshoe kidney, accessory renal arteries, and ectopic origin of renal artery can affect the EVAR. If the aortic neck length distal to the lowest accessory or renal artery meets the criteria for the device IFU, EVAR can still be pursued. Occasionally a small accessory renal artery (diameter less than 2.5 mm) may be covered during EVAR if it supplies a small amount of renal parenchyma. The largest series of outcomes of accessory renal artery coverage during EVAR was studied by Greenberg et al.[88] A total 426 patients who underwent EVAR were identified; accessory renal artery was noted in 69 patients. A total of 35 patients with accessory renal covered versus 29 patients with accessory renal preservation. Renal infarction occurred in 84% of kidneys that had accessory renal artery covered. It is important to note that there was no significant decline in renal function between the two groups and no difference in need for antihypertensive drugs, secondary interventions, and rate of endoleak. Patients with a horseshoe kidney can undergo successful EVAR with careful preoperative CT planning despite the anatomical challenges[89,90] (**Figure 23-12**).

FDA-Approved Devices for EVAR (Figure 23-13)

1. Ancure device (Guidant, Menlo Park, California) withdrawn from US market since 2003
2. Medtronic Endurant, Endurant II Aorta-Uni-Iliac (AUI) stent graft system, Talent, and AneuRx (Medtronic Corp., Minneapolis, Minnesota)

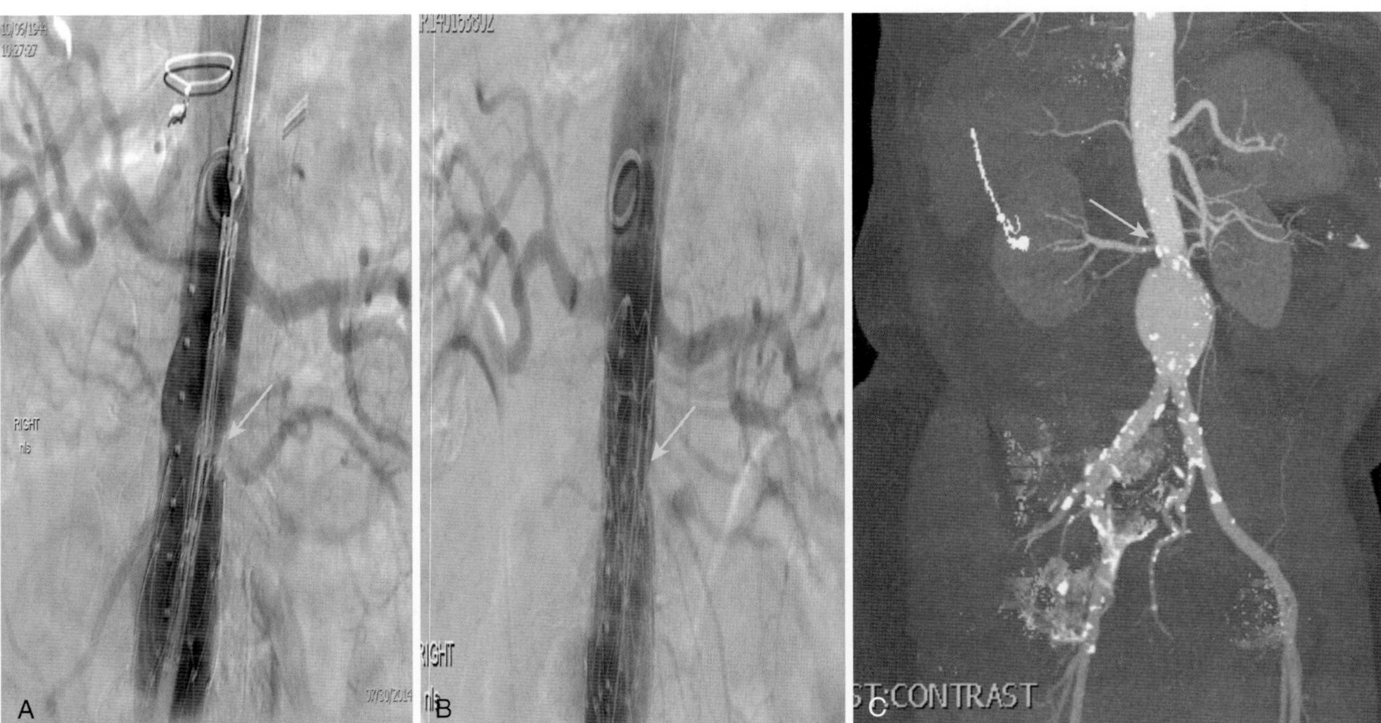

FIGURE 23-12 **A** and **B,** show accessory renal artery covered during EVAR. **C,** Low origin of right renal artery in a patient with abdominal aortic aneurysm (AAA).

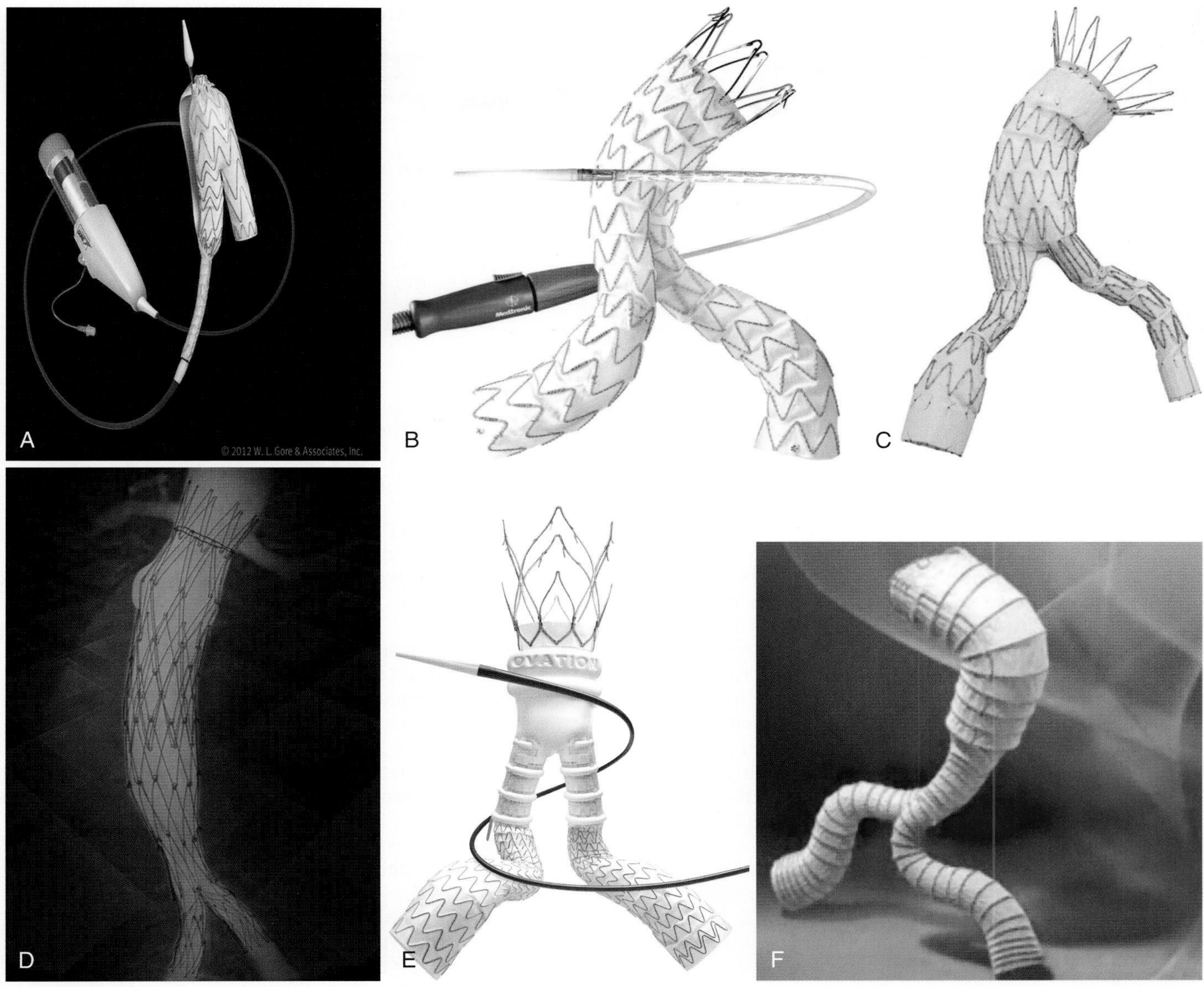

FIGURE 23-13 EVAR devices approved by FDA. **A,** Gore Excluder (W.L. Gore and Associates, Inc., Flagstaff, Ariz.). **B,** Medtronic Endurant II (Medtronic Corp, Minneapolis, Minn.). **C,** Zenith Flex AAA endograft (Cook Medical Inc., Bloomington, Ind.). **D,** Endologix AFX and VELA System (Endologix Inc., Irvine, Calif.). **E,** OVATION abdominal stent graft system (Trivascular Inc., Santa Rosa, Calif.). **F,** Aorfix Flexible AAA Stent Graft System (Lombard Medical Inc., Irvine, Calif.).

3. Gore Excluder and Gore C3 delivery system for Excluder (W.L. Gore and Associates, Inc., Flagstaff, Arizona)
4. Zenith Flex AAA endograft and Zenith Fenestrated AAA endovascular graft (with adjunctive Zenith Alignment stent) (Cook Medical Inc., Bloomington, Indiana)
5. Endologix Powerlink System, AFX, and VELA proximal endograft system (Endologix Inc., Irvine, California)
6. OVATION abdominal stent graft system (Trivascular Inc., Santa Rosa, California)
7. Aorfix flexible stent graft system (Lombard Medical Inc., Framingham, Massachusetts)

Most of the EVAR devices are modular two pieces or a three-piece system, except for Endologix Powerlink System (Endologix Inc., Irvine, California), which is a unibody bifurcated device. The basic EVAR stent graft has four components:

- Delivery system
- Main body of the graft or aortic unibody
- Graft limbs/iliac extensions
- Aortic cuffs and extensions

The majority of the grafts rely on distal fixation at iliac artery and proximal fixation at the infrarenal or suprarenal aorta. The Endologix (Endologix Inc., Irvine, California) relies on anatomical fixation at distal aortic bifurcation and active seal with the graft material. The OVATION (Trivascular Inc., Santa Rosa, California) device provides a seal by hollow rings in the fabric that are expanded by polymer injection after deployment (**Table 23-3**).

Fenestrated Stent Grafts and Physician-Modified Grafts for Complex Aneurysms

The evolution of EVAR to manage complex aneurysms involving the visceral arteries led to the development of fenestrated endovascular stent grafts (f-EVAR). The lack of adequate proximal neck diameters, length, angulations,

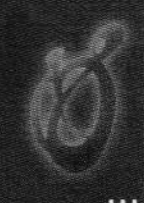

TABLE 23-3 FDA-Approved Available EVAR Devices with Graft Material, Stent Support Individual Characteristics

EVAR DEVICE	GRAFT MATERIAL	STENT SUPPORT	INFRARENAL OR SUPRARENAL	ANCHOR HOOKS
Medtronic Endurant II, Talent, AneuRx	Polyester weave	Nitinol stents outside	Suprarenal and infrarenal	Yes
Gore Excluder	ePTFE	Nitinol stents	Infrarenal	No
COOK Zenith	Polyester weave	Stainless steel stents outside	Suprarenal	Yes
Endologix AFX	STRATA (PTFE)	Cobalt chromium endoskeleton	Suprarenal and infrarenal	No
OVATION	PTFE	Nitinol	Suprarenal	Yes
Aorfix	Woven polyester	Nitinol wire	Infrarenal	Yes

taper, reverse taper, or visceral artery involvement can limit the use of traditional EVAR in up to 40% of patients.[91] Greenberg et al. reported the utilization of branched endograft for thoracoabdominal aneurysms.[92] In this prospective study involving 406 patients with thoracoabdominal aneurysms, 227 patients with juxtarenal aneurysms were noted. The patients who underwent endovascular approach were matched against those undergoing open surgical repair. The short-term mortality and paraplegic rates were similar at 30 days. In the endovascular group late ruptures were noted to be in 0.8% of patients at 18 months. Four patients died due to device component separation, aneurysm rupture proximal to endovascular repair, and failed surgical polyester graft distal to the repair. The fenestrated branch patency for those patients who received reinforcement using a balloon expandable covered stent was 97.8% at 15 months. The study demonstrated technical feasibility of the procedure and low mortality and morbidity.

Greenberg et al. evaluated the results of Zenith endovascular fenestrated stent graft for 30 patients with a short neck and mean aneurysm diameter of 61 mm. The study was conducted at five centers over a period of 1 year. The implant was successful in all patients, there were no aneurysm-related deaths and no rupture. A total of six renal-related events including stenosis, occlusions, and infracts were seen and one patient had device migration. **Figure 23-14** shows a case of fenestrated graft used in an AAA with short neck using the VENTANA system (Endologix Inc., Irvine, California).

Physician-Modified Grafts for Complex Aneurysms

In cases of complex aneurysms such as short neck, reverse taper, or large diameter of the neck greater than 32 mm, physicians may opt to modify the graft to perform EVAR. Such modifications may involve on table fenestration of the graft using a cautery based on preplanning CT scan imaging (**Figure 23-15**).

Step-by-Step Deployments of EVAR Stent Graft (Video 23-2)

Case

An 84-year-old patient with a history of chronic tobacco use for 50 years, one pack per day, presents with incidental finding of large abdominal aneurysm of 7.0 cm noted at an ultrasound screening program. The age, co-morbidities, and patient preference were considered and EVAR was planned. A Gore C3 delivery system for Excluder (W.L. Gore and Associates, Inc., Flagstaff, Arizona) was chosen based on iliac dimensions and low profile of the device (**Figure 23-16**).

The step-by-step deployment of EVAR stent graft is:

1. Under MAC patient was given conscious sedation.
2. Bilateral CFA access was obtained with an ultrasound guidance and micro-puncture needle (described previously).
3. Bilateral preclose technique was used with the ProGlide closure device (described previously).
4. An 18 Fr sheath was placed via the right CFA under fluoroscopy and heparin was given to keep activated clotting time above 250 seconds.
5. A pigtail catheter was placed via the contralateral CFA and bilateral renal arteries were marked on the screen.
6. The main body of the device chosen was placed via the 18 Fr sheaths below the left renal artery and the device was deployed.
7. The contralateral limb was cannulated with a wire and catheter.
8. The contralateral limb length was measured from the gate of the limb to the hypogastric artery using a marker pigtail catheter.
9. The contralateral limb was deployed using a 12 Fr sheath.
10. The graft overlap and proximal and distal ends were dilated with a molding aortic balloon.
11. Final angiogram showed successful exclusion of the aneurysm with no endoleak.
12. The bilateral common femoral artery preclose sutures were approximated to obtain hemostasis.

Patient was ambulated at 6 hours postprocedure and monitored overnight prior to discharge at 24 hours. The patient will be followed in the vascular clinic at 30 days, 6 months, and 1 year with CT scan.

Complications

Most common intraoperative complications are related to vascular access such as iliac rupture, vessel dissections, occlusions, and embolization. Iliac artery rupture can be lethal to the patient if not immediately recognized and treated. Iliac artery rupture can be managed with an endovascular approach. A contralateral aortic balloon tamponade and immediate placement of covered stent or graft to seal the perforation can be life saving. If the rupture cannot

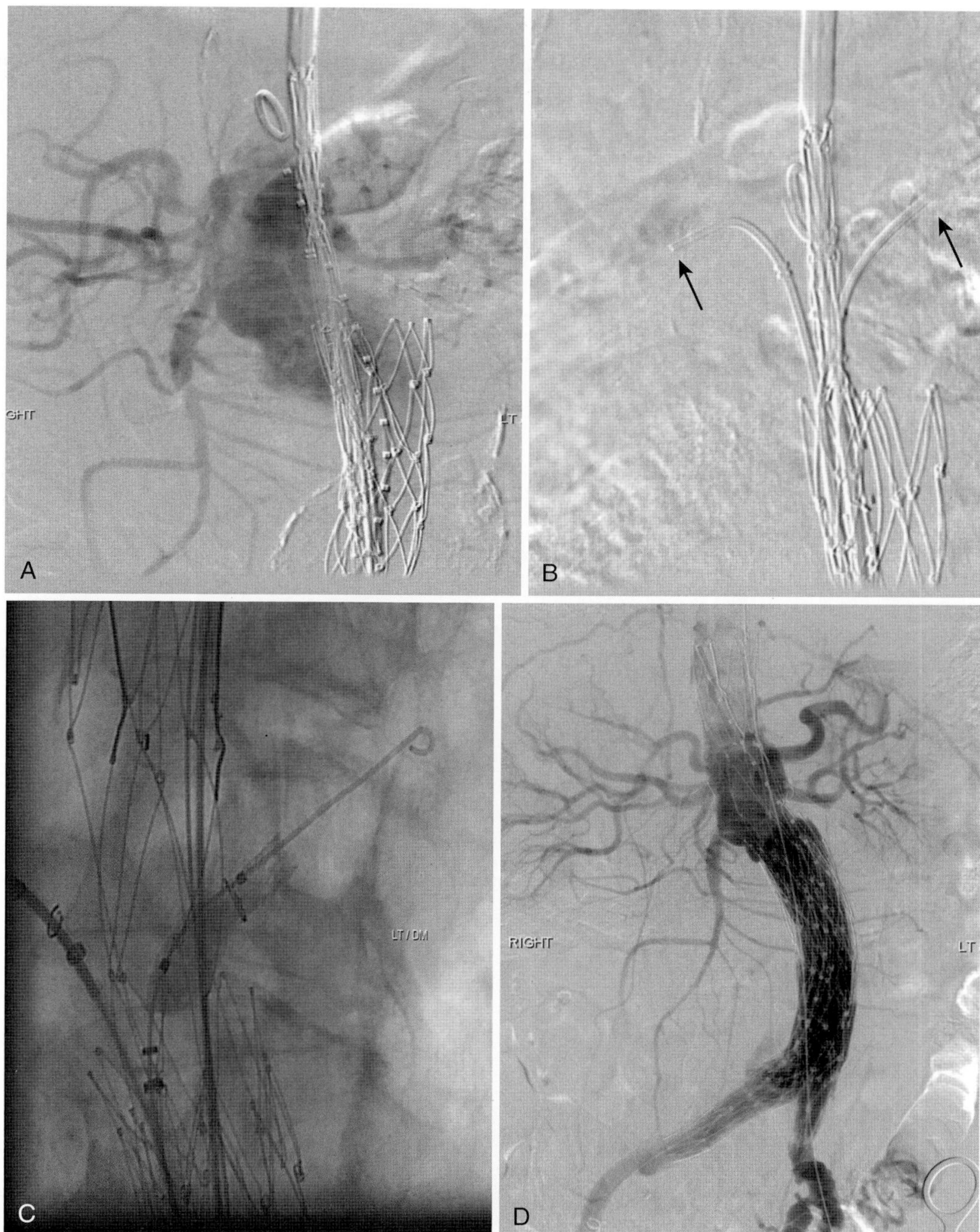

FIGURE 23-14 A case of fenestrated graft used in an abdominal aortic aneurysm (AAA) with short neck using the VENTANA system (Endologix Inc., Irvine, Calif.). **A,** Angiogram shows a short neck. **B,** Cannulation of bilateral renal artery. **C,** Deployment of suprarenal portion of the graft. **D,** Final angiogram to show patency of the renal artery.

be contained or controlled, emergency surgical repair may be be needed (**Figure 23-17**). Arterial occlusion, stenosis, and dissection are usually treated with endovascular balloon dilatation or stent placement. Rarely an iliac vessel occlusion or flow-limiting dissection may require bifurcated EVAR limb conversion to an aorta uni-limb stent graft and a femoral-femoral bypass. Significant atheroembolism requires embolectomy with adjuvant stenting and rarely femoral-distal arterial bypass. The other early complications are intraoperative myocardial infarction, arrhythmias, renal artery embolization, or inadvertent partial or full coverage of renal artery.

Endoleak

Endoleak can occur immediately (Type I and Type III) after procedure or develop in a few months to a few years (Type II and Type IV) after an EVAR. An endoleak permits flow from native aorta into the aneurysmal sac and poses the threat for continued AAA enlargement and future rupture. The Type I and III leaks should be immediately addressed before the patient leaves the endovascular or operating room. Type II and IV endoleak are usually detected during CT scan follow-up and can be treated electively. Late endoleak threatens the durability of EVAR due to persistent blood flow and resultant pressure in the aneurysm sac.

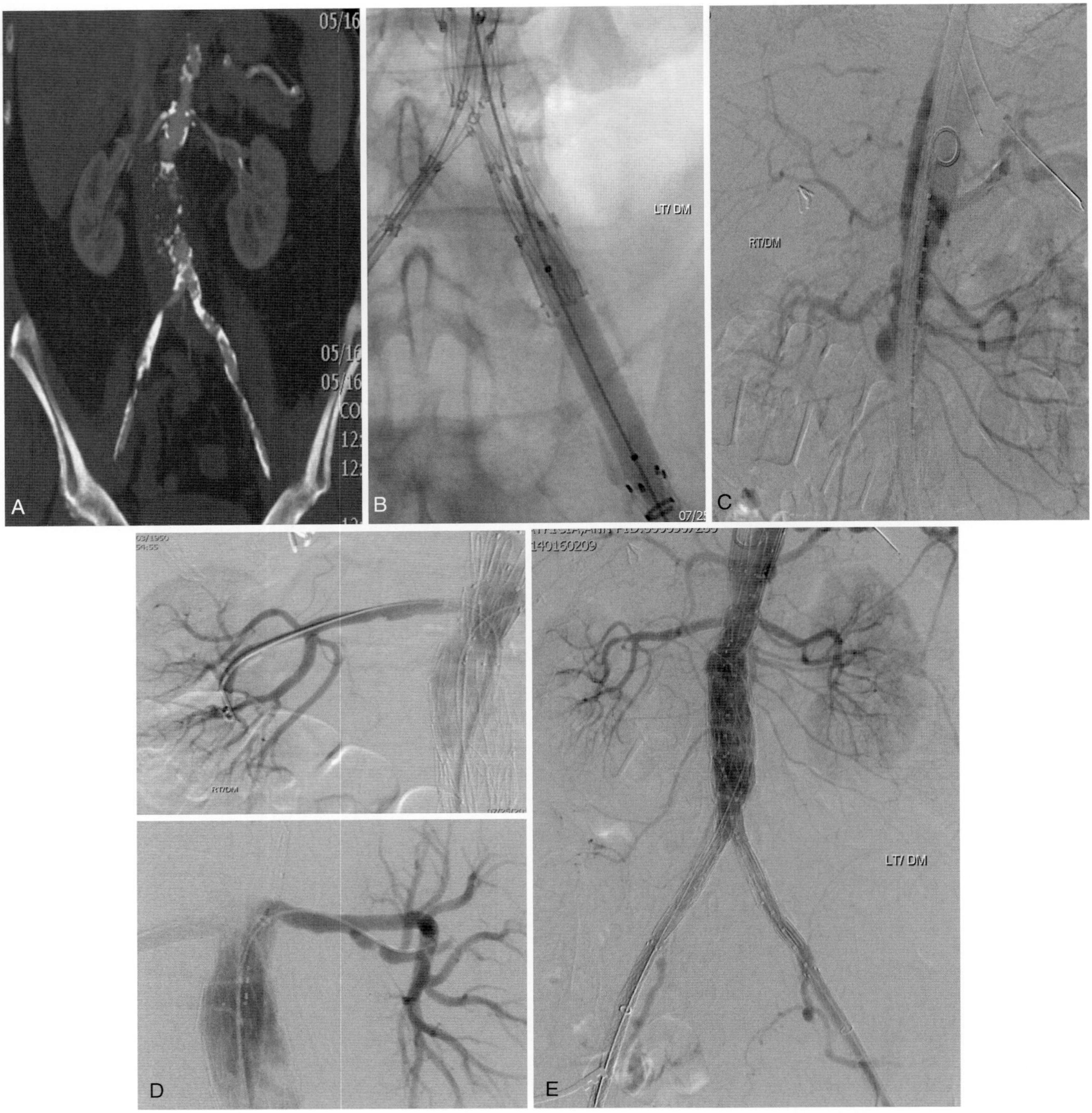

FIGURE 23-15 A case example of bilateral renal artery on table fenestration. **A,** Abdominal aortic aneurysm (AAA) with a short neck <5 mm and reverse taper. **B,** Placement of Endologix main body. **C,** A thoracic Cook TX 2 piece is used for fenestration. **D,** Left and right renal artery fenestration. **E,** Final angiogram.

CT scan is considered the gold standard for detecting and categorization of endoleak, although ultrasound and MR angiogram are being studied as well.[93] The various types of endoleak according to the site and origin of blood flow are described in management and follow-up of EVAR[94] (**Table 23-4**).

Type I Endoleak

Type I endoleak occurs due to inadequate or poor sealing of the endograft at the proximal or distal attachment sites. The antegrade blood flow from systemic pressure results in continued sac enlargement and increases the risk of rupture. Hence, conservative management has no role for Type I endoleak; most of these should be identified and treated at the time of EVAR implantation. The proximal endoleak often occurs due to hostile neck anatomy, less than ideal dimensions, and poor patient selection.[95] A molding balloon inflation at the proximal attachment site can help in sealing the Type I endoleak and if this maneuver fails careful evaluation of the infrarenal neck portion may

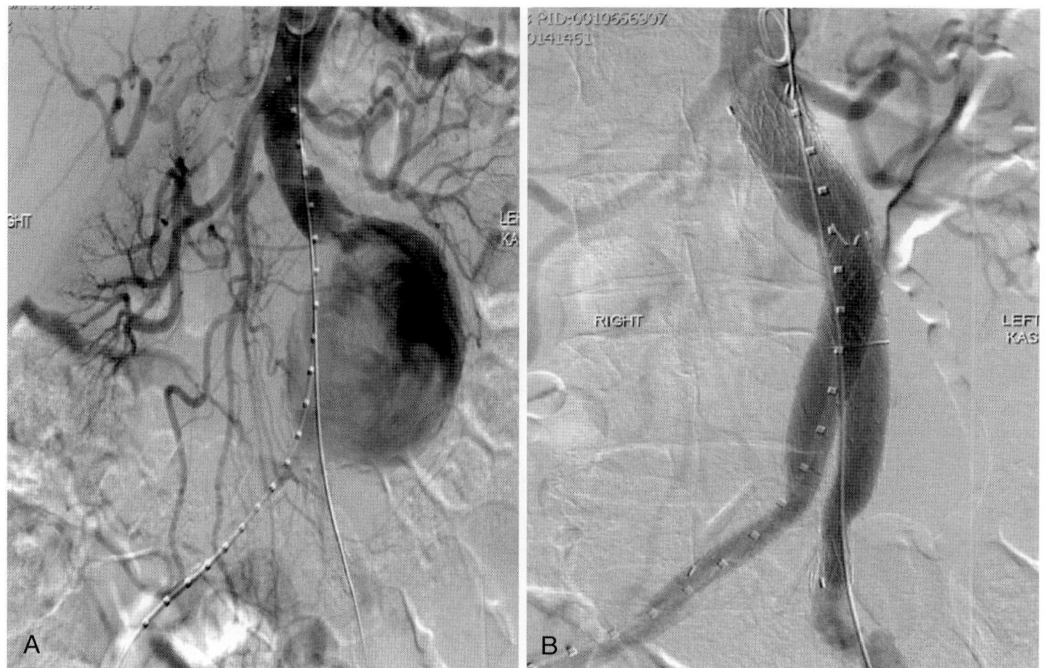

FIGURE 23-16 **A** and **B,** A case of an 80-year-old patient with a large abdominal aortic aneurysm (AAA) of 7.0 cm treated with EVAR.

reveal room for additional aortic cuff placement. Persistent Type I endoleak due to graft not well opposed at the neck can be treated with a Palmaz stent (Cordis, Miami Lakes, Florida) placed at the renal artery level extending to infrarenal neck.[96] Failure of endovascular techniques to correct the endoleak will require open repair[97] (**Figure 23-18**).

Type II Endoleak

Type II endoleak can occur due to retrograde perfusion of the aneurysm. The retrograde flow is usually from patent lumbar arteries, iliac-lumbar collaterals, or patent inferior mesenteric artery via marginal artery of Drummond. Type II leaks are commonly noted in early postoperative CT imaging in up to 10% to 20% of cases. The majority (up to 80%) of these Type II leaks have shown to spontaneously resolve within 6 months of the graft implant.[98,99] Type II endoleaks are low pressure and slowly enlarge the aneurysmal sac over several years and hence have a low likelihood of rupture. The indications for intervention of Type II endoleak are aneurysmal sac expansion and persistent endoleak (**Figure 23-19**). Various techniques and treatment options for Type II endoleak management are described in the literature [100] as follows:

- Coil embolization of the inflow and outflow source of iliac-lumbar collaterals pathway, and the origin of inferior mesenteric artery via the marginal artery of Drummond
- CT- or fluoroscopy-guided direct aneurysmal sac puncture and placement of polymer material in the sac
- Trans-graft puncture using laser and placement of glue or polymer material into the aneurysmal sac
- Laparoscopic ligation of lumbar branches

Type III Endoleak

Type III endoleaks are due to endograft fabric tear or separation of the device components leading to high pressure leak and aneurysmal enlargement or rupture. Improper sizing of iliac limbs can lead to kink in the graft and subsequent device separation can result in Type III endoleak. Aggressive ballooning and instrumentation can lead to iatrogenic graft material tear and subsequent endoleak (**Figure 23-20**). If Type III leaks are noted during the implant they should be corrected with the use of additional limb or cuff immediately. Some of the Type III endoleak is seen during late (4-10 years) follow-up on CT scanning. Such late leaks are usually due to progressive enlargement of the neck or the aneurysmal sac, resulting in migration of the limb and separation of the components.

Type IV Endoleak

This occurs mainly from older graft material with porosity allowing slow oozing of the blood into the aneurysm sac. The recent improvements in the graft material and design have largely eliminated such leaks. Type IV endoleak can be treated with realignment of the graft with newer stent graft with fabric that does not allow porosity.

Endotension

Endotension is pressurization of the aneurysm sac in the absence of endoleak. The exact etiology of endotension is unknown. The transmission of pressure from aorta to aneurysm sac via thrombus layered between the aortic wall and the stent graft is one of the mechanisms for endotension.[101] The sac pressure measurement can be performed by selective catheterization of superior mesenteric artery, inferior mesenteric artery, or internal iliac artery to demonstrate endotension.[102] A specific concise radiofrequency sensor (EndoSensor: Cardio-MEMS Inc., Atlanta, Georgia) has been developed and used in the clinical setting. APEX, a multicenter clinical trial, demonstrated accurate measurement of the sac pressure in 93% of patients.[103]

EVAR Limb Occlusion

Early models of endograft with unsupported limbs caused limb occlusion or stenosis in about 24% of implants. The risk

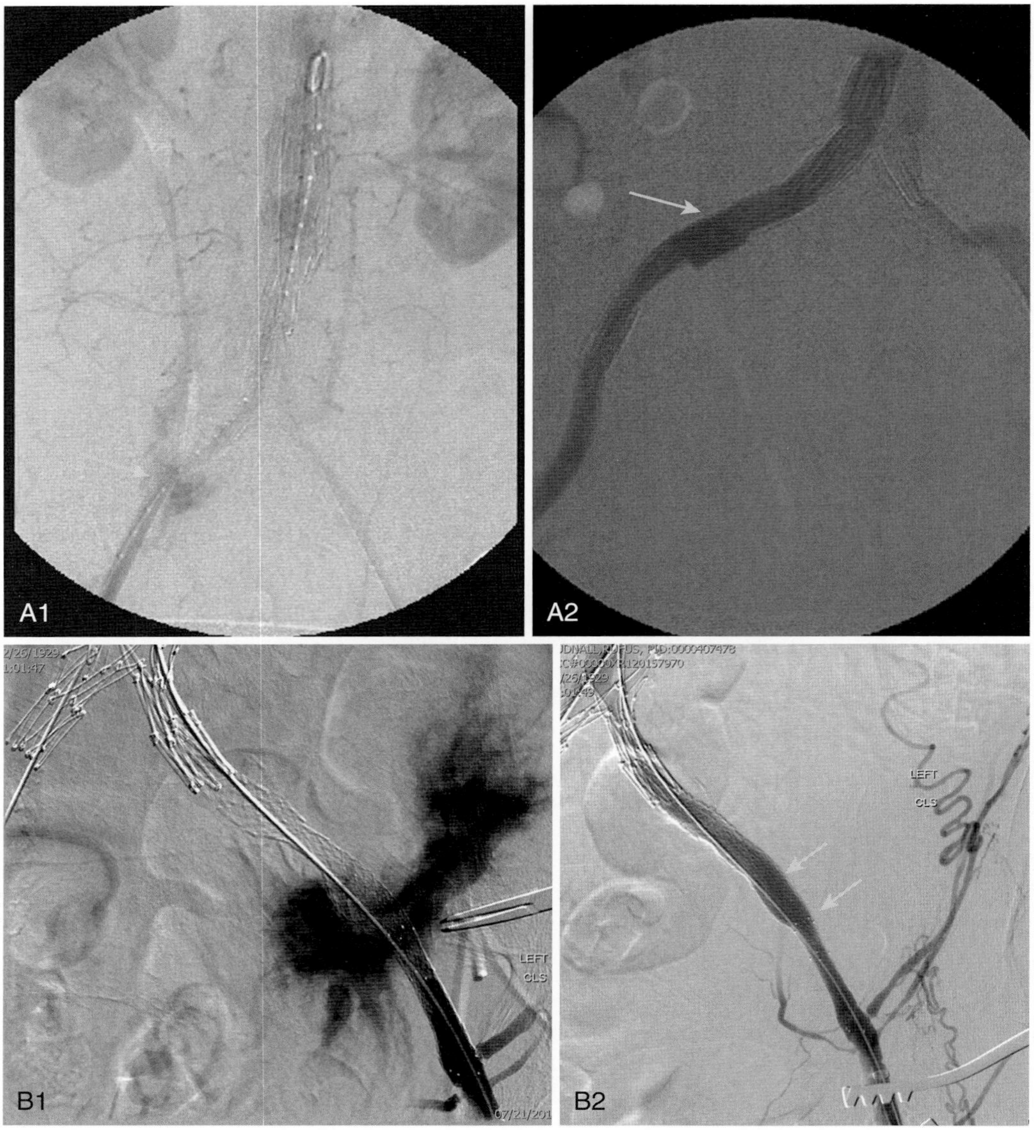

FIGURE 23-17 Complication: The external iliac rupture during EVAR treated with a **(A)** stent graft limb and a **(B)** covered stent at follow-up.

TABLE 23-4 The Endoleak Classification, Features, and Treatment Options

CLASSIFICATION	FEATURES	TREATMENT
Type I	Proximal or distal graft attachment zone	Proximal or distal extension or cuff Embolization in case of patent hypogastric artery
Type II	Patent lumbar vessels or inferior mesenteric artery	Conservative Coil embolization in case of sac expansion
Type III	Graft component separation or graft erosion	Secondary endograft
Type IV	Graft porosity	Conservative

factors that are identified to develop iliac limb occlusions after EVAR are unsupported endografts, small diameter of the iliac artery, pre-existing iliac stenosis, and extension of the graft into EIA.[104] The occluded limbs or stenosis can be treated with an endovascular approach such as stenting with self-expanding stents.[105] During EVAR implantation, if endograft limb stenosis or occlusion or kinking is noted additional evaluation such as IVUS is helpful.[105,106] Limb thrombosis occurs during the early period of postimplant follow-up (2 months) in the majority of patients.[105,106] The clinical presentation includes acute limb ischemia, new onset limb or buttock claudication, and atypical leg pains. Thromboses of limbs can be managed with endovascular techniques such as catheter-directed thrombolysis and adjunctive stenting. Surgical approach involves thrombectomy and, in some cases, femoral-femoral bypass (**Figure 23-21**).

Endovascular Stent Graft Migration

The graft migration is usually noted during CT scan follow-up after EVAR. The graft can migrate cranial or caudal based on involvement of the iliac limbs or aortic main body. The incidence of graft migration is 15% to 45% based on follow-up and definition of migration distance.[107] Despite the use of endovascular stent graft, the proximal aorta and iliac artery distal to the graft dilates and

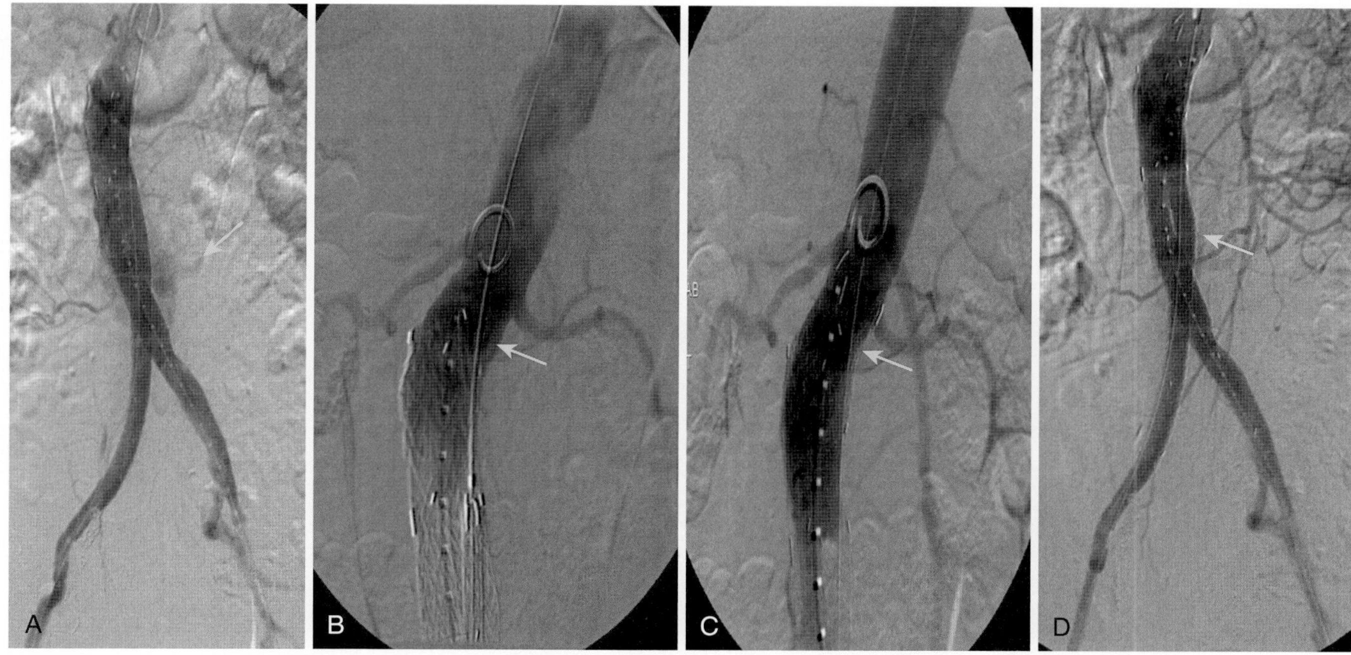

FIGURE 23-18 Type I endoleak and endovascular management. **A,** Type 1 endoleak. **B,** The infrarenal neck shows graft migration. **C,** Additional aortic cuff placed in the infrarenal portion. **D,** Final angiogram showing no further endoleak.

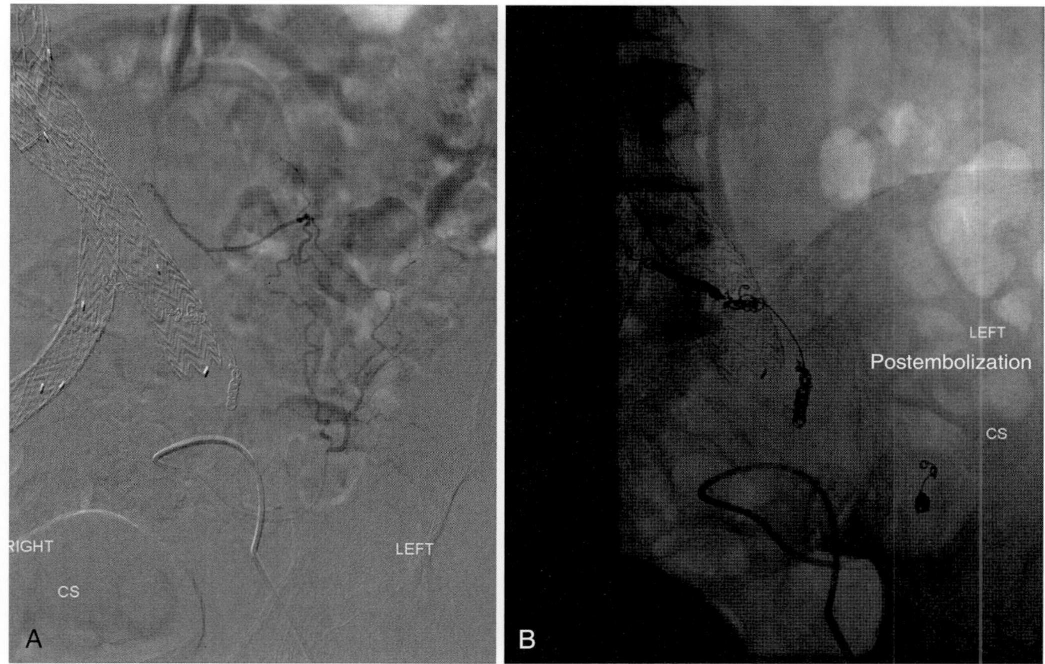

FIGURE 23-19 **A** and **B,** Type II endoleak treated with coil embolization of lumbar collaterals.

facilitates graft migration. Some of the risk factors for endograft migration are baseline AAA dimension greater than 5.5 cm and aneurysmal neck dilatation of greater than 10%.[108] The mean age for graft migration is 1 year and 6 months and half of these migrations need revascularization.[107,108] Various techniques to treat graft migration are placement of aortic cuffs, limb extenders, and reinforcement with Palmaz stent. If endovascular approach fails and the aneurysm continues to grow, open surgical approach may be necessary. Various modifications to the endovascular grafts such as suprarenal stents, hooks, sealing rings, and distal aorta fixation devices have reduced the risk of graft migration (**Figure 23-22**).

Postimplantation Syndrome

A few patients after the implantation of endovascular graft develop elevated white cell count and fever.[109] A work up for infectious etiology in these patients is usually negative. Such patients may also have high C-reactive protein (CRP) levels but the clinical significance is unknown.[110] Conservative

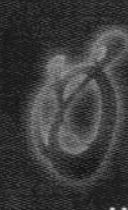

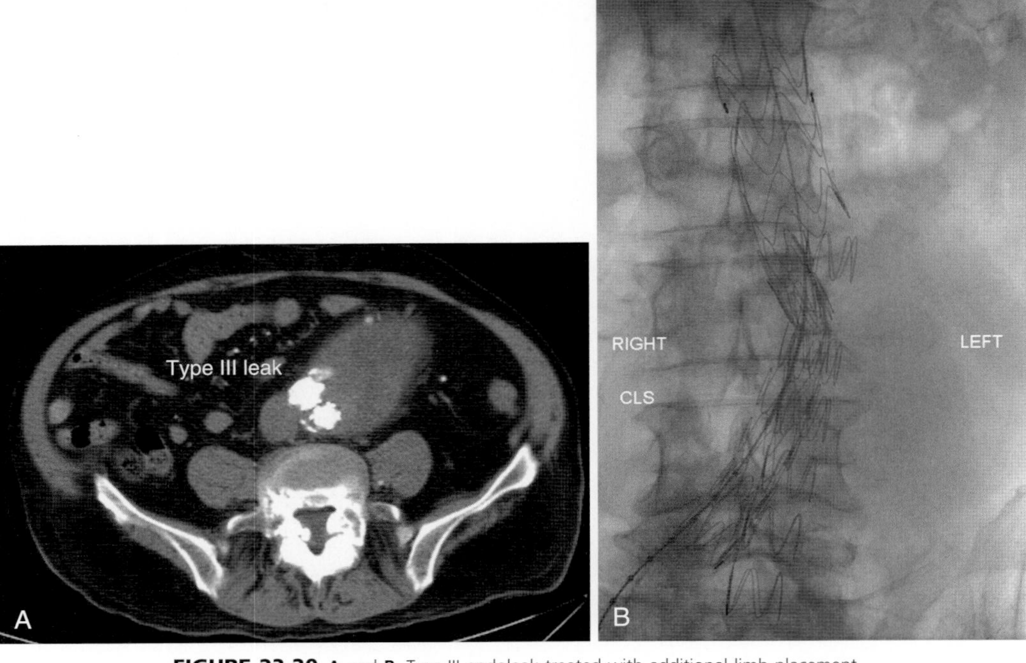

FIGURE 23-20 **A** and **B,** Type III endoleak treated with additional limb placement.

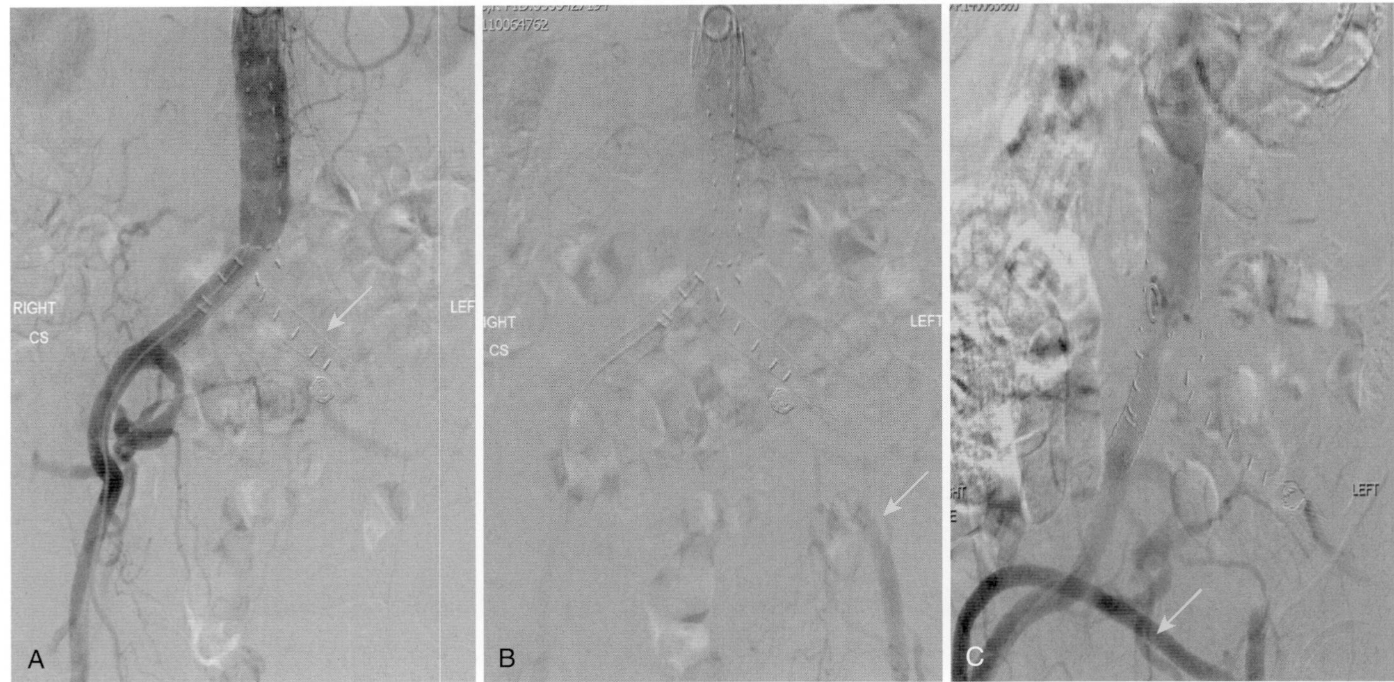

FIGURE 23-21 EVAR patient with limb occlusion due to **(A)** unsupported left graft. **B,** Common femoral artery (CFA) reconstitution **(C)** treated with femoral-femoral bypass.

management is sufficient in most cases of postimplantation syndrome. Persistent fevers, malaise, and positive cultures need aggressive work up and treatment.

Contraindications to EVAR

Most contraindications are based on suitability of AAA anatomy and EVAR device specifications. If the AAA anatomy in every aspect is outside the IFU for any of the device use, EVAR in these patients is contraindicated. EVAR in such patients increases the risk for complications and poor outcomes on follow-up such as endoleak, device migration, and increased secondary interventions. EVAR is performed to prevent rupture and prolong life; any condition that limits life expectancy to less than 6 months is a

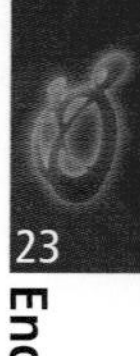

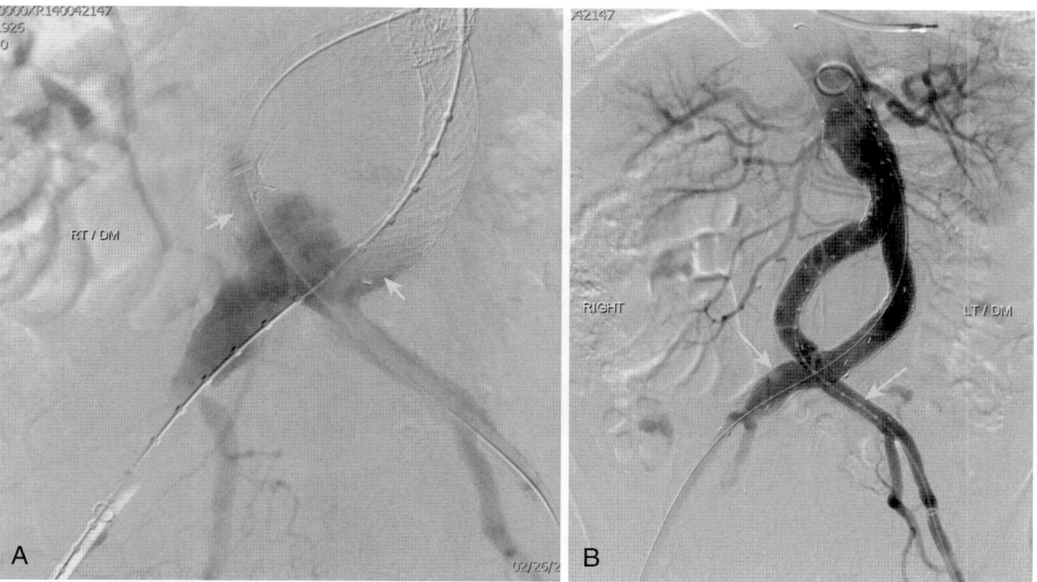

FIGURE 23-22 Migration of distal limbs cranial into the aneurismal neck 6 years after implantation. **A,** The two iliac limbs are inside the aneurysmal sac. **B,** The two iliac limbs are extended into the common iliac artery (CIA).

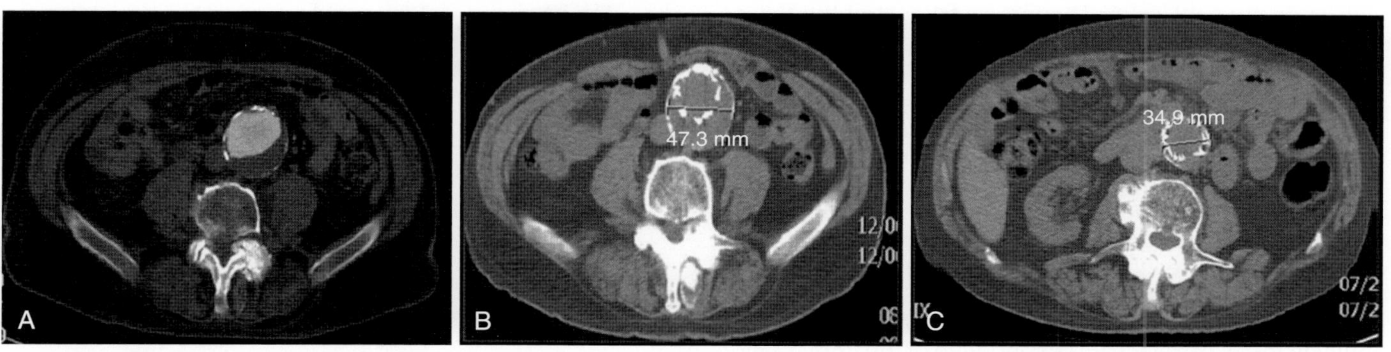

FIGURE 23-23 **A,** Abdominal aortic aneurysm (AAA) at baseline 5.2 cm. **B,** EVAR follow-up at 30 days and **(C)** at 6 months showing shrinkage of size.

relative contraindication for elective EVAR. The implanting team of physicians should always be cognizant of patient's cognitive function and quality of life, and these two factors should be considered prior to EVAR. In-depth unbiased discussion with the family and patient with a focus on the patient's best interest can be helpful in these situations. Presence of an active systemic infection is a high risk for seeding the endoprosthesis and thus may be considered a relative contraindication for EVAR. However, EVAR for a large symptomatic mycotic aneurysm in a patient with significant co-morbidities may benefit in the short-term. Patients with high-grade celiac and superior mesenteric stenosis are dependent on the inferior mesenteric artery to provide perfusion to the large bowel. In these cases EVAR and resultant coverage of the inferior mesenteric artery may result in acute mesenteric ischemia or ischemic bowel and thus may be a relative contraindication for EVAR (**Figure 23-16**).

Surveillance After EVAR

Surveillance and follow-up of patients with EVAR are very important due to late complications such as endoleak, graft migration, graft thrombosis, limb occlusion, distal embolization, limb ischemia, structural endograft failure, delayed aneurysm growth, and rupture. Patients with EVAR thus need lifelong surveillance to diagnose, identify impending graft failure, and if amenable, treat with endovascular, or surgical, or hybrid approach (**Figure 23-23**).

The recommended standard of care EVAR surveillance includes serial contrast CT scans at 1, 6, and 12 months, and yearly thereafter. These recommendations were based on the regimen in the clinical trials and approval process by regulatory agency such as FDA. Some of these surveillance regimens may be impractical and concerns are contrast-induced nephropathy, cumulative dangers of radiation exposure over a lifetime, and high costs.[111,112]

Noll et al. in a long-term follow-up study of EVAR patients identified that surveillance regimens account for 30% to 35% of total costs of EVAR.[113] Sternbergh et al. in a 5-year follow-up of US Zenith multicenter trial identified an improved long-term freedom from aneurysm-related morbidity in the absence of endoleak at 1 month and 1 year.[114] EVAR surveillance thus needs a CT scan follow-up at intervals mentioned above to provide optimal EVAR results.

CONCLUSIONS

Endovascular repair of aortic aneurysm is a safe treatment option for patients with symptomatic AAA and

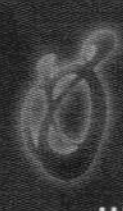

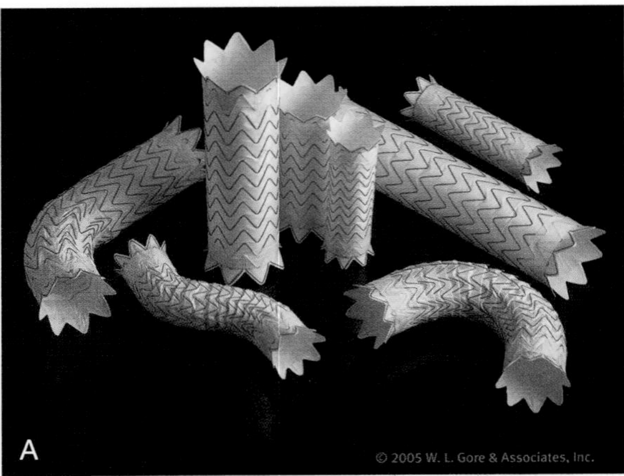

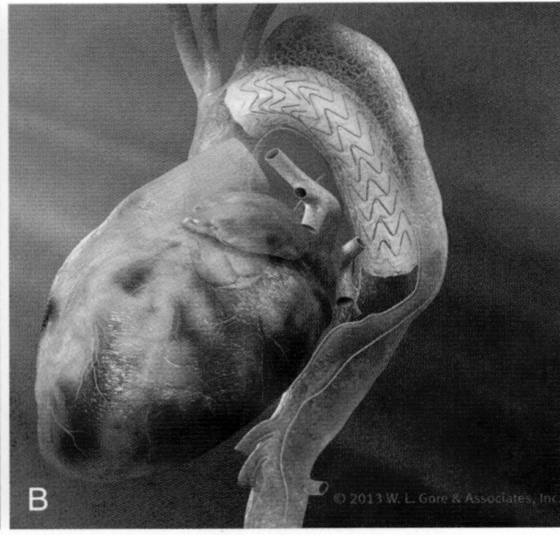

FIGURE 23-24 **A** and **B,** TEVAR device approved by FDA. Gore TAG thoracic endoprosthesis. (W.L. Gore and Associates, Inc., Flagstaff, Ariz.).

asymptomatic AAA >5.5 cm. EVAR offers the advantage of lower perioperative morbidity, mortality, shorter length of stay in the hospital, and early mobilization compared with open surgical repair. The increased cost of the device, surveillance, early and late complications, and secondary interventions should be considered in all patients undergoing EVAR. Lifelong surveillance with periodic CT scans can identify and treat late complications.

The decision between open surgical repairs versus EVAR for an AAA must be made by a cardiovascular team in a nonbiased manner. The patient and family member should be educated on natural history, risk of rupture, mortality, and morbidity of each procedure in a detailed fashion to assist them in the decision process. Patient selection for EVAR based on the age, co-morbidities, AAA anatomy suitability in terms of device IFU, experience of the implantation team, hospital experience, and hospital capacity to perform and follow-up are pivotal in providing optimal outcomes. EVAR should be performed at centers that have demonstrated an in-hospital mortality of less than 3% and primary conversion to open surgical repair of less than 2% for elective cases.

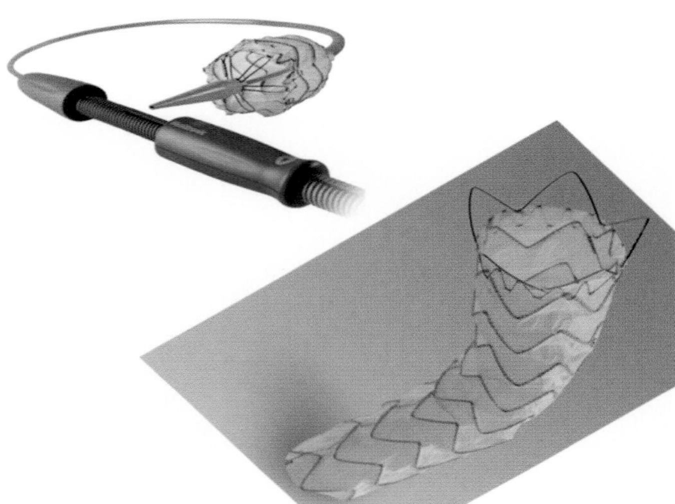

FIGURE 23-25 TEVAR device approved by FDA. Medtronic Talent device. (Medtronic Inc., Santa Rosa, Calif.).

B. Thoracic Endovascular Aortic Repair (TEVAR)

BACKGROUND

Thoracic endovascular aortic repair (TEVAR) was first performed by Dake et al. in 1992 at Stanford University Medical School.[115] The early devices were comprised of stainless steel stents with fabric Dacron material sutured as sleeve and delivered via 24 Fr sheath delivery systems. TEVAR is the preferred choice to treat thoracic aortic aneurysms (TAA) compared with open repair due to reduced perioperative mortality and morbidity.[116] TEVAR was originally developed to treat TAA; however other pathologies such as aortic transection, dissection, intramural hematoma, and penetrating ulcer are also being treated.[117] The advances in technology have enabled the low-profile devices with options to preserve flow into the aortic branches such as the subclavian artery.

DEVICES

There are four devices that are FDA approved for treatment of descending thoracic aorta aneurysms (DTAA) (**Figures 23-24 to 23-28**):

1. Medtronic Talent, Valiant, and Captiva (Medtronic Corp., Sunnyvale, California)
2. Gore TAG device (W.L. Gore and Associates, Flagstaff, Arizona)
3. Cook Zenith Tx1 and Tx2 endografts (Cook Medical, Bloomington, Indiana)
4. Relay thoracic stent graft with plus delivery system (Bolton Medical Inc., Sunrise, Florida)

INDICATIONS FOR TEVAR

TEVAR indications include all symptomatic DTAA and asymptomatic DTAA that are twice the size of the adjacent

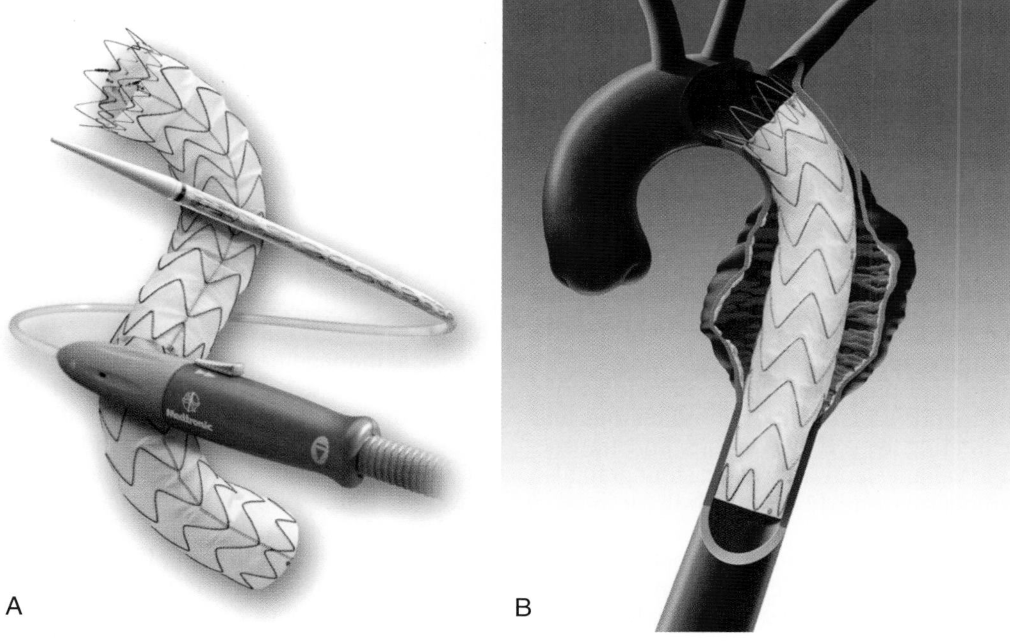

FIGURE 23-26 **A** and **B**, TEVAR device approved by FDA. Medtronic Valiant device. (Medtronic Inc., Santa Rosa, Calif.).

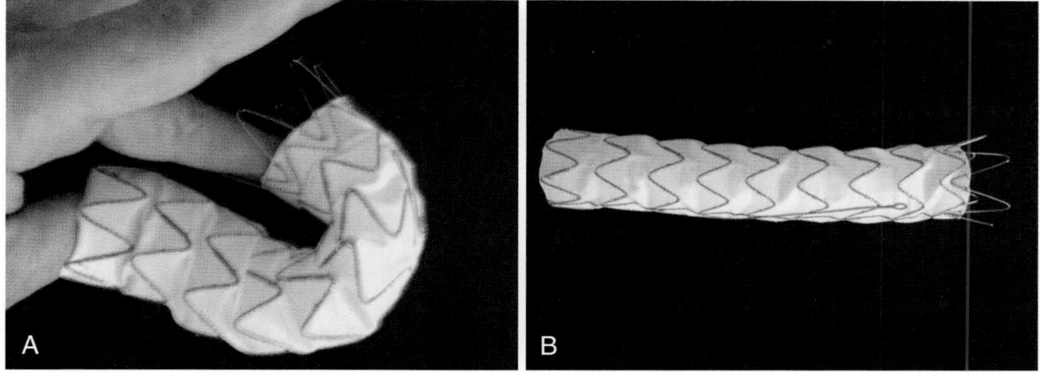

FIGURE 23-27 **A** and **B**, TEVAR device approved by FDA. Relay thoracic device. (Bolton Medical Inc., Sunrise, Fla.).

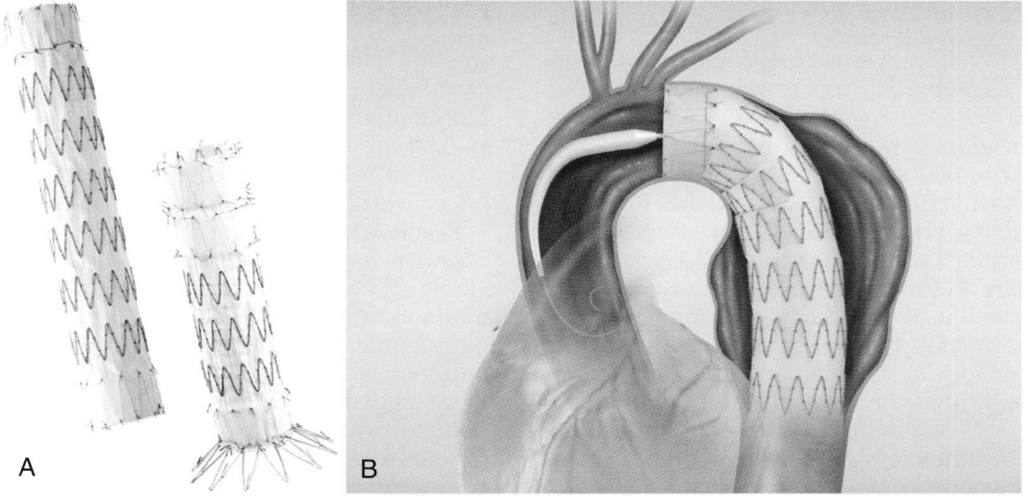

FIGURE 23-28 **A** and **B**, TEVAR device approved by FDA. Cook TX 2 thoracic device. (Cook Medical Inc., Bloomington, Ind.).

TABLE 23-5 Clinical Indications for Thoracic Endovascular Aortic Repair

Symptomatic	Descending thoracic aortic aneurysm, Type B dissection, thoracic aortic transection, and pseudoaneurysm
Asymptomatic	Thoracoabdominal aneurysm >6.0 cm
	Rapid growth of 0.5 cm in 6 months
	Type B dissection, thoracic aortic transection, and pseudoaneurysm

aorta or greater than 6 cm. There must be sufficient landing zones with normal aortic dimension for the stent graft to provide adequate apposition to aortic walls.

Gore TAG thoracic endoprosthesis (W.L. Gore and associates, Inc., Flagstaff, Arizona) has additional indications and FDA approval for treating Type B dissections and transections. The Medtronic Valiant Captiva thoracic stent graft also has additional indications and FDA approval for Type B dissections.

The emerging indications for other aortic pathology are dissection involving the arch vessel, coarctation, and pseudoaneurysms.[118] Mycotic thoracic aneurysms can be treated temporarily with TEVAR; however open surgery is still required in many cases[119] (**Table 23-5**).

CLINICAL DATA FOR TEVAR

Early Experience

Dake and colleagues reported on the safety, feasibility, and effectiveness of TEVAR in 13 patients over a 2-year period.[120] The aortic pathology that was treated included atherosclerotic aneurysm, aortic dissections, anastomotic aneurysm, and pseudoaneurysms with a mean diameter of 6.1 cm. The procedure was successful in all patients with complete thrombosis of the aneurysm around the graft in 12 patients, and 2 patients needed additional stent grafts. There were no deaths, paraplegia, stroke, distal embolization, or infection at one-year follow-up.

Aneurysmal Disease

Gore TAG investigators reported the results of a multicenter trial comparing the endovascular versus open surgical repair of DTAA.[121] A total of 140 patients from 17 sites received Gore TAG thoracic endografts (W.L. Gore and Associates, Flagstaff, Arizona). The perioperative mortality in the TEVAR versus open surgical group was 2.1% versus 11.7% ($p < 0.01$). At 30 days there was a lower incidence of complications in the TEVAR group versus open surgical group: respiratory failure (4% vs. 20%), spinal cord ischemia (4% vs. 14%), and renal insufficiency (1% vs. 13%). The mean length of ICU stay and hospital stay were shorter in the TEVAR group. The endovascular group did have a higher incidence of peripheral vascular complications, re-interventions, and endoleak of 6% and 9% at 1 and 2 years. There was no difference in mortality at 2 years between the two groups.

VALOR II (evaluation of the clinical performance of the valiant thoracic stent graft system in the treatment of DTAA of degenerative etiology in subjects who are candidates for endovascular repair) investigators performed a nonrandomized, prospective trial at 24 clinical sites and enrolled 160 patients.[122] The outcomes of VALOR II were compared with VALOR (evaluation of the Medtronic vascular talent thoracic stent graft system for the treatment of TAA) that had 195 patients enrolled with similar enrollment criteria. TEVAR was successful in 96.3% of the patients and at 30 days the perioperative mortality was 3.1%, major adverse events were seen in 38.1%, paraplegia in 0.6%, paraperesis in 1.9%, and stroke in 2.5% of patients. At 1 year, the aneurysm-related mortality was 4%, graft migration was seen in 2.9%, and endoleak in 13% of patients. In addition, at 1 year there were no ruptures, loss of stent graft patency, or conversion to open surgery.

Type B Aortic Dissection

Acute aortic dissection is associated with considerable mortality and morbidity irrespective of surgical approach or medical management.[123] Dake et al. studied the safety, effectiveness, and feasibility of TEVAR in patients with acute aortic dissections.[124] A total of 19 patients were included, 4 patients with Type A dissection and 15 patients with Type B dissections of the descending thoracic aorta. Dissections involved aortic branches, and 7 patients had symptomatic compromise of branch vessels. The procedure was successful in all patients with complete and partial thrombosis of the false lumen in 15 and 4 patients, respectively. There were 3 deaths at 1 month and none at 13 months follow-up.

Investigation of stent grafts in patients with Type B aortic dissection (INSTEAD-XL) evaluated a total of 140 patients with Type B aortic dissection.[125] A total of 72 patients previously randomized to medical treatment were enrolled to TEVAR versus medical treatment alone for 68 patients. The risk of aorta-specific mortality (6.9% vs. 19.3%; $p = 0.04$), all-cause mortality (11.1% vs. 19.3%; $p = 0.13$), and disease progression (27.5% vs. 46.1%; $p = 0.04$) was noted to be lower in the TEVAR group compared with the medically treated patients at 5 years. TEVAR was associated with false lumen thrombosis in 90.6% of patients. In the United States, the STABLE trial is examining TEVAR for uncomplicated dissections using the COOK (Cook Inc., Bloomington, Indiana) thoracic endovascular stent graft.

Since the FDA approval for use of stent grafts for TEVAR in 2005, the number of cases with endograft implants for thoracic disease has increased exponentially. Physician-modified novel techniques such as carotid to subclavian bypass and graft fenestration have facilitated TEVAR in these complex cases.[126-128]

A metaanalysis of patients who had traumatic thoracic aortic transections by Tang et al., analyzed 699 procedures published in 33 articles.[129] TEVAR was performed in 370 patients and 329 patients had open surgical repair. There was no difference in technical success between the two groups. The mortality rate was significantly lower in the TEVAR group (7.6% vs. 15.2%; $p = 0.0076$), and stroke (0.85% vs. 5.3%; $p = 0.0028$), and rates of paraplegia (0% vs. 5.6%; $p < 0.001$). The peripheral vascular complications, such as iliac artery injury, were high in the endovascular group.

Results of a multicenter, prospective trial of thoracic endovascular aortic repair for blunt thoracic aortic injury (RESCUE) was a multicenter, nonrandomized prospective trial conducted at 20 centers.[130] A total of 50 patients with blunt thoracic injury who underwent TEVAR were enrolled and followed for five years. The procedure was successful in all patients and the 30-day mortality rate was 8%. The nonfatal adverse outcomes related to TEVAR were seen in 12% of patients. There were no events of spinal cord injury or cerebrovascular accidents and no patient required conversion to open surgical repair.

Ruptured Thoracic Aortic Aneurysm

Gopaldas and colleagues identified 923 patients who had undergone repair for ruptured TAA.[131] Among these patients, 364 had TEVAR and 559 underwent open surgical repair. Patients who underwent TEVAR were older and had higher co-morbidities compared with open repair patients. The short-term outcomes of mortality, complications, and failure to rescue were similar between the two groups. TEVAR patients did have a greater chance of routine discharge. The smaller the size of the hospital was a predictor of complications, mortality, and failure to rescue in the open group compared with TEVAR. The study concluded that TEVAR may be a viable alternative to open repair in small-size hospitals where surgical expertise may be lacking for ruptured TAAs.

ENDOVASCULAR TECHNIQUE FOR TEVAR

Imaging for TEVAR

A 0.9- to 3-mm slice CT scan with contrast that includes chest, abdomen, and pelvis is pivotal in case planning for TEVAR. A 3D reconstruction of images is desirable to evaluate the aortoiliac pathology. A MRA, conventional angiogram, and IVUS are all acceptable imaging modalities and can be complementary. A thorough evaluation of iliac dimensions for suitability of large-bore access should be performed at baseline.

Aortic Arch Anatomy

The anatomical knowledge of five zones in the arch of the aorta can help in preplanning a successful TEVAR case are as follows (**Figure 23-29**):

Zone 0: Area proximal to the innominate artery.

Zone 1: Area between the innominate artery and the left common carotid artery.

Zone 2: Area between the left common carotid artery and left subclavian artery.

Zone 3: Area between the left subclavian artery and distal aorta at 2 cm.

Zone 4: The area of thoracic aorta >2 cm from the left subclavian artery.

Aortic Arch Vessel Revascularization and Stent Graft Coverage

The aortic arch vessels, especially the left subclavian and left common carotid arteries, may need to be covered by the graft if the proximal landing zone is less than 2 cm in order to achieve an adequate seal. The anatomical knowledge of the cerebral vessels to determine the dominant vertebral artery and circle of Willis is essential prior to intentional left subclavian artery coverage with a stent graft. The options include carotid-to-left subclavian artery bypass, carotid-to-carotid artery bypass, or arch vessel debranching. The most common arch vessel involved is the left subclavian artery and a left subclavian-to-carotid artery bypass is recommended for dominant left vertebral artery, patient with left internal mammary artery (LIMA) to left anterior descending artery bypass, direct origin of the left vertebral artery from aortic arch, and a patent left upper-extremity arteriovenous dialysis fistula.

Physician-modified TEVAR can be performed wherein the graft is intentionally placed across the subclavian artery and a laser-assisted fenestration of the graft is performed via the brachial artery. The origin of the left subclavian artery can be stented to preserve flow to the left arm, LIMA, and left vertebral artery.

Spinal Drainage

Indications for pre-TEVAR cerebrospinal drainage include the need for extensive coverage of the descending thoracic aorta, multiple pieces of endovascular graft, previous AAA repair, coverage of left subclavian artery, and aortic dissection with visceral or lower extremity malperfusion. Pre-TEVAR cerebrospinal fluid drainage and monitoring for 24 hours to 48 hours can reduce the risk of paraplegia and improve mortality.[132]

Vascular Access

TEVAR patients should have suitable iliac dimensions to accommodate large-bore sheaths and grafts. If the CFA has atherosclerosis and calcification, it will warrant a femoral cutdown rather than a percutaneous approach. If the EIA demonstrates dense calcification, stenosis, small caliber, and tortuosity then iliac conduits may be beneficial.

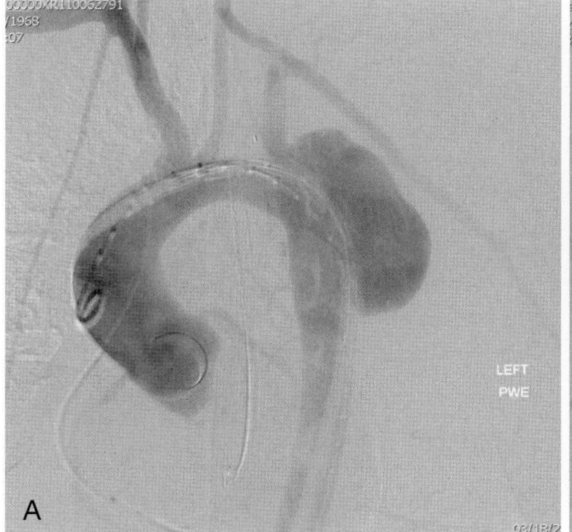

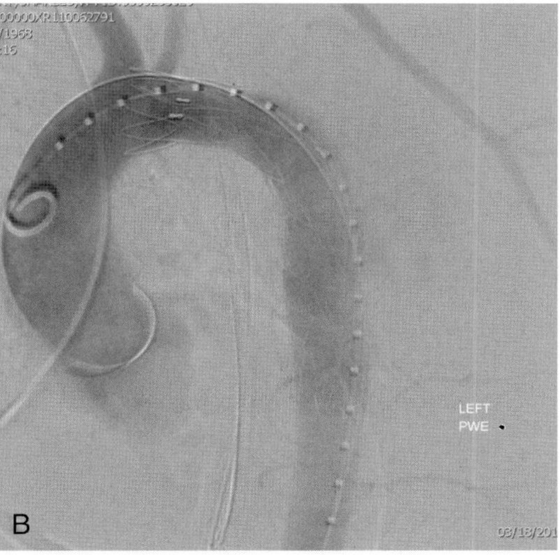

FIGURE 23-29 **A** and **B**, TEVAR for pseudoaneurysm in patient with previous coarctation repair.

Perioperative Risk

A perioperative risk factor assessment can be beneficial in reducing the risk of perioperative cardiovascular events. A multidisciplinary approach to patient care involving endovascular operators, vascular surgery, cardiothoracic surgery, and anesthesia should be used to optimize clinical outcomes.

Anesthesia

General anesthesia, spinal, and MAC can be used for TEVAR, based on the cardiopulmonary status.

Operating Theater

TEVAR cases should ideally be performed in large hybrid endovascular suites that have fixed fluoroscopy imaging. The imaging system should have a large screen image intensifier with digital subtraction, road mapping, and fluoroscopy save options. The air exchange in the room should not only suffice for a femoral cutdown, but also for iliac artery repair or aorta exposure and control, if needed. The hybrid room should be large enough for endovascular, surgical, and anesthesia equipment and personnel. Ceiling-mounted digital monitors for continuous vital signs monitoring are optimal.

Contraindications

Patient

TEVAR for an elective TAA patient with a life expectancy of less than 6 months, active sepsis, or an infected aneurysm.

Aortic Arch and Distal Seal Zone

In TAA patients with significant thrombus, tortuosity, and calcification, the graft delivery may be impeded and the proximal seal may be affected. Distal aorta dimensions at the landing zone that are too large may not allow an adequate distal seal.

Iliac Access

A small caliber iliac artery with calcification and severe atherosclerosis poses a risk for rupture and prevents graft delivery.

Aortic Branches

If the aortic branches are involved, they may prevent adequate perfusion to visceral organs and cerebral vessels.

Complications

Vascular access complications during TEVAR include bleeding, hematoma, a retroperitoneal bleed, and infection. The large-bore sheaths for TEVAR can pose a risk of iliac rupture. Inadvertent coverage of arch vessels during TEVAR can lead to myocardial infarction, endoleak, stroke, and death.

Step-by-Step Deployment of TEVAR Grafts

1. General, MAC, or epidural anesthesia is administered.
2. The common femoral artery cutdown or Preclose Pro-Glide (Abbott Laboratories, Menlo Park, California) is achieved to accommodate large-bore thoracic stent grafts.
3. Anticoagulation with heparin is preferred to achieve an activated clotting time of >150 seconds; in patients with a heparin allergy, bivalirudin may be used.
4. A stiff 0.035-inch wire, such a Lunderquist wire (Cook Medical Group Inc., Bloomington, Indiana), is placed with a catheter support across the aortic arch with the curved wire tip in the ascending aorta close to the aortic root.
5. A contralateral femoral or radial access is obtained and a 6 Fr sheath with a pigtail catheter is placed in the aortic arch. This access aids in pre- and post-TEVAR imaging, and IVUS if needed.
6. The device or sheath is placed over the 0.035-inch wire and all device advancements, especially across the iliac arteries, must be visualized under fluoroscopy.
7. The tip of the TEVAR graft is placed at the proximal end of the seal zone. In order to minimize device movement with the heartbeat, cardiac arrest can be achieved with adenosine injection or right heart pacing at 160 beats to 180 beats per minute. A systolic blood pressure (BP) less than 100 mm Hg can aid in precise graft deployment.
8. The post-dilatation is performed with a molding balloon at the proximal and distal seal zones.
9. The pigtail catheter is withdrawn over a wire and the graft is cannulated with the pigtail catheter into the ascending aorta.
10. A final angiogram should be performed to evaluate for exclusion of the aneurysm, endoleak, and complications, such a perforation, dissection, or branch vessel closure.
11. Vascular access management with closure of the cutdown or approximation of the Preclose sutures should be performed.

Postimplant Care and Discharge

If a spinal drain is used, patients are observed for 48 hours to 72 hours. If stable, the drain is clamped and subsequently removed. If no spinal drain was used and the patient is stable, TEVAR patients can be discharged at 24 to 48 hours.

Surveillance

Patients should be evaluated at 1 week for a femoral access site check for a hematoma, seroma, and suture removal (if a cutdown had been performed). At 30 days, a CT scan with contrast should be performed to evaluate the aneurysm for shrinkage and endoleaks. If there is no endoleak and no further increase in size, the CT scan should be repeated at 6 months and at 1 year thereafter.

Case

A 48-year-old male was seen for back pain with a history of repair of coarctation at age 9 months and 9 years. Patient also had plain old balloon angioplasty of the coarctation of the aorta at age 18 years. A CTA of the chest, abdomen, and pelvis showed an aortic pseudoaneurysm measuring 6 cm of the descending aorta distal to the left subclavian artery. The proximal landing zone measured 1.5 cm. A left subclavian artery-to-carotid bypass was performed. TEVAR was performed with percutaneous access using a Medtronic CAPTIVA (Medtronic Inc., Menlo Park, California) to exclude the pseudoaneurysm. The patient had spinal drainage for 48 hours and was discharged home at 72 hours, following an uneventful hospital course (**Figure 23-29**).

CONCLUSIONS

TEVAR can be safely performed with low morbidity and mortality for patients with symptomatic or asymptomatic TAA greater than 6 cm, aortic transaction, and Type

B dissection. Other indications include a ruptured TAA, pseudoaneurysm, and penetrating ulcer. Patient selection, with special attention to vascular access and branch vessel involvement, can reduce complications. A multidisciplinary approach to evaluate TEVAR patients and follow-up can optimize outcomes.

References

1. Johnston KW, Rutherford RB, Tilson MD, et al: Suggested standards for reporting on arterial aneurysms. Ad hoc committee on reporting standards, society for vascular surgery and north american chapter, international society for cardiovascular surgery. *J Vasc Surg* 13:452–458, 1991.
2. Lederle FA, Johnson GR, Wilson SE, et al: Relationship of age, gender, race, and body size to infrarenal aortic diameter. *J Vasc Surg* 26:595–601, 1997.
3. Singh K, Bonaa KH, Jacobsen BK, et al: Prevalence of and risk factors for abdominal aortic aneurysms in a population-based study. *Am J Epidemiol* 154:236–244, 2001.
4. Lederle FA, Johnson GR, Wilson SE, et al: Rupture rate of large abdominal aortic aneurysms in patients refusing or unfit for elective repair. *JAMA* 287:2968–2972, 2002.
5. Jones K, Brull D, Brown LC, et al: Interleukin-6 and the prognosis of abdominal aortic aneurysms. *Circulation* 103:2260–2265, 2001.
6. Dieter RS: Transluminal endovascular stent-grafting of aortic dissections and aneurysms: a concise review of the major trials. *Clin Cardiol* 24:358–363, 2001.
7. Sakalihasan N, Limet R, Defawe OD: Abdominal aortic aneurysm. *Lancet* 365:1577–1589, 2005.
8. Singh K, Bonaa KH, Jacobsen BK, et al: Prevalence of and risk factors for abdominal aortic aneurysms in a population-based study: the Tromso Study. *Am J Epidemiol* 154:236–244, 2001.
9. Powell JT, Greenhalgh RM: Clinical practice. Small abdominal aortic aneurysms. *N Engl J Med* 348:1895–1901, 2003.
10. Lederle FA, Johnson GR, Wilson SE, et al: Prevalence and associations of abdominal aortic aneurysm detected through screening. *Ann Intern Med* 126:441–449, 1997.
11. Lederle FA, Johnson GR, Wilson SE, et al: The aneurysm detection and management study screening program: validation cohort and final results. Aneurysm detection and management Veterans affairs cooperative study investigators. *Arch Intern Med* 160:1425–1430, 2000.
12. Bengtsson H, Ekberg O, Aspelin P, et al: Ultrasound screening of the abdominal aorta in patients with intermittent claudication. *Eur J Vasc Surg* 3:497–502, 1989.
13. Cabellon S, Jr, Moncrief CL, Pierre DR, et al: Incidence of abdominal aortic aneurysms in patients with atheromatous arterial disease. *Am J Surg* 146:575–576, 1983.
14. Diwan A, Sarkar R, Stanley JC, et al: Incidence of femoral and popliteal artery aneurysms in patients with abdominal aortic aneurysms. *J Vasc Surg* 31:863–869, 2000.
15. Hinchliffe RJ, Macierewicz JA, Hopkinson BR: Endovascular repair of inflammatory abdominal aortic aneurysm. *J Endovasc Ther* 9:277, 2002.
16. Lindeman JH, Ashcroft BA, Beenakker JW, et al: Distinct defects in collagen microarchitecture underlie vessel-wall failure in advanced abdominal aneurysms and aneurysms in Marfan syndrome. *Proc Natl Acad Sci U S A* 107(2):862–865, 2010.
17. Taniyasu N, Tokunaga H: Multiple aortocaval fistulas associated with a ruptured abdominal aneurysm in a patient with Ehlers-Danlos syndrome. *Japan Circ J* 63(7):564–566, 1999.
18. Stanley BM, Semmens JB, Lawrence-Brown M, et al: Endoluminal repair of mycotic thoracic aneurysms. *J Endovasc Ther* 10:511–515, 2003.
19. Berchtold C, Eibl C, Seelig MH, et al: Endovascular treatment and complete regression of an infected abdominal aortic aneurysm. *J Endovasc Ther* 9:543–548, 2002.
20. Dieter RA, Jr, Blum AS, Pozen TJ, et al: Endovascular repair of aortojejunal fistula. *Int Surg* 87:83–86, 2002.
21. Nevitt MP, Ballard DJ, Hallett JW, Jr: Prognosis of abdominal aortic aneurysms. A population-based study. *N Engl J Med* 321(1):9–14, 1989.
22. Johansson G, Nydahl S, Olofsson P, et al: Survival in patients with abdominal aortic aneurysms. Comparison between operative and nonoperative management. *Eur J Vasc Surg* 4:497–502, 1990.
23. Gadowski GR, Pilcher DB, Ricci MA: Abdominal aortic aneurysm expansion rate: effect of size and beta-adrenergic blockade. *J Vasc Surg* 19:727–731, 1994.
24. Bengtsson H, Bergqvist D, Ekberg O, et al: Expansion pattern and risk of rupture of abdominal aortic aneurysms that were not operated on. *Eur J Surg* 159:461–467, 1993.
25. Hirsch AT, Haskal ZJ, Hertzer NR, et al: ACC/AHA 2005 practice guidelines for the management of patients with peripheral arterial disease (lower extremity, renal, mesenteric, and abdominal aortic): a collaborative report from the American association for vascular surgery/society for vascular surgery, society for cardiovascular angiography and interventions, society for vascular medicine and biology, society of interventional radiology, and the ACC/AHA task force on practice guidelines (writing committee to develop guidelines for the management of patients with peripheral arterial disease): endorsed by the American association of cardiovascular and pulmonary rehabilitation; national heart, lung, and blood institute; society for vascular nursing; trans-atlantic inter-society consensus; and vascular disease foundation. *Circulation* 113:e463–e654, 2006.
26. Elefteriades JA: Beating a sudden killer. *Sci Am* 293(2):64–71, 2005.
27. Aggarwal S, Qamar A, Sharma V, et al: Abdominal aortic aneurysm: a comprehensive review. *Exp Clin Cardiol* 16(1):11–15, 2011.
28. Chervu A, Clagett GP, Valentine RJ, et al: Role of physical examination in detection of abdominal aortic aneurysms. *Surgery* 117:454–457, 1995.
29. US Preventive Services Task Force: *Guide to Clinical Preventive Services*, ed 2, Baltimore, 1996, Williams & Wilkins, p 67.
30. LaRoy LL, Cormier PJ, Matalon TA, et al: Imaging of abdominal aortic aneurysms. *AJR Am J Roentgenol* 152:785–792, 1989. US Preventive Services.
31. Petersen MJ, Cambria RP, Kaufman JA, et al: Magnetic resonance angiography in the preoperative evaluation of abdominal aortic aneurysms. *J Vasc Surg* 21:891–898, 1995.
32. Rydberg J, Kopecky KK, Johnson MS, et al: Endovascular repair of abdominal aortic aneurysms assessment with multislice CT. *AJR* 177:607–614, 2001. Van der Laan M, Milner R, Blankensteijn JD. Preprocedural imaging.
33. Marston WA, Ahlquist R, Johnson Jr, G, et al: Misdiagnosis of ruptured abdominal aortic aneurysms. *J Vasc Surg* 16:17–22, 1992.
34. Akkersdijk GJ, van Bockel JH: Ruptured abdominal aortic aneurysm: initial misdiagnosis and the effect on treatment. *Eur J Surg* 164:29–34, 1998.
35. Baxter BT, McGee GS, Flinn WR, et al: Distal embolization as a presenting symptom of aortic aneurysms. *Am J Surg* 160:197–201, 1990.
36. Szilagyi DE, Smith RF, DeRusso FJ, et al: Contribution of abdominal aortic aneurysmectomy to prolongation of life. *Ann Surg* 164:678–699, 1966.
37. Brewster DC, Cronenwett JL, Hallett Jr, JW, et al: Guidelines for the treatment of abdominal aortic aneurysms. Report of a subcommittee of the joint council of the American association for vascular surgery and society for vascular surgery. *J Vasc Surg* 37:1106–1117, 2003.
38. Cronenwett JL, Sargent SK, Wall MH, et al: Variables that affect the expansion rate and outcome of small abdominal aortic aneurysms. *J Vasc Surg* 11:260–268, 1990.
39. Parodi JC, Palmaz JC, Barone HD: Transfemoral intraluminal graft implantation for abdominal aortic aneurysms. *Ann Vasc Surg* 5:491–499, 1991.
40. White GH, Yu W, May J, et al: A new nonstented balloon-expandable graft for straight or bifurcated endoluminal bypass. *J Endovasc Surg* 1:16–24, 1994.
41. Ivancev K, Malina M, Lindblad B, et al: Abdominal aortic aneurysms: experience with the Ivancev-Malmo endovascular system for aorto-monoiliac stent-grafts. *J Endovasc Surg* 4:242–251, 1997.
42. Ohki T, Veith FJ, Sanchez LA, et al: Varying strategies and devices for endovascular repair of abdominal aortic aneurysms. *Semin Vasc Surg* 10:242–256, 1997.
43. Yusuf SW, Whitaker SC, Chuter TA, et al: Emergency endovascular repair of leaking aortic aneurysm. *Lancet* 344:1645, 1994.
44. May J, White GH, Yu W, et al: Current comparison of endoluminal versus open repair in the treatment of abdominal aortic aneurysms: analysis of 303 patients by the life table method. *J Vasc Surg* 27:213–221, 1998.
45. Schwarze ML, Shen Y, Hemmerich J, et al: Age-related trends in utilization and outcome of open and endovascular repair for abdominal aortic aneurysm in the United States, 2001–2006. *J Vasc Surg* 50:722–729, 2009.
46. Schanzer A, MD, Messina L, MD: Two decades of endovascular abdominal aortic aneurysm repair: enormous progress with serious lessons learned. *J Am Heart Assoc.* 1:e000075, 2012.
47. Schwarze ML, Shen Y, Hemmerich J, et al: Age-related trends in utilization and outcome of open and endovascular repair for abdominal aortic aneurysm in the United States, 2001-2006. *J Vasc Surg* 50:722–729, 2009.
48. De Bruin JL, Baas AF, Buth J, et al: Long-term outcome of open or endovascular repair of abdominal aortic aneurysm. *N Engl J Med* 362:1881–1889, 2010.
49. Greenhalgh RM, Brown LC, Powell JT, et al: United Kingdom EVAR trial investigators. Endovascular versus open repair of abdominal aortic aneurysm. *N Engl J Med* 362:1863–1871, 2010.
50. The United Kingdom EVAR Trial Investigators: Endovascular aneurysm repair and outcome in patients unfit for open repair of abdominal aortic aneurysm (EVAR trial 2): randomized controlled trial. *The Lancet* 365(9478):2187–2192, 2005.
51. Lederle FA, Freischlag JA, Kyriakides TC, et al: Open versus endovascular repair (OVER) veterans affairs cooperative study group. outcomes following endovascular vs. open repair of abdominal aortic aneurysm: a randomized trial. *JAMA* 302:1535–1542, 2009.
52. Rydberg J, Kopecky KK, Johnson MS, et al: Endovascular repair of abdominal aortic aneurysms assessment with multislice CT. *AJR* 177:607–614, 2001.
53. Chaikof EL, Lin PH, Brinkman WT, et al: Endovascular repair of abdominal aortic aneurysms risk stratified outcomes. *Ann Surg* 235:833–841, 2002.
54. Elisha S, Nagelhout J, Heiner J, et al: Anesthesia case management for endovascular aortic aneurysm repair. *AANA J* 82(2):145–152, 2014.
55. Franz R, Hartman J, Wright M: Comparison of anesthesia technique on outcomes of endovascular repair of abdominal aortic aneurysms: a five-year review of monitored anesthesia care with local anesthesia vs. general or regional anesthesia. *J Cardiovasc Surg (Torino)* 52(4):567–577, 2011.
56. Rolls AE, Riga CV, Rudarakanchana N, et al: Planning for EVAR: the role of modern software. *J Cardiovasc Surg (Torino)* 55(1):1–7, 2014. Review.
57. Mann K, Sim I, Ali T, et al: Removing the need for crossmatched blood in elective EVAR. *Eur J Vasc Endovasc Surg* 43(3):282–285, 2012.
58. Mayer D, Rancic Z, Pfammatter T, et al: Logistic considerations for a successful institutional approach to the endovascular repair of ruptured abdominal aortic aneurysms. *Vascular* 18(2):64–70, 2010.
59. Maleux G, MD, PhD, Koolen M, MD, Heye S, MD: Complications after endovascular aneurysm repair. *Semin Intervent Radiol* 26(1):3–9, 2009.
60. Chaikof EL, Brewster DC, Dalman RL, et al: The care of patients with an abdominal aortic aneurysm: the society for vascular surgery practice guidelines. *J Vasc Surg* 50(8S):1S–49S, 2009.
61. Kritpracha B, Pigott JP, Russel TE, et al: Bell-bottom aortoiliac endografts: an alternative that preserves pelvic blood flow. *J Vasc Surg* 35:874–881, 2002.
62. Huang Y, Gloviczki P, Duncan AA, et al: Common iliac artery aneurysm: expansion rate and results of open surgical and endovascular repair. *J Vasc Surg* 47:1203–1211, 2008.
63. Antoniou GA, Nassef AH, Antoniou SA, et al: Endovascular treatment of isolated internal iliac artery aneurysms. *Vascular* 19:291–300, 2011.
64. Murphy EH, MD, Woo EY, MD: Endovascular management of common and internal iliac artery aneurysms: how iliac branch grafting may become a first-line treatment option. *Endovascular Today* 2012, 76-81.
65. http://www.medtronic.com/your-health/abdominal-aortic-aneurysm/important-safety-information/index.htm#talent. [Accessed on August 19, 2014].
66. Mehta M, Veith FJ, Ohki T, et al: Unilateral and bilateral hypogastric artery interruption during aortoiliac aneurysm repair in 154 patients: a relatively innocuous procedure. *J Vasc Surg* 33:S27–S32, 2001.
67. Geraghty PJ, Sanchez LA, Rubin BG, et al: Overt ischemic colitis after endovascular repair of aortoiliac aneurysms. *J Vasc Surg* 40:413–418, 2004.
68. Dadian N, Ohki T, Veith FJ, et al: Overt colon ischemia after endovascular aneurysm repair: the importance of microembolization as an etiology. *J Vasc Surg* 34:986–996, 2001.
69. Cynamon J, Lerer D, Veith FJ, et al: Hypogastric artery coil embolization prior to endoluminal repair of aneurysms and fistulas: buttock claudication, a recognized but possibly preventable complication. *J Vasc Interv Radiol* 11:573–577, 2000.
70. Lee WA, Nelson PR, Berceli SA, et al: Outcome after hypogastric artery bypass and embolization during endovascular aneurysm repair. *J Vasc Surg* 44:1162–1169, 2006.
71. Huang Y, Gloviczki P, Duncan AA, et al: Common iliac artery aneurysm: expansion rate and results of open surgical and endovascular repair. *J Vasc Surg* 47:1203–1211, 2008.
72. Friedman SG, Wun H: Hypogastric preservation with Viabahn stent graft during endovascular aneurysm repair. *J Vasc Surg* 54:504–506, 2011.
73. Lobato AC: Sandwich technique for aortoiliac aneurysms extending to the internal iliac artery or isolated common/internal iliac artery aneurysms: a new endovascular approach to preserve pelvic circulation. *J Endovasc Ther* 18:106–111, 2011.
74. Kotsis T, Tsanis A, Sfyroeras G, et al: Endovascular exclusion of symptomatic bilateral common iliac artery aneurysms with preservation of an aneurysmal internal iliac artery via a reverse-U stent-graft. *J Endovasc Ther* 13:158–163, 2006.
75. van Groenendael L, Zeebregts CJ, Verhoeven EL, et al: External-to-internal iliac artery endografting for the exclusion of iliac artery aneurysms: an alternative technique for preservation of pelvic flow? *Catheter Cardiovasc Interv* 73:156–160, 2009.
76. Eisenack M, Umscheid T, Tessarek J, et al: Percutaneous endovascular aortic aneurysm repair: a prospective evaluation of safety, efficiency, and risk factors. *J Endovasc Ther* 16:708–713, 2009.
77. Manunga JM, Gloviczki P, Oderich GS, et al: Femoral artery calcification as a determinant of success for percutaneous access for endovascular abdominal aortic aneurysm repair. *J Vasc Surg* 58:1208–1212, 2013.
78. Mousa AY, Campbell JE, Broce M, et al: Predictors of percutaneous access failure requiring open femoral surgical conversion during endovascular aortic aneurysm repair. *J Vasc Surg* 58:1213–1219, 2013.
79. Torsello GB, Kasprzak B, Klenk E, et al: Endovascular suture versus cutdown for endovascular aneurysm repair: a prospective randomized pilot study. *J Vasc Surg* 38:78–82, 2003.

80. Dalainas I, Nano G, Casana R: Tealdi Dg Dg. mid-term results after endovascular repair of abdominal aortic aneurysms: a four-year experience. *Eur J Vasc Endovasc Surg* 27:319–323, 2004.
81. Fernandez JD, Craig JM, Garrett Jr, HE, et al: Endovascular management of iliac rupture during endovascular aneurysm repair. *J Vasc Surg* 50(6):1293–1299, 2009.
82. Peterson BG, Matsumura JS: Creative options for large sheath access during aortic endografting. *J Vasc Interv Radiol* 19(6 Suppl):S22–S26, 2008.
83. Lee WA, Brown MP, Nelson PR, et al: Midterm outcomes of femoral arteries after percutaneous endovascular aortic repair using the Preclose technique. *J Vasc Surg* 47:919–923, 2008.
84. Lee WA, Brown MP, Nelson PR, et al: Total percutaneous access for endovascular aortic aneurysm repair ("Preclose" technique). *J Vasc Surg* 45:1095–1101, 2007.
85. Elsenack M, Umscheid T, Tesserek J, et al: Percutaneous endovascular aortic aneurysm repair: a prospective evaluation of safety, efficiency, and risk factors. *J Endovasc Ther* 16:708–713, 2009.
86. Mousa AY, Campbell JE, Broce M, et al: Predictors of percutaneous access failure requiring open femoral surgical conversion during endovascular aortic aneurysm repair. *J Vasc Surg* 58(5): 1213–1219, 2013.
87. Krajcer Z, Matos JM: Totally percutaneous endovascular abdominal aortic aneurysm repair: 30-day results from the independent access-site closure study of the PEVAR trial. *Tex Heart Inst J* 40(5):560–561, 2013.
88. Greenberg JI, Dorsey C, Dalman RL, et al: Long-term results after accessory renal artery coverage during endovascular aortic aneurysm repair. *J Vasc Surg* 56(2):291–296, 2012, discussion 296-7. [Epub 2012 Apr 4].
89. Chaudhuri A: Exclusion of an infrarenal AAA with coincident horseshoe kidney and renovascular anomalies is feasible using a standard stent-graft. *Eur J Vasc Endovasc Surg* 41(5):654–656, 2011. [Epub 2011 Feb 25].
90. Tan TW, MD, Farber A, MD, FACS, FICA: Percutaneous endovascular repair of abdominal aortic aneurysm with coexisting horseshoe kidney: technical aspects and review of the literature. *Int J Angiol* 20(4):247–250, 2011.
91. Carpenter JP, Baum RA, Barker CF, et al: Impact of exclusion criteria on patient selection for endovascular abdominal aortic aneurysm repair. *J Vasc Surg* 34:1050–1054, 2001.
92. Greenberg R, Eagleton M, Mastracci T: Branched endografts for thoracoabdominal aneurysms. *J Thorac Cardiovasc Surg* 140(6 Suppl):S171–S178, 2010.
93. Stavropoulos SW, Chandragundla SR: Imaging techniques for detection and management of endoleaks after endovascular aortic aneurysm repair. *Radiology* 243:641–655, 2007.
94. White GH, Yu W, May J, et al: Endoleak as a complication of endoluminal grafting of abdominal aortic aneurysms: classification, incidence, diagnosis and management. *J Endovasc Surg* 4:152–168, 1997.
95. AbuRahma AF, Campbell JE, Mousa AY, et al: Clinical outcomes for hostile versus favorable aortic neck anatomy in endovascular aortic aneurysm repair using modular devices. *J Vasc Surg* 54(1):13–21, 2011.
96. Kim JK, Noll RE, Jr, Tonnessen BH, et al: A technique for increased accuracy in the placement of the "giant" Palmaz stent for treatment of type IA endoleak after endovascular abdominal aneurysm repair. *J Vasc Surg* 48:755–757, 2008.
97. Varcoe RL, Laird MP, Frawley JE: A novel alternative to open conversion for type 1 endoleak resulting in ruptured aneurysm. *Vasc Endovascular Surg* 42:391–393, 2008.
98. Chuter TA, Faruqi RM, Sawhney R, et al: Endoleak after endovascular repair of abdominal aortic aneurysm. *J Vasc Surg* 34:98–105, 2001.
99. Brewster DC, Jones JE, Chung TK, et al: Long-term outcomes after endovascular abdominal aortic aneurysm repair: the first decade. *Ann Surg* 244:426–438, 2006.
100. Jonker FH, Aruny J, Muhs BE: Management of type II endoleaks: preoperative versus postoperative versus expectant management. *Semin Vasc Surg* 22:165–171, 2009.
101. Naoki T, Tetsuji F, Yuji K, et al: Endotension following endovascular aneurysm repair. *Vascular Medicine* 13:305–331, 2008.
102. Lin PH, Bush RL, Katzman JB, et al: Delayed aortic aneurysm enlargement due to endotension after endovascular abdominal aortic aneurysm repair. *J Vasc Surg* 38:840–842, 2003.
103. Ohki T, Ouriel K, Silveria PG, et al: Initial results of wireless pressure sensing for EVAR: the APEX trial—acute pressure measurement to confirm aneurysm sac exclusion. *J Vasc Surg* 45:236–242, 2007.
104. Carroccio A, Faries PL, Morrissey NJ, et al: Predicting iliac limb occlusions after bifurcated aortic stent grafting: anatomic and device-related causes. *J Vasc Surg* 36:679–684, 2002.
105. Parent EN, III, Godziachvili V, Meier GH, et al: Endograft limb occlusion and stenosis after ANCURE endovascular abdominal aneurysm repair. *J Vasc Surg* 35:686–690, 2002.
106. Powell A, Fox LA, Benenati JF, et al: Postoperative management: buttock claudication and limb thrombosis. *Tech Vasc Intervent Radiol.* 4:232–235, 2001.
107. Cao P, Verzini F, Zannetti S, et al: Device migration after endoluminal abdominal aortic aneurysm repair: analysis of 113 cases with a minimum follow-up period of two years. *J Vasc Surg* 35: 229–235, 2002.
108. Conners MS, III, Sternbergh WC, III, Carter G, et al: Endograft migration one to four years after endovascular abdominal aortic aneurysm repair with the AneurRx device: a cautionary note. *J Vasc Surg* 36:476–484, 2002.
109. Storck M, Scharrer-Palmer R, Kapfer X, et al: Does a postimplantation syndrome following endovascular treatment of aortic aneurysms exist? *Vasc Surg* 35:23–29, 2001.
110. Dieter RS, MD, Laird JR, MD: Endovascular Abdominal Aortic Aneurysm Repair Chapter 52 · Endovascular Abdominal Aortic Aneurysm Repair. 1-11, 2007.
111. Alsac JM, Zarins CK, Heikkinen MA, et al: The impact of aortic endografts on renal function. *J Vasc Surg* 41:921–930, 2005.
112. Brenner DJ, Hall EJ: Computed tomography—an increasing source of radiation exposure. *N Engl J Med* 357:2277–2284, 2007.
113. Noll Jr, RE, Tonnessen BH, Mannava K, et al: Long-term follow-up cost after endovascular aneurysm repair. *J Vasc Surg* 46:9–15, 2007.
114. Sternbergh WC, 3rd, Greenberg RK, Chuter TA, et al: Redefining postoperative surveillance after endovascular aneurysm repair: recommendations based on 5-year follow-up in the US Zenith multicenter trial. *J Vasc Surg* 48:278–284, 2008.
115. Dake MD, Kato N, Mitchell RS, et al: Endovascular stentgraft placement for the treatment of acute aortic dissection. *N Engl J Med* 340:1546–1552, 1999.
116. Murad MH, Rizvi AZ, Malgor R, et al: Comparative effectiveness of the treatments for thoracic aortic transection. *J Vasc Surg* 53(1):193–199, e1–21, 2011.
117. Clough RE, Mani K, Lyons OT, et al: Endovascular treatment of acute aortic syndrome. *J Vasc Surg* 54(6):1580–1587, 2011.
118. Dagenais F, Shetty R, Normand JP, et al: Extended applications of thoracic aortic stent grafts. *Ann Thorac Surg* 82:567–572, 2006.
119. Vallejo N, Picardo NE, Bourke P, et al: The changing management of primary mycotic aortic aneurysms. *J Vasc Surg* 54(2):334–340, 2011.
120. Dake MD, Miller DC, Semba CP, et al: Transluminal placement of endovascular stent-grafts for the treatment of descending thoracic aortic aneurysms. *N Engl J Med* 331(26):1729–1734, 1994.
121. Bavaria JE, Appoo JJ, Makaroun MS, et al: Endovascular stent grafting versus open surgical repair of descending thoracic aortic aneurysms in low-risk patients: a multicenter comparative trial. *J Thorac Cardiovasc Surg* 133(2):369–377, 2007.
122. Fairman RM, Tuchek JM, Lee WA, et al: Pivotal results for the medtronic valiant thoracic stent graft system in the VALOR II trial. *J Vasc Surg* 56(5):1222–1231, 2012.
123. Trimarchi S, Nienaber CA, Rampoldi V, et al: Role and results of surgery in acute type B aortic dissection: insights from the international registry of acute aortic dissection (IRAD). *Circulation* 114(1 Suppl):I357–I364, 2006.
124. Dake MD, Kato N, Mitchell RS, et al: Endovascular stent-graft placement for the treatment of acute aortic dissection. *N Engl J Med* 340(20):1546–1552, 1999.
125. Nienaber CA, Kische S, Rousseau H, et al: Endovascular repair of type B aortic dissection: long-term results of the randomized investigation of stent grafts in aortic dissection trial. *Circ Cardiovasc Interv* 6(4):407–416, 2013.
126. Svensson LG, Kouchoukos NT, Miller DC, et al: Expert consensus document on the treatment of descending thoracic aortic disease using endovascular stent-grafts. *Ann Thorac Surg* 85(1 Suppl):S1–S41, 2008.
127. Mikhail P, Hess PJ, Jr, Klodell CT, et al: Closure of type I endoleaks and landing zone preparation of the thoracic aorta. *Ann Thorac Surg* 85(2):e9–e11, 2008.
128. Patel PJ, Grande W, Hieb RA: Endovascular management of acute aortic syndromes. *Semin Intervent Radiol* 28(1):10–23, 2011.
129. Tang GL, Tehrani HY, Usman A, et al: Reduced mortality, paraplegia, and stroke with stent graft repair of blunt aortic transections: a modern meta-analysis. *J Vasc Surg* 47(3):671–675, 2008.
130. Khoynezhad A, Azizzadeh A, Donayre CE, et al: Results of a multicenter, prospective trial of thoracic endovascular aortic repair for blunt thoracic aortic injury (RESCUE trial). *J Vasc Surg* 57(4):899–905, 2013.
131. Gopaldas RR, Dao TK, LeMaire SA, et al: Endovascular versus open repair of ruptured descending thoracic aortic aneurysms: a nationwide risk-adjusted study of 923 patients. *J Thorac Cardiovasc Surg* 142(5):1010–1018, 2011.
132. Cheung AT, Weiss SJ, McGarvey ML, et al: Interventions for reversing delayed-onset postoperative paraplegia after thoracic aortic reconstruction. *Ann Thorac Surg* 74(2):413–419, 2002, discussion 420–421.

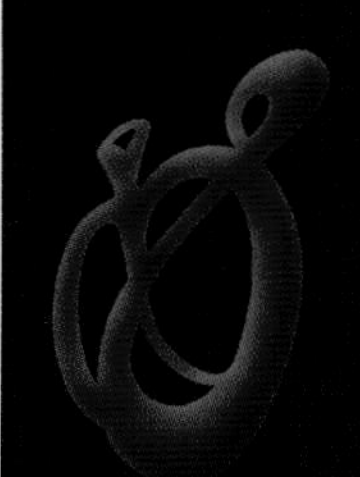

PART IV CEREBROVASCULAR INTERVENTION

24 Carotid and Vertebral Intervention

William A. Gray

Carotid Intervention

THE DATA

When discussing the clinical data for outcomes in carotid artery stenting (CAS), there are several important outcomes to be detailed: periprocedural (30 day) safety, which is composed of death, all stroke, and myocardial infarction; 1-year stroke prevention efficacy composed of ipsilateral stroke rates from 30 to 365 days; and durability, which is measured by restenosis >70% to 80% in severity and/or the need for repeat revascularization. All of these will necessarily be measured against carotid artery endarterectomy (CEA), the standard of care for carotid bifurcation disease requiring intervention.

Although the first reports of endovascular approaches to carotid artery disease were employed in nonatherosclerotic lesions and date back to the early 1980s,[1] the use of stents to augment angioplasty results did not come into routine use until the mid- to late 1990s. When studied in the first large-scale, multicenter, Carotid and Vertebral Artery Transluminal Angioplasty Study started in 1995 (CAVATAS), balloon angioplasty was used alone in 75% of the trial participants randomized to endovascular approach for symptomatic carotid disease, with the last 25% of this enrollment employing stent implantation.[2] The results of the U.K.-based CAVATAS suggested no short-term differences in safety and clinical efficacy between CEA and carotid angioplasty. But two important caveats to that conclusion are warranted. First, the restenosis rate in the angioplasty group was higher than CEA likely related to that lack of a stent scaffold in the majority of cases. Second, while the results between groups were not different, the rates (~10%) of 30-day death and stroke were higher than the standards established by the North American Symptomatic Carotid Endarterectomy Trial (NASCET) for symptomatic lesions[3]—and not a good showing for either approach. Importantly, not only were stents not used in the majority of patients but emboli protection devices (EPD) were still not developed and therefore not employed at all in CAVATAS, thus making these results largely irrelevant in today's era of "modern" CAS with standard EPD.

While CAS with EPD was introduced around 1999, the full penetration of this technology was not realized in Europe (EU) until several years later and was more delayed in the United States. The earlier approval of the technology in Europe did not translate into a deep pool of experienced operators capable of contributing expertly to studies of CAS and CEA early in the decade, when the EU trials were under way. In fact, of the three EU randomized trials, all in symptomatic patients, examining the relative safety and efficacy of these two treatments—Endarterectomy Versus Stenting in patients with Symptomatic Severe carotid Stenosis (EVA-3S), Stent-Protected Angioplasty versus Carotid Endarterectomy (SPACE), and International Carotid Stenting Study (ICSS)—two were severely cofounded by gross CAS operator inexperience, both on an absolute basis and relative to the CEA trial surgeon experience, making the results highly problematic.[4-6] Additionally confounding all three of these studies was the failure to include and/or routinely measure myocardial infarction (MI) as an endpoint, in spite of ample data demonstrating that MI in the perioperative period has significant long-term mortality implications for the patient.[7] Equally problematic, EPD were not mandated in any of the studies from the outset, although after a significant number of strokes had already occurred with CAS in EVA-3S in the first ~80 patients, EPD was finally made standard.

As a result of these and other construct and conduct issues within these EU trials, many of which can be ascribed to their premature initiation in an underdeveloped and novel therapy, their results are both predictable and unfortunate in that they are not helpful in determining the place of CAS in symptomatic patient management today. The French EVA-3S study was the first to report its data in 2006 and had to be halted early after approximately 500 patients due to safety concerns in the CAS arm. The primary endpoint of 30-day death and stroke was 3.9% in the CEA arm and 9.6% in the CAS arm. The second trial to report was the German SPACE (2007), which was also stopped early when a prespecified interim analysis at 1200 patients suggested the need for roughly another 1200 patients at the same event rates to reach a statistically meaningful endpoint, at which point the government funding agency withdrew support; nevertheless there was no difference detected in the 30-day endpoint of death and stroke between CEA and CAS, 6.3% versus 6.8%, respectively (EPD) was used only 27% of the time). Last to report was the U.K.-based ICSS trial, which reported an interim nonprimary endpoint in 2008 demonstrating more outcome events with CAS (8.5%) than CEA (5.2%) but which ultimately reported its 3-year primary endpoint of disabling stroke and death demonstrating no differences between the two therapies.

The progression of study followed a different course in the United States than in Europe. After several reports of reasonable outcomes in CAS in high surgical risk patients using off-label devices, including tracheobronchial stents (which had delivery systems long enough to reach the carotid from the transfemoral route), device development including dedicated nitinol stents and EPD got under way.[8,9] Subsequently, the Food and Drug Administration (FDA) Investigational Device Exemption (IDE) approval process dictated that studies would need to be compared with CEA. Because the procedural safety profile of CAS using EPD had not been fully established,[10] the comparator group was mandated to be those patients who were deemed to require CEA but were at high risk for the operation by virtue of either anatomic or physiologic co-morbidities. These conditions are listed in **Table 24-1**. The first U.S. trial to use these inclusion criteria was the randomized Stenting and Angioplasty with Protection in Patients at High Risk for Endarterectomy study (SAPPHIRE),[11] which tested the Precise carotid stent and the Angioguard filter EPD (Cordis/Johnson and Johnson, Freemont, California). SAPPHIRE turned out to be the only multicenter prospective examination of CEA in this high surgical risk cohort, which had largely been excluded from the landmark CEA trials such as the NASCET, the Asymptomatic Carotid Atherosclerosis Study (ACAS), and the Asymptomatic Carotid Surgery Trial (ACST). Unfortunately, the SAPPHIRE trial did not go to completion, as it didn't enroll a patient in its last 6 months, felt to likely be due to the availability of other competitive non-randomized IDE studies that guaranteed the interested subjects would get CAS. These other, single-arm, studies used objective performance criteria (OPC) to compare the CAS outcomes to and were constructed from a literature review of CEA outcomes in high surgical risk patients in the various categories of surgical risk (e.g., lung disease, congestive heart failure, prior CEA, etc.). They then weighted contributions according to the actual percentage of each category enrolled in the specific trial. While this may seem like an inexact science, in fact the high-risk surgical arm of SAPPHIRE had roughly the same 1-year outcomes that were modeled using the OPC method, which validated this approach; this method became the de facto standard for device trials in CAS for both IDE stent approval and 510(k) EPD clearance.

Although it was not able to be completed, the SAPPHIRE study nevertheless enrolled enough subjects to demonstrate that in a mixed population of symptomatic and asymptomatic patients at high surgical risk for CEA CAS was noninferior to CEA in the primary endpoint of 30-day death, stroke, and MI plus ipsilateral stroke and death to 1 year with trends favoring CAS (**Figure 24-1**).

The next high surgical risk population CAS study completed and reporting data was the ARCHeR trial,[12] which tested the Acculink stent and Accunet EPD system (Abbott Vascular, Santa Clara, California) and was the first single-arm study to compare to an OPC. The ARCHeR study 30-day

TABLE 24-1 High-Risk Factors for CEA

HIGH-RISK CATEGORY	CRITERIA
Age (y)	>80
Severe cardiac dysfunction	NYHA Class III/IV chronic heart failure
	Left ventricular ejection fraction <30%
	Open heart surgery within 6 weeks
	MI within 4 weeks
	NYHA Class III/IV angina
	Cardiac stress test positive for ischemia
Severe renal dysfunction	End-stage renal failure on dialysis
Severe chronic lung disease	Chronic oxygen therapy
	$pO_2 \leq 60$ mm Hg
	Baseline hematocrit ≥50%
	FEV_1 or DLCO ≤50% of predicted
Anatomic co-morbidities	Prior cervical radiation therapy
	Previous ipsilateral carotid endarterectomy
	C2 or higher carotid bifurcation
	Contralateral carotid occlusion
	Contralateral laryngeal nerve palsy
	Presence of a tracheostomy
	Common carotid artery lesion(s) below the clavicle

From **www.cms.gov/Regulations-and-Guidance/Guidance/Transmittals/downloads/R77NCD.pdf**.
C2, Second cervical vertebra; *DLCO,* diffusing capacity of lung for carbon monoxide; *FEV_1,* forced expiratory volume in 1 s; *MI,* myocardial infarction; *NYHA,* New York Heart Association; *pO_2,* partial oxygen pressure.

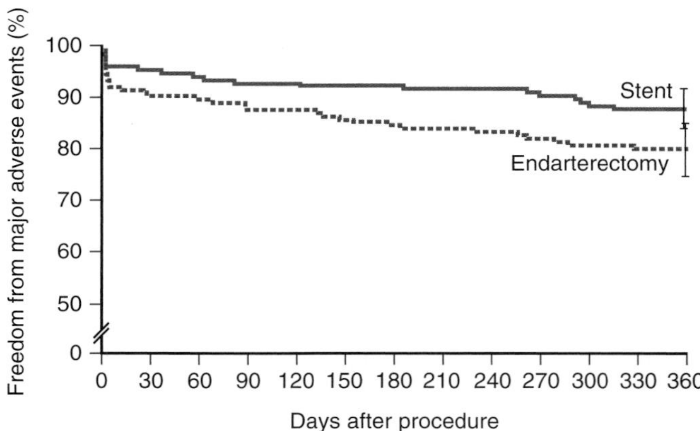

FIGURE 24-1 Freedom from major adverse events at 1 year in the SAPPHIRE trial. The intention-to-treat analysis rate of event-free survival is 87.8% for CAS and 79.9% for CEA, p = 0.053. *(Redrawn with permission from Yadav JS, Wholey MH, Kuntz RE, et al: Stenting and angioplasty with protection in patients at high risk for endarterectomy investigators. Protected carotid-artery stenting versus endarterectomy in high-risk patients. N Engl J Med 351:1493–1501, 2004.)*

TABLE 24-2 Summary of U.S. IDE CAS Device Trials

IDE TRIAL	*N* (CAS)	YEAR OF FDA ACTION	STENT SYSTEM APPROVAL/EPD 510(K) CLEARANCE	POSTMARKET SURVEILLANCE STUDY
ARCHeR	581	2004	Acculink PMA approval Accunet 510(k) clearance	CAPTURE (*N*—4225) CAPTURE (*N*—6361) CHOICE (*N*—19,000)
SECURITY	305	2005	Xact PMA approval Emboshield 510(k) clearance	EXACT (*N*—2145) CHOICE
SAPPHIRE	565	2006	Precise PMA approval Angioguard 510(k) clearance	CASES-PMS (*N*—1493) SAPPHIRE WW (*N*—15,000)
CABERNET	488	2006	Nexstent PMA approval FilterWire Carotid 510(k) clearance	None
CREATE	419	2006 2007	Protégé Carotid PMA approval SpiderFX Carotid 510(k) clearance	CREATE PAS (*N*—3500)
MaVErIC	449	2007	Exponent PMA approval GuardWire Carotid 510(k) clearance	None
PROTECT	320	2008	Emboshield NAV6 510(k) clearance	CHOICE
BEACH	480	2008	Wallstent Carotid PMA approval FilterWire EX System clearance	CABANA (*N* —1097)
EPIC	237	2008	Fibernet 510(k) clearance	None
EMBOLDEN	250	2009	GORE Embolic Filter clearance	None
EMPIRE	245	2009	Gore Flow Reversal 510(k) clearance	FREEDOM (planned *N*—5000)
ARMOUR	228	2009	Mo.Ma 510(k) clearance	None
CREST	1131	2011	Acculink PMA extension	CANOPY (planned *N*—1200)

From Gray WA, Verta P: The impact of regulatory approval and Medicare coverage on outcomes of carotid stenting. Catheter Cardiovasc Interv 83:1158–1166, 2014.
CAS, Carotid artery stenting.

death, stroke, and MI plus ipsilateral stroke to 1 year was 8.3%, the upper limit of the 95% confidence interval (CI) of which was able to satisfy the OPC endpoint estimate of 14.4%. This study led to FDA approval for this carotid stent system, the first in the United States, in 2004. Thereafter, a series of single-arm studies led to FDA approval, or clearance, for a variety of stents and filters, respectively, which are listed in **Table 24-2**. It is noteworthy that no device tested for use in CAS in the United States has failed to establish safety and efficacy by FDA standards.

As a condition of approval for each device tested, the FDA mandated postmarket surveillance registries of approximately 1500 patients to assess devices for any rare or unanticipated events not seen in the smaller pivotal studies, as well as the ability to transfer the technology into the nontrial setting. These single-arm prospective multicenter studies, replete with independent procedural and 30-day neurologic assessment, along with independent clinical event committees, were voluntarily extended by the device manufacturers and have yielded high-quality data from real-world settings from hundreds of sites and operators. The same comparable volume and quality of data—high or standard surgical risk—has not been paralleled in the CEA experience and provides a great deal of unique insight into the evolution of CAS U.S. outcomes, to be discussed further on. These studies, among them CAPTURE (Carotid ACCULINK/ACCUNET Post Approval Trial to Uncover Unanticipated or Rare Events),[13] CAPTURE 2,[14] EXACT (Emboshield and Xact),[15] SAPPHIRE WW,[16] and CHOICE (carotid stenting for high surgical risk patients; evaluating outcomes through the collection of clinical evidence),[17] have studied tens of thousands of patients across hundreds of U.S. operators and sites and have consistently demonstrated that CAS outcomes in the high surgical risk population of patients meets or exceeds the American Heart Association (AHA) guidelines for both symptomatic and asymptomatic patients (**Figure 24-2**).

In the background (2000–2008), while these pivotal and postmarket trials were being completed and conducted in high-risk surgical patients, the National Institutes of Health/ National Heart, Lung, and Blood Institute and Abbott Vascular sponsored the large (2500 subject) Carotid Revascularization Endarterectomy versus Stenting Trial (CREST),[18] which was originally designed to randomize symptomatic patients with standard risk for surgery to either CEA or CAS in 1:1 ratio. As contrasted to the aforementioned European studies, CREST mandated the use of EPD, included MI as a component of the primary endpoint, and insisted on qualified operators. The strict qualification criteria for both surgical and endovascular operators used to select sites resulted in over 50% of endovascular applications being rejected[19] and led to a slower than anticipated ramp up of the number of study sites from 2000 to 2004 since there were few U.S. sites with an adequate qualifying volume of CAS activity. Due to new data from the ACST trial published in 2004 demonstrating an advantage of immediate over deferred CEA in patients with asymptomatic carotid lesions, along with an effort to boost the slower than anticipated enrollment, asymptomatic patients were included in 2005 and the study completed in 2008. The final population was roughly evenly divided between symptomatic and asymptomatic subjects.

CREST demonstrated no differences between CEA and CAS for the primary composite endpoint of 30-day death, stroke, and MI, plus ipsilateral stroke to 4 years (7.2% vs. 6.8%; $p = 0.51$) in the intention-to-treat analysis (ITT) (**Figure 24-3**). In the ITT analysis, periprocedural event rates were

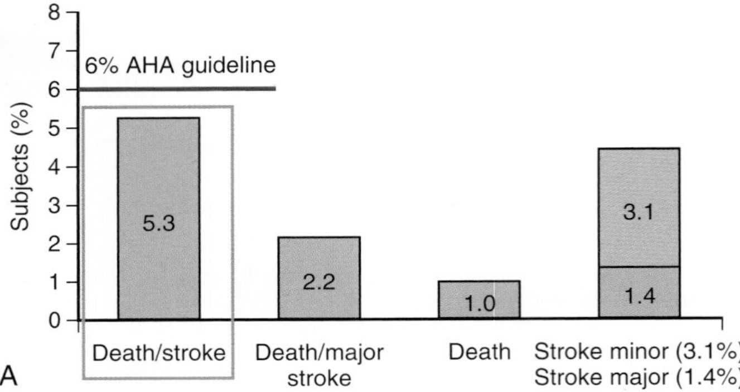

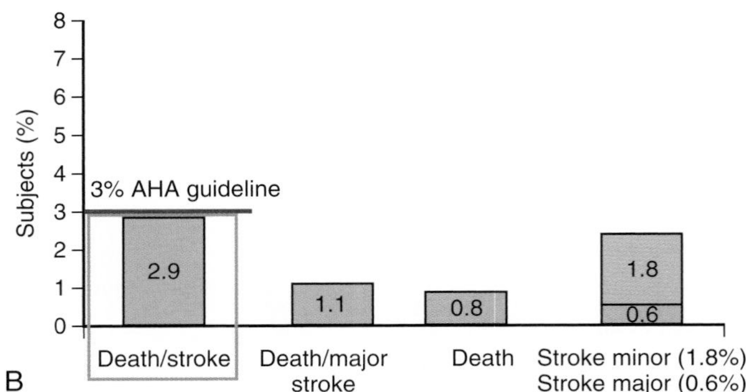

FIGURE 24-2 Combined outcomes from CAPTURE and EXACT single-arm studies in high surgical risk patients satisfying AHA goals for 30-day outcomes. **A,** In symptomatic patients. **B,** In asymptomatic patients. *AHA,* American Heart Association. *(Redrawn with permission from Gray WA, Chaturvedi S, Verta P: Investigators and the Executive Committee's thirty-day outcomes for carotid artery stenting in 6320 patients from 2 prospective, multicenter, high surgical-risk registries. Circ Cardiovasc Interv 2:159–166, 2009.)*

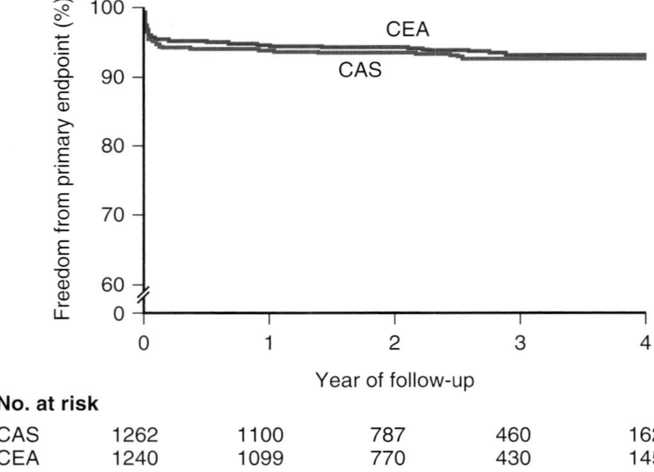

No. at risk

	0	1	2	3	4
CAS	1262	1100	787	460	162
CEA	1240	1099	770	430	145

FIGURE 24-3 Primary endpoint outcomes for CEA and CAS in standard surgical risk combined symptomatic and asymptomatic patients in CREST demonstrating no difference between the therapies. *CAS,* Carotid artery stenting; *CEA,* artery endarterectomy. *(Redrawn with permission from: Brott TG, Hobson RW 2nd, Howard G, et al: CREST Investigators Stenting versus endarterectomy for treatment of carotid-artery stenosis. N Engl J Med 363:11–23, 2010.)*

the lowest reported for CEA and CAS in a multicenter randomized controlled trial setting. Within these 30-day composite outcomes, there were small differences noted between the therapies: CEA had roughly twice the number of MIs (1.1% vs. 2.3%; p = 0.03) and CAS had roughly twice the number of strokes (4.1% vs. 2.3%; p = 0.01), the difference being related to the incidence of minor strokes; major strokes were not different between CAS and CEA. While the trial was not powered to assess these individual components, they serve as hypothesis-generating observations and opportunity for outcome improvements. In CREST, the long-term outcomes such as stroke prevention effectiveness, vessel patency, and target lesion revascularization were the same between the two treatment arms, observations that reinforced those also seen in the SPACE and ICSS studies.[20,21]

The short-term competitive safety profile of CAS was combined with similar comparable longer term durability with CEA represents a unique profile in endovascular intervention. Most, if not all, other endovascular interventions are attractive alternatives to surgery because they can have immediate and similar therapeutic importance to the patient without nearly the morbidity associated with the parallel surgical approach (such as with abdominal aortic aneurysm repair or lower extremity bypass), but generally suffer from a lack of competitive durability (such as SFA stents). In CAS, the long-term durability and stroke prevention being spot on with CEA means that its value and attractiveness really come down to matching the acute safety profile of periprocedural stroke and death in CEA (which is quite good). If short-term safety outcomes can be matched, then the avoidance of nuisance complications like cranial nerve injury and access site re-operation become the only real differentiating features between CEA and CAS.

In a separate per protocol analysis (PP) presented to the FDA as part of a successful application for extension of indication (to standard surgical risk patients) of the study devices by the co-sponsor of the study (Acculink stent and Accunet filter, Abbott Vascular), several other findings were observed.[22] First, whereas a best-fit line in the ITT analysis appeared to demonstrate an advantage of CEA over CAS in octogenarians, a direct FDA assessment of this cohort in the PP analysis found that although the adverse outcomes were indeed higher in octogenarians, there were no differences between CEA and CAS in this group (**Figure 24-4**). Conversely, CAS was found to be safer in the under 60-year-old population.

Second, a follow-up assessment of all patients with minor stroke due to either CEA or CAS demonstrated no differences in the mean severity of neurologic and functional deficit at 1 month and 6 months as measured by National Institutes of Health Stroke Scales (NIHSS) and modified Rankin scale (MRS), suggesting that the CAS minor strokes, while more numerous, ultimately had very little lasting clinical impact (**Figure 24-5**). This confirmed similar findings from previous smaller studies that demonstrated that patients with CAS-related minor stroke were likely to have an NIHSS of 0 or 1 by 1 year.[12] These clinical observations are further bolstered by MRI data from ICSS that show that while there is a higher frequency of new but asymptomatic diffusion-weighted imaging (DWI) abnormalities after CAS compared with CEA, in fact the volume of abnormalities is similar.[23] Not only are there fewer but larger CEA-associated defects than CAS in ICSS, the CEA lesions were more likely to convert from acute to persisting lesions (RR, 0.4; 95% CI, 0.2–0.8; p = 0.007).[24] The clinical implication of these findings is unclear but seems to support the data on the increase in minor stroke events seen in CREST with CAS compared with CEA, but the relative lack of persistent symptoms.

The CREST PP analysis also found that there appeared to be an important trend of outcome improvement within the

CAS operators over the 8 years of the study enrollment (**Figure 24-6**), but that there was no similar trend within the CEA operators. These observations were not surprising given the 60-year experience with CEA and stable techniques and established patient selection criteria at the start of the study, but for CAS the lack of even FDA-approved and dedicated devices until the fourth year of the study.

This last finding in CREST, the improvements in CAS outcomes within the trial, cannot entirely be explained by the experience accrued within the trial, since the average

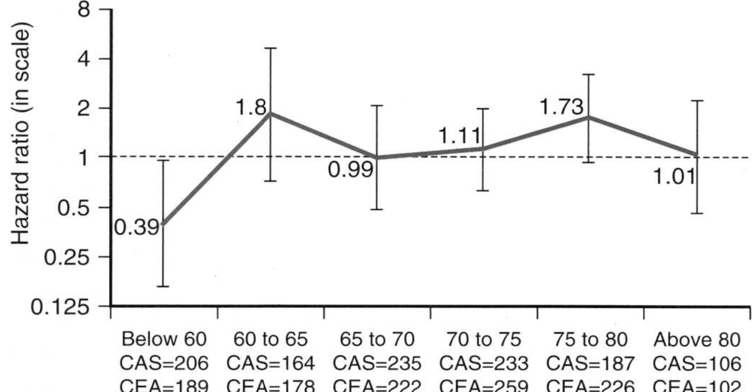

FIGURE 24-4 FDA analysis of age-related outcomes of CAS and CEA from the CREST trial presented with y-axis correctly assigned as logarithmic. *CAS,* Carotid artery stenting; *CEA,* artery endarterectomy. *(Redrawn with permission from Gray WA, Simonton CA, Verta P: Overview of the 2011 Food and Drug Administration Circulatory System Devices Panel meeting on the ACCULINK and ACCUNET Carotid Artery Stent System. Circulation 125:2256–2264, 2012.)*

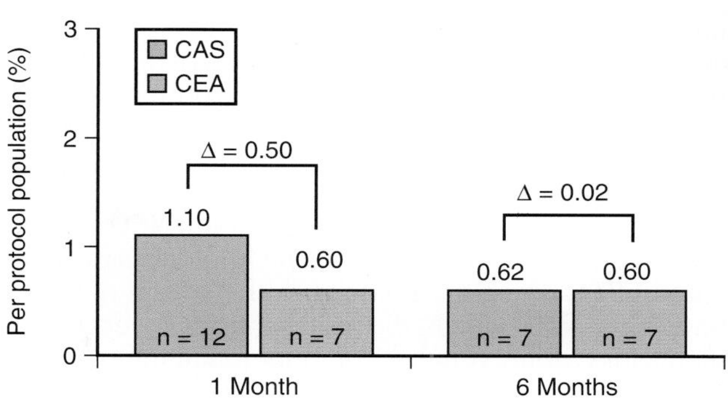

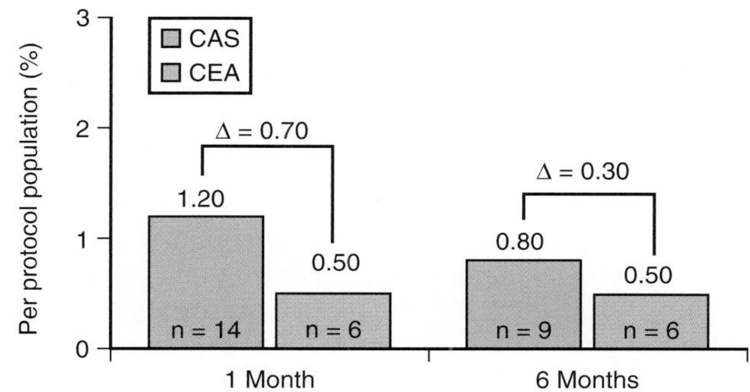

FIGURE 24-5 Outcomes of subjects experiencing a minor stroke related to either CAS or CEA. **A,** National Institutes of Health Stroke Scale (NIHSS). **B,** Modified Rankin Scale (mRS). *CAS,* Carotid artery stenting; *CEA,* artery endarterectomy. *(Redrawn with permission from Gray WA, Simonton CA, Verta P: Overview of the 2011 Food and Drug Administration Circulatory System Devices Panel meeting on the ACCULINK and ACCUNET Carotid Artery Stent System. Circulation 125:2256–2264, 2012.)*

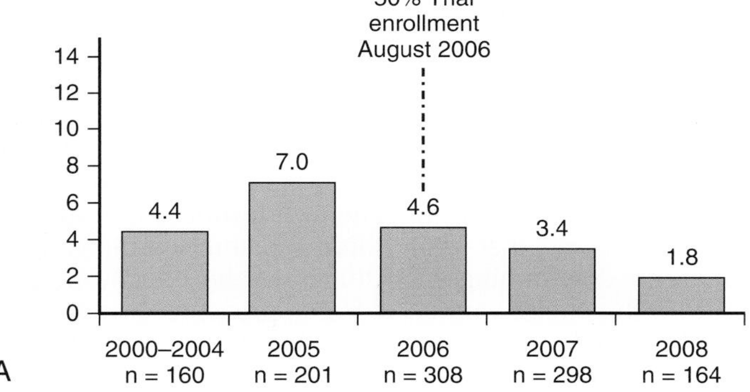

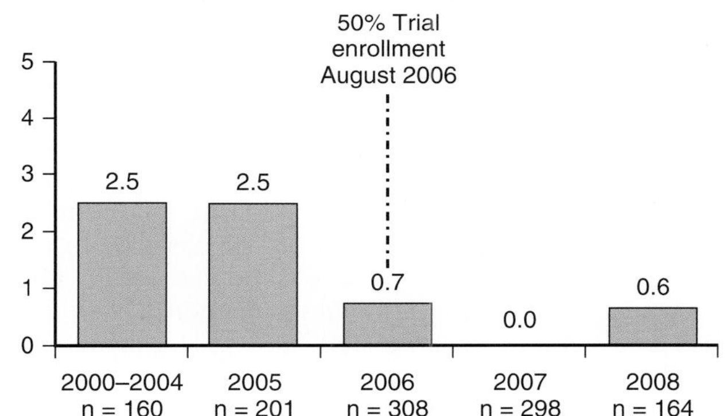

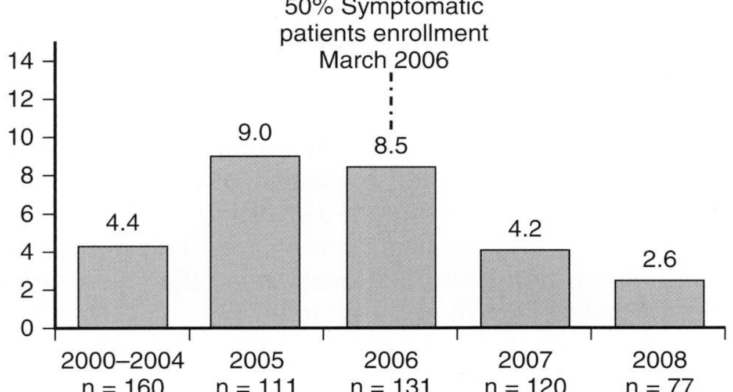

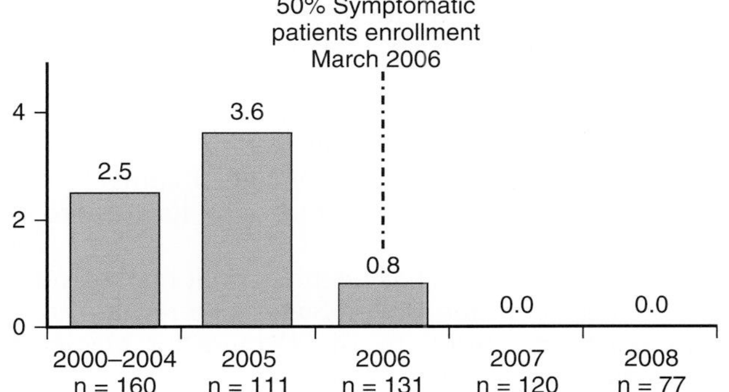

FIGURE 24-6 Outcome improvement demonstrated within the later phases of CREST in the CAS arm. *CAS,* Carotid artery stenting. *(Redrawn with permission from Gray WA, Simonton CA, Verta P: Overview of the 2011 Food and Drug Administration Circulatory System Devices Panel meeting on the ACCULINK and ACCUNET Carotid Artery Stent System. Circulation, 125:2256–2264, 2012.)*

number of CAS cases performed by interventionalists was around six. This is where an intersection of the unique reimbursement hurdles delaying a fuller adoption of CAS as an alternative to CEA or medical therapy requires comment for a fuller understanding of the therapy and its outcomes and status. Specifically, carotid intervention has been under a restrictive national coverage decision (NCD) since the 1980s as a result of a negative technology assessment of carotid PTA, which did not foresee the advent of CAS at the time. This NCD, which did not support coverage or payments for carotid, vertebral, or intracranial intervention, was modified in the early 2000s to allow for research in CAS, and then again in 2005 following FDA approval of the first CAS systems. This second NCD modification extended coverage to patients with high surgical risk with recent symptoms, which represents a small (estimated to be 10% to 15%) fraction of the overall population of patients requiring carotid intervention. The 2005 NCD also allowed for coverage of CAS postmarket registries mandated as a condition of FDA approval that were subsequently extended by the sponsors voluntarily to explore other scientific queries, and that ultimately allowed greater patient access to and operator activity in, CAS. During the time of this coverage of registry activity a great deal was learned and published about the technique and patient selection related to CAS that have been reflected in this chapter and have accrued to the benefit of patients not just in the United States. A recent analysis of the past decade of CAS outcomes strongly backs the concept that CAS outcome improvement seen in CREST was the result of FDA approval (2004) and CMS reimbursement (2005), which supported a much broader and deeper parallel CAS experience outside of CREST, gained primarily in the postmarket studies.[22] These studies allowed the treatment and study of over 50,000 patients in the last half of the decade which generated high-quality prospective 30-day data across hundreds of sites and unparalleled in any CEA experience. This volume of activity dwarfs the first half of the decade when a few small (generally <400 patients) trials in only a few sites, and a few operators, provided the only experience for CAS using EPD in this country. This marked increase in the number of CAS cases being done in the second half of the decade resulted in dramatic improvements in not only the IDE trial results across stent systems but also within the same stent and EPD systems (**Figure 24-7**).

In retrospect, much of the failure of the European trials to have adequate experience in their operators can be explained by the era in which they were both planned and executed; had the studies been done in the second half of the decade rather than the first, the results may have been appreciably different for analogous reasons. Similarly, had the CREST trial enrollment not lagged—the last 4 years of the trial (2005 to 2008) enrolled the significant majority of subjects—as a result of the lack of adequate operator experience due to the enforcement of stringent operator selection criteria, then outcomes may have more closely paralleled the EU's.

Unfortunately, there has been a recent marked reduction of CAS activity in the United States as a result of a unique and persistent refusal by the Centers for Medicare and Medicaid Services (CMS) to expand coverage to devices approved or cleared by the FDA as safe and effective in spite of a number of national coverage determination processes and opportunities to do so. Given the data on outcome improvement in the United States with volume activity that have just been discussed, this has real implications not only for patient access to care but also the quality of their outcomes. It also may make recruitment of qualified sites for CAS research problematic as well as put a damper on spending for technology improvements that can further safeguard patient outcomes.

As has been detailed, the clinical event rates for CAS and CEA are quite low, a happy fact for patients and referring/treating physicians alike; however, this is an unfortunate fact for researchers seeking to compare outcomes across therapies or to improve outcomes within therapies since it means that very large trials are required to assess differences. As an example, an intervention that seeks to demonstrate a 1% difference in outcomes in stroke would mean several thousand patients, and recruitment for trials of this size—even with brisk enrollment—can take close to a decade by which time the technology or method can be obsolete. So in addition to the "classic" clinical outcome measures listed, attempts to define objective but nonclinical differences in techniques and equipment have used surrogate markers of safety. These have primarily centered around the detection—the microembolic signals detected on transcranial Doppler (TCD)—or consequence—new lesions seen on serial magnetic resonance diffusion weighted imaging (MR-DWI)—of microemboli. The former method is confounded by the lack of reliable ability to distinguish gaseous from solid emboli, which means that presumably innocuous microbubbles released from moving devices through sheaths, unsheathing filters and stents, and even contrast injection are counted among potentially harmful ones; even still, it can be useful in characterizing potentially vulnerable stages of the procedure even if it is a bit more difficult to use in a comparative way.[24] In the case of the latter technique, it is preferred since these overwhelmingly clinically silent imaging findings—the result of the edema indicative of cellular ischemia—are counted with consistency and are frequent enough to be used to distinguish both between therapies (i.e., CAS and CEA) and within (e.g., differences among EPD systems) requiring a relatively small number of patients.[25] It should nevertheless be emphasized that while these markers will likely have utility in determining such things as the effectiveness of EPD, or the effects various access approaches or tools have on these measures of microembolism, there has yet to be a clinical correlate directly linked to these strictly image-based findings. That said, the low but real rate of minor stroke excess seen in CAS as compared with CEA, especially in symptomatic patients, appears to roughly parallel in a proportional way the consistent excess in MR-DWI lesions noted postprocedure. Therefore, both intuitively and on a semi-empiric basis, the reduction of MR-DWI lesions is desirable.

Last, while there are several publications reporting the effects of CAS on subtle measures of cognition using the outcomes of neuropsychometric testing,[26,27] the results have been mixed and far from conclusive, likely related to the difficulty in administering these tests reliably and multiple confounders, known and unknown.

THE PROCEDURE

The endovascular management of obstructive atherosclerotic bifurcation carotid disease is practiced by multiple

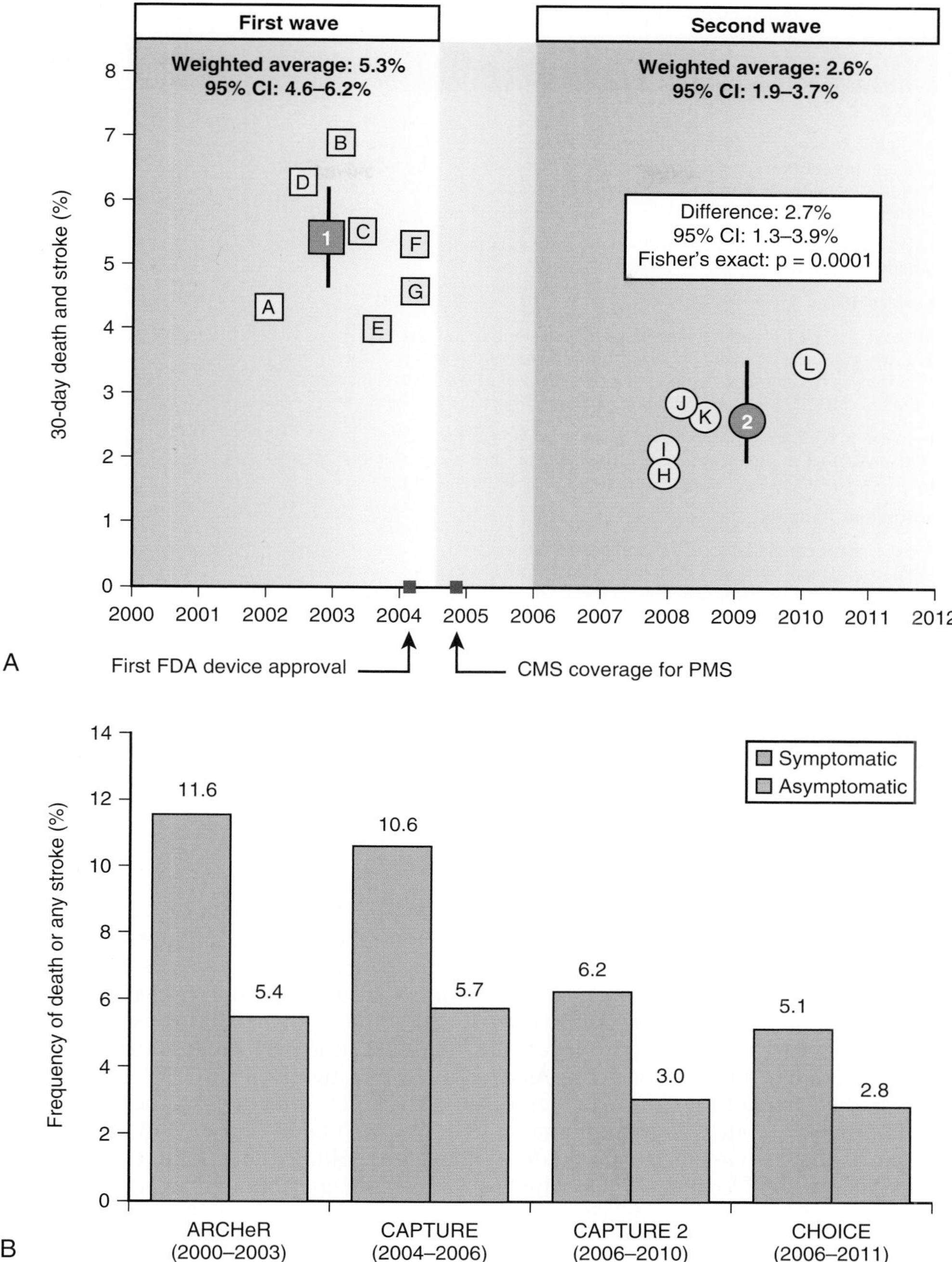

FIGURE 24-7 **A,** Improvement in outcomes among U.S. IDE trials testing different CAS systems demonstrates a halving of complication rates with the approval of device and commensurate increase in clinical procedural volumes. **B,** Similar outcome improvements over the same time period using a single CAS system. *CAS,* Carotid artery stenting. *(Redrawn with permission from Gray WA, Simonton CA, Verta P: Overview of the 2011 Food and Drug Administration Circulatory System Devices Panel meeting on the ACCULINK and ACCUNET Carotid Artery Stent System. Circulation 125:2256–2264, 2012.)*

specialties—interventional cardiology, vascular surgery, neurointerventional radiology, and interventional neurology—and so mandates a confluence of disparate skill sets and understanding of both the disease process as well as the exceptionality of the procedure. This section will endeavor to communicate the relevant elements of endovascular carotid intervention important to performing it expertly and safely.

The predicate of surgical plaque removal—carotid endarterectomy (CEA)—of atherosclerotic bifurcation carotid disease has been performed for over 60 years[28] and has been demonstrated to reduce future stroke in both symptomatic and asymptomatic patients as compared with deferred therapy.[3,29-31] While acknowledging that these trials lacked a programmed, monitored, and modern medical therapy component, they nevertheless represent the highest quality data available (prospective, randomized, controlled, multicenter) to both direct clinical decision making and, in the case of CAS, use as a comparator for the standard of care. As was seen in the first half of this carotid section, the progression of carotid testing and therapy has always been predicated on a comparison, direct or indirect, to CEA.

The carotid artery and associated atherosclerotic plaque are unique not only as pathophysiologic determinants of

TABLE 24-3 Summary of Multidisciplinary Guidelines on the Management of Carotid Disease

INDICATION	RECOMMENDATION	LEVEL OF EVIDENCE
Symptomatic High Surgical Risk		
Among patients with symptomatic severe stenosis (>70%) in whom the stenosis is difficult to access surgically, medical conditions are present that greatly increase the risk of surgery, or when other specific circumstances exist, such as radiation-induced stenosis or restenosis after CEA, CAS may be considered when performed by an experienced operator.	Class IIa	B
It is reasonable to choose CAS over CEA when revascularization is indicated in patients with neck anatomy unfavorable for arterial surgery.	Class IIa	B
Symptomatic Average Surgical Risk		
CAS is indicated as an alternative to CEA for symptomatic patients at average or low risk of complications associated with endovascular intervention when the diameter of the lumen of the internal carotid artery is reduced by >70% as documented by noninvasive imaging or >50% as documented by catheter angiography and the anticipated rate of periprocedural stroke or mortality is <6%.	Class I	B
CAS is indicated as an alternative to CEA for symptomatic patients at average or low risk of complications associated with endovascular intervention when the diameter of the lumen of the internal carotid artery is reduced by >70% by noninvasive imaging or >50% by catheter angiography.	Class I	B
Asymptomatic High Surgical Risk Patients		
Selection of asymptomatic patients for carotid revascularization should be guided by an assessment of co-morbid conditions, life expectancy, and other individual factors and should include a thorough discussion of the risks and benefits of the procedure with an understanding of patient preferences.	Class I	C
It is reasonable to choose CAS over CEA when revascularization is indicated in patients with neck anatomy unfavorable for arterial surgery.	Class IIa	B
Asymptomatic Average Surgical Risk Patients		
Prophylactic CAS might be considered in highly selected patients with asymptomatic carotid stenosis (minimum 60% by angiograph, 70% by validated Doppler ultrasound), but its effectiveness compared with medical therapy alone in this situation is not well established.	Class IIb	B

From White CJ: Carotid artery stenting. J Am Coll Card 64:722–731, 2014.
CAS, Carotid artery stenting; *CEA,* artery endarterectomy.

clinical ischemic syndrome but also in their response to intervention, surgical or endovascular. On the first point, it is only in the small minority of cases that symptoms related to carotid stenosis are due to an actual reduction in distal blood flow, as contrasted with all other atherosclerotic stenoses that create their associated clinical syndromes via restriction in distal bed perfusion—chronic or acute. As a further demonstration of its distinctive nature, an acute occlusion of the carotid artery can often be asymptomatic. All of these characteristic aspects are related to the maintenance of distal perfusion by the circle of Willis, which although complete in less than half the population, nevertheless provides perfusion adequate enough to avoid symptoms in many cases.[32] As regards the second point, the carotid bifurcation plaque, in the significant majority of lesions, is reliably and discretely localized within ~2 cm of the bifurcation. This fact is a result of the flow dynamics within the carotid bulb that set up a flow-eddy responsible for lesion generation,[33] and this allows for its easy and routine surgical removal—not true in many other atherosclerotic vascular territories. In addition, the durability of carotid intervention is unmatched in the arterial circulation: long-term rates of restenosis requiring re-intervention for both CEA and CAS are similar and low—1% to 2% per year.[18] In the case of standard (not eversion) CEA, enlargement of the arteriotomy with a patch is associated with lower rates of restenosis especially in women,[34] whereas in CAS no definitive association with residual stenosis or sex and long-term patency has been shown. Understanding these two unique qualities of the carotid bifurcation drives decision making in the procedural components of CAS.

Although an in-depth exploration of the subject is largely beyond the scope of an interventional chapter on CAS, it is important to at least acknowledge the indications for carotid intervention in general terms, and for CAS specifically, and that some of them are in evolution or testing. These were codified in a 2011 multi-society guidelines document that the following distillation references[35] (**Table 24-3**).

In clinical practice, symptomatic patients with stenosis >70% are offered CEA or CAS without delay since it appears that any salutary effect of intervention is greatest in the first 2 to 4 weeks, although women have a particularly rapid drop-off in the benefit after the first 2 weeks.[36] For the symptomatic patient with stenosis between 50% to 70%, which is a small fraction of the affected population, the benefit is less and these cases should be taken on a case-by-case basis, and a determined search for other potential causes of a cerebrovascular event should be considered (i.e., occult atrial fibrillation).[37] In asymptomatic patients, most operators will not offer an intervention unless the lesion is at least greater than 70% to 80% in combination with a life-expectancy of at least 5 years. This is because the natural history of the unmolested asymptomatic carotid plaque has neurological event rates of roughly 2% to 3% per year,[30] and the risk of CEA or CAS must be "amortized" over a sufficient time period so as to provide a clinically meaningful improvement for the patient. The most recent data available for the 30-day risk for both CEA and CAS suggest that the stroke and death rate is between 1.5% and 2.0%,[18,38] nearly half what it was in some of the landmark, now legacy, CEA studies (ACAS and ACST). Nevertheless, a great deal of speculation has arisen that improved modern medical therapy may have lowered the above rates of stroke in the asymptomatic patient in observational settings such that intervention may no longer be justified[39,40]; however, the only randomized data that exist support CEA and, by extension, CAS. The CREST 2 trial is intended to examine this question by randomizing asymptomatic patients with severe carotid stenosis to either optimized medical therapy or intervention with CEA or CAS. Finally, it is important to acknowledge that CAS has not yet been tested directly versus medical therapy in either the symptomatic or asymptomatic populations; any proposed benefit of CAS is extrapolated primarily from its trial comparisons to CEA.

The performance of the CAS procedure has some variability depending on the type of embolic protection that is used, but otherwise it can be divided into the following steps: establish access, place EPD, balloon dilation (prestent and poststent), stent placement, retrieval of embolic protection. Each step has to be considered within the anatomic and clinical environment at hand, the latter of which can be quite dynamic at times. Although it takes less than 7 to 10 minutes of EPD dwell time to perform a CAS well, more than most other endovascular procedures (save some neurointerventions), performing a successful CAS requires careful planning and unbroken attention during that short but intense time, due to the potentially catastrophic neurological outcomes from even a small error or lapse in method or judgment. In addition to the above technical considerations, the stent pharmacology (control of anticoagulation preprocedure and postprocedure medications), vascular access, hemodynamic and neurological shifts, etc., must all be successfully managed, typically mandating a broad and deep preparedness to do so by not just the operator but the larger care team.

In uncomplicated CAS, some practitioners feel comfortable discharging patients on the same day given the very low rates of overall complications. This appears to be a reasonable, though aggressive, strategy of patient management; however, it will potentially miss late stroke identification, which although numerically very small, requires an independent evaluation up to 24 hours post procedure.

Lesion Considerations

Lesion assessment is a very important component of procedural planning, and proper lesion selection can lead to improved patient outcomes. To start with, using the appropriate method to determine the angiographic lesion severity and thus the indication for CAS in the first place is critical. Although there are several methods (e.g., European Carotid Surgery Trial method [ECST]),[41] the one on which landmark trial data are based and therefore accepted in the United States is the NASCET criteria.[42] In this method, the angiographic lesion minimum lesion diameter (MLD) in the worst projection is used as the numerator and the distal ICA where the vessel stops tapering as the reference segment in the denominator (**Figure 24-8**). If the NASCET criteria are strictly adhered to and the presumed, and typical, distal ICA reference diameter is 5.0 to 5.5 cm, then in an asymptomatic patient the lesion MLD will be ~1 to 1.5 mm (which equals a 70% to 80% lesion). It is useful to bear this rule of thumb in mind since it is easy for the eye to be drawn to the CCA/carotid bulb and overestimate the true diameter stenosis.

Beyond the stenosis severity, there are lesion qualities that must be assessed prior to considering or performing CAS, including filling defects consistent with thrombus, degree and pattern of calcification, length of lesion, and associated tortuosity/angulation. Although some operators report successful CAS in the presence of thrombus (and have advocated proximal protection in these situations), and lesions producing recent cerebrovascular symptoms almost certainly have some degree of thrombus even if not identified

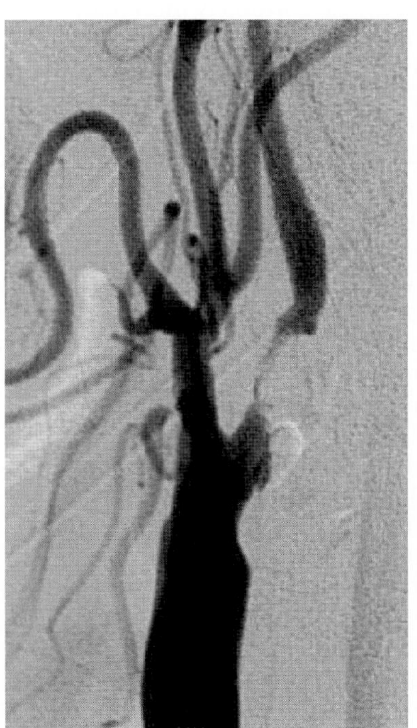

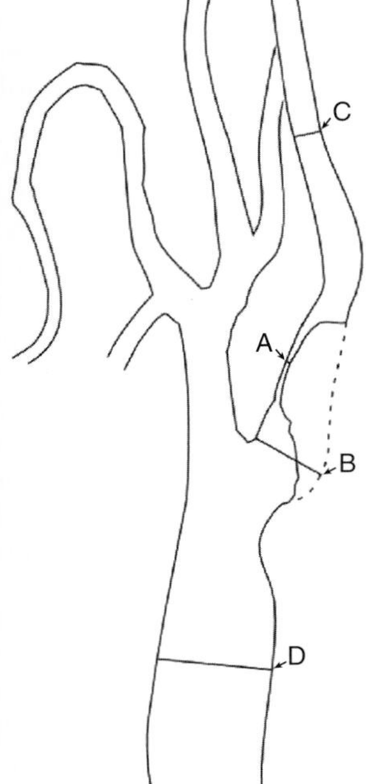

MEASUREMENT of STENOSIS

NASCET

$$1-\frac{A}{C}\times 100 = \%\text{ Stenosis}$$

ECST

$$1-\frac{A}{B}\times 100 = \%\text{ Stenosis}$$

CC

$$1-\frac{A}{D}\times 100 = \%\text{ Stenosis}$$

FIGURE 24-8 The NASCET method of carotid stenosis determination. *(From Higashida RT, Meyers PM, Phatouros CC, et al: Technology Assessment Committees of the American Society of Interventional and Therapeutic Neuroradiology and the Society of Interventional Radiology. Reporting standards for carotid artery angioplasty and stent placement. J Vasc Interv Radiol 15:421–422, 2004.)*

TABLE 24-4 Carotid Artery Stent Patient and Procedural Factors Likely to Be Associated with Adverse Procedural Outcomes

MEDICAL CO-MORBIDITY	ANATOMICAL CRITERIA	PROCEDURAL FACTOR
Elderly (>75/80 yrs)	Type III aortic arch	Inexperienced operator/center
Symptom status	Vessel tortuosity	EPD not used
Bleeding risk/ hypercoagulable state	Heavy calcification	Lack of femoral access
Severe aortic stenosis	Lesion-related thrombus	Time delay to perform procedure from onset of symptoms
Chronic kidney disease	Echolucent plaque	
Decreased cerebral reserve	Aortic arch atheroma	

From White CJ: Carotid artery stenting. J Am Coll Card 64:722–731, 2014.
EPD, Emboli protection devices.

angiographically, generally speaking visible thrombus has been a contraindication for CAS in a patient with a surgical alternative. Heavy calcification, especially in a circumferential pattern, is associated with stent under-expansion and stent delivery system entrapment along with the potential for more pronounced hemodynamic instability and is considered a relative contraindication to CAS. Poorer outcomes have been associated with diffuse, long lesions and those requiring multiple stents[43] and should be approached with caution. Last, angulation that is suboptimally located at or just distal to the bifurcation can lead to difficulty with wire/filter/stent transit and can make filter retrieval difficult (**Table 24-4**). The experienced operator will elect to reconsider CAS in favor of CEA or medical therapy when faced with one or multiple of these attributes and in that way will deliver the best outcomes for the patient, with the understanding that these therapies are clearly complementary, not competitive.

Access

Access to the common carotid artery (CCA) via the common femoral artery is typically achieved using a 6 Fr straight sheath with exceptions noted below, although outside of the United States guide catheters with preformed shapes are also available for use. Some stent devices have smaller delivery system calibers that may allow for 5 Fr sheath use, and while these may be attractive from both radial and femoral access perspectives, the trade-off can be a significant loss of guide stability and support. If proximal protection is to be employed, it is done with a specialized 9 Fr catheter that has an occlusion balloon on its tip and the capacity to place a second occlusion balloon into the ECA. Some operators practice radial artery access for CAS as an alternative to femoral access in order to avoid/minimize both access site complications but also aortic arch interaction.[44] Last, since it has been demonstrated that up to ~35% of strokes associated with CAS may be related to an aortic arch source liberated while establishing access,[45] so direct carotid access has been proposed as an alternative to transfemoral CAS. A commercial system (Silk Road Medical, Sunnyvale, California), which also employs a high flow reversal system not requiring external carotid occlusion to establish the proximal protection, has developed on the plausible logic—and early data—that arch avoidance leads to fewer magnetic resonance imaging diffusion-weighted (MR-DWI) lesions—a marker of cellular edema resulting from cell death—and ultimately fewer strokes.[46] At the current time this system requires a small surgical incision in the proximal CCA to establish access, but may at some point become a percutaneous option.

Arch anatomy, proximal CCA tortuosity, or disease and lesion location will individually or in combination determine both the difficulty of CCA cannulation and sheath placement as well as the method used to gain access. In straightforward anatomy, a support wire is ultimately positioned into the ECA by way of a diagnostic catheter that is advanced into the ECA over a softer wire first. The interventional sheath is then substituted for the diagnostic catheter and the procedure can begin. If the carotid bifurcation is involved with significant occlusive disease making wire passage into the ECA dangerous or anatomically prohibitive, an alternative method involves placing a support wire shaped with a tight pigtail-style curve in the CCA just below the bifurcation and advancing the sheath over that arrangement. As long as there is enough CCA length, this method can be safe and effective in establishing access, but in shorter CCAs it is possible not to have enough wire support in place to allow sheath placement.

If there is significant CCA tortuosity, then access can be challenging in a number of different ways. First, negotiating a wire, followed by even a diagnostic catheter into the CCA, can be problematic. Second, even if a sheath can be successfully placed it can result in associated changes in the more distal vessel (i.e., displacing the proximal tortuosity more distally) in a vessel that is ultimately fixed between two points in its proximal origin (aorta) and distal terminus (petrous carotid), which can make later procedural steps (filter or stent placement) difficult, risky, or impossible. Last, and especially when working in the right CCA, if a reasonably coaxial position of the sheath in the CCA cannot be established due to tortuosity, then dissection of the CCA due to catheter tip trauma becomes a distinct possibility as well.

If the aortic arch is heavily involved with atherosclerosis, then even the most expert catheter manipulation can lead to embolic complications. There are also anatomical arch variants, the most common (~25%) and relevant of which is a bovine origin of the left CCA (i.e., originating from the innominate trunk), which can often be further retroflexed and lead to difficulty in cannulation and/or a stable coaxial position (**Figure 24-9**). In addition, the aorta can elongate and rotate with age and in the case of the aortic arch, pinned between the sternum and the spine, an exaggerated "hump" or apex is established along with the proximal displacement of the great vessels. These changes are categorized into three types:

Type I arch is normal with the great vessels arising from a normally shaped apex.

Type II arch has a proximal displacement of the great vessels with a moderately peaked arch.

Type III arch has an accentuated peak and marked proximal displacement of the great vessels.

These functionally appear to arise from the ascending aorta (**Figure 24-10**). These arch challenges require more aggressively shaped catheters such as the Simmons catheter (Cook, Bloomington, Indiana) and typically multiple attempts with multiple tools until the correct combination of catheters are found, all of which can lead to greater risk

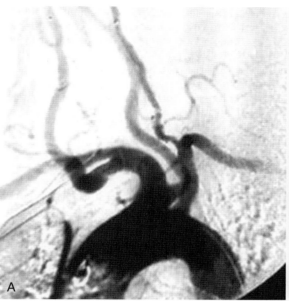

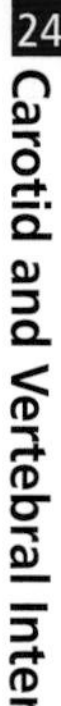

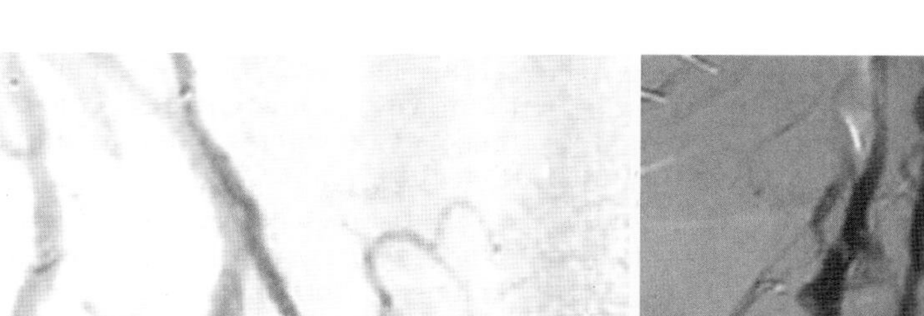

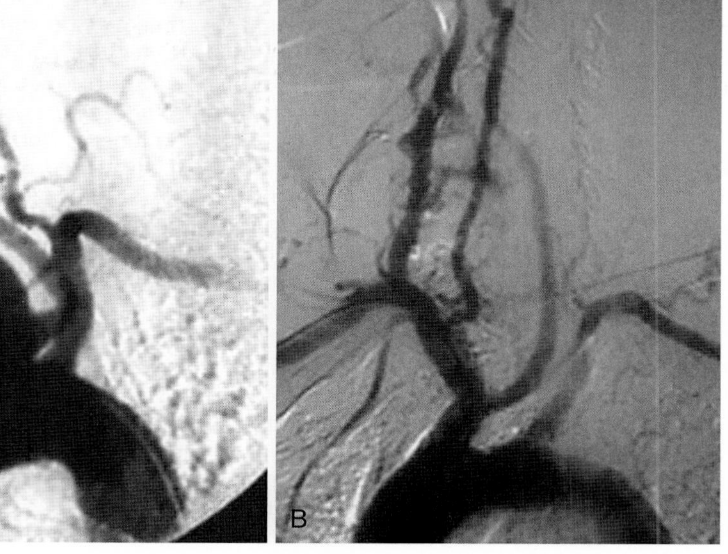

FIGURE 24-9 Examples of bovine arch variation anatomy demonstrating the origin of the left CCA from the innominate trunk. In addition, in the first panel there is additional tortuosity in both the right and left CCA. *CCA,* Common carotid artery. *(From Liapis CD, Efthimios D, Avgerinos D, Chatziioannou A: The aortic arch: markers, imaging, and procedure planning for carotid intervention. Cath Lab Digest 17:6, 2009.)*

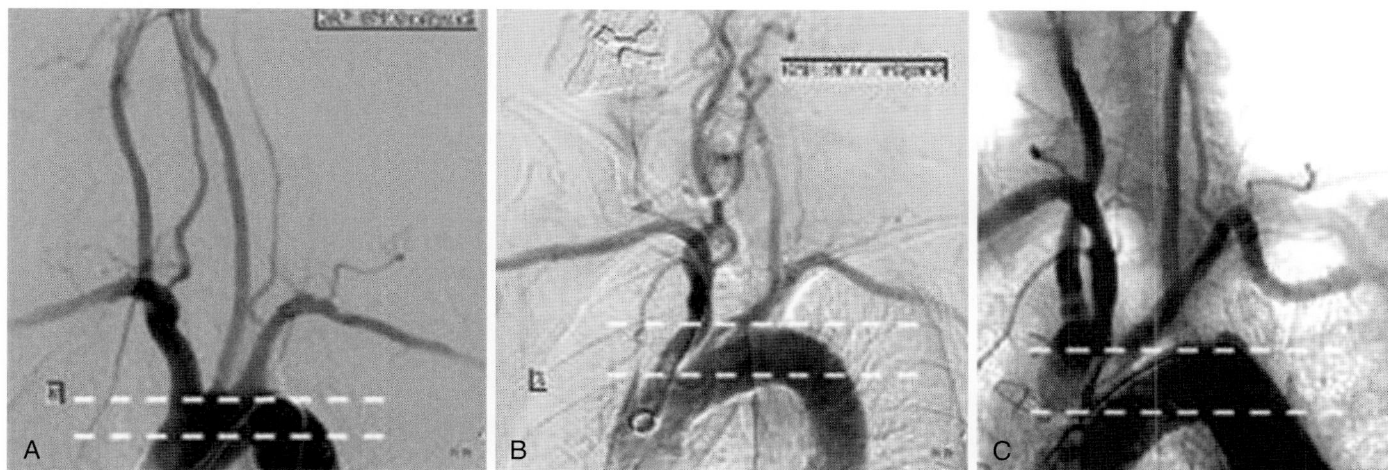

FIGURE 24-10 **A,** Type I aortic arch with great vessels arising from the apex. **B,** Type II aortic arch with moderate proximal displacement of the great vessels. **C,** Type III aortic arch with severe proximal displacement of the great vessels. *(From Liapis CD, Efthimios D, Avgerinos D, Chatziioannou A: The aortic arch: markers, imaging, and procedure planning for carotid intervention. Cath Lab Digest 17:6, 2009.)*

of embolic complication (**Table 24-5**). In fact, some speculate that adverse outcomes in octogenarians are likely due to the difficulty in overcoming the greater incidence of age-related aortic distortion. Therefore, many operators will insist on cross-sectional imaging (CTA or MRA) as part of the preprocedural planning to better assess risk and appropriateness of the CAS option.

When the above listed access challenges occur in isolation but not in the extreme, they have a reasonable chance of being safely overcome by an experienced and skilled operator. However, when they occur in the extreme, or in combination, establishing safe access via femoral or radial access can be impossible or highly risky and should be abandoned in favor of medical therapy, direct carotid access CAS, or CEA, assuming the patient is eligible. Always in the operator's mind should be the preprocedural estimation of stroke risk, which is no longer accurate once the specific

TABLE 24-5 Markers of Aortic Arch Anatomic Features Determining Difficulty with Carotid Access

	FAVORABLE	UNFAVORABLE
Arch elongation	Type I and type II	Type III
Arch vessel	Separate origins of three configurations	Bovine variation arch branches (left carotid access)
Arch calcification	No or a trace of	Luminal irregularity or calcium shadowing diffuse calcification
Arch vessel origin stenosis	<50%	>50%

From Liapis CD, Efthimios D, Avgerinos D, Chatziioannou A: The aortic arch: markers, imaging, and procedure planning for carotid intervention. Cath Lab Digest 17:6, 2009.

anatomic access difficulties are uncovered. This change in procedural risk should cause a reconsideration of the recommendation of CAS in the first place. A determined and unsuccessful, but uncomplicated, attempt at access should not be considered in any way a failure; quite the opposite, it demonstrates good clinical and procedural judgment.

Embolic Protection

Once access is achieved, embolic protection needs to be established. EPD comes in two basic varieties depending on their placement relative to the lesion: distal, with the intent of either blocking (occlusion balloons, which are not used with any frequency any more but were in fact the first available form of EPD) or capturing (filters) any debris that might be liberated during the course of the CAS procedure, or proximal, with the intent of stagnating or reversing carotid flow so that no liberated debris can even achieve cranial travel. There are various styles of filter construction, the qualities of which can be divided into their type of support frame, such as full, partial, and hoop. Their means of actuation since all filters are placed through the lesion in a constrained low-profile (e.g., outer sheath withdrawal, slideable coaxial mechanism), fixed wire versus bare wire, and more detailed features like the number, size, and pattern of pores (which determine flow dynamics), filter membrane materials (e.g., polyethylene terephthalate, ePTFE), tip crossing profiles, etc. (**Figure 24-11**). In difficult anatomy, the bare wire systems Emboshield NAV 6 (Abbott Vascular, Santa Clara, California) and Spider Rx (Covidien, Mansfield, Massachusetts) have the advantage of being able to negotiate tortuous anatomy with a free wire first without having the burden of the filter frame to stiffen the system and lessen the performance of the wire. Since clinical event rates in CAS are low, a randomized head-to-head comparison on outcomes between filters would require several thousand patients to demonstrate a difference and has yet—and will likely never be—performed. Further, any retrospective analyses of filter outcomes are generally not only underpowered but also suffer from potential selection bias.[47]

The most representative comparative data on filters available come from high-quality prospective, high surgical risk, large, all-comer registries where operators did generally not have a choice of EPD. Although stents were also different (more on that later, but suffice to say that there is no measurable effect regarding differential stent outcomes either), there was no difference in outcomes between filters in demographically similar and contemporaneously treated cohorts of several thousand patients.[15] Therefore the choice of filter type will typically be based on operator comfort, anatomic considerations, and experience with one or multiple devices. If the operator volume is relatively low, most will select a workhorse EPD and use it almost exclusively (Video 24-1).

Proximal protection comes in two main varieties: flow cessation (Mo.Ma device, Medtronic, Minneapolis, Minnesota) and flow reversal (Neuro Protection System, WL Gore, Flagstaff, Arizona, and the MICHI System, Silk Road Medical, Sunnyvale, California) (**Figure 24-11**). The Medtronic and

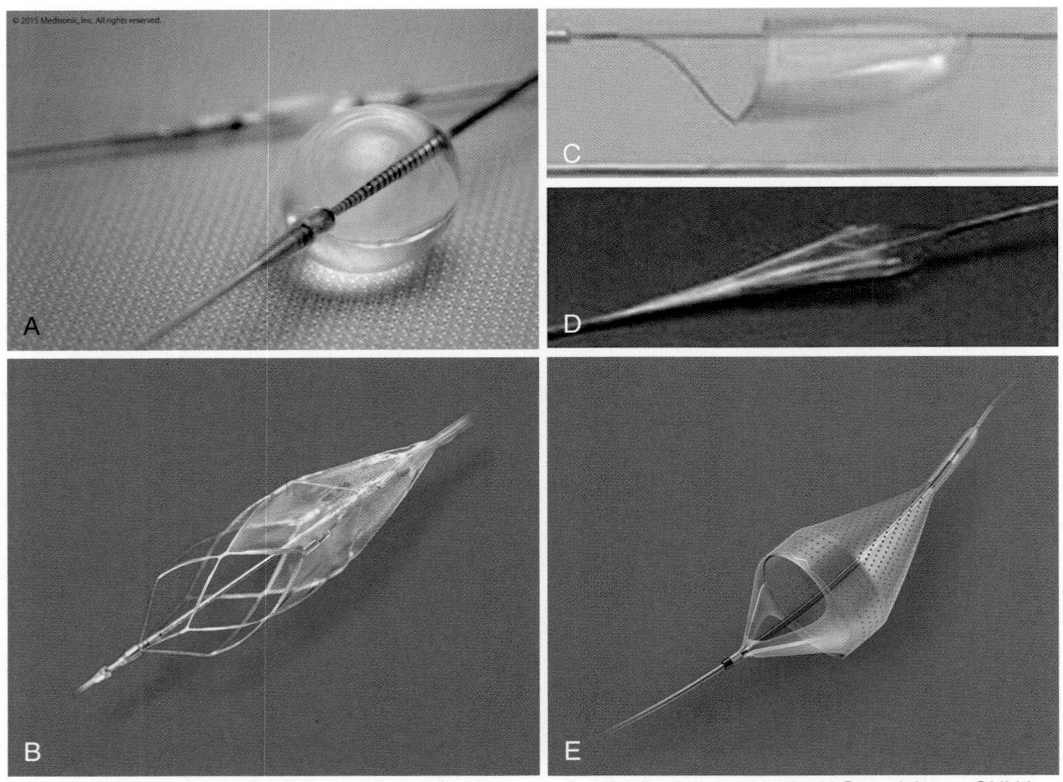

For distribution outside the U.S. and Japan ONLY.
Illustrations are artist renditions.
Not drawn to scale.
Courtesy of Abbott Vascular.

AP2937993-OUS Rev. A

For distribution outside the U.S. and Japan ONLY.
Illustrations are artist renditions.
Not drawn to scale.
Courtesy of Abbott Vascular.

AP2937994-OUS Rev. A

FIGURE 24-11 Various forms of distal embolic protection devices. **A,** GuardWire (Medtronic). **B,** Accunet. *(Courtesy Abbott Vascular. © 2013 Abbott. All rights reserved.)* **C,** FilterWire EZ (Boston Scientific). **D,** Rubicon (Rubicon Medical). **E,** Emboshield. *(Courtesy Abbott Vascular. © 2013 Abbott. All rights reserved.)* *(**C** and **D,** From Dr. Jonathan D. Marmur,* ***www.marmur.com/carotid-artery-stenting.html****).*

Gore devices seek to recapitulate the surgical management of flow during CEA and hence similar embolic protection, by occluding both the ECA and CCA using soft, volume-based, elastomeric balloons placed in each location. This prevents antegrade flow (CCA balloon) and retrograde flow (ECA balloon), both of which result in no flow into the distal circulation. The Gore device creates an arteriovenous shunt to maintain a continuous reversal of flow into the venous circulation (via femoral vein) through a large filter. The Medtronic device maintains flow cessation, and the static column of blood that results, and any material released during the procedure, is then cleared through multiple aspirations at the end of the procedure until the sieved material is clear of debris. Both transfemoral devices appear to result in slightly lower rates of stroke in both their pivotal trials as well as in a meta-analysis,[48-50] although a similarly low rate of complication was seen with a second-generation distal filter device.[51] Supporting the possibility of differential protection, however, are randomized data suggesting lower rates of MR-DWI abnormalities using transfemoral proximal protection.[52] The Silk Road device, as mentioned previously, is surgically placed directly into the CCA so that arch manipulation is unnecessary (**Figure 24-12**). Because it has a high-flow capacity due to specifically engineered side-arm tubing connections and large-bore venous return tubing (it is also meant to be a flow-reversal system), there is no need to occlude the ECA separately. This allows for a smaller sheath size since CCA occlusion is established via a surgical loop, and there is no need to pass an ECA balloon.

Use of proximal protection devices delivered from the femoral access site generally require a 9 Fr sheath, and once balloon occlusion with the device is established there is only a continuous carotid stump pressure reflective of intracerebral hemodynamics but not the usual continuous systemic intraarterial pressure available to monitor intraprocedural carotid body–mediated fluctuations in blood pressure. Some labs preferring not to rely on intermittent cuff pressure for monitoring purposes and will upsize to a 10 Fr femoral access sheath so that systemic pressure can be monitored continuously through a separate transducer. Regardless of 9 Fr or 10 Fr sheath sizing, preprocedural planning of access management and closure is an important component of successful procedure and will involve the usual intersection of closure devices and anticoagulant strategies.

Later in this section we will discuss the predictors and management of neurological and hemodynamic intraprocedural and postprocedural events, some of which are related to flow reversal or even cessation. In addition, the potential clinical differences between distal and proximal strategies in terms of the protection provided the patient will be explored in later sections (Video 24-2).

Stent

Stent selection for CAS has been the topic of some debate and not a little controversy for nearly a decade and pivots on the concept that the stent is, in general, a provocative and not protective component of the procedure. This concept has been supported by imaging that has demonstrated plaque protrusion through stent struts following CAS.[53] Specifically, the openings between stent struts, termed *cells,* reduce the ability of the stent to completely trap the atherosclerotic material behind the metal structure. When discussing cells and carotid stents, definitions and terminology are important. All but one approved carotid stent is laser cut from a slotted tube of nitinol according to a preset pattern. Early, and some current, stent patterns had continuous connectors forming the cells, termed *closed cell.* This makes the stent stiff and nonconforming with the vessel wall, which is fine for reasonably straight vasculature but problematic in the tortuous anatomy, where it could impose significant vasculature kinking. In order to make these stents less rigid and more conformable some of the connectors were removed, which created the "open-cell" stent (**Figure 24-13**). For the one woven carotid stent (Wallstent, Boston Scientific Corporation, Marlborough, Massachusetts), which is made from elgiloy (Co-Cr-Ni alloy), the cells are by definition closed, albeit variable in size. Furthermore, there are two relevant terms used to describe the cells of a stent: free cell area and maximum circular unsupported surface area (MCUSA). The first term refers to the open area outlined by the stent struts, which will always be smaller for closed-cell stents (**Figure 24-13**), and the second can be thought of as referring to the maximum size of a pellet that could fit through a cell (**Figure 24-14**), which in fact does not vary much according to cell type, the two measurements being only loosely related to each other (**Figures 24-15** and **24-16**), and many believe that the latter term is the more relevant measure of emboligenic potential.

Nevertheless, some practitioners have posited that closed-cell stent dimensions offer better trapping function of the stent and lessen the likelihood of an embolic complication causing stroke. Advocates of this view also point to data that appear to demonstrate a significant frequency of postprocedural stroke,[45] most of it in the first 24 hours, minor in severity, and nonhemorrhagic in nature, as support for a continued emboligenic hazard from the stent. To the contrary, transcranial Doppler monitoring of CAS post procedure does not support continued embolization; in fact, no embolic signals are reported.[54] In addition, there are those who believe (this author included) that in fact the "late" strokes that are noted are actually events that occur intraprocedurally but are either not detected or do not manifest until after the procedure. Giving credence to the first theory is the repeated observation that a neurologist will detect subtle strokes that the operators generally miss,[55,56] and this evaluation is typically done the day following the procedure, hence the late detection of the original procedural stroke. The second theory is at least in part supported by the practice of purposely allowing the patient's blood pressure to become elevated by withholding medications on the day of the procedure in order to counter any vigorous hypotensive occurrence during the procedure. Medications are then reinstituted and blood pressure controlled; if a minor event occurs intraprocedurally the permissive hypertension could mask it by increasing collateralization, only to become evident when the collateral flow is reduced as blood pressure normalizes. This phenomenon has been documented to occur and is therefore also a tenable explanation for delayed notification of stroke following CAS.[57]

Moreover, definitive clinical data supporting a differential outcome effect of stent type is lacking. Remembering that to demonstrate any material clinical differences in CAS would require several thousand prospectively randomized patients, all the data—on both sides of the argument—generally fall far short. One of the first reports was from Bosiers et al.[58] who retrospectively analyzed over 3000 patients from four interventional sites in Europe, and found worse outcomes according to free cell area among symptomatic, but not asymptomatic, patients. However, this

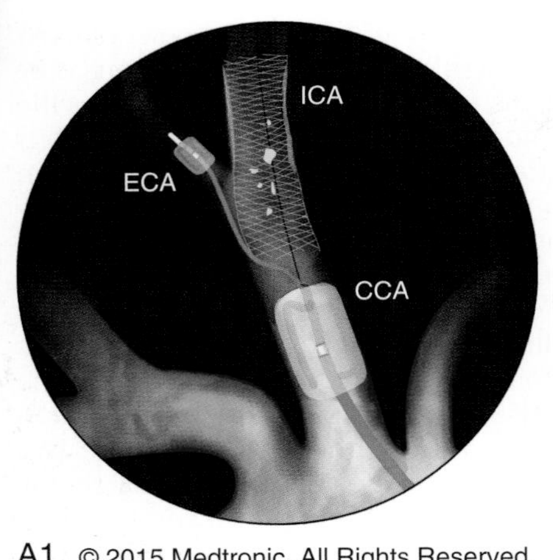

A1

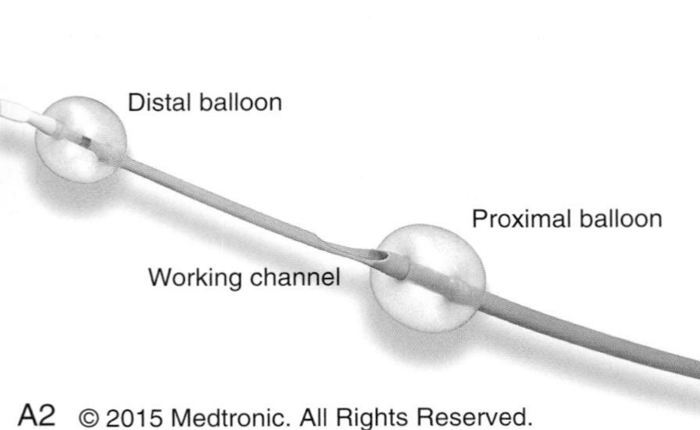

A2

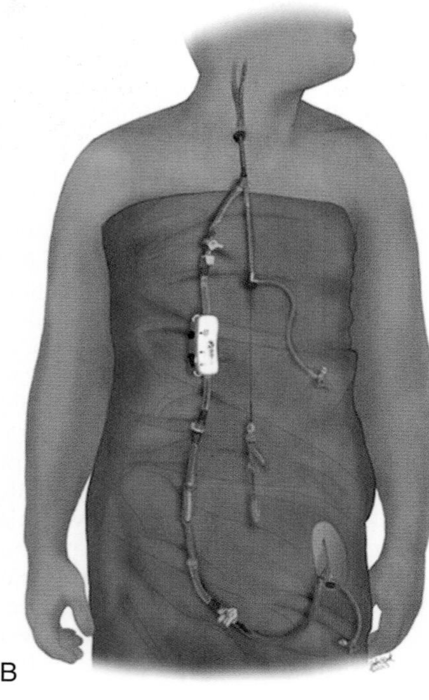

B

FIGURE 24-12 **A,** Medtronic Mo.Ma device. **B,** Silk Road Medical direct carotid access Michi system. *(**A,** © 2015 Medtronic. All Rights Reserved. **B,** From* **www.columbianeurosurgery.org/2013/09/meyers-sees-first-patients-in-roadster-trial.***)*

analysis was not propensity-adjusted, and was therefore subject to significant selection bias. Moreover, the vast majority of closed-cell stents were Wallstents, which comprised >2/3 of the stents used, out of a total of seven stent types. This disproportionate use of one stent type has several implications, including small sample sizes in the remaining stent groups and that no statement regarding class effect related to cell type can legitimately be made. There have been several other retrospective studies, some propensity-adjusted, that have not shown any differences in outcomes by stent type.[59,60] Last, the most voluminous and least biased by selection or ascertainment are the data from the high surgical risk single-arm contemporaneously run prospective postmarket U.S. studies, CAPTURE 2 and EXACT, which demonstrated no outcome differences between the closed-cell Xact and the open-cell Acculink stents.[15]

The observations that even the smallest cell area in current stents are a relatively large 2 mm^2 have led to the development of mesh-covered open-cell stents. In this manner, the flexibility of an open-cell stent can be combined with maximal plaque coverage: the mesh "cell size" is in the 0.25 mm^2 range. Possible trade-offs to this approach include the potential for an increase in stent thrombosis (a rare event with current stents) and/or possible changes in long-term stent patency. A trial in the United States is currently under way to test the WL Gore (Flagstaff, Arizona) version of this stent, and two other manufacturers also have mesh-covered stents in human testing outside the United States.

Other selection decisions related to the stent involve tapered versus straight shapes, without data to differentiate outcomes, and stent length that ranges from 2 to 4 cm. All current stents fit through a 6 Fr sheath, a minority through a 5 Fr sheath. Once selected, the technical aspects of stent implantation are relatively straightforward. The lesion is generally centered within the chosen stent length so as to provide a reasonably disease-free zone 0.5 to 1.0 cm at the proximal and distal margins. This centering function is especially relevant when using the hybrid Cristallo stent (center closed-cell, proximal and distal open-cell—not approved in the United States) so as to place the closed-cell section over the bulk of the lesion. In most cases, except in post-CEA restenosis, the lesion will involve the carotid bifurcation since the flow-eddy there creates the lesion in the first place even if the most severe aspect of the lesion is more distal; therefore every effort should be made to cover the bifurcation with the stent in order to assure that the potential for plaque rupture there is reduced as well. If there is significant tortuosity in the vessel, an open-cell stent will provide for much less vessel kinking after deployment and is typically chosen. Stent localization in an angulated or tortuous vessel is done so as not to accentuate the straightening effect, which can lead to vessel kinking, even by a more flexible open-cell stent, by not placing the edge of the stent at the junction of a straight and turned segment. Finally, there does not appear to be a penalty for stent length in terms of acute thrombosis or long-term patency so longer stents (up to 4 cm) are generally chosen in order to assure lesion coverage and minimize geographic miss.

Balloon Dilation

Balloon dilation during CAS is generally done both before (predilation) and after (postdilation) stent implantation. Predilation balloons are generally undersized (2 to 4 mm) and also longer (3 to 4 cm) than the lesion so as to minimize balloon slippage. Given that the average human mid-distal internal carotid artery (ICA) ranges between 5.0 and 5.5 cm, and the CCA and carotid bulb are always larger, the undersized predilation balloon will only interact with the lesion and not the remaining vessel so no unintended vessel trauma is inflicted. Some operators have employed specialty balloons (e.g., cutting, scoring, etc.) in calcified lesions, but there are no data supporting this practice and the risk of

Example of a “closed cell design stent”: Free cell area is marked black

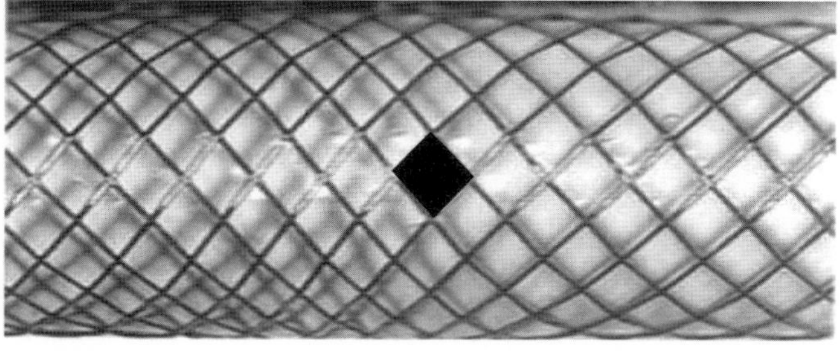

A

Example of an “open cell design stent”: Free cell area is marked black

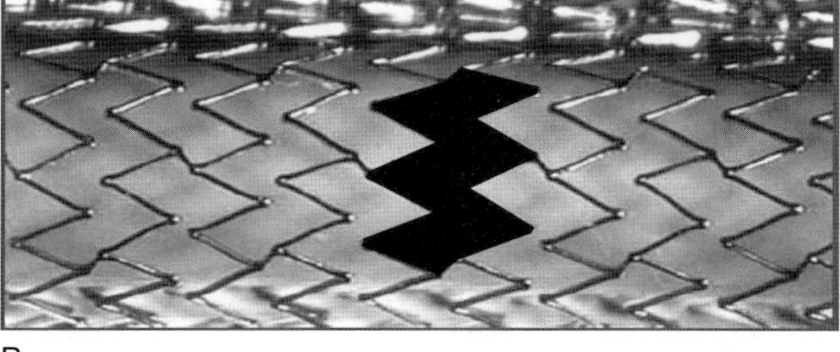

B

FIGURE 24-13 **A,** Closed-cell stent. **B,** Open-cell stents. *(From Schillinger M, Gschwendtner M, Reimers B, et al: Does carotid stent cell design matter? Stroke 39:905–909, 2008.)*

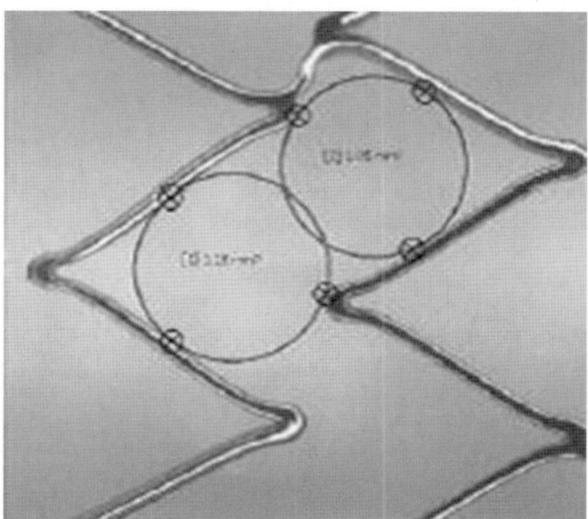

FIGURE 24-14 Illustration of maximal circular unsupported area (MCUSA) or "largest fitted-in circle." *(Reused with permission from Müller-Hülsbeck S, Schäfer PJ, Charalambous N, et al: Comparison of carotid stents: an in-vitro experiment focusing on stent design. J Endovasc Ther 16:168–177, 2009.)*

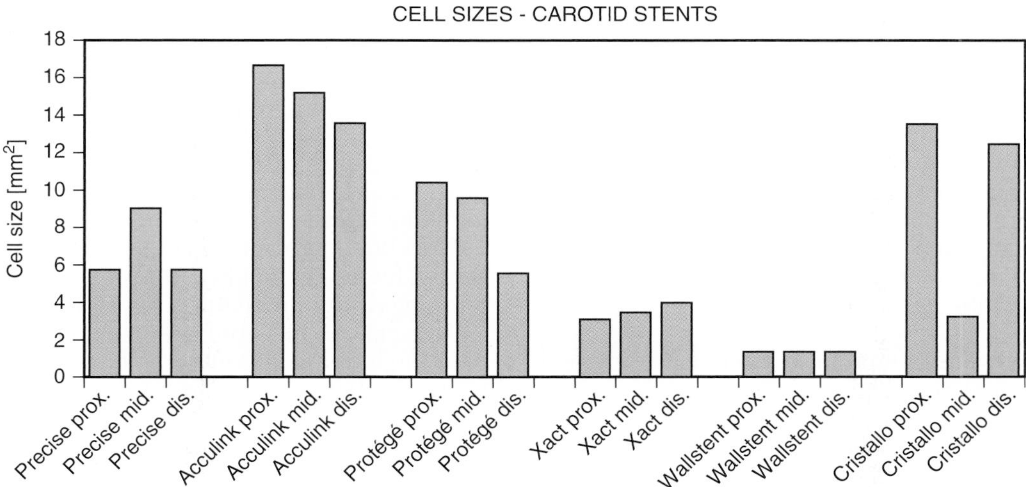

FIGURE 24-15 Relationship between free cell area. The Wallstent and the Xact stent are closed cell, and the Cristallo is a hybrid stent with open cells on the proximal and distal ends. *(Redrawn with permission from Müller-Hülsbeck S, Schäfer PJ, Charalambous N, et al: Comparison of carotid stents: an in-vitro experiment focusing on stent design. J Endovasc Ther 16:168–177, 2009.)*

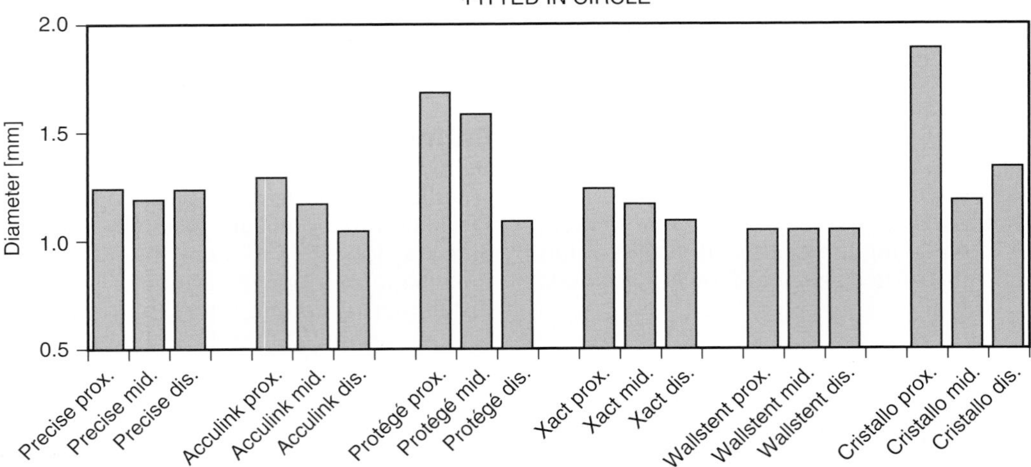

FIGURE 24-16 The characterization of carotid stents by their largest fitted-in circle demonstrating minimal differences among most of them. Note that the Cristallo stent is not approved for use in the United States. *(Redrawn with permission from Müller-Hülsbeck S, Schäfer PJ, Charalambous N, et al: Comparison of carotid stents: an in-vitro experiment focusing on stent design. J Endovasc Ther 16:168–177, 2009.)*

carotid perforation—rare in CAS—may be increased. However, there may be reasonable logic supported by reports of safety and early efficacy to use these specialty balloons to treat in-stent restenosis.[61-63] Postdilation balloons are usually not sized bigger than 5.0 mm in diameter and 2 cm in length since anything larger is unnecessary to achieve stenosis resolution given the aforementioned standard ICA size and can potentially create more emboligenic risk.

There have been modifications to the predilation and postdilation algorithm, each with its own logic, but neither with much data support. Some operators will choose not to predilate the lesion, preferring instead to primarily place the stent and then postdilate. This is considered time saving and so reduces filter dwell, or flow-reversal/cessation, time. Others, including this operator, prefer to fully predilate with a 4.0-mm balloon, then stent, and assess for the need to postdilation. A residual stenosis of less than 30% is generally not postdilated and occurs in roughly half of the cases we perform. The rationales for this approach are the following:

- Predilation is generally not associated with clinical or angiographic complication.
- There are no convincing data that a minor residual stenosis after CAS leads to worse acute or long-term outcomes and that the 4.0-mm balloon is likely to produce an adequate, stand-alone CAS result in resistant lesions.
- Most of the anecdotal reports of the occurrence of intraprocedural stroke are during the postdilation phase.
- Transcranial microembolic signal (MES) confirmation that postdilation is the most emboligenic part of the CAS procedure (apart from the stent placement, which is likely related to microbubbles trapped in the stent sheath and released while retracting the sheath during stent deployment).[64]
- When hemodynamic compromise occurs in CAS, it is usually the result of postdilation.

There may be other reasons to perform postdilation beyond reducing residual stenosis, including difficulty in passing the retrieval catheter for the filter, which can be due to stent struts in an open-cell stent that have not "laid-down" or a leading edge of any stent that needs to be better opposed to the vessel wall. Of course, hemodynamic perturbations already extant after stent placement will also modify any postdilation strategy.

Hemodynamic Management

CAS can produce both bradycardia and hypotension via stimulation of the carotid sinus by balloon dilation, stent implantation, or both. The bradycardia is a usually short-lived, vagal-mediated, parasympathetic response that typically resolves with balloon depressurization/deflation; it can typically be managed with atropine, and long-term increase in permanent pacemaker placement is not reported. The placement of a prophylactic temporary pacemaker is occasionally warranted in patients with critical aortic stenosis or severe cardiomyopathy with residual nonrevascularized ischemic coronary lesions, since in neither patient is loss of coronary circulation tolerated and may be irrecoverable.

Alternatively, hypotension is mediated through a sympathetic medullary pathway that can result in profound venodilation that, with or without accompanying bradycardia, can cause a significant and dramatic drop in blood pressure. Depending on the definition used, the incidence of significant hypotension is usually defined as the need for prolonged pressor support ranging from 14% to 51%.[65-70] Although previously thought to be a benign procedural occurrence if managed promptly, newer data suggest that it may be associated with an increased number of new lesions on MR-DWI.[71] Patients with bulky, calcified lesions involving the carotid bulb are thought to be at most risk of developing procedural hypotension[72] and this may in fact be a confounding feature as regards the finding of MR-DWI lesions.

Procedural hypotension is best managed before it starts by withholding antihypertensive medications on the morning of the procedure. This, along with patient anxiety, will typically result in preprocedural blood pressures greater than 160 mm, and it is important to resist treating the hypertension acutely, as precipitous falls in systolic blood pressure of up to 80 to 100 mm can occur within seconds of dilation or stent placement. Another preventative strategy is to make certain that the patient is not dehydrated (given the venodilatory mechanism described previously), which can often be the case as patients will have been nothing by mouth (NPO) for several hours/overnight prior to CAS. In most cases, the patient will tolerate at least a 250- to 500-cc intravenous bolus preprocedure, and it is our custom to do so.

Once the patient becomes hypotensive, preparation and rapid action are key. Nursing staff should be in-serviced as to all potential consequences of CAS, medication should be drawn and ready for administration, and a well-functioning intravenous ensured. A check of nursing preparedness prior to postdilation balloon inflation is always a good idea. Atropine and neosynephrine injectables are typical acute treatment choices, and dopamine drip (which can address both bradycardia and hypotension) should be mixed and ready as needed. Rapid administration of normal saline or lactated Ringer's is an important component of treatment as well. The procedural hypotension should be able to be recovered within 1 to 2 minutes, at least temporarily (prolonged pressor drips are occasionally required) and the operator will need to consider whether any further procedural steps are required to complete the CAS and wrap up in an expeditious fashion. Other causes of hypotension (e.g., access site hemorrhage) should always be kept in mind as well. The hypotension related to CAS can be considered an acquired autonomic dysfunction, and for this reason many operators will prefer to use a closure device for the access site whenever possible and will push for early ambulation—even if pressor support is present/required—as prolonged bedrest can extend the time of the hypotensive period.

As problematic as procedural bradycardia and hypotension can be, the persistence of hypertension after carotid revascularization can be equally important and needs to be managed appropriately and aggressively. Hypertension may persist for a variety of reasons, including prior CEA, which denervates the carotid body and largely obviates any response, primary lesion location away from the bulb, variability in lesion responsiveness, etc. Regardless, the hypertension should be quickly brought under control as it is believed to be a contributor to cerebral hemorrhage, especially in isolated vascular territories (i.e., poorly collateralized) and/or recently or repetitively symptomatic patients. In addition to re-instituting the preprocedural antihypertensive medication regimen, many labs will temporize using intravenous beta-blockers as heart rate allows and intravenous nitroglycerin (NTG) for immediate hypertension control. However, longer term administration of NTG can be problematic owing not only to rapid tachyphylaxis but also the side effect of headache, which can be confusing as intracranial hemorrhage is a concern in this at-risk population and may be difficult to distinguish. Some operators will prefer an intravenous calcium channel blocker (e.g., nicardipine) as first-line management of blood pressure, which provides predictable control but is not associated with confounding symptomatic side effects.

Neurological Management

This section is dedicated to the management of neurological changes when they occur as part of the procedure. The patient undergoing CAS can have neurological symptoms for a variety of reasons, and rapid diagnosis can be important in the correct management. The majority of neurological symptoms will be related to a proximal or embolic slowing or interruption of flow causing hypoperfusion and cerebral ischemia. Before addressing the management of these more common presentations, it is worth noting that patients, although quite infrequently, will have a partial or generalized seizure when even a short predilation balloon inflation interrupts blood flow, with focal symptoms persisting after flow restoration due to a Todd's paralysis, giving the impression of possible embolic complication.

When employing proximal protection of any variety, antegrade flow is purposefully interrupted or reversed. Mean stump pressure readings above 40 mm Hg will usually be sufficient to maintain cerebral perfusion. However, symptoms of intolerance may be seen at pressures lower than 30 to 40 mm Hg. Subtle symptoms include slowness to respond to commands or questions, yawning, agitation, or lowered level of consciousness. More overt symptoms may include focal neurological signs, generalized seizures, or loss of consciousness. A high index of suspicion can allow the operator to reduce or eliminate symptoms of intolerance. If systemic blood pressure is raised then cerebral collateral perfusion can be further recruited/enabled and should be one of the first maneuvers attempted in low-grade intolerance. If this maneuver is not successful in mitigating symptoms or if they worsen, then releasing the proximal CCA balloon occlusion and restoring flow are indicated but only after the column of blood (in the case of flow cessation) is cleared. It is possible in some patients to precondition the cerebral circulation with intermittent occlusion such that successively longer interruptions in flow can be tolerated. In most cases the procedure can be completed in less than 5 minutes with good preparation, so usually intolerance is not an issue to CAS except in the most extreme cases. In cases of absolute intolerance, a filter EPD can be deployed through the proximal protection sheath system and the protected procedure completed this way. A corollary cause of neurological symptoms can occur when a no-flow situation arises due to a filter that has become occluded with debris, fibrin, or both. In these cases, it is especially important to suction and clear the static column of blood below the filter because it almost certainly contains meaningful and harmful debris.

Although there are no randomized studies to prove the efficacy of EPD in preventing stroke, both anecdotal experience and meta-analyses suggest that they are indeed protective, almost certainly for major embolic complications, with very little downside risk[73-75] (**Figure 24-17**). These observations are counterposed with nonclinical imaging data suggesting that there are greater numbers of asymptomatic MR-DWI abnormalities with the use of filters—possibly

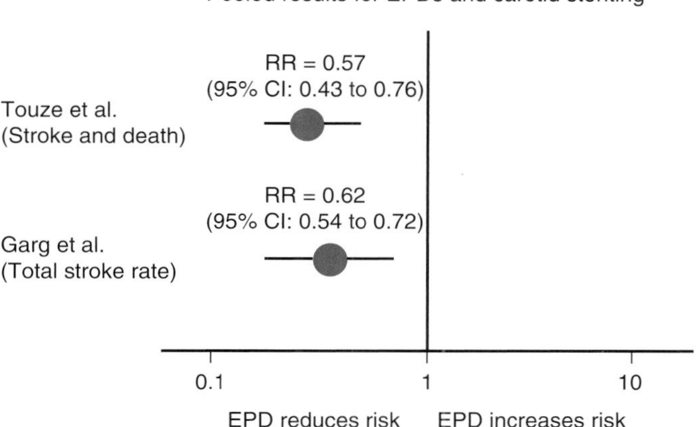

FIGURE 24-17 Results of summary data from meta-analyses of the clinical utility of EPD use in CAS. *CAS,* Carotid artery stenting; *EPD,* emboli protection devices. *(Redrawn with permission from White CJ: Carotid artery stenting. J Am Coll Card 64:722–731, 2014.)*

related to the embolization of microbubbles released when the sheath is withdrawn to deploy the filter.[76] Nevertheless, embolic complications can still occur when loss of filtration occurs due to lack of wall opposition (e.g., when a filter is positioned on a vessel bend point, etc.) or after the filter is removed as discussed previously. Intraprocedural embolic complications can manifest immediately as a focal sign or may be masked by the permissive hypertension associated with CAS as mentioned previously. However, should immediate symptoms arise and be confirmed by angiography to be due to embolism, a relatively straightforward decision tree can be followed. Armed with the knowledge that most minor strokes, defined as a change in the NIHSS of less than four, will resolve within 30 days with little or no disability, then the site of embolic occlusion can be managed appropriately.[12,22] A proximal intracranial vessel occlusion will generally produce major stroke symptoms and requires immediate neurointerventional management and extraction of the offending material. However, more distal occlusions (M3 or M4) will more likely (but not always) be associated with lesser symptomatology that is also likely to largely resolve, and since their retrieval can be problematic and potentially risky, the decision to attempt intracranial manipulations is generally tempered. The role of pharmacological treatment with intraarterial/systemic thrombolytics or GPIIb/IIIa platelet inhibitors has not been defined in distal embolization following CAS associated with a neurological syndrome.

Pharmacology

Although there are no data to drive pre- and postprocedural pharmacology, the accepted standard is to initiate dual-antiplatelet therapy with clopidogrel and aspirin at least 3 days ahead of the procedure or to give a loading dose of clopidogrel several hours ahead of the procedure. Dual therapy is continued for 30 days, although shorter durations (~2 weeks) have been employed in cases where the need for early cardiac surgery was present. The carotid artery is a high-flow vessel supplying a low-resistance cerebral circulation, and the medium-diameter stents used for CAS rarely thrombose; when they do it generally occurs acutely at the time of implant and is thought to be related to the biology of the plaque (i.e., intraplaque contents) although the adequacy of pharmacology has also been suggested.[77,78] Intraprocedural anticoagulation is also not driven by data but more by convention, with recommended activated clotting times of >250 to 300 seconds, with the most susceptible component of the procedure to inadequate anticoagulation is likely the filter. Anticoagulation can be achieved using either heparin or bivalirudin; there is an ongoing blinded multicenter study randomizing endovascular procedures between the two drugs that will assess outcomes in a reasonably sized cohort of CAS patients. Prior, smaller, single-center, and nonrandomized data support that the use of bivalirudin appears to be at least as safe as heparin.[79]

CONCLUSIONS

CAS is a relatively young interventional field, having been practiced with dedicated approved equipment for approximately a decade, although under a restricted U.S. coverage environment. Nevertheless, a great deal of improvement in outcomes has been documented, most likely related to the accumulated knowledge regarding technique and patient selection. Future directions will include efforts to reduce nonclinical but likely meaningful surrogates such as MR-DWI with improvements in stent construction, access techniques and sites, and EPD strategies. These improvements will almost certainly accrue to the benefit of our patients.

References

1. Bockenheimer SA, Mathias K: Percutaneous transluminal angioplasty in arteriosclerotic internal carotid artery stenosis. *AJNR Am J Neuroradiol* 4(3):791–792, 1983.
2. Endovascular versus surgical treatment in patients with carotid stenosis in the Carotid and Vertebral Artery Transluminal Angioplasty Study (CAVATAS): a randomised trial. *Lancet* 357(9270):1729–1737, 2001.
3. North American Symptomatic Carotid Endarterectomy Trial Collaborators: Beneficial effect of carotid endarterectomy in symptomatic patients with high-grade carotid stenosis. *N Engl J Med* 325:445–453, 1991.
4. Mas JL, Chatellier G, Beyssen B, et al: EVA-3S Investigators. Endarterectomy versus stenting in patients with symptomatic severe carotid stenosis. *N Engl J Med* 355(16):1660–1671, 2006.
5. SPACE Collaborative Group, Ringleb PA, Allenberg J, et al: 30 day results from the SPACE trial of stent-protected angioplasty versus carotid endarterectomy in symptomatic patients: a randomised non-inferiority trial. *Lancet* 368(9543):1239–1247, 2006.
6. International Carotid Stenting Study investigators, Ederle J, Dobson J, et al: Carotid artery stenting compared with endarterectomy in patients with symptomatic carotid stenosis (International Carotid Stenting Study): an interim analysis of a randomised controlled trial. *Lancet* 375(9719):985–997, 2010.
7. Stilp E, Baird C, Gray WA, et al: An evidence-based review of the impact of periprocedural myocardial infarction in carotid revascularization. *Catheter Cardiovasc Interv* 82(5):709–714, 2013.
8. Diethrich EB, Ndiaye M, Reid DB: Stenting in the carotid artery: initial experience in 110 patients. *J Endovasc Surg* 3(1):42–62, 1996.
9. Yadav JS, Roubin GS, Iyer S, et al: Elective stenting of the extracranial carotid arteries. *Circulation* 95(2):376–381, 1997.
10. Alberts MJ: Results of a multicenter prospective randomized trial of carotid artery stenting vs carotid endarterectomy. *Stroke* 32:325, 2001.
11. Yadav JS, Wholey MH, Kuntz RE, et al, Stenting and Angioplasty with Protection in Patients at High Risk for Endarterectomy Investigators: Protected carotid-artery stenting versus endarterectomy in high-risk patients. *N Engl J Med* 351(15):1493–1501, 2004.
12. Gray WA, Hopkins LN, Yadav S, et al: Protected carotid stenting in high surgical-risk patients: the ARCHeR results. *J Vasc Surg* 44(2):258–268, 2006.
13. Gray WA, Yadav JS, Verta P, et al: The CAPTURE registry: results of carotid stenting with embolic protection in the post approval setting. *Catheter Cardiovasc Interv* 69(3):341–348, 2007.
14. Gray WA, Rosenfield KA, Jaff MR, et al: Influence of site and operator characteristics on carotid artery stent outcomes: analysis of the CAPTURE 2 (Carotid ACCULINK/ACCUNET Post Approval Trial to Uncover Rare Events) clinical study. *JACC Cardiovasc Interv* 4(2):235–246, 2011.
15. Gray WA, Chaturvedi S, Verta P, et al: Thirty-day outcomes for carotid artery stenting in 6320 patients from 2 prospective, multicenter, high surgical-risk registries. *Circ Cardiovasc Interv* 2(3):159–166, 2009.
16. Massop D, Dave R, Metzger C, et al: Stenting and angioplasty with protection in patients at high-risk for endarterectomy: SAPPHIRE Worldwide Registry first 2,001 patients. *Catheter Cardiovasc Interv* 73(2):129–136, 2009.
17. Shishehbor MH, Venkatachalam S, Gray WA, et al: Experience and outcomes with carotid artery stenting: an analysis of the CHOICE (carotid stenting for high surgical-risk patients; evaluating outcomes through the collection of clinical evidence) study. *JACC Cardiovasc Interv* 7(11):1307–1317, 2014. pii S1936-8798.
18. Brott TG, Hobson RW, 2nd, Howard G, et al: CREST Investigators Stenting versus endarterectomy for treatment of carotid-artery stenosis. *N Engl J Med* 363(1):11–23, 2010.
19. Hobson RW, 2nd, Howard VJ, Roubin GS, et al: Credentialing of surgeons as interventionalists for carotid artery stenting: experience from the lead-in phase of CREST. *J Vasc Surg* 40(5):952–957, 2004.
20. Eckstein HH, Ringleb P, Allenberg JR, et al: Results of the Stent-Protected Angioplasty versus Carotid Endarterectomy (SPACE) study to treat symptomatic stenoses at 2 years: a multinational, prospective, randomised trial. *Lancet Neurol* 7(10):893–902, 2008.
21. Mas JL, Trinquart L, Leys D, et al: Endarterectomy Versus Angioplasty in Patients with Symptomatic Severe Carotid Stenosis (EVA-3S) trial: results up to 4 years from a randomised, multicentre trial. *Lancet Neurol* 7(10):885–892, 2008.
22. Gray WA, Simonton CA, Verta P: Overview of the 2011 Food and Drug Administration circulatory system devices panel meeting on the ACCULINK and ACCUNET carotid artery stent system. *Circulation* 125(18):2256–2264, 2012.
23. Gensicke H, Zumbrunn T, Jongen LM, ICSS-MRI Substudy Investigators: Characteristics of ischemic brain lesions after stenting or endarterectomy for symptomatic carotid artery stenosis: results from the International Carotid Stenting Study-magnetic resonance imaging substudy. *Stroke* 44(1):80–86, 2013.
24. Chen CI, Iguchi Y, Garami Z, et al: Analysis of emboli during carotid stenting with distal protection device. *Cerebrovasc Dis* 21(4):223–228, 2006.
25. Rostamzadeh A1, Zumbrunn T, Jongen LM, et al: Predictors of acute and persisting ischemic brain lesions in patients randomized to carotid stenting or endarterectomy; ICSS-MRI Substudy Investigators. *Stroke* 45(2):591–594, 2014.
26. Gaudet JG, Meyers PM, McKinsey JF, et al: Incidence of moderate to severe cognitive dysfunction in patients treated with carotid artery stenting. *Neurosurgery* 65(2):325–329, 2009.
27. Plessers M, Van Herzeele I, Vermassen F, et al: Neurocognitive functioning after carotid revascularization: a systematic review. *Cerebrovasc Dis Extra* 4(2):132–148, 2014.
28. Eastcott H: Reconstruction of internal carotid artery in a patient with intermittent attacks of hemiplegia. *Lancet* 264:994–996, 1954.
29. Executive Committee for the Asymptomatic Carotid Atherosclerosis Study: Endarterectomy for asymptomatic carotid artery stenosis. *JAMA* 273:1421–1428, 1995.
30. Halliday A, Mansfield A, Marro J, et al: Prevention of disabling and fatal strokes by successful carotid endarterectomy in patients without recent neurological symptoms: randomised controlled trial. *Lancet* 363(9420):1491–1502, 2004.
31. Halliday A, Harrison M, Hayter E, et al: 10-year stroke prevention after successful carotid endarterectomy for asymptomatic stenosis (ACST-1): a multicentre randomised trial. *Lancet* 376(9746):1074–1084, 2010.
32. Henderson RD, Eliasziw M, Fox AJ, et al: Angiographically defined collateral circulation and risk of stroke in patients with severe carotid artery stenosis. *Stroke* 31(1):128–132, 2000.
33. Ku DN, Giddens DP, Zarins CK, et al: Pulsatile flow and atherosclerosis in the human carotid bifurcation. Positive correlation between plaque location and low oscillating shear stress. *Arteriosclerosis* 5:293–302, 1985.

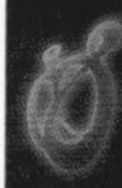

34. Ouriel K, Green RM: Clinical and technical factors influencing recurrent carotid stenosis and occlusion after endarterectomy. *J Vasc Surg* 5(5):702–706, 1987.
35. Brott TG, Halperin JL, Abbara S, et al: 2011 ASA/ACCF/AHA/AANN/AANS/ACR/ASNR/CNS/SAIP/SCAI/SIR/SNIS/SVM/SVS guideline on the management of patients with extracranial carotid and vertebral artery disease: executive summary: a report of the American College of Cardiology Foundation/American Heart Association Task Force on Practice Guidelines, and the American Stroke Association, American Association of Neuroscience Nurses, American Association of Neurological Surgeons, American College of Radiology, American Society of Neuroradiology, Congress of Neurological Surgeons, Society of Atherosclerosis Imaging and Prevention, Society for Cardiovascular Angiography and Interventions, Society of Interventional Radiology, Society of NeuroInterventional Surgery, Society for Vascular Medicine, and Society for Vascular Surgery Developed in Collaboration With the American Academy of Neurology and Society of Cardiovascular Computed Tomography. *J Am Coll Cardiol* 57:1002–1044, 2011.
36. Rothwell PM, Eliasziw M, Gutnikov SA, et al, Carotid Endarterectomy Trialists Collaboration: Effect of endarterectomy for symptomatic carotid stenosis in relation to clinical subgroups and to the timing of surgery. *Lancet* 363:915–924, 2004.
37. Barnett HJM, Taylor DW, Eliasziw M, et al: Benefit of carotid endarterectomy in symptomatic patients with moderate and severe stenosis. North American Symptomatic Carotid Endarterectomy Trial Collaborators. *N Engl J Med* 339:1415–1425, 1998.
38. Matsumura JS, Gray W, Chaturvedi S, et al: Results of carotid artery stenting with distal embolic protection with improved systems: protected carotid artery stenting in patients at high risk for carotid endarterectomy (PROTECT) trial. *J Vasc Surg* 55(4):968–976, 2012.
39. Abbott AL: Medical (nonsurgical) intervention alone is now best for prevention of stroke associated with asymptomatic severe carotid stenosis: results of a systematic review and analysis. *Stroke* 40(10):e573–e583, 2009.
40. Marquardt L, Geraghty OC, Mehta Z, et al: Low risk of ipsilateral stroke in patients with asymptomatic carotid stenosis on best medical treatment. *Stroke* 41, 2010.
41. European Carotid Surgery Trialists' Collaborative Group: Randomised trial of endarterectomy for recently symptomatic carotid stenosis: final results of the MRC European Carotid Surgery Trial (ECST). *Lancet* 351:1379–1387, 1998.
42. Moneta GL, Edwards JM, Chitwood RW, et al: Correlation of North American Symptomatic Carotid Endarterectomy Trial (NASCET) angiographic definition of 70% to 99% internal carotid artery stenosis with duplex scanning. *J Vasc Surg* 17(1):152–157, 1993.
43. Gray WA, Yadav JS, Verta P, et al: The CAPTURE registry: predictors of outcomes in carotid artery stenting with embolic protection for high surgical risk patients in the early post-approval setting. *Catheter Cardiovasc Interv* 70(7):1025–1033, 2007.
44. Etxegoien N, Rhyne D, Kedev S, et al: The transradial approach for carotid artery stenting. *Catheter Cardiovasc Interv* 80(7):1081–1087, 2012.
45. Fairman R, Gray WA, Scicli AP, et al: The CAPTURE registry: analysis of strokes resulting from carotid artery stenting in the post approval setting: timing, location, severity, and type. *Ann Surg* 246(4):551–556, 2007.
46. Leal I, Orgaz A, Flores Á, et al: A diffusion-weighted magnetic resonance imaging-based study of transcervical carotid stenting with flow reversal versus transfemoral filter protection. *J Vasc Surg* 56(6):1585–1590, 2012.
47. Loghmanpour NA, Siewiorek GM, Wanamaker KM, et al: Assessing the impact of distal protection filter design characteristics on 30-day outcomes of carotid artery stenting procedures. *J Vasc Surg* 57(2):309–317, 2013.
48. Clair DG, Hopkins LN, Mehta M, et al: Neuroprotection during carotid artery stenting using the GORE flow reversal system: 30-day outcomes in the EMPiRE Clinical Study. *Catheter Cardiovasc Interv* 77(3):420–429, 2011.
49. Ansel GM, Hopkins LN, Jaff MR, et al: Safety and effectiveness of the INVATEC MO.MA proximal cerebral protection device during carotid artery stenting: results from the ARMOUR pivotal trial. *Catheter Cardiovasc Interv* 76(1):1–8, 2010.
50. Bersin RM, Stabile E, Ansel GM, et al: A meta-analysis of proximal occlusion device outcomes in carotid artery stenting. *Catheter Cardiovasc Interv* 80(7):1072–1078, 2012.
51. Matsumura JS, Gray W, Chaturvedi S, et al: Results of carotid artery stenting with distal embolic protection with improved systems: protected carotid artery stenting in patients at high risk for carotid endarterectomy (PROTECT) trial. *J Vasc Surg* 55(4):968–976, 2012.
52. Montorsi P, Caputi L, Galli S, et al: Microembolization during carotid artery stenting in patients with high-risk, lipid-rich plaque. A randomized trial of proximal versus distal cerebral protection. *J Am Coll Cardiol* 58(16):1656–1663, 2011.
53. de Donato G, Setacci F, Sirignano P, et al: Optical coherence tomography after carotid stenting: rate of stent malapposition, plaque prolapse and fibrous cap rupture according to stent design. *Eur J Vasc Endovasc Surg* 45(6):579–587, 2013.
54. Censori B, Camerlingo M, Casto L, et al: Carotid stents are not a source of microemboli late after deployment. *Acta Neurol Scand* 102(1):27–30, 2000.
55. Rothwell PM, Slattery J, Warlow CP: A systematic review of the risks of stroke and death due to endarterectomy for symptomatic carotid stenosis. *Stroke* 27(2):260–265, 1996.
56. Chaturvedi S, Aggarwal R, Murugappan A: Results of carotid endarterectomy with prospective neurologist follow-up. *Neurology* 55(6):769–772, 2000.
57. Tan KT, Cleveland TJ, Berczi V, et al: Timing and frequency of complications after carotid artery stenting: what is the optimal period of observation? *J Vasc Surg* 38(2):236–243, 2003.
58. Bosiers M, de Donato G, Deloose K, et al: Does free cell area influence the outcome in carotid artery stenting? *Eur J Vasc Endovasc Surg* 33(2):135–141, 2007.
59. Schillinger M1, Gschwendtner M, Reimers B, et al: Does carotid stent cell design matter? *Stroke* 39(3):905–909, 2008.
60. Grunwald IQ, Reith W, Karp K, et al: Comparison of stent free cell area and cerebral lesions after unprotected carotid artery stent placement. *Eur J Vasc Endovasc Surg* 43(1):10–14, 2012.
61. Bendok BR, Roubin GS, Katzen BT, et al: Cutting balloon to treat carotid in-stent stenosis: technical note. *J Invasive Cardiol* 15:227–232, 2003.
62. Tamberella MR, Yadav JS, Bajzer CT, et al: Cutting balloon angioplasty to treat carotid in-stent stenosis. *J Invasive Cardiol* 16:133–135, 2004.
63. Shah QA, Georgiadis AL, Suri MF, et al: Cutting balloon angioplasty for carotid in-stent restenosis: case reports and review of the literature. *J Neuroimaging* 18:428–432, 2008.
64. Antonius Carotid Endarterectomy, Angioplasty and Stenting Study Group: Transcranial Doppler monitoring in angioplasty and stenting of the carotid bifurcation. *J Endovasc Ther* 10(4):702–710, 2003.
65. Dangas G, Laird JR, Jr, Satler LF, et al: Postprocedural hypotension after carotid artery stent placement: predictors and short- and long-term clinical outcomes. *Radiology* 215:677–683, 2000.
66. Gupta R, Abou-Chebl A, Bajzer CT, et al: Rate, predictors, and consequences of depression after carotid artery stenting. *J Am Coll Cardiol* 47:1538–1543, 2006.
67. Park BD, Divinagracia T, Madej O, et al: Predictors of clinically significant postprocedural hypotension after carotid endarterectomy and carotid angioplasty with stenting. *J Vasc Surg* 50:526–533, 2009.
68. Qureshi AI, Luft AR, Sharma M, et al: Frequency and determinants of postprocedural hemodynamic instability after carotid angioplasty and stenting. *Stroke* 30:2086–2093, 1999.
69. Lavoie P, Rutledge J, Dawoud MA, et al: Predictors and timing of hypotension and bradycardia after carotid artery stenting. *AJNR Am J Neuroradiol* 29:1942–1947, 2008.
70. Altinbas A1, Algra A, Bonati LH, et al, ICSS Investigators: Periprocedural hemodynamic depression is associated with a higher number of new ischemic brain lesions after stenting in the International Carotid Stenting Study-MRI Substudy. *Stroke* 45(1):146–151, 2014.
71. Matsukawa H, Fujii M, Uemura A, et al: Pathology of embolic debris in carotid artery stenting. *Acta Neurol Scand* doi: 10.1111/ane.12303, 2014. [Epub ahead of print].
72. Gupta R, Abou-Chebl A, Bajzer CT, et al: Rate, predictors, and consequences of hemodynamic depression after carotid artery stenting. *J Am Coll Cardiol* 47(8):1538–1543, 2006.
73. Macdonald S: The evidence for cerebral protection: an analysis and summary of the literature. *Eur J Radiol* 60(1):20–25, 2006.
74. Garg N, Karagiorgos N, Pisimisis GT, et al: Cerebral protection devices reduce periprocedural strokes during carotid angioplasty and stenting: a systematic review of the current literature. *J Endovasc Ther* 16:412–427, 2009.
75. Touze E, Trinquart L, Chatellier G, et al: Systematic review of the perioperative risks of stroke or death after carotid angioplasty and stenting. *Stroke* 40:e683–e693, 2009.
76. Macdonald S, Evans DH, Griffiths PD, et al: Filter-protected versus unprotected carotid artery stenting: a randomised trial. *Cerebrovasc Dis* 29(3):282–289, 2010.
77. Xiromeritis K1, Dalainas I, Stamatakos M, et al: Acute carotid stent thrombosis after carotid artery stenting. *Eur Rev Med Pharmacol Sci* 16(3):355–362, 2012.
78. Köklü E, Arslan S, Yüksel IO, et al: Acute carotid artery stent thrombosis due to dual antiplatelet resistance. *Cardiovasc Intervent Radiol* 2014. [Epub ahead of print].
79. Schneider LM, Polena S, Roubin G, et al: Carotid stenting and bivalirudin with and without vascular closure: 3-year analysis of procedural outcomes. *Catheter Cardiovasc Interv* 75(3):420–426, 2010.

Intracranial Intervention and Acute Stroke

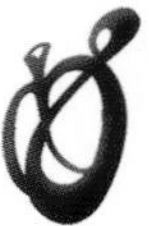

Alex Abou-Chebl

INTRODUCTION

The management of cerebrovascular disease has often lagged behind the advances made in the management of cardiovascular disease. However those same technological advances in cardiovascular devices have facilitated the development of dedicated neurovascular devices, which have resulted in a narrowing of the treatment gap. Still there remain major differences primarily due to anatomical and physiological differences between the coronary and cerebral vasculatures.

CEREBROVASCULAR DISEASE

Epidemiology

There are approximately 800,000 strokes each year in the United States.[1,2] Of these, more than 83% to 85% are ischemic strokes; the remaining 15% to 17% of strokes are hemorrhagic.[1,2] Of the former, 70% are large cerebral vessel occlusions and the remainder are so-called small vessel strokes (i.e., lacunar strokes).[3] Spontaneous intracerebral hemorrhage (ICH), otherwise known as parenchymal hemorrhage, accounts for roughly two thirds of hemorrhagic strokes while spontaneous (nontraumatic) subarachnoid hemorrhage (SAH) accounts for the remainder and is caused by ruptured cerebral aneurysms.[1,2] Stroke mortality has been declining due to advances in medical treatment and prevention and stroke currently ranks as the fourth leading cause of death in the United States, although it remains as the second leading cause worldwide.[2] However, stroke remains the leading cause of adult disability in the United States.[4]

What makes stroke unique, as compared with coronary artery disease (CAD) for example, is that it can be caused by a multitude of different pathological processes. Unlike acute myocardial infarction, which is overwhelmingly caused by ruptured coronary artery atherosclerotic plaques, stroke can be ischemic or hemorrhagic. Ischemic stroke can be caused by cardiac embolism (20%), cervical-cranial large vessel atherosclerosis (20%), lipohyalinosis-associated lacunar stroke (25%-30%), unknown causes (25%-30%), or a variety of rare causes (5%) (e.g., arterial dissection, vasculitis, migraine, hypercoagulable states, mitochondrial encephalopathies, etc.).[5,6] Coronary disease and stroke share similar risk factors but hypertension stands out as the major risk factor.[2,7] Hypertension is the major cause of parenchymal (nonaneurysmal) ICH as well as lacunar strokes. Populations at increased risk for ischemic stroke include African-Americans, patients with diabetes mellitus, men, and the elderly.[7,8]

Clinical Manifestations

The clinical manifestations of stroke are highly varied and can range from asymptomatic to catastrophic. The exact manifestation is dependent on the location of the stroke, the volume of the brain affected, the rapidity of insult onset, the underlying health of the brain, the adequacy of brain collaterals in the case of ischemic injury, patient age, as well as a multitude of systemic, serological, and genetic factors. Generally speaking, stroke consists of the painless loss of neurological function except in the case of aneurysmal SAH, which is classically associated with an instantaneous and severe headache.[9] Parenchymal ICH is associated with headache in about 40% to 50% of patients and the headache tends to be progressive in onset.[10] Both ICH and SAH can be associated with nausea and vomiting along with focal neurological dysfunction.[10] The typical clinical manifestations of ischemic stroke of the anterior circulation (i.e., the carotid artery territory) include unilateral motor and sensory dysfunction and cognitive dysfunction, with or without visual loss. The cognitive dysfunction can consist of confusion but more commonly consists of aphasia (a disturbance of language) if the dominant (usually left) hemisphere is affected. If the nondominant (usually right) hemisphere is affected cognitive dysfunction may manifest with visual-spatial deficits and hemi-neglect. Alteration of consciousness is atypical in anterior circulation strokes unless the stroke is massive and if found early on suggests that an ICH is the cause rather than ischemia. Posterior circulation (i.e., vertebrobasilar territory) strokes manifest with crossed sensory-motor deficits typically associated with diplopia, severe dysarthria, gait imbalance, ataxia, and vertigo. Profound and deep alteration of consciousness (i.e., stupor or coma) is much more likely than in anterior circulation strokes.

The majority of large ischemic strokes affect the middle cerebral artery (MCA) territory for several reasons. The bilateral MCAs supply the majority of the cerebral hemispheres and are effectively the terminations of the ICAs, which carry 80% of cerebral blood flow. Additionally, the cervical ICAs are the most common site of extracranial cerebral atherosclerosis.

Transient neurological deficits may also occur and can herald a permanent event.[11,12] These transient ischemic attacks (TIAs) are clinically defined by complete resolution of the neurological deficits within 24 hours; longer events are classified as strokes. Modern imaging (i.e., magnetic resonance diffusion weighted imaging), however, has shown that events lasting hours are very often associated with permanent injury.[13] Most true TIAs will last 5 minutes to a couple of hours. These events are most often associated with large vessel processes such as left atrial thrombi in atrial fibrillation, cervical internal carotid artery stenosis, or intracranial stenosis. The other etiologies described above may all manifest with TIA, including ICH (rarely). Therefore a TIA is a true medical emergency and requires the same thorough evaluation that a patient presenting with stroke would receive.[14]

Diagnostic Evaluation

The diagnostic evaluation of the patient presenting with cerebrovascular disease is aimed at limiting the potential for permanent neurological injury. As can be surmised from the above discussion of the heterogeneous pathogenic mechanisms and varied clinical manifestations of stroke, a simple cookbook or algorithmic approach to all stroke patients is not feasible. However, there are many published guidelines that can facilitate the process.[9,15-18] Generally speaking, the first step, after the basic ABC's of resuscitation and neurological examination, is to differentiate an ischemic event from a hemorrhagic event. This is essential because one may mimic the other and the major and most dreaded side effect of all therapy for ischemia is ICH and vice versa. To accomplish this, a noncontrast computerized tomography (CT) scan of the brain should be performed to evaluate the brain parenchyma and its surroundings.[16] Magnetic resonance imaging (MRI) has much greater sensitivity and specificity than CT but is time consuming and, except in some research institutions, is inadequate in the ultra-early phases of ICH. An evaluation of the cerebral vasculature should also be performed evaluating the entirety of the cerebral vascular tree, from aortic arch to the intracranial vessels.[16] Both CT- and MRI-based noninvasive angiographic techniques (i.e., CTA and MRA) are available and have their benefits and drawbacks. Catheter cerebral angiography with digital subtraction (DSA) remains the gold standard for evaluating the vasculature. A cardiac evaluation (electrocardiography, echocardiography) along with a variety of laboratory studies may also be warranted.[14,15]

THE CEREBRAL VASCULATURE

The brain and cerebral circulation have several unique characteristics and are histologically different from other vessels in the body. Shortly after penetrating the skull base (~1 cm) the cerebral arteries lose the external elastic lamina and the tunica muscularis and adventitia thin considerably. As a consequence they become significantly more fragile and prone to injury during interventional procedures. Furthermore, after penetrating the dura matter the arteries enter the subarachnoid space that overlies the surface of the brain. Any injury that results in vessel rupture or perforation (e.g., dissection) can lead to catastrophy because the resultant SAH and/or ICH can result in a rapid and marked elevation of intracranial pressure (ICP) leading to either herniation or reduction/cessation of cerebral blood flow. The elevated ICP and its consequences are difficult to manage pharmacologically and sometimes require emergent neurosurgical decompression. Another important consideration is that embolization or occlusion of distal branches or perforators, even if nearly microscopic, can result in major disability. Finally, the cerebral vessels are also extremely tortuous and prone to vasospasm. For example, the internal carotid arteries (ICAs) have 180-degree turns in their cavernous segments. The proximal segments of the intracranial ICA run through the densest bone in the human body, the petrous bone, and are subsequently anchored within the cavernous sinus and the layers of the leathery dura matter. These factors, combined with their fragility, make the navigation of endovascular devices intracranially particularly difficult and potentially hazardous.

The brain is supplied blood by the paired ICA and vertebral arteries (VAs). The ICAs are branches of the common carotid artery and have no extracranial branches. Their first important intracranial branch is the ophthalmic artery. Shortly thereafter they (variable) give off the posterior communicating artery (PCom), which is the major anterior-posterior circulation collateral. They then give off the very important anterior choroidal artery before dividing into the MCA and anterior cerebral arteries (ACAs) (**Figure 25-1**). The VAs are the first branches of the subclavian arteries and have many muscular branches in the neck as well as collaterals to the spinal cord. They enter the foramen magnum and join together to form the single basilar artery (BA) after giving off the (usually) large posterior inferior cerebellar artery. The BA has numerous perforators and branches supplying the pons, midbrain, and remainder of the cerebellum (**Figure 25-1**). The BA then divides into the bilateral posterior cerebral arteries (PCAs), which supply the occipital lobes. The PCom joins the ipsilateral PCA and in combination with the bilateral ICA, bilateral ACA, and single anterior communicating artery (ACom) complete the Circle of Willis. The Circle is an inherent source of collaterals and (when present) can completely supply CBF to the territory of an occluded ICA or BA. Unfortunately, a complete Circle exists in only 25% to 40% of humans.[19,20]

There are essential perforating arteries that emanate from the MCA, BA, and PCA trunks (**Figure 25-1**). These vessels supply critical structures and, although small (50-200 μm), their occlusion can cause major and disabling neurological deficits. These vessels are at risk of occlusion during intracranial interventions, especially if they were the etiology of the presenting symptoms. Furthermore, they are particularly vulnerable to wire perforation. They arise from the dorsal (superiorly in anterior-posterior view) aspect of the MCA and (posteriorly in anterior-posterior view) BA.

ACUTE ISCHEMIC STROKE TREATMENT

Current acute stroke therapies include intravenous (IV) tissue plasminogen activator (tPA), which is effective in both small and large vessel strokes and endovascular therapy (EVT), which is used for large vessel strokes. The former was approved in 1996 by the Food and Drug Administration (FDA) based mainly upon the results of the National Institute of Neurologic Disorders and Stroke (NINDS) study.[21] More

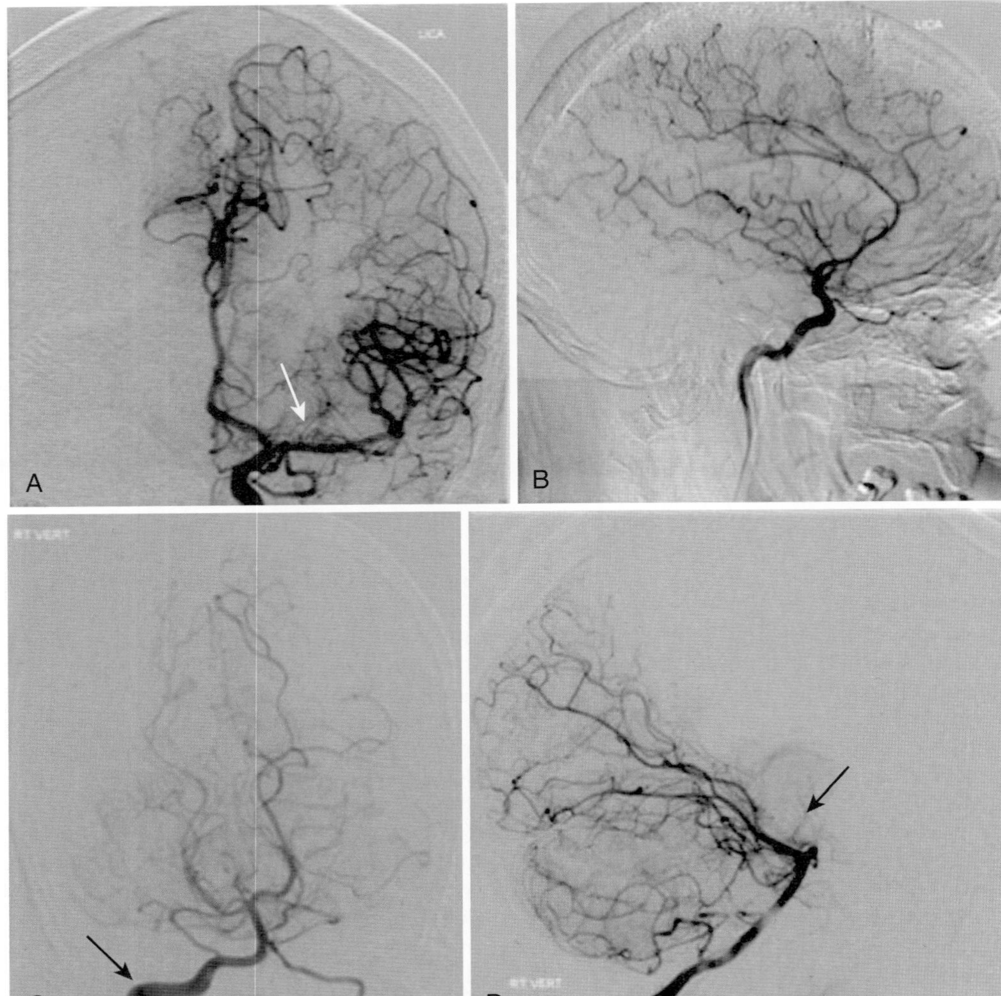

FIGURE 25-1 A selective left internal carotid angiogram shows normal intracranial branching pattern. The perforators (lenticulostriates) emanating from the middle cerebral artery trunk are easily identified *(arrow)* in the anterio-posterior view **(A)**. They are not visible in the lateral view **(B)** but the cortical branches of the middle cerebral and anterior cerebral arteries are well visualized. In **(C)**, a right vertebral artery injection in the steep anterio-posterior view shows the basilar artery and its branches well: note the dominant right vertebral artery *(arrow)*. A lateral projection of a vertebral artery angiogram **(D)** shows the many small perforating branches emanating posteriorly from the basilar artery trunk as well as superiorly *(arrow)* from the basilar artery apex and posterior cerebral arteries.

than a decade later, on average, only 5% to 10% of patients with ischemic stroke receive IV-tPA treatment.[22-24] The major limiting factors are the strict criteria for the administration of IV-tPA, in particular the narrow time window for administration of only 3 hours from clear symptom onset.[25] Furthermore, IV-tPA is poorly effective at recanalizing larger vessels.[26,27] The middle cerebral artery (MCA) recanalization rate is approximately 30% while the larger ICA is successfully recanalized in <10% of cases.[26,27] Consequently, EVT has been studied as an adjunctive/alternative treatment for large vessel acute ischemic stroke. Endovascular therapy (AKA Intraarterial thrombolysis [IAT]) is not an FDA-approved treatment. The only FDA-approved treatment for acute ischemic stroke (IS) remains IV-tPA.[18]

The indications for EVT are evolving and since there is no approved EVT for stroke, there is a great deal of variability between practitioners in the field with regards to the indications.[16,28] In general, patients with acute IS presenting less than 4.5 hours meeting criteria should be offered IV-tPA, and EVT should be offered to all others, and to those who refuse IV-tPA. It is important to note that treatment with IV-tPA does not reduce stroke mortality and patients with large vessel occlusions,[29,30] large thrombus burden (i.e., thrombi longer than 8 mm),[31] and those with more severe strokes respond less well to IV thrombolysis.[32] For these patients EVT may be considered as an (unproven) alternative to IV thrombolysis.[33] In one observational study of 112 patients with hyperdense middle cerebral artery (MCA) sign, half of whom received IV-tPA and the other EVT, favorable outcome was doubled and risk of death reduced by two thirds in patients treated with EVT.[34]

The traditional time window for EVT is up to 6 hours for thrombolysis and 8 hours for mechanical embolectomy.[16] The duration of ischemia is a leading predictor of neurological outcome, but with modern penumbral imaging selection of patients for EVT may be time-independent (see further on).[35-38]

Patients must also have a significant clinical deficit that warrants intervention since mild deficits (i.e., National Institutes of Health Stroke Score [NIHSS] <4) are less likely to be associated with a visible proximal large arterial occlusion; such milder strokes have an excellent prognosis on average even without treatment.[39] On the other end of the spectrum patients with severe strokes (NIHSS >20) generally do not benefit as much from treatment. Multimodal imaging techniques such as perfusion imaging may help select patients with major deficits who have small infarct cores and large penumbral zones who may still benefit from treatment. [35,36] A recent prospective cohort study (Diffusion and Perfusion Imaging Evaluation for Understanding Stroke Evolution Study 2 [DEFUSE 2]) tested whether an MRI perfusion-based definition of target mismatch (TMM) could appropriately detect who would benefit from EVT within 12 hours of stroke onset.[40] Of the 99 patients with perfusion imaging, 78 had a TMM, and 42 of whom were treated beyond the 6-hour time window. With recanalization and a TMM there was an odds ratio (OR) of 8.5 for good neurological outcomes in patients treated >6 hours along with a 2.9 OR for those treated <6 hours, compared with those without a TMM. Importantly, no reperfusion led to infarct growth and patients without a TMM did not benefit from recanalization (OR 0.2; $p = 0.004$). Unfortunately there is a paucity of level 1 evidence on the use of and parameters for defining penumbra with these techniques. An alternative is to select patients using the Alberta Stroke Program Early CT score (ASPECTS): a 10-point scale with 10 representing a normal CT and 0 a complete infarct of the entire MCA territory.[41] A baseline ASPECTS score of ≥8 is an excellent predictor of clinical response to treatment.[41]

The contraindications for IAT are generally any that would increase the risk of ICH. A history of spontaneous ICH or an untreated ruptured aneurysm or arteriovenous malformation are contraindications to thrombolysis although mechanical embolectomy may be performed in selected patients. A history of dementia, unless mild, should be a contraindication as those patients have a low probability of recovering. Relative contraindications are active anticoagulation with any class of anticoagulant, including antiplatelet agents; one small study has shown that mechanical embolectomy may be safe.[42]

Techniques

Intraarterial Thrombolysis

A coordinated team approach is essential to the efficient, rapid, and safe implementation of endovascular therapy. Multiple concurrent events must be coordinated and everyone on the team should know in advance what their duties are. For example, while one is prepping and draping, someone else is readying the thrombolytic agents, while another is manging the medical needs of the patient. A cart containing all of the stroke specific devices should be brought into the suite if necessary to avoid delays searching for devices. Although practices vary, an 8 Fr sheath should be inserted into the femoral artery (a radial approach is feasible but has its own challenges, especially if a balloon occlusion guide catheter is to be used). Alternatively a 6 Fr sheath can be inserted. Ideally a 6 Fr guide catheter should then be quickly tracked into the vessel of interest. Although arch variants (e.g., common origin of the innominate and left common carotid artery or a bovine arch) are not uncommon (25%-30% of patient) and may make selective cannulation difficult, taking time to perform an arch angiogram can waste precious minutes.[43] In practice most patients will have a CTA performed during the initial assessment and all such scans should always include the aortic arch and great vessels that can be of great help in planning for unusual anatomy or ostructions.

For anterior circulation strokes a common carotid artery (CCA) injection should be performed, and then if safe to do so a selective internal carotid artery (ICA) injection should be performed. For posterior circulation (i.e., vertebrobasilar [VB]) strokes, the dominant VA (generally the left, which is easier to cannulate) should be gently injected. All angiography should be performed in standard biplanar views (AP and lateral) using digital subtraction angiography (DSA). It is important to use a large field of view to visualize the entire inner table of the skull. Angiography should include the entirety of the arterial, capillary, and venous phases. Besides the identification of the occlusion and contraindications to thrombolysis (e.g., arteriovenous malformation) an assessment of collateral blood flow is essential since the presence of robust collaterals is a marker for clinical benefit and their absence is a harbinger of poor outcomes and probable futility.[44,45] Full angiography of the other cerebral vessels is greatly discouraged especially if non-invasive imaging (i.e., CTA or MRA) is available and can be performed after recanalization is achieved, if necessary.

Any unnecessary delay in initiation of therapy should be avoided but if there are no collaterals seen on the ipsilateral injection it is reasonable to quickly inject the other vessels because a complete absence of collaterals is a grave prognostic sign and recanalization therapy should be reconsidered.[44-46]

The periprocedural use of antithrombotics is variable and only one study (PROACT I) has studied this aspect, although it was in the setting of intra-arterial thrombolysis with pro-urokinase.[39] In that trial, a high-dose heparin regimen was associated with excessive risk of ICH and the low-dose regimen (2000 U heparin bolus followed by 500 U/hr up to 4 hours) was found to be safer and has effectively been adopted by many in the field.

Stable access to the symptomatic vessel was one of the most important factors that determined procedural success but advancements in catheter design and manufacturing have made this less of an issue. Still sheath and guide catheter choice remains important. In most patients with straight cervical vessels a a short sheath and a 6 Fr neuroguide catheter (e.g., Envoy XB, Cordis Inc., Miami, Florida) advanced into the distal cervical ICA or V2 segment of the VA will provide adequate support for most therapeutic devices. In cases with severely tortuous great vessels or steeply angulated aortic arches, a modified approach utilizing a long 6-8 Fr sheath with the tip in the distal common carotid or subclavian arteries may be necessary for stable access. The newer generation of highly deliverable guide catheters such as the Neuron Max (Penumbra Inc., Alameda, California) provide stable access while being highly deliverable even intracranially.

The next step is to advance a microcatheter to the site of occlusion. This is most commonly performed over a soft-tipped hydrophillic 0.014-inch wire. Wire advancement and placement is one of the riskier aspects of neuro-interventions due to the aforementioned fragility of the cerebral vessels. Great care and advanced knowledge of the anatomy and variations are neceesary. The wire tip must not cannulate the small perforators arising from the superior MCA or posterior BA walls to avoid perforation or occlusion. The occlusion should be crossed with the wire with careful attention to the course of the tip while avoiding any tip deflection. The catheter can then be advanced into or past the thrombus. In most cases mechanical embolectomy will be performed, therefore the catheter needs to be advanced at least 2-3 cm distal to the distal most aspect of the thrombus. This can be gleaned from careful angiography noting the retrograde pial collateral flow, which will often reach the distal aspect of the occlusion or ideally from the preprocedure CTA. Some operators like to perform microcatheter angiography to document the exact location of the occlusion. This has been associated with an increased risk of ICH and may waste precious time that could be better used to achieve recanalization.

Some operators will then infuse thrombolytic agents distal to the clot. This has fallen out of the favor in the modern era of mechanical embolectomy but is an option in selected individuals with distal occlusions in which mechanical approaches may not be feasible. There is a great variability in the thrombolytic agents used for IAT. The agents that have been used include t-PA, streptokinase, retiplase, urokinase, as well as recombinant pro-urokinase (rpro-UK).[39,47-56] Streptokinase is no longer used due to an excessive risk of hemorrhage. The PROACT II trial studied a fixed dose infusion of rpro-UK over 2 hours directly into the MCA; unfortunately while the trial was positive the clinical benefit in PROACT II was not profound.[39] Even though the initiation of recanalization therapy in PROACT II was approximately within 5.3 hours from stroke onset, recanalization occurred well past the 6 hour window in many patients due to the mandate for a 2-hour infusion. Most operators, including the author, advocate a more rapid infusion of thrombolytics to be given in aliquots every 5-10 minutes. The author also advocates for an adjustment of the dose of thrombolytic so as to use the lowest effective dose to decrease the risk of ICH which has been associated with thromboytic dosage.[57]

The following factors are associated with a higher risk of ICH therefore warranting lower doses of thrombolytics: older age especially >80 years old, presenting blood pressure >185/110, hyperglycemia, long duration of ischemia >4-6 hours, the presence of early infarct signs on pretreatment CT or MRI, and the presence of any other confounders such as the infusion of GPIIb/IIIa inhibitors. The lowest possible dose of all antithrombotic and fibribolytic agents should be used to the decrease the risk of ICH. Generally thrombolytics are reserved for those with distal thrombi not amenable to mechanical embolectomy devices or those who fail such interventions. Maneuvers such as wire manipulation of the thrombus have been described but are mostly ineffective and there are no prospective data supporting their use as they were prohibited in PROACT II.[39]

Combination treatment with thrombolytics and GPIIb/IIIa antagonists has some potential advantages and has been described in small series.[55,58,59] Anecdotally the combination may be most effective in cases of atherosclerotic occlusions, thrombosis complicating endovascular procedures or cases of artery to artery embolism due to endothelial injury (e.g., dissection, ruptured plaque, etc.). GPIIb/IIIa antagonists may have a role if emergency stent implantation is necessary. The use of these agents is very poorly studied and has been associated with ICH; furthermore there is no indication for continuous infusion as is the practice in acute myocardial infarction due to a very high rate of intracranial hemorrhage.[60]

Combined IV/IA Thrombolysis

Intravenous tPA can be rapidly initiated without the need to wait for the EVT team or vascular lab to be available. Therefore an approach of IV thrombolysis followed by IAT has been described and studied in the IMS (Interventional Management of Stroke) trials. IMS I (a phase I feasibility and safety trial) combined IV and IA tPA and the follow-up IMS II added the MicroLys US infusion catheter (EKOS Inc., Bothell, Washington) to the combined IV/IA approach. In the IMS II treatment arm the ORs of attaining an mRS ≤2 were 1.74 and 2.82 compared with tPA and placebo-treated subjects, respectively.[61]

The IMS III trial was a randomized controlled trial that enrolled 656 patients (out of a planned 900) treated within 3 hours of stroke onset with NIHSS ≥10 who were randomized to receive IV-tPA alone versus IV-tPA followed by EVT.[62] The latter consisted largely of IA-tPA (80%) followed in order of frequency by the Merci Retriever (Stryker Inc., Kalamazoo, Michigan) (29%), and Penumbra (Penumbra Inc., Alameda, California) (16%), EKOS (6.6%), and Solitaire (Covidien/EV3 Inc.) (1.5%). The study was stopped prematurely for reasons of futility without any safety concerns. Analysis of enrolled patients did not show a significant difference in good outcomes between the IV only versus IV/EVT group, although trends in favor of the combined approach were noted in patients presenting with NIHSS >20. Symptomatic ICH rates and mortality did not differ between groups, indicating that the combined approach is as safe as IV-tPA alone. There was a strong correlation between recanalization success and outcomes. The limitations of IA-tPA and first-generation embolectomy devices were highlighted by the fact that in the endovascular therapy arm there was only a 44% thrombolysis in cerebral infarction (TICI) 2b/3 rate. Furthermore, initiation of EVT was generally very slow with a mean IV-tPA to groin puncture time of 82 min. These findings underscore the critical importance of complete and rapid recanalization. IMS III did not require proof of vascular occlusion at enrollment but in a prespecified subgroup analysis of patients with baseline CTA confirming a large vessel occlusion, there was a 6% higher rate of good outcomes in favor of the combined treatment, particularly in patients with ICA occlusion (23% in the IV/IA group vs. 5% in the IV-only group; $p = 0.14$).

At this time therefore there are no data to support a combined IV/IA strategy in IV-tPA eligible patients; however, in IMS III, patients were randomized to EVT before completion of the IV infusion so those results may not be strictly applicable to failed IV-tPA patients. To complicate matters there is no consensus on what constitutes IV-tPA "failure."[63] There are some data that recanalization, if it occurs, will occur within 1 hour of tPA infusion, therefore it is reasonable to consider EVT if patients do not recanalize or improve clinically within 1 hour of receiving IV-tPA.[64]

Mechanical Embolectomy

Despite the fact that thrombolysis, both IV and IA, has been proven effective, it has significant limitations. The speed of recanalization and recanalization efficacy are the primary limitations. Pharmacological thrombolysis is based on the assumption that all thrombi/emboli are similar and are equally amenable to thrombolysis. In reality thrombi/emboli may be composed of different components (platelets, fibrin, cholesterol debris, etc.) and are of widely varied sizes and volumes. Furthermore thrombolysis may be contraindicated under certain circumstances due to an increased risk of systemic bleeding (e.g., gastrointestinal)) or intracerebral hemorrhage (e.g., head trauma). Mechanical embolectomy removes many of these limitations due to the lack of a systemic and persistent pharmacological effect. Anecdotal reports using a variety of devices and snares designed for foreign body removal were first reported in the late 1990s.[65,66] Since that time dedicated devices have been developed and tested. The major advantage of this approach is the potential to achieve recanalization in a few minutes rather than 1 to 2 hours or longer. There are some theoretical disadvantages primarily an increased risk of vascular injury and dissection.[67]

The technique of mechanical embolectomy varies depending on the device being used. Currently, the stent-trievers are the dominant devices and their use is markedly simpler than the older (Merci Retriever and Penumbra) devices. The approach is exactly like the IAT approach with two major differences. The first is that mechanical embolectomy is most effective with proximal flow arrest and aspiration. Therefore once the site of occlusion has been confirmed angiographically the 5 Fr diagnostic catheter or 6 Fr guide catheter are exchanged for an 8 Fr or 9 Fr balloon occlusion guide catheter (e.g., Merci). The lesion is crossed with the microcatheter and microwire but device-specific microcatheters must be used. The wire is removed and then the embolectomy device is delivered to the site of occlusion with about half of the device deployed distal to the thrombus and the remainder within the thrombus (**Figure 25-2**). Angiographic confirmation of appropriate device deployment is then performed, which should show restoration of antegrade flow through the occluded segment as the tines of the stent push the thrombus aside. The device is left

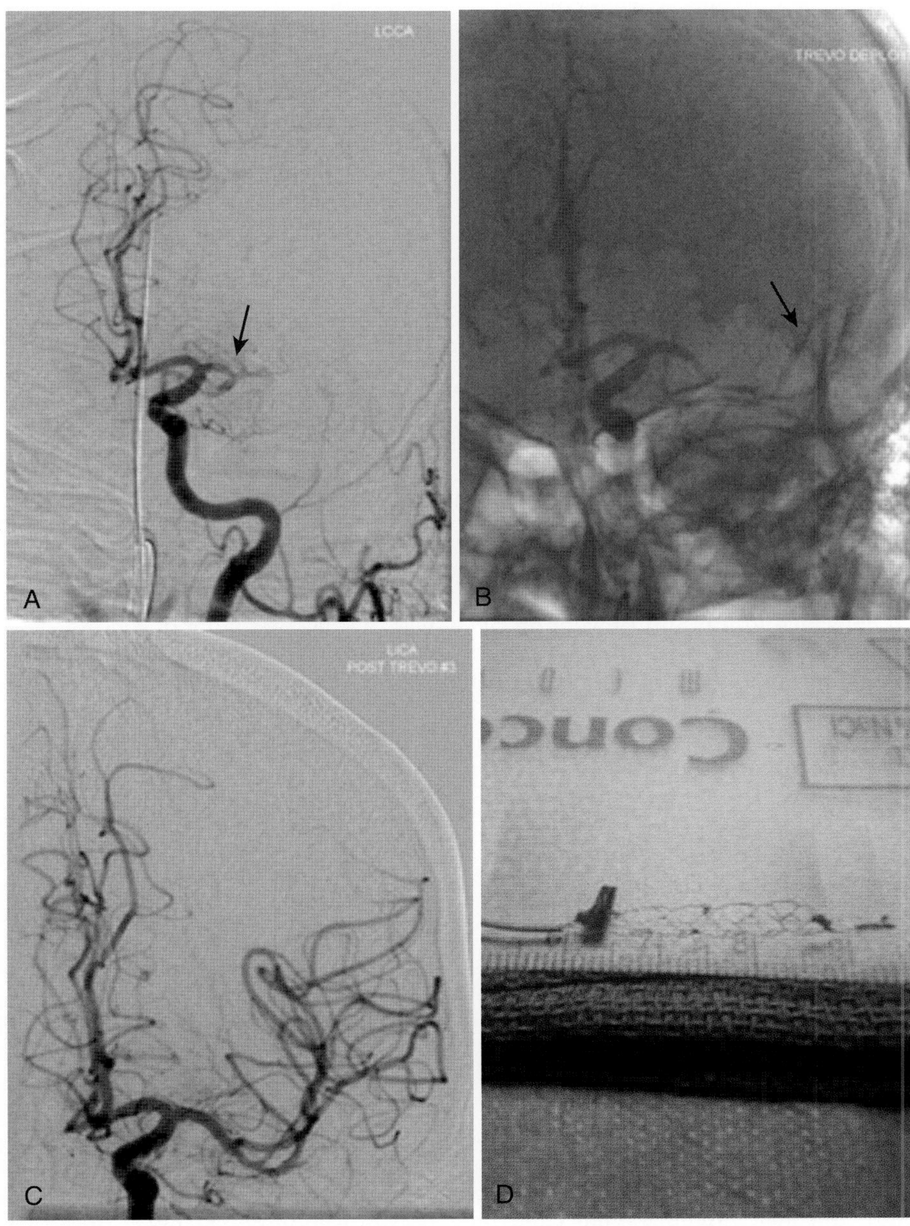

FIGURE 25-2 A left common carotid artery injection in the anterio-posterior view **(A)** shows a complete left middle cerebral artery occlusion *(arrow)* in a patient who failed to recanalyze with intravenous tPA. A Trevo stent-triever device was deployed in the middle cerebral artery with half deployed distally in a secondary branch (*arrow* in **B** points to device tip). Following the third pass with the device there was complete recanalization **(C)** and the thrombus was ensnared in the device **(D)**.

deployed for 3 to 10 minutes. Then with the balloon on the guide catheter inflated to occlude antegrade flow, the device is slowly withdrawn (while still deployed) while aspiration on the central lumen of the balloon guide catheter is performed. This creates retrograde flow in the parent vessel and facilitates thrombus extraction. The device can be reprepped and utilized for more passes as needed.

Balloon Angioplasty and Stenting

In several large Japanese series angioplasty has been reported to be very effective with recanalization rates near 90%.[68,69] Those series have also reported lower rates of ICH compared with IAT (3% vs. >10%). These results may not be generalizable since intracranial atherosclerosis is the leading cause of ischemic stroke in Japanese and Asian populations and angioplasty may be particularly effective, as it is in the coronary arteries, under such circumstances.[70] Still angioplasty has sometimes been effective even with non-atherosclerotic occlusions[58,71,72] and is generally performed with gentle balloon inflation using an undersized coronary balloon. The author recommends angioplasty in cases of likely thrombotic occlusion (e.g., the presence of calcification at the site of occlusion, especially in patients of African-American or Asian descent without atrial fibrillation); this approach is anecdotal and it needs to be validated prospectively.

Stenting has also been reported to be highly effective particularly in cases of cervical internal carotid artery atherosclerotic occlusion.[73-75] There has only been one prospective study of stenting in AIS in which 20 patients were treated with a self-expanding stent. That study demonstrated a TIMI 2/3 recanalization rate of 100% with a 5% sICH rate.[76] Sixty percent of the patients had a good neurological outcome. As with angioplasty, stenting may be especially effective for cervical ICA atherosclerotic occlusions; the major drawback is the increased risk of ICH due to the need for dual antiplatelet therapy.[75,77] The benefits of successful stenting include the possibility of improving flow rapidly even if the angiographic result is less than optimal. Another potential benefit is the definitive treatment of the underlying causative lesion and prevention of acute or subacute stroke recurrence. The drawbacks of emergent intracranial stenting include vessel injury, especially if the stent is oversized. Since most AIS patients will not be taking dual antiplatelet agents if stents are implanted GPIIb/IIIa receptor antagonists may be necessary but there are only anecdotal reports of their use in this setting.

It is worth re-emphasizing that stroke is heterogeneous and it is the author's belief that treatment should be tailored to the needs of every individual, for example, intracranial stenting in an elderly patient with tortuous and heavily calcified vessels may be associated with a high likelihood of complications and primary angioplasty or thrombolysis may be safer approaches. The goal of rapid recanalization must not come at cost of ICH. The technique of intracranial stenting is discussed in the section below on Intracranial Angioplasty and Stenting.

Clinical Outcomes

Although there have been numerous series of IAT reported they shared in common only two qualities, they were a series of patients who had ischemic stroke and who were treated with intra-arterially delivered thrombolytics. They differed greatly in patient selection, duration of ischemia, occlusion location, stroke etiology, the endovascular approaches, and the pharmacological agents used. Individually most of these series suggested that IAT is effective at recanalization and that patients derived clinical benefit. Unfortunately a meta-analysis suggested there was no net benefit with pharmacological IAT.[53]

Only one randomized trial of IAT has been completed and published, the Prolyse in Acute Cerebral Thromboembolism (PROACT) II trial.[39] PROACT II evaluated the recanalization and clinical efficacy of rpro-UK in acute ischemic stroke. In that trial patients who had MCA occlusion of <6 hours duration, without CT evidence of infarct greater than one third of the MCA territory, were randomized to an infusion directly into the MCA of a fixed dose (9 mg) of rpro-UK over 2 hours or placebo. Mechanical clot disruption was not permitted.[78,79] All patients received 2000 units of unfractionated heparin followed by 500 U/hr for a total of 4 hours. Treatment was associated with a 15% absolute benefit (58% relative benefit) in the 90 day modified Rankin Scale ($p = 0.04$). In the treatment group the TIMI 2 or 3 recanalization rate was 66% at 2 hours (vs. 18% for the placebo group); unfortunately the TIMI 3 rate was only 19% in the treatment arm.[80]

In PROACT II the treatment group symptomatic ICH risk was 10% but only 2% in the control patients. This symptomatic ICH rate compared favorably with the rates in the major IV-tPA trials (6% in the NINDS trial, 9% in ECASS II, and 7% in ATLANTIS).[21,79,81] Despite the positive results of the PROACT II trial the FDA did not grant approval, so IA thrombolysis remains an investigational treatment. Intra-arterial thrombolysis had become the standard of care at many academic medical centers until the advent of the newer mechanical embolectomy devices.

A second randomized trial of IAT was the Japanese Middle Cerebral Artery Embolism Local Fibrinolytic Intervention Trial (MELT) of intra-arterial urokinase for <6 hour MCA occlusion.[82] It was stopped after enrolling 114 patients because of IV-tPA approval in Japan. The primary endpoint of mRS ≤2 was not significantly different and the rate of sICH was 9%. A preplanned secondary analysis showed that recovery to normal or near normal (mRS ≤1) was significantly higher in the treatment group (42.1% vs. 22.8%; $p = 0.045$).

The accepted time window for the initiation of IAT has been 6 hours from stroke onset in the anterior (ICA and MCA) circulation. Anecdotal reports have suggested that the time window in the VB circulation may be longer.[49,83] Some investigators have treated patients including those with anterior circulation strokes well beyond the traditional time windows, suggesting that time is not the absolute determinant of EVT success. In one series of 55 consecutive EVT patients selected by perfusion imaging with a mean NIHSS of 19.7 ± 5.7, 21 were treated on average within 18.6 ± 16.0 hours from stroke onset while the other 34 patients were treated on average 3.4 ± 1.6 hours from stroke onset.[37] Recanalization rates (82.8% vs. 85.7%; p = NS) and the rates of good neurological outcome (41.2% vs. 42.9%; p = NS) were similar. What was most encouraging was that the risk of symptomatic ICH was also comparable between the early and late treatment groups (8.8% vs. 9.5%; p = NS). The duration of ischemia was not a predictor of poor outcome or death. A larger multicenter, retrospective study confirmed these results in 237 anterior circulation stroke patients

TABLE 25-1 Contraindications to Intravenous Thrombolysis

Computerized tomography findings of lobar, subdural, intraventricular, or subarachnoid hemorrhage
History of intracerebral hemorrhage
Cerebral arterio-venous malformation or giant thrombosed cerebral aneurysm*
Brain tumor (meningioma not included)
Computerized tomography evidence of acute >1/3 middle cerebral artery territory
Infarct or large ischemic core on perfusion imaging†
Uncontrolled hypertension >185/110 mm Hg (despite medical intervention)
Unknown stroke duration or duration >4.5 hours
Thrombocytopenia <100,000
Bleeding diathesis or internal bleeding within 21 days
International normalized ratio (INR) >1.7
History of advanced Alzheimer's disease or amyloid angiopathy†
Seizure at stroke onset (unless an acute arterial occlusion is documented)
Recent surgery or trauma within 14 days
Intracranial or spinal surgery, head trauma, or stroke within 3 months
Age >80 years old‡
History of prior stroke and diabetes‡
Any anticoagulant use regardless of INR‡

*Unruptured, incidental, nonthrombosed aneurysms are not a contraindication.
†Relative contraindication.
‡Contraindications for thrombolysis between 3 hours to 4.5 hours from stroke onset.

treated with IAT on average 15 ± 11.2 hours after stroke onset.[38] In that study patients were also selected based on either CT- or MRI-based perfusion imaging. Ninety-day good clinical outcomes and mortality were 45% and 21.5%, respectively. Remarkably sICH occurred in 8.9%. Although both of these series were retrospective and need to be confirmed with prospective studies, these data suggest that patients with salvageable brain tissue and severe clinical deficits should be considered for EVT regardless of stroke duration.

Endovascular therapy has several potential advantages as compared to IV thrombolysis; chief among which are the longer time window and increased recanalization efficacy. Additionally EVT may be safer in situations where there is an increased risk of hemorrhage such as recent (<2 weeks) thoracic or abdominal surgery, extra-cerebral hemorrhage, arterial puncture in a noncompressible site, as well as in patients being treated with systemic anticoagulation (**Table 25-1**). Mechanical embolectomy is the safest approach in such patients but even IAT may be safer due to the fact that lower doses of local thrombolytics may be given.[4,42,84,85]

Mechanical embolectomy with the MERCI clot retriever received FDA approval 10 years ago on the basis of the single arm MERCI study.[67] That trial of 151 patients included patients treated within 3-8 hours of stroke onset and only evaluated the safety and feasibility of mechanical embolectomy. The clot burden in the MERCI study was on average greater than that in the PROACT II and MELT trials since all comers, including ICA occlusion, were enrolled; and although the IV tPA trials did not assess for arterial occlusion the mean NIHSS in MERCI was far greater consistent with more large vessel occlusions. Device-only recanalization (TIMI 2-3) was achieved in 46% but with adjunctive thrombolysis it increased to 60.3%. A good outcome (mRS ≤2) was achieved in 27.7% of patients and 43.5% were deceased by 90 days. Most informative was that the symptomatic ICH was only 7.8%, which was only slightly greater than the 6% seen with IV tPA. Therefore since the MERCI trial proved the safety of the device the FDA granted approval for "clot removal" not for stroke treatment.

The follow-up Multi MERCI trial was another multicenter single-arm trial of the first generation MERCI retrievers and the second-generation retriever with the added goal of exploring the technical efficacy and safety of embolectomy in patients with "failed" IV thrombolysis.[63] Twenty-nine percent of patients had "failed" IV-tPA and 34.8% received intraprocedural IA thrombolytics. Device-only recanalization was noted in 55% but was 68% with adjunctive thrombolysis. The clinical results were similar to MERCI with a good outcome in 36% and 34% mortality. The rate of sICH was 9.8%. Much has been made of the relatively poor clinical outcomes in these trials compared with the outcomes in the randomized IV-tPA trials. Those are inappropriate comparisons, however, since the MERCI trials had patients with more severe strokes, larger thrombus burdens, and longer durations of ischemia. These trials were not designed or powered to show clinical efficacy; rather they were designed to show effectiveness in clot removal. Since they have been proven effective at clot removal and recanalization, which is the most effective treatment for stroke it has been assumed that they are effective at stroke treatment.

The MERCI Registry, the largest prospective registry of mechanical embolectomy, included 1000 "real-world" patients. It had no predefined exclusion criteria (Jovin T, Oral Presentation, ISC, February 2011, Los Angeles, California). The Registry patients were treated later than in the earlier studies, approximately 17% were treated beyond 8 hours from stroke onset. Recanalization was achieved in 80.1% of patients but only 31.6% had good outcomes and 33.4% died. Recanalization was the best predictor of good outcomes (mRS ≤2) but with an age disparity: compared with <60 year olds, patients >79 had an approximately half the probability of achieving a good outcome despite recanalization and 40% mortality. On the other hand there was no possibility (0%) of a good outcome if there was no recanalization. Mortality with successful recanalization in those <60 was 15%. With complete recanalization good neurological outcomes (70% vs. 10%) and mortality (<15% vs. 40-50%) were better in those with NIHSS <16 compared with those with NIHSS >25, respectively. The sICH rate was 7% overall but was lower with successful recanalization (5.4% with TICI flow grade of 3% compared to 9.2% if the final TICI grade was 0-1).[86] Predictors of good outcome in a multivariate analysis included baseline NIHSS (OR 0.88; $p < 0.0001$), age (OR 0.95; $p < 0.0001$), and successful revascularization defined as TICI 2a-3 (OR 4.02; $p < 0.0001$).

The second FDA approved device was the Penumbra (Penumbra Inc., Alameda, California) clot extraction device. Its clot extraction efficacy was validated in a 125-patient study with an 8-hour time window.[87] Revascularization success (TIMI 2-3) and 90-day good outcomes were achieved in 81.6% and 25% of patients, respectively. Ninety-day mortality was 32.8% with 11.2% sICH. There was a trend for benefit with successful recanalization.

The poor clinical outcomes, and too often incomplete revascularization with these earlier devices, led to the development of a new class of devices designed to be safer and more effective. The so-called stent-trievers, or stent retrievers, combine the benefits of stenting (immediate flow restoration) with embolectomy devices (clot extraction) without leaving a stent permanently in the vessel (**Figure 25-2**). Two randomized, noninferiority trials have been published comparing the recanalization and clinical efficacy of stent retrievers versus the MERCI retrievers in patients treated within 8 hours of stroke onset. The Solitaire With the Intention For Thrombectomy (SWIFT) trial tested the Solitaire device, and TREVO 2 tested the Trevo (Stryker Inc., Kalamazoo, Michigan) device.[88,89] Enrollment in the SWIFT trial was halted after 113 patients were enrolled when a pre-planned interim analysis showed a major benefit of Solitaire over the MERCI device. The primary efficacy outcome of TIMI 2 or 3 flow was achieved more often with Solitaire (61% vs. 24%; OR 4.87; p <0.0001).[88] In addition good neurological outcome (58% vs. 33%; OR 2.78; p = 0.0001) and 90-day mortality (17% vs. 38%; OR 0.34; p = 0.0001) were more favorable in the Solitaire group. The sICH rate was significantly lower with Solitaire (2% vs. 11%; OR 0.14; p = 0.057).

The TREVO 2 trial results were similar with 178 patients randomized.[89] Recanalization (TICI 2 or greater) was higher with Trevo (86% vs. 60%; OR 4.22; p <0.0001) as was good clinical outcome (40% vs. 22%; OR 2.39; p = 0.013). There was no difference in sICH (7% vs. 9%; OR 0.75; p = 0.78) or 90-day mortality (33% vs. 24%; OR 1.61; p = 0.18). The trials differed in some endpoint definitions and there was a difference in sICH and good outcomes. At this time there are insufficient data to differentiate between stent retrievers, although their superiority over the older MERCI device seems to be real. Certainly the speed of recanalization with the stent retrievers in general is a major advantage (e.g., time to achievement of recanalization from guide catheter placement was 36 minutes with Solitaire vs. 52 minutes with MERCI; p = 0.038).[88] Both the Solitaire and Trevo devices received FDA clearance for clot removal and are currently the defacto devices used by most centers performing EVT. As of this writing two randomized trials of mechanical embolectomy + medical therapy (including IV tPA if appropriate) vs. medical therapy alone have been halted due to "overwhelming efficacy." Although the full trial results are not yet available the expectation is that mechanical embolectomy with stentrievers will become the standard of care treatment for large vessel occlusion within 12 hours of stroke onset.

Peri-procedural Management

The medical management of patients peri-procedurally has not been well studied during EVT. While basic measures such as supporting the airway and maintaining oxygenation are standard, other variables are not.[16] The use of general anesthesia during EVT appears to be associated with worse neurological outcomes and increased mortality.[90-93] However if patients are comatose, are unable to handle secretions, or maintain their airway the risk of not performing endotracheal intubation is likely far greater than the potential harm; otherwise all patients should be kept awake during EVT. Since the cerebral vessels are richly innervated they are quite sensitive to manipulation and the resultant headache may be an important sign of impending vessel injury.[94]

An equally critical issue is blood pressure control. In the setting of ischemia cerebral autoregulation results in maximal arterial and arteriolar vasodilation distal to the site of occlusion, as a result cerebral blood flow (CBF) becomes directly proportional to mean arterial pressure. Consequently blood pressure elevation results in an increase in CBF and an increased risk of ICH, conversely lower pressures decrease CBF exacerbating the ischemia.[95,96] It is therefore critical to keep blood pressure moderately elevated except in patients who have a very high risk for ICH or those with ongoing myocardial infarction for example.[16] Although there are no validated guidelines the generally recommended range is 150-185 mm Hg.[16] After a successful intervention blood pressure should be lowered into the normal range immediately to avoid the cerebral hyperperfusion syndrome.

Post-operatively patients should be transferred to a neurological intensive care until stable.[16] Headache and a change in neurological status should warrant immediate neurological assessment and an emergent CT scan. The care of stroke patients in dedicated neurological units and by stroke specialists have been associated with decreased mortality and improved clinical outcomes.[18]

ISCHEMIC STROKE PREVENTION

Intracranial Angioplasty and Stenting

Intracranial atherosclerosis (ICAD) causes 8% to 10% of ischemic strokes in the United States.[97-100] The exact prevalence is unknown since many patients with the condition are asymptomatic, noninvasive imaging is nonspecific, and there is limited pathological analysis. The deferential diagnosis of intracranial stenosis includes vasculitis, dissection, embolism undergoing recanalization, moyamoya arteriopathy, postradiation arteriopathy, and infectious vasculitides.[101] Cerebral ischemia is caused primarily by limitation of flow as well as by vessel thrombosis and occlusion with or without distal embolization.

Treatment for ICAD has been generally inadequate. The Warfarin-Aspirin for Symptomatic Intracranial Disease (WASID) trial demonstrated that even with medical therapy (warfarin or 1300 mg of aspirin) the recurrent stroke rate was as high as 22% annually in patients with an angiographic stenosis between 70% to 99% in severity.[98,102] Surgical bypass has proved to be ineffective in a randomized trial and endarterectomy is very difficult to perform.[103] Endovascular therapy has emerged as a feasible and potentially highly effective means of treating patients with ICAD. The primary goal of endovascular therapy is to improve flow through the stenosis; while desirable, a perfect angiographic result is not necessary since the cerebral vessels are so fragile, the pursuit of such a goal may lead to dissection, arterial rupture, or ICH. The latter is often catastrophic and not amenable to treatment in this setting. This concept is of paramount importance, especially compared with the goals of epicardial coronary intervention, for which there are data supporting a more "aggressive" endpoint.

Indications and Patient Selection

The primary indication for intracranial stenting is the presence of a symptomatic intracranial atherosclerotic stenosis that has not responded to optimal medical therapy (OMT). Treatment of asymptomatic stenoses is not recommended and is generally not performed because the risk of TIA, or stroke, is thought to be low. In patients with symptomatic, angiographically proven >50% intracranial stenoses measured via the WASID method, the risk of recurrent stroke is approximately 12% annually regardless of treatment with aspirin or warfarin.[102] However, in those who have a >70% stenosis the risk of stroke is approximately 22% annually[104] and these patients are the ideal candidates for intracranial intervention. Importantly, the patient's symptoms should be attributable to the territory distal to the stenotic segment, rather than due to the territory of a perforator arising from the stenosis.[105] Anecdotally, patients presenting with perforator ischemia have a high likelihood of complete perforator occlusion with subsequent infarction. Recently symptomatic patients, especially those with a large or disabling infarct, may have an increased risk of ICH.[106,107] Unless the need is pressing, some have advocated delaying treatment for 6 weeks or more in these patients.[108] Patients should also be selected with functional imaging to assess cerebrovascular reserve (i.e., collateral competence) since those patients with impaired reserve have the highest risk of stroke with medical therapy and may derive the most benefit from intervention.[105,109] Cerebrovascular reserve can be assessed with acetazolamide single photon emission CT (SPECT), breath-holding transcranial Doppler ultrasound (TCD) studies, acetazolamide perfusion CT, or positron emission tomography (PET) scanning.

Lesion characteristics are also important in patient selection and although the data on this subject are limited, it is the author's belief that the same risk factors for complications with coronary percutaneous interventions are also applicable for intracranial interventions.[105,110] Lesion length, eccentricity, calcification, and angulation, as well as small vessel size, proximity to a bifurcation, and large adjacent branches are all risk factors for complications. Given the fragility of the cerebral vessels these factors are even more relevant than in the thicker, more muscular coronary arteries.

The last but equally important selection criterion is the feasibility of balloon and stent delivery to the lesion. This is now less of an issue with the availability of the self-expanding cerebral stent systems but it remains important.[111] Vessel tortuosity, especially of the ICA or VA, can be so severe that guide catheters cannot be delivered into the parent artery and can even prevent balloon catheter delivery. The risk of vessel dissection or intracranial artery perforation is great in such cases. The author's approach is to not intervene if a stent is unlikely to be delivered safely in case there is vessel dissection or abrupt closure after PTA necessitating provisional stenting.

Clinical Manifestation

The clinical features of ICAD are varied. The most common presentation is ischemia but the specific symptoms depend on which vessel is involved and the eloquence of the brain region affected. TIAs often precede a stroke in patients with ICAD.[112] The stenoses may also cause hemodynamic symptoms that are stereotyped, recurrent, and may be precipitated by drops in systemic mean arterial pressure brought on by upright posture.[113] Symptoms may also be attributable to emboli into distal small branches; these typically cause mild deficits that can be transient or stereotyped and recurrent.[113,114] In patients with MCA or BA trunk stenoses the atherosclerotic involvement of the origins of perforators can occur. These perforator syndromes that have typical features and are often stereotyped are important to recognize as they may not be amenable to endovascular therapy.[115] Patients may also present with symptoms due to a combination of one of these mechanisms.[116]

Techniques

Patients who meet the indications for intracranial intervention should be adequately pretreated with a dual antiplatelet regimen consisting of aspirin and clopidogrel. Use of other agents is unproven and is discouraged. Balloon angioplasty alone may be performed using treatment with a single agent if necessary. Anecdotal experience suggests that confirmation of adequate platelet inhibition preprocedure will decrease ischemic complications. A full understanding of each patient's cerebrovascular anatomy is essential and can be gleaned by noninvasive imaging such as CT angiography (CTA) or magnetic resonance angiography (MRA), but thorough, multiplanar digital subtraction angiography (DSA) is also essential for understanding the anatomy, lesion configuration, sources of collateral flow, and the presence of other pathologies or anatomical variants. An important consideration is maintenance of side-branch patency, especially at bifurcations, and this is where thorough angiography is essential. Complex techniques like y-stenting, kissing-stents, etc., are generally not feasible, and if technically achievable, are likely to be associated with a high-risk of vessel perforation and death. Therefore a thorough knowledge of cerebrovascular anatomy and eloquence of the brain tissue served by a particular branch are essential in deciding which branch(s) it is safe to jail with a stent. Plaque-shifting, snow-plowing, etc., may all occur and should be anticipated with steps taken to avoid them if possible.

A femoral approach is preferred, especially for MCA and ICA procedures, but brachial or radial access may be considered for vertebrobasilar interventions if there is severe and unfavorable innominate, subclavian, or vertebral artery angulation. Heparin is given to achieve an activated clotting time (ACT) between 250 to 300 seconds. Routine use of GPIIb/IIIa receptor antagonists is not recommended. A 6 Fr guide catheter, with or without an intermediate catheter, should be placed distally in the cervical ICA or distal V2 segment of the VA if safe and feasible. If there is severe tortuosity then advancing a 6 Fr to 8 Fr sheath into the common carotid or subclavian arteries should be considered to provide additional support for the guide catheter. The lesion should then be crossed with a soft microwire with an atraumatic tip such as a Synchro or Transcend (Stryker Inc., Kalamazoo, Michigan). The guidewire should be advanced with great care to avoid cannulating small branches or perforators and this is best performed with roadmapping technology. For terminal ICA and MCA treatment the wire should be passed into the second or proximal third-order MCA branches and for VB treatment one of the PCA is adequate. Throughout the procedure a thorough angiographic assessment must be performed to exclude distal embolization, branch occlusion, dissection, or perforation.

The author recommends that these procedures be performed under local rather than general anesthesia, so as to permit frequent intraoperative neurological assessments.[94,117] Headache can be an important marker for impending vessel injury and should prompt a reassessment of wire position, balloon inflation rate and pressure, amount of force being used to deliver a stent, etc. Such maneuvers may avert disaster.[94]

No randomized data have shown superiority of stenting over angioplasty but similar to coronary disease intervention, stenting has been generally preferred.[118,119] The author's approach is to predilate the lesion with an undersized over-the-wire balloon; undersizing is essential as oversizing can lead to vessel rupture or dissection (**Figure 25-3**).[108] This approach permits adequate sizing of the vessel and observation of lesion response to angioplasty, as well as the

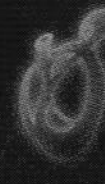

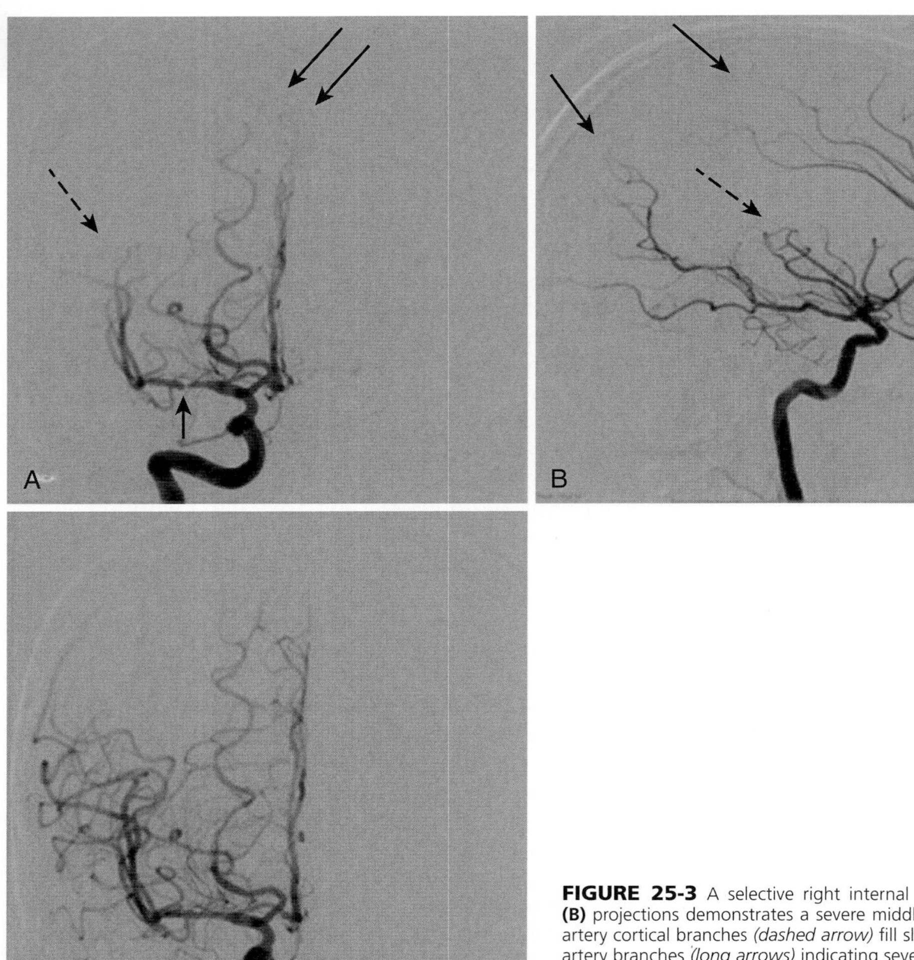

FIGURE 25-3 A selective right internal carotid angiogram in the anterio-posterior **(A)** and lateral **(B)** projections demonstrates a severe middle cerebral artery stenosis *(short arrow)*. The middle cerebral artery cortical branches *(dashed arrow)* fill slower than the anterior cerebral and (fetal) posterior cerebral artery branches *(long arrows)* indicating severe flow-limitation. Following stenting with a 2.75 mm stent, there is normalization of antegrade flow **(C)** with a marked, but not complete, normalization of the vessel lumen.

development of pain. A headache with submaximal balloon inflation suggests that the patient's vessel may not tolerate a stent much larger than the predilation balloon or that inflation rates need to be slower.[94] Nitroglycerin (200-400 μg) may then be given through the guide catheter before angiography to obtain the best size of the vessel. Depending on the circumstances, if there is an excellent result following PTA, with <30% residual stenosis, stenting may not be necessary. Otherwise, stenting should be considered with a stent sized no larger than the smallest normal segment into which the stent will be placed and with the minimal length needed to cover the lesion or angioplasty segment. Stenting of the ICA terminus or the vertebrobasilar junction is particularly difficult due to big step-off in size of the vessels. At those locations a self-expanding stent may be preferred, if there is a big size discrepancy between parent vessel and the branch.

The most challenging aspect of these procedures is stent delivery.[117] The latest generation of cobalt-chromium coronary stents has proven to be highly deliverable but in 8% to 10% of patients even these stents cannot be delivered safely, especially through the severe angulation of the cavernous carotid artery.[120] Better guide catheter support, exchanging for medium support wires, buddy wires, and other "tricks" may sometimes facilitate stent delivery.[121] Very stiff wires should never be used in the intracranial vessels. Throughout, close observation of the patient and monitoring for headache should be carried out.[94]

There are two stents that have been developed specifically for the cerebral vasculature. The balloon expandable Neurolink (Guidant Corp.) stent, was evaluated in a 43-patient trial (SSYLVIA)[122] and was highly deliverable, but it demonstrated a high restenosis rate of 32.4%. It is not approved in the United States. The more recent device, the Wingspan stent (Stryker Inc.) is a self-expanding, nitinol, highly flexible and deliverable stent. It received FDA approval under a humanitarian device exemption (HDE) following a prospective single arm 45 patient study.[123] Although highly deliverable, the clinical results with Wingspan have not been as good as expected (see further on). Therefore, the ideal device for the treatment of intracranial stenosis is yet to be developed. It is the author's opinion that the clinician must decide on a case-by-case basis which device to use, and it is also important to discuss the options with the patient beforehand, clearly explaining any off-label use and that the Wingspan system is the only FDA-approved device.

Postdilation is rarely needed unless a self-expanding stent is used; however, it must be noted that the instructions for use of the Wingspan stent warn against postdilation. Based on the author's (anecdotal) experience, postdilation of the Wingspan is almost always needed to avoid a very small residual lumen; as always a slightly undersized compliant balloon should be used. The procedure may be terminated after a final neurological assessment and a thorough evaluation of multiplanar angiograms.

Embolism and thrombosis are the most likely causes of ischemia during angioplasty and stenting, but dissection and vasospasm may also occur and cause symptoms. If a new neurological deficit is found during the intervention, an immediate cerebral angiogram of the likely culprit vessel should be performed in multiple orthogonal planes and reviewed closely. If a large vessel occlusion is seen (e.g., ICA, MCA trunk, or first order branch occlusion), or if the patient has a severe neurological deficit, then EVT must be rapidly performed following the approach described earlier but with the following precautions: the stent-retriever systems should be avoided if a stent is already deployed, as they can become ensnared and fibrinolytics, and GPIIb/IIIa antagonists should be used with extreme caution in patients with recent stroke or profound hypertension, due to the risk of cerebral hyperperfusion syndrome. The latter can lead to fatal ICH.[124-126] Cerebral vasospasm is very common and is commonly transient, asymptomatic, and generally does not require treatment but if severe may be treated with nitroglycerin, verapamil, or cardene.

If there is any deterioration, and angiography does not show an occlusion, an expanding ICH should be suspected and intraoperative CT should be performed immediately. If there is frank extravasation of contrast on angiography, immediate blood pressure reduction, heparin reversal, and transfusion of coagulation factors and platelets should be performed. Temporary balloon occlusion should be considered. Rarely, therapeutic embolization and vessel sacrifice may be needed to save the patient's life. For the most part, there is no treatment for ICH and SAH and what treatment exists is either ineffective or associated with a high risk of ischemia, and few patients survive an ICH despite all of the measures mentioned.[127] Prevention and treatment of cerebral hyperperfusion are aggressive blood pressure control postoperatively, ideally to SBP <120 mm Hg or even lower.[128]

Close observation of neurological status and monitoring of blood pressure are critical postoperatively as described above following acute stroke EVT. Dual antiplatelet therapy should be continued for at least 30 days, but the author's approach is to continue them for 6 to 12 months (1-2 years for a drug-eluting stent [DES]) or until a follow-up angiogram confirms that there is no restenosis.[120] This is very controversial because of the lack of long-term safety data and the presence of evidence that dual therapy increases the risk of ICH in some stroke patients.[129,130]

Clinical Outcomes

Up until recently the only data available were those from retrospective series of patients treated with balloons or balloon expandable coronary stents. The outcomes from those series have been highly variable because of differences in patient selection, technique, operator experience, and a lack of adequate angiographic and clinical follow-up.[101] Therefore, no firm conclusions regarding long-term safety, efficacy, and durability could be drawn from those data. Most studies reported 30-day stroke, ICH, and death rates of 8% to 20%, but some reported rates as high as 50%, with an average rate of 10% to 12%.[94,107,108,131-143] The author and others have reported on the limited use of DES for intracranial stenoses, with excellent success. However, the ultimate safety of this approach remains unclear.[133,144]

Two registries of real world experience with the Wingspan stent system have been published. The first of those studies included 78 patients with a major periprocedural complication rate of 6.1%. However, in-stent restenosis (≥50% narrowing) was seen in 34.5% of patients and the stent thrombosis rate was 4.1%.[145] The largest prospective registry included 129 patients with symptomatic 70% to 99% stenoses. The technical success rate was 96.7% with a 30-day stroke/death rate of 9.6%.[146] Restenosis was seen in 24.5% of those who underwent follow-up imaging. When compared with the event rates in patients on medical therapy in the WASID trial beyond 3 months, the recurrent event rate was lower for those stented. Restenosis rates appear to be high with the Wingspan stent and its management is generally repeat angioplasty.[147]

The largest registry of angioplasty and stenting ever published retrospectively reviewed the outcomes of 670 treated lesions in 637 patients from five international centers.[148] The majority 454 (68%) were treated with balloon expandable stents and the remainder received a self-expanding stent. The 30-day periprocedural complication rate was 6.1% and was similar between the types of stents. Treatment within 24 hours of the presenting stroke was a major predictor of complications (OR 4.0; 95% CI, 1.7-6.7; $p < 0.007$). As expected, focal lesions were associated with lower perioperative events (OR 0.31; 95% CI, 0.13-0.72; $p < 0.001$). Midterm restenosis rates were lower in patients with a lower post-treatment residual stenosis (OR 0.97; 95% CI, 0.95-0.99; $p < 0.006$) and in patients treated with balloon expandable (20%) versus self-expanding stents (28%).

The only published randomized trial data of intracranial stenting comes from the Stenting and Aggressive Medical Management for Preventing Recurrent Stroke in Intracranial Arterial Stenosis (SAMMPRIS) trial.[106] That trial randomized 451 patients with a recently symptomatic 70% to 99% stenosis to either OMT or OMT plus angioplasty and stenting with the Wingspan stent system. The trial was stopped early after a planned interim analysis showed that the 30-day stroke:death rate was 14.7% with angioplasty and stenting, but only 5.8% with OMT ($p = 0.002$).[106] The 30-day risk of angioplasty and stenting was approximately twice as high as previously assumed and the 30-day risk under OMT alone was approximately half of predicted.[102,145,146] Although SAMMPRIS was the best and largest trial to date, it had significant limitations.[105,149] The major limitations included the following:

1. Inclusion of patients who had not failed OMT and who were many days or weeks from the primary event, creating selection bias for patients who would do well with OMT.
2. The operators did not have to have experience with the Wingspan stent or with treatment of ICAD.
3. Patients were not selected based on the presence of decreased flow reserve.
4. Patients with perforator ischemia were enrolled, thus increasing the risk of complications (the majority of ischemic complications were due to perforator occlusion), and with minimal potential for benefit.
5. The procedures were performed under general anesthesia, thus preventing assessment of neurological status, or pain, and resulting in a high number of wire perforations and ICH.[105,149]

The only other randomized trial (Vitesse Intracranial Stent Study for Ischemic Therapy [VISSIT]) was stopped early due to futility and the results have not been published or presented.[150] That trial was of a novel balloon expandable stent (Pharos Vitesse stent [Codman Inc.]) designed for the neurovasculature. Other than the issue of deliverability, there are many reasons that balloon expandable stents may be preferred for ICAD, much like coronary PTCA.[148] However, given the SAMMPRIS data, the current medical-legal environment, and the fact that Wingspan is the only FDA-approved device, the use of balloon expandable stents is problematic.

There are very limited long-term follow-up data. The only series reporting long-term follow-up included 53 patients with 69 arterial lesions treated with a mix of angioplasty, bare-metal stents, and DES[120] who were followed for up to 7 years (median 24 months). The 30-day death:stroke rate was 10.1%, with only one death. The 2-year stroke/death/TIA rate was 15.9%, significantly lower than the 22% to 23% annual rate of stroke expected with medical therapy. One-year restenosis was 15.9%, 18.2% of which were symptomatic. Restenosis was associated with vessel size <2.5 mm (hazard ratio [HR] = 4.78; 95% CI, 1.35-16.93) and interventions performed in the setting of an acute stroke (HR = 6.36; 95% CI, 1.78-22.56).

CONCLUSIONS

Acute ischemic stroke due to large vessel occlusion can be effectively treated endovascularly, but the outcomes are highly dependent on appropriate patient selection. The newest generation of mechanical embolectomy devices is highly effective at achieving rapid recanalization in embolic stroke. Emergent angioplasty and stenting may be effective in cases of atherosclerotic occlusion. Due to the lack of efficacy and durability data from prospective, randomized clinical trials, intracranial stenting remains investigational and should be used only in carefully selected patients who have failed medical therapy and only after thorough evaluation of their clinical presentation, vascular anatomy, and the presence of impaired cerebrovascular reserve. There is a pressing need for prospective clinical trials of both procedures.

References

1. Lloyd-Jones D, Adams RJ, Brown TM, et al: Executive summary: Heart disease and stroke statistics—2010 update: a report from the American Heart Association. *Circulation* 121:948–954, 2010.
2. Roger VL, Go AS, Lloyd-Jones DM, et al: Heart disease and stroke statistics—2011 update: a report from the American Heart Association. *Circulation* 123:e18–e209, 2011.
3. Bozzao L, Fantozzi LM, Bastianello S, et al: Ischaemic supratentorial stroke: angiographic findings in patients examined in the very early phase. *J Neurol* 236:340–342, 1989.
4. Sacco RL, Benjamin EJ, Broderick JP, et al: American Heart Association Prevention Conference. IV. Prevention and rehabilitation of stroke. Risk factors. *Stroke* 28:1507–1517, 1997.
5. Sacco RL, Boden-Albala B, Gan R, et al: Stroke incidence among white, black, and hispanic residents of an urban community: The Northern Manhattan Stroke Study. *Am J Epidemiol* 147:259–268, 1998.
6. Adams Jr, HP, Bendixen BH, Kappelle LJ, et al: Classification of subtype of acute ischemic stroke. Definitions for use in a multicenter clinical trial. TOAST. Trial of org 10172 in acute stroke treatment. *Stroke* 24:35–41, 1993.
7. Arnold M, Halpern M, Meier N, et al: Age-dependent differences in demographics, risk factors, co-morbidity, etiology, management, and clinical outcome of acute ischemic stroke. *J Neurol* 255:1503–1507, 2008.
8. Sacco RL, Boden-Albala B, Abel G, et al: Race-ethnic disparities in the impact of stroke risk factors: The Northern Manhattan Stroke Study. *Stroke* 32:1725–1731, 2001.
9. Mayberg MR, Batjer HH, Dacey R, et al: Guidelines for the management of aneurysmal subarachnoid hemorrhage. A statement for healthcare professionals from a special writing group of the Stroke Council, American Heart Association. *Circulation* 90:2592–2605, 1994.
10. Mohr JP, Caplan LR, Melski JW, et al: The Harvard Cooperative Stroke Registry: a prospective registry. *Neurology* 28:754–762, 1978.
11. Rothwell PM, Giles MF, Flossmann E, et al: A simple score (ABCD) to identify individuals at high early risk of stroke after transient ischaemic attack. *Lancet* 366:29–36, 2005.
12. Johnston SC: Short-term prognosis after a TIA: a simple score predicts risk. *Cleve Clin J Med* 74:729–736, 2007.
13. Easton JD, Saver JL, Albers GW, et al: Definition and evaluation of transient ischemic attack: a scientific statement for healthcare professionals from the American Heart Association/American Stroke Association Stroke Council; Council on Cardiovascular Surgery and Anesthesia; Council on Cardiovascular Radiology and Intervention; Council on Cardiovascular Nursing; and the Interdisciplinary Council on Peripheral Vascular Disease. The American Academy of Neurology affirms the value of this statement as an educational tool for neurologists. *Stroke* 40:2276–2293, 2009.
14. Johnston SC, Albers GW, Gorelick PB, et al: National Stroke Association recommendations for systems of care for transient ischemic attack. *Ann Neurol* 69:872–877, 2011.
15. Furie KL, Kasner SE, Adams RJ, et al: Guidelines for the prevention of stroke in patients with stroke or transient ischemic attack: a guideline for healthcare professionals from the American Heart Association/American Stroke Association. *Stroke* 42:227–276, 2011.
16. Adams Jr, HP, del Zoppo G, Alberts MJ, et al: Guidelines for the early management of adults with ischemic stroke: a guideline from the American Heart Association/American Stroke Association Stroke Council, Clinical Cardiology Council, Cardiovascular Radiology and Intervention Council, and the Atherosclerotic Peripheral Vascular Disease and Quality of Care Outcomes in Research Interdisciplinary Working Groups: The American Academy of Neurology affirms the value of this guideline as an educational tool for neurologists. *Stroke* 38:1655–1711, 2007.
17. Broderick JP, Adams Jr, HP, Barsan W, et al: Guidelines for the management of spontaneous intracerebral hemorrhage: a statement for healthcare professionals from a special writing group of the Stroke Council, American Heart Association. *Stroke* 30:905–915, 1999.
18. Adams Jr, HP, Brott TG, Furlan AJ, et al: Guidelines for thrombolytic therapy for acute stroke: a supplement to the guidelines for the management of patients with acute ischemic stroke. A statement for healthcare professionals from a special writing group of the Stroke Council, American Heart Association. *Circulation* 94:1167–1174, 1996.
19. Li Q, Li J, Lv F, et al: A multidetector CT angiography study of variations in the circle of Willis in a Chinese population. *J Clin Neurosci* 18:379–383, 2011.
20. Macchi C, Lova RM, Miniati B, et al: The circle of Willis in healthy older persons. *J Cardiovasc Surg (Torino)* 43:887–890, 2002.
21. The National Institute of Neurological Disorders and Stroke rt-PA Stroke Study Group: Tissue plasminogen activator for acute ischemic stroke. *N Engl J Med* 333:1581–1587, 1995.
22. Hsia AW, Edwards DF, Morgenstern LB, et al: Racial disparities in tissue plasminogen activator treatment rate for stroke: a population-based study. *Stroke* 42:2217–2221, 2011.
23. Eissa A, Krass I, Bajorek BV: Optimizing the management of acute ischaemic stroke: a review of the utilization of intravenous recombinant tissue plasminogen activator (tPA). *J Clin Pharm Ther* 37:620–629, 2012.
24. Kleindorfer D, Lindsell CJ, Brass L, et al: National US estimates of recombinant tissue plasminogen activator use: Icd-9 codes substantially underestimate. *Stroke* 39:924–928, 2008.
25. Katzan IL, Hammer MD, Hixson ED, et al: Utilization of intravenous tissue plasminogen activator for acute ischemic stroke. *Arch Neurol* 61:346–350, 2004.
26. Wolpert SM, Bruckmann H, Greenlee R, et al: Neuroradiologic evaluation of patients with acute stroke treated with recombinant tissue plasminogen activator. The rt-PA Acute Stroke Study Group. *AJNR Am J Neuroradiol* 14:3–13, 1993.
27. Saqqur M, Uchino K, Demchuk AM, et al: Site of arterial occlusion identified by transcranial doppler predicts the response to intravenous thrombolysis for stroke. *Stroke* 38:948–954, 2007.
28. Meyers PM, Schumacher HC, Higashida RT, et al: Indications for the performance of intracranial endovascular neurointerventional procedures: a scientific statement from the American Heart Association Council on Cardiovascular Radiology and Intervention, Stroke Council, Council on Cardiovascular Surgery and Anesthesia, Interdisciplinary Council on Peripheral Vascular Disease, and Interdisciplinary Council on Quality of Care and Outcomes Research. *Circulation* 119:2235–2249, 2009.
29. Kharitonova T, Ahmed N, Thoren M, et al: Hyperdense middle cerebral artery sign on admission CT scan—prognostic significance for ischaemic stroke patients treated with intravenous thrombolysis in the safe implementation of thrombolysis in stroke international stroke thrombolysis register. *Cerebrovasc Dis* 27:51–59, 2009.
30. De Silva DA, Brekenfeld C, Ebinger M, et al: The benefits of intravenous thrombolysis relate to the site of baseline arterial occlusion in the Echoplanar Imaging Thrombolytic Evaluation Trial (EPITHET). *Stroke* 41:295–299, 2010.
31. Riedel CH, Zimmermann P, Jensen-Kondering U, et al: The importance of size: successful recanalization by intravenous thrombolysis in acute anterior stroke depends on thrombus length. *Stroke* 42:1775–1777, 2011.
32. Saver JL, Yafeh B: Confirmation of tPA treatment effect by baseline severity-adjusted end point reanalysis of the NINDS-tPA stroke trials. *Stroke* 38:414–416, 2007.
33. Del Zoppo GJ, Saver JL, Jauch EC, et al: Expansion of the time window for treatment of acute ischemic stroke with intravenous tissue plasminogen activator: a science advisory from the American Heart Association/American Stroke Association. *Stroke* 40:2945–2948, 2009.
34. Mattle HP, Arnold M, Georgiadis D, et al: Comparison of intraarterial and intravenous thrombolysis for ischemic stroke with hyperdense middle cerebral artery sign. *Stroke* 39:379–383, 2008.
35. Lansberg MG, Thijs VN, Bammer R, et al: The MRA-DWI mismatch identifies patients with stroke who are likely to benefit from reperfusion. *Stroke* 39:2491–2496, 2008.
36. Davis SM, Donnan GA, Parsons MW, et al: Effects of alteplase beyond 3 h after stroke in the Echoplanar Imaging Thrombolytic Evaluation Trial (EPITHET): a placebo-controlled randomised trial. *Lancet Neurol* 7:299–309, 2008.
37. Abou-Chebl A: Endovascular treatment of acute ischemic stroke may be safely performed with no time window limit in appropriately selected patients. *Stroke* 41:1996–2000, 2010.
38. Jovin TG, Liebeskind DS, Gupta R, et al: Imaging-based endovascular therapy for acute ischemic stroke due to proximal intracranial anterior circulation occlusion treated beyond 8 hours from time last seen well: retrospective multicenter analysis of 237 consecutive patients. *Stroke* 42:2206–2211, 2011.
39. Furlan A, Higashida R, Wechsler L, et al: Intra-arterial prourokinase for acute ischemic stroke. The PROACT II study: a randomized controlled trial. Prolyse in Acute Cerebral Thromboembolism. *JAMA* 282:2003–2011, 1999.
40. Lansberg MG, Straka M, Kemp S, et al: MRI profile and response to endovascular reperfusion after stroke (DEFUSE 2): a prospective cohort study. *Lancet Neurol* 11:860–867, 2012.
41. Hill MD, Rowley HA, Adler F, et al: Selection of acute ischemic stroke patients for intra-arterial thrombolysis with pro-urokinase by using aspects. *Stroke* 34:1925–1931, 2003.
42. Nogueira RG, Smith WS: Safety and efficacy of endovascular thrombectomy in patients with abnormal hemostasis: pooled analysis of the Merci and Multi Merci trials. *Stroke* 40:516–522, 2009.
43. Natsis KI, Tsitouridis IA, Didagelos MV, et al: Anatomical variations in the branches of the human aortic arch in 633 angiographies: clinical significance and literature review. *Surg Radiol Anat* 31:319–323, 2009.
44. Ribo M, Flores A, Rubiera M, et al: Extending the time window for endovascular procedures according to collateral pial circulation. *Stroke* 42:3465–3469, 2011.
45. Liebeskind DS, Tomsick TA, Foster LD, et al: Collaterals at angiography and outcomes in the interventional management of stroke (IMS) III trial. *Stroke* 45:759–764, 2014.
46. Kim JJ, Fischbein NJ, Lu Y, et al: Regional angiographic grading system for collateral flow: correlation with cerebral infarction in patients with middle cerebral artery occlusion. *Stroke* 35:1340–1344, 2004.
47. The Multicenter Acute Stroke Trial—Europe Study Group: Thrombolytic therapy with streptokinase in acute ischemic stroke. *N Engl J Med* 335:145–150, 1996.
48. Arnold M, Schroth G, Nedeltchev K, et al: Intra-arterial thrombolysis in 100 patients with acute stroke due to middle cerebral artery occlusion. *Stroke* 33:1828–1833, 2002.

49. Barnwell SL, Clark WM, Nguyen TT, et al: Safety and efficacy of delayed intraarterial urokinase therapy with mechanical clot disruption for thromboembolic stroke. *AJNR Am J Neuroradiol* 15:1817–1822, 1994.
50. Brekenfeld C, Remonda L, Nedeltchev K, et al: Endovascular neuroradiological treatment of acute ischemic stroke: Techniques and results in 350 patients. *Neurol Res* 27(Suppl 1):S29–S35, 2005.
51. Chang KC, Hsu SW, Liou CW, et al: Intra-arterial thrombolytic therapy for acute intracranial large artery occlusive disease in patients selected by magnetic resonance image. *J Neurol Sci* 297:46–51, 2010.
52. Tountopoulou A, Ahl B, Weissenborn K, et al: Intra-arterial thrombolysis using rt-pa in patients with acute stroke due to vessel occlusion of anterior and/or posterior cerebral circulation. *Neuroradiology* 50:75–83, 2008.
53. Mandava P, Kent TA: Intra-arterial therapies for acute ischemic stroke. *Neurology* 68:2132–2139, 2007.
54. del Zoppo GJ, Ferbert A, Otis S, et al: Local intra-arterial fibrinolytic therapy in acute carotid territory stroke. A pilot study. *Stroke* 19:307–313, 1988.
55. Qureshi AI, Harris-Lane P, Kirmani JF, et al: Intra-arterial reteplase and intravenous abciximab in patients with acute ischemic stroke: an open-label, dose-ranging, phase I study. *Neurosurgery* 59:789–796, 2006.
56. Qureshi AI, Ali Z, Suri MF, et al: Intra-arterial third-generation recombinant tissue plasminogen activator (reteplase) for acute ischemic stroke. *Neurosurgery* 49:41–48, 2001.
57. Yokogami K, Nakano S, Ohta H, et al: Prediction of hemorrhagic complications after thrombolytic therapy for middle cerebral artery occlusion: value of pre- and post-therapeutic computed tomographic findings and angiographic occlusive site. *Neurosurgery* 39:1102–1107, 1996.
58. Abou-Chebl A, Bajzer CT, Krieger DW, et al: Multimodal therapy for the treatment of severe ischemic stroke combining GPIIb/IIIa antagonists and angioplasty after failure of thrombolysis. *Stroke* 36:2286–2288, 2005.
59. Lee DH, Jo KD, Kim HG, et al: Local intraarterial urokinase thrombolysis of acute ischemic stroke with or without intravenous abciximab: a pilot study. *J Vasc Interv Radiol* 13:769–774, 2002.
60. Adams Jr, HP, Effron MB, Torner J, et al: Emergency administration of abciximab for treatment of patients with acute ischemic stroke: Results of an international phase iii trial: abciximab in emergency treatment of stroke trial (abestt-ii). *Stroke* 39:87–99, 2008.
61. IMS II Trial Investigators: The interventional management of stroke (IMS) II study. *Stroke* 38:2127–2135, 2007.
62. Broderick JP, Palesch YY, Demchuk AM, et al: Endovascular therapy after intravenous t-PA versus t-PA alone for stroke. *N Engl J Med* 368:893–903, 2013.
63. Smith WS, Sung G, Saver J, et al: Mechanical thrombectomy for acute ischemic stroke: final results of the Multi Merci trial. *Stroke* 39:1205–1212, 2008.
64. Ribo M, Alvarez-Sabin J, Montaner J, et al: Temporal profile of recanalization after intravenous tissue plasminogen activator: selecting patients for rescue reperfusion techniques. *Stroke* 37:1000–1004, 2006.
65. Wikholm G: Mechanical intracranial embolectomy. A report of two cases. *Interv Neuroradiol* 4:159–164, 1998.
66. Chopko BW, Kerber C, Wong W, et al: Transcatheter snare removal of acute middle cerebral artery thromboembolism: technical case report. *Neurosurgery* 46:1529–1531, 2000.
67. Smith WS, Sung G, Starkman S, et al: Safety and efficacy of mechanical embolectomy in acute ischemic stroke: results of the Merci trial. *Stroke* 36:1432–1438, 2005.
68. Nakano S, Iseda T, Yoneyama T, et al: Direct percutaneous transluminal angioplasty for acute middle cerebral artery trunk occlusion: an alternative option to intra-arterial thrombolysis. *Stroke* 33:2872–2876, 2002.
69. Yoneyama T, Nakano S, Kawano H, et al: Combined direct percutaneous transluminal angioplasty and low-dose native tissue plasminogen activator therapy for acute embolic middle cerebral artery trunk occlusion. *AJNR Am J Neuroradiol* 23:277–281, 2002.
70. Sacco RL, Kargman DE, Gu Q, et al: Race-ethnicity and determinants of intracranial atherosclerotic cerebral infarction. The Northern Manhattan Stroke Study. *Stroke* 26:14–20, 1995.
71. Ringer AJ, Qureshi AI, Fessler RD, et al: Angioplasty of intracranial occlusion resistant to thrombolysis in acute ischemic stroke. *Neurosurgery* 48:1282–1288, 2001.
72. Qureshi AI, Siddiqui AM, Suri MF, et al: Aggressive mechanical clot disruption and low-dose intra-arterial third-generation thrombolytic agent for ischemic stroke: a prospective study. *Neurosurgery* 51:1319–1327, 2002.
73. Gupta R, Vora NA, Horowitz MB, et al: Multimodal reperfusion therapy for acute ischemic stroke: factors predicting vessel recanalization. *Stroke* 37:986–990, 2006.
74. Zaidat OO, Wolfe T, Hussain SI, et al: Interventional acute ischemic stroke therapy with intracranial self-expanding stent. *Stroke* 39:2392–2395, 2008.
75. Abou-Chebl A, Vora N, Yadav JS: Safety of angioplasty and stenting without thrombolysis for the treatment of early ischemic stroke. *J Neuroimaging* 19:139–143, 2009.
76. Levy EI, Siddiqui AH, Crumlish A, et al: First food and drug administration-approved prospective trial of primary intracranial stenting for acute stroke: saris (stent-assisted recanalization in acute ischemic stroke). *Stroke* 40:3552–3556, 2009.
77. Jovin TG, Gupta R, Uchino K, et al: Emergent stenting of extracranial internal carotid artery occlusion in acute stroke has a high revascularization rate. *Stroke* 36:2426–2430, 2005.
78. Larrue V, von Kummer RR, Muller A, et al: Risk factors for severe hemorrhagic transformation in ischemic stroke patients treated with recombinant tissue plasminogen activator: a secondary analysis of the European-Australasian Acute Stroke Study (ECASS II). *Stroke* 32:438–441, 2001.
79. Hacke W, Kaste M, Fieschi C, et al: Randomised double-blind placebo-controlled trial of thrombolytic therapy with intravenous alteplase in acute ischaemic stroke (ECASS II). Second European-Australasian Acute Stroke Study investigators. *Lancet* 352:1245–1251, 1998.
80. Tomsick T: TIMI, TIBI, TICI: I came, I saw, I got confused. *AJNR Am J Neuroradiol* 28:382–384, 2007.
81. Albers GW, Clark WM, Madden KP, et al: Atlantis trial: Results for patients treated within 3 hours of stroke onset. Alteplase thrombolysis for acute noninterventional therapy in ischemic stroke. *Stroke* 33:493–495, 2002.
82. Ogawa A, Mori E, Minematsu K, et al: Randomized trial of intraarterial infusion of urokinase within 6 hours of middle cerebral artery stroke: the Middle Cerebral Artery Embolism Local Fibrinolytic Intervention Trial (MELT) Japan. *Stroke* 38:2633–2639, 2007.
83. Hoffman AI, Lambiase RE, Haas RA, et al: Acute vertebrobasilar occlusion: treatment with high-dose intraarterial urokinase. *AJR Am J Roentgenol* 172:709–712, 1999.
84. Chalela JA, Katzan I, Liebeskind DS, et al: Safety of intra-arterial thrombolysis in the postoperative period. *Stroke* 32:1365–1369, 2001.
85. Katzan IL, Masaryk TJ, Furlan AJ, et al: Intra-arterial thrombolysis for perioperative stroke after open heart surgery. *Neurology* 52:1081–1084, 1999.
86. Higashida RT, Furlan AJ, Roberts H, et al: Trial design and reporting standards for intra-arterial cerebral thrombolysis for acute ischemic stroke. *Stroke* 34:e109–e137, 2003.
87. Penumbra Pivotal Stroke Trial Investigators: The penumbra pivotal stroke trial: safety and effectiveness of a new generation of mechanical devices for clot removal in intracranial large vessel occlusive disease. *Stroke* 40:2761–2768, 2009.
88. Saver JL, Jahan R, Levy EI, et al: Solitaire flow restoration device versus the Merci retriever in patients with acute ischaemic stroke (SWIFT): a randomised, parallel-group, non-inferiority trial. *Lancet* 380:1241–1249, 2012.
89. Nogueira RG, Lutsep HL, Gupta R, et al: Trevo versus Merci retrievers for thrombectomy revascularisation of large vessel occlusions in acute ischaemic stroke (TREVO 2): a randomised trial. *Lancet* 380:1231–1240, 2012.
90. Abou-Chebl A, Lin R, Hussain MS, et al: Conscious sedation versus general anesthesia during endovascular therapy for acute anterior circulation stroke: preliminary results from a retrospective, multicenter study. *Stroke* 41:1175–1179, 2010.
91. Davis MJ, Menon BK, Baghirzada LB, et al: Anesthetic management and outcome in patients during endovascular therapy for acute stroke. *Anesthesiology* 116:396–405, 2012.
92. Gupta R: Local is better than general anesthesia during endovascular acute stroke interventions. *Stroke* 41:2718–2719, 2010.
93. Molina CA, Selim MH: General or local anesthesia during endovascular procedures: sailing quiet in the darkness or fast under a daylight storm. *Stroke* 41:2720–2721, 2010.
94. Abou-Chebl A, Krieger DW, Bajzer CT, et al: Intracranial angioplasty and stenting in the awake patient. *J Neuroimaging* 16:216–223, 2006.
95. Ahmed N, Nasman P, Wahlgren N: Effect of intravenous nimodipine on blood pressure and outcome after acute stroke. *Stroke* 31:1250–1255, 2000.
96. Ahmed N, Wahlgren N, Brainin M, et al: Relationship of blood pressure, antihypertensive therapy, and outcome in ischemic stroke treated with intravenous thrombolysis: retrospective analysis from Safe Implementation of Thrombolysis in Stroke-International Stroke Thrombolysis Register (SITS-ISTR). *Stroke* 40:2442–2449, 2009.
97. Sacco RL, Kargman DE, Zamanillo MC: Race-ethnic differences in stroke risk factors among hospitalized patients with cerebral infarction: the Northern Manhattan Stroke Study. *Neurology* 45:659–663, 1995.
98. Thijs VN, Albers GW: Symptomatic intracranial atherosclerosis: outcome of patients who fail antithrombotic therapy. [comment]. *Neurology* 55:490–497, 2000.
99. Wityk RJ, Lehman D, Klag M, et al: Race and sex differences in the distribution of cerebral atherosclerosis. *Stroke* 27:1974–1980, 1996.
100. Feldmann E, Daneault N, Kwan E, et al: Chinese-white differences in the distribution of occlusive cerebrovascular disease. *Neurology* 40:1541–1545, 1990.
101. Yadav JS, Abou-Chebl A: Intracranial angioplasty and stenting. *J Interv Cardiol* 22:9–15, 2009.
102. Chimowitz MI, Lynn MJ, Howlett-Smith H, et al: Comparison of warfarin and aspirin for symptomatic intracranial arterial stenosis. *N Engl J Med* 352:1305–1316, 2005.
103. Failure of extracranial-intracranial arterial bypass to reduce the risk of ischemic stroke. Results of an international randomized trial. The EC/IC Bypass Study Group. *N Engl J Med* 313:1191–1200, 1985.
104. Kasner SE, Chimowitz MI, Lynn MJ, et al: Predictors of ischemic stroke in the territory of a symptomatic intracranial arterial stenosis. *Circulation* 2006.
105. Abou-Chebl A, Steinmetz H: Critique of "stenting versus aggressive medical therapy for intracranial arterial stenosis" by Chimowitz et al in the New England Journal of Medicine. *Stroke* 43:616–620, 2012.
106. Chimowitz MI, Lynn MJ, Derdeyn CP, et al: Stenting versus aggressive medical therapy for intracranial arterial stenosis. *N Engl J Med* 365:993–1003, 2011.
107. Gupta R, Schumacher HC, Mangla S, et al: Urgent endovascular revascularization for symptomatic intracranial atherosclerotic stenosis. *Neurology* 61:1729–1735, 2003.
108. Connors JJ, III, Wojak JC: Percutaneous transluminal angioplasty for intracranial atherosclerotic lesions: evolution of technique and short-term results. *J Neurosurg* 91:415–423, 1999.
109. Liebeskind DS, Cotsonis GA, Saver JL, et al: Collaterals dramatically alter stroke risk in intracranial atherosclerosis. *Ann Neurol* 69:963–974, 2011.
110. Mori T, Fukuoka M, Kazita K, et al: Follow-up study after intracranial percutaneous transluminal cerebral balloon angioplasty. *AJNR Am J Neuroradiol* 19:1525–1533, 1998.
111. Jiang WJ, Cheng-Ching E, Abou-Chebl A, et al: Multi-center analysis of stenting in symptomatic intracranial atherosclerosis. *Neurosurgery* 2011.
112. Ovbiagele B, Cruz-Flores S, Lynn MJ, et al: Early stroke risk after transient ischemic attack among individuals with symptomatic intracranial artery stenosis. *Arch Neurol* 65:733–737, 2008.
113. Hinton RC, Mohr JP, Ackerman RH, et al: Symptomatic middle cerebral artery stenosis. *Ann Neurol* 5:152–157, 1979.
114. Adams HP, Gross CE: Embolism distal to stenosis of the middle cerebral artery. *Stroke* 12:228, 1981.
115. Caplan LR: Intracranial branch atheromatous disease: a neglected, understudied, and underused concept. *Neurology* 39:1246–1250, 1989.
116. Caplan LR, Hennerici M: Impaired clearance of emboli (washout) is an important link between hypoperfusion, embolism, and ischemic stroke. *Arch Neurol* 55:1475–1482, 1998.
117. Jiang WJ, Yu W, Du B, et al: Wingspan experience at Beijing Tiantan hospital: New insights into the mechanisms of procedural complication from viewing intraoperative transient ischemic attacks during awake stenting for vertebrobasilar stenosis. *J Neurointerv Surg* 2:99–103, 2010.
118. Foley DP, Serruys PW: Provisional stenting—stent-like balloon angioplasty: evidence to define the continuing role of balloon angioplasty for percutaneous coronary revascularization. *Semin Interv Cardiol* 1:269–273, 1996.
119. Knight CJ, Curzen NP, Groves PH, et al: Stent implantation reduces restenosis in patients with suboptimal results following coronary angioplasty. *Eur Heart J* 20:1783–1790, 1999.
120. Mazighi M, Yadav JS, Abou-Chebl A: Durability of endovascular therapy for symptomatic intracranial atherosclerosis. *Stroke* 39:1766–1769, 2008.
121. Lee TH, Choi CH, Park KP, et al: Techniques for intracranial stent navigation in patients with tortuous vessels. *AJNR Am J Neuroradiol* 26:1375–1380, 2005.
122. SSYLVIA Study Investigators: Stenting of Symptomatic Atherosclerotic Lesions in the Vertebral or Intracranial Arteries (SSYLVIA): Study results. *Stroke* 35:1388–1392, 2004.
123. Bose A, Hartmann M, Henkes H, et al: A novel, self-expanding, nitinol stent in medically refractory intracranial atherosclerotic stenoses: the Wingspan study. *Stroke* 38:1531–1537, 2007.
124. Reigel MM, Hollier LH, Sundt TM, Jr, et al: Cerebral hyperperfusion syndrome: a cause of neurologic dysfunction after carotid endarterectomy. *J Vasc Surg* 5:628–634, 1987.
125. Abou-Chebl A, Yadav JS, Reginelli JP, et al: Intracranial hemorrhage and hyperperfusion syndrome following carotid artery stenting: risk factors, prevention, and treatment. *J Am Coll Cardiol* 43:1596–1601, 2004.
126. Meyers PM, Higashida RT, Phatouros CC, et al: Cerebral hyperperfusion syndrome after percutaneous transluminal stenting of the craniocervical arteries. *Neurosurgery* 47:335–343, discussion 343–335, 2000.
127. Khatri R, Ansar M, Sultan F, et al: Requirements for emergent neurosurgical procedures among patients undergoing neuroendovascular procedures in contemporary practice. *AJNR Am J Neuroradiol* 33:465–468, 2012.
128. Abou-Chebl A, Reginelli J, Bajzer CT, et al: Intensive treatment of hypertension decreases the risk of hyperperfusion and intracerebral hemorrhage following carotid artery stenting. *Catheter Cardiovasc Interv* 69:690–696, 2007.
129. Diener HC, Bogousslavsky J, Brass LM, et al: Aspirin and clopidogrel compared with clopidogrel alone after recent ischaemic stroke or transient ischaemic attack in high-risk patients (MATCH): Randomised, double-blind, placebo-controlled trial. *Lancet* 364:331–337, 2004.
130. Bhatt DL, Flather MD, Hacke W, et al: Patients with prior myocardial infarction, stroke, or symptomatic peripheral arterial disease in the CHARISMA trial. *J Am Coll Cardiol* 49:1982–1988, 2007.
131. Rasmussen PA, Perl J, Barr JD, et al: Stent-assisted angioplasty of intracranial vertebrobasilar atherosclerosis: an initial experience. *J Neurosurg* 92:771–778, 2000.
132. Alazzaz A, Thornton J, Aletich VA, et al: Intracranial percutaneous transluminal angioplasty for arteriosclerotic stenosis. *Arch Neurol* 57:1625–1630, 2000.
133. Abou-Chebl A, Bashir Q, Yadav JS: Drug-eluting stents for the treatment of intracranial atherosclerosis: initial experience and midterm angiographic follow-up. *Stroke* 36:e165–e168, 2005.

134. Weber W, Mayer TE, Henkes H, et al: Stent-angioplasty of intracranial vertebral and basilar artery stenoses in symptomatic patients. *Eur J Radiol* 55:231–236, 2005.
135. Kim DJ, Lee BH, Kim DI, et al: Stent-assisted angioplasty of symptomatic intracranial vertebrobasilar artery stenosis: feasibility and follow-up results. *AJNR Am J Neuroradiol* 26:1381–1388, 2005.
136. Higashida RT, Meyers PM, Connors JJ, III, et al: Intracranial angioplasty & stenting for cerebral atherosclerosis: a position statement of the American Society of Interventional and Therapeutic Neuroradiology, Society of Interventional Radiology, and the American Society of Neuroradiology. *AJNR Am J Neuroradiol* 26:2323–2327, 2005.
137. Jiang WJ, Wang YJ, Du B, et al: Stenting of symptomatic m1 stenosis of middle cerebral artery: an initial experience of 40 patients. *Stroke* 35:1375–1380, 2004.
138. Abou-Chebl A, Krieger D, Bajzer C, et al: Intracranial angioplasty and stenting in the awake patient. *Stroke* 34:2003.
139. Lee JH, Kwon SU, Lee JH, et al: Percutaneous transluminal angioplasty for symptomatic middle cerebral artery stenosis: Long-term follow-up. *Cerebrovasc Dis* 15:90–97, 2003.
140. Marks MP, Wojak JC, Al-Ali F, et al: Angioplasty for symptomatic intracranial stenosis: Clinical outcome. *Stroke* 37:1016–1020, 2006.
141. Mori T, Kazita K, Chokyu K, et al: Short-term arteriographic and clinical outcome after cerebral angioplasty and stenting for intracranial vertebrobasilar and carotid atherosclerotic occlusive disease. *AJNR Am J Neuroradiol* 21:249–254, 2000.
142. Mori T, Mori K, Fukuoka M, et al: Percutaneous transluminal cerebral angioplasty: serial angiographic follow-up after successful dilatation. *Neuroradiology* 39:111–116, 1997.
143. Lylyk P, Cohen JE, Ceratto R, et al: Angioplasty and stent placement in intracranial atherosclerotic stenoses and dissections. *AJNR Am J Neuroradiol* 23:430–436, 2002.
144. Gupta R, Al-Ali F, Thomas AJ, et al: Safety, feasibility, and short-term follow-up of drug-eluting stent placement in the intracranial and extracranial circulation. *Stroke* 37:2562–2566, 2006.
145. Fiorella D, Levy EI, Turk AS, et al: US multicenter experience with the Wingspan stent system for the treatment of intracranial atheromatous disease: periprocedural results. *Stroke* 38:881–887, 2007.
146. Zaidat OO, Klucznik R, Alexander MJ, et al: The NIH registry on use of the Wingspan stent for symptomatic 70-99% intracranial arterial stenosis. *Neurology* 70:1518–1524, 2008.
147. Levy EI, Turk AS, Albuquerque FC, et al: Wingspan in-stent restenosis and thrombosis: incidence, clinical presentation, and management. *Neurosurgery* 61:644–650, 2007.
148. Jiang WJ, Cheng-Ching E, Abou-Chebl A, et al: Multicenter analysis of stenting in symptomatic intracranial atherosclerosis. *Neurosurgery* 70:25–30, 2012.
149. Abou-Chebl A: Intracranial stenting with Wingspan: still awaiting a safe landing. *Stroke* 42:1809–1811, 2011.
150. Zaidat OO, Castonguay AC, Fitzsimmons BF, et al: Design of the Vitesse Intracranial Stent Study for Ischemic Therapy (VISSIT) trial in symptomatic intracranial stenosis. *J Stroke Cerebrovasc Dis* 22:1131–1139, 2013.

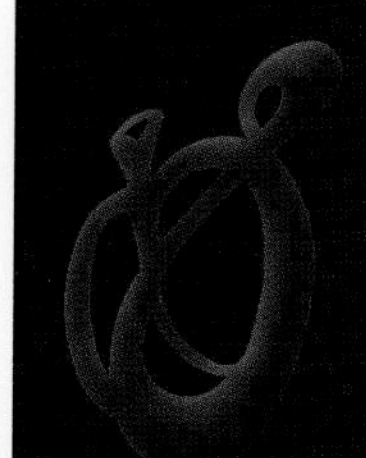

PART V

VENOUS INTERVENTION

26 Interventional Management of Lower Extremity Deep Vein Thrombosis and Pulmonary Embolism

Akhilesh K. Sista and Suresh Vedantham

INTRODUCTION

Venous thromboembolic disease (VTE), comprised of deep vein thrombosis (DVT) and pulmonary embolism (PE), is morbid, expensive, and potentially fatal. It ranks as the third most common cardiovascular disease, and consumes significant health care dollars.[1] Over the past several decades, the management of DVT and PE for many patients has been altered by the introduction of catheter-based therapies. Considerable data has been generated for these techniques during this time, although randomized trials are few. This chapter is divided into two sections, one discussing lower extremity DVT and the second describing the interventional management of pulmonary embolism. The DVT section will review epidemiology, medical management, the post-thrombotic syndrome and its prevention, and both the conservative and interventional management of established post-thrombotic syndrome. Section 2 will discuss the epidemiology, categorization, and escalation options for acute pulmonary embolism, with a focus on the evolving role of catheter-based techniques.

Section 1: Lower Extremity Deep Vein Thrombosis

Acute Deep Vein Thrombosis

Epidemiology and Pulmonary Embolus Prevention

It is estimated that 350,000 to 600,000 acute symptomatic DVTs are diagnosed per year in the United States, out of which up to 250,000 are a new diagnosis in the lower extremity. Given the 100,000 to 180,000 individuals who die of pulmonary embolism,[1] the treatment for DVT has traditionally focused on the prevention of PE through anticoagulation.[2] Since the focus of this chapter is the interventional management of VTE, an in-depth discussion of anticoagulation will not be provided here. Briefly, the majority of patients will be initiated on a parenteral regimen (e.g., unfractionated heparin, a low-molecular-weight heparin [LMWH], fondaparinux) and transitioned to an oral vitamin K antagonist (warfarin) for a minimum of 3 months, with the duration of therapy based on multiple factors, the most important being the presence or absence of reversible provoking factors. Patients with active cancer appear to derive the most benefit from extended LMWH therapy.[3,4] Recently, the oral factor X inhibitor rivaroxaban was FDA approved for the treatment of VTE, and it has gained traction given its convenience and apparent equal efficacy compared with warfarin.[5] If rivaroxaban is used, antecedent heparin therapy is not needed. However, rivaroxaban does not yet have an antidote, which can be problematic should bleeding occur, and the longitudinal experience physicians have had with warfarin for many years is lacking.

IVC Filters

When anticoagulation is contraindicated or fails, inferior vena cava (IVC) filters are frequently inserted to prevent large thrombi from traveling to the lungs. These two scenarios are relative indications for filter placement per societal guidelines.[2] Filters may also be placed in the setting of a hemodynamically significant pulmonary embolus in a patient with limited cardiopulmonary reserve who would poorly tolerate additional emboli. The placement of IVC filters for perioperative prophylaxis in patients who are deemed to be at high risk for VTE (e.g., patients with prior history of VTE who will be immobilized after surgery for a prolonged period) is controversial at present, with little substantiating data for or against. While filters are effective at preventing pulmonary embolism, they may be associated with a number of complications, including perforation, migration, fracture, and caval thrombosis/stenosis.[6] The PREPIC (Prevention du Risque d'Embolie Pulmonaire par Interruption Cave) study from the late 1990s indicated that in DVT patients who can be anticoagulated, filters reduce the rate of PE but increase the rate of DVT, resulting in a similar rate of VTE to patients not receiving filters.[7] Thus, insertion of a filter should be performed only after a thorough evaluation of the short-term and long-term risks and benefits. Moreover, when IVC filtration is no longer indicated, every effort should be made to remove the filter if safe to do so.

IVC filters may be retrievable or permanent. No data adequately compares the merits of one versus the other, but retrievable filters are being more frequently placed because of the potential ability to remove them at a later date and thus avoid some of the complications listed above. When selecting a retrievable filter brand, consideration of (1) the time window for planned retrieval and (2) the filter's track record in terms of extent of use and documented migrations/fractures/embolizations is worthwhile. Several new designs are entering the market in an attempt to overcome some of the complications associated with retrievable filters, but no formal recommendation can be made based on current data (Video 26-1). The insertion can be performed via the internal jugular vein, common femoral vein, or arm vein (brachial, basilic, or cephalic) if the delivery sheath is low profile. Care must be taken to ensure the appropriate orientation of the device if the same kit is used for a jugular or femoral insertion. Especially in the absence of prior cross-sectional imaging, venography prior to insertion provides some valuable information. The size of the cava, position of the renal veins, presence of caval thrombus, caval duplication, and variant anatomy such as a circumaortic renal vein can all be detected. If possible, venography should be performed from the left common iliac vein, as a duplicated cava can be detected most commonly from this position. Megacava is defined as a diameter greater than 28 mm; this finding is rare, and it is important to rule out a flattened cava by performing cavography at multiple obliquities. If one is found, only filters capable of filling the entire diameter, such as a bird's nest filter, should be deployed. If standard caval anatomy and size are present, the filter should be deployed inferior to the renal vein insertions to avoid trapped clot from propagating into the renal veins. In the event of caval duplication, two filters may be necessary (**Figure 26-1**). A circumaortic renal vein may require a suprarenal filter, given that it can act as a bypass circuit if the filter is inserted below its more cranial insertion. Post-deployment venography ensures proper positioning and may be useful for later retrieval.

As mentioned previously, given the later complications of IVC filters, the need for filtration should be reassessed at periodic time points after insertion if a retrievable filter was used; the optimal time frame for removal is within 4 to 6 weeks of placement. With time, filters can become embedded in the wall of the cava and more difficult to extract. At the time of retrieval, venography should be performed to exclude significant clot within the filter. In the absence of this, retrieval may proceed. A ubiquitous feature of currently available retrievable filters is a "hook" at the top or bottom that can be engaged with a snare. The venous access site (femoral vs. jugular) depends on filter design; however, most filters have the hook at the cranial aspect, necessitating a jugular approach. Once the snare grasps the hook, an appropriately sized sheath (typically between 10 and 12 Fr) can be advanced over the filter to collapse it, and the filter is then pulled through the sheath out the body (Video 26-2).

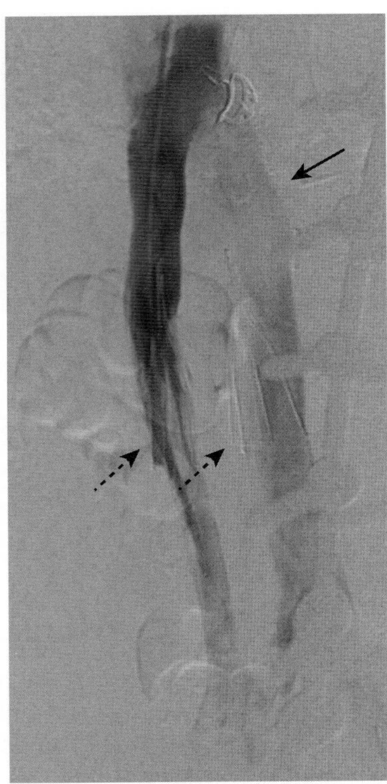

FIGURE 26-1 Inferior vena cavagram demonstrating a duplicated IVC *(solid arrow)*. Note subtracted IVC filters *(dashed arrows)* in both the main and duplicated IVC.

The Post-Thrombotic Syndrome

The traditional view of treating DVT with anticoagulation to prevent pulmonary embolism needs modification because of the growing awareness of the post-thrombotic syndrome (PTS). In spite of anticoagulation, ~40% of individuals suffering an acute symptomatic DVT experience some version of this disease. PTS is a constellation of chronic symptoms and signs in the affected limb that includes daily pain, swelling, aching, paresthesia, fatigue, and heaviness that worsen as the day progresses and in the standing position. Severe manifestations include stasis dermatitis, venous claudication, and ulceration (**Figure 26-2**). The post-thrombotic syndrome has been shown to adversely affect quality of life and self-perception, and the individual and societal costs (both direct medical and indirect loss of work) are significant.[8-14] Thus, any strategy that can prevent or reduce the severity of PTS needs to be examined.

The development of PTS following a proximal DVT is thought to be secondary to a combination of obstruction and valvular damage. While incompletely understood, the pathogenesis is related to an inflammatory leukocytic infiltration and cytokine release in response to acute thrombus that ultimately results in clot organization and wall thickening in the event of incomplete thrombus clearance.[15-18] The narrowed lumen causes outflow obstruction, and in

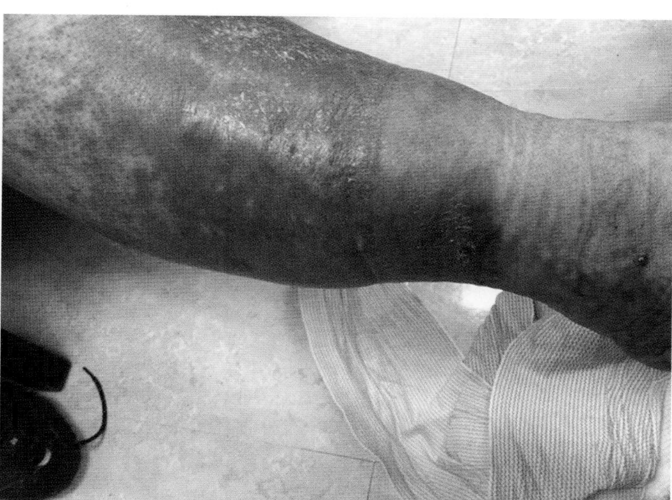

FIGURE 26-2 Severe PTS, with edema, hyperpigmentation, and healed ulcers.

combination with damaged valves, results in venous hypertension and dilation of more peripheral uninvolved deep and superficial veins.[19-22] Ultimately, the venous hypertension and reflux cause edema, calf pump dysfunction, tissue hypoxia, subcutaneous fibrosis, and ulceration.[23-26]

Several factors have been identified that place a patient at higher risk for developing the post-thrombotic syndrome. These include recurrent ipsilateral DVT (2.6-fold increased risk),[8] subtherapeutic anticoagulation (2.5-fold increased risk),[27] and iliofemoral (iliac and/or common femoral vein) DVT (50% incidence of PTS).[28,29] Minor risk factors include advanced age, obesity, and female gender. The main lesson is that a patient presenting with an iliofemoral DVT needs to receive meticulous anticoagulation therapy and monitoring to prevent recurrent DVT and PTS. It should be noted, however, that even with this approach, the rate of PTS in this population is unacceptably high.

Preventing the Post-Thrombotic Syndrome: Beyond Anticoagulation

Until recently, elastic compression stockings (ECS) were considered standard of care in the prevention of PTS, given two randomized single-center studies that demonstrated a reduction in PTS with their daily use.[30,31] However, the recently completed placebo-controlled, double-blind, randomized controlled multicenter SOX trial, which was more than twice as large as the two previous studies combined, demonstrated an equally high rate of PTS in the ECS group as the "sham" stocking group.[32] Thus, the best evidence suggests that ECS therapy does not prevent PTS and the recommendation to use compression stockings will likely come under scrutiny. However, a case-by-case approach may be appropriate to control PTS symptoms during long-term follow-up—if stockings provide symptomatic relief and there are no contraindications (e.g., peripheral arterial disease, skin hypersensitivity), the patient may certainly use them.

Given the high incidence of PTS following a symptomatic proximal DVT in spite of therapeutic anticoagulation, thromboreductive strategies, ranging from systemic thrombolysis to surgical embolectomy to catheter-directed techniques, have been trialled. These more aggressive strategies are predicated on the "open-vein" theory, which maintains that restoring patency to a thrombosed vein makes that vein less susceptible to re-thrombosis, reflux, and the pathophysiologic process leading to post-thrombotic syndrome. There is significant evidence to support the open-vein theory. Prandoni et al. noted higher 2-year rates of PTS in patients who had residual thrombus at 6 months.[22] Hull et al. found a strong correlation between the amount of residual thrombus and recurrent VTE,[33] which, as stated above, correlates with higher rates of PTS. Taking the lessons of small studies examining systemic thrombolysis and surgical embolectomy, aggressive thrombus clearance resulted in lower rates of PTS (albeit at the cost of higher morbidity and bleeding rates).[34-36]

From these experiences, catheter-directed therapy has emerged with the possibility of offering comparable or greater efficacy with less morbidity and bleeding. This approach allows for intra-thrombus injection of lytic to allow for greater clot penetration. The rationale stems from studies that have demonstrated that nonocclusive thrombi are much more likely to be lysed than occlusive thrombi when systemic thrombolytics are administered.[37] In essence, when the lytic drug is capable of reaching thrombus, it has a greater likelihood of lysing it. In contrast to directed intravenous lytic infusion (placing a catheter peripheral to a thrombus and infusing a lytic drug), image-guided catheter-directed intra-thrombus infusion has shown greater efficacy and safety.[38-40]

Endovascular Thrombus Removal Techniques

Catheter-based therapies have evolved considerably over the past two decades to minimize complications and maximize efficacy and patient comfort. Under the umbrella of endovascular thrombus removal is the following: catheter-directed thrombolysis (CDT), percutaneous mechanical thrombectomy (PMT), and pharmacomechanical catheter-directed thrombolysis (PCDT). The procedural details of these variant techniques and their results are discussed below.

CDT refers to the placement of a multi-sidehole infusion catheter into the thrombus with subsequent infusion of a lytic drug over a period of time. Access is gained most commonly into the popliteal vein under ultrasound guidance. After a guidewire and catheter traverse the clot, venography is performed to delineate thrombus extent. Next, an appropriately sized multi-sidehole infusion catheter is positioned within the clot, and an infusion is begun at a rate of 50 to 100 cc/hour of recombinant tissue plasminogen activator (rt-PA, maximum 1 mg/hr), reteplase (0.25-0.5 U/hr), or tenecteplase (0.25 mg/hr). It should be noted that none of these are FDA approved for DVT lysis. Infusion on average lasts between 6 and 24 hours, after which the patient is brought back to the interventional suite for repeat venography. If an underlying obstructive lesion is identified in the deep pelvic veins, it is commonly stented to reduce the incidence of recurrent thrombosis and improve outflow and symptomatology.[41]

In a multicenter registry conducted in the late 1990s, the major bleeding rate from CDT was found to be 11%.[39] Since then, limiting the hourly rt-PA dose, reducing the heparin to "subtherapeutic" levels (e.g., partial thromboplastin time 1.2-1.7 times control), and routinely using ultrasound guidance have reduced the major bleed rate to 2% to 4%.[42-44] Ultrasound-assisted thrombolysis has emerged relatively recently to theoretically speed the time to lysis and improve lytic drug efficacy; however, the technology is yet unproven in its ability to do either of these compared with standard infusion, and further studies are needed.[45,46]

Percutaneous mechanical thrombectomy refers to clot removal from the venous lumen. The rationale is that partial thrombus reduction with a mechanical device will create a flow channel and increase the surface area for endogenous thrombolysis. Through either a 7 or 8 Fr catheter or using a specialized device, thrombus is aspirated from the obstructed vein. Results have been fairly disappointing without the addition of a thrombolytic agent, and clot manipulation carries the risk of embolism and valvular damage.[41]

Pharmacomechanical catheter-directed thrombolysis (PCDT) (**Figure 26-3**) is a combination of the above techniques that uses both mechanical methods and lytic drugs to achieve thrombus reduction. The mechanical portion both reduces thrombus burden and achieves faster and more robust intrathrombus dispersion of the lytic drug, while the lytic component reduces the risk of embolism and results in more complete lysis. First-generation PCDT is the serial use of CDT and PMT, in which one of the techniques is used first, and the second is used subsequently. Either method requires two separate sessions with an infusion of lytic drug in between. First-generation PCDT has been shown to reduce the dose of lytic drug required, reduce hospitalization length, and cost.[47] More recently, PCDT has evolved to include techniques that enable very rapid drug dispersion, often permitting single-session DVT treatment. Two such methods include the "power-pulse" technique using the AngioJet (Bayer Healthcare) and "isolated thrombolysis" with the Trellis (Covidien). With the Angiojet in "power-pulse"

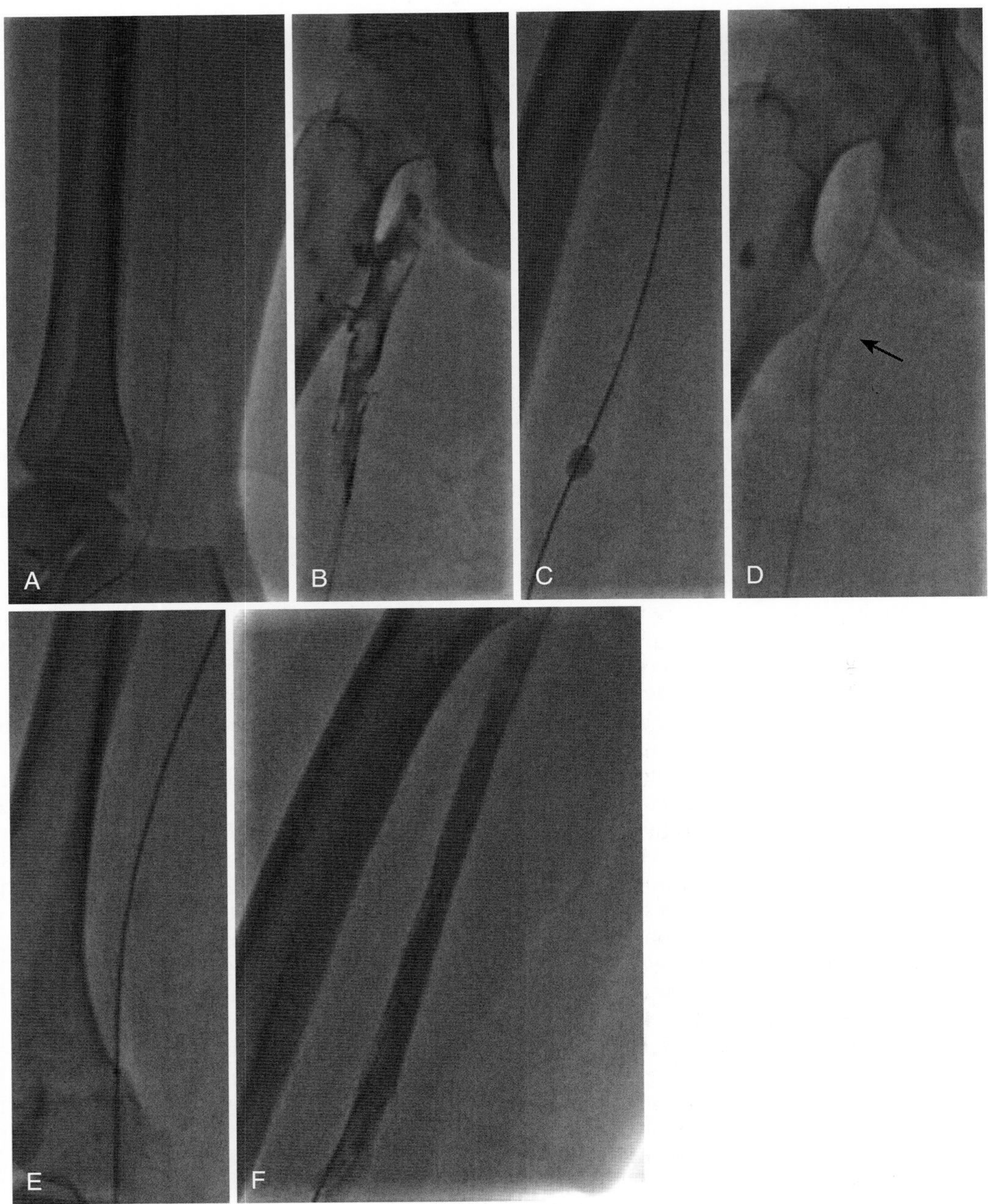

FIGURE 26-3 PCDT. **A,** Posterior tibial vein access (performed under ultrasound guidance). **B,** Acute thrombus in the femoral vein extending into the common femoral vein. **C, D,** Trellis device infusing lytic and macerating thrombus with a sinusoidal wire *(arrow)* within the catheter between the proximal and distal **(D)** balloons. **E,** Placement of an infusion catheter across the thrombus. **F,** Venographic appearance after 20 hours of lytic infusion, demonstrating near 100% thrombus clearance.

TABLE 26-1 Patient Selection for Catheter-Based Treatment of Acute Lower Extremity DVT

	Bleeding Risk		
DVT PRESENTATION	LOW	MODERATE	HIGH
Proximal DVT with limb threat	Yes	Yes	Possibly, with surgical consultation
IVC thrombus	Yes	Yes	No
DVT symptom progression or thrombus progression on anticoagulation	Yes	Possibly	No
Iliofemoral DVT to prevent PTS	Usually yes	No	No

DVT, Deep vein thrombosis; *IVC,* inferior vena cava; *PTS,* post-thrombotic syndrome.

mode, the diluted thrombolytic is forcefully injected into the thrombus and allowed to dwell for 20 to 30 minutes. The setting is then switched to "aspiration," and the catheter is run along the length of the thrombus to remove thrombus fragments. The Trellis consists of a multi-sidehole catheter flanked by two balloons that isolate the thrombus. A rotating wire is introduced coaxially that macerates and distributes lytic throughout the thrombus. At the end of the infusion, thrombus aspiration can be accomplished through the device itself or a separate aspiration catheter.[48-51] Approximately 50% of patients can be treated in this manner without a subsequent period of lytic infusion.

Patient Selection (Table 26-1)

The decision of whether to proceed with thrombolysis is based on a risk-benefit analysis, where the risk is primarily bleeding. Acute limb-threat, caval thrombus, and thrombus extension/worsening symptoms in spite of adequate anticoagulation have lower thresholds for intervention to minimize short-term mortality and morbidity from the thrombus itself. If none of these is present, the decision to lyse is normally based upon the desire to prevent PTS and alleviate severe symptoms of the acute DVT, if present. Thus, a patient with a reasonable life expectancy, low likelihood of bleeding, and an iliofemoral DVT (which, as stated above, has the strongest association with PTS) is a good candidate for intervention. A young, healthy, and active individual may elect to undergo thrombolysis in the setting of a highly symptomatic femoropopliteal DVT, although the outcomes of lytic therapy in this patient subgroup have not been separately reported.

Outcomes and Data (Table 26-2)

Numerous studies have been performed on outcomes associated with endovascular thrombus removal that show improved PTS and venous patency rates. It should be noted that significant methodological flaws exist for each, however, including small sample size, lack of randomization, single-center experience, and lack of objective measures of PTS. Comerota et al. conducted a multicenter registry and found improved rates of PTS and quality of life in the treated group.[52] AbuRahma et al. performed a nonrandomized comparison of treated and untreated groups and found better 5-year symptoms and venous patency.[53] Elsharawy et al. conducted a single-center randomized trial that showed higher venous patency rates and less reflux in the catheter-treated group.[54]

Most recently, the multicenter randomized controlled CaVenT study (Long-Term Outcome After Additional Catheter-Directed Thrombolysis Versus Standard Treatment for Acute Iliofemoral Deep Vein Thrombosis) was completed in Norway and showed a 26% relative risk reduction in those who received CDT. This study was limited by its modest sample size (n = 189) and the use of an older technique (CDT).[55] The ongoing NIH-sponsored ATTRACT trial (Acute Venous Thrombosis: Thrombus Removal With Adjunctive Catheter-Directed Thrombolysis) seeks to definitively answer the primary question of whether PCDT should be a first-line therapy for the treatment of symptomatic proximal DVT to prevent PTS.[56]

TABLE 26-2 Catheter-Directed Thrombolysis: Comparative Studies

STUDY	DESIGN	OUTCOME
Comerota (2000)[52]	Multicenter registry	Reduction in PTS, improved physical functioning
AbuRahma (2001)[53]	Prospective nonrandomized	Improved patency and freedom from symptoms
Elsharawy (2002)[54]	Randomized single-center	Higher return to normal venous function
CaVenT (2012)[55]	Multicenter randomized trial	Significant improvement in 2 year rate of PTS
ATTRACT (ongoing)[56]	Multicenter randomized trial	Pending

PTS, Post-thrombotic syndrome.

Chronic Deep Vein Thrombosis

Chronic venous insufficiency is costly and morbid, with venous ulcers alone costing $3 billion per year and resulting in the loss of 2 million working days per year.[57] Historical data suggest that PTS accounts for at least ~12% of chronic venous insufficiency cases.[58] As alluded to in the previous section, incomplete thrombus clearance and organization result in endothelialized channels that partially recanalize the vein. The robustness of this recanalization and collateral formation determines whether the patient will develop PTS. Most patients present with mild-moderate PTS, while a minority present with severe PTS/ulcer formation.

Patient Workup

Pertinent data to gather include a history of VTE, trauma, IVC filter placement, dialysis catheter placement, a family history of VTE, or malignancy. The duration and severity of symptoms should also be documented; a sudden exacerbation may represent an acute thrombotic episode. Recording an objective measurement of disease severity with a Villalta score and/or a CEAP score establishes a baseline (**Table 26-3**). A photograph of the affected limb(s) and calf and

TABLE 26-3 CEAP and Villalta Classifications

"C" or "Clinical" Definition of CEAP Classification
C0: No signs of venous disease
C1: Telangiectasias/reticular veins
C2: Varicocities
C3: Edema
C4a: Venous eczema/hyperpigmentation
C4b: Lipodermatosclerosis
C5: Healed ulcer
C6: Active ulcer
Villalta Scale*
Symptoms
Cramps
Itching
Pins and needles
Leg heaviness
Pain
Signs
Pretibial edema
Skin induration
Hyperpigmentation
Venous ectasia
Redness
Pain during calf compression
Ulceration

CEAP, Clinical-ediology-anatomy-pathophysiology; *PTS,* post-thrombotic syndrome.
*Each symptom/sign graded from 0 to 3, with 0 = none and 3 = severe. Score >5 = PTS. Ulceration = automatic severe PTS.

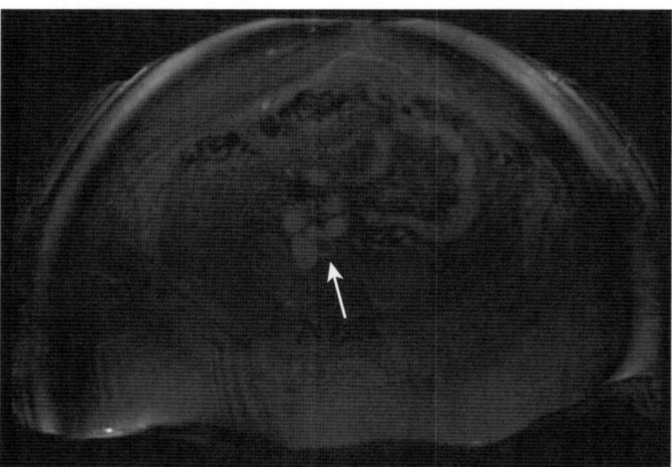

FIGURE 26-4 Magnetic resonance imaging of the pelvis demonstrating a central thrombus in the left common iliac vein.

thigh circumferences can be added to the baseline assessment. Understanding the anatomic extent of the post-thrombotic veins is essential for treatment planning; Doppler sonography can assess up to the peripheral external iliac vein, but visualizing pelvic veins and the IVC requires cross-sectional imaging (magnetic resonance venography or computed tomography, **Figure 26-4**).

Noninterventional Management of PTS

Several measures can be taken to optimize a patient with existing PTS. First, the anticoagulation status should be assessed, and all efforts should be made to prevent re-thrombosis, including prolonged anticoagulation if appropriate and safe. Compression stockings and pneumatic compression devices may provide symptomatic relief.[2,59,60] Weight loss, smoking cessation, and exercise[61] should be encouraged to minimize symptoms. Optimal wound care for those suffering from venous ulcers includes compression, analgesics, anti-inflammatories, lymphedema therapy, surgical debridement, and antibiotics if necessary.

Endovascular Intervention in the Setting of Established PTS

Prior to endovascular recanalization techniques, surgical bypass was the primary means of improving flow in these patients. Now, it is reserved for those who fail endovascular treatment.[62] Patients who are being considered for endovascular recanalization should obtain a full set of labs (complete blood count, international normalized ratio (INR), and basic metabolic profile). Recanalization should be performed with the patient fully anticoagulated to avoid thrombosis during and after the procedure. Additional patient factors to consider are the ability to tolerate moderate sedation for a prolonged period of time and the ability to lie flat or prone. If these are in question, an anesthesiology consult is warranted. If a patient is not on anticoagulation, he or she should be a candidate for it given that some length of anticoagulation in a post-thrombotic patient is necessary following the placement of endovenous stents.

Interventional Techniques to Recanalize Post-Thrombotic Deep Veins

As mentioned above, knowing the extent of thrombosis/stenosis and the etiology is essential for interventional planning and goals. Three common scenarios will be discussed—IVC and iliac occlusion secondary to an embedded IVC filter, iliofemoral chronic thrombosis, and femoropopliteal chronic thrombosis.

Caval stenosis or occlusion secondary to an embedded IVC filter occurs at a rate of approximately 1% to 2%.[6] The mechanism is unclear, but is thought to be a combination of organized thrombus and a fibrotic response to the metallic elements of the filter.[63] It is also unclear how long it takes this process to develop, and why it occurs in some individuals but not in most. However, it can result in significant bilateral PTS. Filter removal, if it can be performed safely, should be attempted prior to recanalization. Because the filter is commonly embedded, extraction is not simple, and may require advanced endovascular techniques, including the loop-snare technique, excimer-laser-assisted removal, and grasping forceps.[64,65] While a centered filter with a hook is easier to grasp with a snare,[66] the filter can be so strongly adhered to the caval wall that the hook may bend or the snare may break. In these instances, laser assistance may be helpful to lyse fibrous tissue between the filter metal and the cava. If the hook cannot be grasped, the loop-snare technique may allow the interventionalist to center the filter and sheath over it. Grasping forceps are useful in this scenario as well. It is important to note that while these techniques are generally safe, complications including caval perforation and fragment embolization have been encountered.[67] Once the filter has been removed, wire access across the stenosis or occlusion is the next essential step (**Figure 26-5**). Usually, the combination of a stiff and potentially hydrophilic guiding catheter and hydrophilic guidewire is able to traverse the stenosis successfully. After wire access is achieved, angioplasty to facilitate the introduction of stent catheters can be performed if necessary, especially in very tight stenoses or long-standing occlusions. Stents are then deployed and post-angioplastied. Typical caval stent sizes

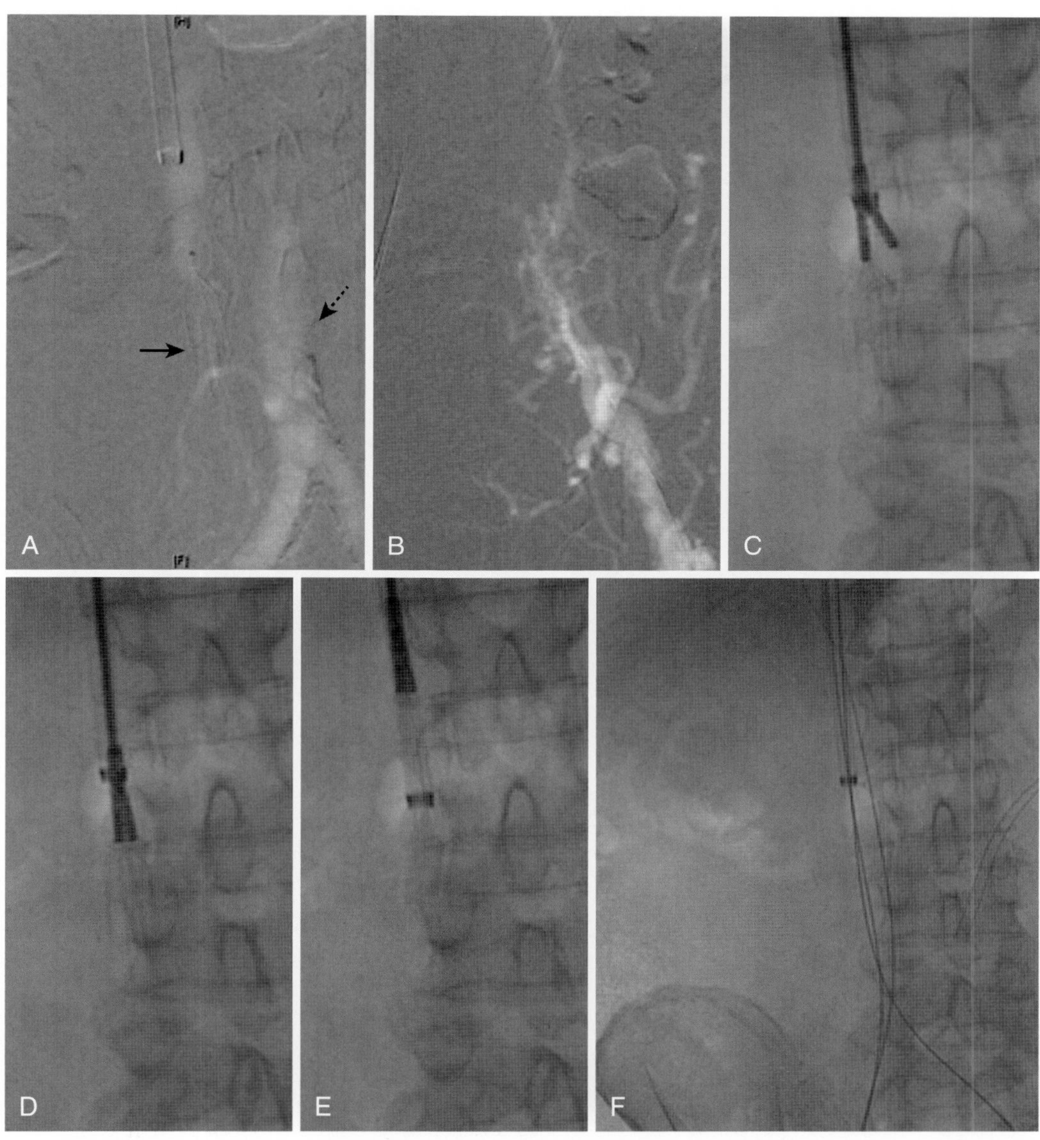

FIGURE 26-5 **A,** Inferior vena cavagram with carbon dioxide as a contrast agent (because of renal insufficiency) showing no flow below a chronically embedded IVC filter *(solid arrow)*. Incidentally, a small AV fistula outlines the aorta *(dashed arrow)*, likely seen because of the low viscosity of carbon dioxide. **B,** Left common iliac venography shows no flow into the IVC with marked collateralization. **C-E,** Retrieval of the chronically embedded filter using forceps. **F,** Successful wire placement across obstructed iliocaval segments.

Continued

range in diameter from 20 to 24 mm. Self-expanding metallic stents with good radial strength effectively open the cava. In particularly recalcitrant lesions or with in-stent occlusions, balloon expandable stents may be necessary. Frequently, the chronic thrombosis extends into both iliac veins, necessitating "kissing" iliac stents into the IVC stent. Common iliac stent sizes range from 14 mm to 18 mm; self-expanding nitinol or stainless steel stents work well.

Iliofemoral occlusions from a prior DVT frequently require a popliteal puncture, since the thrombosis extends to the common femoral vein and the femoral vein as well. These iliofemoral occlusions may have been the result of a May-Thurner lesion or one of its variants (**Figure 26-6**). Classic May-Thurner results from compression of the left common iliac vein by the pulsating right common iliac artery anteriorly and the vertebral body posteriorly. This chronic compression leads to intraluminal webs and fibrous bridging that narrow the lumen and predispose to thrombosis and venous hypertension. While up to 25% to 30% of the population has been shown to have this anatomically, it is unclear why some develop symptoms and most are asymptomatic.[68] Regardless, treating an iliofemoral occlusion may require stenting up to and possibly into the IVC to open the May-Thurner compression. Routine puncture of the femoral vein along the thigh should be avoided, given the difficulty of compressing it against a bony structure and the theoretically higher potential for a postoperative hematoma. Obtaining wire access across the occluded iliofemoral segment is often the most challenging part of the case and, as mentioned above, is most frequently accomplished with the combination of a hydrophilic wire and strong support catheter. Occasionally more vigorous techniques, such as sharp recanalization, are required (**Figure 26-7**).[69] Once wire access is obtained, stenting is performed as discussed above. The stents need to extend to a segment of open flow; while routine stenting of the femoral vein should be avoided due to historically low patency rates, it may be necessary on occasion in order to

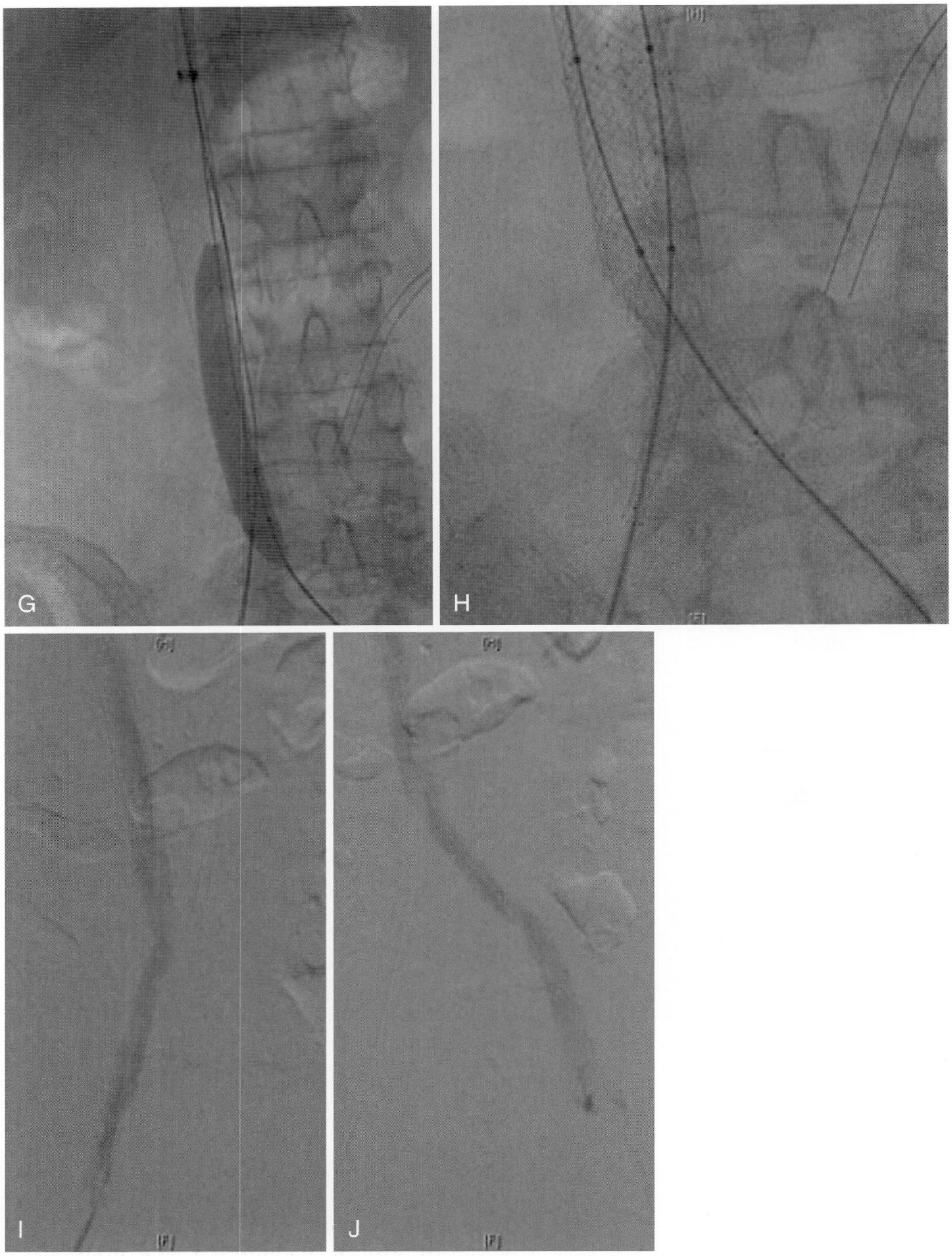

FIGURE 26-5, cont'd G, Intra-stent angioplasty after deployment of a self-expanding IVC stent. H, Deployment of bilateral kissing iliac stents. I, J, Completion venography with dilute contrast demonstrating brisk flow through stented iliac veins and IVC with resolution of collaterals.

obtain flow into the iliac stents. If the femoral vein is occluded, extending the stents into the profunda femoral vein may be necessary.

Treating chronic femoropopliteal disease in the absence of iliac obstruction is more controversial. While thought to confer a much lower risk of PTS,[10] chronic femoropopliteal disease can result in bothersome symptoms, especially to active individuals. For these patients, attempted recanalization using angioplasty can be attempted, but the long-term results are unknown, and given the significant recoil of a fibrotic post-thrombotic vein, the valvular damage it has already sustained, and the possibility of re-thrombosis, more data need to be gathered before routine use of this technique can be recommended.

Most individuals will need at least a short duration of anticoagulation following a recanalization, most commonly for 3 months. Antiplatelet agents, including aspirin and clopidogrel, can be added to aid in stent patency. The duration of therapy is not established, and varies between practitioners.

Complications and Outcomes

Given that interventions are being performed in the venous system, significant bleeding is rare, especially given that

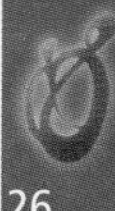

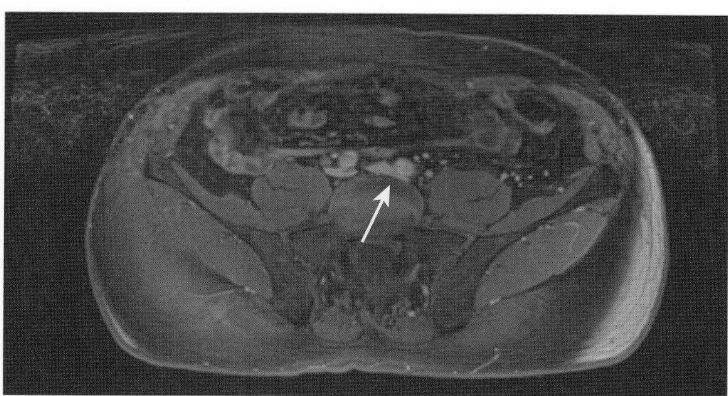

FIGURE 26-6 Magnetic resonance imaging of the pelvis demonstrating compression of the left common iliac vein *(arrow)* between the left common iliac artery and vertebral body (May-Thurner variant).

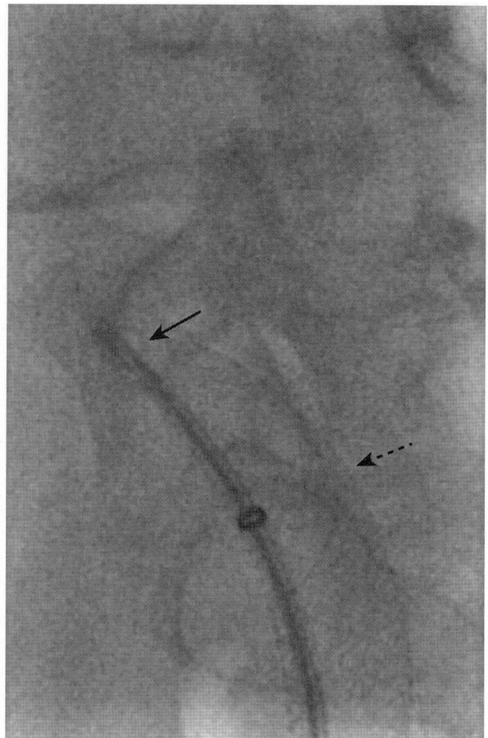

FIGURE 26-7 Sharp recanalization through a chronically occluded stent *(dashed arrow)* with the back end of a stiff wire *(solid arrow)*.

recanalization is being performed in areas with very slow or no flow. Access site oozing is fairly common, especially given the intra- and postprocedural anticoagulation necessary to keep the recanalized segments open. However, it can usually be controlled with manual compression. Patients may experience significant pain during and after the procedure in the stented and angioplastied regions. Stent migration is rare, and in experienced hands should not occur if the stents are sized appropriately. Patients should be cautioned that the procedure may not be technically successful, especially in long-standing occlusions, and that re-intervention may be necessary given that between 15% and 40% of patients who undergo such procedures require a repeat procedure within 4 years.[70,71]

Primary patency for stents deployed in post-thrombotic veins is approximately 70%, while primary assisted and secondary patencies are as high as 90% to 95%.[72] Clinical outcomes are most prominent for patients with more severe disease (C4-C6 in the CEAP classification), with greater than 50% resolution of venous dermatitis and ulcers after endovascular treatment.[73] A single-center study demonstrated an 80% complete or partial response to endovascular techniques (both deep and superficial) in patients with established PTS.[70] However, it should be noted that robust, prospective, controlled studies are not available and that patients in the above series were highly selected.

Section 2: Acute Pulmonary Embolism

Epidemiology and Classification

Pulmonary embolism kills between 100,000 to 180,000 people in the United States per year, with a case fatality rate of 15%.[74,75] While the low-risk patients have <1% mortality and are well treated with heparin alone, patients with massive or submassive PEs have 20% to 50% and 3% to 9% mortality rates, respectively, in spite of full anticoagulation.[76,77] The poorer outcomes in these subgroups have prompted clinicians to consider escalating therapy via intravenous thrombolytics, catheter-directed techniques, and/or surgical embolectomy.

The American Heart Association (AHA) issued a guidance document in 2011 that defined the terms "massive," "submassive," and "low-risk."[77] A massive pulmonary embolism is one that causes sustained hypotension (<90 mm Hg systolic for >15 minutes) or requires pressor support. A submassive pulmonary embolism is one that causes right heart strain, dysfunction, or ischemia. Echocardiography is essential for stratification, as it detects right ventricular pathology. Elevations in basic natriuretic peptide (BNP) or troponin also qualify a PE as being submassive. Specific EKG changes also can put a patient is the submassive category. Low-risk PE is defined as having no associated hypotension or right heart pathology.

Treatment Escalation for Massive Pulmonary Embolism

Given the high mortality rates for this classification, most physicians and guidance documents agree that treatment escalation is prudent.[2,77] The best treatment has not been established, however, because strong data are lacking. Systemic thrombolytics have been associated with a lower composite endpoint of death and recurrent PE in a metaanalysis conducted in 2004.[78] However, it is also associated with a 20% major bleeding rate.[79] Surgical embolectomy is a viable option either as a rescue treatment for failed systemic thrombolysis or as a primary therapy for a patient in extremis.[80-83] Studies analyzing surgical embolectomy are nonrandomized and underpowered, making analysis of its benefit inconclusive; however, the ability to add extracorporeal membrane oxygenation (ECMO) in the operating room allows for advanced care of massive PE patients with the gravest prognosis.

Catheter-directed techniques offer several potential advantages. First, the morbidity and potential mortality associated with a sternotomy in a hemodynamically unstable patient is avoided. Second, in a patient with a high risk of bleeding from systemic lysis, flow can be restored with little or no thrombolytic agent. In a metaanalysis conducted by Kuo et al., catheter-directed massive PE treatment resulted in an 86% survival to discharge.[84] It should be noted that the

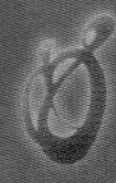

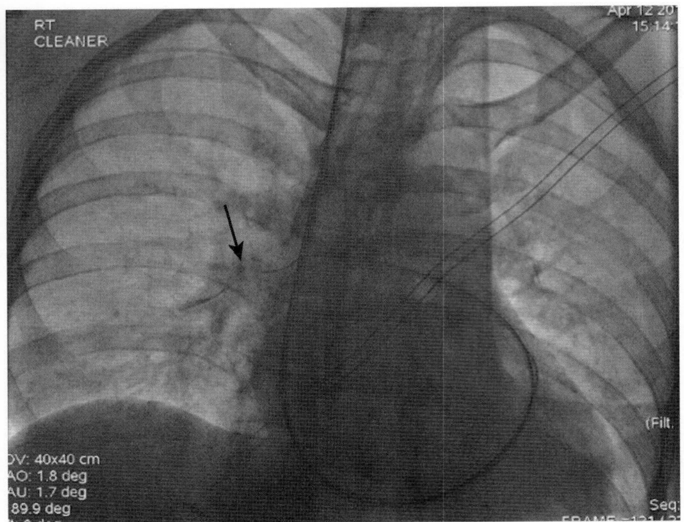

FIGURE 26-8 Mechanical clot maceration with a rotating thrombectomy device *(arrow)* in a patient with a massive pulmonary embolism.

studies comprising this metaanalysis were most commonly retrospective without control arms, and that publication bias could reduce reporting of patients with poor outcomes. Nonetheless, it demonstrated the potential of catheter-based techniques to play a role in massive PE. The endovascular strategy in the setting of massive PE is to restore flow through the pulmonary artery to improve left-sided filling pressures. Thus, mechanical clot maceration (**Figure 26-8**) and aspiration in combination with local delivery of a thrombolytic effectively reduces clot burden. Maceration can be accomplished by rotating a pigtail catheter within the thrombus or by using an automated mechanical device. Aspiration is typically performed through a 7 to 10 Fr catheter. Lacing the thrombus with a lytic agent can be used in conjunction, even in a patient who has a high risk of bleeding or a preexisting bleed, given the low dose and local administration. If the patient is a candidate, prolonged lytic infusion following these mechanical maneuvers can dramatically reduce thrombus burden.

Treatment Escalation for Submassive Pulmonary Embolism

The submassive group, representing up to 40% of acute PEs, is particularly challenging for clinicians, because there are considerable differences of opinion regarding if, when, and how treatment escalation should occur. On the one hand, patients with submassive PEs are normotensive and therefore momentarily compensated. On the other, they have evidence of right heart strain, dysfunction, and/or ischemia, all of which are associated with higher mortality.[85,86] In essence, whether a patient will stabilize on heparin alone or will spiral toward progressive obstruction of the pulmonary arterial bed and exceed the threshold of right ventricular tolerance is nearly impossible to predict. Moreover, there is concern about the development of chronic pulmonary hypertension in those patients with substantial residual clot burden who are treated with heparin alone.[87-89] Compounding the complexity of escalating treatment in this subgroup is the fact that each strategy carries risk, invasiveness, inconvenience, and/or added costs. Society guideline documents do not give strong recommendations, reflecting the paucity of evidence to support one treatment over another.[2,77] Clearly, if a treatment or approach emerges that is low risk, convenient, and efficacious, that treatment would be utilized for most submassive PE patients given the disease's volatility.

Surgical embolectomy has been explored in the setting of submassive PE, but given its considerable morbidity and the relative stability of a submassive patient, it is infrequently the first-line treatment.[90] On the other hand, intravenous thrombolytics have been studied in this population. Two randomized trials have demonstrated a net benefit in the primary endpoint of death or heroic resuscitative measures at early time points in the group treated with intravenous thrombolytics plus anticoagulation compared with the anticoagulation-alone group.[91,92] In one of these studies, however, a statistically significant increase in intracranial hemorrhage was observed.[92] Catheter-directed thrombolysis attempts to improve the safety profile of thrombolytic delivery by administering the agent directly into the thrombus, allowing for lower doses over a longer period of time. A small randomized trial (ULTIMA [Prospective, Randomized, Controlled Study of Ultrasound Accelerated Thrombolysis for the Treatment of Acute Pulmonary Embolism]) that evaluated ultrasound-assisted catheter-directed thrombolysis (EKOS Corporation, Bothell, WA) demonstrated better immediate and 3-month right ventricular function in the catheter-treated group than the heparin-only group, with no major or intracranial bleeding.[93] The SEATTLE II study (Prospective, Single-Arm, Multi-Center Trial of Ekosonic Endovascular System and Activase for Treatment of Acute Pulmonary Embolism), which enrolled 150 patients in a single-arm design, found a statistically significant reduction in the RV/LV ratio 48 hours after initiation of ultrasound-assisted catheter-directed thrombolysis in the setting of massive and submassive PE with no intracranial or fatal bleeding.[94] As this technology is now FDA-approved for use for PE, it will likely play a larger role in the management of PE.

The ideal candidate for catheter-directed PE lysis has central thrombus through which an infusion catheter can be placed (**Figure 26-9**). If the clot is too peripheral such that the catheter cannot be embedded within the thrombus, alternative strategies should be considered. Procedurally, venous access can be from the common femoral vein or internal jugular vein. Pulmonary arterial pressure measurements should be performed to establish a baseline and to determine the injection rate for angiography. Angiography can be performed from the main pulmonary artery or the right and left main branches; the latter allows for better delineation of the clot burden and location. A wire is then guided through the clot, over which a multi-sidehole infusion catheter is advanced into the thrombus. A bolus of thrombolytic can be given, after which an infusion is begun. If bilateral emboli are present, a second infusion catheter can be placed on the contralateral side. During the infusion, heparin should be continued; while some argue that subtherapeutic doses should be used to reduce the risk of bleeding, others maintain that the real mortality associated with submassive PE that decompensates deserves full anticoagulation.

Patient Follow-Up

Patients with massive and submassive pulmonary emboli should continue to be followed as outpatients following discharge from their acute event. Repeat echocardiography

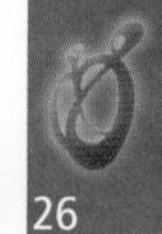

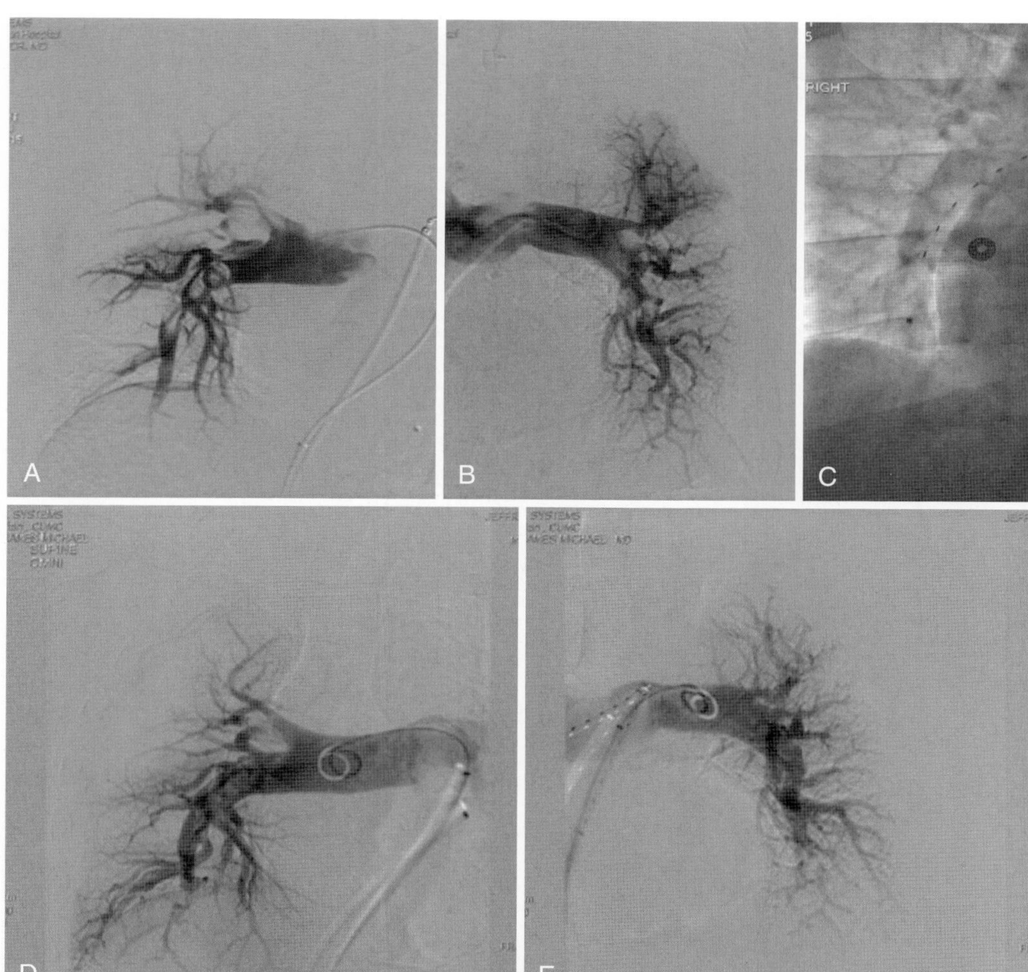

FIGURE 26-9 Right **(A)** and left **(B)** pulmonary angiograms demonstrating thrombus in the right upper and lower lobe branches and left lingular and lower lobe branches. **C,** Placement of bilateral ultrasound-assisted infusion catheters into lower lobe thrombi. Infusion occurred over 20 hours. Right **(D)** and left **(E)** pulmonary angiograms after lytic infusion demonstrating markedly improved perfusion. The pulmonary systolic pressure was reduced from 56 mm Hg to 36 mm Hg.

can document persistent right ventricular dysfunction or the development of pulmonary hypertension. Cardiopulmonary rehabilitation and appropriate pulmonary hypertension treatment can be initiated as necessary. A multidisciplinary team including hematologists, cardiologists, interventionalists, and pulmonologists ensures optimal care for these patients. The duration and type of anticoagulation can be monitored, and if an IVC filter was placed during the hospitalization, it can be removed if appropriate and feasible.

CONCLUSIONS

Venous thromboembolic disease carries significant morbidity and mortality in the short term and has long-term consequences, both in the form of PTS and chronic pulmonary hypertension. While anticoagulation alone is appropriate for a majority of these patients, more aggressive management/treatment escalation should be considered for a subset of PE and DVT patients. The treatment algorithms for these patients will continue to evolve as data emerge regarding the relative strengths and weaknesses of the various treatment options. Catheter-directed therapy in particular will likely play an important role given its promising efficacy and safety thus far.

References

1. Meissner MH: Indications for platelet aggregation inhibitors after venous stents. *Phlebology* 28(Suppl 1):91–98, 2013.
2. Kearon C, Akl EA, Comerota AJ, et al: Antithrombotic therapy for VTE disease: antithrombotic therapy and prevention of thrombosis, 9th ed: American College of chest physicians evidence-based clinical practice guidelines. *Chest* 141(2 Suppl):e419S–e494S, 2012.
3. Lee AY, Levine MN, Baker RI, et al: Low-molecular-weight heparin versus a coumarin for the prevention of recurrent venous thromboembolism in patients with cancer. *N Engl J Med* 349(2):146–153, 2003.
4. Meyer G, Marjanovic Z, Valcke J, et al: Comparison of low-molecular-weight heparin and warfarin for the secondary prevention of venous thromboembolism in patients with cancer: a randomized controlled study. *Arch Intern Med* 162(15):1729–1735, 2002.
5. Investigators E, Bauersachs R, Berkowitz SD, et al: Oral rivaroxaban for symptomatic venous thromboembolism. *N Engl J Med* 363(26):2499–2510, 2010.
6. Angel LF, Tapson V, Galgon RE, et al: Systematic review of the use of retrievable inferior vena cava filters. *J Vasc Interv Radiol* 22(11):1522–1530 e3, 2011.
7. Decousus H, Leizorovicz A, Parent F, et al: A clinical trial of vena caval filters in the prevention of pulmonary embolism in patients with proximal deep-vein thrombosis. Prevention du Risque d'Embolie Pulmonaire par Interruption Cave Study Group. *N Engl J Med* 338(7):409–415, 1998.
8. Kahn SR, Shrier I, Julian JA, et al: Determinants and time course of the postthrombotic syndrome after acute deep venous thrombosis. *Ann Intern Med* 149(10):698–707, 2008.
9. Beyth RJ, Cohen AM, Landefeld CS: Long-term outcomes of deep-vein thrombosis. *Arch Intern Med* 155(10):1031–1037, 1995.
10. Kahn SR, Shbaklo H, Lamping DL, et al: Determinants of health-related quality of life during the 2 years following deep vein thrombosis. *J Thromb Haemost* 6(7):1105–1112, 2008.
11. Caprini JA, Botteman MF, Stephens JM, et al: Economic burden of long-term complications of deep vein thrombosis after total hip replacement surgery in the United States. *Value Health* 6(1):59–74, 2003.
12. Phillips T, Stanton B, Provan A, et al: A study of the impact of leg ulcers on quality of life: financial, social, and psychologic implications. *J Am Acad Dermatol* 31(1):49–53, 1994.
13. Bergqvist D, Jendteg S, Johansen L, et al: Cost of long-term complications of deep venous thrombosis of the lower extremities: an analysis of a defined patient population in Sweden. *Ann Intern Med* 126(6):454–457, 1997.
14. Olin JW, Beusterien KM, Childs MB, et al: Medical costs of treating venous stasis ulcers: evidence from a retrospective cohort study. *Vasc Med* 4(1):1–7, 1999.
15. Roumen-Klappe EM, Janssen MC, Van Rossum J, et al: Inflammation in deep vein thrombosis and the development of post-thrombotic syndrome: a prospective study. *J Thromb Haemost* 7(4):582–587, 2009.

16. Shbaklo H, Holcroft CA, Kahn SR: Levels of inflammatory markers and the development of the post-thrombotic syndrome. *Thromb Haemost* 101(3):505–512, 2009.
17. Wakefield TW, Myers DD, Henke PK: Role of selectins and fibrinolysis in VTE. *Thromb Res* 123(Suppl 4):S35–S40, 2009.
18. Deroo S, Deatrick KB, Henke PK: The vessel wall: a forgotten player in post thrombotic syndrome. *Thromb Haemost* 104(4):681–692, 2010.
19. Caps MT, Manzo RA, Bergelin RO, et al: Venous valvular reflux in veins not involved at the time of acute deep vein thrombosis. *J Vasc Surg* 22(5):524–531, 1995.
20. Markel A, Manzo RA, Bergelin RO, et al: Valvular reflux after deep vein thrombosis: incidence and time of occurrence. *J Vasc Surg* 15(2):377–382; discussion 83–84, 1992.
21. Shull KC, Nicolaides AN, Fernandes e Fernandes J, et al: Significance of popliteal reflux in relation to ambulatory venous pressure and ulceration. *Arch Surg* 114(11):1304–1306, 1979.
22. Prandoni P, Frulla M, Sartor D, et al: Vein abnormalities and the post-thrombotic syndrome. *J Thromb Haemost* 3(2):401–402, 2005.
23. Meissner MH, Manzo RA, Bergelin RO, et al: Deep venous insufficiency: the relationship between lysis and subsequent reflux. *J Vasc Surg* 18(4):596–605; discussion 6–8, 1993.
24. Nicolaides AN, Hussein MK, Szendro G, et al: The relation of venous ulceration with ambulatory venous pressure measurements. *J Vasc Surg* 17(2):414–419, 1993.
25. Welkie JF, Comerota AJ, Katz ML, et al: Hemodynamic deterioration in chronic venous disease. *J Vasc Surg* 16(5):733–740, 1992.
26. Araki CT, Back TL, Padberg FT, et al: The significance of calf muscle pump function in venous ulceration. *J Vasc Surg* 20(6):872–877; discussion 8–9, 1994.
27. Johnson BF, Manzo RA, Bergelin RO, et al: Relationship between changes in the deep venous system and the development of the postthrombotic syndrome after an acute episode of lower limb deep vein thrombosis: a one- to six-year follow-up. *J Vasc Surg* 21(2):307–312; discussion 13, 1995.
28. van Dongen CJ, Prandoni P, Frulla M, et al: Relation between quality of anticoagulant treatment and the development of the postthrombotic syndrome. *J Thromb Haemost* 3(5):939–942, 2005.
29. Douketis JD, Crowther MA, Foster GA, et al: Does the location of thrombosis determine the risk of disease recurrence in patients with proximal deep vein thrombosis? *Am J Med* 110(7):515–519, 2001.
30. Brandjes DP, Buller HR, Heijboer H, et al: Randomised trial of effect of compression stockings in patients with symptomatic proximal-vein thrombosis. *Lancet* 349(9054):759–762, 1997.
31. Prandoni P, Lensing AW, Prins MH, et al: Below-knee elastic compression stockings to prevent the post-thrombotic syndrome: a randomized, controlled trial. *Ann Intern Med* 141(4):249–256, 2004.
32. Kahn SR, Shbaklo H, Shapiro S, et al: Effectiveness of compression stockings to prevent the post-thrombotic syndrome (the SOX Trial and Bio-SOX biomarker substudy): a randomized controlled trial. *BMC Cardiovasc Disord* 7:21, 2007.
33. Hull RD, Marder VJ, Mah AF, et al: Quantitative assessment of thrombus burden predicts the outcome of treatment for venous thrombosis: a systematic review. *Am J Med* 118(5):456–464, 2005.
34. Plate G, Akesson H, Einarsson E, et al: Long-term results of venous thrombectomy combined with a temporary arterio-venous fistula. *Eur J Vasc Surg* 4(5):483–489, 1990.
35. Goldhaber SZ, Buring JE, Lipnick RJ, et al: Pooled analyses of randomized trials of streptokinase and heparin in phlebographically documented acute deep venous thrombosis. *Am J Med* 76(3):393–397, 1984.
36. Goldhaber SZ, Meyerovitz MF, Green D, et al: Randomized controlled trial of tissue plasminogen activator in proximal deep venous thrombosis. *Am J Med* 88(3):235–240, 1990.
37. Meyerovitz MF, Polak JF, Goldhaber SZ: Short-term response to thrombolytic therapy in deep venous thrombosis: predictive value of venographic appearance. *Radiology* 184(2):345–348, 1992.
38. Schwieder G, Grimm W, Siemens HJ, et al: Intermittent regional therapy with rt-PA is not superior to systemic thrombolysis in deep vein thrombosis (DVT)–a German multicenter trial. *Thromb Haemost* 74(5):1240–1243, 1995.
39. Mewissen MW, Seabrook GR, Meissner MH, et al: Catheter-directed thrombolysis for lower extremity deep venous thrombosis: report of a national multicenter registry. *Radiology* 211(1):39–49, 1999.
40. Semba CP, Dake MD: Iliofemoral deep venous thrombosis: aggressive therapy with catheter-directed thrombolysis. *Radiology* 191(2):487–494, 1994.
41. Vedantham S, Thorpe PE, Cardella JF, et al: Quality improvement guidelines for the treatment of lower extremity deep vein thrombosis with use of endovascular thrombus removal. *J Vasc Interv Radiol* 17(3):435–447; quiz 48, 2006.
42. Grunwald MR, Hofmann LV: Comparison of urokinase, alteplase, and reteplase for catheter-directed thrombolysis of deep venous thrombosis. *J Vasc Interv Radiol* 15(4):347–352, 2004.
43. Shortell CK, Queiroz R, Johansson M, et al: Safety and efficacy of limited-dose tissue plasminogen activator in acute vascular occlusion. *J Vasc Surg* 34(5):854–859, 2001.
44. Sugimoto K, Hofmann LV, Razavi MK, et al: The safety, efficacy, and pharmacoeconomics of low-dose alteplase compared with urokinase for catheter-directed thrombolysis of arterial and venous occlusions. *J Vasc Surg* 37(3):512–517, 2003.
45. Baker R, Samuels S, Benenati JF, et al: Ultrasound-accelerated vs standard catheter-directed thrombolysis–a comparative study in patients with iliofemoral deep vein thrombosis. *J Vasc Interv Radiol* 23(11):1460–1466, 2012.
46. Parikh S, Motarjeme A, McNamara T, et al: Ultrasound-accelerated thrombolysis for the treatment of deep vein thrombosis: initial clinical experience. *J Vasc Interv Radiol* 19(4):521–528, 2008.
47. Kim HS, Patra A, Paxton BE, et al: Adjunctive percutaneous mechanical thrombectomy for lower-extremity deep vein thrombosis: clinical and economic outcomes. *J Vasc Interv Radiol* 17(7):1099–1104, 2006.
48. Cynamon J, Stein EG, Dym RJ, et al: A new method for aggressive management of deep vein thrombosis: retrospective study of the power pulse technique. *J Vasc Interv Radiol* 17(6):1043–1049, 2006.
49. Hilleman DE, Razavi MK: Clinical and economic evaluation of the Trellis-8 infusion catheter for deep vein thrombosis. *J Vasc Interv Radiol* 19(3):377–383, 2008.
50. Lin PH, Zhou W, Dardik A, et al: Catheter-direct thrombolysis versus pharmacomechanical thrombectomy for treatment of symptomatic lower extremity deep venous thrombosis. *Am J Surg* 192(6):782–788, 2006.
51. O'Sullivan GJ, Lohan DG, Gough N, et al: Pharmacomechanical thrombectomy of acute deep vein thrombosis with the Trellis-8 isolated thrombolysis catheter. *J Vasc Interv Radiol* 18(6):715–724, 2007.
52. Comerota AJ, Throm RC, Mathias SD, et al: Catheter-directed thrombolysis for iliofemoral deep venous thrombosis improves health-related quality of life. *J Vasc Surg* 32(1):130–137, 2000.
53. AbuRahma AF, Perkins SE, Wulu JT, et al: Iliofemoral deep vein thrombosis: conventional therapy versus lysis and percutaneous transluminal angioplasty and stenting. *Ann Surg* 233(6):752–760, 2001.
54. Elsharawy M, Elzayat E: Early results of thrombolysis vs anticoagulation in iliofemoral venous thrombosis. A randomised clinical trial. *Eur J Vasc Endovasc Surg* 24(3):209–214, 2002.
55. Enden T, Haig Y, Klow NE, et al: Long-term outcome after additional catheter-directed thrombolysis versus standard treatment for acute iliofemoral deep vein thrombosis (the CaVenT study): a randomised controlled trial. *Lancet* 379(9810):31–38, 2012.
56. Vedantham S, Goldhaber SZ, Kahn SR, et al: Rationale and design of the ATTRACT Study: a multicenter randomized trial to evaluate pharmacomechanical catheter-directed thrombolysis for the prevention of postthrombotic syndrome in patients with proximal deep vein thrombosis. *Am Heart J* 165(4):523–530 e3, 2013.
57. Raffetto JD: Inflammation in chronic venous ulcers. *Phlebology* 28(Suppl 1):61–67, 2013.
58. Heit JA, Rooke TW, Silverstein MD, et al: Trends in the incidence of venous stasis syndrome and venous ulcer: a 25-year population-based study. *J Vasc Surg* 33(5):1022–1027, 2001.
59. Ginsberg JS, Magier D, Mackinnon B, et al: Intermittent compression units for severe post-phlebitic syndrome: a randomized crossover study. *CMAJ* 160(9):1303–1306, 1999.
60. O'Donnell MJ, McRae S, Kahn SR, et al: Evaluation of a venous-return assist device to treat severe post-thrombotic syndrome (VENOPTS). A randomized controlled trial. *Thromb Haemost* 99(3):623–629, 2008.
61. Kahn SR, Shrier I, Shapiro S, et al: Six-month exercise training program to treat post-thrombotic syndrome: a randomized controlled two-centre trial. *CMAJ* 183(1):37–44, 2011.
62. Jost CJ, Gloviczki P, Cherry Jr, KJ, et al: Surgical reconstruction of iliofemoral veins and the inferior vena cava for nonmalignant occlusive disease. *J Vasc Surg* 33(2):320–327; discussion 7–8, 2001.
63. Rimon U, Bensaid P, Golan G, et al: Optease vena cava filter optimal indwelling time and retrievability. *Cardiovasc Intervent Radiol* 34(3):532–535, 2011.
64. Kuo WT, Odegaard JI, Rosenberg JK, et al: Excimer laser-assisted removal of embedded inferior vena cava filters: a single-center prospective study. *Circ Cardiovasc Interv* 6(5):560–566, 2013.
65. Stavropoulos SW, Dixon RG, Burke CT, et al: Embedded inferior vena cava filter removal: use of endobronchial forceps. *J Vasc Interv Radiol* 19(9):1297–1301, 2008.
66. Oh JC, Trerotola SO, Dagli M, et al: Removal of retrievable inferior vena cava filters with computed tomography findings indicating tenting or penetration of the inferior vena cava wall. *J Vasc Interv Radiol* 22(1):70–74, 2011.
67. Hill DA, Goldstein N, Kuo EY: Vena cava filter fracture with migration to the pulmonary artery. *Ann Thorac Surg* 95(1):342–345, 2013.
68. Kibbe MR, Ujiki M, Goodwin AL, et al: Iliac vein compression in an asymptomatic patient population. *J Vasc Surg* 39(5):937–943, 2004.
69. Razavi MK, Hansch EC, Kee ST, et al: Chronically occluded inferior venae cavae: endovascular treatment. *Radiology* 214(1):133–138, 2000.
70. Nayak L, Hildebolt CF, Vedantham S: Postthrombotic syndrome: feasibility of a strategy of imaging-guided endovascular intervention. *J Vasc Interv Radiol* 23(9):1165–1173, 2012.
71. Raju S, Neglen P: Percutaneous recanalization of total occlusions of the iliac vein. *J Vasc Surg* 50(2):360–368, 2009.
72. Neglen P, Hollis KC, Olivier J, et al: Stenting of the venous outflow in chronic venous disease: long-term stent-related outcome, clinical, and hemodynamic result. *J Vasc Surg* 46(5):979–990, 2007.
73. Raju S, Darcey R, Neglen P: Unexpected major role for venous stenting in deep reflux disease. *J Vasc Surg* 51(2):401–408; discussion 8, 2010.
74. Beckman MG, Hooper WC, Critchley SE, et al: Venous thromboembolism: a public health concern. *Am J Prev Med* 38(4 Suppl):S495–S501, 2010.
75. White RH: The epidemiology of venous thromboembolism. *Circulation* 107(23 Suppl 1):I4–I8, 2003.
76. Goldhaber SZ, Visani L, De Rosa M: Acute pulmonary embolism: clinical outcomes in the International Cooperative Pulmonary Embolism Registry (ICOPER). *Lancet* 353(9162):1386–1389, 1999.
77. Jaff MR, McMurtry MS, Archer SL, et al: Management of massive and submassive pulmonary embolism, iliofemoral deep vein thrombosis, and chronic thromboembolic pulmonary hypertension: a scientific statement from the American Heart Association. *Circulation* 123(16):1788–1830, 2011.
78. Wan S, Quinlan DJ, Agnelli G, et al: Thrombolysis compared with heparin for the initial treatment of pulmonary embolism: a meta-analysis of the randomized controlled trials. *Circulation* 110(6):744–749, 2004.
79. Fiumara K, Kucher N, Fanikos J, et al: Predictors of major hemorrhage following fibrinolysis for acute pulmonary embolism. *Am J Cardiol* 97(1):127–129, 2006.
80. Ahmed P, Khan AA, Smith A, et al: Expedient pulmonary embolectomy for acute pulmonary embolism: improved outcomes. *Interact Cardiovasc Thorac Surg* 7(4):591–594, 2008.
81. Aymard T, Kadner A, Widmer A, et al: Massive pulmonary embolism: surgical embolectomy versus thrombolytic therapy–should surgical indications be revisited? *Eur J Cardiothorac Surg* 43(1):90–94; discussion 4, 2013.
82. Kadner A, Schmidli J, Schonhoff F, et al: Excellent outcome after surgical treatment of massive pulmonary embolism in critically ill patients. *J Thorac Cardiovasc Surg* 136(2):448–451, 2008.
83. Zarrabi K, Zolghadrasli A, Ostovan MA, Azimifar A. Short-term results of retrograde pulmonary embolectomy in massive and submassive pulmonary embolism: a single-center study of 30 patients. *Eur J Cardiothorac Surg* 40(4):890–893, 2011.
84. Kuo WT, Gould MK, Louie JD, et al: Catheter-directed therapy for the treatment of massive pulmonary embolism: systematic review and meta-analysis of modern techniques. *J Vasc Interv Radiol* 20(11):1431–1440, 2009.
85. Sanchez O, Trinquart L, Colombet I, et al: Prognostic value of right ventricular dysfunction in patients with haemodynamically stable pulmonary embolism: a systematic review. *Eur Heart J* 29(12):1569–1577, 2008.
86. Becattini C, Vedovati MC, Agnelli G: Prognostic value of troponins in acute pulmonary embolism: a meta-analysis. *Circulation* 116(4):427–433, 2007.
87. Kline JA, Steuerwald MT, Marchick MR, et al: Prospective evaluation of right ventricular function and functional status 6 months after acute submassive pulmonary embolism: frequency of persistent or subsequent elevation in estimated pulmonary artery pressure. *Chest* 136(5):1202–1210, 2009.
88. Sharifi M, Bay C, Skrocki L, et al: Moderate pulmonary embolism treated with thrombolysis (from the "MOPETT" Trial). *Am J Cardiol* 111(2):273–277, 2013.
89. Stevinson BG, Hernandez-Nino J, Rose G, et al: Echocardiographic and functional cardiopulmonary problems 6 months after first-time pulmonary embolism in previously healthy patients. *Eur Heart J* 28(20):2517–2524, 2007.
90. Leacche M, Unic D, Goldhaber SZ, et al: Modern surgical treatment of massive pulmonary embolism: results in 47 consecutive patients after rapid diagnosis and aggressive surgical approach. *J Thorac Cardiovasc Surg* 129(5):1018–1023, 2005.
91. Konstantinides S, Geibel A, Heusel G, et al: Heparin plus alteplase compared with heparin alone in patients with submassive pulmonary embolism. *N Engl J Med* 347(15):1143–1150, 2002.
92. Konstantinides SV, Meyer G: Single-bolus tenecteplase plus heparin compared with heparin alone for normotensive patients with acute pulmonary embolism who have evidence of right ventricular dysfunction and myocardial injury: rationale and design of the Pulmonary Embolism Thrombolysis (PEITHO) trial. *Am Heart J* 163(1):33–U51, 2012.
93. Kucher N, Boekstegers P, Müller O, et al: Randomized controlled trial of ultrasound-assisted catheter-directed thrombolysis for acute intermediate-risk pulmonary embolism. *Circulation* 2013. CIRCULATIONAHA. 113.005544.
94. ACC.14: the 63rd annual scientific session of the American College of Cardiology. 2014.

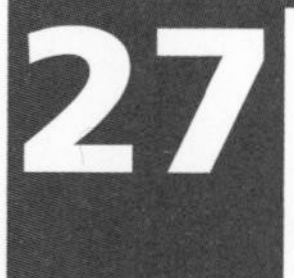

Management of Chronic Venous Insufficiency

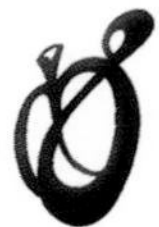

Nicolas W. Shammas

EPIDEMIOLOGY AND RISK FACTORS OF CHRONIC VENOUS DISEASE

Chronic venous disease (CVD) is a condition that affects the superficial and deep venous systems resulting in venous hypertension and a cascade of biochemical and vessel wall changes that lead to a spectrum of pathologies ranging from telangiectasias to venous stasis ulcerations. Chronic venous insufficiency (CVI) is an advanced form of CVD, generally presenting with lower extremity edema, trophic skin changes, and venous ulcerations. This chronic condition has often been neglected by providers because of its chronic and subtle progression and the lack of emphasis on its clinical presentation and pathophysiology within the general medical education curriculum. Unfortunately, CVI has a major impact on society, negatively affecting the quality of life of patients and consuming large health care dollars and resources.

CVD is highly prevalent in the United States and western Europe but its true prevalence is unknown because of variability in the definition of the disease and methodology of evaluation. An estimated 25 million people in the United States have chronic venous disease, with 2 million to 6 million having CVI, and nearly 500,000 have venous stasis ulceration.[1] In the Edinburgh Vein Study, a cross-sectional study of a random sample of 1566 subjects, the prevalence of telangiectasias and reticular veins was approximately 80% and 85%, varicose veins 40% and 16%, and ankle edema 7% and 16% in men and women, respectively.[2] Various studies have shown that the prevalence of varicose veins ranged from 2% to 56% in men and 1% to 60% in women.[3] This prevalence increases with age. In the Edinburgh study, the overall prevalence of venous reflux by duplex ultrasound was 9.4% of men and 6.6% of women but rose to 21.2% in men and 12.0% in women over the age of 50.[4] Similarly trophic skin changes seem to increase with age with a prevalence of 1.8% in young women 30 years to 39 years of age, and 20.7% in women over the age of 70 years.[5] Finally, venous ulcers occur in approximately 1% of the general population and also increase with age.[2,6,7]

The incidence of CVD or its occurrence within a defined period of time has been evaluated in the Framingham Study.[8] Every second year and over a period of 16 years, subjects were examined for the appearance of varicose veins. The 1-year incidence rate of varicose veins was found to be 1.97% for men and 2.6% for women. In the Edinburgh Vein Study[9] the annual incidence rate in developing varicose veins was 1.4%, with incidence rates similar in men and women.

Several studies have suggested that women have a higher incidence of CVD but this has not been shown in more recent studies.[9,10] Women are likely to be more aware of their varicose veins and therefore are more likely to participate in studies leading to a selection bias. Also, age-adjusted prevalence of CVD in females has not been consistently performed in studies. In addition, pregnancy is a risk factor for CVD and is likely to bias the overall prevalence of CVD against women. Race has also been linked to CVD. In the San Diego Population Study, CVD was less prevalent in Blacks and Asians when compared with subjects of European origin.[11] Another study showed that English women are five times at risk of CVD than Egyptian women.[12] Furthermore, other risk factors have been linked to CVD and they include obesity,[9,13] standing occupation,[14] pregnancy,[15] heredity,[15] and prior history of limb trauma. In the Edinburgh Vein Study[9] subjects with a family history of venous disease were more likely to develop varicose veins (odds ratio [OR] 1.75). Also, in the same study obesity was associated with an age-adjusted OR of 3.58 with the development of CVI. In another study,[14] multivariate logistic regression analysis showed that female gender (OR 2.2), increasing age (OR 2.2 to 2.8), a reported positive family history for

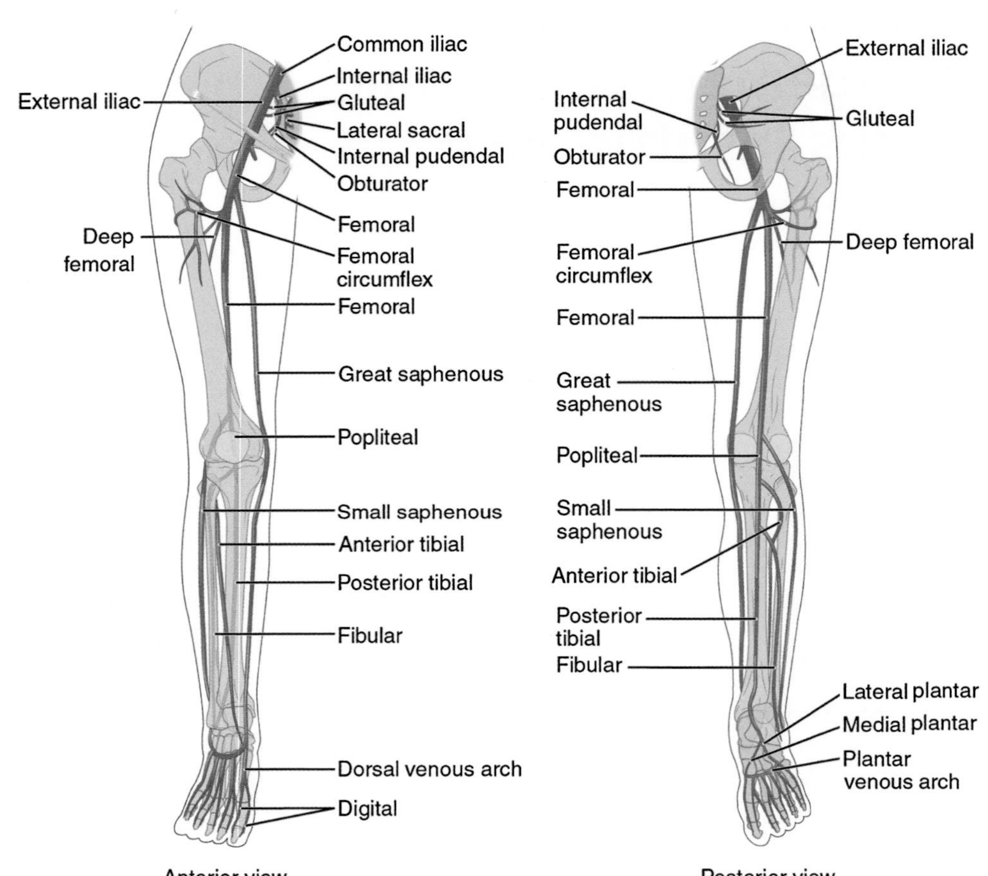

FIGURE 27-1 Anterior and posterior view of the major veins that drain the lower limb. *(Reused with permission from OpenStax CNX. "Circulatory Pathways." Figure: Major veins serving the lower limbs.* **http://cnx.org/content/m46646/latest/***.)*

varicose veins (OR 4.9), increasing number of births (OR 1.2 to 2.8), standing posture at work (OR 1.6), and higher weight (OR 1.2) and height (OR 1.4) were independent predictors of varicose veins.

CVI has a significant direct and indirect socioeconomic burden on society. In the United States, venous ulcerations resulted in a loss of 2 million workdays per year.[16] In France and Sweden, 2.24 billion euros and 73 million euros were spent per year for the treatment of CVI, respectively.[17,18] A study from Germany found that inpatient and outpatient direct costs were 250 million euros and 234 million euros, respectively, loss of working days costs were 270 million euros, and drug costs were 207 million euros.[19] The presence of venous ulcerations also impacted on quality of life substantially with more than 20% of ulcers remained not healed within 2 years follow-up.[20] These ulcers have been responsible for early retirement of 12.5% of workers with this condition.[21]

VENOUS ANATOMY AND PHYSIOLOGY

Treatment of chronic venous insufficiency requires a good understanding of normal venous anatomy and physiology. The veins of the lower limbs are divided into the superficial venous system, the deep venous system, and the perforator veins, connecting the superficial and deep veins at various levels from the foot to the gluteal area (**Figure 27-1**). The superficial venous system is located within the superficial compartment surrounded anteriorly by the hyperechoic saphenous fascia and posteriorly by the muscular fascia. Within the saphenous compartment reside the saphenous veins, accompanying arteries, and saphenous nerves. A saphenous vein exiting the saphenous compartment is better described as a tributary. The superficial veins of the lower limbs are numerous and interconnected in a network that eventually empties into two primary trunks that feed into the deep venous system: the great saphenous vein (GSV), and the small saphenous vein (SSV). These superficial veins connect to the deep system at the level of the common femoral vein for the GSV and quite often the popliteal vein for the SSV. Also, several perforators connect these superficial systems and their tributaries to the deep system. When discussing anatomy of the venous system, it is important to adhere to the current international nomenclature that has been adopted by the Union Internationale de Phlebologie (UIP) and is currently in use.[22,23] Below is an anatomic description of the venous system of the lower limbs from this consensus meeting.

Superficial Veins of the Lower Limb

Great Saphenous Vein

The great saphenous vein (GSV) is the longest and main superficial vein of the lower limb. It begins at the medial end of the arch as a continuation of the medial marginal vein of the foot. It ascends slightly anteriorly to the medial malleolus and continues anteromedially in the lower leg before it takes a short posterior course behind the medial condyle of the tibia at the level of the knee. In the lower thigh it ascends anterolaterally, then takes a medial course to below the inguinal ligament, passing through the cribriform fascia

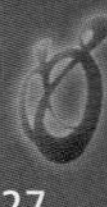

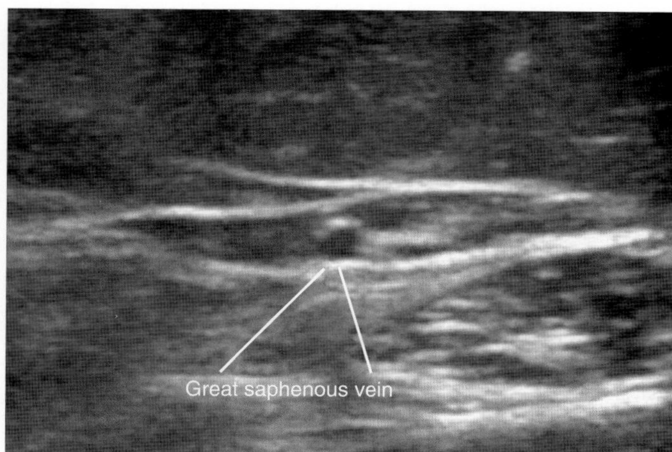

FIGURE 27-2 Great saphenous vein located within the saphenous compartment. The "Egyptian eye" is seen. The superficial fascia is the upper eyelid, the deep fascia is the lower eyelid, and the lumen of the GSV is the iris.

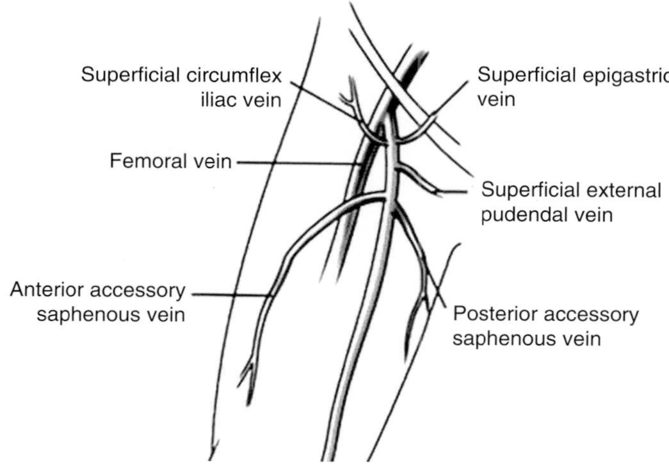

FIGURE 27-3 Proximal tributaries of the great saphenous vein.

that covers the fossa ovalis to join the common femoral vein (CFV) at the saphenofemoral junction (SFJ). The GSV is located within the saphenous compartment. The latter has been compared with the "Egyptian eye" when seen on a transverse scan by B-mode ultrasound (**Figure 27-2**). The superficial fascia is the upper eyelid, the deep fascia is the lower eyelid, and the lumen of the GSV is the iris. Outside the "eye," the saphenous trunk is called a superficial tributary even though it can still play the role of a main axial superficial vein. There are several anatomic variations to the GSV; it can be a single GSV within the "eye" and no large tributary, rarely two parallel GSV within the same compartment (true duplication), or a single GSV in the proximal thigh, and at various distances exit the "eye" to become a large subcutaneous tributary (present in about 30% of the time). Large tributaries running parallel to the entire length of the GSV outside the saphenous compartment can also be present and enter the GSV at different levels.

There are several valves in the GSV ranging from 8 to 20 in number. They are mostly located at the junctions with other veins. A constant terminal valve in the GSV is located 1 mm to 2 mm distal to the SFJ. Often, a preterminal valve is seen 2 cm distal to the terminal valve and delineates the distal limit of the SFJ area. At the SFJ, a confluence of proximal veins is seen and includes the superficial epigastric vein, superficial circumflex iliac vein, and external pudendal vein (**Figure 27-3**). Their clinical importance is in their ability to transmit retrograde flow into the GSV despite a competent terminal valve. Also, the GSV receives many tributary veins; some may be large, including the anterior accessory saphenous vein (AASV) (present in 41% of subjects and entering the GSV within 1 cm of the SFJ), and posterior accessory saphenous vein (PASV), often entering the GSV distal to the preterminal valve at variable distance. In addition, the anterior thigh circumflex vein ascends obliquely into the anterior thigh and enters either the GSV or the AASV; the posterior thigh circumflex vein ascends obliquely into the posterior thigh and may originate from the thigh extension of the small saphenous vein (SSV), directly from the SSV, or from the lateral vein plexus, and enters the GSV. The lateral extension of the SSV into the thigh that connects with the posterior circumflex vein is often called the vein of Giacomini (**Figure 27-4**).

Anterior Accessory Saphenous Vein

The AASV enters laterally the GSV just below the SFJ. Close to the SFJ both AASV and GSV often share the same saphenous compartment. The AASV, however, has its own saphenous eye more distally and can be distinguished from the GSV by the "alignment" sign where it runs anterior and parallel to the GSV and in line with the femoral artery and femoral vein.

Posterior Accessory Saphenous Vein

The PASV ascends parallel and posterior to the GSV within its own fascial compartment. It is not always easily found and it connects at various lengths with the GSV below the SFJ area. The PASV can be present above or below the knee. The below-the-knee segment that connects to the GSV is called Leonardo's vein, or posterior arch vein, and is present in approximately 27% of subjects.

Small Saphenous Vein (SSV)

The small saphenous vein (SSV) is a continuation of the lateral marginal foot vein and ascends behind the lateral malleolus to the posterior aspect of the calf in between the medial and lateral heads of gastrocnemius muscle. The SSV lies within the interfascial compartment across its length. On transverse duplex ultrasound, the SSV appears within the "eye," similar to the GSV. Proximally, it is within a triangular compartment outlined by the superficial fascia anteriorly, and the lateral and medial heads of the gastrocnemius muscle laterally and medially, respectively. The SSV generally terminates in the popliteal vein at the saphenopopliteal junction (SPJ) but not always (**Figure 27-5**). The SPJ is mostly located within 2 cm to 4 cm above the knee crease but this can significantly vary. The SSV continues into the thigh as the thigh extension (TE). TE is present in 95% of subjects and is intrafascial in position within a triangular compartment defined by the superficial fascia anteriorly, the semitendinous muscle medially, and the biceps femoris muscle laterally. The TE may end in the inferior gluteal vein, connected via a sciatic perforator or posterolateral thigh perforator to the femoral vein, or connected to the GSV via the posterior thigh circumflex vein. Both the TE of the SSV together with the posterior thigh circumflex vein that empties into the GSV are described as the vein of Giacomini.

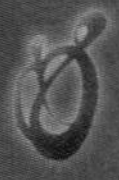

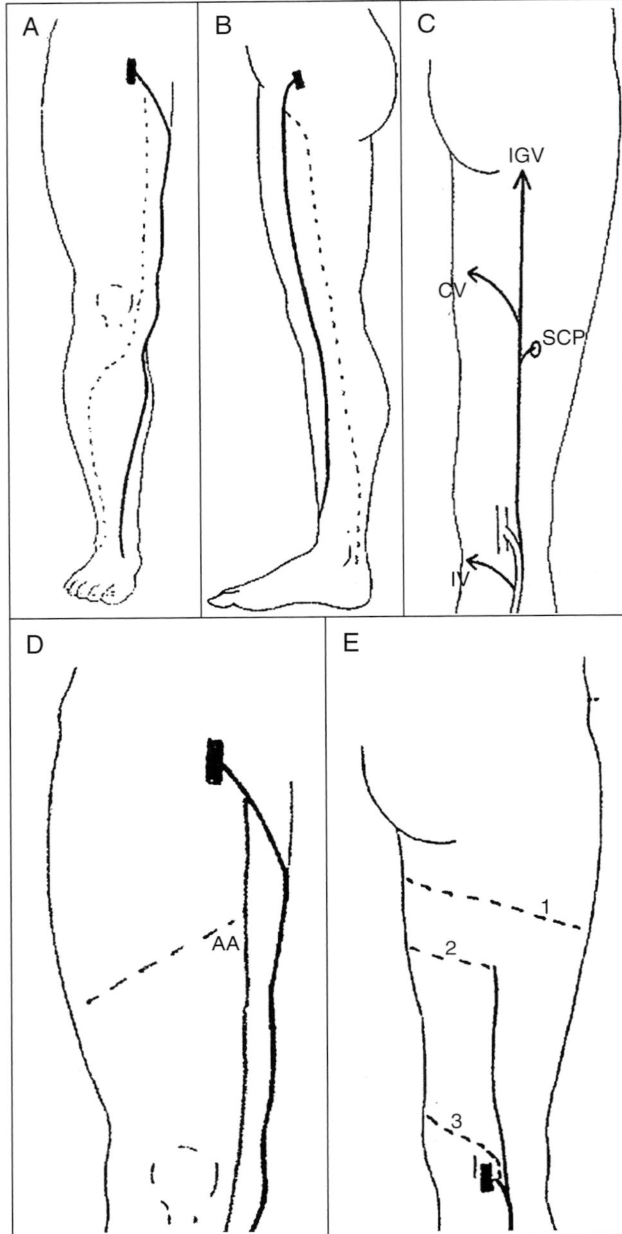

FIGURE 27-4 Course of the anterior accessory vein, posterior accessory vein, and thigh extension of the small saphenous vein. **A,** The course of the anterior accessory great saphenous vein *(dotted line)* is parallel and more anterior to the great saphenous vein *(black line)*. **B,** The course of the posterior accessory great saphenous vein *(dotted line)* is parallel and more posterior with respect to the great saphenous vein *(black line)*. **C,** The cranial extension of the small saphenous vein *(black line)* ends in the inferior gluteal vein (IGV) and can be connected to a sciatic perforator (ScP), or to the great saphenous vein via the posterior thigh circumflex vein (CV). One or more intersaphenous veins (IV) connect the small and great saphenous veins at the calf. **D,** The anterior thigh circumflex vein *(dashed line)* ascends obliquely in the anterior thigh to reach the anterior accessory great saphenous vein (AA) or the great saphenous vein. **E,** The posterior thigh circumflex vein *(dashed lines)* originates from the lateral venous plexus (1), or from the cranial extension of the small saphenous vein (2), or directly from the small saphenous vein (3). It courses obliquely in the posterior thigh toward the great saphenous vein. *(Reused with permission from Caggiati A, Bergan J, Gloviczki, P et al. Nomenclature of the veins of the lower limbs: an international interdisciplinary consensus statement. J Vasc Surg 36(2):416–422, 2002.* **www.jvascsurg.org/article/S0741-5214(02)00070-8/abstract.***)*

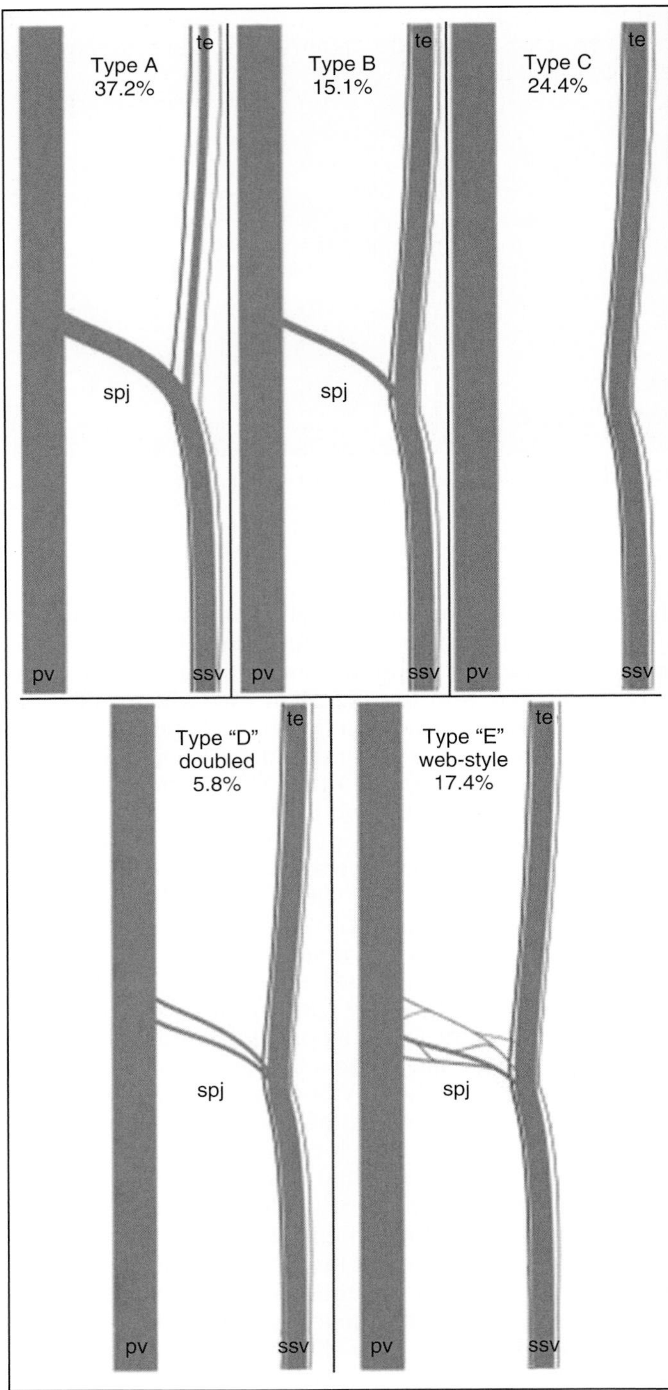

FIGURE 27-5 Anatomic variations of the small saphenous vein. Types A, B, C are labeled according to the UIP-consensus; Type "D" representing a doubled saphenopopliteal junction, and Type "E" representing a web-style saphenopopliteal junction. *PV,* Popliteal vein; *SSV,* short saphenous vein; *TE,* thigh extension. *(Reused with permission from Schweighofer G, Mühlberger D, Brenner E: The anatomy of the small saphenous vein: fascial and neural relations, saphenofermoral junction, and valves. J Vasc Surg 51(4):982–989, 2010.* **www.jvascsurg.org/article/S0741-5214(09)01829-1/fulltext.***)*

The gastrocnemius veins may merge with the SSV to empty into the popliteal vein or they could empty directly into the popliteal vein near the SPJ. Like the GSV, there is a terminal valve in the SSV close to the popliteal vein and a preterminal valve generally located below the TE of the SSV.

Perforators of the Lower Limb

The superficial veins are connected to the deep veins via the perforator veins (**Table 27-1**) that penetrate the deep fascia. More than 40 perforator veins have been described. The perforators are located at several levels in the lower limb: foot, ankle, lower leg, knee, thigh, and gluteal area (**Figure 27-6**). From a historic point of view, they have been named after individuals who described them. Descriptive terms to their location are preferred and have been widely adopted, as follows:

- The perforators of the foot (venae perforantes pedis) are described into dorsal, medial, lateral, and plantar foot perforators.
- The ankle perforators (venae perforantis tarsalis) are the medial, anterior, and lateral ankle perforators.
- The perforators of the leg (venae perforantes cruris) are separated into four main groups:
  - Medial leg perforators (paratibial and posterior tibial). The paratibial perforators connect the GSV or its tributaries to the posterior tibial vein (PTV) and the posterior tibial perforators connect below the knee PASV to the PTV. These perforators are indicated by their location as upper, middle, and lower.
  - Anterior leg perforators connect the anterior tributaries of the GSV to the anterior tibial veins (ATV).
  - Lateral leg perforators connect veins of the lateral venous plexus to the peroneal veins.
  - Perforators of the posterior leg (medial gastrocnemius perforators, lateral gastrocnemius perforators, intergemellar perforators (connecting the SSV to the soleal veins) and para-Achillean perforators (connecting the SSV to the peroneal veins).
- The perforators of the knee (venae perforantes genus) are designated as medial, lateral, suprapatellar, infrapatellar, and popliteal fossa knee perforators.
- The perforators of the thigh (venae perforantes femoris) are separated into the following:
  - Medial thigh (perforators of the femoral canal and inguinal perforators) connecting the GSV or its tributaries to the femoral vein
  - Anterior thigh
  - Lateral thigh
  - Posterior thigh (posteromedial, sciatic perforators, posterolateral) and pudendal perforators
- The perforators of the gluteal muscles (venae perforantes glutealis) are divided in superior, mid, and lower perforators.

TABLE 27-1 Perforator Groups and Subgroups in the Lower Limb

PERFORATOR GROUPS	SUBGROUPS
Foot	Dorsal, plantar, lateral, medial
Ankle	Anterior, medial, and lateral
Leg	Medial (paratibial and posterior tibial) [GSV or tributaries to PTV] Anterior [GSV tributaries to ATV] Lateral [lateral venous plexus to peroneal] Posterior (medial and lateral gastrocnemius, intergemellar [SSV to soleal]) Para-achillean [SSV to peroneal]
Knee	Medial, lateral, suprapatellar, infrapatellar, popliteal fossa
Thigh	Medial (femoral canal, inguinal), anterior, lateral, posterior (posteromedial, sciatic, posterolateral, pudendal)
Gluteal	Superior, mid, lower

ATV, Anterior tibialis vein; *GSV,* greater saphenous vein; *PTV,* posterior tibialis vein; *SSV,* small saphenous vein; [...] indicates the superficial to deep vein connections of the perforator veins.

Deep Venous System

The deep venous system is located below the muscular fascia in the deep compartment. It is comprised of axial veins and intramuscular veins. The deep venous system eventually receives all venous flow that empties in the right atrium. The main axial veins are the popliteal vein (PV) that

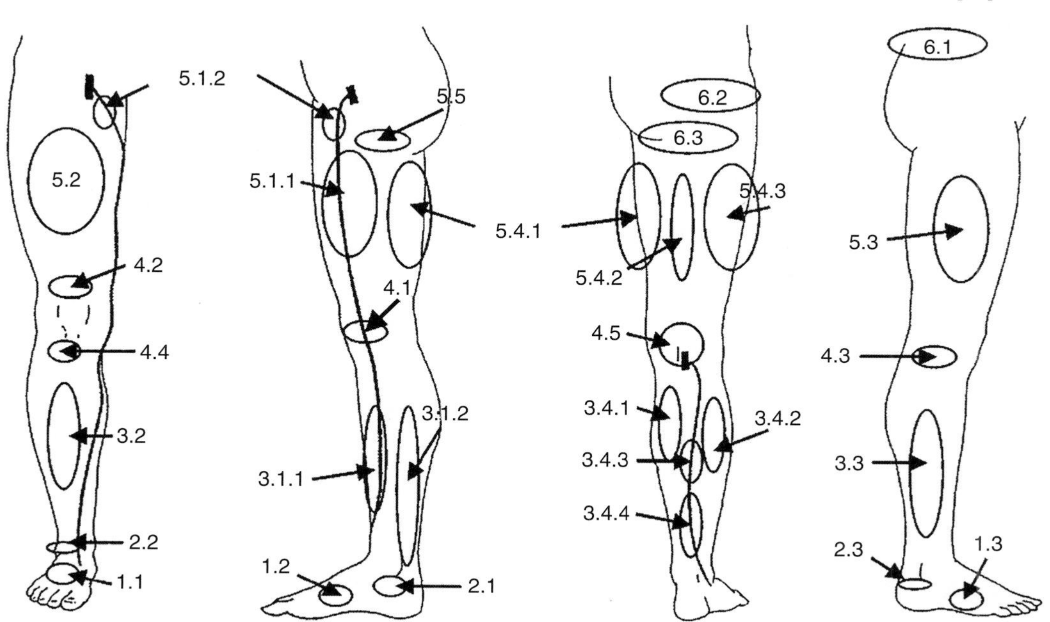

FIGURE 27-6 Main groups of popliteal veins (PVs).
Foot 1.1, dorsal foot; 1.2, medial foot; 1.3, lateral foot.
Ankle 2.1, medial ankle; 2.2, anterior ankle; 2.3, lateral ankle.
Leg 3.1.1, paratibial; 3.1.2, posterior tibial; 3.2, anterior leg; 3.3, lateral leg; 3.4.1, medial gastrocnemius; 3.4.2, lateral gastrocnemius; 3.4.3, intergemellar; 3.4.4, para-achillean.
Knee 4.1, medial knee; 4.2, suprapatellar; 4.3, lateral knee; 4.4, infrapatellar; 4.5, popliteal fossa.
Thigh 5.1.1, the femoral canal; 5.1.2, inguinal; 5.2, anterior thigh; 5.3, lateral thigh; 5.4.1, posteromedial thigh; 5.4.2, sciatic; 5.4.3, posterolateral thigh; 5.5, pudendal.
Gluteal 6.1, superior gluteal; 6.2, midgluteal; 6.3, lower gluteal. *(Reused with permission from Caggiati A, Bergan J, Gloviczki P, et al: Nomenclature of the veins of the lower limbs: an international interdisciplinary consensus statement. J Vasc Surg 36(2):416–422, 2002.* **www.jvascsurg.org/article/S0741-5214(02)00070-8/abstract.***)*

becomes the femoral vein (FV) above the knee when it passes through the adductor canal then the common femoral vein (CFV) as it joins the deep femoral vein (DFV) at the groin level. The CFV leads to the iliac veins, then the inferior vena cava to the right atrium.

Intramuscular venous sinusoids coalesce and form the venous plexi within the soleal and gastrocnemius calf muscles. These gastrocnemius lateral and medial veins connect to form an extramuscular trunk that travels 1 cm to 4 cm into the popliteal fossa and empties directly into the popliteal vein, or into the SSV at the level of the SPJ, or simultaneously into both popliteal and SSV. The soleus veins unite into one or several main trunks and terminate in either the PTV or the peroneal vein. The term *sural veins* refers to the lateral and medial gastrocnemius veins, soleal vein, and intergemellar vein, which courses deep to the SSV between the heads of the gastrocnemius muscles.

Physiology of the Venous System

The venous system functions as a large reservoir storing about 70% of the blood in a subject. It also serves as a low-flow, low-pressure conduit moving venous blood to the heart. Flow into the venous system travels against gravity and therefore a series of muscle pumps and valves are built in to assist in this flow. Predominantly calf muscle contraction and to a lesser extent foot and thigh muscles increase fascial compartment pressures, compressing the intramuscular veins and venous plexi in the calf and driving venous flow upward against gravity. Negative intrathoracic pressure also assists in the process of forward flow. A series of unidirectional bicuspid valves are present in the lower limb and superficial venous systems that continue to ensure a forward flow of blood to the heart against gravity.[24] Valves are also present at the perforators that prevent flow from the deep system back into the superficial system. The CFV typically has one valve. The inferior vena cava and common iliac veins have no valves. Infrequently, a valve can be seen in the external iliac vein. The infrainguinal veins have several valves located at different levels but most seem to concentrate at the knee level and below.

The resting standing venous pressure is approximately 80 to 90 mm Hg. Following ambulation, the muscle contraction moves the venous flow forward emptying the venous system and dropping the pressure to 15 to 30 mm Hg. When muscle relaxation occurs the venous system refills slowly (more than 20 seconds) from arterial inflow into the superficial and deep veins, distending the veins and allowing the valves (**Figure 27-7**) to open, creating a single pipe of fluid with a pressure at the ankle equal to the height of the column of blood. In a competent valve system, contraction of the muscle leads to quick emptying of the veins with no refluxing of flow backward, and a quick drop of pressure in the venous system typically more than 50% decrease from the resting standing pressure.[25]

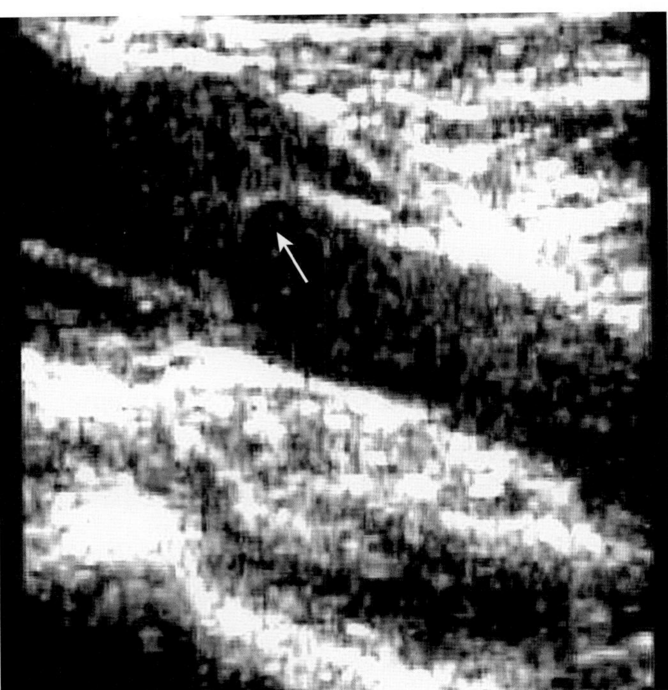

FIGURE 27-7 Venous valve *(arrow)*.

ETIOLOGY AND PATHOPHYSIOLOGY OF CHRONIC VENOUS INSUFFICIENCY

The main pathophysiologic mechanism of CVI is high venous pressure in the lower extremity due to failure in keeping venous upward flow toward the heart. This can result from backward reflux of venous flow through incompetent valves in the deep or superficial venous systems, or the perforators that connect both. Venous obstruction in the deep system can also impede venous flow and contribute to high venous pressure. In addition, muscular dysfunction can also contribute to reducing forward venous flow and along with reflux becomes an important risk factor for venous ulceration. When valve incompetence is present, the backward flow of blood to the lower veins contributes to raising the venous pressure faster to resting level (in less than 10-20 seconds). Also the drop of venous pressure in an incompetent valve system with ambulation is blunted and venous pressure remains higher than 50% its resting value.[25] The constant high venous pressure in the lower limb is ultimately responsible for venous microangiopathy and subsequently the development of signs and symptoms of chronic venous insufficiency.

Valve incompetence in the superficial veins may be due to primary valve failure or weakness in the vessel wall. Secondary causes of valve incompetence can be trauma, hormonal effects, thrombophlebitis, or high pressure.[26] There are several potential sources of reflux from the deep system into the superficial system via incompetent perforators, or incompetent SPJ, or SFJ. Also reflux can be transmitted from the GSV, perineal veins, and thigh perforators to the SSV via the Giacomini vein, or backward from the SPJ to the GSV, or the veins of the posterior aspect of the thigh via the same system.[22] The deep system could also develop significant reflux mostly due to obstruction, partial or complete. This can be related to deep vein thrombosis (DVT), stenosis, or extrinsic compression. Compression of the iliac vessels can produce obstruction to upward venous flow resulting in high venous pressure leading to vein dilation, and reflux. Iliac extrinsic compression is quite often an underestimated cause of CVD and a high index of suspicion is needed to correctly identify this problem.[27] Finally, muscle pump dysfunction is a contributor to venous ulcerations in patients with venous reflux. Reflux in conjunction with muscle pump failure is a significant risk factor for developing venous ulcers. The presence of good muscle pump function lessens the chance of ulcerations in patients with severe reflux, and the presence of poor muscle function can increase the risk of ulceration, even when minimal reflux is present.[28,29]

Venous microangiopathy is the result of high venous pressure transmitted to the microvasculature of the lower legs. In its mild form, CVI results in an increase in transcapillary diffusion of sodium fluorescein (NaF), a marker of leak in the capillary bed seen early in the disease process and is accompanied by an increase in pericapillary space (halo). As CVI progresses and becomes more severe, capillary thromboses occur, leading to a reduced capillary density and a reduction in transcutaneous oxygen tension (tcpO2), particularly at the ulcer rim. The remaining capillaries become more elongated and tortuous. They become more permeable because of the stretching of their inter-endothelial pores. Larger molecules can exit the capillaries into the extracapillary space, leading to chronic inflammation and edema and eventually skin trophic changes and ulcerations. Also, in the severe stages of CVI, there is a destruction of the lymphatic capillary network and an increase in the permeability of the remaining lymphatic fragments suggesting lymphatic microangiopathy.[30] Dysfunction of local nerve fibers also occurs.

There are several hypotheses on how microangiopathy leads to venous ulcerations. Browse and colleagues[31] proposed the fibrin cuff theory, which centers on the leak of fibrinogen into the pericapillary space. This results in pericapillary fibrin cuffs that were thought to be a barrier for diffusion of oxygen. Fibrin cuffs, however, are not a specific finding for venous ulceration and were found not to impair oxygen diffusion significantly.[30] Another theory is the trapping of leukocytes in the capillaries, or postcapillary venules with subsequent release of their inflammatory mediators and proteolytic enzymes leading to endothelial injury.[32] Finally, trapping of leaked growth factors in the pericapillary space is thought to prevent their ability to participate in the healing of damaged capillary bed.[33]

EVALUATION AND CLASSIFICATION OF THE PATIENT WITH CHRONIC VENOUS INSUFFICIENCY

Chronic venous disease (CVD) presents with a spectrum of pathologies ranging from telangiectasia to skin hyperpigmentation to venous ulcers. The term *CVI* is generally used for patients with an advanced form of CVD generally presenting with symptoms and signs of lower extremity edema, trophic skin changes, and venous ulcerations.

The initial evaluation of a patient with CVI starts with a comprehensive history and physical examination.[34] Symptoms of CVI include heaviness, achiness, tightness, itching, muscle cramps, involuntary movements of the limb, and tingling. These worsen when patients are standing and improve when the feet are elevated at heart level. Patients' symptoms are worse as the day progresses and generally mild or fewer symptoms are noted in the morning prior to standing out of bed. The interference of symptoms with daily activity and the response to prior treatment such as compression garments should be documented. Risk factors for developing CVD should be identified, such as advanced age, a higher weight and height, standing occupation, heredity, prior injury, surgeries or trauma, history of DVT, multiple pregnancies, and ethnic background. A past history of early childhood varicose veins is important to note as it may be related to some rare congenital blood vessel malformations such as in Klippel–Trénaunay–Weber syndrome.[35] Providers need to keep in mind other sources of pain that may mimic CVI, including tendinitis, arthritis, neuropathy, or arterial insufficiency. Careful history and examination should help in identifying these etiologies.

The physical examination should be performed in a warm, well-lit room and when the patient is standing. The entire leg needs to be checked starting from the inguinal area to the foot, and findings of abnormal veins, skin changes, or ulcerations need to be well documented on a drawing showing the anterior, posterior, medial, and lateral parts of the leg. Palpation over the GSV, SSV, SFJ, and SPJ may reveal additional varicosities, subcutaneous cords, or areas of indurations not visible with inspection only. Palpation of the SFJ with cough can reveal a thrill that indicates reflux at this level (cough impulse test). Also, a tap on the GSV distally while palpating the SFJ area may allow the feeling of a transmitted pulse to the SFJ indicating GSV distention. The opposite is true with a tap on the SFJ, allowing a feeling of transmitted pulse to the distal GSV indicating reflux (the tap test).[36] These tests, however, lack good sensitivity in identifying reflux at the SFJ. The Brodie-Trendelenburg test can help identify perforator reflux into the GSV. The patient's leg is elevated 45 degrees and blood is massaged up the leg from the foot. A tourniquet is then applied proximally close to the groin area. The patient is then allowed to stand up. If no dilation of the lower leg veins is seen after 20 to 30 seconds, perforator valves are likely to be competent. If after releasing the tourniquet, the veins in the leg distend quickly, this indicates that the superficial venous system is incompetent. This test is highly sensitive but poorly specific in identifying superficial and perforator reflux.[36] Another test that can be performed in the office is the Perthes test. A tourniquet is placed below the knee in a standing position. The patient is asked to raise the heel 10 times. If varicosities empty, this indicates that the perforators of the lower superficial venous system are competent and reflux is likely cranial to the tourniquet. On the other hand, if more distention occurs to the varicosities of the lower leg, this indicates that reflux is present in the deep perforators below the knee. The presence of severe pain in the calf with raising the heel repetitively could indicate the presence of DVT. These physical maneuvers have been widely replaced with duplex ultrasound to the lower leg that has a higher accuracy in identifying the presence and location of the reflux.

Once the examination and history are obtained, disease needs to be classified based on its clinical presentation. The Clinical, Etiologic, Anatomic, and Pathophysiology (CEAP) classification system was developed at the American Venous Forum annual meeting in 1994, and revised in 2004.[34] The physical findings are divided into seven clinical manifestations ranging from no visible findings of CVD to active venous ulcerations. Given the progression of CVD, the classification also reflects the natural clinical progression of this disease. The etiologic, anatomic and pathophysiologic classifications require additional anatomic and functional testing that will be discussed later. The CEAP classification is described in **Table 27-2** and clinical manifestations are shown in **Figures 27-8 to 27-11**.

The venous clinical severity score (VCSS)[37] (**Table 27-3**) was designed to complement the CEAP score and to provide

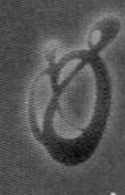

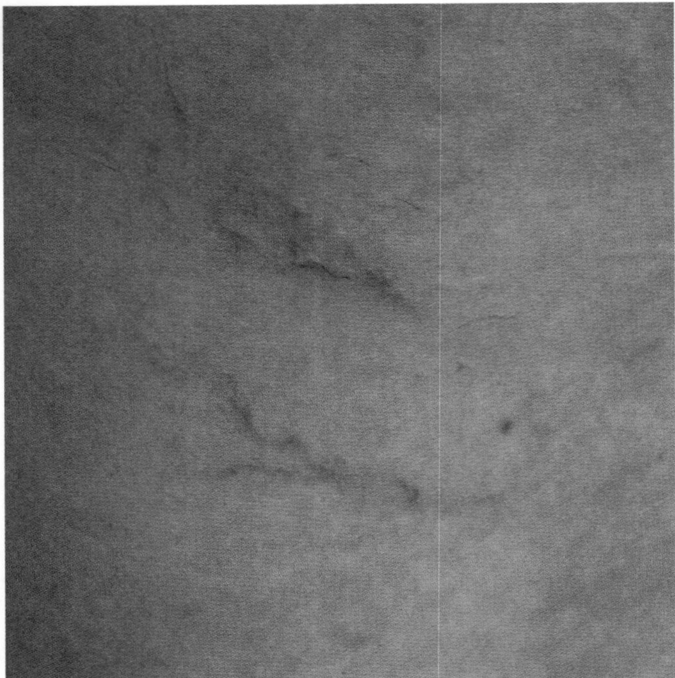

FIGURE 27-8 CEAP Class I with telangiectasias (spider veins).

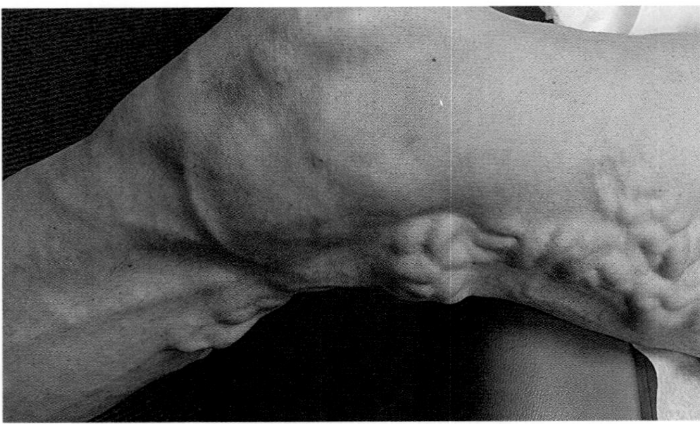

FIGURE 27-9 CEAP Class II with large varicosities.

TABLE 27-2 Clinical Manifestations Classes Per CEAP Classification

GRADE	DESCRIPTION
C 0	No visible or palpable signs of venous disease
C 1	Superficial telangiectasias (intradermal, less than 1 mm, flat, red vessels) or reticular veins (subdermal, 1-3 mm, flat, bluish) or venulectasias (rise above skin, 1-2 mm, blue)
C 2	Varicose veins (diameter more or equal 3 mm)
C 3	Ankle edema
C 4	Changes in skin and subcutaneous tissue
	C4a: Pigmentation or eczema
	C4b: Lipodermatosclerosis or atrophie blanche
C 5	Healed venous ulcer
C 6	Active venous ulcer

CEAP, Clinical, etiologic, anatomic, pathophysiologic classification.

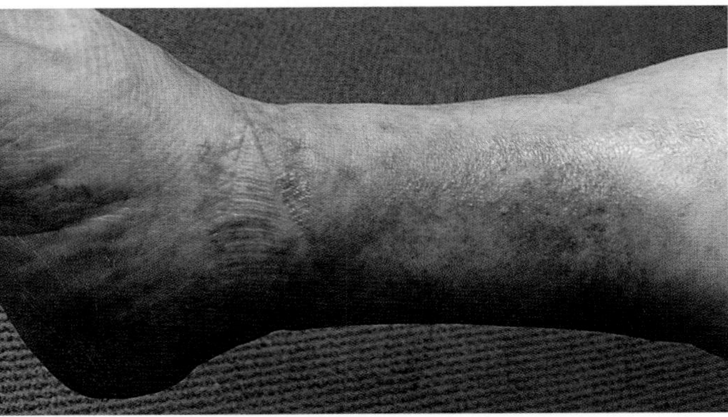

FIGURE 27-10 CEAP Class IVb with skin hyperpigmentation and atrophie blanche changes.

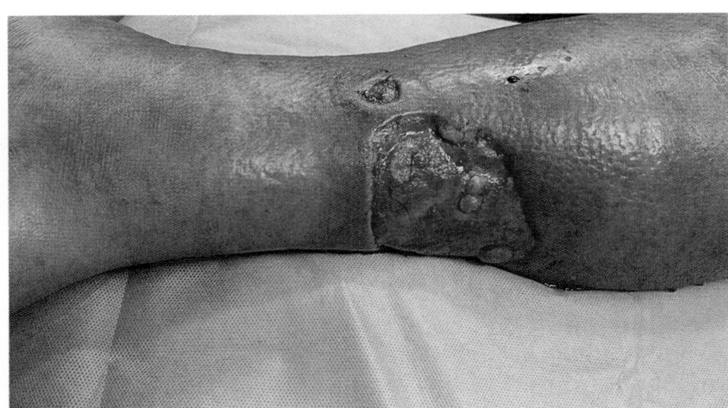

FIGURE 27-11 CEAP Class VI with nonhealing venous ulcer.

a method to serially assess the severity of disease over time, and in response to a treatment. The advantage of the VCSS is that it is dynamic and is able to capture changes in disease severity whereas the CEAP class is descriptive and static, particularly in its advanced classes (IV to VI).

The venous severity score (VSS) is another scoring system that grades disease severity and is sum score of multiple other scoring systems including VCSS, Venous Segmental Disease Score (VSDS), and Venous Disability Score (VDS).[38] Other scoring systems are present and one should adopt a scoring system that complements the CEAP score in order to be able to assess longitudinal changes in patients' symptoms and signs of CVI either naturally or after intervention.

ANATOMIC AND PHYSIOLOGIC TESTING OF CHRONIC VENOUS INSUFFICIENCY

There are several anatomic and physiologic tests that can be utilized to diagnose and understand the etiology of chronic venous insufficiency. The most practical and commonly used test in an office setting is the duplex venous ultrasound (DU) and to a lesser extent plethysmography.

Duplex Venous Ultrasound of the Lower Limb

Duplex venous ultrasound (DU) is likely to be the most widely used technique in the diagnosis of venous disorders, including DVT and superficial venous disease. This section will focus on the use of DU in the diagnosis and management of patients with chronic superficial venous disease. An

TABLE 27-3 Venous Clinical Severity Score (VCSS)

ATTRIBUTE	ABSENT = 0	MILD = 1	MODERATE = 2	SEVERE = 3
Pain	None	Occasional pain or other discomfort	Daily pain or other discomfort	Daily pain or discomfort, limits most regular daily activities
Varicose veins ≥3 mm in diameter	None	Scattered, includes corona phlebectatica	Confined to calf or thigh	Involves calf and thigh
Edema	None	Limited to foot and ankle	Extends above ankle but below knee	Extends to knee and above
Pigmentation	None or focal	Limited to perimalleolar area	Diffuse over lower third of calf	Above lower third of calf
Inflammation	None	Limited to perimalleolar area	Diffuse over lower third of calf	Above lower third of calf
Induration	None	Limited to perimalleolar area	Diffuse over lower third of calf	Wider distribution above lower third of calf
Number of active ulcers	0	1	2	≥3
Duration of longest active ulcer	None	<3mo	>3 mo but <1 yr	Not healed for >1 yr
Size of largest active ulcer	None	Diameter <2 cm	Diameter 2 to 6 cm	Diameter >6 cm
Compression therapy	Not used	Intermittent use of stockings	Wears stockings most days	Full compliance: stockings

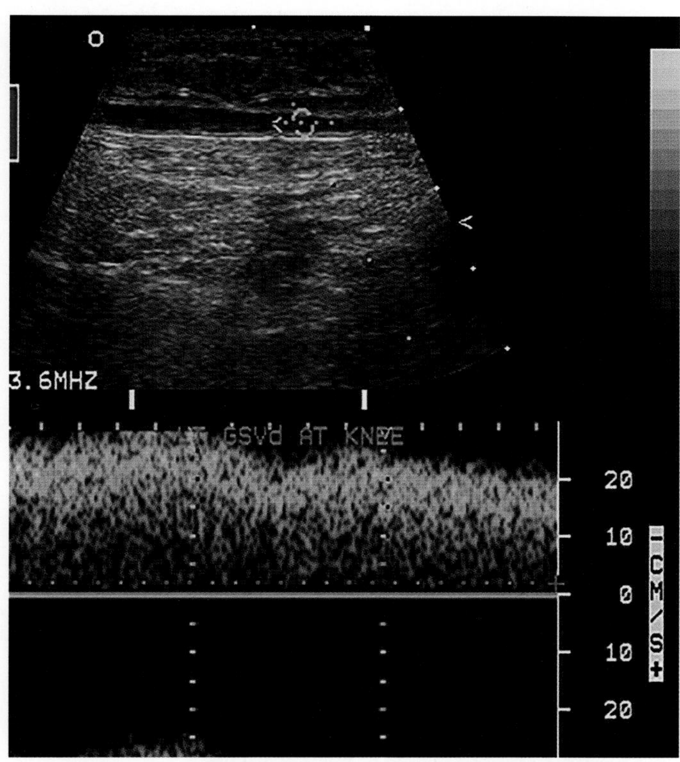

FIGURE 27-12 Spectral Doppler showing reflux in the great saphenous vein.

evaluation of the deep venous system is routinely performed when assessing superficial venous reflux to rule out coexistent DVT, assess for deep venous reflux, and assist in the diagnosis of potential iliac obstructive disease.[39]

Spectral Doppler flow is utilized to determine the degree of reflux in the superficial venous and deep venous systems (**Figure 27-12**). Reflux in the deep venous system is evaluated in the supine position with the head elevated 10 degrees to 15 degrees. Evaluation of the superficial venous system needs to be performed in the standing position with distal augmentation and with the patient standing with the weight mostly on the contralateral leg. The heel of the leg under examination should be flat on the floor to avoid calf muscle contraction during the test. The cutoff for abnormal retrograde flow is greater than 500 ms in the superficial system and deep calf veins but greater than 1000 ms in the femoropopliteal vein. Reflux in the perforator vein is abnormal if it is more than 350 ms[40] but the cutoff for clinical intervention is more than 500 ms. Reflux is best reported in seconds rather than graded in severity as mild, moderate, or severe as the correlation with the severity of disease is not standardized, and is variable. Initially, the SSV is interrogated, including its relationship to the popliteal vein. The thigh extension of the SSV will also need to be identified along with its termination. Next, the GSV and its tributaries are evaluated. In approximately 2% of the time, there is a duplicate GSV.[41] Reflux and GSV sizes are measured at the level of the SFJ, mid thigh, and above and below the knee. Mapping the AASV and the PASV follows the GSV. Furthermore, tributaries at least 50% the size of the native saphenous veins are mapped.[42] Finally, perforators' veins are mapped, which is particularly important in patients with healed and nonhealed venous ulcerations. An extensive mapping of perforators is less useful. Perforators large enough to be more than 3.5 mm in diameter and with reflux more than 500 ms are of particular importance in patients with venous ulcerations as these perforators are typically the target for therapeutic intervention. The mapping data are then compiled into a diagram that will be utilized for diagnostic and therapeutic intervention.

DU can also identify other pathologies, including aneurysms, tumors, or presence of Baker's cyst in the popliteal fossa. In addition, it helps monitoring the success of endovenous ablative procedures and in the progression of reflux in symptomatic patients. Guidelines of the American Venous Forum on duplex ultrasound scanning in patients with venous reflux indicate that DU is recommended as the first diagnostic test for all patients with suspected CVI. DU is also indicated for follow-up after successful endovenous ablation procedure if symptoms have recurred. Routine application of DU, however, after successful ablation and with no symptoms' recurrence is not indicated.

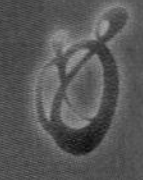

Plethysmography

Plethysmography provides functional information that is complementary to DU in the management of CVI.[43,44] Plethysmography is a test that quantitatively measures blood volume changes within the leg. Air plethysmography (AP) is a convenient and inexpensive test that uses an air-filled long cuff to measure fluctuations in leg volume. In AP, the patient starts in a supine position. The leg being examined is raised up at 45 degrees for 5 minutes to cause venous emptying. An air-filled cuff is then placed below the knee and inflated at 6 mm Hg. The patient is then placed in the standing position and the leg veins are allowed to fill via arterial influx and venous reflux. Maximum venous volume (VV) (mL) is then recorded. The time to fill 90% of the VV is determined (VFT90) (seconds). A venous filling index (VFI) is then calculated (VV/VFT90 [mL per sec]). The patient is then asked to flex the ankle to contract the calf muscle. The volume of blood ejected is recorded (EV). The ejection fraction (EF) of the calf muscle contraction is then calculated (EF = EV/VV*100). After the VV is restored, 10 consecutive tip-toe movements are done. Residual volume (RV) is determined from time zero. Residual volume fraction (RVF) is then calculated using the formula RV/VV*100 (**Figure 27-13**).

VFI correlates with the clinical severity of CVI through Class 2 of the CEAP classification.[45,46] Clinical deterioration beyond Class 2 does not correlate with further deterioration of hemodynamics. VFI over 5 mL per second correlates with deep venous and perforator reflux,[44] and more than 7 mL per second identifies the risk of "critical" deep venous reflux likely to be predictive of venous ulceration.[47] VFI is also a predictor of multisystem reflux (deep, superficial, and perforator).[48] VFI of 6.68 mL per second correlated with triple-system incompetence, whereas a VFI of 4.5 correlates with a dual-system incompetence. The number of incompetent system increases with clinical severity of disease. In general, however, all AP parameters are poor predictors for severe disease or ulcerations.[44] EF and RVF are good indicators of calf muscle function but they rarely influence the clinical severity of disease and do not discriminate between different types of reflux.[44]

TREATMENT OF SUPERFICIAL CHRONIC VENOUS INSUFFICIENCY

CVI is a progressive disease.[49] Treatment of all sources of reflux is important to reduce symptoms and obtain a successful outcome. Initially it was thought that reflux is always descending, starting at the level of the common femoral vein or the SFJ and progressing distally. Several studies, however, indicate that vessel wall changes may occur at any level, causing segmental reflux with no junctional or proximal reflux.[50,51] In fact, reflux develops in most people at the knee or the calf level with no involvement of the saphenous junctions.[52] Younger patients less than 30 years of age have several refluxing tributaries of saphenous or nonsaphenous veins and statistically less involvement of the junctions compared with patients over the age of 60. In this study, 44% of varicose limbs also had a normal saphenous vein.[53] In addition, retrograde reflux is seen from the vein of Giacomini into the GSV leading to GSV reflux with no SFJ involvement. Finally, refluxing perforators into the superficial veins may occur, leading to segmental saphenous reflux.

Superficial venous reflux quite often coexists with deep venous reflux. Segmental deep venous reflux can be induced

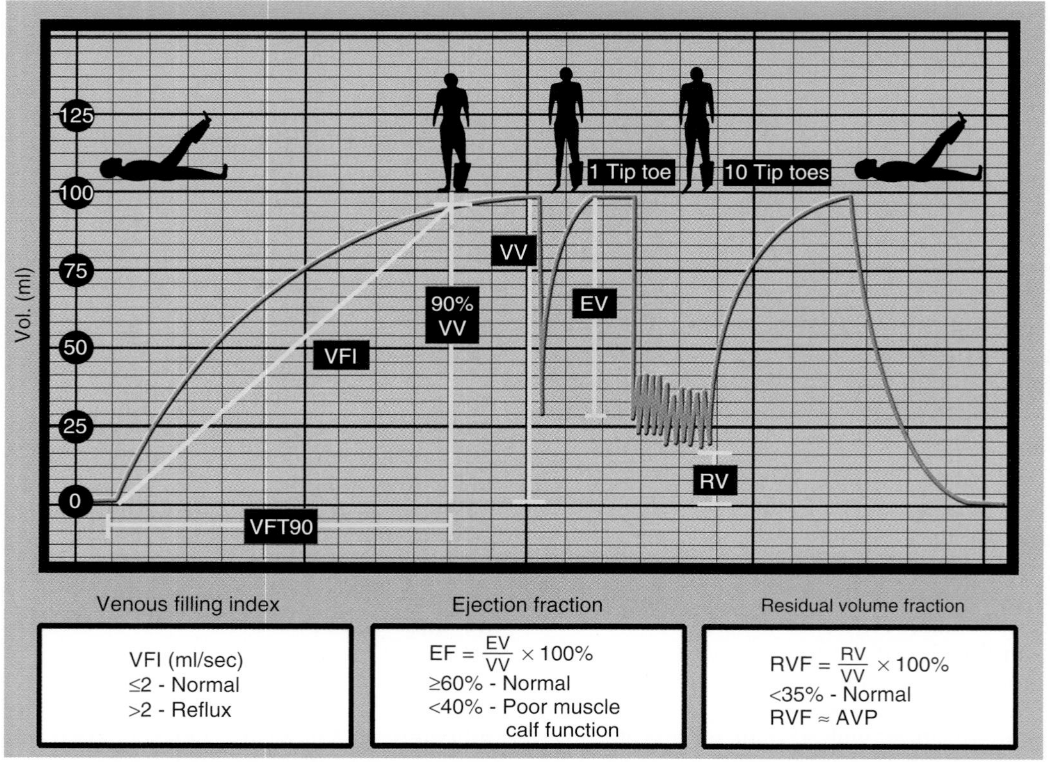

FIGURE 27-13 Air plethysmogram. VFI = VV/VFT90 (mL per sec). The ejection fraction (EF) of the calf muscle contraction is = EV/VV*100. Residual volume fraction (RVF) is = RV/VV*100. *EF,* ejection fraction; *EV,* volume of blood ejected; *RV,* residual volume; *RVF,* residual volume fraction; *VFI,* venous filling index; *VFT90,* time to fill 90% of the VV (/sec); *VV,* venous volume. *(Reused with permission from J Physiol 374(Suppl):1P–16P, 1986, page 11P, figure 1B, Wileyonline Publication.)*

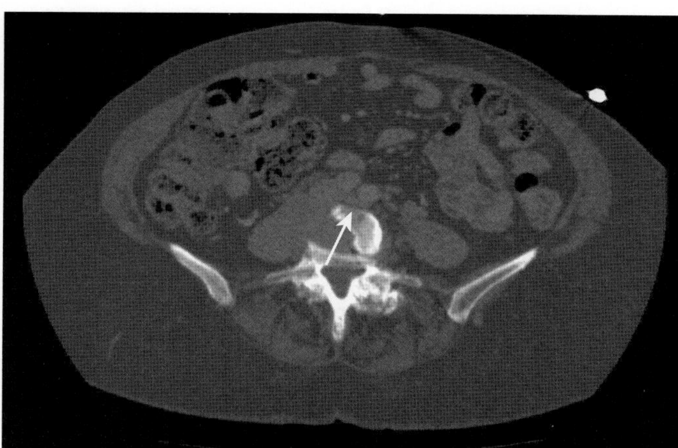

FIGURE 27-14 Left common iliac vein compression by the right iliac artery consistent with May-Thurner syndrome.

by reflux from incompetent veins draining into the deep system.[54,55] In one study, ablation of incompetent superficial venous reflux eliminates coexistent incompetence in the deep venous system in 94% of patients (Sales CM, 1996). Also, complete GSV surgical stripping significantly reduced deep venous reflux on postoperative DU, whereas incomplete stripping of refluxing GSV was associated with the development of new deep vein reflux on follow-up.[56] When significant swelling in the lower legs or ulcerations cannot be explained by the degree of reflux seen in the superficial veins, iliac venous compression needs to be ruled out. Furthermore, in case of unilateral swelling with combined deep and superficial venous reflux, DVT and/or pelvic venous compression syndrome need to be ruled out prior to superficial venous ablation (**Figure 27-14**) (Videos 27-1 and 27-2). The presence of DVT with no axial flow in the femoropopliteal vein or severe iliac compression should be considered a contraindication to ablate the superficial vein. Finally, venous claudication, particularly with an increase in venous pressure by three times the normal with exercise compared with the contralateral leg, should raise suspicion for an iliac compression syndrome.[57] A decrease in phasicity at the level of the common femoral vein in the affected leg compared with the contralateral common femoral vein should raise suspicion for a venous compression syndrome.[58] Computed tomography with venous filling phase (CTV) or magnetic resonance venography (MRV) may confirm the diagnosis. The most reliable test, however, in identifying iliac venous compression is the intravascular ultrasound.

The treatment of superficial venous reflux can range from graded compression therapy, which is generally the first-line treatment, followed by ablative or surgical stripping of the refluxing superficial veins if symptoms persist. Later in this chapter is a description of various therapies for superficial venous reflux and CVI.

Compression Therapy

Compression therapy is effective in reducing the symptoms of discomfort, swelling, and ulcerations in patients with chronic venous insufficiency. Historically, this method of treatment has been used since antiquity[59] and remains the standard of care in the initial treatment of patients with venous insufficiency. Its aim is to reduce capacity and pressure within the venous system of the lower limbs, reduce edema by accelerating venous return, and aid in venous ulceration healing. This can be achieved with bandages, compression stockings, or dynamic intermittent compression. Compression therapy is indicated for all classes of the CEAP grading system and for patients with lymphedema. Also, quite often compression therapy is used for DVT prophylaxis and for post-DVT management to reduce post-thrombotic syndrome.[60]

Prior to initiating compression therapy, patients need to be ruled out for severe peripheral arterial disease. An ankle brachial index (ABI) of less than 0.5 should be considered a contraindication to compression bandages or stockings. A reduced compression pressure needs to be considered for patients with moderate reduction in their ABI (0.5 to 0.7).[61] Compression pressures are classified into mild (less than 20 mm Hg), moderate (20 to less than 40 mm Hg), strong (40 to less than 60 mm Hg), and very strong (60 mm Hg or more).[62] The worse the symptoms, the higher the pressure needed. Typically strong, more than 40 mm Hg compression is used for patients with venous ulcerations when tolerated and with no contraindication. There has been some debate, however, about the optimal pressure needed to achieve the desired clinical outcome in patients with leg discomfort and edema. A metaanalysis of randomized controlled trials comparing stockings with ankle pressure of 10 to 20 mm Hg versus more than 20 mm Hg showed no added benefit of the higher pressure versus the lower pressure in these categories. Pressure less than 10 mm Hg was ineffective in alleviating symptoms.[63] Recently, the concept of upward progressive compression was introduced. Compression stockings can be upward progressive (pressure highest at calf), or degressive (pressure highest at the ankle). In one randomized trial upward progressive compression was more effective at 3 months in improving pain or heaviness in the legs without the development of DVT or ulcerations.[64]

Compression therapy, whether using bandages or stockings, can be elastic (high pressure at rest, less pressure with muscle contraction) or rigid/inelastic (low pressure at rest, high pressure with muscle contraction). In addition it can be single or multilayered. If multilayered, it can be a combination of elastic and inelastic support. In general, bandages are used during the active phase of treatment (lymphedema, ulcerations, excessive swelling) or in patients that cannot tolerate or are not capable of applying compression stockings. The pressure applied by the bandages is variable and operator dependent. Compression stockings provide reliable pressure and are generally applied for prevention of symptoms and edema, or to prevent progression of disease to ulceration. Comparative effectiveness data between below-the-knee and above-the-knee compression stockings are lacking. In addition to static compression, dynamic compression has been used along with manual lymphatic drainage to treat primary and secondary lymphedema.[59] Dynamic compression uses sequential inflation and deflation to enhance venous return and improve edema. They are effective in patients who cannot tolerate stockings or bandages, or have limited muscular function or severe arterial disease.[62]

Endovascular Heat Ablative Therapies

Endovascular ablative therapies consist of thermal and nonthermal ablation methods. Thermal (or endovascular heat ablation [EVHA]) is a highly effective technique in ablating

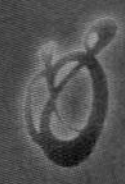

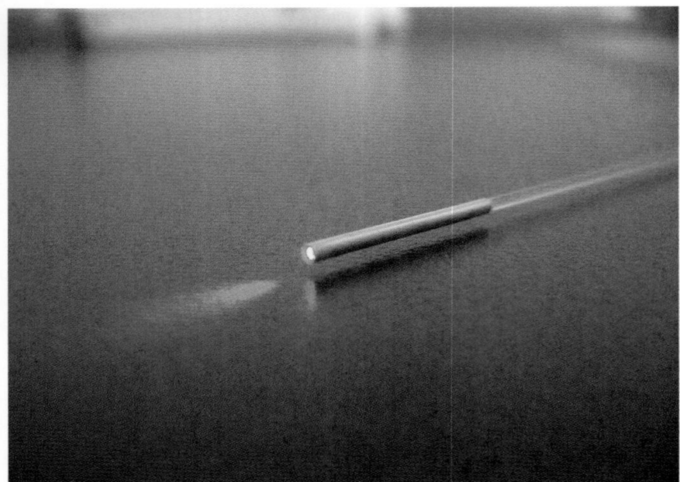

FIGURE 27-15 Laser energy seen at the tip of the NeverTouch gold-tip fiber. *(Courtesy Angiodynamics.)*

refluxing saphenous veins. It is an office-based procedure with minimal complications and a quick patient's recovery. EVHA has largely replaced surgical stripping. It consists of either endovascular laser ablation (EVLA) or endovascular radiofrequency ablation (EVRA). Steam Ablation is also a thermal ablative method available in Europe but not yet approved in the United States.

Endovascular Laser Ablation

EVLA exerts its action via thermal injury to the vessel wall, the mechanism of which is still not very well defined.[65] Current lasers use a continuous energy delivery system instead of the pulsed method of the older generation. The extent of transmitted energy from the laser (**Figure 27-15**) to the vessel wall depends on several factors. Some of these factors include the power settings (watts or joules per seconds), velocity of pullback of the laser fiber (cm per seconds), and vessel diameter. Other factors may include wavelength of the laser, fiber contact with vessel wall, and the type of fibers used (covered versus noncovered), but these need to be more validated in controlled studies. Frequently, the linear endovenous energy density (LEED, or joules per cm) is reported with laser ablative therapy and is essentially a reflection of the amount of energy released per cm of vessel treated. The LEED is derived from the laser power and the velocity of pullback of the fiber (laser power/velocity of pullback = LEED). Therefore, a low energy at low pullback speed may result in the same LEED as a high energy at high pullback velocity. For unified reporting in the case of continuous energy lasers, reporting the LEED alone without reporting the speed of pullback or the laser power would render comparative conclusions among different lasers potentially misleading.[66]

The energy transfer of the laser is generally to either the red blood cells or water in the vessel wall depending on the laser wavelength. Vessel wall water has a higher affinity to higher wavelength lasers (1319 nm, 1320 nm, and 1470 nm) whereas red blood cells have a higher affinity to shorter wavelength lasers (810 nm, 940 nm, and 980 nm). Energy can be transmitted by direct vessel contact with the laser hot tip (using older generation pulsed lasers with bare fibers and a common cause of perforation), boiling steam bubbles mediated by red blood cells with shorter wavelength lasers, and heat conduction.[66] It is speculated that higher wavelength lasers with covered tip fibers have the ability to generate the desired LEED (joules per cm) with less power and less direct contact with the vessel wall and therefore, they have less ecchymosis and discomfort.[67,68] The importance of the wavelength needs to be further validated. However, using the same LEED and power, one study suggested that the 1320 nm had less ecchymosis and pain on follow-up then the 810-nm laser.[69] It is speculated that higher wavelength lasers are likely to cause heat-induced vessel wall damage by fibrosis and scarring whereas the shorter wavelength lasers cause red blood cell destruction and thrombosis. Current studies indicate that the optimal LEED needed for effective ablation is between 60 to 100 J/cm for effective ablation.[70-72] In some studies, however, lower LEEDs (20 to 30 J/cm) have been reported to be effective with the 1470-nm laser.[67]

Compared with surgical ligation and stripping, abolishment of reflux and improvement in quality of life were similar with the laser with more postoperative hematomas seen with surgery and more bruises with the laser. In the same study, a slightly higher reopening of great saphenous vein is seen with the laser compared with surgery at 2 years.[73]

Endovascular Radiofrequency Ablation

Radiofrequency ablation (RF), also called Venefit Targeted Endovenous Therapy (formerly known as the VNUS Closure procedure), is performed using the Covidien ClosureFast catheter (Covidien, Minnesota), inserted under tumescent local anesthetic into the GSV or SSV. The RF energy causes thermal injury to the vein wall and results in vessel wall inflammation, fibrosis, and closure. The mechanism by which RF generates heat is resistive to the tissue that is in direct contact with the electrode. Heat is then conducted to deeper tissue, causing endothelial denudation, denaturation of collagen, and obliteration of the vein with a fibrotic seal. Minimal thrombus or coagulum is formed.[74]

RF ablation is very effective in closure of the GSV, SSV, or perforators. It compares favorably with surgical ablation with less pain and a faster recovery as was shown in the prospective randomized study of endovenous radiofrequency obliteration versus ligation and vein stripping study (EVOLVeS). In this study and at 2 years follow-up, RF closure of GSV was statistically similar to surgical ligation and stripping with the majority of GSV remained closed, and 41% became undetectable because of progressive shrinkage.[75] Compared with EVLA, EVRA has less ecchymosis and pain in the first 2 to 3 weeks after the treatment, which is particularly true for the early laser generation. A recent study,[76] however, continued to show less postoperative discomfort and faster return to work and normal activities with RF ablation, compared with EVLA in a patient population randomized predominantly to the 1470-nm laser versus RF. Irrespective, both treatment modalities were effective at 1 year with only 5.8% and 4.8% of GSV were patent with the laser and the radiofrequency modalities, respectively.[76]

Complications of RF ablation include discomfort, vagal reaction, dysrhythmia, saphenous nerve pain, paresthesia, skin burn, hematoma, thrombophlebitis, DVT (less than 1%),[77] and infection. Paresthesia is usually mild and transient but can occur in 2% to 23% of patients. Endovenous heat induced thrombosis (EHIT) (**Figure 27-16**) involving

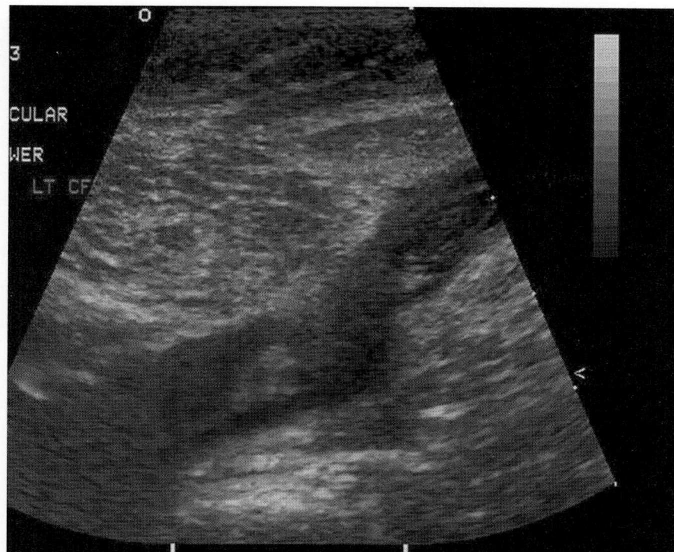

FIGURE 27-16 Heat induced thrombosis (HIT) extending into the deep system from the great saphenous vein (GSV).

the SFJ and SPJ is rarely associated with pulmonary embolization. An increasing ablation distance peripheral to the SFJ (from 2 to 2.5 cm) could result in a reduced rate of EHIT.[78] Other risk factors for EHIT include thrombophilia, use of anesthesia with delayed ambulation postprocedure, and poor ablation technique. Typically, thrombi not extending into the deep system are treated conservatively and closely followed-up with DU to ensure spontaneous resolution or no progression into the deep venous system. If a thrombus is extending into the deep system, treatment with anticoagulation is recommended with close follow-up using serial DU until thrombus resolution.

Steam Ablation

EVSA is a recently developed technique by CermaVein (France) to ablate saphenous veins using heated steam at 120° C. EVSA is done under tumescent anesthetic delivering steam pulsation across a saphenous vein using a small catheter and a steam generator. One advantage of CermaVein EVSA is the small size and flexibility of the catheters that can negotiate saphenous vein tortuosity. Experimental models suggest that 1 steam pulse per cm is likely to create heterogenous results and is insufficient for vein ablation whereas 2 to 3 pulses per cm seem to be adequate.[79,80] Also, experimental data suggest histopathologic changes after EVSA similar to EVLA and EVRA, with high vein wall destruction and low perivenous wall damage.[81] The experience with EVSA remains limited at this time.

Nonthermal Ablative Therapies

Nonthermal ablative methods include sclerotherapy (liquid or foam, ultrasound, or nonultrasound guided), catheter-assisted balloon sclerotherapy (CABS), ClariVein or mechanochemical endovenous ablation (MOCA), and cyanoacylate adhesive. The development of nonthermal ablation methods aims to reduce discomfort and heat-related complications that may result from EVHA such as pain, discomfort from applying the tumescent anesthetic, skin burns, and nerve injury, particularly the sural nerve during SSV ablations.

Sclerotherapy

Sclerotherapy is a technique that utilizes a sclerosing agent injected with a fine needle directly into the vein. It is effective in ablating smaller spider and reticular veins but also used for ablating deeper (done under ultrasound guidance) saphenous veins, nonsaphenous tributaries, or incompletely treated saphenous veins. Sclerotherapy is also used for the treatment of persistent incompetent perforators following treatment of SSVs to enhance healing of venous ulceration.[82] The sclerosing agent can be in liquid (generally utilized for the small spider or reticular veins) or foam (for the larger deeper veins). Sclerotherapy with ultrasound guidance for incompetent truncal and tributary varicose veins was shown to be highly effective.[83,84] Foam sclerotherapy has several advantages to liquid therapy, including the need for smaller volume of sclerosing agent, lack of dilution with blood, better visibility with ultrasound, and homogenous distribution in the injected vein.[85]

Sclerotherapy causes intimal inflammation and thrombus formation leading to fibrous tissue and obliteration of the injected vein. Sclerotherapy is contraindicated when the following is present:

- History of allergy to the sclerosant
- Pregnancy
- Lymphedema
- Thromboembolic risk (prior history of DVT, pulmonary embolus, active cancer, thrombophilia, or active superficial vein thrombosis)
- Known symptomatic intracardiac right to left shunt
- History of neurologic events following prior sclerotherapy treatments
- Relative contraindications include history of multiple drug and nondrug allergies with anaphylaxis and history of migraine headaches with aura.

Complications of sclerotherapy are as follows:

1. Neurosensorial (migraine, transient blurred vision, transient ischemic attack and stroke [0.01%], and sensory and motor nerve damage [0.2%])
2. Local (tissue necrosis, superficial thrombophlebitis [4.4%], veno-arterial reflex vasospasm in adjacent arterioles, swelling and edema [0.5%], pigmentation [10% to 30%], telangiactic matting [15% to 24%], and skin irritation)
3. Systematic (anaphylaxis, DVT (1% to 3%), and pulmonary embolization)[86-90]

There are several sclerosing agents[91] available (**Table 27-4**), including detergents: sodium tetradecyl sulfate, polidocanol and sodium morrhuate; osmotic agents: hypertonic solution and sodium chloride solution with dextrose (Sclerodex); and chemical irritants: chromated glycerin and polyiodinated iodine. The most commonly used ones are polidocanol, sodium tetradecyl sulfate, hypertonic solution, and chromated glycerin. Polidocanol causes less pigmentation, necrosis, and pain than sodium tetradecyl sulfate. Different concentrations are used for different vein sizes. Typically the lowest appropriate concentration is used, and a low injection pressure is applied. Avoiding infiltration is important to reduce the chance of hyperpigmentation and skin necrosis. Hypertonic solution causes significant pain and marked staining. Chromated glycerin[92] is widely used in Europe. It also causes pain with injection but its main

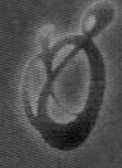

TABLE 27-4 Commonly Used Sclerosing Agents

GENERIC NAME	COMMERCIAL NAME	CONCENTRATION	INDICATIONS	SIDE EFFECTS
Polidocanol (laureth-9) (FDA approved)	Asclera	For spider veins 0.5% For reticular veins 1% Use 0.1 to 0.3 mL per injection and no more than 10 mL per session	Uncomplicated spider (≤1 mm) or reticular veins (1-3 mm) Not studied for veins ≥3 mm	Irritation, hematoma, discoloration, pain, pruritis, warmth, neovascularization, thrombosis
Polidocanol (FDA approved)	Varithena	Administered via a single cannula into the lumen of the target incompetent trunk veins or by direct injection into varicosities Use up to 5 mL per injection and no more than 15 mL per session Once activated, injectable foam delivering a 1% solution	Incompetent GSVs, accessory saphenous veins, and visible varicosities of the GSV system above and below the knee	Irritation, hematoma, discoloration, hyperpigmentation, pain, pruritus, warmth, thrombosis, necrosis, neovascularization anaphylaxis, dyspnea, vasculitis, palpitations, TIA/stroke, migraine, fainting, confusion, urticaria
Sodium tetradecyl sulfate (FDA approved)	Sotradecol	1% and 3% solutions Inject 0.5 mL followed by observation for several hours before additional injections Keep dose small using 0.5 to 2 mL (preferably 1 mL maximum) for each injection Maximum single treatment not to exceed 10 mL	Small uncomplicated varicose veins of the lower extremities (with competent valves) Do not use in acute superficial thrombophlebitis; valvular or deep vein incompetence; large superficial veins communicating to deeper veins; cellulitis; allergic conditions; infections; asthma; neoplasm; or Buerger disease	Irritation, hematoma, discoloration, pain, pruritis, warmth, neovascularization, thrombosis including DVT and pulmonary embolus, tissue necrosis with extravasation, anaphylaxis, urticaria, asthmatic reaction
Morrhuate sodium (FDA approved)	Scleromate	Small or medium veins 50 to 100 mg (1 to 2 mL of 5% injection) Large veins, 150 to 250 mg (3 to 5 mL) May be repeated at 5-day to 7-day intervals.	Uncomplicated varicose veins with competent valves Contraindicated if hypersensitivity to fatty acids; DVT; superficial thrombophlebitis; allergic conditions; infections; or asthma	Thrombosis (DVT, pulmonary embolism), valvular incompetency, vascular collapse, drowsiness, headache, dizziness, urticaria, nausea, burning at injection site, weakness, asthma
Hypertonic saline (not approved in United States as a sclerosing agent)	Hypertonic saline 23.4%	23.4% for reticular veins, 11.7% for spider veins	Treatment of reticular veins and spider veins Not for treatment of larger veins	Pain, burning, leg cramps, tissue necrosis, hemosiderin staining
72% chromated glycerin (no FDA approval in United States)	Sclermo	Maximum recommended dose is 10 mL per session (concentrations from 25% to 100% have been used outside U.S.)	Spider and reticular veins	Pain upon injection (often compounded with lidocaine), highly allergenic, could lead to ureteral colic and hematuria.

FDA, Food and Drug Administration; *GSV*, great saphenous veins; *TIA*, transient ischemic attack.

advantage is the rare occurrence of hyperpigmentation, telangiectactic matting, and necrosis.

Catheter-Assisted Balloon Sclerotherapy

Catheter-assisted balloon sclerotherapy (CABS) uses a targeted approach to deliver sclerotherapy to a particular segment of the GSV. Using a double lumen catheter inserted in the GSV, a balloon is inflated at the tip of the catheter, which stops the blood flow. The second lumen is utilized to inject and aspirate the sclerosing agent. Early studies have shown a 90% closure rate of the GSV using this technique and with no serious side effects at 6 months follow-up.[93] More data are needed to determine how this technique compares with the more established techniques of EVLA and EVRA.

ClariVein or Mechanochemical Endovenous Ablation

Mechanochemical endovenous ablation (MOCA) uses the ClariVein catheter (Vascular Insights), which allows mechanical injury to the vessel coupled with the administration of a sclerosing agent. Using this technique, tumescent anesthetic is not required. The ClariVein catheter is positioned within the saphenous vein under ultrasound guidance and the distal tip positioned 2 cm distal to the SFJ. A metal wire with a small ball at the tip runs through the catheter and induces vein wall injury by rotating at 3500 rpm for 2 to 3 seconds. The sclerosing agent is infused simultaneously with the wire rotation. Data suggest that this technique is effective in obliterating the GSV. In one study, 87% of GSV were closed at 6 weeks follow-up and with an improvement in venous clinical severity score (VCSS).[94] In another study of 29 patients, primary closure was achieved in 96.7% of patients at 6 months follow-up. MOCA was also applied in SSV successfully.[95] In a study of 50 patients, the 1-year ablation success rate was 94% and with no major complications. Also the VCSS was reduced significantly.[96] Complications of this procedure included localized ecchymosis, induration at access site and superficial thrombophlebitis with no nerve injury, DVT, or necrosis.[96] At this time the effectiveness of this technique is uncertain in larger-diameter veins. Also, it is unclear how anticoagulation can affect the outcome of this procedure.

Cyanoacrylate Adhesive

Cyanoacrylate adhesive (Sapheon, Inc., Santa Rosa, California) is a tissue adhesive that polymerizes on contact with anionic substances such as blood or plasma and induces an inflammatory damage to the vein wall.[97] The adhesive eventually undergoes resorption and is replaced with fibrous tissue.The delivery of cyanoacrylate does not require tumescent anesthetic. Early data suggest complete occlusion of the GSV in 92% of patients with significant improvement in VCSS scores.[98] Cyanoacrylate glue is not Food and Drug Administration (FDA) approved and data are still needed to determine its safety and efficacy compared with current approved ablation techniques

Phlebectomy

Phlebectomy is the removal of varicose veins using microsurgical techniques by creating sequential 2-mm skin incisions along the course of the vein followed by its extraction with a hook.Robert Muller,a dermatologist from Switzerland in the mid-1950s, refined this technique. It is carried out under local anesthetic on an outpatient basis. This technique needs to be avoided in patients with skin infections near the phlebectomy site, severe lower extremity edema, and in patients on anticoagulation, or who have thrombophilia.[99] In this technique, the veins are marked preoperatively in the standing position. Phlebectomy should be performed first below the knee when done in the setting of EVHA, or ligation and stripping of either the GSV or SSV. It is recommended, however, that phlebectomy be performed several weeks after treating the GSV or SSV.[99] Complications of phlebectomy includes infection, induration, hyperpigmentation and tattooing, hypopigmentation (incision site), keloid tissue, swelling, ischemia, tissue necrosis, bleeding, superficial thrombophlebitis, DVT, edema, nerve damage, and neuroma.[99,100]

Surgical Vein Stripping

Surgical stripping and ligation (S&L) has been widely replaced with endovascular vein obliteration. It is generally performed under local or general anesthesia and is an outpatient procedure. One or more incisions are made over the large varicosities; the vein is tied off and removed using a stripper. A recent randomized trial showed that EVLA and S&L were similar in clinical and ultrasound recurrences of varicose veins at 2 years follow-up. In this study, 121 patients were randomized to EVLA versus S&L of the GSV from the SFJ. Recurrence of varicose veins occurred in 26% and 37% of EVLA and surgery, respectively (not significant). The sources of reflux were also the same in both groups.[101] In addition, in another randomized trial of EVLA, ultrasound-guided sclerotherapy, and S&L, EVLA was superior to ultrasound-guided sclerotherapy and equally effective to S&L in obliterating the GSV at 1 year.[102] In addition, in a recent randomized trial EVRA was compared with S&L and showed that EVRA had early advantages over S&L with quicker recovery, less pain scores, and an earlier return to work.The magnitude of the differences became less between 1 week and 4 months follow-up.[103] Predictors of recurrent varicose veins after S&L appear to be the presence of neovascularization, incompetent superficial vessel in the thigh, or incompetent SFJ at 2 years follow-up postoperatively. Recurrence of varicosities was associated with a worse Aberdeen Varicose Vein Symptom Severity Score (AVVSSS).[104]

Pharmacologic Management of Chronic Venous Insufficiency

There are several mechanisms postulated as the cause of symptoms and structural changes in patients with CVI. Venous wall tension and hypoxia of the venous wall are likely to be underlying mechanisms for generating pain in the early phases of venous insufficiency. Hemorheological disorders with increased blood viscosity are likely to worsen the hypoxic injury to the vessel wall, which triggers an inflammatory reaction leading also to pain and restlessness. Venous pressures along with increase in capillary permeability due to inflammation lead to edema. Eventually, the inflammatory reaction triggered by oxygen free radicals and leukocyte-endothelial interaction lead to the release of multiple inflammatory mediators, growth factors, and proteolytic enzymes that may be directly responsible for the structural and permanent damage seen in patients with CVI. Although the mainstay of treatment is to reduce venous pressures and obliterate refluxing veins, pharmacological management may have a role in the management of these patients.[105]

There is no current standard in the use of phlebotropic drugs in the management of CVI. These drugs are currently not approved in the United States for treating CVI but have been in use as alternative therapy in Europe for treating CVI:

a. Benzopyrones
   i. α-Benzopyrones. 5,6-Benzo-[α]-pyrone (also known as coumarin) increases proteolysis by activating tissue macrophages.[106] Protein removal allows a steady reduction in edema and inflammation.[107] Coumarin is not an anticoagulant like 4-hydroxycoumarins, which also belong to the same class.
   ii. Chromenones (flavonoids or γ-benzopyrones). This includes micronized purified flavonoid fraction (MPFF) (Daflon), diosmin, diosmethin, rutin, oxerutins, and others. MPFF contains 90% diosmin. It reduces inflammation by inhibiting endothelial activation. In randomized trials, MPFF shortened the time for ulcer healing and reduced edema and symptoms of reflux. In addition, it may delay the reflux and the appearance of varicosities.[108] In addition, oxerutins were shown to be significantly better than placebo in controlling symptoms and objective findings of chronic venous hypertension.[109]

b. Saponosides

   Horse-chestnut extracts (aesculus hippocastanum). Randomized trials have shown that horse-chestnut extract is effective in reducing symptoms of edema comparably to compression stockings and significantly better than placebo.[105,110-112] The long-term effectiveness and safety is not yet clear but short-term use seems to be safe and reasonably well tolerated with improvement in patient's symptoms.

c. Synthetic products

   These include calcium dobesilate, benzarone, and naftazone. Dobesilate reduces capillary permeability and platelet aggregation with an increase in endothelium-dependent relaxation secondary to nitric oxide synthesis.[113] A metaanalysis of randomized trials suggested that dobesilate is more effective than placebo in improving night cramps, paresthesias, and swelling with higher

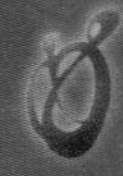

efficacy in patients with more severe disease.[114] A recent double-blind multicenter trial showed that dobesilate improves quality of life at 12-month follow-up but was not significantly different from placebo at 3 months.[115] Naftazone has been shown by the French Venous Naftazone trial group[116] to reduce disability and leg swelling from uncomplicated symptomatic varicose veins in women.

ENDOVASCULAR MANAGEMENT OF VENOUS ULCERATIONS

Venous ulcerations account for 60% to 80% of ulcers seen in the lower extremity.[117] The incidence is higher in women than men (20.4 vs. 14.6 per 100,000 person-years) and increases with age. The incidence of venous ulceration has not changed substantially since 1981.[118] An early conservative approach with high compression bandages or stockings is currently the first line of therapy. The 24-week healing rate with compression alone was 65%.[119] The duration of the ulcer and the size are high predictors to complete healing and to the time to heal. Smaller and more recent ulcers tend to heal more frequently, and in a shorter duration of time (ulcers less than 5 cm^2, 72% healed at a mean time of 7.5 weeks; ulcers more than 5 cm^2, 40% healed at 9.8 weeks; ulcers less than 1-year duration, 64% healed, and those more than 3 years, 24% healed).[120]

The combination of compression stockings with surgical treatment of refluxing veins resulted in a reduction in 12-month recurrence of venous ulcerations compared with compression therapy alone (12% vs. 28%; p <0.0001).[119] At 24 weeks the healing rate, however, was statistically similar between the two strategies (65% vs. 65%).[119] In another randomized trial, however, the healing rate was faster after surgical treatment followed by 20 mm Hg to 30 mm Hg elastic compression stockings compared with foam dressing, zinc oxide, and an inelastic bandage. Healing occurred at 31 days with surgery and 63 days with compression alone. In addition, at 3 years follow-up, the recurrence rate was reduced with surgery to 9% versus 38% in the compression group (p <0.05) with a better improvement in the quality of life in the surgical group.[120] Several surgical approaches to treat refluxing veins and perforators have been developed, including ligation and stripping for the saphenous veins, and endoscopic and open subfascial division of incompetent perforating veins.[103,121] Currently endovascular techniques are increasingly more utilized and largely replacing the surgical options.

Refluxing perforators are highly prevalent in venous ulcers and have been linked to the formation of chronic ulcerations[122] (**Figure 27-17**). Perforators are an important therapeutic target in patients with venous ulcers. Currently perforators larger or equal to 3.5 mm and with a minimum of 0.5 seconds reflux located at the ulcer,[123] or refluxing via tributaries to the ulcer are a target for treatment when conservative management or ablation of the SSVs has failed in healing the ulceration. Treatment of the refluxing truncal saphenous veins may lead to healing of ulcerations without treatment of perforators.[124,125] It is prudent to treat refluxing saphenous veins first along with compression therapy and wound management prior to perforators' ablation. For medial ulcers, the focus needs to be on the posterior tibial perforators, and for lateral malleolar ulcerations on the lateral calf and ankle perforators.[126] Endovascular techniques have emerged as an effective treatment of refluxing perforators. These include radiofrequency,[126,127] laser ablation,[128] or ultrasound-guided foam sclerotherapy.[129]

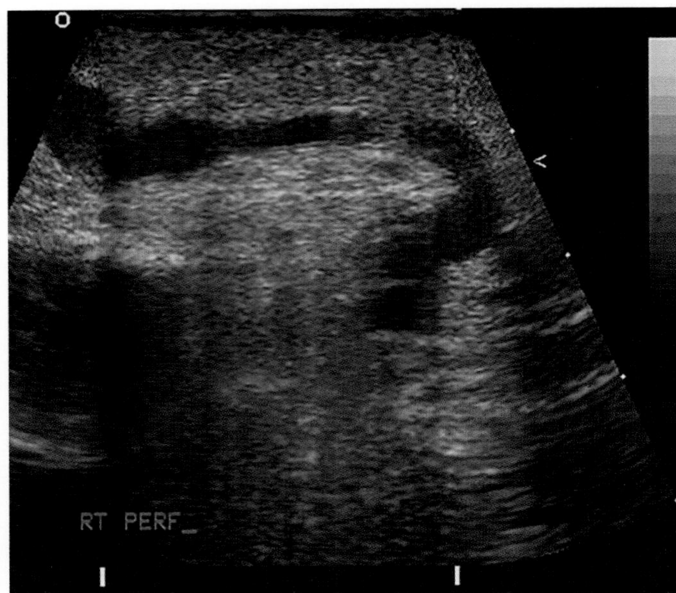

FIGURE 27-17 Right posterior tibial perforator.

The endovascular management of patients with venous ulcerations should focus on evaluating the deep system. It is important to rule out DVT or proximal venous obstruction. Abnormal spectral Doppler flow in one common femoral vein compared with the other should raise suspicion of proximal venous obstruction. In select patients, CTV or MRV is needed to rule out proximal venous compression. Predictors of failure following treatment of refluxing perforators should raise suspicion for abnormal proximal venous flow.[130] In addition, identifying proximal venous obstruction and treating it in patients with deep venous reflux may be sufficient to alleviate the symptoms and achieve the desired outcome from the treatment with no adverse effect on the deep reflux.[131]

DEEP VENOUS VALVES

Deep venous valve dysfunction has been the subject of considerable research. Currently there is no consensus on treating the deep venous valves. Deep venous valve reflux can contribute to the development of progressive chronic venous insufficiency leading to ulcerations and disability. Treatment of the deep venous valves is a target in patients with advanced symptoms of ulceration and impaired quality of life.

An open surgical technique to treat the femoral vein valves has been described in a select group of patients with postphlebitic syndrome.[132] In this procedure the valve underwent primary repair with a "series of tucking sutures and shortening the cusp."[133] Ulcer healing was accomplished in 90% of patients. A modification on this open technique is external venous valve repair (transcommisural valvuloplasty), which was described in a series of 179 patients with significant improvement of pain and swelling, and cumulative ulcer recurrence-free interval of 63% at 30 months.[133] This technique involved "placing transluminal sutures along the valve attachment lines, which simultaneously closed the valve attachment angle and also tightened the valve cusps."

Complications included bleeding, venothromboembolic disease, and infections. Another surgical approach in patients with damaged, nonrepairable valves (post-DVT) was valve transposition from the profunda femoris, axillary, or saphenous veins using vein substitution techniques,[134] or the use of cryopreserved valve to the femoropopliteal vein.[135] A high failure rate was seen with the cryovalves, including acute rejection and early and late occlusion. Patent and competent cryovalves at 24 months were 41% and 27%, respectively. There was no change in pain relief or degree of swelling. Ulcers recurrence-free rate at 36 months was 50%. Finally, the construction of neovalve[136] in the deep venous system seems to improve reflux and healing at a median follow-up of 5 months.[137] This data need to be duplicated in a larger sample and be sustained on longer follow-up. Successful treatment of deep venous refluxing valves with no repair options (as seen in end-stage venous insufficiency or post-thrombotic cases) has so far been in autogenous valve transfer using surgical techniques.[138] There have not been any successful options for transplanting allograft or xenograft valves despite pretreatment of the valve with various methods to reduce its immunogenicity prior to implantation.

Transcatheter deep valve repair is a nonsurgical approach that is currently under intense investigation and remains well in its very early stages. In a goat animal model,[139] endoscopic harvesting of a valve-containing segment of external jugular vein, sutured within a self-expanding Wallstent, was compressed and delivered through a 12 Fr sheath to the contralateral external jugular vein. At 6 weeks, the valve remained intact and five of the six valves were competent. To date, this observation has not been translated into a clinical application. In an ovine model,[140] percutaneous autogenous venous valves (PAVVs) from harvested jugular veins were mounted on a stent template and delivered into the contralateral jugular vein using a percutaneous femoral approach. On 3-month follow-up, 8 out of 9 valves were intact and nonthickened and were free of thrombus. Recently, and in a sheep model,[141] a segment of vein from the internal jugular with a venous valve was mounted on a circumferential barbed stent and deployed into the contralateral internal jugular vein. At 6 months, there was no thrombus, tilting, migration, or incompetence in these valves. On the other hand, using a valve-containing vein segment harvested from a bovine jugular vein preserved in glutaraldehyde and mounted on a balloon expandable stent in six lambs in the inferior vena cava yielded total occlusions of these valves in 2 months.[142] It is unclear whether this was the result of barotrauma of the balloon expandable stent, the xenograft material, or the bulk of metal on the stent.[138] The percutaneous outcomes were similar to surgery. The autograft seems to have the most reliable success when implanted percutaneously or surgically.

Several valve designs are currently in research with a particular focus on tissue-engineered valves. Prosthetic valves fabricated by electrospinning and consisting of polyurethane fiber scaffolds,[143] autologous cell-derived tissue engineered venous valves (TEVVs) on fully biodegradable scaffolds,[144] and porcine small intestinal submucosa (SIS) bioprosthetic valves with endothelial progenitor outgrowth cells as a source of endothelialization.[145] Venous PercValve with eNitinol membranes are also currently in development. NiTi or nitinol is a nickel-titanium alloy, biologically inert, has shape memory, and could be made in ultrathin membranes (eNitinol) that are flexible enough to be used in valve development.[146] Finally, improvements are ongoing on the stent delivery system with no barbs on the stents to minimize vessel wall injury,[147] and with minimal metal struts exposed to the circulation.

CONCLUSIONS

There has been less emphasis on the venous system in general medical education. Over 25 million people in the United States suffer from progressive chronic venous disease that eventually leads to venous hypertension, venous insufficiency, hyperpigmentation, and disabling venous ulcerations. The venous anatomy and physiology is complex and understanding it is important to correctly identify and treat superficial venous disease. Different safe and effective percutaneous methods have evolved in treating the superficial venous system, and surgical vein stripping is now infrequently performed. A complex relationship exists between the superficial and deep venous system. A full evaluation of the patient is important and a detailed mapping to the venous circulatory network is required for an effective therapeutic strategy. Percutaneous valve transplantation to the deep venous system may become an important future therapy in symptomatic patients with deep venous reflux.

References

1. White JV, Ryjewski C: Chronic venous insufficiency. *Perspect Vasc Surg Endovasc Ther* 17:319–327, 2005.
2. Evans CJ, Fowkes FGR, Ruckley CV, et al: Prevalence of varicose veins and chronic venous insufficiency in men and women in the general population: Edinburgh Vein Study. *J Epidemiol Community Health* 53:149–153, 1999.
3. Robertson L, Evans C, Fowkes FG: Epidemiology of chronic venous disease. *Phlebology* 23:103–111, 2008.
4. Ruckley CV, Evans CJ, Allan PL, et al: Chronic venous insufficiency: clinical and duplex correlations. The Edinburgh Vein Study of venous disorders in the general population. *J Vasc Surg* 36:520–525, 2002.
5. Coon WW, Willis PW, Keller JB: Venous thromboembolism and other venous disease in the Tecumseh community health study. *Circulation* 48:839–846, 1973.
6. Kurz X, Kahn SR, Abenhaim L, et al: Chronic venous disorders of the leg: epidemiology, outcomes, diagnosis and management. Summary of an evidencebased report of the VEINES task force. Venous Insufficiency Epidemiologic and Economic Studies. *Int Angiol* 18:83–102, 1999.
7. Moffatt CJ, Franks PJ, Doherty DC, et al: Prevalence of leg ulceration in a London population. *QJM* 97:431–437, 2004.
8. Brand FN, Dannenberg AL, Abbott RD, et al: The epidemiology of varicose veins: the Framingham study. *Am J Prev Med* 4:96–101, 1988.
9. Robertson L, Lee AJ, Evans CJ, et al: Incidence of chronic venous disease in the Edinburgh Vein Study. *J Vasc Surg Venous Lymphat Disord* 1:59–67, 2013.
10. Casarone MR, Belcaro G, Nicolaides AN, et al: Real epidemiology of varicose veins and chronic venous disease: the San Valentino Vascular Screening Project. *Angiology* 53:119–130, 2002.
11. Criqui MH, Jamosmos M, Fronek A, et al: Chronic venous disease in an ethnically diverse population: the San Diego Population Study. *Am J Epidemiol* 158:448–456, 2003.
12. Mekky S, Schilling RSF, Walford J: Varicose veins in women cotton workers. An epidemiological study in England and Egypt. *BMJ* 2:591–595, 1969.
13. Lee AJ, Evans CJ, Allan PL, et al: Lifestyle factors and the risk of varicose veins: Edinburgh Vein Study. *J Clin Epidemiol* 56:171–179, 2003.
14. Laurikka JO, Sisto T, Tarkka MR, et al: Risk indictors for varicose veins in forty to sixty-year-olds in the Tampere Varicose Vein Study. *World J Surg* 26:648–651, 2002.
15. Chiesa R, Marone EM, Limoni C, et al: Demographic factors and their relationship with the presence of CVI signs in Italy: the 24-cities cohort study. *Eur J Vasc Endovasc Surg* 30:674–680, 2005.
16. McGuckin M, Waterman R, Brooks J, et al: Validation of venous leg ulcer guidelines in the United States and United Kingdom. *Am J Surg* 183:132–137, 2002.
17. Lafuma A, Fagnani F, Peltier-Pujol F, et al: Venous disease in France: an unrecognized public health problem [in French]. *J Mal Vasc* 19:185–189, 1994.
18. Dinkel R: Venous disorders, a cost intensive disease. *Phlebology* 26:164–168, 1997.
19. Tennvall GR, Andersson K, Bjellerup M, et al: Treatment of venous leg ulcers can be better and cheaper. Annual costs calculation based on an inquiry study. *Lakartidningen* 101:1506–1513, 2004.
20. Callam MJ, Harper DR, Dale JJ, et al: Chronic ulcer of the leg: clinical history. *BMJ* 294:1389–1391, 1987.
21. Da Silva A, Navarro MF, Batalheiro J: The importance of chronic venous insufficiency: various preliminary data on its medico-social consequences. *Phlebologie* 45:439–443, 1992.
22. Cavezzi A, Labropoulos N, Partsch H, et al: Duplex ultrasound investigation of the veins in chronic venous disease of the lower limbs–UIP consensus document. Part II. Anatomy. *Eur J Vasc Endovasc Surg* 31:288–299, 2006.
23. Caggiati A, Bergan JJ, Gloviczki P, et al: International interdisciplinary consensus committee on venous anatomical terminology. Nomenclature of the veins of the lower limbs: an international interdisciplinary consensus statement. *J Vasc Surg* 36:416–422, 2002.
24. Mozes G, Carmichael SW, Gloviczki P: Development and anatomy of the venous system. In Gloviczki P, Yao JS, editors: *Handbook of Venous Disorders*, ed 2, New York, NY, 2001, Arnold, pp 11–24.
25. Eberhardt RT, Raffetto JD: Chronic venous insufficiency. *Circulation* 111:2398–2409, 2005.

26. Burnand KG: The physiology and hemodynamics of chronic venous insufficiency of the lower limbs. In Gloviczki P, Yao JS, editors: *Handbook of Venous Disorders*, ed 2, New York, NY, 2001, Arnold, pp 49–57.
27. Neglén P, Thrasher TL, Raju S: Venous outflow obstruction: an underestimated contributor to chronic venous disease. *J Vasc Surg* 38:879–885, 2003.
28. Araki CT, Back TL, Padberg FT, et al: The significance of calf muscle pump function in venous ulceration. *J Vasc Surg* 20:872–877, 1994.
29. Christopoulos D, Nicolaides AN, Cook A, et al: Pathogenesis of venous ulceration in relation to the calf muscle pump function. *Surgery* 106:829–835, 1989.
30. Franzeck UK, Haselbach P, Speiser D, et al: Microangiopathy of cutaneous blood and lymphatic capillaries in chronic venous insufficiency (CVI). *Yale J Biol Med* 66:37–46, 1993.
31. Browse NL, Burnand KG: The cause of venous ulceration. *Lancet* 2:243–245, 1982.
32. Coleridge-Smith PD, Thomas P, Scurr JH, et al: Causes of venous ulceration: a new hypothesis? *Br Med J* 296:1726–1727, 1988.
33. Falanga V, Eaglstein WH: The trap hypothesis of venous ulceration. *Lancet* 341:1006–1008, 1993.
34. Eklöf B, Rutherford RB, Bergan JJ, et al: American Venous Forum International Ad Hoc Committee for Revision of the CEAP Classification. Revision of the CEAP classification for chronic venous disorders: consensus statement. *J Vasc Surg* 40:1248–1252, 2004.
35. Jacob AG, Driscoll DJ, Shaughnessy WJ, et al: Klippel-Trénaunay syndrome: spectrum and management. *Mayo Clin Proc* 73:28–36, 1998.
36. Kim J, Richards S, Kent PJ: Clinical examination of varicose veins–a validation study. *Ann R Coll Surg Engl* 82:171–175, 2000.
37. Vasquez MA, Rabe E, McLafferty RB, et al: American Venous Forum Ad Hoc Outcomes Working Group. Revision of the venous clinical severity score: venous outcomes consensus statement: special communication of the American Venous Forum Ad Hoc Outcomes Working Group. *J Vasc Surg* 52:1387–1396, 2010.
38. Rutherford RB, Padberg FT, Jr, Comerota AJ, et al: Venous severity scoring: an adjunct to venous outcome assessment. *J Vasc Surg* 31:1307–1312, 2000.
39. Fowler B, Zygmunt J, Ramirez H, et al: Venous insufficiency evaluation with duplex scanning. *J Vasc Ultrasound* 38(1):1–7, 2014.
40. Labropoulos N, Tiongson J, Pryor L, et al: Definition of venous reflux in lower extremity veins. *J Vasc Surg* 38:793–798, 2003.
41. Labropolous N, Kokkosis A, Spentzouris G, et al: The distribution and significance of varicosities in the saphenous trunks. *J Vasc Surg* 51:96–103, 2010.
42. Zygmunt J, Pichot O, Dauplaise T: *Practical phlebology: Venous Ultrasound*, London, 2013, CRC Press.
43. Hirai M, Naiki K, Nakayama R: Chronic venous insufficiency in primary varicose veins evaluated by plethysmographic technique. *Angiology* 42:468–472, 1991.
44. Criado E, Farber MA, Marston WA, et al: The role of air plethysmography in the diagnosis of chronic venous insufficiency. *J Vasc Surg* 27:660–670, 1998.
45. Welkie JF, Comerota AJ, Kerr RP, et al: The hemodynamics of venous ulceration. *Ann Vasc Surg* 6:1–4, 1992.
46. Belcaro G, Labropoulos N, Christopoulos D, et al: Noninvasive tests in venous insufficiency. *J Cardiovasc Surg (Torino)* 34:3–11, 1993.
47. Harada R, Katz ML, Comerota A: A noninvasive screening test to detect "critical" deep venous reflux. *J Vasc Surg* 22:532–537, 1995.
48. Ibegbuna V, Delis KT, Nicolaides AN: Haemodynamic and clinical impact of superficial, deep and perforator incompetence. *Eur J Vasc Endovasc Surg* 31:535–541, 2006.
49. Labropoulos N, Leon L, Kwan S, et al: Study of the venous reflux progression. *J Vasc Surg* 41:291–295, 2005.
50. Psaila JV, Melhuish J: Vasoelastic properties and collagen content of the long saphenous vein in normal and varicose veins. *Br J Surg* 76:37–40, 1989.
51. Elsharawy MA, Naim MM, Abdelmaguid EM, et al: Role of saphenous vein wall in the pathogenesis of primary varicose veins. *Interact Cardiovasc Thorac Surg* 6:219–224, 2007.
52. Labropoulos N, Giannoukas AD, Delis K, et al: Where does venous reflux start? *J Vasc Surg* 26:736–742, 1997.
53. Caggiati A, Rosi C, Heyn R, et al: Age-related variations of varicose veins anatomy. *J Vasc Surg* 44:1291–1295, 2006.
54. Somjen GM, Royle JP, Fell G, et al: Venous reflux patterns in the popliteal fossa. *J Cardiovasc Surg (Torino)* 33:85–91, 1992.
55. Sales CM, Bilof ML, Petrillo KA, et al: Correction of lower extremity deep venous incompetence by ablation of superficial reflux. *Ann Vasc Surg* 10:186–189, 1996.
56. MacKenzie RK, Allan PL, Ruckley CV, et al: The effect of long saphenous vein stripping on deep venous reflux. *Eur J Vasc Endovasc Surg* 28:104–107, 2004.
57. Mussa FF, Peden EK, Zhou W, et al: Iliac vein stenting for chronic venous insufficiency. *Tex Heart Inst J* 34:60–66, 2007.
58. Sanford DA, Kelly D, Rhee SJ, et al: Importance of phasicity in detection of proximal iliac vein thrombosis with venous duplex examination. *J Vasc Ultrasound* 35:150–152, 2011.
59. Felty CL, Rooke TW: Compression therapy for chronic venous insufficiency. *Semin Vasc Surg* 18:36–40, 2005.
60. Kakkos SK, Daskalopoulou SS, Daskalopoulos ME, et al: Review on the value of graduated elastic compression stockings after deep vein thrombosis. *Thromb Haemost* 96:441–445, 2006.
61. Marston W, Vowden K: Compression therapy: a guide to safe practice. In *European Wound Management (EWMA) Position Document. Understanding Compression Therapy*, London, 2003, MEP Ltd, pp 11–17.
62. World Union of Wound Healing Societies (WUWHS): *Principles of Best Practice: Compression in Venous Leg Ulcers. A Consensus Document*, London, 2008, MEP Ltd.
63. Amsler F, Blättler W: Compression therapy for occupational leg symptoms and chronic venous disorders—a meta-analysis of randomised controlled trials. *Eur J Vasc Endovasc Surg* 35:366–372, 2008.
64. Couzan S, Leizorovicz A, Laporte S, et al: A randomized double-blind trial of upward progressive versus degressive compressive stockings in patients with moderate to severe chronic venous insufficiency. *J Vasc Surg* 56:1344–1350, 2012.
65. Vuylsteke ME, Mordon SR: Endovenous laser ablation: a review of mechanisms of action. *Ann Vasc Surg* 26:424–433, 2012.
66. Malskat WSJ, Poluektova AA, van der Geld CWM, et al: Endovenous laser ablation (EVLA): a review of mechanisms, modeling outcomes, and issues for debate. *Lasers Med Sci* 29:393–403, 2014.
67. Almeida J, Mackay E, Javier J, et al: Saphenous laser ablation at 1470 nm targets the vein wall, not blood. *Vasc Endovascular Surg* 43:467–472, 2009.
68. Schwarz T, Von Hodenberg E, Furtwangler C, et al: Endovenous laser ablation of varicose veins with the 1470-nm diode laser. *J Vasc Surg* 51:1474–1478, 2010.
69. Mackay EG, Almeida JI, Raines JK Do different laser wavelengths translate into different patient experiences? *Endovascular Today* 45-48, 2006.
70. Timperman PE, Sichlau M, Ryu RK: Greater energy delivery improves treatment success of endovenous laser treatment of incompetent saphenous veins. *J Vasc Interv Radiol* 15:1061–1063, 2004.
71. Theivacumar NS, Dellagrammaticas D, Beale RJ, et al: Factors influencing the effectiveness of endovenous laser ablation (EVLA) in the treatment of great saphenous vein reflux. *Eur J Vasc Endovasc Surg* 35:119–123, 2008.
72. Pannier F, Rabe E, Maurins U: First results with a new 1470-nm diode laser for endovenous ablation of incompetent saphenous veins. *Phlebology* 24:26–30, 2009.
73. Christenson JT, Gueddi S, Gemayel G, et al: Prospective randomized trial comparing endovenous laser ablation and surgery for treatment of primary great saphenous varicose veins with a 2-year follow up. *J Vasc Surg* 52:1234–1241, 2010.
74. Roth SM: Endovenous radiofrequency ablation of superficial and perforator veins. *Surg Clin North Am* 87:1267–1284, 2007.
75. Lurie F, Creton D, Eklof B, et al: Reprinted article "Prospective randomized study of endovenous radiofrequency obliteration versus ligation and vein stripping (EVOLVeS): two-year follow up." *Eur J Vasc Endovasc Surg* 42(Suppl 1):S107–S113, 2011.
76. Rasmussen LH, Lawaetz M, Bjoern L, et al: Randomized clinical trial comparing endovenous laser ablation, radiofrequency abaltion, foam sclerotherapy and surgical stripping for great saphenous varicose veins. *Br J Surg* 98:1079–1087, 2011.
77. Marsh P, Price BA, Holdstock J, et al: Deep vein thrombosis (DVT) after venous thromboablation techniques: rates of endovenous heat-induced thrombosis (EHIT) and classical DVT after radiofrequency and endovenous laser ablation in a single centre. *Eur J Vasc Endovasc Surg* 40:521–527, 2010.
78. Sadek M, Kabnick LS, Rockman CB, et al: Increasing ablation distance peripheral to the saphenofemoral junction may result in a diminished rate of endothermal heat-induced thrombosis. *J Vasc Surg Venous Lymphat Disord* 1:257–262, 2013.
79. van den Bos RR, Milleret R, et al: Proof-of-principle study of steam ablation as novel thermal therapy for saphenous varicose veins. *J Vasc Surg* 53:181–186, 2010.
80. van Ruijven PW, van den Bos RR, Alazard LM, et al: Temperature measurements for dose-finding in steam ablation. *J Vasc Surg* 53:1454–1456, 2011.
81. Thomis S, Verbrugghe P, Milleret R, et al: Steam ablation versus radiofrequency and laser ablation: an in vivo histological comparative trial. *Eur J Vasc Surg* 46:378–382, 2013.
82. Pang KH, Bate GR, Darvall KA, et al: Healing and recurrence rates following ultrasound-guided foam sclerotherapy of superficial venous reflux in patients with chronic venous ulceration. *Eur J Vasc Endovasc Surg* 40:790–795, 2010.
83. Rathbun S, Norris A, Morrison N, et al: Performance of endovenous foam sclerotherapy in the USA for the treatment of venous disorders: ACP/SVM/AVF/SIR quality improvement guidelines. *Phlebology* 29:76–82, 2014.
84. Nael R, Rathbun S: Effectiveness of foam sclerotherapy for the treatment of varicose veins. *Vasc Med* 15:27–32, 2010.
85. Weiss RA, Sadick NS, Goldman MP, et al: Post-sclerotherapy compression: controlled comparative study of duration of compression and its effects on clinical outcome. *Dermatol Surg* 25:105–108, 1999.
86. Cavezzi A, Parsi K: Complications of foam sclerotherapy. *Phlebology* 27(Suppl 1):46–51, 2012.
87. Peterson JD, Goldman MP: An investigation of side-effects and efficacy of foam-based sclerotherapy with carbon dioxide or room air in the treatment of reticular leg veins: a pilot study. *Phlebology* 27:73–76, 2012.
88. Peterson JD, Goldman MP, Weiss RA, et al: Treatment of reticular and telangiectatic leg veins: double-blind, prospective comparative trial of polidocanol and hypertonic saline. *Dermatol Surg* 38:1322–1330, 2012.
89. Guex JJ, Allaert FA, Gillet JL, et al: Immediate and midterm complications of sclerotherapy: report of a prospective multicenter registry of 12,173 sclerotherapy sessions. *Dermatol Surg* 31:123–128, 2005.
90. Parsi K: Paradoxical embolism, stroke and sclerotherapy. *Phlebology* 27:147–167, 2012.
91. Parsons ME: Sclerotherapy basics. *Dermatol Clin* 22:501–508, 2004.
92. Kern P, Ramelet AA, Wutschert R, et al: Single-blind, randomized study comparing chromated glycerin, polidocanol solution, and polidocanol foam for treatment of telangiectatic leg veins. *Dermatol Surg* 30:367–372, 2004.
93. Broderson JP, Geismar U: Catheter-assisted vein sclerotherapy: a new approach for sclerotherapy of the greater saphenous vein with a double-lumen balloon catheter. *Dermatol Surg* 33:469–475, 2007.
94. Van Eekeren RRJP, Boersma D, Elias S, et al: Endovenous mechanochemical ablation of great saphenous vein incompetence using the ClariVein device: a safety study. *J Endovasc Ther* 18:328–334, 2011.
95. Elias S, Raines JK: Mechanochemical tumescentless endovenous ablation: final results of the initial clinical trial. *Phlebology* 27:67–72, 2012.
96. Boersma D, van Eekeren RRJP, Werson DAB, et al: Mechanochemical endovenous ablation of small saphenous vein insufficiency using the ClariVein Device: one-year results of a prospective series. *Eur J Vasc Endovasc Surg* 45:299–303, 2013.
97. Wang YM, Cheng LF, Li N: Histopathological study of vascular changes after intra-arterial and intravenous injection of N-butyl-2-cyanoacrylate. *Chin J Dig Dis* 7:175–179, 2006.
98. Almeida J, et al Cyanoacrylate glue great saphenous vein ablation: preliminary 180-day follow-up of a first-in-man feasibility study of a no-compression-no-local-anesthesia technique. Presented: American Venous Forum 24th Annual Congress, 2012; Orlando, FL, USA.
99. Olivencia JA: Complications of ambulatory phlebectomy: review of 1,000 consecutive cases. *Dermatol Surg* 23:51–54, 1997.
100. Kabnick LS, Ombrellino M: Ambulatory phlebectomy. *Semin Intervent Radiol* 22:218–224, 2005.
101. Rasmussen LH, Bjoem L, Lawaetz M, et al: Randomized clinical trial comparing endovenous laser ablation with stripping of the great saphenous vein: cllinical outcome and recurrence after 2 years. *Eur J Vasc Endovasc Surg* 39:630–635, 2010.
102. Biemans AA, Kockaert M, Akkersdijk GP, et al: Comparing endovenous laser ablation, foam sclerotherapy and conventional surgery for great saphenous varicose veins. *J Vasc Surg* 58:727–734, 2013.
103. Lurie F, Creton D, Eklof B, et al: Prospective randomized study of endovenous radiofrequency obliteration (closure procedure) versus ligation and stripping in a selected patient population (EVOLVeS Study). *J Vasc Surg* 38:207–214, 2003.
104. Winterborn RJ, Foy C, Earnshaw JJ: Causes of varicose vein recurrence: late results of a randomized controlled trial of stripping the long saphenous vein. *J Vasc Surg* 40:634–639, 2004.
105. Perin M, Ramelet AA: Pharmacologic treatment of primary chronic venous disease: rationale, results and unanswered questions. *Eur J Vasc Endovasc Surg* 41:117–125, 2011.
106. Casley-Smith JR, Morgan RG, Piller NB: Treatment of lymphedema of the arms and legs with 5,6-Benzo-[α]-pyrone. *N Engl J Med* 329:1158–1163, 1993.
107. Casley-Smith JR, Gaffney RM: Excess plasma proteins as a cause of chronic inflammation and lymphoedema: quantitative electron microscopy. *J Pathol* 133:243–272, 1981.
108. Katsenis K: Micronized purified flavonoids fraction (MPFF): a review of its pharmacologic effects, therapeutic efficacy, and benefits in the management of chronic venous insufficiency. *Curr Vasc Pharmacol* 3:1–9, 2005.
109. Petruzzellis V, Troccoli T, Candiani C, et al: Oxerutins (Venoruton): efficacy in chronic venous insufficiency—a double blind randomized controlled study. *Angiology* 53:257–263, 2002.
110. Diehm C, Vollbrecht D, Amendt K, et al: Medical edema protection-clinical benefit in patients with chronic deep vein incompetence. *Vasa* 21:188–192, 1992.
111. Diehm C, Trampisch HJ, Lange S, et al: Comparison of leg compression stocking and oral horse-chestnut seed extract therapy in patients with chronic venous insufficiency. *Lancet* 347:292–294, 1996.
112. Ramelet AA: Daflon 500 mg: symptoms and edema clinical update. *Angiology* 56(Suppl 1):S25–S32, 2005.

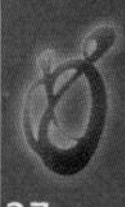

113. Tejerina T, Ruiz E: Calcium dobesilate: pharmacology and future approaches. *Gen Pharmacol* 31:357–360, 1998.
114. Ciapponi A, Laffaire E, Roqué M: Calcium dobesilate for chronic venous insufficiency: a systematic review. *Angiology* 55:147–154, 2004.
115. Martínez-Zapata MJ, Moreno RM, Gich I, et al; for the Chronic Venous Insufficiency Study Group: A randomized, double-blind multicentre clinical trial comparing the efficacy of calcium dobesilate with placebo in the treatment of chronic venous disease. *Eur J Vasc Endovasc Surg* 35(3):358–365, 2008.
116. Vayssairat M: Placebo-controlled trial of naftozone in women with primary uncomplicated symptomatic varicose veins. *Phlebology* 12:17–20, 1997.
117. Callam MJ: Prevalence of chronic leg ulceration and severe chronic venous disease in western countries. *Phlebology* 7(Suppl 1):6–12, 1992.
118. Heit JA, Rooke TW, Silverstein MD, et al: Trends in the incidence of venous stasis syndrome and venous ulcer: a 25-year population-based study. *J Vasc Surg* 1151:159–162, 2001.
119. Barwell JR, Davies CE, Deacon J, et al: Comparison of surgery and compression with compression alone in chronic venous ulceration (ESCHAR study): randomised controlled trial. *Lancet* 363:1854–1859, 2004.
120. Zamboni P, Cisno C, Marchetti F, et al: Minimally invasive surgical management of primary venous ulcers vs. compression treatment: a randomized clinical trial. *Eur J Vasc Endovasc Surg* 25:313–318, 2003.
121. Pierik EG, van Urk H, Hop WC, et al: Endoscopic versus open subfascial division of incompetent perforating veins in the treatment of leg ulceration: a randomized trial. *J Vasc Surg* 26:1049–1054, 1997.
122. O'Donnell TF: The role of perforators in chronic venous insufficiency. *Phlebology* 25:3–10, 2010.
123. Gloviczki P, Comerota AJ, Dalsing MC, et al: Society for Vascular Surgery; American Venous Forum. The care of patients with varicose veins and associated chronic venous diseases: clinical practice guidelines of the Society for Vascular Surgery and the American Venous Forum. *J Vasc Surg* 53(5 Suppl):2S–48S, 2011.
124. Bello M, Scriven M, Hartshorne T, et al: Role of superficial venous surgery in the treatment of venous ulceration. *Br J Surg* 86:755–759, 1999.
125. Marrocco CJ, Atkins MD, Bohannon WT, et al: Endovenous ablation for the treatment of chronic venous insufficiency and venous ulcerations. *World J Surg* 34:2299–2304, 2010.
126. Lawrence PF, Alktaifi A, Rigberg D, et al: Endovenous ablation of incompetent perforating veins is effective treatment for recalcitrant venous ulcers. *J Vasc Surg* 54:737–742, 2011.
127. Marsh P, Price BA, Holdstock JM, et al: One-year outcomes of radiofrequency ablation of incompetent perforator veins using the radiofrequency stylet device. *Phlebology* 25:79–84, 2010.
128. Proebstle TM, Herdemann S: Early results and feasibility of incompetent perforator vein ablation by endovenous laser treatment. *Dermatol Surg* 33:162–168, 2007.
129. Elias S, Peden E: Ultrasound-guided percutaneous ablation for the treatment of perforating vein incompetence. *Vascular* 15:281–289, 2007.
130. Hingorani AP, Ascher E, Marks N, et al: Predictive factors of success following radio-frequency stylet (RFS) ablation of incompetent perforating veins (IPV). *J Vasc Surg* 50:844–848, 2009.
131. Raju S, Darcey R, Neglén P: Unexpected major role for venous stenting in deep reflux disease. *J Vasc Surg* 51:401–408, 2010.
132. Kistner RL: Surgical repair of the incompetent femoral vein valve. *Arch Surg* 110:1336–1342, 1975.
133. Raju S, Berry MA, Neglén P: Transcommissural valvuloplasty: technique and results. *J Vasc Surg* 32:969–976, 2000.
134. Kistner RL, Masuda E, Lurie F: Valvuloplasty in primary venous insufficiency. In Bergan JJ, Bunke-Paquette N, editors: *The Vein Book*, ed 2, 2014, Oxford University Press, pp 486–498.
135. Neglen P, Raju S: Venous reflux repair with cryopreserved vein valves. *J Vasc Surg* 37:552–557, 2003.
136. Maleti O, Perrin M: Reconstructive surgery for deep vein reflux in the lower limbs: techniques, results and indications. *Eur J Vasc Endovasc Surg* 41:837–848, 2011.
137. Lugli M, Guerzoni S, Garofalo M, et al: Neovalve construction in deep venous incompetence. *J Vasc Surg* 49:156–162, 2009.
138. Dalsing MC: Prosthetic venous valves. In Bergan JJ, Bunke-Paquette N, editors: *The Vein Book*, ed 2, 2014, Oxford University Press, pp 499–504.
139. Ofenloch JC, Chen C, Hughes JD, et al: Endoscopic venous valve transplantation with a valve-stent device. *Ann Vasc Surg* 11:62–67, 1997.
140. Pavcnik D, Yin Q, Uchida B, et al: Percutaneous autologous venous valve transplantation: short-term feasibility study in an ovine model. *J Vasc Surg* 46:338–345, 2007.
141. Phillips MN, Dijkstra ML, Khin NY, et al: Endovenous valve transfer for chronic deep venous insufficiency. *Eur J Vasc Endovasc Surg* 46:360–365, 2013.
142. Boudjemline Y, Bonnet D, Sidi D, et al: Is percutaneous implantation of a bovine venous valve in the inferior vena cava a reliable technique to treat chronic venous insufficiency syndrome? *Med Sci Monit* 10:BR61–BR66, 2004.
143. Moriyama M, Kubota S, Tashiro H, et al: Evaluation of prosthetic venous valves, fabricated by electrospinning, for percutaneous treatment of chronic venous insufficiency. *J Artif Organs* 14:294–300, 2011.
144. Weber B, Robert J, Ksiazek A, et al: Living engineered valves for transcatheter venous valve repair. *Tissue Eng Part C Methods* 2013. [Epub ahead of print].
145. Jones CM, Hinds MT, Pavcnik D: Retention of an autologous endothelial layer on a bioprosthetic valve for the treatment of chronic deep venous insufficiency. *J Vasc Interv Radiol* 23:697–703, 2012.
146. Levi DS, Kusnezov N, Carman GP: Smart materials applications for pediatric cardiovascular devices. *Pediatr Res* 63:552–558, 2008.
147. de Borst GJ, Moll FL: Percutaneous venous valve designs for treatment of deep venous insufficiency. *Eur J Vasc Endovasc Surg* 46:360–365, 2013.

28 Hemodialysis Access Intervention

John A. Bittl

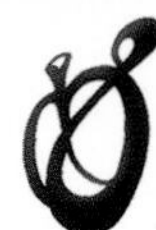

INTRODUCTION

The primary purpose of vascular access is to facilitate hemodialysis for as long as possible at minimal risk of complications. To achieve this goal, vascular surgeons primarily use vascular accesses created from native tissue, but when suitable autogenous components are not available, prosthetic arteriovenous grafts are preferred over tunneled catheter systems.

The creation of hemodialysis fistulas and grafts has become one of the most common types of vascular surgery in the United States, accounting for 40% to 50% of the operative volume in some programs.[1] Because the primary patency of hemodialysis fistulas and long-term patency of hemodialysis grafts is low, interventional therapies now play a prominent role in the health care of hemodialysis patients.

This chapter defines the pathophysiology of hemodialysis access failure, reviews the success rates for endovascular treatments, and uses color figures and videos to illustrate the catheter-based approaches for treating failing and thrombosed fistulas and grafts.

EPIDEMIOLOGY AND PREVALENCE OF STAGE V KIDNEY DISEASE

Survival

More than one in 1000 patients in the United States now has end-stage renal disease (ESRD), and 80% of these individuals undergo hemodialysis. The overall annual mortality rate for patients on hemodialysis exceeds 20%.[2] The mortality rate for elderly patients during the first year after initiation of dialysis is 58%.[3] Almost 40% of patients with ESRD have concomitant coronary artery disease,[4] and the overall annual rate of myocardial infarction for patients on hemodialysis exceeds 10%. In the hemodialysis population, the 1-year mortality rate after myocardial infarction exceeds 50%.[5]

Hemodialysis

The number of patients with ESRD requiring renal replacement therapy (RRT) exceeded 340,000 in 2006,[6] and by the year 2020, the number of patients with ESRD is expected to be 750,000.[6] The United States hemodialysis program now comprises more than 6% of the entire Medicare budget.[6] The growing prevalence of ESRD can be attributed primarily to changing demographics and the under-treatment of hypertension, diabetes, and chronic kidney disease (CKD) in the general population. Functioning hemodialysis access is critical for patients with ESRD.

VASCULAR ANATOMY

Nomenclature

The selection of a surgical site for hemodialysis access is based on evidence favoring the creation of an autogenous hemodialysis access ("fistula") whenever possible, before resorting to the creation of prosthetic arteriovenous access with polytetrafluoroethylene (PTFE) or other synthetic materials ("graft'), in compliance with the "Fistula First" policy established in the United States[7] and in other countries.[8] The proportion of hemodialysis patients with fistulas has been increasing in the United States. In one report, the proportion of patients on hemodialysis with autogenous fistulas increased from 48 ± 4% to 62 ± 4% between 1999 and 2007.[9]

The identification of a specific site for permanent access creation is based on venous (**Figure 28-1**) and arterial anatomy (**Figure 28-2**), according to the practice favoring the nondominant arm before the dominant arm, the forearm before the upper arm, and the upper extremity before the lower extremity.[7]

Autogenous Arteriovenous Accesses

A fistula is surgically created when a native inflow artery is directly anastomosed with a native outflow vein. A common

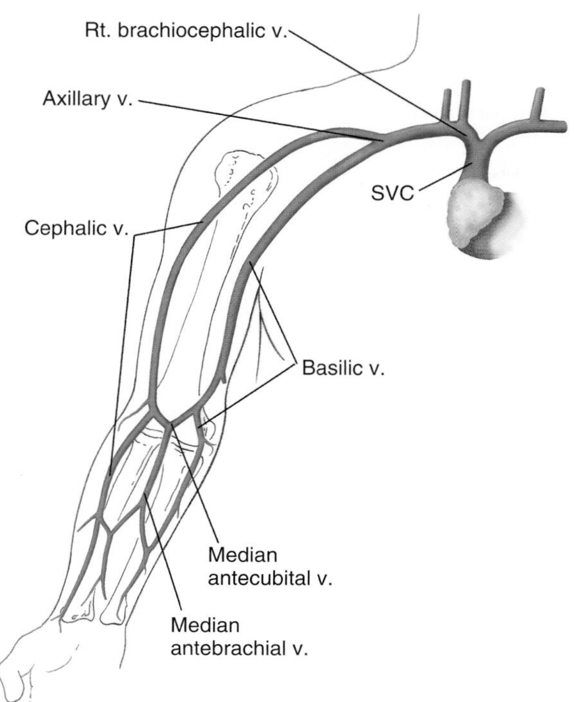

FIGURE 28-1 Venous anatomy of the upper extremity. *(Reprinted with permission from the author and Elsevier Inc. Bittl JA: Catheter interventions for hemodialysis fistulas and grafts. JACC Cardiovasc Interv 3:1–11, 2010.)*

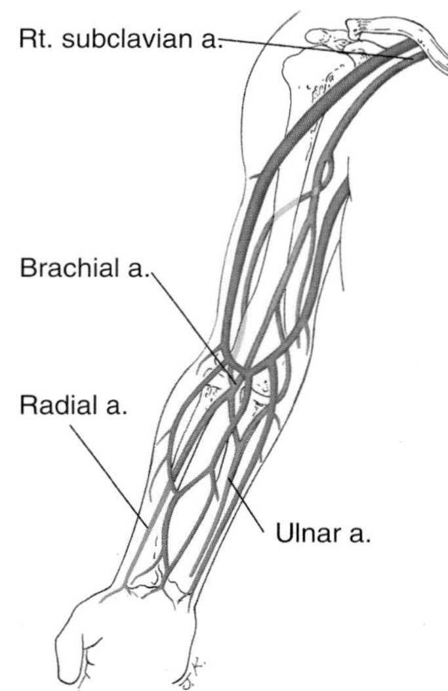

FIGURE 28-2 Arterial and venous anatomy of the upper extremity. *(Reprinted with permission from the author and Elsevier Inc. Bittl JA: Catheter interventions for hemodialysis fistulas and grafts. JACC Cardiovasc Interv 3:1–11, 2010.)*

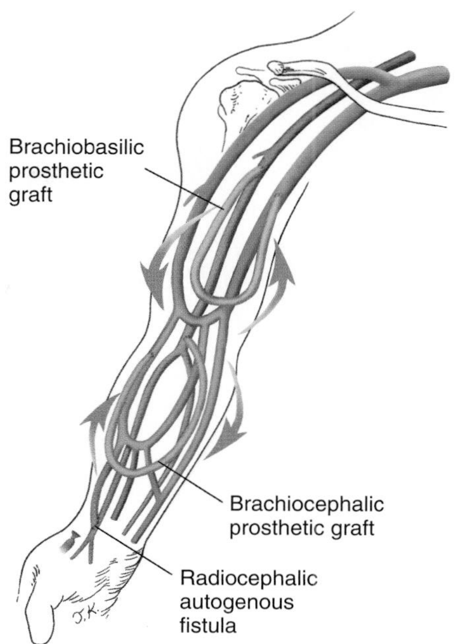

FIGURE 28-3 Access anatomy of the upper extremity. A radial-cephalic fistula *(small distal arrows)* is created by an end-to-side anastomosis between the cephalic vein and the radial artery, with ligation of the distal stump of the cephalic vein. A brachial-cephalic graft in the forearm *(large arrows)* requires the surgical interposition of a polytetrafluoroethylene (PTFE) loop using end-to-side connections. A brachial-basilic graft in the upper arm *(larger arrows)* requires the surgical insertion of a PTFE loop using end-to-side connections. *(Reprinted with permission from the author and Elsevier Inc. Bittl JA: Catheter interventions for hemodialysis fistulas and grafts. JACC Cardiovasc Interv 3:1–11, 2010.)*

configuration at the wrist involves an end-to-side anastomosis between the radial artery and the cephalic vein, creating the Brescia-Cimino radial-cephalic fistula (**Figure 28-3**). Another common configuration in the upper arm entails mobilization and tunneling of the basilic vein laterally and superficially for an end-to-side anastomosis with the brachial artery, creating a transposed brachial-basilic fistula.

Prosthetic Arteriovenous Accesses

A prosthetic arteriovenous access is constructed by surgically interposing a segment of PTFE between a native artery and a native vein in either a straight or looped configuration. Loop grafts are favored over straight grafts because they increase the length of the graft amenable to needle entry. The most common graft patterns include the brachial-cephalic configuration in the forearm (**Figure 28-3**) or the brachial-basilic configuration in the upper arm (**Figure 28-3**).

In the forearm, the radial-cephalic autogenous access and the brachial-cephalic prosthetic access are the favored configurations (**Figure 28-3**), with the outflow in both instances carried by the cephalic vein. This follows a medial-to-lateral course, continues along the lateral aspect of the arm, traverses the pectoral groove, and anastomoses with the axillary vein and then becomes the subclavian vein.

In the upper arm, the brachial-basilic autogenous access and the brachial-basilic prosthetic graft are common configurations, with the outflow in both instances carried by the basilic vein. This follows a lateral-to-medial course and continues in a straight line into the axillary vein, subclavian vein, and thence into the central circulation (**Figure 28-3**). In the thigh, the superficial femoral artery-greater saphenous vein configuration is preferred, with venous outflow following a lateral-to-medial course (**Figure 28-4**).

Anatomic Variants

A few anatomic variations are commonly encountered. Alternative patterns for prosthetic grafts include the brachial-basilic graft in the forearm that has a lateral-to-medial course, and the brachial-cephalic graft in the upper arm that has a medial-to-lateral course.

Another configuration in the forearm consists of the proximal radial artery anastomosed in a side-to-side manner with the median antebrachial vein, producing a double-outlet

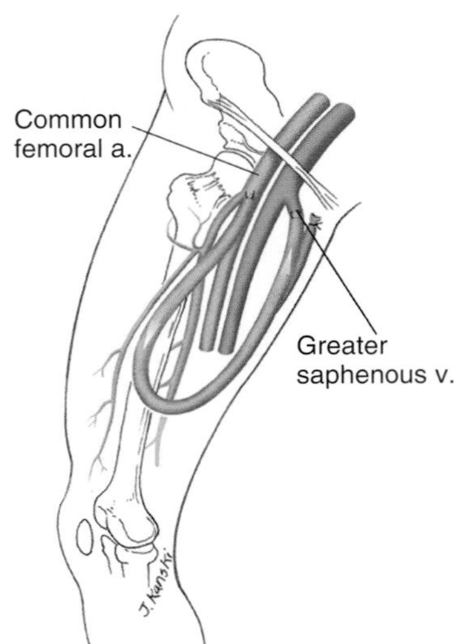

FIGURE 28-4 Access anatomy of the thigh. Creation of a thigh graft involves the surgical placement of a polytetrafluoroethylene (PTFE) loop connected end-to-side with superficial femoral artery and end-to-end with the greater saphenous vein.

TABLE 28-1 Pathophysiology of Access Failure

Primary failure of new fistulas
• Inflow (anastomotic) stenosis
• Failure to undergo hypertrophy
Failure of old fistulas and grafts
• Isolated venous or outflow anastomotic stenosis
• Thrombosis

configuration coursing proximally and distally from the arteriovenous anastomosis.[11] Another type of "double-outlet" access is the radial-cephalic fistula that drains into the basilic vein, a desirable variant that reduces the risk of thrombosis when one limb develops an outflow stenosis.

PATHOGENESIS OF ACCESS FAILURE

Two modes of failure commonly affect fistulas and grafts (**Table 28-1**), and both types of failure are amenable to interventional treatment. An autogenous fistula has a greater chance for long-term patency than a prosthetic arteriovenous graft, but the primary patency of fistulas remains low because of the lack of suitable anatomy in many cases and the inability to achieve adequate hypertrophy. Fewer than 50% of fistulas mature adequately to allow reliable hemodialysis.[12-16] When fistulas mature adequately and have been successfully used for hemodialysis, they fail after a median of 3 to 7 years.[17-19]

Patients who are not candidates for fistulas can have prosthetic grafts constructed from PTFE. Although the primary patency of such prosthetic grafts exceeds 80%[1] prosthetic accesses fail after a median lifetime of only 12 to 18 months.[17-20]

Failure to Mature

An anastomotic arteriovenous stenosis in a newly created fistula restricts inflow and prevents fistula hypertrophy.[21-23] Low primary patency rates may improve slightly after successful angioplasty of the inflow stenosis or surgical revision so that secondary patency rates at 1 year are 10% to 20% higher than primary patency rates.[12,24]

The failure of autogenous fistulas to mature is a more common problem in diabetic patients and in the elderly. The patency of upper-arm brachial-cephalic and transposed basilic vein fistulas in diabetic patients at 18 months (78%) may be significantly better than that of forearm fistulas (33%).[25]

Stenosis Development in Mature Accesses, with or without Thrombosis

About 50% of failing accesses contain thrombus, but thrombosis is the primary cause of failure in less than 1% of cases.[10] In almost every case, a culprit stenosis restricts flow, produces stasis, and ultimately causes thrombosis. In chronically used fistulas and grafts, high pressures and flow in the thin-walled outflow vein raise shear stress and trigger fibromuscular hyperplasia.[26,27] When the hyperplasia is exuberant, a severe stenosis appears, reduces flow, and precipitates thrombosis.

The success of catheter-based treatments of access thrombosis requires delineating and treating the culprit stenosis that initiated the pathologic process of stasis and thrombosis. Stenoses can occur anywhere in the dialysis access, but the most common site in 47% to 65% of cases involves the anastomosis between the prosthetic graft and the outflow vein.[28-30] Other sites for stenosis formation include a nonanastomotic location within a peripheral outflow vein in 37% to 53%, the graft itself in 38% to 50%, central veins in 3% to 20%, and multiple sites in 31% to 59%.[28,30] Fistulas contain no outflow anastomosis, but like grafts, they are nonetheless susceptible to stenosis formation in the "arterialized" outflow vein.

The bulk of the thrombus that occurs secondarily within a clotted access is typically red thrombus, which is rich in fibrin and red cells and easily extracted with rheolytic methods or pulse-spray thrombolysis. The platelet-rich white clot at the arterial inflow anastomosis is usually resistant to rheolytic or thrombolytic methods and may require mechanical removal with Fogarty thrombectomy.[31]

Primary thrombosis of chronically used hemodialysis accesses occurs rarely. It may occur unpredictably and unavoidably after major surgery, myocardial infarction, or sepsis associated with hypotension or hyperfibrinogenemia. Other causes of primary access thrombosis are excessive postdialysis access compression, hyperviscosity from hemoconcentration, polycythemia, or hypovolemia. When primary thrombosis of an access occurs without an identifiable pathogenic stenosis or if it occurs in the setting of a hypercoagulable state such as Factor V Leiden or the antiphospholipid syndrome,[32] chronic anticoagulation with warfarin is recommended.

No medical therapy has been identified that prevents the development of a venous outflow stenosis or an arterial inflow stenosis. Although several randomized trials of antiplatelet agents have been reported, none has shown clear success in preventing access thrombosis[33-35] or improving maturation rates. In a randomized trial of 877 patients,[14] clopidogrel was associated with similar maturation rates as placebo (38% vs. 40%). In a separate randomized trial of 649 patients,[15] however, dipyridamole was modestly better than placebo in achieved primary unassisted patency of autogenous arteriovenous fistulas at 1 year (28% vs. 23%).

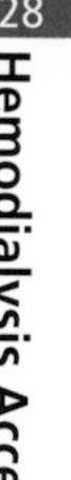

DIAGNOSTIC EVALUATION

The National Kidney Foundation-Dialysis Outcomes Quality Initiative (NKF-DOQI) document recommends establishing an organized program to identify failing fistulas and grafts.[36]

Monitoring

Access integrity can be assessed with regular bedside examinations and an assessment of dialysis adequacy. The history or physical examination may suggest the presence of an inflow or outflow obstruction. Increased postdialysis bleeding suggests the development of an outflow stenosis.

The presence of a focal and short high-pitched bruit suggests the presence of an obstruction, whereas a continuous medium-pitched bruit similar to the continuous murmur of a patent ductus arteriosus, associated with a prominent thrill along an easily palpable and ballotable course in the subcutaneous tissue, is evidence of normal access function. A soft bruit and inconspicuous thrill over a recently created, slowly maturing, hypoplastic radial-cephalic fistula may indicate the presence of an anastomotic inflow stenosis. On the other hand, prominent access pulsation may signify elevated pressure caused by an outflow stenosis. Multiple aneurysmal segments in the distribution of a large, serpiginous access used for many years may indicate long-standing high pressures within the access. Marked arm edema, sometimes producing peau d'orange, usually indicates dual venous obstruction (cephalic and basilic) or a subclavian vein stenosis or occlusion.

Infected accesses may be difficult to diagnose. Mild isolated erythema without tenderness or edema is usually not a sign of infection, but fever and leukocytosis as signs of infection may be masked in uremic patients. Signs of infection include cellulitis, fluctuance, skin breakdown, or purulent discharge. Access infection is a contraindication to interventional treatment because sepsis may ensue when infected thrombus is agitated.

Surveillance

Surveillance refers to the performance of noninvasive testing of access structure and function. Measurements of intra-access flow and static venous dialysis pressures provide evidence of access adequacy. The finding of rising pressures of more than 150 mm Hg at a constant flow of 200 mL/min on hemodialysis may indicate the presence of an outflow stenosis. Estimating the recirculation fraction using urea concentrations or clinical parameters such as body weight, volume status, or serum potassium concentration may indicate incomplete dialysis. These are probably relatively late predictors of hemodialysis access failure and become abnormal at the time of impending thrombosis.

Repeat ultrasonographic studies may identify early stenosis formation before physical signs are apparent,[37] but the cost of noninvasive methods and the uncertain benefits of pre-emptive graft intervention are tempering enthusiasm for noninvasive surveillance.[36]

Diagnostic Testing

Diagnostic testing refers to the performance of angiographic procedures to define access anatomy and hemodynamics. The generic term "fistulogram" refers to the angiographic study of either an autogenous arteriovenous fistula or a prosthetic arteriovenous graft. A significant stenosis is defined angiographically by the presence of a 50% diameter stenosis and clinically by bleeding or thrombus formation. A successful endovascular intervention is the ability to complete at least one dialysis session via the treated access. The definition of patency duration is the time from intervention to referral for repeat intervention, vascular surgery, or placement of a temporary dialysis catheter because of a failing or thrombosed access.

Hemodynamic measurements made during catheter-based intervention can be important to assess procedural success. The ideal systolic pressure of an access should be less than 50 mm Hg, and the optimal ratio of systolic pressure in the access to systolic systemic pressure should be 0.30 to 0.40.[28,38] Modest elevations of venous pressures to 60 mm Hg caused by central vein stenoses or occlusions can cause limb edema. If treatment normalizes pressures, edema may improve within one to two days.

CATHETER-BASED TREATMENT OF FAILING ACCESSES

Indications

A fistulogram is indicated on an emergency, urgent, or semi-elective basis when hemodialysis cannot be successfully carried out or when there is evidence from monitoring or surveillance to suggest that thrombosis is imminent (**Table 28-2**). Emergency indications for catheter-based treatment include refractory access bleeding, hyperkalemia, volume overload, or refractory hypertension associated with a failing or thrombosed access. An urgent indication within 24 hours of diagnosis and within 48 hours of most recent dialysis session for endovascular treatment is access thrombosis that may avoid the need for temporary catheter placement. A semi-elective indication for angiography is the finding of a malfunctioning but nonthrombosed dialysis access (**Table 28-2**), which should be referred within 48 hours of discovery because thrombosis may be imminent.

Contraindications to percutaneous treatment include graft infection, a central right-to-left shunt, or pulmonary hypertension (**Table 28-3**). A relative contraindication to catheter-based therapy is thrombosis of a new fistula or graft within 30 days of creation or surgical revision. In this situation, thrombosis has likely arisen from a technical problem or unfavorable biology not amenable to catheter-based therapy.

TABLE 28-2 Indications for Invasive Evaluation of Failing or Thrombosed Dialysis Accesses

Delayed maturation of hypoplastic fistula
Access thrombosis
Increased postdialysis bleeding
Absent or decreased thrill
Absent bruit or pulse
Change in bruit from continuous medium pitch to short high pitch
New prominent pulsation over access
Pseudoaneurysm
Recurrent access needle thrombosis
Repeated difficulty initiating hemodialysis
Decreased dialysis efficiency
Increased dialysis time
Increasing pressure in return line at constant flow
Peripheral edema in graft extremity
Increased recirculation fraction >20%

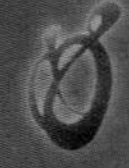

TABLE 28-3 Contraindications to Endovascular Treatment of Thrombosed Dialysis Accesses

Right-to-left intracardiac shunt
Pulmonary hypertension
Infected access
Recent surgical revision (within ~30 days)

TABLE 28-4 Four-Step Approach

1. Thrombectomy of outflow and inflow segments
2. Percutaneous transluminal angioplasty of venous outflow stenosis
3. Fogarty thrombectomy of adherent clot at the arterial inflow anastomosis
4. Angiography of central veins

4-Step Procedure for Thrombosed Accesses

A 4-step procedure is applicable for thrombosed fistulas and grafts (**Table 28-4**). This is based on the understanding of the pathophysiology of access failure discussed previously. The procedures outlined here define an approach that can be performed by interventional cardiologists, nephrologists, or radiologists with predictably high success.[10,39]

Before the procedure, information should be gathered about the etiology of ESRD, concurrent illnesses, access history, and indications (**Table 28-2**) or contraindications (**Table 28-3**). Physical examination should focus on the presence of volume overload and adequacy of circulation in the access extremity (e.g., Allen test). The measurement of the serum potassium level should be made if a dialysis session has been missed. Patients treated chronically with warfarin or the new oral anticoagulants do not need to have their medications held before a fistulogram. Intravenous lines should not be placed in any potential venous site for future access creation, but hand veins ipsilateral to an access site are permissible sites.[36]

Many physicians administer aspirin 325 mg orally before the procedure, but this can be omitted or replaced with clopidogrel in patients allergic to aspirin. Many interventionalists give heparin intravenously in a dose of 5000 U if there is evidence of access thrombosis. Lower doses of heparin can be considered or heparin can be omitted altogether if the risk of bleeding or perforation is increased, as in recently created thin-walled fistulas. Antibiotic prophylaxis with cephalothin 1 g intravenously is commonly recommended. If an allergy to cephalosporins exists, vancomycin 1 g intravenously can be substituted and given over 1 hour.

Thrombectomy

De-clotting is the first step in treating a thrombosed access. This is achieved by entering the occluded fistula or graft near existing needle "tracks" with a percutaneous 18-gauge needle or a 4 Fr micropuncture set (Cook, Inc., Bloominton, Indiana), inserting guidewires in both the inflow and outflow directions, and placing two 6 Fr sheaths (**Figure 28-5**). It is important to avoid puncturing the back wall of the graft, because an extrinsic hematoma may compress the access. Upon entering a thrombosed access, no flashback will be seen. No contrast should be injected into a thrombosed access, because thrombus near injected contrast will embolize. Successful entry into a thrombosed access is easily confirmed by smooth guidewire advancement.

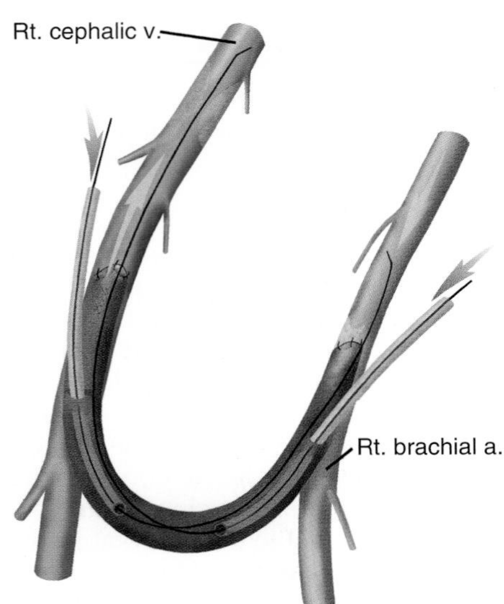

FIGURE 28-5 Cross-sheath method. A 6 Fr sheath is inserted into the access near the arterial-inflow anastomosis and directed into the direction of the outflow, and a 7 Fr sheath is inserted into the access near the venous-outflow in the direction of the inflow. Guidewires are advanced in the direction of the inflow and outflow under fluoroscopic guidance. No contrast is injected into a thrombosed access. *(Reprinted with permission from the author and Elsevier Inc. Bittl JA: Catheter interventions for hemodialysis fistulas and grafts. JACC Cardiovasc Interv 3:1–11, 2010.)*

After two 6 Fr sheaths are placed within the access, one in the direction of the venous outflow and one in the direction of the arterial inflow, the sheath tips face each other but do not overlap. Two 150-cm 0.018-inch V-18 hydrophilic control wires (Boston Scientific Medi-Tech, Miami, Florida) are advanced under fluoroscopic guidance without contrast injection (Video 28-1). If it is difficult to identify or advance the wire beyond the outflow stenosis or to enter the inflow artery, a 65-cm 5 Fr multipurpose A1 catheter (Cordis, Miami Lakes, Florida) may enhance torque control.

Several thrombectomy devices are available, including the dedicated AngioJet AVX rheolytic thrombectomy catheter (Possis Medical, Minneapolis, Minnesota), pulse-spray infusion catheters (Cook, Inc., Bloomington, Indiana), pulse-spray side-slit catheters (Angiodynamics, Inc., Glens Falls, New York), the Amplatz thrombectomy device (Microvena, White Bear Lake, Minnesota), the Arrow-Tretola percutaneous thrombectomy device (Arrow International, Reading, Pennsylvania), and the Gelbfish Endo-Vac device (Neovascular Technology, New York, New York). Thrombectomy is carried out first in the outflow (**Figure 28-6** and Video 28-1) and inflow directions (**Figure 28-7** and Video 28-2). After flow is achieved, the access sheaths are flushed with heparinized saline, and angiography can be performed to identify the culprit stenosis (Video 28-3).

Nonthrombosed fistulas and grafts are treated with an abbreviated approach. A diagnostic fistulogram can usually be obtained through a 4 Fr micropuncture catheter placed in either direction. The catheter should be directed toward the inflow if the fistula is hypoplastic. The catheter should be directed toward the outflow if the access has been chronically used for hemodialysis and demonstrates signs of increased pressure. When a stenosis is identified, angioplasty can be carried out through the 4 Fr micropuncture sheath using a coronary balloon (Maverick, Boston Scientific, Natick, Massachusetts) or through 4 Fr or 5 Fr sheaths using

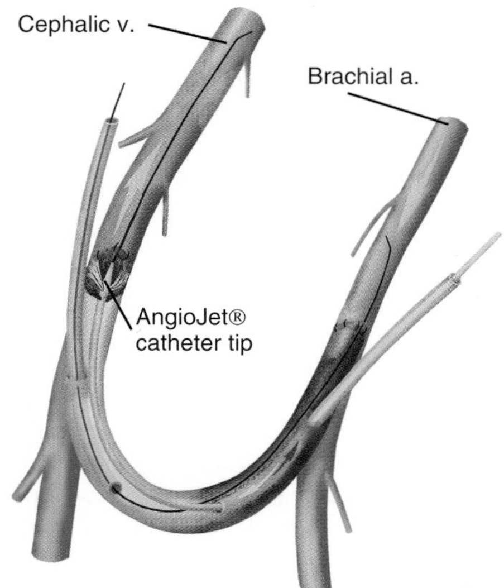

FIGURE 28-6 Rheolytic thrombectomy of venous outflow. *(Reprinted with permission from the author and Elsevier Inc. Bittl JA: Catheter interventions for hemodialysis fistulas and grafts. JACC Cardiovasc Interv 3:1–11, 2010.)*

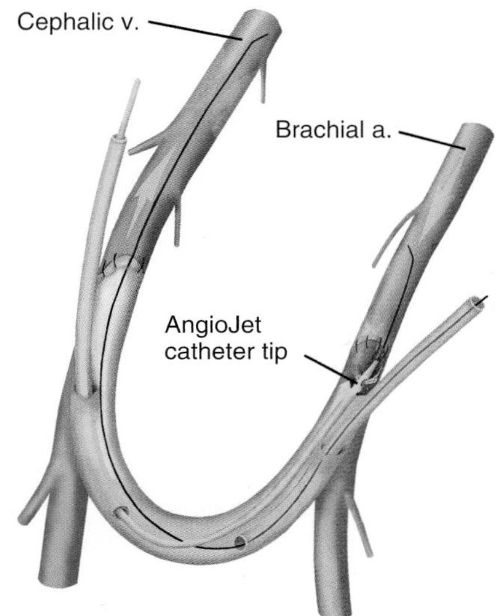

FIGURE 28-7 Rheolytic thrombectomy of arterial inflow. *(Reprinted with permission from the author and Elsevier Inc. Bittl JA: Catheter interventions for hemodialysis fistulas and grafts. JACC Cardiovasc Interv 3:1–11, 2010.)*

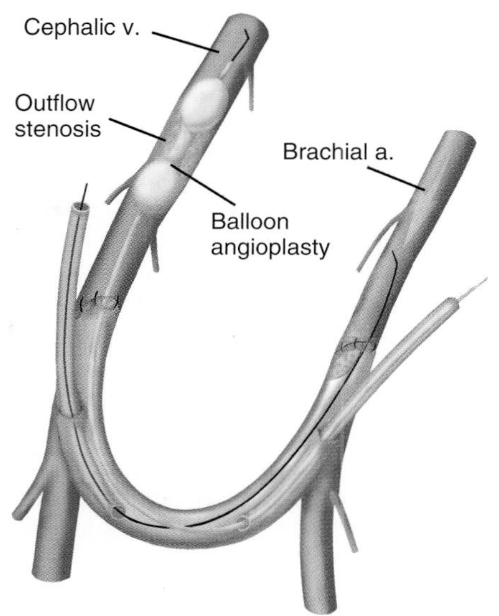

FIGURE 28-8 Balloon dilatation of outflow stenosis. The outflow stenosis is commonly found at or near the venous outflow anastomosis but can be encountered anywhere in the peripheral vein. *(Reprinted with permission from the author and Elsevier Inc. Bittl JA: Catheter interventions for hemodialysis fistulas and grafts. JACC Cardiovasc Interv 3:1–11, 2010.)*

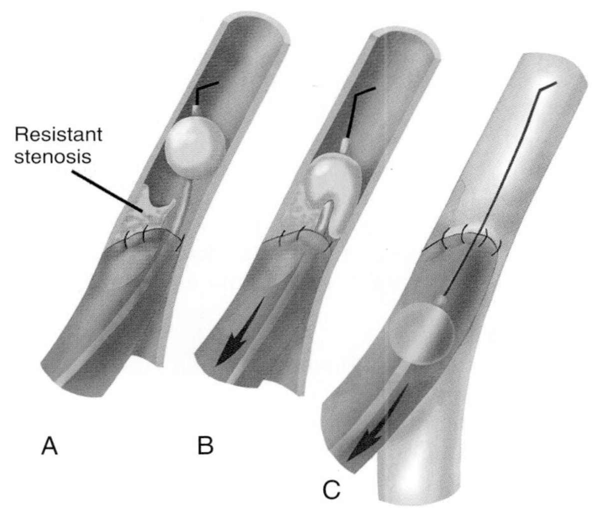

FIGURE 28-9 Fogarty embolectomy. The balloon catheter is inflated **(A)**, pulled back to the thrombus **(B)**, and forcefully withdrawn to mechanically dislodge the resistant inflow stenosis **(C)**. *(Reprinted with permission from the author and Elsevier Inc. Bittl JA: Catheter interventions for hemodialysis fistulas and grafts. JACC Cardiovasc Interv 3:1–11, 2010.)*

peripheral monorail balloons (Sterling, Boston Scientific Medi-Tech, Miami, Florida). If ultrahigh-pressure balloons are needed, however, larger sheaths may be required.

Angioplasty, Stenting, or Stent-Grafting of Stenosis

The second step involves identification (Video 28-3) and angioplasty of the culprit outflow stenosis with 4-mm to 10-mm balloons (**Figure 28-8**). The venous stenoses tend to be fibrotic, are resistant to dilatation, and occasionally require pressures greater than 20 atmospheres (Video 28-4). High-pressure, noncompliant balloons (Conquest or Dorado, Bard Peripheral Vascular Inc., Tempe, Arizona) with rated burst pressures of 20 to 24 can be used to achieve an adequate result (Video 28-5). Cutting balloons (Boston Scientific) can be used when high-pressure balloons are unsuccessful,[40,41] but the use of peripheral cutting balloons in one study was associated with an increased risk of rupture.[42] Stents are usually reserved for severe recoil, venous perforations, or stenoses in surgically inaccessible veins, but the use of stent grafts will likely increase in an effort to reduce restenosis.[43]

Fogarty Embolectomy

The third step involves Fogarty thrombectomy using an over-the-wire 4 Fr Thru-Lumen embolectomy catheter (Edwards Lifesciences, Irvine, California) to extract resistant thrombus at the arterial inflow (**Figures 28-9**). The maneuver is usually immediately successful (Video 28-6).

Central Venous Angiography

The fourth step entails venography of the entire venous outflow and central veins to exclude the presence of a central venous stenosis (Video 28-7). In the central circulation, critical stenoses or occlusions of the subclavian vein, which are commonly caused by prior catheter placement, or pacemaker or defibrillator leads, can be diagnosed when filling of the large axillary vein terminates abruptly and is associated with a medusa-like network of collaterals draining into the internal jugular vein.

If treatment of a central-vein stenosis is recommended, it requires large-diameter devices such as the XXL balloon (Boston Scientific Medi-Tech, Natick, Massachusetts), Atlas balloon (Bard), or SMART Control stent (Cordis, Miami, Florida) up to 14 mm in diameter (Videos 28-8 to 28-14). However, treatment of incidental central vein stenoses remains controversial. Levit et al.[44] evaluated the success of pre-emptive angioplasty or stenting for central venous stenoses ipsilateral to hemodialysis accesses in 35 patients who underwent 86 angiograms over a 6-year period. Angioplasty or stenting of asymptomatic stenoses was associated with more rapid stenosis progression and escalation of lesions than the strategy of watchful waiting.

OUTCOMES

Success Rates

The acute success rate for endovascular treatment depends on access type and failure mode. Catheter-based treatment of thrombosed fistulas ranges from 78% to 87%[10,28,39]; the treatment of thrombosed grafts ranges from 93% to 96%.[10,28,39]

Six-month patency rates after endovascular treatment range from 61% to 66%, and the 1-year patency rates range from 38% to 41%.[28,45] Fistulas have longer median patencies than grafts,[28,46] unless thrombosis has occurred, because the presence of thrombosis reduces the long-term patency for all accesses and eliminates the fistula advantage.

Complications

Complications from endovascular treatment of dialysis access failure are rare but usually mild and controllable. Iatrogenic hematomas are categorized by severity.[47] Grade I hematomas are minor and nonflow limiting, whereas Grade II hematomas are large and flow limiting. Grade III hematomas are massive, associated with pulsatile extravasation or free perforation. Free-flowing rupture usually requires firm compression and placement of a Viabahn Endoprosthesis (W.L. Gore and Associates, Flagstaff, Arizona), Fluency Plus tracheobronchial stentgraft (Bard Peripheral Vascular), or polyethylene teryltolate-covered stent (WallGraft, Boston Scientific, Natick, Massachusetts) after upsizing to an 11 Fr sheath (Videos 28-15 to 28-21). Pinhole perforations can usually be controlled by manual compression alone or with suture placement.[42] Massive perforations, like massive pseudoaneurysms (Video 28-22), may require surgical repair.

Several studies have reported the risk of major complications during catheter-based treatment of malfunctioning hemodialysis accesses. In one series,[48] venous rupture occurred in 40 of 2414 procedures (1.7%). Wallstents (Boston Scientific, Natick, Massachusetts) were successful in 28 of 37 cases, but a leak was still visible at the end of the intervention in 11 cases. A covered Cragg EndoPro stent (MinTec, La Ciotat, France) was needed in one case, and surgical drainage was required for one patient. In another series,[49] venous rupture occurred in 12 of 579 procedures (2.1%). Stents were successful in 10 of 12 patients. In another series of 23 patients with venous rupture,[50] the use of Wallstents led to a patency rate of 26% at 180 days.

In another series of 1242 procedures,[42] venous rupture or perforation occurred in 11 (0.9%) patients. No patient with a rupture or perforation died or required emergency or urgent surgical repair. Two of 11 patients (18.2%) required transfusions, 8 of 11 patients (72.7%) required stenting, and 6 of 8 patients (75.0%) who needed stenting received covered stents to achieve hemostasis. Rupture led to access thrombosis within 30 days in 9 of 11 cases (82%). Multivariable logistical regression analysis suggested that using a balloon catheter more than 2 mm larger than the diameter of the hemodialysis access or using peripheral cutting balloons increased the risk of rupture or perforation.[42]

Other complications include catheter or device breakage requiring retrieval with snares. Arterial embolization requires Fogarty thrombectomy or surgical treatment. Pulmonary embolism is rare after endovascular treatment of thrombosed accesses. No scintigraphic evidence of pulmonary embolism was seen in a systematic evaluation after various catheter-based approaches to treat thrombosed dialysis accesses.[51]

NEWER APPROACHES

Several experimental methods are under investigation to enhance the long-term patency of arteriovenous grafts by targeting intimal hyperplasia in the venous outflow. External beam radiation has been tried, but in a small series of patients this was unable to reduce the likelihood of repeat restenosis.[52] The concept of endothelial cell seeding of PTFE grafts was based on the concept that these cells form a biologically active lining to reduce the release from flowing blood of mitogens for vascular smooth muscle cells. Lining of PTFE grafts with anti-CD34 antibodies, which can bind bone marrow-derived CD34(+) endothelial progenitor cells with the potential to proliferate and differentiate into mature endothelial cells in an experimental model, resulted in almost complete endothelialization of the grafts but paradoxically increased neointimal hyperplasia at the graft-vein anastomosis.[53]

Stent Grafts

Haskal and colleagues randomized 190 hemodialysis patients with venous anastomotic stenoses to undergo either balloon angioplasty alone or placement of a nitinol PTFE stent graft (Flair, Bard Peripheral Vascular, Tempe, Arizona). At 6 months, the primary endpoints of target lesion patency (51% vs. 23%; $p < 0.001$) and access patency (38% vs. 20%; $p = 0.008$) were greater in the stent-graft group than in the balloon-angioplasty group. A potential drawback of the study was the 81% higher likelihood of access thrombosis in the stent-graft group than in the angioplasty group (odds ratio [OR] 1.81; 95% confidence interval [CI] 0.93-3.51). As a salvage procedure, however, the placement of stent grafts preserves accesses that have failed multiple balloon procedures (Videos 28-23 to 28-26).

Interventional Nephrology

The relatively new specialty of interventional nephrology has transformed the referral of hemodialysis patients for angiographic procedures. The emergence of interventional nephrology has been associated with the routine (self-) referral of functioning fistulas and grafts for angiography and pre-emptive angioplasty, but the practice remains controversial. The Vascular Access Work Group[54] has concluded that as a preventive strategy, "there is considerable debate concerning whether PTA interventions improve long-term outcomes."

Pre-emptive Angiography

Several studies have evaluated the ability of pre-emptive angioplasty to prevent access thrombosis, but results have been mixed. Positive reports include a small study[55] of 21 patients with prosthetic arteriovenous accesses that had not previously clotted or required intervention, in which pre-emptive angioplasty reduced the risk of thrombosis from 44% to 10% per 100 patients-years ($p = 0.01$). Another small study[56] reported that prophylactic angioplasty ($n = 32$) was superior to the standard treatment of fistulas ($n = 30$) in reducing the thrombosis rate from 25% to 16% per 100 patient-years.[56] Tessitore and colleagues[57] evaluated the cost effectiveness of access blood-flow measurements and pre-emptive angioplasty in 159 patients and observed that a threefold increase in the number of angiographic procedures offset a 77% reduction in thrombosis events and a 65% reduction in fistula loss, thus defining an "economically dominant therapy" (i.e., cost-saving).

Several randomized studies have suggested that pre-emptive angioplasty fails to prevent access thrombosis. A prospective randomized trial of 64 patients monitored with monthly static venous-to-systolic blood pressure ratios compared prophylactic angioplasty with the strategy of delayed invasive management at the time of thrombosis and observed similar rates of thrombosis and access loss.[58] Another randomized trial[59] of 112 patients compared monthly access blood-flow measurements with standard surveillance and reported that the greater number of interventions performed in the surveillance group than in the control group did not reduce the rate of access thrombosis (41% vs. 51% per 100 patient-years, p = not significant).

A recent economic analysis[9] suggested that pre-emptive percutaneous transluminal angioplasty (PTA) produced a decline in access thrombosis from 27.6 to 22.0 events per 100 patient-years ($p < 0.029$) at a net cost of $34,586 per 100 patient-years and an incremental cost-effectiveness ratio of $6177 per thrombosis event avoided. This appeared to be less economically appealing than increasing the proportion of fistulas in the hemodialysis population.

Salvage of Hypoplastic Fistulas

In newly placed but hypoplastic fistulas, balloon angioplasty of a stenosis at the arterial-venous anastomosis can successfully allow a small unusable fistula (Video 28-27) to undergo adaptive remodeling (Video 28-28).[23] When fistulas or grafts have recurrent venous outflow stenoses that require frequent balloon angioplasty procedures, surgical excision with end-to-end repair may be recommended. Several studies have reported that nonmaturing arteriovenous fistulas can be salvaged. Surgical ligation of tributaries, superficialization procedures, or revision of anastomoses can salvage a significant number of hypoplastic fistulas that fail to mature adequately.[60] Secondary surgical or interventional procedures for nonmaturing autogenous fistulas improve the success rate by at least ten percentage points.[13]

CONCLUSIONS

Catheter-based therapies have been a major advance for treating thrombosed and failing hemodialysis fistulas and grafts. Successful in more than 80% of cases, catheter-based therapies have obviated the need for placing temporary catheters or consuming precious venous conduits. Future studies are required to reduce the risk of stenosis formation and to define the optimal role of pre-emptive angiography and intervention in the growing and vulnerable population of patients with ESRD who undergo hemodialysis.

References

1. Weiswasser JM, Sidawy AN: Strategies of arteriovenous dialysis access. In Rutherford RB, editor: *Vascular Surgery*, ed 6, Philadelphia, 2005, Elsevier Saunders, pp 1669–1676.
2. US Renal Data System: USRDS 2004 annual data report: Atlas of End-Stage Renal Disease in the United States. *Am J Kidney Dis* 45(Suppl 1):S1–S280, 2005.
3. Kurella Tamura M, Covinsky KE, Chertow GM, et al: Functional status of elderly adults before and after initiation of dialysis. *N Engl J Med* 361:1539–1547, 2009.
4. Chueng AK, Sarnak MJ, Yan G, et al: Cardiac diseases in maintenance hemodialysis patients: results of the HEMO study. *Kidney Int* 65:2380–2389, 2004.
5. Herzog CA, Ma JZ, Collins AJ: Poor long-term survival after acute myocardial infarction among patients on long-term dialysis. *N Engl J Med* 339:799–805, 1998.
6. Collins AJ, Foley RN, Herzog C, et al: Excerpts from the United States Renal Data System 2007 annual data report. *Am J Kidney Dis* 51(Suppl 1):S1–S320, 2008.
7. Vascular Access 2006 Work Group: NKF-DOQI clinical practice guidelines for vascular access, update 2006. *Am J Kidney Dis* 48(Suppl 1):S176–S306, 2006.
8. Ohira S, Naito H, Amono I, et al: 2005 Japanese Society for Dialysis Therapy guidelines for vascular access construction and repair for chronic hemodialysis. *Ther Apher Dial* 10:449–462, 2006.
9. Bittl JA, Cohen DJ, Seek MM, et al: Econcomic analysis of angiography and preemptive angioplasty to prevent hemodialysis-access thrombosis. *Catheter Cardiovasc Interv* 75:14–21, 2010.
10. Bittl JA: Catheter interventions for hemodialysis fistulas and grafts. *JACC Cardiovasc Interv* 3:1–11, 2010.
11. Bruns SD, Jennings WC: Proximal radial artery as inflow site for native arteriovenous fistula. *J Am Coll Surg* 197:58–63, 2003.
12. Asif A, Gadalean FN, Merrill D, et al: Inflow stenosis in arteriovenous fistulas and grafts: a multicenter, prospective study. *Kidney Int* 67:1986–1992, 2005.
13. Berman SS, Gentile AT: Impact of secondary procedures in autogenous arteriovenous fistula maturation and mainenance. *J Vasc Surg* 34:866–871, 2001.
14. Dember LM, Beck GJ, Allon M, et al: Effect of clopidogrel on early failure of arteriovenous fistulas for hemodialysis: a randomized controlled trial. *JAMA* 299:2164–2171, 2008.
15. Dixon BS, Beck GJ, Vazquez MA, et al: Effect of dipyridamole plus aspirin on hemodialysis graft patency. *N Engl J Med* 360:2191–2201, 2009.
16. Patel ST, Hughes J, Mills JL, Sr: Failure of arteriovenous fistula maturation: an unintended consequence of exceeding Dialysis Outcome Quality Initiative guidelines for hemodialysis access. *J Vasc Surg* 38:439–445, 2003.
17. Huber MS, Mooney JF, Madison J, et al: Use of a morphologic classification to predict clinical outcome after dissection from coronary angioplasty. *Am J Cardiol* 68:467–471, 1991.
18. Perera GB, Mueller MP, Kubaska SM, et al: Superiority of autogenous arteriovenous hemodialysis access: maintenance of function with fewer secondary interventions. *Ann Vasc Surg* 18:66–73, 2004.
19. Schwartz C, McBrayer C, Sloan J, et al: Thrombosed dialysis grafts: comparison of treatment with transluminal angioplasty and surgical revision. *Radiology* 194:337–341, 1995.
20. Schwab SJ: Vascular access for hemodialysis. *Kidney Int* 55:2078–2090, 1999.
21. Beathard GA, Arnold P, Jackson J, et al: Aggessive treatment of early fistula failure. *Kidney Int* 64:1487–1494, 2003.
22. Achkar K, Nassar GM: Salvage of a severely dysfunctional arteriovenous fistula with a strictured and occluded outflow tract. *Semin Dial* 18:336–342, 2005.
23. Bittl JA, von Mering GO, Feldman RL: Adaptive remodeling of hypoplastic hemodialysis fistulas salvaged with angioplasty. *Catheter Cardiovasc Interv* 73:974–978, 2009.
24. Hodges TC, Fillinger MF, Zwolak RM, et al: Longitudinal comparison of dialysis graft access methods: risk factors for failure. *J Vasc Surg* 26:1009–1019, 1997.
25. Hakaim A, Nalbandian M, Scott T: Superior maturation and patency of primary brachiocephalic and transposed basilic vein arteriovenous fistulae in patients with diabetes. *J Vasc Surg* 27:154–157, 1998.
26. Swedberg SH, Brown BG, Sigley R, et al: Intimal fibromuscular hyperplasia at the venous anastomosis of PTFE grafts in hemodialysis patients. Clinical, immunocytochemical, light and electron microscopic assessment. *Circulation* 80:1726–1736, 1989.
27. Roy-Chaudhury P, Kelly BS, Miller MA, et al: Venous neointimal hyperplasia in polytetrafluoroethylene dialysis grafts. *Kidney Int* 59:2325–2334, 2001.
28. Bittl JA, Feldman RL: Prospective assessment of hemodialysis access patency after percutaneous intervention: Cox proportional hazards analysis. *Catheter Cardiovasc Interv* 66:309–315, 2005.
29. Kanterman RY, Vesely TM, Pilgram TK, et al: Dialysis access grafts: anatomic location of venous stenosis and results of angioplasty. *Radiology* 195:1995.
30. Beathard GA: Angioplasty for arteriovenous grafts and fistulae. *Semin Nephrol* 22:202–210, 2002.
31. Valji K: Transcatheter treatment of thrombosed hemodialysis access grafts. *AJR Am J Roentgenol* 164:823–829, 1995.
32. Knoll GA, Wells PS, Young D, et al: Thrombophilia and the risk for hemodialysis vascular access thrombosis. *J Am Soc Nephrol* 16:1108–1114, 2005.
33. Domoto DT, Bauman JE, Joist JH: Combined aspirin and sulfinpyrazone in the prevention of recurrent hemodialysis vascular access thrombosis. *Thromb Res* 62:737–743, 1991.
34. Kaufman JS, O'Connor TZ, Zhang JH, et al: Randomized controlled trial of clopidogrel plus aspirin to prevent hemodialysis access graft thrombosis. *J Am Soc Nephrol* 14:2313–2321, 2003.
35. Sreedhara R, Himmelfarb J, Lazarus JM, et al: Anti-platelet therapy in graft thrombosis: results of a prospective, randomized double-blind study. *Kidney Int* 45:1477–1483, 1994.
36. Anonymous: NKF-K/DOQI clinical practice guidelines for vascular access: update 2000. *Am J Kidney Dis* 37:S137–S181, 2001.
37. Malik J, Slavikova M, Svobodova J, et al: Regular ultrasonographic screening significantly prolongs patency of PTFE grafts. *Kidney Int* 67:1554–1558, 2005.

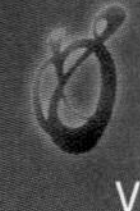

38. Lilly RZ, Carlton D, Barker J, et al: Predictors of arteriovenous graft patency after radiologic intervention in hemodialysis patients. *Am J Kidney Dis* 37:945–953, 2001.
39. Beathard GA, Litchfield T: Effectiveness and safety of dialysis vascular access procedures performed by interventional nephrologists. *Kidney Int* 66:1622–1632, 2004.
40. Bittl JA, Feldman RL: Cutting balloon angioplasty for undilatable venous stenoses causing dialysis graft failure. *Catheter Cardiovasc Interv* 58:524–526, 2003.
41. Vesely TM, Siegel JB: Use of the peripheral cutting balloon to treat hemodialysis-related stenoses. *J Vasc Interv Radiol* 16:1593–1603, 2005.
42. Bittl JA: Venous rupture during percutaneous treatment of hemodialysis fistulas and grafts. *Catheter Cardiovasc Interv* 74:1097–1101, 2009.
43. Haskal ZJ, Trerotola S, Dolmatch B, et al: Stent graft versus balloon angioplasty for failing dialysis-access grafts. *N Engl J Med* 362:494–503, 2010.
44. Levit RD, Cohen RM, Kwak A, et al: Asymptomatic central venous stenosis in hemodialysis patients. *Radiology* 238:1051–1056, 2006.
45. Beathard GA: Percutaneous transvenous angioplasty in the treatment of vascular access stenosis. *Kidney Int* 42:1390–1397, 1992.
46. Woods JD, Turenne MN, Strawderman RL, et al: Vascular access survival among incident hemodialysis patients in the United States. *Am J Kidney Dis* 30:50–57, 1997.
47. Beathard GA: Management of complications of endovascular dialysis access procedures. *Semin Dial* 16:309–313, 2003.
48. Raynaud AC, Angel CY, Sapoval MR, et al: Treatment of hemodialysis access rupture during PTA with Wallstent implantation. *J Vasc Interv Radiol* 9:437–442, 1998.
49. Sofocleous CT, Schur I, Koh E, et al: Percutaneous treatment of complications occurring during hemodialysis graft recanalization. *Eur J Radiol* 47:237–246, 2003.
50. Funaki B, Szymski GX, Leef JA, et al: Wallstent deployment to salvage dialysis graft thrombolysis complicated by venous rupture: early and intermediate results. *AJR Am J Roentgenol* 169:1435–1437, 1997.
51. Petronis JD, Regan F, Briefel G, et al: Ventilation-perfusion scintigraphic evaluation of pulmonary clot burden after percutaneous thrombolysis of clotted hemodialysis access grafts. *Am J Kidney Dis* 34:207–211, 1999.
52. Parikh S, Nori D, Rogers D, et al: External beam radiation therapy to prevent postangioplasty dialysis access restenosis: a feasibility study. *Cardiovasc Radiat Med* 1:36–41, 1999.
53. Rotmans JI, Heyliger JMM, Verhagen HJM, et al: In vivo seeding using anti-CD34 antibodies successfully accelerates endotheliazation but stimulates intimal hyperplasia in porcine arteriovenous expanded polytetrafluoroethylene grafts. *Circulation* 112:12–18, 2005.
54. Vascular Access 2006 Work Group: NKF-DOQI clinical practice guidelines for vascular access, update 2006: clinical practice recommendations for guideline 4: detection of access dysfunction: monitoring, surveillance, and diagnostic testing. *Am J Kidney Dis* 48(Suppl 1):S269–S270, 2006.
55. Martin LG, MacDonald MJ, Kikeri D, et al: Prophylactic angioplasty reduces thrombosis in virgin ePTFE arteriovenous dialysis grafts with greater than 50% stenosis: subset analysis of a prospectively randomized study. *J Vasc Interv Radiol* 10:389–396, 1999.
56. Schwab SJ, Oliver MJ, Suhocki P, et al: Hemodialysis arteriovenous access: detection of stenosis and response to treatment by vascular access blood flow. *Kidney Int* 59:358–362, 2001.
57. Tessitore N, Bedogna V, Poli A, et al: Adding access blood flow surveillance to clinical monitoring reduces thrombosis rates and costs, and improves fistula patency in the short term: a controlled cohort study. *Nephrol Dial Transplant* 23:3578–3584, 2008.
58. Dember LM, Holmberg EF, Kaufman JS: Randomized controlled trial of prophylactic repair of hemodialysis arteriovenous graft stenosis. *Kidney Int* 66:390–398, 2004.
59. Moist LM, Churchill DN, House AA, et al: Regular monitoring of access flow compared with monitoring of venous pressure fails to improve graft survival. *J Am Soc Nephrol* 14:2645–2653, 2003.
60. Gelabert HA, Freischlag JA: Angioaccess. In Rutherford RB, editor: *Vascular Surgery*, ed 4, Philadelphia, 2000, W.B. Saunders Co., pp 1466–1477.

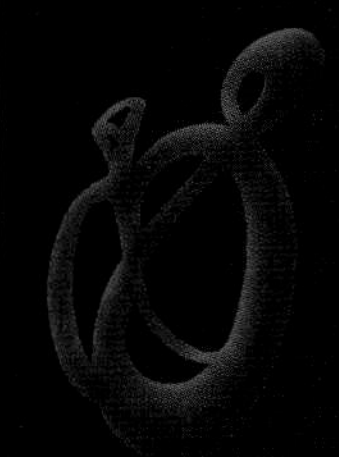

PART VI

STRUCTURAL HEART INTERVENTION

29 Aortic Valvuloplasty and Transcatheter Aortic Valve Replacement

Susheel K. Kodali, Darshan Doshi, and Martin B. Leon

INTRODUCTION

Balloon aortic valvuloplasty (BAV) was developed as one of the first minimally invasive approaches to treat symptomatic severe aortic stenosis (AS). Alain Cribier first described the procedure in 1986 in a case series of three patients with severe calcific aortic stenosis.[1] While the procedure was initially intended to be a minimally invasive alternative to surgical aortic valve replacement (SAVR), recognition of a high procedural complication rate, early restenosis, and lack of a mortality benefit eventually limited its overall utility.

Transcatheter aortic valve replacement (TAVR) or implantation (TAVI) has become a viable and durable therapy for patients with severe AS who have been deemed "inoperable" or "high-risk" for conventional SAVR. Since Alain Cribier first described the TAVR procedure in 2002,[2] it is estimated that more than 125,000 procedures have been successfully performed worldwide in over 750 centers. During the past decade, procedural success, patient safety, and valve performance have improved dramatically due to technology enhancements, technique refinements, better patient selection, and a greater understanding of early and late clinical outcomes.

This chapter reviews the following: techniques for BAV; outcomes and complications with BAV; current indications for BAV; newer BAV technology; historical perspectives of TAVR; techniques for implantation of transcatheter valves; current and expanded clinical TAVR indications; updated TAVR clinical trial results; complications of TAVR; and an overview of the next generation of TAVR devices.

BALLOON AORTIC VALVULOPLASTY

Procedural Considerations

BAV is a procedure in which one or more balloons are placed across a stenotic valve and inflated to fracture the calcified aortic valve leaflets. The procedure results in separation of the commissures and stretching of the aortic valve annulus. The immediate hemodynamic results include an increase in aortic valve area (although rarely greater than 1.0 cm^2) and a reduction of the transvalvular gradient. Despite only modest changes in the valve parameters, the procedure can lead to meaningful, albeit short-term, symptomatic improvement in patients.

The BAV procedure can be performed via a retrograde or an antegrade approach. The retrograde approach is more commonly utilized and involves access via the femoral artery with a 10 Fr to 14 Fr sheath. Anticoagulation is typically achieved with heparin dosing to achieve an activated clotting time (ACT) >250 but bivalirudin can be used in patients with heparin allergy. An extra-stiff guidewire (0.035 inch) is utilized for the procedure and is required for stabilization of the balloon during inflation and deflation. Care must be taken to position the wire with a gentle curve in the left ventricular (LV) apex to avoid the risk of ventricular perforation. Typically, a slightly undersized balloon, ~1 mm smaller than the annulus, is used to minimize risk of annular rupture while maximizing results. If an adequate result is not obtained with initial inflation, a larger balloon sized to the annulus may be used. The various balloons available (Zymed, Tyshack, Cristal) have different profiles and compliance curves and are typically inflated manually. Rapid ventricular pacing (160 to 180 bpm) via a temporary transvenous pacemaker can be utilized to stabilize the balloon during inflation by reducing forward cardiac output. Care must be taken to avoid prolonged pacing runs, which may cause ischemia and hemodynamic compromise. Vascular closure can be achieved by manual compression or the "preclose" technique with the Abbott Vascular Perclose device (Abbott Vascular Inc., California).

The antegrade transvenous approach has also been utilized for BAV and requires creation of a transcirculatory loop from the femoral vein to the ascending aorta via a transseptal puncture. An Inoue balloon (Toray, Tokyo, Japan) or a traditional valvuloplasty balloon can be used. One advantage of the Inoue balloon is the shape, which allows the waist of the balloon to fit the aortic valve annulus while the larger distal bulbous portion stretches the aortic leaflets more fully into the sinuses of Valsalva. Also, with one 26-mm balloon, multiple inflations can be performed at sizes ranging from 20 to 26 mm while assessing hemodynamic results in between. The potential benefits of the antegrade approach are reduced vascular complications, reduction of stroke, and greater increase in post-BAV area.[3] However, it is more technically demanding given the need for a transseptal puncture and the subsequent looping of the guidewire in the LV apex.

Outcomes

The two largest registries that have evaluated BAV are the National Heart, Lung, and Blood Institute (NHLBI) and the Mansfield Scientific registries. The NHLBI registry evaluated 674 BAV patients immediately post procedure and up to 3 years later.[4,5] High complication rates and in-hospital mortality were reported in this registry, with a 25% complication rate and a 3% mortality rate within the first 24 hours. The most common complication was the need for a transfusion in 20% due to vascular access issues. The cumulative cardiovascular mortality rate before discharge was 8%. Overall survival was 55% at 1-year, 35% at 2-year, and 23% at 3-year follow-up. Recurrent hospitalization (64%) and early restenosis were common. Echocardiography at 6 months demonstrated restenosis from the postprocedural valve area of 0.78 to 0.65 cm^2.

The Mansfield Scientific Aortic Valvuloplasty Registry contained 492 patients and demonstrated comparable results.[6] Approximately 20.5% of patients had complications after the procedure, with a 4.9% 24-hour mortality rate and a 7.5% mortality rate during the index hospital stay. Restenosis was also demonstrated to be nearly ubiquitous.

Although improved patient selection and technical improvements have led to a modest decrease in complication rates over the past 20 years, postprocedural morbidity remains high.[7,8] In a contemporary series of 262 high-risk surgical or inoperable AS patients,[7] the most common complications after BAV were intraprocedural death (1.6%); stroke (1.99%); coronary occlusion (0.66%); severe aortic regurgitation (1.3%); need for permanent pacemaker (0.99%); severe vascular complication (6.9%)—perforation (1.6%), ischemic leg (2.6%), pseudoaneurysm (1.99%), arterial-venous fistula (0.66%); acute kidney injury (11.3%); and new hemodialysis (0.99%). At approximately 6 months, there was a 50% mortality rate, and restenosis was evident as early as a few days postprocedure.

Given the frequency of these complications, their prompt identification and management are imperative. Despite smaller sheaths, vascular complications remain frequent and operators must have the skill set to manage them utilizing endovascular techniques with covered stents and prolonged balloon inflations. The most devastating complication for patients remains cerebrovascular injury, which occurs in 1% to 2% of patients.[7,8] The etiology is typically atheroembolism from the ascending aorta or calcific embolism from the valve. The use of embolic protection devices in the future may further mitigate these complications.

Indications

The 2014 American College of Cardiology (ACC)/American Heart Association (AHA) guidelines[9] on valvular heart disease specify that BAV might be reasonable (Class IIB recommendation) as a bridge to SAVR or TAVR in patients with severe AS. In the prior 2006 ACC/AHA valve guidelines,[10] BAV was given a Class IIB recommendation for palliation in patients with co-morbidities that prevent aortic valve replacement, but this recommendation was removed in the 2014 guidelines owing to a lack of evidence. The updated 2012 European Society of Cardiology (ESC) and the European Association for Cardio-Thoracic Surgery (EACTS) valve guidelines[11] also give a Class IIB recommendation for BAV as a bridge to SAVR or TAVR in hemodynamically unstable patients who are at high risk for surgery or in patients with symptomatic AS who require urgent major non-cardiac surgery. However, the ESC guidelines also state that BAV may be considered for palliation in patients unfit for SAVR or TAVR, but do not designate a formal class recommendation.

While BAV can be utilized as a bridge to TAVR in patients who are at extreme risk, it has also been utilized as a selection strategy for TAVR and SAVR in patients with severe AS but with other potential causes of their symptoms such as severe lung disease. Temporary improvement in symptoms after BAV would support aortic stenosis as the cause, and replacement of the aortic valve would be warranted. And last, BAV has been used to temporize patients with acute

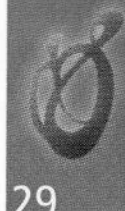

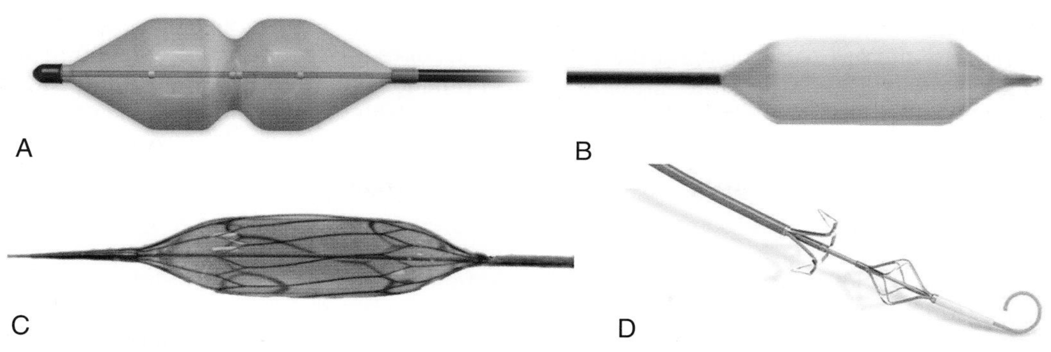

FIGURE 29-1 Next generation valvuloplasty devices. A, V8 Aortic Valvuloplasty Balloon Catheter (InterValve, Plymouth, Minn.). **B,** TRUE™ Dilatation Balloon Catheter (Bard, Burlingame, Calif.). (© 2015 C. R. Bard, Inc. Used with permission. Bard and TRUE are trademarks and/or registered trademarks of C. R. Bard, Inc.). **C,** Balloon aortic valvuloplasty (BAV) investigational device image courtesy of AngioScore, Inc. This product has not been registered or approved by the FDA or any other regulatory entity. **D,** Leaflex Catheter System (Pi-Cardia, Beit Oved, Israel).

hemodynamic failure while formulating a decision between SAVR, TAVR, and medical therapy.

Next Generation BAV Devices

With the advent of TAVR, there has been renewed interest in BAV. Several new devices have now been developed with the hope of improving both the safety and efficacy of BAV as a stand-alone procedure, as well as improving preparation (predilatation) for subsequent TAVR. Four such devices are the InterValve V8 (InterValve, Plymouth, Minnesota), Bard TRUE™ dilatation balloon catheter (Bard Medical, Burlingame, California), the CardioSculpt scoring balloon (AngioScore, Fremont, California), and the Pi-Cardia LeafLex system (Pi-Cardia, Beit Oved, Israel)[12] (**Figure 29-1**).

The InterValve V8 (**Figure 29-1A**) and Bard TRUE™ balloon (**Figure 29-1B**) are Food and Drug Administration (FDA) approved and available for use. Both of these devices attempt to address limitations of the current devices. The InterValve V8 has a dumbbell shape, which allows it to lock into the valve anatomy and limit balloon movement. The waist of the balloon is 5 to 7 mm less than the proximal and distal bulbous segments of the balloon, and this shape is maintained throughout inflation. The proximal bulb allows for hyperextension of the leaflets into the sinus to enhance valve opening, and the smaller waist reduces the risk of annular dissection. Furthermore, a rapid balloon inflation and deflation time minimizes ischemic time and hypotension. The balloon comes in 22-, 24-, 26-, and 28-mm sizes. Bard TRUE™ dilatation balloon catheter is made of Kevlar composite balloon material with a precisely reproduced size and shape. It has also been designed for fast inflation and deflation, rewrapping, and puncture resistance. The balloon comes in sizes 20, 22, 24, and 26 mm × 4.5 cm length.

The CardioSculpt BAV (**Figure 29-1C**) and the Pi-Cardia LeafLex system (**Figure 29-1D**) are two devices undergoing investigation. The CardioSculpt device is a scoring balloon, which consists of a balloon encased in a nitinol scoring element. In theory, it also allows for better seating and stability of the device. Also the balloon has rapid deflation times and excellent rewrap, reducing deflated device profile. The Pi-Cardia LeafLex system is not a balloon but a catheter that delivers mechanical shock waves to fracture calcium within the aortic valve. This allows for increased leaflet compliance with an increase in aortic valve area. Clinical results from both these devices may demonstrate their efficacy and potential role in patients.

TRANSCATHETER AORTIC VALVE REPLACEMENT (IMPLANTATION)—GENERAL CONCEPTS

Historical Perspectives and Unmet Clinical Need

During the past 50 years, the standard of care for symptomatic AS has been SAVR, which in most patients is associated with prolonged survival, improved symptoms, and few procedural complications. However, both the risks and the recovery after SAVR are less favorable in elderly AS patients, especially those with multiple co-morbidities, including prior cardiac surgery, chronic lung disease, peripheral vascular disease, prior stroke, renal failure, coronary artery disease, and frailty.[13] In addition, there are anatomic factors, such as porcelain aorta and chest wall deformities, that increase the risk of conventional SAVR. For these reasons, it is estimated that at least one-third of patients with symptomatic severe AS are either not candidates or are denied surgical therapy.[14] This has prompted investigation into alternative less invasive catheter-based approaches such as BAV and TAVR. From the mid-1980s to the mid-1990s, BAV was selectively used in high-risk AS patients, but as previously discussed, the recognition of procedural complications, prohibitive early restenosis, and lack of mortality benefit relegated the use of BAV to a small clinical niche: either palliative therapy or as a bridge to definitive valve replacement.[1,15]

The first catheter-based aortic valve replacement was performed in 1965 by Davies in a canine model for the temporary relief of aortic insufficiency.[16] Andersen performed the first contemporary transcatheter aortic valve replacement procedure using a stent-based porcine bioprosthesis in pigs in 1992.[17] The first implantation of a transcatheter valve in a human was performed by Bonhoeffer in 2000 involving the percutaneous replacement of a pulmonary valve in a right-ventricle to pulmonary-artery prosthetic conduit, using a bovine jugular valve to treat a 12-year-old boy with severe stenosis and regurgitation of the valved prosthesis.[18] Cribier's first-in-human landmark TAVR procedure in 2002 was undertaken as a last resort in a patient with cardiogenic shock, failed BAV, and multiple co-mordibities.[2] Since that time, TAVR has become the standard of care in patients who are "inoperable" and is an important alternative in patients who are high risk for surgery, with more than a dozen different device variations either commercially available or under active investigation.[19]

Clinical Indications

In the current ESC/EACTS and ACC/AHA guidelines for the management of valvular heart disease,[9,11] it is recommended that the following patients be considered for TAVR procedures: patients with severe, symptomatic, calcific stenosis of a trileaflet aortic valve who have aortic and vascular anatomy suitable for TAVR, an expected survival >12 months, and surgical risk assessment by a multidisciplinary heart team indicating the following:

1. A prohibitive surgical risk as defined by an estimated 50% or greater risk of mortality or irreversible morbidity at 30 days or other factors such as frailty, prior chest wall radiation therapy, porcelain aorta, severe hepatic or pulmonary disease
2. A high surgical risk with an expected 30-day mortality at least 15%, as an alternative to SAVR

All other indications for TAVR, including moderate surgical risk patients and bioprosthetic valve failure are currently under active investigation. It is notable that in the past several years with improved TAVR clinical outcomes and next generation TAVR systems, there has been a general downshifting of the risk strata, largely outside the United States, such that traditionally lower risk patients are being considered acceptable candidates for TAVR, especially in older patients (>80 years old), with one or two co-morbidities.

Heart Team Model and Risk Assessment

Given the complexity regarding the management of elderly patients with severe AS, a collaborative heart team model is essential for appropriate patient selection and subsequent care. This multidisciplinary team consists of experienced cardiac surgeons, interventional cardiologists, imaging specialists, heart failure specialists, cardiac anesthesiologists, intensivists, neurologists, geriatricians, nurses, and social workers. The coordinated approach of the heart team results in more comprehensive patient evaluations, facilitated gathering of essential data, improved communication with patients and families, superior decision making, and ultimately, better clinical outcomes. The importance of the heart team model is emphasized in both the European and the US TAVR guidelines.[9,11]

Several different surgical risk algorithms are utilized by heart teams for the selection of patients for TAVR. The two most common risk assessment tools are the Society of Thoracic Surgeons (STS) score and the logistic EuroSCORE.[20,21] The STS score is derived from outcomes data of 24 covariates in 67,292 patients undergoing isolated SAVR in the United States, while the logistic EuroSCORE is derived from 12 covariates from 14,799 patients undergoing all forms of cardiac surgery in Europe. While both have been shown to be accurate for estimating risk (i.e., 30-day surgical mortality) in low-risk patients with AS, their accuracy is far less precise in higher risk patients.[22,23] The two scores differ predominantly in the covariates utilized in the respective models and in the populations studied. It is generally acknowledged that the STS score is more accurate at estimating SAVR mortality in higher risk populations. There is reasonable consensus that an STS score ≥8 is deemed to be high risk for SAVR and that these patients should also be considered for TAVR. While both the STS and logistic EuroSCORE can aid in the selection of patients for TAVR, they serve as only one aspect of the selection process and should be utilized in the context of the entire clinical picture.

Several important concepts relevant to risk assessment for TAVR require further consideration. In the unique patient population currently screened for possible TAVR (elderly patients with co-morbidities or anatomic limitations), many risk factors are not represented in the standard risk scores, including frailty, dementia, hepatic disease, and anatomic factors (e.g., porcelain aorta or "hostile" chest). These ignored or under-represented co-morbidities must be considered by the heart team during risk assessment. At the extreme end of the risk spectrum are the so-called futile AS patients, wherein there is little hope of meaningful quality of life and/or limited life expectancy (e.g., untreatable malignancy or severe dementia), despite successful TAVR therapy. Although this may be a difficult societal conundrum, it is the responsibility of the heart team to thoughtfully identify these patients, such that TAVR may be sensitively withheld as a treatment option. Importantly, surgical risk is a continuum and the categorization of risk status into discrete groups is somewhat arbitrary and depends on definitions that are changing over time and may be different in the rarified confines of a clinical trial versus real-world community standards. Finally, since the predictors of early and late outcomes after TAVR are different compared with SAVR, specific risk assessment models for TAVR would be clinically useful and are being actively evaluated.

Anatomic Screening and Need for Multimodality Imaging

The information gathered during multimodality anatomic screening should be utilized to make an informed judgment on the candidacy of a patient for TAVR and in the overall management of patients with AS. The salient imaging data needed for comprehensive TAVR screening include (1) confirmation of the diagnosis of tri-leaflet, calcific, and severe valvular AS; (2) determination of left ventricular size and function; (3) coronary artery anatomy; (4) peripheral vasculature of sufficient size and suitability for catheter access and prosthesis delivery; and (5) geometry, measurement, and calcium patterns of the left ventricular outflow tract, proximal aorta, and the aortic annulus for appropriate device selection. Imaging for anatomic screening consists of a combination of echocardiography, angiography, and multi-slice computed tomography (MSCT).

Echocardiography is clearly the gold standard for assessing the etiology and severity of AS. Other important anatomic findings best determined by echocardiography are left ventricular mass, size, and function; right ventricular size and function; and other valvular lesions (especially mitral and tricuspid regurgitation). Usually, transthoracic echocardiography is sufficient, but in some patients with difficult imaging planes transesophageal echocardiography is preferred. Coronary angiography is crucial in every patient to determine the need for concomitant revascularization, given the frequent co-existence of coronary artery disease and AS. Peripheral angiography is also recommended to assess tortuosity, size, and calcification of the distal aorta, iliac, and femoral vessels. However, MSCT with contrast is the best imaging study to quantitatively measure the lumen dimensions of peripheral arteries and their suitability for a given TAVR system. MSCT is also the recommended imaging study to determine the optimal transcatheter valve size, which may differ depending on the specific transcatheter valve type. These three-dimensional (3D) reproducible measurements of the annulus region using validated algorithms

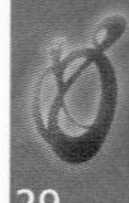

derived from high-quality contrast MSCT have become the global standard modality in selecting the correct valve size. Intraprocedural 3D echocardiography can also be used to confirm the annulus measurements and to assist in valve sizing. MSCT is also helpful in measuring the location and height of the coronary arteries; patterns of calcification in the aortic valve, aorta, and left ventricular outflow tract; and the shape, angulation, and size of the proximal aorta. Much of the success of TAVR and the recent improvements in clinical outcomes have been directly linked to meticulous preprocedural planning using the aforementioned multimodality imaging studies.

Procedural Considerations

TAVR is always performed in a sterile environment, either a catheterization laboratory or an operating room, with fluoroscopic and angiographic digital imaging capabilities. Most recently, there has been a growing interest in using a "hybrid" catheterization laboratory–operating room suite for TAVR. These hybrid procedure rooms combine the advantages of a high-resolution angiographic catheterization lab with the concomitant availability of a sterile environment for surgical management of complications and to facilitate nonpercutaneous alternative access routes.

The presence of cardiac anesthesiology to supervise sedation and analgesia control and to assist with hemodynamic monitoring and management has been an important requirement for TAVR to provide optimal care of these high-risk AS patients. There is growing controversy whether general anesthesia versus monitored anesthesia control (conscious sedation) is necessary or preferred in all or most patients during TAVR procedures. Similarly, the requirement of intraprocedural transesophageal echocardiography in every case has been highly debated. The more traditional approach incorporates general anesthesia with transesophageal echocardiography to help guide the procedure, including confirmation of valve sizing and positioning, assessment of paravalvular regurgitation, and rapid recognition of complications. Nevertheless, an increasing number of TAVR operators prefer a more "minimalist" approach, without general anesthesia and employing only transthoracic echocardiography, as needed. The reasons for this less invasive TAVR strategy are reduced resource consumption, fewer anesthesia-related complications, more rapid patient ambulation, and shorter durations of hospital stay. Thus far, experienced operators adopting this simplified approach have had equivalent procedural outcomes.[24] Perhaps a stratified patient-specific approach is most reasonable, wherein lower risk patients or those with anticipated intubation morbidities (e.g., severe chronic obstructive pulmonary disease [COPD]), can be triaged to the minimalist strategy and the higher risk patients can be managed using a more intense strategy with general anesthesia and transesophageal echocardiography guidance. As sheath sizes decrease and operator experience increases, likely the majority of TAVR worldwide will be performed in catheterization laboratories using conscious sedation.

BALLOON EXPANDABLE VALVES

Technology Overview and Early Access Approaches

All TAVR systems are composed of three integrated components: a support frame (usually metallic), a bioprosthetic tri-leaflet valve, and a delivery catheter. The support frame is crimped onto the delivery catheter immediately prior to valve implantation and is expanded by either retracting a sheath or inflating an underlying balloon. Balloon-expandable TAVR systems (Edwards Lifesciences, Irvine, California) were the earliest used in patients and have undergone several generations of evolution. However, many technology features have remained constant over time, including the tubular-slotted metallic frame geometry, pericardial bioprosthetic valve leaflets sewn to the frame, a fabric "skirt" covering the bottom of the frame, and out-of-body circumferential crimping of the valve and frame assembly onto the delivery catheter. The Cribier-Edwards valve became available in 2004 and was used in many of the early feasibility cases in Europe and the United States. This TAVR system had both 23- and 26-mm valve sizes and a stainless steel frame with an attached equine pericardial trileaflet valve that was directly crimped onto a commercial balloon valvuloplasty catheter. Cribier's first case and many of the earliest cases were performed using an antegrade transfemoral vein approach, wherein after right femoral vein access, a transseptal puncture provided entry to the left heart, followed by positioning a stiff guidewire across both the mitral and aortic valves. Navigating these first generation devices and large-sized catheters with roughened distal edges across the interatrial septum and the tortuous intracardiac anatomy was challenging. The initial antegrade transfemoral vein transseptal access procedures required very experienced operators with advanced skills and resulted in many intraprocedural complications.[25] Specifically, the generation of a large guidewire loop inside the left ventricle, which was required to avoid traction on the anterior mitral valve leaflet, was extremely difficult to maintain throughout the procedure and often resulted in severe mitral regurgitation with hemodynamic collapse.

Difficulties with the unpredictability of the antegrade transseptal approach resulted in modifications of both the access approach and the delivery catheter. A simpler and more familiar access site, typically used with BAV procedures, was the femoral artery with retrograde transaortic entry into the left ventricle. This can be accomplished with direct percutaneous access or through an open surgical exposure of the common femoral artery. Webb and colleagues reviewed their initial experience with the Cribier-Edwards valve via a retrograde transfemoral approach in a case series of 50 patients.[26] For this purpose, a steerable delivery catheter with a deflectable tip was also developed to safely advance the TAVR system within the vasculature and to better align the valve assembly with the central valve orifice. In 2007, the next generation Edwards-SAPIEN (Edwards Lifescience, Irvine, California) transcatheter valve was introduced (**Figure 29-2A**). The major differences included a change from equine to bovine pericardium valve leaflet material, which enabled surgical valve-like consistency in tissue processing (decalcification, thickness, flexibility, and tensile strength), as well as further improvements in the delivery catheter. The third generation SAPIEN XT valve (20-, 23-, 26-, and 29-mm sizes) began clinical evaluations in 2010 and represented a more radical design change of all system components, with a major goal to importantly reduce the overall profile (**Figure 29-2B**). The support frame had less metal and was changed from stainless steel to a thinner cobalt alloy, the valve geometry was modified to allow partial closing in the open position, and the delivery catheter was reduced in diameter by 33% for

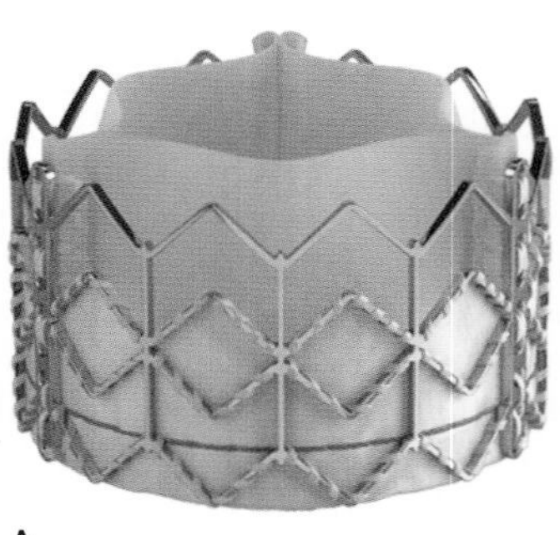
A

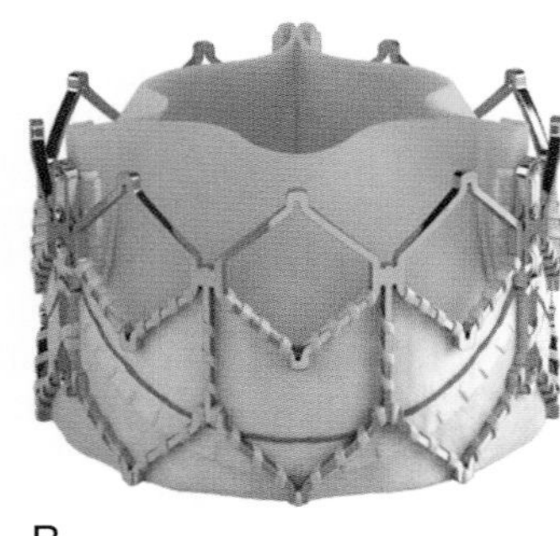
B

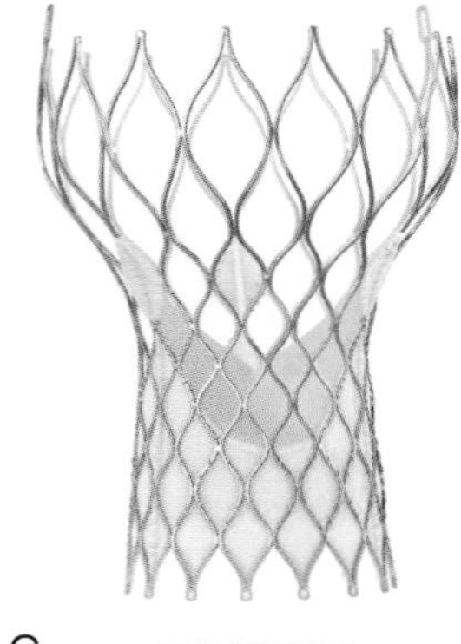
C

FIGURE 29-2 Current generation of transcatheter valves. A, Edwards SAPIEN Valve (Edwards Lifesciences, Irvine, Calif.). **B,** SAPIEN XT (Edwards Lifesciences, Irvine, Calif.). **C,** CoreValve (Medtronic, Minneapolis, Minn. Copyright 2015, Medtronic, Inc.).

all valve sizes, with improved transitions to facilitate advancement and crossing. The marked reduction in system profile was in part due to an endovascular docking maneuver, such that the valve was crimped onto the catheter shaft for arterial entry, and in the descending aorta, the balloon was pulled back underneath the valve for subsequent deployment. The SAPIEN XT is the current commercially available balloon expandable TAVR system in the United States.

Most recently, the fourth generation SAPIEN 3 device (**Figure 29-3A**) has completed enrollment in clinical trials in the United States (PARTNER II registry) and has received CE approval in Europe. The overall system profile has been further reduced, with most valve sizes introduced through a 14 Fr expandable sheath. The frame geometry has been modified with larger cells distally, and in addition to the internal skirt, an external skirt has been added to fill gaps and to prevent paravalvular regurgitation.

Procedural Details for Sapien or Sapien XT Implantation

The typical approach for balloon expandable valve implantation is via the transfemoral approach if arterial access permits. For the current generation Sapien XT, a 16 Fr, 18 Fr, or 20 Fr e-sheath is required for the 23-, 26-, and 29-mm valves, respectively. As noted earlier, procedures are typically performed in a hybrid OR under either general anesthesia or conscious sedation. In addition to fluoroscopy, echocardiography (transthoracic echocardiogram [TTE] or transesophageal echocardiogram [TEE]) should be available for procedural guidance and/or postdeployment assessment. A temporary pacemaker is required for the procedure and is placed at the beginning via the femoral or internal jugular vein. Aortography is performed to identify a coplanar view for valve deployment. It is essential that the nadirs of all three cusps be in the same plane to ensure proper deployment of the valve (Video 29-1). The view can be identified by the preoperative CT scan or though fluoroscopy and aortography.[27] Arterial access for the valve delivery sheath can be obtained either percutaneously or via a surgical cutdown; however, as sheath sizes continue to decrease, the majority of procedures will be done utilizing percutaneous access and closure with the "preclose" technique.[28] In the near future, there may be dedicated closure devices for large vessel access.

The remaining steps of the transfemoral retrograde TAVR procedure are as follows:

1. Placement of the valve delivery sheath after proper dilation of the artery.
2. Guidewire crossing of the stenosed native aortic valve and positioning of a tightly curved Amplatz extra-stiff guidewire in the left ventricular apex.
3. Although some operators are avoiding predilatation, valvuloplasty is usually performed with an under-sized balloon using transient rapid right ventricular pacing at heart rates of 180 beats to 200 beats per minute to minimize pulsatile transaortic flow.
4. Advancement of the steerable delivery catheter and crimped valve assembly through the vasculature to a coaxial position above the native valve.
5. Crossing the native valve, retraction of the sheath, and final positioning in a transvalvar location with approximately 60% to 70% of the prosthesis above the annulus confirmed using coplanar fluoroscopic views +/− transesophageal echo (prosthesis will shorten ~3 mm from the ventricular side during deployment) (Video 29-2).
6. Deployment of the bioprosthetic valve by slow balloon inflation during rapid right ventricular pacing to insure a stable platform (Video 29-3).
7. Assessment of paravalvular regurgitation (by hemodynamics, angiography, and echocardiography).
8. If significant paravalvular aortic regurgitation is present, postdilatation may be performed with addition of 1 to 2 cc of volume to the balloon delivery catheter (postdilatation should not be performed in scenarios where there is increased risk for annular or root injury such as aggressive valve oversizing [>20%] or severe left ventricular outflow tract [LVOT] calcification).
9. Removal of the catheters and suture-based closure of the percutaneous arteriotomy site or surgical repair of the access site.

Alternative Access Approaches

In patients with severe peripheral artery disease and/or marked vessel tortuosity, or concerning pathological anatomy of the ascending aorta, there was a pressing need for an alternative to retrograde transfemoral arterial access. The first important nontransfemoral access site for balloon expandable transcatheter valves was the antegrade transapical approach,[29] wherein the left ventricular apex was exposed via a small left anterolateral intercostal incision (fifth or sixth intercostal space) to expose the left ventricular apex. After purse string or mattress sutures are placed to secure the apex, direct needle puncture allows introduction of a hemostatic sheath into the left ventricle. The valve prosthesis is crimped in the antegrade direction onto the

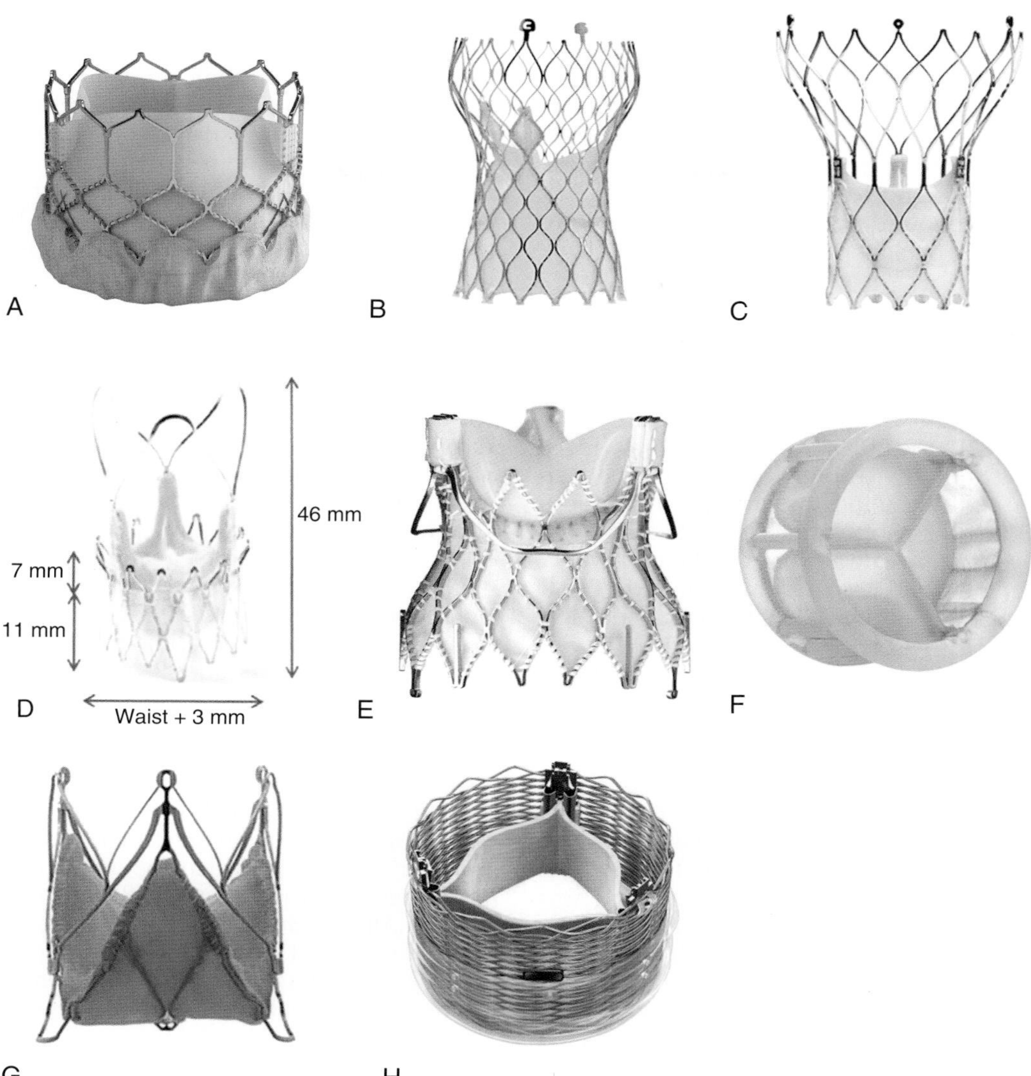

FIGURE 29-3 Next generation of transcatheter valves. A, Sapien 3 (Edwards Lifescience, Irvine, Calif.). **B,** CoreValve Evolut R (Medtronic Inc., Minneapolis, Minn. Copyright 2015, Medtronic, Inc.). **C,** Portico (St. Jude's Medical Inc., St. Paul, Minn.). **D,** Acurate (Symetis Inc., Ecublens, Switzerland); **E,** Engager (Medtronic Inc., Minneapolis, Minn. Copyright 2015, Medtronic, Inc.). **F,** Direct Flow (Direct Flow Medical, Inc., Santa Rosa, Calif.). **G,** JenaValve (JenaValve Inc., Munich, Germany). **H,** Lotus (Boston Scientific Inc., Natick, Mass.).

delivery catheter and is introduced through the sheath to an optimal transannular location, followed by deployment with balloon expansion during rapid right ventricular pacing. Bleeding from the apical entry site is always a concern, and careful surgical closure is required to avoid complications.

The transapical approach was often preferred by surgeon TAVR operators for the following reasons:

- More precise control of transcatheter valve positioning, due to the close proximity of the entry and deployment sites
- Less need for predilatation with valvuloplasty balloons, as the ventricular surfaces of the native aortic valve were less resistant to crossing
- Avoidance of "hostile" proximal ascending aorta pathology
- An early perception of reduced periprocedural strokes

Disadvantages associated with the transapical approach include the possibility of early and late access site bleeding from the left ventricular apex, hemodynamic instability due to placement of a large intraventricular sheath, especially in patients with small hypercontractile ventricles or severe left ventricular dysfunction, the requirement to use general anesthesia in all patients, and the sequelae of a left thoracotomy procedure resulting in increased patient pain and delayed recovery. With the reduced catheter profiles of modern TAVR systems, the need for alternative transapical access has significantly diminished.

In addition to transapical access, other interesting alternative access concepts have been developed for patients with unsuitable anatomy for the standard percutaneous transfemoral technique. For some TAVR systems, there is a preference for the subclavian/axillary artery approach, via surgical cutdown, with either direct access or use of a prosthetic graft to the artery. Recently, the direct aortic approach has become more popular, due to the familiarity with standard surgical procedures involving exposure of the ascending aorta and aortic root cannulation. The direct aortic approach requires an upper hemisternotomy or an upper right parasternal intercostal incision to expose a disease-free portion of the ascending aorta just below the origin of the innominate artery. This retrograde access site is used to insert a short sheath followed by the TAVR delivery system. Other less commonly used access alternatives include direct iliac and distal descending aorta exposure via a retroperitoneal incision for placement of an iliac conduit, direct exposure of a carotid artery, and transcaval access with placement of a sheath from the inferior vena cava to the abdominal aorta followed by closure of the aortotomy hole using implantable occluder devices.

Early Feasibility Trials

After the initial first-in-human experiences with TAVR, four different nonrandomized feasibility studies for balloon expandable Edwards transcatheter valves (Cribier-Edwards or Edwards SAPIEN) were conducted: REVIVE II, REVIVAL II, PARTNER EU, and TRAVERCE.[30-33] These feasibility registries demonstrated that TAVR could successfully be performed in a safe and efficacious manner in high-risk AS patients, and affirmed the short- to intermediate-term durability of the first generation Edwards transcatheter valves.

The earliest feasibility trial was the multicenter REVIVE II registry, which consisted of 106 patients in Canada and Europe who underwent retrograde transfemoral-TAVR with the Cribier-Edwards valve. The nearly concurrent US transfemoral REVIVAL II registry comprised another 55 similar high-risk patients. In a pooled analysis of the two trials,[34] TAVR was attempted in 161 patients with successful valve deployment in 142 (88.2%). Thirty-day major adverse events were 18.6%, with 18 (11.2%) deaths, 5 (3.1%) myocardial infarctions, and 7 (4.3%) cerebrovascular events. Adverse vascular events occurred in 15.5% of patients, and 4.9% needed permanent pacemakers. The 1-year survival was 73.8% and multivariate analysis demonstrated that prior coronary artery bypass surgery, baseline NYHA class, and procedural vascular complications were strong predictors of 1-year mortality. A subsequent transapical REVIVAL II feasibility study with the Edwards SAPIEN valve was initiated with 40 patients in the United States.[32] There was higher than anticipated valve migration or embolization (12.5%); mortality and strokes were 17.5% and 5.5% at 30 days and 36% and 9% at 6 months. This small early study demonstrated that while transapical TAVR was feasible, it was associated with significant morbidity and mortality, perhaps in part due to the increased co-morbidities in the patients ineligible for transfemoral vascular access.

The European-based PARTNER EU feasibility study with the Edwards SAPIEN valve included concurrent transapical and transfemoral patient cohorts.[31] This registry consisted of 130 patients, of whom 61 patients underwent transapical and 69 underwent transfemoral TAVR. Overall, successful valve deployment was 95.4% in the transapical patients and 96.4% in the transfemoral patients. In transapical patients, mortality was 18.8% at 1 month and 50.7% at 1 year, compared with 8.2% at 1 month and 21.3% at 1 year in the transfemoral patients. At 1 year, improvement in NYHA class was observed in 78.1% of surviving transapical patients and in 84.8% of transfemoral patients. In addition, quality of life, measured using the Kansas City Cardiomyopathy Questionnaire, improved in 73.9% in the transapical group and in 72.7% in the transfemoral group. No evidence of structural valve deterioration was observed during 1-year follow-up. The single arm TRAVERCE trial included 168 European patients who underwent transapical TAVR with either the Cribier-Edwards or the Edwards SAPIEN valve.[33] For the entire group, 95.8% had successful valve implantation; the remainder had valve migration, embolization, or severe valve regurgitation. Overall, mortality at 30 days, 6 months, and 1 year was 15%, 30%, and 37%, respectively. Other outcomes included conversion to conventional surgery in 5.4%, early stroke in 1.2%, and new permanent pacemakers in 6%. Again, there appeared to be higher early and late mortality associated with the transapical approach, but it was difficult to determine if differences in baseline patient characteristics (co-morbidities) or the transapical access route were responsible.

SOURCE and Other Registries

The SAPIEN Aortic Bioprosthesis European Outcome (SOURCE) registry was created to gather clinical outcome data on the Edwards SAPIEN 23- and 26-mm transcatheter valves, for both the transfemoral and transapical approaches, during the early phase of commercialization in Europe[35-38] (**Table 29-1**). At the time, it was the largest single registry of TAVR patients and it was meant to reflect a consecutive case "real-world" experience. The SOURCE registry included 2307 consecutive patients in 37 different centers from 14 different countries and was divided into two cohorts, based on the time of enrollment; cohort 1 were patients enrolled from November 2007 to January 2009, and cohort 2 were patients enrolled from February 2009 to December 2009. Due to the large size of the Edwards SAPIEN TAVR system (outer sheath diameters 8 to 9 mm), the majority of patients (62.7%) were treated using transapical access. The mean logistic EuroSCORE was 27.6% in the transapical group and 23.9% in the transfemoral group, indicating different risk profiles. The mean age of all patients was 81.6 years and 57.8% were women. All data were site reported, there were no core laboratories or formal event adjudication committees, and currently, 2-year follow-up results have been reported.

The 30-day, 1-year, and 2-year all-cause mortality for transapical patients was 11%, 26%, and 34.5%, respectively, and for the transfemoral patients it was 7.6%, 19.9%, and 26.9%, respectively. Most of the late deaths were from noncardiac causes, as the 2-year cardiac mortality was only 12.8% after transapical TAVR and 9.6% after transfemoral TAVR. Increased major bleeding was more frequent in transapical patients (3.9% vs. 2.3%), whereas greater vascular access-related complications were observed in the transfemoral patients (major—11.3% vs. 2.0%; minor—10.4% vs. 1.0%). At 2 years, the rates of all strokes were 5.9% in the transapical group and 5.8% in the transfemoral group, and new pacemakers were needed in 8.7% of transapical and 9.3% of transfemoral patients. Additionally, 1.9% of transapical patients needed a re-intervention of the bioprosthetic valve, compared with 0.5% of transfemoral patients. At 2 years, there was a sustained, similar symptom improvement (reduction in NYHA class in survivors) for both access approaches.

The Multicenter Canadian Study is another real-world registry that sought to capture the early experiences with balloon expandable valves in the Canadian population.[39] The study included 339 patients judged to be nonoperable or at very high surgical risk who underwent either transfemoral or transapical TAVR from January 2005 to June 2009 in six Canadian centers with the Cribier-Edwards, Edwards SAPIEN, or the SAPIEN XT balloon expandable valve. The average age was 81 years, mean Society of Thoracic Surgeons (STS) score was 9.8%, and there was a nearly equal distribution of transapical and transfemoral cases (52% vs.

TABLE 29-1 Major TAVR Registries for Patients with Severe Symptomatic Aortic Stenosis

REGISTRY	VALVE(S) USED	PATIENT* POPULATION	AVERAGE† RISK SCORE	ACCESS	MAJOR ENDPOINTS
SOURCE (Cohort 1 and 2)	ESV 100%	N = 2307 Age 81.6 Females 57.8%	EuroSCORE 26.0%	TF: 60.2% TA: 39.8%	**30 days:** All-cause mortality 9.6% Stroke 4.7% Major vascular complication 5% Major bleeding 3.6% New PPM 7% **1 year:** TF: All-cause mortality 7.5% Stroke 2.9% New PPM 6.7% TA: All-cause mortality 10.9% Stroke 2.5% New PPM 7.1%
Canadian Multicenter	ESV/SXT 100%	N = 339 Age 81 Females 55.2%	STS 9.8%	TF: 48.6% TA: 51.4%	**30 days:** Procedural success rate 93.3% All-cause mortality 10.4% (TF 9.5%, TA 11.3%) Stroke 0.6% (TF 0.6%, TA 0.6%) Major vascular complication 13% (TF 13%, TA 13%) New PPM 4.9% (TF 3.6%, TA 6.2%) **1 year:** TF: All-cause mortality 25%, TA: All-cause mortality 22% **2 year:** TF: All-cause mortality 35%, TA: All-cause mortality 36%
SOURCE XT	SXT 100%	N = 2688 Age 81.7 Females 57.3%	EuroSCORE 20.5%	TF: 62.7% TA: 33.3% TAo: 3.7% TSc: 0.3%	**30 days**: All-cause mortality 6.3% Stroke 2.2% Major vascular complication 14.5% Major bleeding 8% New PPM 9.5% **1 year:** All-cause mortality 19.5% Stroke 6.3% All rehospitalizations 29.4% Moderate or severe PVR 6.2%
PREVAIL (TA and TF)	SXT 100%	TA: N = 212 Age 81.2 Females 29.2%	TA: EuroSCORE 24.1	TF: 60% TA: 40%	**TA 30 days:** All-cause mortality 7.5% Stroke 1.5% Major vascular complications 0.9% New PPM 12% **TA 1 year:** All-cause mortality 17% Stroke 3.1% New PPM 13.1%
		TF: N = 141 Age 83.7 Females 67.4%	TF: EuroSCORE 22.4		**TF 30 days:** All-cause mortality 8.5% Stroke 4.4% Major vascular complication 11.4% New PPM 8.7% **TF 1 year:** All-cause mortality 17% Stroke 6.8% New PPM 13.5%
Piazza et al.	MCV 100%	N = 646 Age 81 Females 54%	EuroSCORE 23%	TF: 100%	**30 day:** Procedural success 97% All-cause mortality 8% Composite of death, stroke, or MI 9.3%

Continued

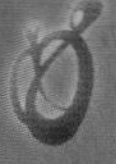

TABLE 29-1 Major TAVR Registries for Patients with Severe Symptomatic Aortic Stenosis—cont'd

REGISTRY	VALVE(S) USED	PATIENT* POPULATION	AVERAGE† RISK SCORE	ACCESS	MAJOR ENDPOINTS
Italian Registry	MCV 100%	N = 659 Age 81 Females 55.8%	EuroSCORE 23%	TF: 90% TSc: 10%	**30 days:** All-cause mortality 5.4% **1 year:** Composite of death, major stroke, MI, and life-threatening bleeding 30.4% All-cause mortality 23.6% **2 year:** Composite of death, major stroke, MI, and life-threatening bleeding 36.5% All-cause mortality 30.3% **3 year:** Composite of death, major stroke, MI, and life-threatening bleeding 40.3% All-cause mortality 34.8%
Australia/NZ Registry	MCV 100%	N = 441 Age 83.9 Females 44.9%	EuroSCORE 17.3%	TF: 88.9% Other: 11.1%	**1 year:** MACCE 22.1% All-cause mortality 12% Stroke 5.8% **2 year:** MACCE 32.9% All-cause mortality 22.1% Stroke 8.2%
ADVANCE	MCV 100%	N = 1015 Age 81.1 Females 50.5%	EuroSCORE 19.4%	N/A	**30 day:** MACCE 8% All-cause mortality 4.5% Stroke 3.0% **1 year:** MACCE 21.2% All-cause mortality 17.9% Stroke 4.5%
UK TAVI	ESV 48%, MCV 42%	N = 870 Age 81.9 Females 47.6%	EuroSCORE 19%	TF: 69% Other: 31%	**30 days**: Procedural success 97% MACCE 10.3% All-cause mortality 7.1% Stroke 4.1% Major vascular complication 6.3% New PPM 16% Moderate/Severe AR 14% **1 year:** All-cause mortality 21% **2 year:** All-cause mortality 26% **Comparison of TF vs. other access:** TF had lower mortality and surgical conversion, but more AR and vascular complications **ESV vs. MCV:** ESV had less AR, need for second valve, and PPM, but greater surgical conversion
FRANCE 2	ESV 67%, MCV 33%	N = 3195 Age 82.7 Females 49%	EuroSCORE 22%	TA: 18% Non-TA: 82%	**30 days:** Procedural success 96.9% All-cause mortality 9.7% **1 year:** All-cause mortality 24% Stroke 4.1% Incidence of all PVR 64.5%

TABLE 29-1 Major TAVR Registries for Patients with Severe Symptomatic Aortic Stenosis—cont'd

REGISTRY	VALVE(S) USED	PATIENT* POPULATION	AVERAGE† RISK SCORE	ACCESS	MAJOR ENDPOINTS
GARY	ESV 53%, MCV 42%, Other 5%	N = 3875 Age 82 Females 56%	EuroSCORE 25%	TA: 30%	**TA 30 days:** All-cause mortality 9.0% **TA 1 year:** All-cause mortality 28.0% Stroke 3.6% New PPM 14.1%
				Non-TA: 70%	**Non-TA 30 days:** All-cause mortality 5.6% **Non-TA 1 year:** All-cause mortality 20.7% Stroke 4.8% New PPM 26.2%
PRAGMATIC	ESV 43%, MCV 57%	N = 793 Age 82 Females 47.2%	EuroSCORE 21%	TF: 100%	**MCV vs. ESV at 30 days:** Procedural success 94% vs. 96% All-cause mortality 7.5% vs. 5.0% Major stroke 3.5% vs. 1.5% Major vascular complication 9.1% vs. 15% Life-threatening bleed 12% vs. 14% PPM 23% vs. 5.9% **MCV vs. ESV at 1 year:** All-cause mortality 17% vs. 14%

AR, Aortic regurgitation; *ESV,* Edwards SAPIEN valve; *MCV,* Medtronic CoreValve; *MI,* myocardial infarction; *PPM,* permanent pacemaker; *PVR,* paravalvular regurgitation; *STS,* Society of Thoracic Surgeons; *SXT,* SAPIEN XT; *TA,* transapical, *TAo;* transaortic; *TAVR,* transcatheter aortic valve replacement; *TF,* transfemoral; *TSc,* transsubclavian.
*For patient population, the age listed is the approximate average age of the population studied in any particular trial.
†For European trials, the logistic EuroSCORE is given, whereas for North American trials, the STS score is given.

48%). Long-term outcomes including nearly 4 years of systematic follow-up results have been published.[40]

The procedural success was 93.3%, 30-day all-cause mortality was 10.4% (transfemoral—9.5%, transapical—11.3%), and 30-day strokes were 2.3% (transfemoral—3%, transapical—1.7%). Patients with either porcelain aorta (18%) or frailty (25%) exhibited 30-day outcomes similar to the rest of the study population, and porcelain aorta patients tended to have a better survival at 1 year. At a mean follow-up of 42 months, 55.5% of patients had died, and the causes of late death were noncardiac in 59.2%, cardiac in 23.0%, and unknown in 17.8%. Predictors of late mortality were chronic obstructive pulmonary disease, chronic kidney disease, chronic atrial fibrillation, and frailty. A mild nonclinically significant decrease in valve area was seen at 2-year follow-up, but no further reduction in valve area was observed during the later follow-up evaluations (mean 3.5 years). No late changes in paravalvular regurgitation and no cases of structural valve failure were observed during the extended follow-up period.

The lower profile SAPIEN XT TAVR system was studied in three registries—PREVAIL TA, PREVAIL TF, and SOURCE XT.[41-45] The PREVAIL TA registry included 212 patients undergoing TAVR via transapical access and the PREVAIL TF registry included 141 patients with transfemoral access. All-cause mortality was 7.5% and 17% at 30 days and 1 year in the transapical cohort and 8.5% and 17% at 30 days and 1 year in the transfemoral cohort. Other outcomes including stroke, myocardial infarction (MI), and acute kidney injury were also similar between the two approaches, although major vascular complications were higher in the transfemoral patients.

The SOURCE XT registry enrolled 2688 patients in 93 centers from 17 European countries between July 2010 and October 2011.[42,45] Vascular access in the trial was not limited to transfemoral and transapical, but also included a small number of direct aortic access cases (3.7%). Unlike the original SOURCE registry, SOURCE XT included standardized valve academic research consortium (VARC) endpoint definitions, core laboratories, and an independent clinical events committee.[46] Compared with SOURCE, patients in the SOURCE XT registry had a lower logistic EuroSCORE (overall, 20.4%), a significant minority (28%) did not have general anesthesia during the procedure, and due to the smaller delivery systems, patients were more likely to be treated using the transfemoral access route (62.7%).

All-cause mortality was lower in SOURCE XT than in the previous SOURCE registries: 6.3% at 30 days and 19.5% at 1 year (cardiac mortality 10.8% at 1 year). Importantly, vascular complications were no longer associated with increased mortality, due to improved management strategies and fewer major events. Periprocedural (within 48 hours) and 1-month strokes were 2.2% and 6.3% and the need for periprocedural pacemakers was 5.7%. The frequency of moderate or severe paravalvular regurgitation was only 5.5% at 1 month and 6.2% at 1 year. There was dramatic symptom improvement in survivors at 1 year and all-cause mortality at 1 year was better in women ($p = 0.008$) and in patients with a lower logistic EuroSCORE (<15% vs. ≥15%; $p = 0.003$). The 1-year mortality was almost double in the transapical versus the transfemoral patients (27.2% vs. 15.0%) and multivariate analysis clearly indicated that transapical access was a strong predictor of 1-year mortality (hazard ratio [HR] 1.64; 95% confidence interval [CI], 1.28, 2.09; $p < 0.0001$).

The PARTNER Trial

The Placement of Aortic Transcatheter Valves (PARTNER) trial is the seminal trial that demonstrated the safety and efficacy of TAVR for high-risk and inoperable AS patients and set the benchmark for all subsequent TAVR device approval trials[47-53] (**Figure 29-4A**) (**Table 29-2**). PARTNER

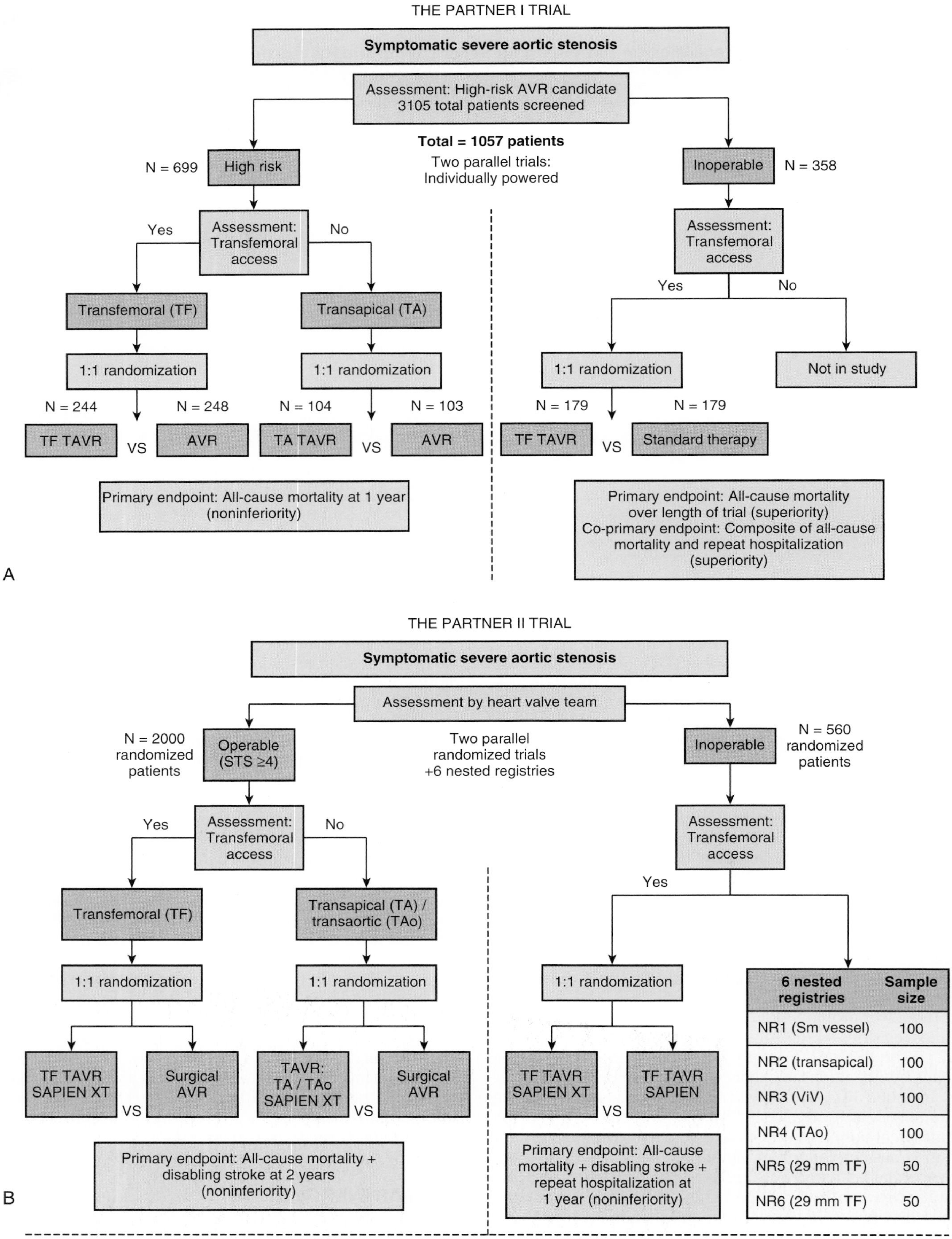

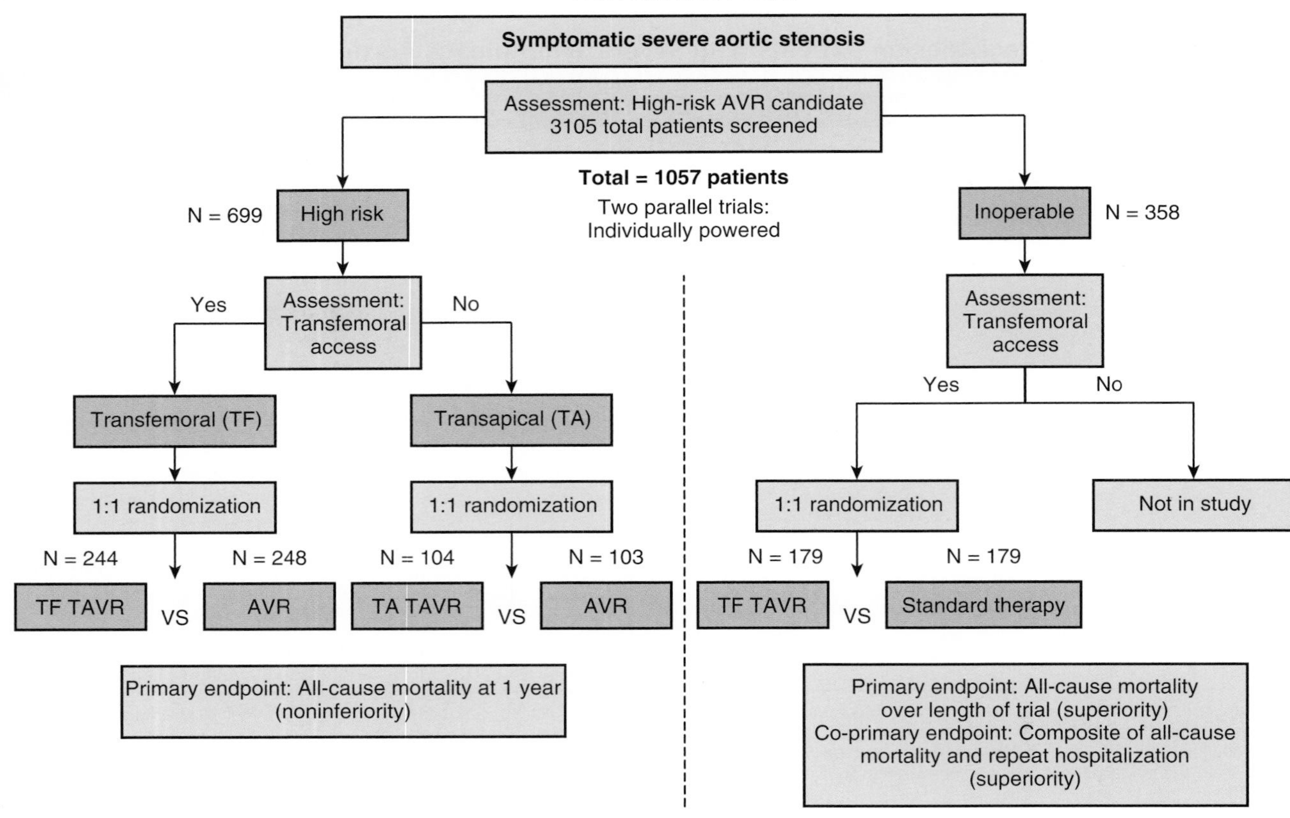

THE PARTNER I TRIAL
Symptomatic severe aortic stenosis
Assessment: High-risk AVR candidate
3105 total patients screened
Total = 1057 patients
Two parallel trials:
Individually powered
N = 699
High risk
Inoperable
N = 358
Yes
Assessment:
Transfemoral
access
No
Transfemoral (TF)
Transapical (TA)
1:1 randomization
1:1 randomization
N = 244
N = 248
N = 104
N = 103
TF TAVR
VS
AVR
TA TAVR
VS
AVR
Primary endpoint: All-cause mortality at 1 year
(noninferiority)
A
Assessment:
Transfemoral
access
Yes
No
1:1 randomization
Not in study
N = 179
N = 179
TF TAVR
VS
Standard therapy
Primary endpoint: All-cause mortality
over length of trial (superiority)
Co-primary endpoint: Composite of all-cause
mortality and repeat hospitalization
(superiority)
THE PARTNER II TRIAL
Symptomatic severe aortic stenosis
Assessment by heart valve team
N = 2000
randomized
patients
Operable
(STS ≥4)
Two parallel
randomized trials
+6 nested registries
Inoperable
N = 560
randomized
patients
Yes
Assessment:
Transfemoral
access
No
Transfemoral (TF)
Transapical (TA) /
transaortic (TAo)
1:1 randomization
1:1 randomization
TF TAVR
SAPIEN XT
VS
Surgical
AVR
TAVR:
TA / TAo
SAPIEN XT
VS
Surgical
AVR
Primary endpoint: All-cause mortality +
disabling stroke at 2 years
(noninferiority)
B
Assessment:
Transfemoral
access
Yes
1:1 randomization
TF TAVR
SAPIEN XT
VS
TF TAVR
SAPIEN
Primary endpoint: All-cause
mortality + disabling stroke +
repeat hospitalization at
1 year (noninferiority)
6 nested registries
Sample size
NR1 (Sm vessel) 100
NR2 (transapical) 100
NR3 (ViV) 100
NR4 (TAo) 100
NR5 (29 mm TF) 50
NR6 (29 mm TF) 50

FIGURE 29-4 Study designs for randomized controlled TAVR trials. *AVR,* Aortic valve replacement; *NR,* nested registry; *PARTNER,* Placement of Aortic Transcatheter Valves trial; *STS,* Society of Thoracic Surgery risk score; *SURTAVI,* surgical replacement and transcatheter aortic valve implantation; *TA,* transapical; *TAo,* transaortic; *TAVI,* transfemoral aortic valve replacement; *TF,* transfemoral; *ViV,* valve-in-valve. **A,** The trial design of the PARTNER trial is shown with cohort A (high surgical risk) on the left and cohort B (inoperable) on the right. **B,** The trial design of the PARTNER II trial is shown with cohort A (intermediate surgical risk) on the left and cohort B (inoperable) on the right, as well as the six nested registries.

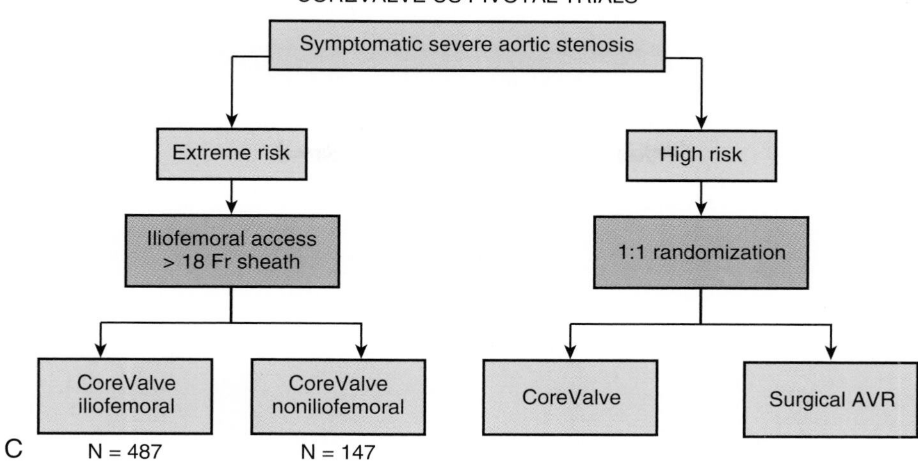

FIGURE 29-4, cont'd **C,** The trial design of the CoreValve US Pivotal Trial is shown with the "extreme-risk" group on the left and "high-risk" group on the right.

TABLE 29-2 TAVR Randomized Controlled Trials for Patients with Severe Symptomatic Aortic Stenosis

TRIAL	PRIMARY VALVE STUDIED	TREATMENT ARMS	POPULATION STUDIED	MAJOR STUDY RESULTS
PARTNER 1A 1-Year Outcomes	Edwards SAPIEN balloon-expandable valve	TAVR vs. SAVR	High-risk surgical candidates (STS ≥ 10%) N = 699	**30 day:** All-cause mortality 3.4% vs. 6.5% (p = 0.07) Stroke 4.6% vs. 2.4% (p = 0.12) Major vascular complications 11% vs. 3.2% (p < 0.001) Major bleeding 9.3% vs. 19.5% (p < 0.001) Atrial fibrillation 8.6% vs. 16% (p = 0.006) **1 year**: All-cause mortality 23% vs. 26.8% (p = NS) Stroke 6.0% vs. 3.2% (p < 0.08)
PARTNER 1A 2-Year Outcomes	Edwards SAPIEN balloon-expandable valve	TAVR vs. SAVR	High-risk surgical candidates (STS ≥ 10%) N = 699	All-cause mortality 33.9% vs. 35% (p = NS) Stroke 7.7% vs. 4.9% (p = NS)
PARTNER 1A 3-Year Outcomes	Edwards SAPIEN balloon-expandable valve	TAVR vs. SAVR	High-risk surgical candidates (STS ≥ 10%) N = 699	All-cause mortality 44.2% vs. 44.8% (p = NS) Stroke 8.2% vs. 9.3% (p = NS)
PARTNER 1B 1-Year Outcomes	Edwards SAPIEN balloon-expandable valve	TAVR vs. standard therapy	Inoperable patients N = 358	**30 day:** All-cause mortality 5.0% vs. 2.9% (p = NS) Stroke 5.0% vs. 1.1% (p = 0.06) Vascular complications 16% vs. 1.1% (p < 0.001) **1 year:** All-cause mortality 31% vs. 51% (p < 0.001) Death or hospitalization 43% vs. 72% (p < 0.001) NYHA ≥ III 25% vs. 58% (p < 0.001)
PARTNER 1B 2-Year Outcomes	Edwards SAPIEN balloon-expandable valve	TAVR vs. standard therapy	Inoperable patients N = 358	All-cause mortality 43% vs. 68% (p < 0.001) Cardiac mortality 31% vs. 62% (p < 0.001) Stroke 13.8% vs. 5.5% (p = 0.01) Rehospitalization 35% vs. 73% (p < 0.001)
PARTNER 1B 3-Year Outcomes	Edwards SAPIEN balloon-expandable valve	TAVR vs. Standard therapy	Inoperable patients N = 358	All-cause mortality 80.9% vs. 54.1% (p < 0.001) Cardiac mortality 74.5% vs. 41.4% (p < 0.001) Rehospitalization 75.5% vs. 42.3% (p < 0.001)
PARTNER 2A	Edwards SAPIEN XT balloon-expandable valve	TAVR vs. SAVR	Intermediate-risk surgical candidates (STS ≥ 4%) N = 2000	Enrollment completed; currently in the follow-up period

Continued

TABLE 29-2 **TAVR Randomized Controlled Trials for Patients with Severe Symptomatic Aortic Stenosis—cont'd**

TRIAL	PRIMARY VALVE STUDIED	TREATMENT ARMS	POPULATION STUDIED	MAJOR STUDY RESULTS
PARTNER 2B	Edwards SAPIEN XT balloon-expandable valve	TAVR with SAPIEN XT vs. SAPIEN	Inoperable patients N = 358	**30 day:** All-cause mortality, disabling stroke, or rehospitalization 17% vs. 15.3% (p = NS) Major vascular events 9.6% vs. 15.5% (p = 0.04) Procedural: Less anesthesia time, aborted procedures, multiple valve implants, and need for hemodynamic support with SAPIEN XT **1 year:** All-cause mortality, disabling stroke, or rehospitalization 33.9% vs. 34.7% (p = NS) All-cause mortality 22.5% vs. 23.7% (p = NS) Disabling stroke 4.5% vs. 4.6% (p = NS) Rehospitalization 19% vs. 17.4% (p = NS)
CoreValve Pivotal Trial Extreme Risk	Medtronic self-expanding CoreValve	Iliofemoral TAVR with CoreValve (Standard therapy comparison arm removed after results of PARTNER 1B)	Inoperable patients N = 471	**30 day:** All-cause mortality or major stroke 9.3% All-cause mortality 7.9% Major stroke 2.4% Moderate to severe PVR 11.5% NPP 22.2% **1 year:** All-cause mortality or major stroke 25.5% All-cause mortality 24.0% Major stroke 4.1% Moderate to severe PVR 4.1% (no severe PVR) NPP 27.1%
CoreValve Pivotal Trial High Risk	Medtronic self-expanding CoreValve	SAVR vs. TAVR	High-risk surgical candidates (STS ≥ 10%) N = 699	**30 day:** All-cause mortality 4.5% vs. 3.3% (p = NS) MACCE 10.4% vs. 7.7% (p = NS) Major stroke 3.1% vs. 3.9% (p = NS) **1 year:** All-cause mortality 19.1% vs. 14.2% (p = NS) MACCE 27.3% vs. 20.4% (p = 0.03) Major stroke 7.0% vs. 5.8% (p = NS)
SURTAVI	Medtronic self-expanding CoreValve	SAVR vs. TAVR	Intermediate-risk surgical candidates (STS ≥ 4% ≤ 10%) N = 2000	Completing enrollment and entering follow-up period
CHOICE	Edward SAPIEN XT/ Medtronic self-expanding CoreValve	Balloon-expandable valves vs. self-expanding valves	High-risk surgical candidates (STS ≥ 10%) N = 241	**Procedural:** All-cause mortality 0% vs. 0% (p = NS) Implant ≥2 valves 0.8% vs. 5.8% (p = 0.03) Device success 95.8% vs. 77.5% (p < 0.001) **30 day:** All-cause mortality 4.1% vs. 5.1% (p = NS) Combined safety endpoint 18.2% vs. 23.1% (p = NS) Stroke 5.8% vs. 2.6% (p = NS) NPP 17.3% vs. 37.6% (p = 0.001)

NYHA, New York Heart Association; *PVR,* paravalvular regurgitation; *SAVR,* surgical aortic valve replacement; *STS,* Society of Thoracic Surgeons risk score; *TAVR,* transcatheter aortic valve replacement.

was the first multi-center, randomized controlled trial of TAVR compared with accepted standard therapies in carefully defined patient populations. The results of this trial ultimately led to the approval of the Edwards SAPIEN valve by the U.S. Food and Drug Administration (FDA) and has informed the worldwide cardiology community of the benefits and concerns of TAVR as an important new therapy for patients with AS.

During the course of PARTNER development and enrollment, it became clear that more robust standardized clinical trial processes were necessary to assess study outcomes in patients with AS. The Valve Academic Research Consortium (VARC) was convened in 2009, including representatives from surgical and cardiology societies in Europe and the United States, prominent Academic Research Organizations, the FDA, and several expert consultants.[46,54] Standardized endpoint definitions for all important clinical outcomes were carefully developed and published in the first consensus document in 2011. Thereafter, upon testing these definitions in clinical trial settings, several additions and revisions were published as the VARC-2 consensus document in 2012. This dynamic process of creating optimal and standardized endpoint definitions has strengthened the TAVR evidence-based medicine effort and VARC definitions were immediately incorporated into the PARTNER trials.

The purpose of the PARTNER trial was to study the Edwards-SAPIEN TAVR system in discrete high-surgical-risk patients using rigorous clinical trial methodologies (randomization vs. control therapies, core laboratories, adjudicated and carefully defined clinical events, etc.). PARTNER began enrollment in 2007 and included 1057 patients (of 3105 screened patients) with severe AS (defined as an aortic valve area <0.8 cm^2 or aortic valve area index <0.5 cm^2/m^2, and a mean aortic valve gradient >40 mm Hg, or a peak aortic jet velocity >4.0 m/sec), and cardiac symptoms (NYHA Class II or greater) in two parallel randomized trials in whom conventional SAVR was associated with high or prohibitive risk. Patients were divided into two cohorts[47,48]:

- **Cohort A:** those who were not considered to be suitable candidates for surgery because they had co-existing conditions that would be associated with a predicted probability of 50% or more of either death by 30 days after surgery or a serious irreversible condition.
- **Cohort B:** those who were considered to be candidates for surgery despite being at high surgical risk, defined by an STS risk score of 10% or higher or the presence of co-existing conditions that would be associated with a predicted risk of death by 30 days after surgery of 15% or higher.

In the inoperable cohort, 358 patients were randomly assigned (1:1) to either transfemoral TAVR or to standard therapy (medical therapy with or without adjunctive BAV). In the high-risk cohort, 699 patients were randomly assigned (1:1) to either transfemoral TAVR or SAVR (244 vs. 248 patients) or, if the peripheral vascular anatomy was not suitable to accommodate the large sheaths, transapical TAVR or SAVR (104 vs. 103 patients). The primary endpoint for both cohorts was all-cause mortality, with cohort B powered for superiority versus standard therapy over the course of the trial and cohort A powered for noninferiority versus SAVR at 1 year. In both studies, the follow-up was at least 1 year in all patients before assessing the primary endpoint results and other outcomes. Thus far, findings from PARTNER have been presented with 5-year follow-up for the inoperable cohort[53] and with 3-year follow-up for the high-risk cohort.[52]

Patients in the inoperable cohort averaged 83 years old, more than half were female, mean STS score was 11.7%, multiple co-morbidities were prevalent (including frailty and COPD), >90% had NYHA functional Class III or Class IV symptoms, and ~80% received BAV (at least once) in the standard therapy arm. The primary endpoint analysis at 1 year indicated a reduction in all-cause mortality from 50.8% with standard therapy to 30.7% after transfemoral TAVR ($p < 0.0001$; **Figure 29-5A**); the number needed to treat was only 5 patients.[47] This dramatic reduction in mortality was sustained over time with landmark analyses indicating incremental TAVR mortality benefits up to 3 years (**Figure 29-5B**).[49,51,53] Importantly, in standard therapy patients who did not receive crossover to TAVR (allowed after 1 year) or out-of-protocol valve replacement, there was only one survivor at 5 years, which recapitulates the dire prognosis of "untreated" severe AS. Improved mortality after TAVR was demonstrated in all age groups, although limited in patients with the highest baseline STS scores (>15%).[53] Other benefits associated with TAVR therapy in these inoperable patients included significant reductions in rehospitalizations and improved cardiac symptoms with significant quality-of-life enhancement.[47,49,51,53,55] Notable complications associated with TAVR therapy were:

- Major vascular complications and bleeding associated with the large delivery catheters
- Increased strokes (6.7% vs. 1.7%)
- Paravalvular regurgitation

After the index hospitalization, there was no continuous hazard of increased strokes in the TAVR subgroup.[51,53] Echocardiography core laboratory analyses showed after TAVR an improvement in left ventricular function, regression of left ventricular hypertrophy, a sustained increase in aortic valve areas with a decrease in transvalvular gradients, and no worsening of paravalvular aortic regurgitation. There were no signs of structural valve deterioration during the current 5 years of follow-up.

PARTNER patients in the high-risk cohort were also elderly (mean age: 84 years), the majority were male (57%), the mean STS score was 11.7%, and >90% had NYHA functional Class III or Class IV symptoms. There was a slight mortality benefit at 30 days with TAVR compared with SAVR (intention-to-treat analysis: 3.4% vs. 6.5%, $p = 0.07$), but the primary 1-year mortality endpoint was similar in both groups (24.2% with TAVR vs. 26.8% with SAVR, $p = 0.44$) and the noninferiority criteria were fulfilled (**Figure 29-5C, D**).[48] As demonstrated in previous studies, the mortality outcomes at 30 days and 1 year were better in patients receiving transfemoral versus transapical TAVR. Thus far, follow-up to 3 years has indicated continued similar mortality in the TAVR and SAVR cohorts.[52] Although strokes at 30 days and 1 year were more frequent with TAVR (30 days: 4.6% vs. 2.4%, $p = 0.12$; 1 year: 6.0% vs. 3.2%, $p = 0.08$), strokes at 3 years were similar for both therapies (TAVR 8.2% vs. SAVR 9.3%, $P_{log\ rank} = 0.76$). Other differences between TAVR and SAVR included increased vascular complications and paravalvular regurgitation with TAVR and increased bleeding events and new-onset atrial fibrillation with SAVR. The need for new permanent pacemakers at 1 month was similar with both therapies (TAVR 6.4%, SAVR 5.0%, $p = 0.44$). Transfemoral TAVR was also associated with reduced intensive care unit and hospital length of stay and earlier symptom benefit (by 30 days), although overall symptom improvement from baseline was equivalent and impressive, with both therapies at 6 months and 1 year.[56] A cost-effectiveness analysis at 1 year indicated that transfemoral TAVR was cost-effective (reduced costs and improved quality adjusted life years) compared with SAVR in the PARTNER randomized high-risk cohort.[56] Echocardiography assessment of valve hemodynamics (gradients and areas) after valve replacement was similar for TAVR and SAVR, but there was significantly greater paravalvular regurgitation in TAVR patients. During follow-up, even mild paravalvular regurgitation after TAVR was associated with a significant increase in late mortality.[50] However, there were no signs of structural valve deterioration at 3 years after either TAVR or SAVR, and the magnitude of paravalvular regurgitation was unchanged after TAVR during follow-up.[52]

Several already published sub-studies from the PARTNER trial are noteworthy. The high frequency of major vascular complications (~15%) in elderly patients (especially women) with frequent peripheral vascular disease and their association with mortality has been highlighted[57] and has stimulated efforts to reduce TAVR system profiles and develop more effective femoral access site closure techniques. Similarly, the importance of bleeding events (early and late), seen more commonly with SAVR than TAVR, was previously under-appreciated, and has been shown to have a significant impact on mortality.[58] A study of gender in PARTNER (high-risk cohort) demonstrated that women

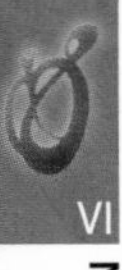

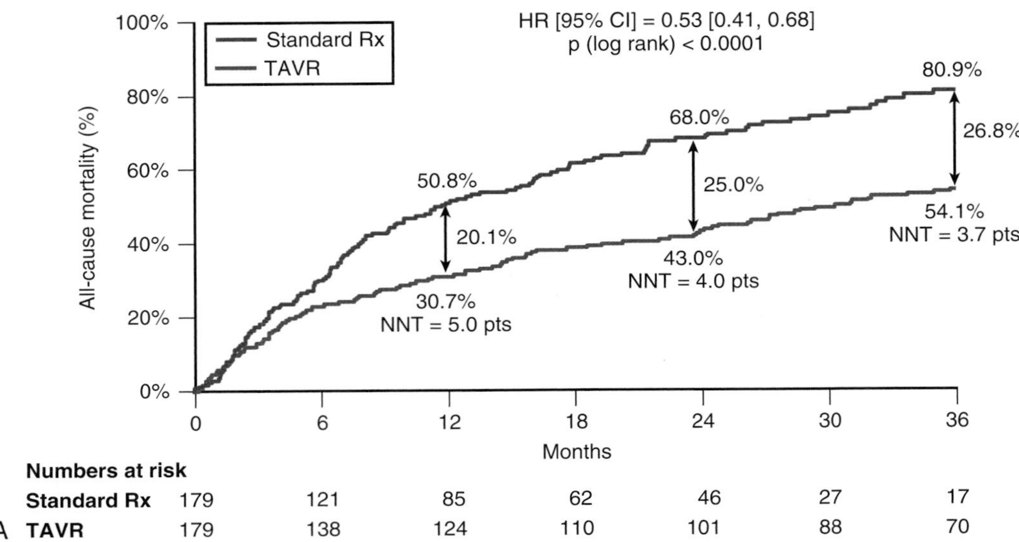

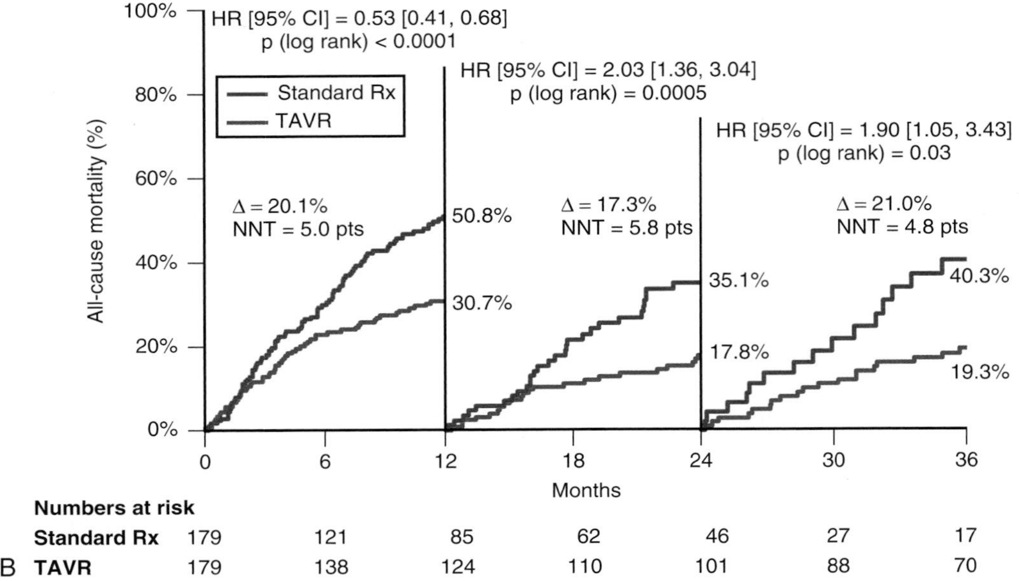

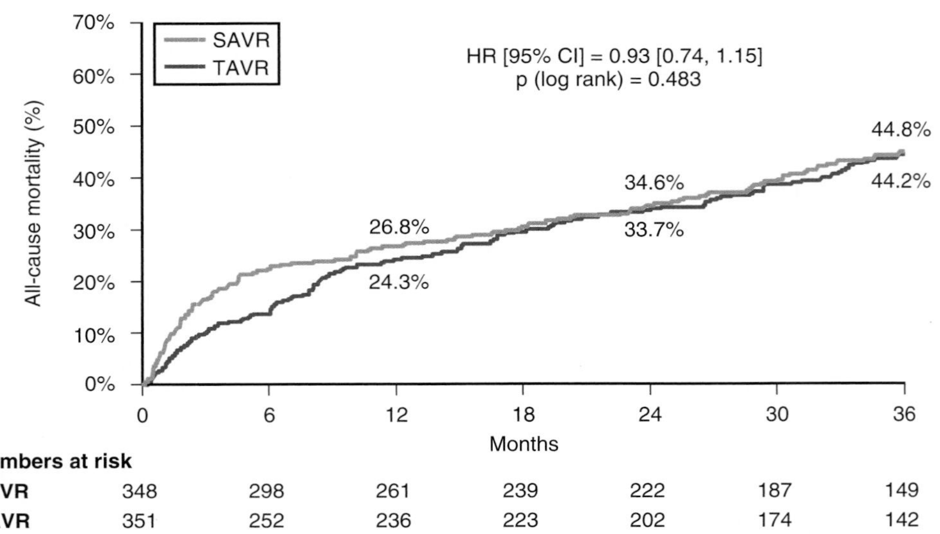

FIGURE 29-5 The 3-year outcomes of the PARTNER trial. A, Cumulative hazard curves of all-cause mortality between patients randomized to TAVR or standard therapy (cohort B). **B,** Landmark analysis for all-cause mortality for cohort B. The left side of the panel demonstrates cumulative mortality in the two groups in the first year of follow-up. The middle portion of the panel shows mortality in the second year of follow-up, conditional upon survival up to 1 year. The right side of the panel shows mortality in the third year of follow-up, conditional upon survival up to 2 years. **C,** Cumulative hazard curves of all-cause mortality between patients randomized to TAVR and surgical AVR (cohort A).

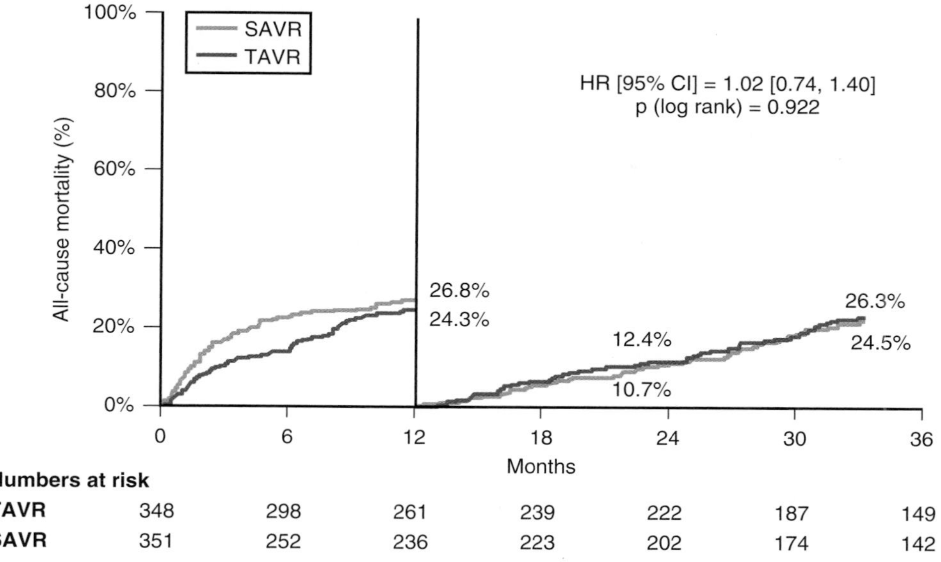

FIGURE 29-5, cont'd **D,** Landmark analysis for all-cause mortality for cohort A. The left side of the panel demonstrates cumulative mortality in the two groups in the first year of follow-up. The right side of the panel shows mortality in the second and third years of follow-up, conditional upon survival up to 1 year.

undergoing TAVR had lower 1-year and 2-year mortality compared with SAVR ($p = 0.05$), which was amplified in the transfemoral patients ($p = 0.02$), whereas there were no mortality differences in men.[59] There also was a significant treatment interaction in diabetic patients in PARTNER; all-cause mortality at 1 year was lower in diabetics after TAVR compared with SAVR (18.0% vs. 27.4%, $P_{log\ rank} = 0.04$), which was consistent among transfemoral and transapical subgroups.[60] Finally, in those patients with preoperative moderate or severe mitral regurgitation, significant improvement in mitral regurgitation severity was shown at 30 days in the majority of patients after either treatment (69.4% after SAVR and 57.6% after TAVR),[61] but preoperative mitral regurgitation was a predictor of late mortality in only the SAVR cohort.

The PARTNER II trial is a multi-component study designed to evaluate the safety and efficacy of the lower profile SAPIEN XT TAVR system under a variety of conditions. The first phase (PARTNER IIB, **Figure 29-4B**) began enrollment in 2010 and was a prospective, multicenter trial in severe AS patients, in the inoperable risk category, from 28 US participating centers. A total of 560 patients and were randomly assigned (1:1) to transfemoral TAVR using either the original Edwards-SAPIEN or the newer SAPIEN XT TAVR systems. The primary endpoint was a nonhierarchical composite of all-cause mortality, disabling stroke, and repeat hospitalization at 1 year, using a noninferiority study methodology. The primary endpoint results have already been presented[62]; 30-day mortality was low in both groups (Edwards SAPIEN 5.1% and SAPIEN XT 3.5%), and the composite outcomes were similar for both treatment cohorts at 1 year (Edwards SAPIEN 34.7% and SAPIEN XT 33.9%). The main advantage of the SAPIEN XT system was the lower profile, which resulted in reduced (compared with Edwards SAPIEN) major vascular complications (from 15.5% to 9.6%, $p = 0.04$), disabling bleeding events (from 12.6% to 7.8%, $p = 0.06$), vascular perforations, and severe dissections.

The second phase of PARTNER II was a large multicenter randomized trial in moderate-risk AS patients, who were defined by an STS score ≥4% (or ≥3% with documented co-morbidities by the heart team) (PARTNER IIA, **Figure 29-4B**). More than 2000 moderate-risk AS patients from more than 50 participating US centers were randomly assigned (1:1) to either transfemoral SAPIEN XT TAVR versus SAVR, or if the peripheral vascular anatomy was not suitable to accommodate the catheters, either transapical or direct aortic SAPIEN XT TAVR versus SAVR. The primary endpoint was a composite of all-cause mortality and disabling stroke at 2 years, using a noninferiority study methodology. In addition, there were a series of nested registries in PARTNER IIB for the purpose of gathering data on various study topics, including the larger 29-mm valve size, the direct aortic access approach, and an aortic valve-in-valve registry for patients with surgical bioprosthesis failure. Most recently (starting in 2013), the PARTNER II trial was expanded to include the newest SAPIEN 3 TAVR system in two large registries: 550 patients who are either high-risk for surgery or are inoperable and 1080 patients who are at moderate risk for SAVR.

SELF-EXPANDING VALVES

Technology Overview

Self-expanding transcatheter valves offer an alternative to the balloon expandable technology described above. The first of these is the CoreValve ReValving system (Medtronic, Inc., Minneapolis, Minnesota), which was acquired by Medtronic in 2009. This design consists of a self-expanding nitinol frame that extends from the LVOT to the aortic root (see **Figure 29-2C**). The frame has three distinct zones:

1. An inflow portion with high radial forces to exclude the native valve and seal the annulus
2. A constrained portion designed to avoid the coronaries
3. An outflow portion that has low radial force to help orient the valve in the aorta

Within the constrained portion of the frame is a sewn porcine pericardial tissue valve, which is designed to be supra-annular. This design allows the valve to remain circular at the coaptation point of the leaflets even in noncircular annular geometries, which in theory, leads to optimized hemodynamics.

The first generation device utilized bovine pericardial tissue and was delivered through a 24 Fr delivery system. The first human CoreValve implant was performed in July 2004 by Jean-Claude Laborde in India on a 62-year-old male with critical AS and multiple co-morbidities.[63] Although the implant was successful, the patient died 4 days later due to multi-organ failure. The second generation device utilized porcine pericardial tissue, thereby reducing the crimped profile and allowing delivery through a 21 Fr sheath. A first-in-human trial with the first and second generation systems demonstrated acute device success of 88% but with an in-hospital mortality rate of 20%.[64] These initial procedures were performed with extracorporeal bypass for support and surgical cutdown for vascular access (common iliac, femoral, or subclavian). The third generation of the device reduced the profile further to 18 Fr, allowing for fully percutaneous delivery without hemodynamic support. Also the frame design was modified to have a broader upper segment, allowing for improved fixation in the ascending aorta. A multicenter study utilizing both the second and third generation devices demonstrated acute device success of 88% with a procedural mortality of 6%.[65] In six patients, valve malpositioning led to urgent conversion to surgical valve replacement. Thirty-day mortality was 12% with a combined MAACE (mortality and major adverse cardiac events) including death, stroke, and MI of 22%. Valve hemodynamics were excellent with significant reduction in mean gradients. Mean aortic regurgitation as assessed by the site based on echo and aortography was unchanged from baseline. No patients had moderate to severe (3+) or severe (4+) aortic regurgitation.

Based on these initial data, the Medtronic CoreValve received CE mark approval in 2007. In 2010, an updated delivery system incorporating the AccuTrak Stability Layer to minimize movement during deployment received CE mark. In January 2014, the device received FDA approval for inoperable patients, which was extended to include high-risk patients in June 2014. The CoreValve ReValving system is currently available in four different sizes: 23, 26, 29, and 31 mm.

The next generation of CoreValve is the Evolut R with EnVeo R delivery system, which received CE mark approval in September 2014[66] (**Figure 29-3B**). The valve promises to have several refinements from the original CoreValve to improve anatomical fit, annular sealing, and durability. The nitinol frame has been designed to confirm better to the annulus across different size ranges, which may reduce the stress on the conduction system and thereby reduce the frequency of permanent pacemakers. The height of the Evolut R frame has also been reduced so that it is approximately 10% shorter than the prior CoreValve. Plus, the pericardial skirt has been extended on the inflow side to improve annular seal and potentially reduce paravalvular regurgitation. Finally, the delivery system has been modified significantly. The valve is recapturable and repositionable until final release. Moreover, the sheath has been integrated into the delivery catheter so that the outer diameter of the entire system is 18 Fr, which is equivalent to a 14 Fr sheath. The valve is currently available in 23-, 26-, and 29-mm sizes but a 31-mm valve will soon be available. Ongoing studies will demonstrate whether these design modifications will improve clinical outcomes following TAVR with the Medtronic CoreValve system.

Procedural Details for CoreValve Implantation

The standard delivery route for CoreValve implantation is via the transfemoral approach, which requires two operators and in general the approach is similar across sites. Although general anesthesia is not required for the procedure (and TAVR is increasingly being done without it), the use of TEE facilitates the assessment and management of paravalvular regurgitation.[67] All patients have a temporary transvenous pacemaker placed at the beginning of the procedure, which is usually left in place for 24 to 48 hours. Typically, it is inserted via the right internal jugular vein to facilitate patient mobilization. The vast majority of procedures are performed percutaneously utilizing the "preclose" technique for vascular closure, but surgical cutdown is utilized in some cases.[28] The fluoroscopic view for valve deployment is identified by performing an aortogram with the pigtail catheter at the base of the noncoronary cusp (Video 29-4). The preoperative computed tomography (CT) scan can be used to identify this view in advance.

The remainder of the procedure consists of the following steps:

1. An 18 Fr delivery sheath is placed from the femoral approach.
2. The aortic valve is crossed and through a pigtail catheter a stiff wire with a preshaped curve is placed in the LV apex.
3. Balloon aortic valvuloplasty with an undersized balloon can be performed at this point but is not necessary.[68]
4. The CoreValve device is advanced across the aortic valve and the fluoroscopic view is adjusted based on the distal marker of the sheath to ensure coaxial deployment of the valve.
5. The valve is positioned so that the first "node" is at the annulus and the valve is slowly unsheathed by rotating the wheel on the delivery catheter.
6. Aortograms are performed as the valve flairs to ensure that device is landing ~4 mm below the annulus (Video 29-5).
7. Ventricular pacing at a rate of 100 bpm to 120 bpm can be performed at this point to stabilize the valve.
8. Once the valve has made annular contact (one third deployed), the valve can be unsheathed to the two-thirds position rapidly (blood pressure can drop at this point due to the prosthesis obstructing outflow).
9. The valve is then released by completely unsheathing the prosthesis (Video 29-6).
10. Assessment of aortic regurgitation is performed by multiple modalities (hemodynamic assessment, aortogram, echocardiogram).[69,70]
11. If significant paravalvular regurgitation is present, post-dilatation can be performed with an appropriately sized balloon, which is typically the minimum diameter of the annulus as measured on 3D reconstructions. However, in the absence of high-risk features for annular rupture, such as severe LVOT calcification, a balloon sized to the mean diameter can be used.

Alternative Access Approaches

For patients without iliofemoral access, the CoreValve prosthesis can be placed via a subclavian or direct aortic approach.[71,72] Currently, no transapical delivery system exists for the CoreValve system. The procedure for implantation via the subclavian artery first requires exposure of the artery in the deltopectoral groove of the anterior chest wall. After placement of purse string sutures, a 6 Fr sheath is introduced into the vessel using a modified Seldinger technique. Next using an exchange catheter, a stiff wire is advanced into the ascending aorta. After successive dilatation of the artery, the 18 Fr delivery system sheath is advanced through the subclavian artery and into the ascending aorta. Insertion of the prosthesis then proceeds in standard fashion. The sheath is withdrawn at the end of the procedure and the purse string suture is tied. Utilization of the subclavian approach requires careful preoperative screening to ensure that the vessel size is adequate (minimal size, 6 mm) and that there is minimal tortuosity and calcification. In cases where there is a patent left internal mammary artery supplying coronary flow, extreme caution should be used, and the minimal vessel size at that level needs to be large enough to allow flow to the mammary even with the sheath in place.

When iliofemoral or subclavian access is not possible for CoreValve insertion, a direct aortic approach can be carried out via a small right anterior thoracotomy or a small right upper "J" hemisternotomy. After gaining exposure to the ascending aorta, pledgeted purse string sutures are placed. Operators must be careful to ensure that there is adequate distance (~7 cm) between the intended puncture site and the aortic valve. A 6 Fr sheath is then inserted within the purse string sutures using a modified Seldinger technique. The aortic valve is then crossed in the standard fashion and a pigtail catheter is advanced into the LV. A stiff wire with a preshaped curve is positioned in the LV apex, and the 6 Fr sheath is exchanged for the 18 Fr delivery sheath. Valve deployment then proceeds in the standard fashion without predilatation of the valve. After deployment of the prosthesis, the purse string sutures are tied under direct vision, and the chest wall is closed is in regular surgical fashion.

Overview of Registry Data and ADVANCE

Several different registries have reported short, intermediate, and long-term outcomes with the third generation CoreValve prosthesis. Piazza et al. first published a multicenter European registry of 646 patients to evaluate performance and outcomes after CE mark approval. Procedural success in this early experience was 97% with a 30-day all-cause mortality of 8%.[73] A subsequent dedicated Italian registry, containing 663 patients from 14 different centers, demonstrated a mortality rate of 5.4% at 30 days, 12.2% at 6 months, and 15.0% at 1 year.[74] Although procedural complications were strongly associated with early mortality at 30 days, co-morbidities and postprocedural paravalvular aortic regurgitation ≥2+ were noted to mainly impact late outcomes between 30 days and 1 year. Recently, outcomes out to 3 years in 181 patients in the Italian registry demonstrate an all-cause mortality rate at 1 year, 2 years, and 3 years of 23.6%, 30.3%, and 34.8%, respectively.[75] Cardiovascular death at 1, 2, and 3 years was 11.2%, 12.1%, and 13.5%, respectively, indicating that the majority of deaths were noncardiac in origin. The actuarial survival free from a composite of death, major stroke, myocardial infarction, and life-threatening bleeding was 69.6% at 1 year, 63.5% at 2 years, and 59.7% at 3 years. While varying degrees of paravalvular leak were observed in a majority of patients, no cases of structural valve deterioration were seen.

A New Zealand and Australia CoreValve-only registry of 441 patients from 10 different centers reported 2-year outcomes.[76] At 1 year and 2 years, the all-cause mortality rates were 12% and 22.1% and the stroke rates were 5.8% and 8.2%, respectively. Permanent pacemaker implantation was required in 28.6% of patients in this registry. These early registries demonstrated that implantation of a CoreValve prosthesis was feasible with high procedural success, and survival was reasonable with appropriate patient selection. In addition, although not adjudicated, these early studies identified important procedural complications.

The largest CoreValve registry to date is the ADVANCE study, which enrolled 1015 patients at 44 centers in 12 countries.[77] There were several unique aspects of this registry. First, all sites were experienced and had performed at least 40 procedures prior to participating. Second, all patients were monitored and the primary endpoints were adjudicated by a clinical events committee. Finally, there was core laboratory assessment of echocardiograms and angiograms. Procedural success in this study was 97.5% but 40 patients (4%) required two valves, primarily due to malposition of the first valve. Thirty-day MAACE, based on Valve Academic Research Consortium (VARC) criteria, was 8.0% with all-cause mortality of 4.5%. The primary endpoint of 1-year MAACE (all-cause mortality, MI, emergent surgery or percutaneous re-intervention, or stroke) was 21.2%. The 1-year all-cause mortality was 17.9% and stroke rate was 4.5%. Survival varied considerably according to baseline EuroSCORE, with lower 1-year survival in patients with a score >20 (76.4%) compared with those with a score <10 (88.9%). Moderate or severe paravalvular regurgitation was seen in 17.9% of patients and its presence was independently associated with higher 1-year mortality [HR 1.63]. Requirements for new permanent pacemaker placement was 26.3% at 30 days and 29.2% at 1 year.

Conduction abnormalities are frequently noted after CoreValve implantation. The frequency of new LBBB has ranged from 35% to 57% in several studies with CoreValve,[78-80] which is significantly higher than the rate seen following Edwards Sapien implantation.[80-82] However, the impact of LBBB on clinical outcomes remains controversial. Although one study did demonstrate increased mortality at 1 year in patients with a new left bundle branch block (LBBB),[81] subsequent studies have failed to corroborate this finding.[79,82,83] Regardless, several reports have shown that patients with new LBBB show lack of improvement in LV function.[82] Requirement for permanent pacemaker implantation in these early registries was significantly higher with CoreValve than with the Sapien transcatheter valves.[84] However, the presence of a new pacemaker does not appear to impact late mortality.[85,86]

CoreValve US Pivotal Trial

The CoreValve US Pivotal Study was designed to compare transcatheter aortic valve replacement (AVR) to standard therapies in patients with severe AS at either high or extreme risk for surgical AVR (**Figure 29-4C**). Initially the study was designed as two separate randomized controlled trials for both "high-risk" and "extreme-risk" groups.[87,88] However, after presentation of the PARTNER cohort B data showing survival benefit with TAVR over medical therapy, it was deemed unethical to randomize patients to medical therapy. Therefore, the study design was changed to a registry of ~500 extreme-risk patients undergoing iliofemoral TAVR with CoreValve compared with an objective performance goal (OPG) derived from seven contemporary BAV studies as well as the medical arm of PARTNER cohort B. In addition,

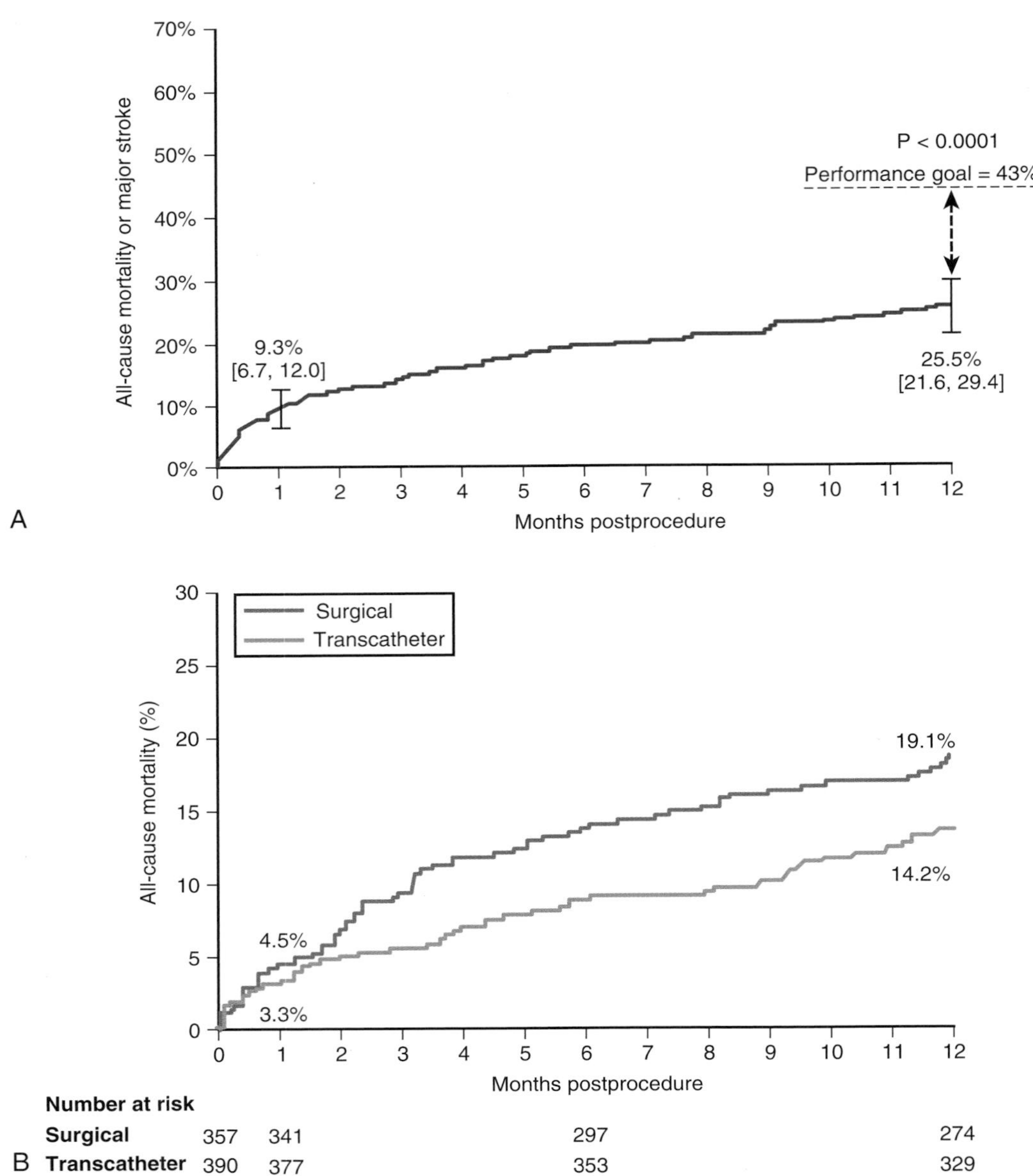

FIGURE 29-6 The 1-year CoreValve US Pivotal Trial. A, Cumulative hazard curve of all-cause mortality or major stroke in extreme-risk patients undergoing TAVR compared with a prespecified objective performance goal. **B,** Cumulative hazard curves of all-cause mortality between high-risk patients randomized to TAVR and surgical AVR.

there was a simultaneous registry of 150 patients who underwent noniliofemoral TAVR. Extreme risk was defined as patients with a >50% chance of mortality or irreversible morbidity with SAVR. Risk assessment was performed by the local heart team and adjudicated on a conference call with members of the trial screening committee. The "high-risk" group was defined by an operative mortality of ≥15%, and the patients in that group were randomized to SAVR or CoreValve TAVR. The primary endpoint for the "extreme-risk" group was all-cause mortality and major stroke at 12 months, while for the "high-risk" group it was all-cause mortality at 12 months.

The Extreme Risk Study enrolled patients at 41 centers in the United States between February 2011 and August 2012.[88] The as-treated population consisted of 489 patients where iliofemoral TAVR was attempted. The patient population was similar to the PARTNER trial: elderly (mean age 83.2), female (52.1%), and high surgical risk (mean STS 10.3%). There was a high frequency of important co-morbidities such as severe lung disease (29.9%), peripheral vascular disease (35.2%), coronary artery disease (81.8%), diabetes mellitus (41.5%), and atrial fibrillation (46.8%). Also for the first time, detailed frailty metrics were collected revealing a much debilitated population. The valve was successfully implanted in 486 patients. The trial met its primary endpoint of all-cause mortality and major stroke at 1 year with a rate of 26.0%, which was significantly lower than the OPG of 43% (**Figure 29-6A**). At 1 month, the rate of stroke was 4.0%, and it remained low over time with a 1-year rate of 7.0%. Other important complications included major vascular (8.2%) and major or life-threatening bleeding (36.7%). Conduction abnormalities were frequent, and new permanent pacemakers were required in 21.6% of patients at 30 days. Valve hemodynamics were excellent with reduction of mean gradient to 8.9 mm Hg with an effective orifice area of 1.9 cm^2 at 12 months. Moderate or severe aortic regurgitation was present in 13.8% of patients at discharge. Only severe aortic regurgitation was associated with increased 1- year mortality. Interestingly, paravalvular regurgitation appeared to decrease over time with 82.8% of patients with moderate paravalvular regurgitation at discharge showing an improvement at 1 year. There was significant improvement in functional status with NYHA class improving by an average in 1.6 ± 0.9 in the treatment population. Based on the safety and efficacy results of this trial, the CoreValve received FDA approval for use for inoperable AS patients in January 2014.

In the CoreValve High-Risk Study, 795 patients were randomized between February 2011 and September 2012 at 45 centers in the United States to receive either TAVR or SAVR.[87] In the surgical arm, 41 patients (10.2%) withdrew after randomization, leaving a total as-treated population of 747 patients (390 TAVR, 357 SAVR). Although the treatment population was elderly (mean age 83.2), STS-PROM was lower than that seen in the PARTNER high-risk cohort (7.4% vs. 11.7%). As noted earlier, risk assessment was performed by the heart team and incorporated the STS-PROM risk score as well as incremental risk factors not accounted for in the risk calculator. In the prespecified as-treated primary analysis, the rate of death from any cause was significantly lower with TAVR than SAVR group (14.2% vs. 19.1%, $p < 0.001$ for noninferiority, one sided $p = 0.04$ for superiority) (**Figure 29-6B**). This was the first trial to demonstrate the superiority of TAVR versus SAVR in high-risk patients. Hierarchical testing of secondary endpoints showed that echocardiographic indices of valve function, quality of life and functional status, were noninferior with TAVR. Unlike in the PARTNER trial, analyses did not show any increased risk of stroke with TAVR, as compared with surgery. Major vascular complications and permanent pacemaker complications were more frequent in the TAVR group while bleeding complications, acute kidney injury, and atrial fibrillation were more common in the surgical group. Based on the strength of the data from the high-risk cohort, the Medtronic CoreValve was approved for use in high-risk patients in June 2014.

"REAL-WORLD" REGISTRIES AND OTHER STUDIES (CHOICE AND TVT REGISTRY)

Several large real-world registries, often serving as national postapproval studies for specific European countries, have studied both balloon expandable and self-expanding TAVR systems. These include the UK-TAVI, FRANCE-2, GARY, PRAGMATIC, and TVT.[89-93] The UK-TAVI Registry prospectively followed 1620 patients undergoing transfemoral or transapical TAVR with the Edwards SAPIEN valve, or transfemoral, or subclavian TAVR with the CoreValve.[89] Mortality in patients undergoing the SAPIEN transapical TAVR approach was higher than with transfemoral at 30 days (11.2% vs. 4.4%, $p < 0.01$), 1 year (28.7% vs. 18.1%), and 2 years (56.0% vs. 43.5%). No mortality differences were found between transfemoral and subclavian TAVR with CoreValve. There were also significant differences in mortality at any time-point between patients treated with SAPIEN (n = 812) and CoreValve (n = 808) prostheses. However, CoreValve-treated patients had a significantly higher rate of new permanent pacemaker implantation (23.1% vs. 7.2%), and grade ≥2 aortic regurgitation assessed by postprocedure echocardiography (13.0% vs. 7.3%).

In the FRANCE-2 registry, 3195 high-risk AS patients (mean age 82 years, logistic EuroSCORE 21.8%) were enrolled at 33 French centers, implanting either SAPIEN (66.9%) or CoreValve (33.1%) TAVR systems (transfemoral 75%, transapical 18%, and subclavian 6%).[90] Overall, the mortality at 30 days and 1 year was 9.7% and 24.0%, respectively. There were no differences among SAPIEN versus CoreValve-treated patients in mortality at any time point or strokes (overall incidence 4.1% at 1 year), but there were more frequent new pacemakers implanted after CoreValve (24.0% vs. 11.8%). In a multivariate model, a higher logistic EuroSCORE, NYHA functional Class III or Class IV symptoms, the use of transapical TAVI, and a greater amount of paravalvular regurgitation were significantly associated with reduced survival.

The German Aortic Valve Registry (GARY) is a comprehensive analysis of consecutive patients with AS treated by either SAVR or TAVR from 78 centers (out of 96 in Germany), initially included 13,860 patients enrolled during 2011.[91] At present, data from in-hospital outcomes[94] and 1-year outcomes[95] have been summarized for 6523 conventional SAVR patients, 3464 patients with SAVR and concomitant coronary artery bypass graft surgery (CABG), 2695 patients with transvascular TAVI, and 1181 patients with transapical TAVI. The in-hospital mortality was 2.1% (SAVR alone) and 4.5% (SAVR + CABG) for patients undergoing conventional surgery, and 5.1% (transvascular TAVI) and 7.7% (transapical TAVI) for patients treated using the newer transcatheter modalities. The stroke frequency was low in all groups: 1.3% SAVR, 1.9% SAVR + CABG, 1.7% transvascular TAVI, and 2.3% transapical TAVI. Patients undergoing catheter-based techniques were significantly older and had higher risk profiles. Using a newly developed German-AV risk score[96] to categorize patients, the outcomes in the highest risk categories were similar for SAVR and transvascular TAVI. The 1-year results from GARY (vital status known in >98% of patients) indicated lower overall mortality after SAVR (6.7% alone and 11.0% + CABG) compared with TAVI (20.7% transvascular and 28.0% transapical), but after stratification into four risk categories, mortality was similar with SAVR and transvascular TAVI in the highest risk patients.

The Pooled-Rotterdam-Milano-Toulouse In Collaboration (PRAGMATIC) registry included 793 patients from four experienced European centers with the explicit purpose of comparing outcomes after transfemoral TAVI with the self-expanding CoreValve (n = 453) versus the balloon expandable SAPIEN and SAPIEN XT (n = 340) transcatheter heart valves.[92] To account for differences in baseline clinical characteristics, propensity score matching was performed and 240 matched patients were identified in each treatment group. At 30 days there were no differences between the two devices in all-cause and cardiovascular mortality, strokes, device success, major vascular complications, or life-threatening bleeding, except for a greater need for permanent pacemakers with the CoreValve than SAPIEN or SAPIEN XT (22.5% vs. 5.9%, $p < 0.001$). At 1 year, there were also no differences in all-cause and cardiovascular mortality.

The Comparison of Balloon-Expandable versus Self-Expandable Valves in Patients Undergoing Transcatheter Valve Replacement (CHOICE) trial is the only randomized control study comparing balloon expandable with self-expanding TAVR systems.[97] CHOICE was an investigator-initiated trial randomizing 241 patients to receive either SAPIEN XT (121 patients) or CoreValve (120 patients) bioprostheses at five different centers in Germany. The study was powered to determine differences in "device success," which was defined by VARC as the composite of successful delivery and deployment in the proper location of a single valve with the "intended" performance (expected effective orifice area and without moderate or severe aortic regurgitation). Although these were described as high-risk AS patients, the mean STS score was only 5.6% in the balloon expandable group and 6.2% in the self-expanding group. There were no differences between the different valve types in mortality, strokes, or other significant procedural complications (major vascular or bleeding events). However, the primary device success endpoint occurred more frequently in balloon expandable versus self-expanding TAVR (95.9% vs. 77.5%, $p < 0.001$). This difference was attributed to a significantly higher frequency of moderate or severe aortic regurgitation (18.3% vs. 4.1%, $p < 0.001$) and a more frequent need for implanting more than one valve (5.8% vs. 0.8%, $p = 0.03$) in the self-expanding valve group. The need for permanent pacemakers was also higher in the self-expanding valve group (37.6% vs. 17.3%, $p = 0.001$).

After TAVR was approved by the USFDA for the treatment of high-risk AS patients, the STS and the ACC jointly developed a comprehensive national postapproval registry, the Transcatheter Valve Therapy (TVT) registry,[93] to meet a condition for Medicare coverage and also to facilitate outcome assessment and comparison with other trials and international registries. This comprehensive registry database harmonized definitions from the surgical STS database and the VARC (1 and 2) initiatives and required long-term follow-up, including quality-of-life assessments. After commercial approval of the Edwards-SAPIEN TAVR system, between November 2011 and May 2013, 7710 patients were enrolled at 224 participating centers in the TVT registry. The risk categories were 20% inoperable patients and 80% high-risk but still operable patients. The mean age was 84 years, 49% were females, and the median STS score was 7%. The most common access site was transfemoral (64%), followed by transapical (29%). In-hospital outcomes included mortality in 5.5%, strokes in 2.0%, dialysis-dependent renal failure in 1.9%, and major vascular injury in 6.4%. At 30 days, in a subset with available data (3133 patients), mortality was 7.6%, strokes were 2.8%, and re-intervention occurred in 0.5% of patients. One-year follow-up in 5980 of these patients was recently presented,[98] and major outcomes were all-cause mortality 26.2% and strokes 3.6%, which were comparable to the results reported from PARTNER. Baseline predictors of 1-year mortality included age, male sex, severe COPD, end-stage renal disease, higher STS scores, and non-transfemoral access site. Although there are many limitations of large registries, the ongoing findings from the TVT registry will be useful to monitor changing patient demographics, clinical outcomes, and generalizability of TAVR in the United States.

NEW CLINICAL INDICATIONS

Once TAVR had become incorporated into the armamentarium of therapies for patients with severe AS, it was predictable that many patients not included in earlier studies, but who were nevertheless at high risk or not candidates for surgical valve replacement, would be considered potential candidates. Thus, preliminary data are accumulating in patients with bicuspid AS, bioprosthetic valve failure, and AS and concomitant coronary disease. Similarly, once TAVR safety and durability concerns have been properly addressed, the exploration of less invasive TAVR in lower risk AS patients has generated considerable controversy. Importantly, the current success of TAVR has been linked to the dual pathways of careful evidence-based clinical research and technology evolution, which should continue to stimulate expansion of TAVR to new clinical indications in the future.

Bioprosthetic Valve Failure

The potential use of TAVR technologies to manage difficult patients with surgical bioprosthetic valve failure has been a consideration for many years. The first case utilizing a transcatheter aortic valve via a percutaneous approach to treat a failing surgical bioprosthesis was reported in 2007 when a CoreValve self-expanding prosthesis was placed inside a degenerated surgical aortic valve in a patient at very high risk for redo SAVR.[99] Subsequently, several case series and small registries have demonstrated the feasibility and safety of transfemoral and transapical valve-in-valve implantation with both self-expanding and balloon expandable transcatheter valves for failing bioprosthetic *aortic* valves (stenosis and regurgitation)[100-104] and balloon expandable valve-in-valves for failing *mitral* bioprostheses.[101,103-106] Moreover, case reports and small series have also emerged in high-risk patients with balloon expandable valve treatment of failed surgical tricuspid bioprostheses[104,105] and failed mitral annuloplasty rings as well.[107] Three requirements for successful valve-in-valve procedures are necessary. First, an intimate understanding of the underlying surgical bioprosthesis is critical for case planning, including the internal valve dimensions (not merely the registered valve size), stented versus stentless, location of the sewing ring, valve leaflets internal or external to the valve frame, and fluoroscopic appearance. Second, advanced imaging with transesophageal echocardiography and MSCT is essential to best delineate anatomic details and quantitative measurements for correct valve sizing. Third, these procedures require advanced operator skills and should only be performed by the most experienced centers and operators to avoid and treat serious complications.

The largest and most comprehensive evaluation of the *aortic* valve-in-valve procedure are the results from the Global Valve-in-Valve registry, which evaluated 202 patients with degenerated surgical bioprosthetic aortic valves from 38 cardiac centers.[101] The mode of bioprosthesis failure was stenosis in 42%, regurgitation in 34%, or combined stenosis and regurgitation in 24%, and implanted TAVR devices were the CoreValve in 61% and the Edwards SAPIEN in 39%. Overall procedural success was 93.1% and the most common adverse procedural outcome was initial device malposition in 15.3% of cases. Ostial coronary obstruction was also more common with the valve-in-valve procedure (3.5%) and seems largely due to the spatial geometry of the surgical valve leaflets inside the aortic sinuses, especially when the leaflets are mounted externally over the stent. High postprocedural valve gradients are common after the valve-in-valve procedure; 28% of patients had ≥20 mm Hg mean gradients after implantation. Although the results of CoreValve versus Edwards SAPIEN devices were generally similar after valve-in-valve procedures, there was a difference with lower post-procedural gradients in smaller surgical bioprostheses (<20-mm diameter) favoring the CoreValve self-expanding prosthesis, perhaps due to the more cranial supra-annular location of the porcine pericardial valve within the frame. At 30 days, overall all-cause mortality was 8.4%, strokes were seen in 2% of patients, and 84% had marked symptom benefit (NYHA functional Class I or Class II). Two worthwhile differences in the valve-in-valve procedures were the low rates of new permanent pacemakers and less severe paravalvular regurgitation; 95% of patients had ≤+1 degree of aortic regurgitation. The expanding TAVR clinical indications of valve-in-valve treatment for bioprosthetic valve failure appear promising, and in the future, surgical strategies of mechanical versus bioprosthetic valve selection for AS patients may be adjusted accordingly.

Moderate-Risk Patients

The expansion of TAVR as an acceptable treatment alternative to a larger segment of the surgical AS population has been the topic of furious debate and has transitioned to clinical reality. Since the introduction of TAVR to Europe in 2007 and the United States in 2011, the definitions of risk strata have "downshifted," such that conventional surgical risk scores have become less relevant than thoughtful decision making about individual patients by the multidisciplinary heart valve team. Whereas previously an STS score of >8% was considered high risk and 4% to 8% moderate risk, in current clinical practice, especially outside the United States, so-called high-risk AS patients are routinely being treated with TAVR, despite STS scores <8%. This is also reflected in several recent clinical trials and large registries. In the high-risk cohort of the CoreValve US Pivotal trial the mean STS score was 7.4%, the median STS score in high-risk and inoperable patients in the TVT registry was 7%, and the mean STS score in the high-risk CHOICE trial was 5.9%. Since risk profiling more logically represents a continuous function rather than dichotomous strata categories, it seems natural that the risk boundaries would downshift with time, as there is a greater confidence in TAVR procedural safety and a better understanding of which patients would most likely benefit. There are two European trials that have carefully studied the results of TAVI in higher versus lower risk AS patients, and as expected, there was a significant reduction in 30-day mortality after TAVI in the lower risk cohorts.[108,109] In addition, there have been three European studies using risk adjustment propensity matching methodologies to compare surgical and TAVI outcomes in moderate-risk AS patients.[110-112] In each of these trials, the 30-day mortality and strokes were similar in SAVR and TAVI patients, and in the two trials with 1-year outcomes, mortality was again similar with both treatment strategies.[113]

Since moderate risk patients constitute approximately one third to one quarter of all surgically eligible AS patients, the definitive recommendation to endorse TAVR as an acceptable alternative to SAVR demands supporting data from rigorous prospective randomized trials. As previously discussed, the balloon expandable SAPIENT XT valve and the self-expanding CoreValve are in the midst of completing two large randomized trials comparing TAVR versus SAVR in moderate-risk patients (PARTNER II, SURTAVI), with the same primary endpoint, a composite of mortality and stroke. Undoubtedly, the more than 4000 patients randomized in these moderate-risk studies will provide further meaningful insights on the value of TAVR in lower risk AS patients.

TAVR for Bicuspid Aortic Valve

An area of ongoing investigation is the use of TAVR in patients with bicuspid aortic valves. The body of evidence on the long-term safety and efficacy in patients with bicuspid aortic valves is markedly limited, as these patients have been uniformly excluded from TAVR trials and registries. Anatomic features intrinsic to bicuspid valves, such as annular eccentricity, high leaflet coaptation, and extensive asymmetric calcification, have led to concerns regarding the risk of TAVR, including valve dislocation, uneven prosthetic expansion, periprosthetic leaks, accelerated leaflet degeneration, coronary obstruction, and annular rupture. These adverse outcomes were reported in other types of stented valves implanted surgically, in which adverse events were common in patients with bicuspid aortic valves but not tricuspid aortic valves.[114]

Nevertheless, given that patients with bicuspid aortic valves comprise over 2% of the general population and of those, over 30% will go on to develop valvular disease,[115] the possibility of TAVR in this subgroup is starting to be explored. Data from single case studies and small cohorts of high and inoperable surgical risk patients have already demonstrated the feasibility of TAVR in this subset.[116-120] Moreover, in a systematic review of the published data regarding TAVR in patients with bicuspid aortic valve, no overall differences in device success, mortality, stroke, or major vascular complications in the short or intermediate term were found when compared with contemporary trials of patients with tricuspid aortic valve stenosis undergoing TAVR.[121] However, a slightly higher rate of paravalvular regurgitation (PVR) (68.5%) was noted in this study, but the vast majority was mild PVR (80%). In a study of 143 patients at 12 European centers with bicuspid aortic valve patients undergoing TAVR, the use of CT for valve sizing compared with echocardiography alone did result in dramatically lower rates of PVR in this population (odds ratio [OR] 0.17; 95% CI, 0.05-0.53; $p = 0.002$),[122] suggesting that routine use of CT in patients with bicuspid aortic valve undergoing TAVR sizing may be necessary.

Thus far, the data appear to be promising for the use of TAVR in bicuspid aortic valve stenosis in high-risk and inoperable patients but more prospective data are needed.

TAVR for Native Aortic Valve Regurgitation

While TAVR has been approved for the treatment of severe aortic valve stenosis in high-risk and inoperable patients, it is also being actively evaluated for the treatment of pure, severe native valve aortic regurgitation (AR). Anatomic challenges for successful TAVR in this patient group include large annular sizes, the lack of calcification for positioning and fixation, and fairly diverse and variable aortic anatomy. Yet, despite these challenges, TAVR for native valve AR has been successfully achieved.

In an Italian, multi-center study of over 1500 patients, approximately 26 patients underwent TAVR with the CoreValve prosthesis for severe aortic regurgitation on the basis of compassionate use after being deemed to be at prohibitive surgical risk.[123] Compared with patients undergoing TAVR for severe AS, the patients with severe AR had a lower rate of device success (79% vs. 96%, $p = 0.006$), along with higher 30-day overall mortality (23% vs. 5.9%; OR 4.22 [3.03-8.28]; $p < 0.001$). In another registry of 43 patients, device success was found to be greater (97.7%), but 8 patients required a second transcatheter valve due to residual PVR. The all-cause 30-day mortality was 9.3% and 21.4% at 12 months. Given the staggeringly poor prognosis of patients with severe aortic regurgitation when treated medically, TAVR with the current generation of transcatheter valves may be a reasonable alternative for inoperable patients.

However, newer TAVR devices, such as the JenaValve, have been specifically developed for the treatment of AR and are under ongoing investigation.[124]

COMPLICATIONS OF TAVR

An essential step in the developmental process and acceptance of a new treatment like TAVR is the elucidation and management of clinically relevant therapy-associated complications. Therefore, considerable effort has been directed to the precise definitions of untoward clinical events, identifying their frequency and possible etiologies and reacting with subsequent procedural or technology enhancements.[125] The main complications related to TAVR are strokes, paravalvular regurgitation, conduction abnormalities, vascular complications and bleeding, and other infrequent but extremely important events such as coronary occlusion or annulus rupture.

Stroke

Stroke remains the most feared and devastating complication associated with TAVR. At present, the 30-day frequency of clinically significant strokes after TAVR varies from 2% to 6% in different studies.[48,49,126-128] In a large meta-analysis involving more than 10,000 patients treated with TAVR,[126] the frequency of both strokes and transient ischemic attacks was 3.3% at 30 days and the associated 30-day mortality was 25.5%, compared with 6.9% 30-day mortality in patients without strokes ($p < 0.001$). Studies have systematically demonstrated that strokes following TAVR peak in the first several days after the procedure, but delayed strokes can occur in the first 2 weeks, and late strokes (after 30 days) are not infrequent in this elderly patient population with frequent atrial fibrillation. The 1-year stroke frequency has been 3.6% to 13.8% after TAVR in different studies and 5.2% in the large meta-analysis. Several studies have indicated that the stroke frequency after TAVR has been declining in recent years due to improved case selection, procedural technique refinements, increased operator experience, and new TAVR systems.[129] There does not appear to be a significant difference in stroke frequency when comparing either balloon expandable versus self-expanding TAVR or transapical versus transfemoral access approaches.[129]

There are multiple potential etiologies of stroke after TAVR. The vast majority of early strokes are due to embolic debris liberated from the aorta, native valve leaflets, or the left ventricle during the course of procedural manipulation of guidewires, balloon catheters, and transcatheter valves. In patients with antecedent cerebrovascular disease, sustained hypotension or hypoperfusion at any point during the procedure, such as during rapid right ventricular pacing, may lead to ischemic infarctions. Another recognized etiology of increased strokes after TAVR is the use of balloon postdilatation after valve deployment for the purpose of lowering the magnitude of paravalvular regurgitation.[127-129] Lastly, up to a third of patients can have new onset atrial fibrillation after TAVR, which may further result in cardioembolic phenomena and strokes.[130]

While the frequency of strokes is relatively low after TAVR, subclinical brain injury is more frequent. Diffusion-weighted magnetic resonance imaging (MRI) studies after TAVR have demonstrated that up to 84% of TAVR patients have new foci of restricted diffusion, consistent with embolic lesions, and more than 75% have multiple foci.[131] However, despite the high frequency of new embolic lesions visualized by MRI, the vast majority of patients with these findings are asymptomatic with no overt clinical sequelae, including no decline in cognitive function, worsening quality of life, or increased 1-year mortality. Nevertheless, the neuroimaging studies are supported by recent findings, which indicate that macroscopic material liberated during TAVR was captured by a dual filter-based cerebral embolic protection device in 75% of the 40 patients studied.[132] Thrombotic material was found in 52% of patients, and tissue fragments compatible with aortic valve leaflet or aortic wall origin were also found in 52% of patients. Currently, there are three different filters or deflectors mounted on delivery catheters designed to protect the brain from intraprocedural embolic debris. Using these devices, small registries have reported some reduction in mean lesion volume after early diffusion-weighted MRI, and more definitive randomized trials are ongoing. Clearly, there are many unanswered questions relating to stroke prevention after TAVR, including the following:

1. Impact of even lower profile TAVR devices and reduced balloon dilation (pre- and post-TAVR)
2. Importance of perfusion deficits on neuroimaging studies and their association with sophisticated measures of neurocognitive function
3. Benefit of rigorous detection and pharmacotherapy management of new onset atrial fibrillation
4. Value of new cerebral protection devices for either systematic or selective use during TAVR

Paravalvular Regurgitation

Unlike SAVR, where PVR is distinctly uncommon, after either balloon expandable or self-expanding TAVR, PVR is frequently observed due to the difficulty in achieving circumferential flush apposition of the metallic support frame with the asymmetric, distorted, and heavily calcified aortic annulus and valve leaflets. The determinants of PVR are a complex interaction of patient characteristics, procedural factors, assessment modality, and valve type. Although the reported frequency and severity of PVR after TAVR vary widely among studies, most agree that some PVR is present in at least 50% of TAVR cases and moderate or severe PVR is present in approximately 10% to 15% of cases.[133-137] The differences in reported frequency of PVR are likely due to the nonstandardized application of imaging assessment technologies (angiography vs. echocardiography vs. cardiac MR) and the imprecision and subjective nature of PVR severity classification schemes. Nevertheless, there is general agreement that moderate or severe PVR after TAVR is detrimental and is associated with increased subsequent mortality.[133,136,138] In the most recent analysis from the PARTNER trial, including 2434 balloon expandable TAVR cases, a multivariate analysis indicated that the presence of moderate or severe PVR (HR, 2.18; 95% CI, 1.57-3.02; $p < 0.001$) and even mild PVR (HR 1.37; 95% CI, 1.14-1.90; $p = 0.012$) was associated with higher 1-year mortality.[136]

Differences in PVR frequency and severity among the various TAVR systems have been studied without definitive resolution. In single center and multi-center registries, comparing the self-expanding CoreValve with the balloon expandable SAPIEN, PVR severity was increased after CoreValve.[139,140] Similarly, in a large meta-analysis including 12,926 patients, the incidence of moderate or severe PVR after CoreValve was 16.0%, whereas after SAPIEN, the

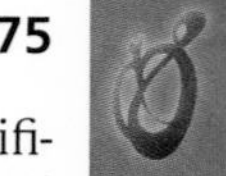

incidence of PVR was 9.1% ($p < 0.005$).[133] These findings were consistent with the previously discussed CHOICE randomized trial,[97] which also indicated that PVR was reduced after SAPIEN compared with CoreValve treatment, based on multi-modality imaging assessments.

In the aforementioned meta-analysis, predictors of significant PVR after TAVR were the valve implantation depth, valve undersizing, and mean Agatston calcium score.[133] These findings underscore the three main etiologies of PVR:

1. Malposition of the transcatheter valve (either too high or too low), causing misalignment of the frame "seal zone" (containing the interior skirt) with the annulus
2. Undersizing the valve relative to the annulus implant dimensions
3. Severe calcification that prevents flush contact with the nondeformable support frame

Both MSCT and echocardiography studies have strongly linked PVR to the overall extent of aorta and valve calcification, asymmetric calcium distribution patterns, and vulnerable calcium locations (aortic wall, valve commissures, left ventricular outflow tract, and valve landing zone).[141-143] Optimal valve sizing has become a critical consideration in TAVR procedural planning to prevent significant PVR.[144,145] Adjunctive imaging with 3D MSCT using standardized image acquisition protocols and analyzed with custom quantitative algorithms provide the most consistent measurements of the aortic annulus for valve sizing, including assessment of annulus geometry, major and minor axis diameters, area, and perimeter. These data are used to select the optimal valve size for a given patient, recognizing that each valve type may differ regarding sizing requirements. Not infrequently, the MSCT images are sub-optimal, and additional measures such as intraprocedural balloon sizing and 3D echocardiography are used in complementary fashion to finalize the correct valve selection.

The assessment of PVR after valve implantation is controversial. Most centers use a combination of hemodynamic evaluations and imaging studies (preferably both aortography and echocardiography). Arguably, intraprocedural transesophageal echocardiography, performed and analyzed by a trained specialist, is the most sensitive imaging study to determine the location and severity of PVR immediately after TAVR. Hemodynamic assessments of AR severity are also helpful, especially calculation of the dimensionless AR index[69] in patients with a stable heart rate. Also, there are data to indicate that for both the balloon expandable and the self-expanding TAVR devices, there can be spontaneous improvement in PVR severity in the first 30 minutes after valve implantation,[146] which should mitigate against the immediate initiation of reparative therapies, unless there is severe hemodynamic compromise. Once significant PVR has developed after TAVR there are limited treatment options. Postdilatation with a carefully sized balloon has been demonstrated to be an effective technique in reducing the degree of PVR in numerous studies,[128,146] but the risks of increasing embolic strokes and excessive trauma to the aortic root and annulus should always be considered. In cases where malposition of the valve causes severe PVR, placement of a second correctly located transcatheter valve (either above or below the first valve) can be curative. In the PARTNER trial, 36.1% of patients with moderate or severe PVR after the Edwards SAPIEN valve required a valve-in-valve procedure. However, the need for a second valve also resulted in a higher 1-year cardiovascular mortality ($p = 0.041$).[147] Lastly, if the PVR is persistent and clinically significant (worsening heart failure) after the index procedure, focal areas of PVR can be repaired using conventional catheter-based implantable occluder devices.

Undoubtedly, the answer to preventing PVR associated with transcatheter valves resides in meticulous assessment of the native valve anatomy with careful valve sizing using MSCT 3D imaging and advanced new TAVR designs with either subannular fixation or space-filling external materials to fill the gaps between the frame and the native valve structures.

Conduction Abnormalities and Arrhythmias

Similar to surgical aortic valve procedures, conduction disturbances occur frequently after TAVR. The pathophysiology of these new conduction disturbances is due to the superficial location of the left bundle branch in the uppermost part of the left ventricular septum and its close proximity to the aortic valve apparatus. New onset LBBB is the most commonly observed conduction disturbance and has been reported to vary from 29% to 65% with the CoreValve bioprosthesis, and from 6% to 18% with the SAPIEN valve.[78,82,148,149] However, approximately half of the patients who develop LBBB post-TAVR have resolution by 30 days. Although one study demonstrated an association between new onset LBBB after TAVR and increased 1-year mortality,[81] multiple other studies[82,83] have indicated similar late mortality in patients with and without new LBBB. Importantly, there have been consistent findings that new LBBB after TAVR is associated with reduced augmentation in left ventricular function and an increased need for new pacemakers.[82,83]

Two large meta-analyses[150,151] have observed a 13% to 15% frequency of new pacemakers after TAVR: approximately 25% after CoreValve implantation and 6% after SAPIEN valves ($p < 0.001$). There are three major predictors of new pacemakers after TAVR, including baseline right bundle branch block, low placement of the transcatheter valve, and a narrowed left ventricular outflow tract (or exaggerated valve oversizing). The higher frequency of pacemakers after CoreValve procedures is likely due to the longer frame length with implantation depth extending farther into the left ventricular outflow tract, creating augmented contact and disruption of the underlying left bundle branch tract. Studies have shown that if the depth of implantation is reduced with the CoreValve, a lower permanent pacemaker rate can be achieved. Due to the high frequency of both new LBBB and the increased need for permanent pacemakers, it is recommended that essentially all CoreValve patients (without baseline pacemakers) be observed with a temporary transvenous pacemaker for 24 to 48 hours after valve implantation. New permanent pacemakers after TAVR have not been associated with increased late mortality, but there have been increased repeat hospitalizations and reduced left ventricular function compared with patients without new pacemakers.[152]

New onset atrial fibrillation has been identified in 18% to 32% of patients after TAVR[47,48,130] and associated predictors were moderate or severe left atrial enlargement and the transapical access route. Limited reports suggest that even brief episodes of new onset atrial fibrillation after TAVR have been associated with an increased risk of both early and late strokes but not cardiac mortality.[130] There is a clear need for more intensive patient arrhythmia monitoring after TAVR and rigorous pharmacotherapy treatment in patients with

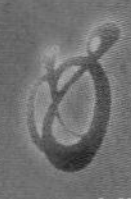

newly discovered atrial fibrillation. Other controversies that bear noting are the increasing use of cardiac resynchronization therapy after TAVR in patients with conduction disturbances and residual heart failure and the need for more sophisticated electrophysiology assessments to better determine the definite need for permanent pacemakers in patients with post-TAVR conduction disturbances.

Vascular Complications and Bleeding

From the earliest TAVR experiences, the frequent occurrence of vascular complications has tainted clinical outcomes, provoked changes in procedural techniques, and driven advances in next generation device development. Depending on the specific definitions applied to vascular complications, the frequency has ranged from 5% to 50% in the literature. The VARC initiatives[46,54] helped to consolidate and clarify these definitions into two main categories: "major" vascular complications, which involved serious injury to the ventricle(s), aorta, or peripheral vessels (such as rupture, perforation, or severe dissection), resulting in compromised flow and/or concerning blood loss (≥4 units) and usually requiring either interventional or surgical corrective repair; and "minor" vascular complications, which included less serious hematomas, dissections, and other vascular events that could be managed usually without deleterious long-lasting clinical outcomes.

The use of larger profile devices (>20 Fr) coupled with an unforgiving anatomic substrate (older patients with frequent peripheral vascular disease) and less experienced operators resulted in 10% to 15% major vascular complications in SOURCE,[36] PARTNER,[47,48] and an early meta-analysis.[125] In PARTNER, 15.3% of patients had major and 11.9% had minor vascular complications within 30 days, including severe dissections (62.8%), perforations (31.3%), and large access-site hematoma (22.9%).[57] Major vascular complications were associated with increased major bleeding, renal failure requiring dialysis, and mortality at both 30 days and 1 year. The only identifiable independent predictors of major vascular complications were female sex[57] and a larger sheath-to-femoral-artery ratio.[153,154] Over time, commensurate with increased operator experience, which resulted in the development of new procedural methods to better secure the vascular access site, and improved techniques to manage vascular complications (e.g., stent grafts),[155] and the emergence of smaller sized TAVR systems,[62] the rates of both major and minor vascular complications declined significantly. Presently, in high-volume TAVR centers specializing in fully percutaneous procedures with access to modern low-profile TAVR devices, the expected frequency of major vascular complications is <5%. Importantly, advanced interventional skills in vascular access, closure, and complication management are absolutely necessary to achieve optimal outcomes.

The critical nature of major bleeding during interventional and surgical procedures and the association with increased subsequent mortality has been highlighted over the past several years. The frequency of major bleeding in PARTNER was 22.7% after SAVR and 11.2% after transfemoral TAVR ($p = 0.0004$), and similarly, the need for any transfusion and ≥4 unit transfusions were increased in the surgical patients.[58] Predictors of major bleeding were different in the SAVR vs. the TAVR patients; baseline hemoglobin was the strongest predictor with SAVR and major vascular complications with TAVR. One-year mortality was two-fold greater with major bleeding after SAVR (with major bleeding 40.5%, without major bleeding 21.2%, $P_{log\ rank} < 0.0001$), whereas there was little change after TAVR (with major bleeding 27.6%, without major bleeding 23.3%, $P_{log\ rank} = 0.55$). Moreover, the incidence, need for transfusion, and long-term impact of major bleeding in the transfemoral TAVR patients decreased with lower patient risk profiles and increased operator experience. Underscoring the importance in recognizing and preventing procedure-related major bleeding, especially after SAVR, among all independent predictors of 1-year mortality in the PARTNER trial (including stroke), major bleeding events had the greatest effect on late mortality (HR 2.36, $p < 0.0001$).[58] Recently, provocative reports have indicated that *late* (>30 days) bleeding after TAVR, most commonly arising from the gastrointestinal tract, and amplified by the presence of atrial fibrillation, resulted in a striking increase in 1-year mortality, raising concerns that a TAVR-associated bleeding diathesis perhaps combined with the effects of adjunctive pharmacotherapy must be further explored in the future.

Other Less Frequent Complications

There are several rare, but nonetheless clinically important, complications associated with TAVR. Among this group of less frequent complications, the two that deserve special mention are coronary artery obstruction and aortic root rupture. Others that have been recently reported are delayed transcatheter valve thrombosis and dynamic left ventricular outflow tract obstruction. Several case reports of late (2 to 12 months after the index procedure) valve thrombosis have been described,[156,157] wherein premature impaired leaflet motion and elevated aortic valve gradients mimicking early structural valve deterioration have responded to chronic systemic anticoagulation using warfarin with normalized leaflet motion. Clearly, in these cases, the thickened and immobile valve leaflets were largely due to unexplained thrombus formation. Another rare complication after TAVR has been the unmasking of dynamic outflow tract obstruction appearing as obstructive hypertrophic cardiomyopathy with hypotension and a "suicide" ventricle, which have been treated with aggressive volume replacement and also with alcohol septal ablation.[158]

Coronary obstruction during TAVR is a rare but dreaded complication due to displacement of the native aortic valve leaflets into the coronary ostia resulting in a sudden pseudo-obstruction with associated clinical sequelae. In a large multicenter TAVR registry (6688 patients), there were 44 cases of symptomatic coronary obstruction (0.66%).[159] Baseline and procedural variables associated with coronary obstruction were older age, female sex, no previous coronary artery bypass graft, the use of a balloon expandable valve, and previous surgical aortic bioprosthesis. The left coronary artery was the most commonly involved (88.6%), and both low-lying coronary ostia and narrowed sinus of Valsalva diameter were associated anatomic factors. Most patients presented with persistent severe hypotension (68.2%) and electrocardiographic changes (56.8%). Percutaneous coronary intervention was attempted in 75% of these cases (successful in 81.8%), and 30-day mortality was 40.9%. In high-risk cases (low lying coronaries and narrowed sinuses), many operators are "protecting" the coronary ostia with placement of guidewires, balloons, and even stents, which can be deployed immediately if coronary obstruction is observed.

Another rare but potentially devastating complication during TAVR is either contained or noncontained rupture of the left ventricular outflow tract, annulus, or aorta. An analysis of anatomic and procedural features of 31 consecutive ruptures (of which 11 were contained peri-aortic hematomas) associated with balloon expandable TAVR was compiled from 16 centers.[160] Patients with root rupture had a higher degree of sub-annular or outflow tract calcification, a higher frequency of ≥20% annular area valve oversizing, and more frequent balloon postdilatation. The typical phenotype of a rupture-prone TAVR patient is a frail, low-BMI female with a heavily calcified aorta, narrowed or effaced aortic sinuses, and receiving chronic corticosteroid therapy. Aortic rupture occurs more frequently with balloon expandable compared with self-expanding TAVR systems. Most cases of noncontained aortic rupture result in immediate or progressive hemodynamic collapse, requiring emergency pericardiocentesis and open surgical repair, usually with poor short-term survival.

NEW TAVR DEVICES

Overview

Despite the success of "first generation" TAVR systems, several device design limitations have been identified that contributed to suboptimal clinical outcomes. Previously, large diameter TAVR delivery sheaths created a significant femoral artery—sheath size mismatch in many patients resulting in major vascular complications and the frequent use of nontransfemoral access sites. In the future, to safely support successful transfemoral access in the vast majority of TAVR-eligible patients (especially women), an outer sheath diameter of less than 18 Fr for all valve sizes is advisable. Smaller TAVR system profiles are also important to negotiate tortuous vascular anatomy, facilitate native valve crossing, minimize trauma to the aorta and the native valve, allow the option of no predilation before deployment, and improve alignment and positioning accuracy during implantation. Another important limitation of early and current TAVR systems is the lack of consistent and precise positioning of the valve at the ideal landing zone, which has resulted in valve malpositioning, obstruction of the coronary arteries (too high placement), interference with the conduction system or the mitral valve (too low placement), and increased PVR (either too high or too low placement). Ideally, a slow and controlled valve deployment, allowing for positioning adjustments before final implantation, is preferred. The availability of partial or complete valve retrieval is being incorporated into many of the newer self-expanding TAVR systems, which provides the operator a "second chance" if the initial attempts at precise positioning were suboptimal. One of the greatest differences between SAVR and TAVR has been the increased frequency and severity of PVR. To address this issue, newer TAVR devices have explored improvements in sub-annular fixation and coaxial alignment, as well as the addition of external space-filling materials to reduce or eliminate incomplete circumferential apposition of the valve frame against the aortic annulus. Finally, durability of the frame and valve itself remains a concern, especially if long-term implants in younger patients are being contemplated. In addition to the balloon expandable SAPIEN 3 and the self-expanding CoreValve EVOLUT R, other new TAVR systems, which are currently available or in early-stage clinical investigations, have attempted to address many of the aforementioned design limitations (**Figure 29-3**).

Self-Expanding TAVR Systems

Most of the new TAVR devices have features of a self-expanding support frame composed of nitinol and deployed using a sheath retraction system.

CENTERA (Edwards Lifescience, Irvine, California) is a "short frame" self-expanding valve, which consists of treated bovine pericardial tissue leaflets attached to a nitinol frame, and is designed to anchor in the annulus. Valve delivery is a fully motorized single-operator system, which is both fully retrievable and compatible with a 14 Fr expandable sheath (**Figure 29-3C**). The Centera TAVR has completed first-in-human studies[161] and a European safety and performance study is currently under way.

PORTICO (St. Jude's Medical Inc., St. Paul, Minnesota); is a recently introduced "long frame" self-expanding TAVR system (**Figure 29-3D**). Although similar in some respects to CoreValve, differentiating features include an intra-annular bovine pericardial valve with a lower porcine pericardial sealing cuff, larger stent cells to improve anatomic conformation and coronary access, and complete retrievability of the valve during deployment. A total of 83 patients were studied in six European centers using the transfemoral system with favorable clinical outcomes, good valve hemodynamics, lower than expected new pacemakers (10.8%), and infrequent moderate or severe PVR (5%).[162] Access alternatives for the Portico TAVR system include transfemoral, subclavian, direct aortic, and a soon to be tested transapical version.

The *ACURATE* (Symetis Inc., Ecublens, Switzerland) valve (**Figure 29-3E**) consists of stabilizing arches in the aorta to maintain coaxial alignment, a supra-annular porcine pericardial valve within a self-expanding upper crown, and a contoured lower crown encircled by a fabric skirt that can be partially re-sheathed (**Figure 29-3E**). The commissures of the stent have a circular radiopaque appearance, which facilitates commissural alignment with the native valve. The lower portion of the frame tends to self-adjust to the geometry of the annulus, which creates a sub-annular fixation zone to reduce PVR. The 28 Fr transapical TA Acurate system was studied in 40 patients with excellent results; low mortality, low PVR, and infrequent need for new pacemakers[163] and the transfemoral version were evaluated in five centers in Brazil and Germany in 80 patients with similar favorable outcomes.[164]

The *ENGAGER* (Medtronic Inc., Minneapolis, Minnesota) TAVR system (**Figure 29-3F**) is currently a transapical device with a self-expanding short nitinol frame and polyester skirt, control arms that are placed outside the native leaflets, a supra-annular bovine pericardial tissue valve, and commissural alignment features. A 125-patient registry in high-risk AS patients indicated good clinical outcomes with very low (<5%) mild, moderate, or severe PVR but frequent new pacemakers (~30%) due to new conduction system abnormalities.[165]

Other TAVR Concepts

The *DIRECT FLOW MEDICAL* (Direct Flow Medical, Inc., Santa Rosa, California) aortic valve is an intra-annular bovine pericardial tissue valve, which is mounted on two inflatable polyester rings (**Figure 29-3G**). The valve system has no metal components and was designed to adapt to the left ventricular outflow tract and the aortic annulus to minimize PVR. During deployment, the rings are filled with saline and contrast and positioning are facilitated by three translation wires. The system is fully repositionable and retrievable, by deflating the rings and reorienting the device. Once the valve is positioned in the optimal location, the saline and contrast mixture in the rings is exchanged for a quick-curing polymer to anchor the valve in place. The Discover trial was conducted at 10 European centers in 100 patients and revealed low mortality and strokes, rare moderate or severe PVR (2%), infrequent new pacemakers, and slightly higher transvalvular gradients compared with other TAVR systems.[166]

The *JENA VALVE* (JenaValve Inc., Munich, Germany) consists of a short self-expanding nitinol frame housing a valve derived from porcine valve material, with a porcine pericardial skirt and an upper crown for stabilization. Arms or "feelers" are positioned behind the native valve leaflets allowing "clipping" of the valve against the lower stent (**Figure 29-3H**). When ideally positioned, there is correct commissural alignment, sparing of the coronary arteries, and an intra-annular position, which avoids the conduction system. The Jupiter multicenter study in 126 patients, all with transapical access, showed very low mortality and strokes, rare PVR, and rare new pacemakers.[167] This device has also been used for patients with predominant aortic regurgitation in a small registry.[124] A transfemoral version of the Jena Valve has begun clinical evaluation in Europe.

The *LOTUS* (Boston Scientific Inc., Natick, Massachusetts) TAVR system is a woven nitinol frame housing an intra-annular bovine pericardial valve, which shortens and locks into position (**Figure 29-3I**). The device is fully retrievable and has an exterior adaptive membrane to reduce PVR. The Reprise II clinical trial enrolled 120 patients at 14 centers in Australia and Europe using the transfemoral SADRA Lotus TAVR system.[168] Clinical outcomes at 30 days revealed all-cause mortality in 4.2%, strokes in 5.9%, moderate or severe PVR in 1%, and pacemakers in 28.6%.

FUTURE DIRECTIONS

TAVR is a breakthrough new technology platform, which has expanded the armamentarium of therapies for patients with AS, especially those who are at high risk for conventional surgery. The multi-disciplinary heart valve team serves as the central vehicle for determining appropriate case selection and directing care for these patients. Thus far, impressive clinical research validation of TAVR has been established via randomized controlled trials and careful registries.

Despite the impressive growth of TAVR, there are many challenges as well as future opportunities for expanding clinical applications and improving patient outcomes. Ultimately, the role of this less invasive form of valve replacement will depend on three unresolved issues:

1. Equivalence or superiority compared with surgery of major clinical endpoints, particularly death and stroke, for designated study populations
2. Further reduction of TAVR procedure-related major complications (e.g., PVR, vascular and bleeding events)
3. Valve durability similar to surgical bioprostheses

If these issues can be resolved in favor of TAVR, it is likely that most patients with severe AS in the future, irrespective of risk profile, can be candidates for TAVR therapy. Exceptions might be on the basis of anatomic considerations, such as true bicuspid aortic valves, AS with concomitant severe coronary disease or other valve lesions, and vascular access contraindications. Other clinical scenarios like surgical bioprosthesis failure (aortic and mitral), severe asymptomatic AS, and low flow–low gradient AS might also benefit from a less invasive valve replacement strategy.

Clinical expansion to lower risk AS patient cohorts will also depend on further procedural adjustments to improve user-friendliness and insure safety. Next generation TAVR systems have already reduced catheter profile substantially, which is necessary to eliminate vascular complications and make a fully percutaneous transfemoral procedure (the preferred approach) available in the great majority of patients. Other procedural enhancements may include reducing the need for either predilation or postdilation, cerebral protection to decrease strokes, improved online adjunctive imaging to refine valve positioning, and reducing the need for general anesthesia. Combined procedures with TAVR—either coronary angioplasty, left atrial appendage closure, or MitraClip edge-to-edge repair for residual moderate or severe MR—are also currently under investigation. Finally, improved adjunctive pharmacotherapy strategies after TAVR require careful exploration in the form of thoughtful clinical trials.

CONCLUSIONS

Clearly, the explosion of new TAVR technology, including worthwhile iterations of first generation devices, has been a major contributor to improved clinical results. Creative new TAVR designs that appear to essentially eradicate PVR and improve positioning accuracy (often with retrieval features) will undoubtedly be commonplace in the forthcoming years. One can easily imagine a time in the near future when 3D bioprinting of the diseased native valve generates true anatomic models for precise case planning experiences to optimize choices of the most appropriate valve designs and sizes for a given patient. The pioneering spirit and vision of Alain Cribier more than a decade ago to provide a new catheter-based alternative treatment for AS has been realized with lofty expectations that future evolution and maturation will render TAVR as the preferred standard therapy for the majority of severe AS patients.

References

1. Cribier A, Savin T, Saoudi N, et al: Percutaneous transluminal valvuloplasty of acquired aortic stenosis in elderly patients: an alternative to valve replacement? *Lancet* 1(8472):63–67, 1986.
2. Cribier A, Eltchaninoff H, Bash A, et al: Percutaneous transcatheter implantation of an aortic valve prosthesis for calcific aortic stenosis: first human case description. *Circulation* 106(24):3006–3008, 2002.
3. Sakata Y, Syed Z, Salinger MH, et al: Percutaneous balloon aortic valvuloplasty: antegrade transseptal vs. conventional retrograde transarterial approach. *Catheter Cardiovasc Interv* 64(3):314–321, 2005.
4. NHLBI Balloon Valvuloplasty Registry Participants: Percutaneous balloon aortic valvuloplasty. Acute and 30 day follow-up results in 674 patients from the NHLBI Balloon Valvuloplasty Registry. *Circulation* 84(6):2383–2397, 1991.
5. Otto CM, Mickel MC, Kennedy JW, et al: Three-year outcome after balloon aortic valvuloplasty. Insights into prognosis of valvular aortic stenosis. *Circulation* 89(2):642–650, 1994.
6. McKay RG: The Mansfield Scientific Aortic Valvuloplasty Registry: overview of acute hemodynamic results and procedural complications. *J Am Coll Cardiol* 17(2):485–491, 1991.
7. Ben-Dor I, Pichard AD, Satler LF, et al: Complications and outcome of balloon aortic valvuloplasty in high-risk or inoperable patients. *JACC Cardiovasc Interv* 3(11):1150–1156, 2010.
8. Eltchaninoff H, Durand E, Borz B, et al: Balloon aortic valvuloplasty in the era of transcatheter aortic valve replacement: acute and long-term outcomes. *Am Heart J* 167(2):235–240, 2014.
9. Nishimura RA, Otto CM, Bonow RO, et al: 2014 AHA/ACC guideline for the management of patients with valvular heart disease: a report of the American College of Cardiology/American Heart Association Task Force on Practice Guidelines. *Circulation* 2014, 48(1):e1–e132.
10. American College of C, American Heart Association Task Force on Practice G, Society of Cardiovascular A, et al: ACC/AHA 2006 guidelines for the management of patients with valvular heart disease: a report of the American College of Cardiology/American Heart Association Task Force on Practice Guidelines (Writing Committee to Revise the 1998 guidelines for the management of patients with valvular heart disease) developed in collaboration with the Society of Cardiovascular Anesthesiologists endorsed by the Society for Cardiovascular Angiography and Interventions and the Society of Thoracic Surgeons. *J Am Coll Cardiol* 48(3):e1–e148, 2006.
11. Vahanian A, Alfieri O, Andreotti F, et al: Guidelines on the management of valvular heart disease (version 2012): the Joint Task Force on the Management of Valvular Heart Disease of the

European Society of Cardiology (ESC) and the European Association for Cardio-Thoracic Surgery (EACTS). *Eur J Cardiothorac Surg* 42(4):S1–S44, 2012.
12. Leon MB: A review of new aortic valvuloplasty systems: InterValve, Loma Vista, CardioSculpt, and Pi-Cardia. In Transcatheter Cardiovascular Therapeutics 25th Annual Scientific Symposium, San Francisco, California, 2013.
13. Connolly HM, Oh JK, Orszulak TA, et al: Aortic valve replacement for aortic stenosis with severe left ventricular dysfunction. Prognostic indicators. *Circulation* 95(10):2395–2400, 1997.
14. Iung B, Cachier A, Baron G, et al: Decision-making in elderly patients with severe aortic stenosis: why are so many denied surgery? *Eur Heart J* 26(24):2714–2720, 2005.
15. Kuntz RE, Tosteson AN, Berman AD, et al: Predictors of event-free survival after balloon aortic valvuloplasty. *N Engl J Med* 325(1):17–23, 1991.
16. Davies H: Catheter-mounted valve for temporary relief of aortic insufficiency. *Lancet* 1(7379):250, 1965.
17. Andersen HR, Knudsen LL, Hasenkam JM: Transluminal implantation of artificial heart valves. Description of a new expandable aortic valve and initial results with implantation by catheter technique in closed chest pigs. *Eur Heart J* 13(5):704–708, 1992.
18. Bonhoeffer P, Boudjemline Y, Saliba Z, et al: Percutaneous replacement of pulmonary valve in a right-ventricle to pulmonary-artery prosthetic conduit with valve dysfunction. *Lancet* 356(9239):1403–1405, 2000.
19. Leon MB, Gada H, Fontana GP: Challenges and future opportunities for transcatheter aortic valve therapy. *Prog Cardiovasc Dis* 56(6):635–645, 2014.
20. Nashef SA, Roques F, Hammill BG, et al: Validation of European System for Cardiac Operative Risk Evaluation (EuroSCORE) in North American cardiac surgery. *Eur J Cardiothorac Surg* 22(1):101–105, 2002.
21. O'Brien SM, Shahian DM, Filardo G, et al: The Society of Thoracic Surgeons 2008 cardiac surgery risk models: part 2—isolated valve surgery. *Ann Thorac Surg* 88(1 Suppl):S23–S42, 2009.
22. Dewey TM, Brown D, Ryan WH, et al: Reliability of risk algorithms in predicting early and late operative outcomes in high-risk patients undergoing aortic valve replacement. *J Thorac Cardiovasc Surg* 135(1):180–187, 2008.
23. Piazza N, Wenaweser P, van Gameren M, et al: Relationship between the logistic EuroSCORE and the Society of Thoracic Surgeons Predicted Risk of Mortality score in patients implanted with the CoreValve ReValving system—a Bern-Rotterdam Study. *Am Heart J* 159(2):323–329, 2010.
24. Babaliaros V, Devireddy C, Lerakis S, et al: Comparison of transfemoral transcatheter aortic valve replacement performed in the catheterization laboratory (minimalist approach) versus hybrid operating room (standard approach): outcomes and cost analysis. *JACC Cardiovasc Interv* 7(8):898–904, 2014.
25. Cribier A, Eltchaninoff H, Tron C, et al: Early experience with percutaneous transcatheter implantation of heart valve prosthesis for the treatment of end-stage inoperable patients with calcific aortic stenosis. *J Am Coll Cardiol* 43(4):698–703, 2004.
26. Webb JG, Chandavimol M, Thompson CR, et al: Percutaneous aortic valve implantation retrograde from the femoral artery. *Circulation* 113(6):842–850, 2006.
27. Kasel AM, Cassese S, Leber AW, et al: Fluoroscopy-guided aortic root imaging for TAVR: "follow the right cusp" rule. *JACC Cardiovasc Imaging* 6(2):274–275, 2013.
28. Sharp AS, Michev I, Maisano F, et al: A new technique for vascular access management in transcatheter aortic valve implantation. *Catheter Cardiovasc Interv* 75(5):784–793, 2010.
29. Lichtenstein SV, Cheung A, Ye J, et al: Transapical transcatheter aortic valve implantation in humans: initial clinical experience. *Circulation* 114(6):591–596, 2006.
30. Kodali SK, O'Neill WW, Moses JW, et al: Early and late (one year) outcomes following transcatheter aortic valve implantation in patients with severe aortic stenosis (from the United States REVIVAL trial). *Am J Cardiol* 107(7):1058–1064, 2011.
31. Lefevre T, Kappetein AP, Wolner E, et al: One year follow-up of the multi-centre European PARTNER transcatheter heart valve study. *Eur Heart J* 32(2):148–157, 2011.
32. Svensson LG, Dewey T, Kapadia S, et al: United States feasibility study of transcatheter insertion of a stented aortic valve by the left ventricular apex. *Ann Thorac Surg* 86(1):46–54, discussion 54–55, 2008.
33. Walther T, Kasimir MT, Doss M, et al: One-year interim follow-up results of the TRAVERCE trial: the initial feasibility study for trans-apical aortic-valve implantation. *Eur J Cardiothorac Surg* 39(4):532–537, 2011.
34. Kodali S: Pooled Analysis with Extended Follow-up from the REVIVE II and REVIVAL II Transfemoral Feasibility Registries. In Transcatheter Cardiovascular Therapeutics 20th Annual Scientific Symposium, Washington, DC, October 12-17, 2008.
35. Thomas M, Schymik G, Walther T, et al: One-year outcomes of cohort 1 in the Edwards SAPIEN Aortic Bioprosthesis European Outcome (SOURCE) registry: the European registry of transcatheter aortic valve implantation using the Edwards SAPIEN valve. *Circulation* 124(4):425–433, 2011.
36. Thomas M, Schymik G, Walther T, et al: Thirty-day results of the SAPIEN aortic Bioprosthesis European Outcome (SOURCE) Registry: a European registry of transcatheter aortic valve implantation using the Edwards SAPIEN valve. *Circulation* 122(1):62–69, 2010.
37. Wendler O, Walther T, Nataf P, et al: Trans-apical aortic valve implantation: univariate and multivariate analyses of the early results from the SOURCE registry. *Eur J Cardiothorac Surg* 38(2):119–127, 2010.
38. Wendler O, Walther T, Schroefel H, et al: Transapical aortic valve implantation: mid-term outcome from the SOURCE registry. *Eur J Cardiothorac Surg* 43(3):505–511, discussion 511–512, 2013.
39. Rodes-Cabau J, Webb JG, Cheung A, et al: Transcatheter aortic valve implantation for the treatment of severe symptomatic aortic stenosis in patients at very high or prohibitive surgical risk: acute and late outcomes of the multicenter Canadian experience. *J Am Coll Cardiol* 55(11):1080–1090, 2010.
40. Rodes-Cabau J, Webb JG, Cheung A, et al: Long-term outcomes after transcatheter aortic valve implantation: insights on prognostic factors and valve durability from the Canadian multicenter experience. *J Am Coll Cardiol* 60(19):1864–1875, 2012.
41. Sack S: The PREVAIL XT (TF and TA) Registries. In Transcatheter Cardiovascular Therapeutics 24th Annual Scientific Symposium, Miami, FL, October 22-26, 2012.
42. Thomas M: The SOURCE Multicenter EU Registries (including XT). In Transcatheter Cardiovascular Therapeutics 24th Annual Scientific Symposium, Miami, FL, October 22-26, 2012.
43. Walther T, Thielmann M, Kempfert J, et al: PREVAIL TRANSAPICAL: multicentre trial of transcatheter aortic valve implantation using the newly designed bioprosthesis (SAPIEN-XT) and delivery system (ASCENDRA-II). *Eur J Cardiothorac Surg* 42(2):278–283, discussion 283, 2012.
44. Walther T, Thielmann M, Kempfert J, et al: One-year multicentre outcomes of transapical aortic valve implantation using the SAPIEN XT valve: the PREVAIL transapical study. *Eur J Cardiothorac Surg* 43(5):986–992, 2013.
45. Windecker S: One-year outcomes from the SOURCE XT post-approval study. In EuroPCR Annual Scientific Symposium, Paris, France, 2013.
46. Leon MB, Piazza N, Nikolsky E, et al: Standardized endpoint definitions for Transcatheter Aortic Valve Implantation clinical trials: a consensus report from the Valve Academic Research Consortium. *J Am Coll Cardiol* 57(3):253–269, 2011.
47. Leon MB, Smith CR, Mack M, et al: Transcatheter aortic-valve implantation for aortic stenosis in patients who cannot undergo surgery. *N Engl J Med* 363(17):1597–1607, 2010.
48. Smith CR, Leon MB, Mack MJ, et al: Transcatheter versus surgical aortic-valve replacement in high-risk patients. *N Engl J Med* 364(23):2187–2198, 2011.
49. Makkar RR, Fontana GP, Jilaihawi H, et al: Transcatheter aortic-valve replacement for inoperable severe aortic stenosis. *N Engl J Med* 366(18):1696–1704, 2012.
50. Kodali SK, Williams MR, Smith CR, et al: Two-year outcomes after transcatheter or surgical aortic-valve replacement. *N Engl J Med* 366(18):1686–1695, 2012.
51. Kapadia SR, Tuzcu EM, Makkar RR, et al: Long-term outcomes of inoperable patients with aortic stenosis randomized to transcatheter aortic valve replacement or standard therapy. *Circulation* 130(17):1483–1492, 2014.
52. Thourani VH: Three-year outcomes after transcatheter or surgical aortic valve replacement in high-risk patients with severe aortic stenosis. In American College of Cardiology Annual Scientific Session, San Francisco, CA, 2013.
53. Kapadia SR: Five-year outcomes of transcatheter aortic valve replacement (TAVR) in "inoperable" patients with severe aortic stenosis: the PARTNER trial. In Transcatheter Cardiovascular Therapeutics 26th Annual Symposium, Washington, DC, 2014.
54. Kappetein AP, Head SJ, Genereux P, et al: Updated standardized endpoint definitions for transcatheter aortic valve implantation: the Valve Academic Research Consortium-2 consensus document. *J Thorac Cardiovasc Surg* 145(1):6–23, 2013.
55. Reynolds MR, Magnuson EA, Lei Y, et al: Health-related quality of life after transcatheter aortic valve replacement in inoperable patients with severe aortic stenosis. *Circulation* 124(18):1964–1972, 2011.
56. Reynolds MR, Magnuson EA, Wang K, et al: Health-related quality of life after transcatheter or surgical aortic valve replacement in high-risk patients with severe aortic stenosis: results from the PARTNER (Placement of AoRTic TraNscathetER Valve) trial (Cohort A). *J Am Coll Cardiol* 60(6):548–558, 2012.
57. Genereux P, Webb JG, Svensson LG, et al: Vascular complications after transcatheter aortic valve replacement: insights from the PARTNER (Placement of AoRTic TraNscathetER Valve) trial. *J Am Coll Cardiol* 60(12):1043–1052, 2012.
58. Genereux P, Cohen DJ, Williams MR, et al: Bleeding complications after surgical aortic valve replacement compared with transcatheter aortic valve replacement: insights from the PARTNER I trial (Placement of Aortic Transcatheter Valve). *J Am Coll Cardiol* 63(11):1100–1109, 2014.
59. Williams M, Kodali SK, Hahn RT, et al: Sex-related differences in outcomes after transcatheter or surgical aortic valve replacement in patients with severe aortic stenosis: insights from the PARTNER trial (Placement of Aortic Transcatheter Valve). *J Am Coll Cardiol* 63(15):1522–1528, 2014.
60. Lindman BR, Pibarot P, Arnold SV, et al: Transcatheter versus surgical aortic valve replacement in patients with diabetes and severe aortic stenosis at high risk for surgery: an analysis of the PARTNER trial (Placement of Aortic Transcatheter Valve). *J Am Coll Cardiol* 63(11):1090–1099, 2014.
61. Barbanti M, Webb JG, Hahn RT, et al: Impact of preoperative moderate/severe mitral regurgitation on 2-year outcome after transcatheter and surgical aortic valve replacement: insight from the Placement of Aortic Transcatheter Valve (PARTNER) trial Cohort A. *Circulation* 128(25):2776–2784, 2013.
62. Leon MB: A randomized evaluation of the SAPIEN XT transcatheter valve system in patients with aortic stenosis who are not candidates for surgery: PARTNER II, inoperable cohort. In American College of Cardiology Annual Scientific Session, San Francisco, CA, 2013.
63. Lal P, Upasani P, Kanwar S, et al: First-in-man experience of percutaneous aortic valve replacement using self-expanding CoreValve prosthesis. *Indian Heart J* 63(3):241–244, 2011.
64. Grube E, Laborde JC, Gerckens U, et al: Percutaneous implantation of the CoreValve self-expanding valve prosthesis in high-risk patients with aortic valve disease: the Siegburg first-in-man study. *Circulation* 114(15):1616–1624, 2006.
65. Grube E, Schuler G, Buellesfeld L, et al: Percutaneous aortic valve replacement for severe aortic stenosis in high-risk patients using the second- and current third-generation self-expanding CoreValve prosthesis: device success and 30-day clinical outcome. *J Am Coll Cardiol* 50(1):69–76, 2007.
66. Piazza N, Martucci G, Lachapelle K, et al: First-in-human experience with the Medtronic CoreValve Evolut R. *EuroIntervention* 9(11):1260–1263, 2014.
67. Oguri A, Yamamoto M, Mouillet G, et al: Clinical outcomes and safety of transfemoral aortic valve implantation under general versus local anesthesia: subanalysis of the French Aortic National CoreValve and Edwards 2 registry. *Circ Cardiovasc Interv* 7(4):602–610, 2014.
68. Grube E, Naber C, Abizaid A, et al: Feasibility of transcatheter aortic valve implantation without balloon pre-dilation: a pilot study. *JACC Cardiovasc Interv* 4(7):751–757, 2011.
69. Sinning JM, Hammerstingl C, Vasa-Nicotera M, et al: Aortic regurgitation index defines severity of peri-prosthetic regurgitation and predicts outcome in patients after transcatheter aortic valve implantation. *J Am Coll Cardiol* 59(13):1134–1141, 2012.
70. Zoghbi WA, Chambers JB, Dumesnil JG, et al: Recommendations for evaluation of prosthetic valves with echocardiography and doppler ultrasound: a report from the American Society of Echocardiography's Guidelines and Standards Committee and the Task Force on Prosthetic Valves, developed in conjunction with the American College of Cardiology Cardiovascular Imaging Committee, Cardiac Imaging Committee of the American Heart Association, the European Association of Echocardiography, a registered branch of the European Society of Cardiology, the Japanese Society of Echocardiography and the Canadian Society of Echocardiography, endorsed by the American College of Cardiology Foundation, American Heart Association, European Association of Echocardiography, a registered branch of the European Society of Cardiology, the Japanese Society of Echocardiography, and Canadian Society of Echocardiography. *J Am Soc Echocardiogr* 22(9):975–1014, quiz 1082–1084, 2009.
71. Moynagh AM, Scott DJ, Baumbach A, et al: CoreValve transcatheter aortic valve implantation via the subclavian artery: comparison with the transfemoral approach. *J Am Coll Cardiol* 57(5):634–635, 2011.
72. Reardon MJ, Adams DH, Coselli JS, et al: Self-expanding transcatheter aortic valve replacement using alternative access sites in symptomatic patients with severe aortic stenosis deemed extreme risk of surgery. *J Thorac Cardiovasc Surg* 148(6):2869–2876, 2014.
73. Piazza N, Grube E, Gerckens U, et al: Procedural and 30-day outcomes following transcatheter aortic valve implantation using the third generation (18 Fr) CoreValve Revalving system: results from the multicentre, expanded evaluation registry 1-year following CE mark approval. *EuroIntervention* 4(2):242–249, 2008.
74. Fiorina C, Barbanti M, De Carlo M, et al: One year clinical outcomes in patients with severe aortic stenosis and left ventricular systolic dysfunction undergoing transcatheteter aortic valve implantation: results from the Italian CoreValve Registry. *Int J Cardiol* 168(5):4877–4879, 2013.
75. Barbanti M, Ussia GP, Cannata S, et al: 3-year outcomes of self-expanding CoreValve prosthesis—the Italian Registry. *Ann Cardiothorac Surg* 1(2):182–184, 2012.
76. Meredith IT: The Australia-New Zealand TAVR Registry. In Transcatheter Cardiovascular Therapeutics 24th Annual Scientific Symposium, Miami, FL, 2012.
77. Linke A: 1-Year outcomes in real-world patients treated with transcatheter aortic valve implantation: the ADVANCE study. In EuroPCR, Paris, France, 2013.
78. Khawaja MZ, Rajani R, Cook A, et al: Permanent pacemaker insertion after CoreValve transcatheter aortic valve implantation: incidence and contributing factors (the UK CoreValve Collaborative). *Circulation* 123(9):951–960, 2011.
79. Testa L, Latib A, De Marco F, et al: Clinical impact of persistent left bundle-branch block after transcatheter aortic valve implantation with CoreValve Revalving System. *Circulation* 127(12):1300–1307, 2013.

80. Franzoni I, Latib A, Maisano F, et al: Comparison of incidence and predictors of left bundle branch block after transcatheter aortic valve implantation using the CoreValve versus the Edwards valve. *Am J Cardiol* 112(4):554–559, 2013.
81. Houthuizen P, Van Garsse LA, Poels TT, et al: Left bundle-branch block induced by transcatheter aortic valve implantation increases risk of death. *Circulation* 126(6):720–728, 2012.
82. Nazif TM, Williams MR, Hahn RT, et al: Clinical implications of new-onset left bundle branch block after transcatheter aortic valve replacement: analysis of the PARTNER experience. *Eur Heart J* 35(24):1599–1607, 2014.
83. Urena M, Mok M, Serra V, et al: Predictive factors and long-term clinical consequences of persistent left bundle branch block following transcatheter aortic valve implantation with a balloon-expandable valve. *J Am Coll Cardiol* 60(18):1743–1752, 2012.
84. van der Boon RM, Nuis RJ, Van Mieghem NM, et al: New conduction abnormalities after TAVI—frequency and causes. *Nat Rev Cardiol* 9(8):454–463, 2012.
85. Buellesfeld L, Stortecky S, Heg D, et al: Impact of permanent pacemaker implantation on clinical outcome among patients undergoing transcatheter aortic valve implantation. *J Am Coll Cardiol* 60(6):493–501, 2012.
86. De Carlo M, Giannini C, Bedogni F, et al: Safety of a conservative strategy of permanent pacemaker implantation after transcatheter aortic CoreValve implantation. *Am Heart J* 163(3):492–499, 2012.
87. Adams DH, Popma JJ, Reardon MJ, et al: Transcatheter aortic-valve replacement with a self-expanding prosthesis. *N Engl J Med* 370(19):1790–1798, 2014.
88. Popma JJ, Adams DH, Reardon MJ, et al: Transcatheter aortic valve replacement using a self-expanding bioprosthesis in patients with severe aortic stenosis at extreme risk for surgery. *J Am Coll Cardiol* 63(19):1972–1981, 2014.
89. Moat NE, Ludman P, de Belder MA, et al: Long-term outcomes after transcatheter aortic valve implantation in high-risk patients with severe aortic stenosis: the U.K. TAVI (United Kingdom Transcatheter Aortic Valve Implantation) Registry. *J Am Coll Cardiol* 58(20):2130–2138, 2011.
90. Gilard M, Eltchaninoff H, Iung B, et al: Registry of transcatheter aortic-valve implantation in high-risk patients. *N Engl J Med* 366(18):1705–1715, 2012.
91. Beckmann A, Hamm C, Figulla HR, et al: The German Aortic Valve Registry (GARY): a nationwide registry for patients undergoing invasive therapy for severe aortic valve stenosis. *Thorac Cardiovasc Surg* 60(5):319–325, 2012.
92. Chieffo A, Buchanan GL, Van Mieghem NM, et al: Transcatheter aortic valve implantation with the Edwards SAPIEN versus the Medtronic CoreValve Revalving system devices: a multicenter collaborative study: the PRAGMATIC Plus Initiative (Pooled-RotterdAm-Milano-Toulouse In Collaboration). *J Am Coll Cardiol* 61(8):830–836, 2013.
93. Mack MJ, Brennan JM, Brindis R, et al: Outcomes following transcatheter aortic valve replacement in the United States. *JAMA* 310(19):2069–2077, 2013.
94. Hamm CW, Mollmann H, Holzhey D, et al: The German Aortic Valve Registry (GARY): in-hospital outcome. *Eur Heart J* 35(24):1588–1598, 2013.
95. Mohr FW, Holzhey D, Mollmann H, et al: The German Aortic Valve Registry: 1-year results from 13,680 patients with aortic valve diseasedagger. *Eur J Cardiothorac Surg* 46(5):808–816, 2014.
96. Kotting J, Schiller W, Beckmann A, et al: German Aortic Valve Score: a new scoring system for prediction of mortality related to aortic valve procedures in adults. *Eur J Cardiothorac Surg* 43(5):971–977, 2013.
97. Abdel-Wahab M, Mehilli J, Frerker C, et al: Comparison of balloon-expandable vs self-expandable valves in patients undergoing transcatheter aortic valve replacement: the CHOICE randomized clinical trial. *JAMA* 311(15):1503–1514, 2014.
98. Holmes DR, Brennan Jm, Rumsfeld JS, et al: One year outcomes from the STS/ACC Transcatheter Valve Therapy (TVT) Registry. In American College of Cardiology Annual Scientific Session, Washington, DC, 2014.
99. Wenaweser P, Buellesfeld L, Gerckens U, et al: Percutaneous aortic valve replacement for severe aortic regurgitation in degenerated bioprosthesis: the first valve in valve procedure using the CoreValve Revalving system. *Catheter Cardiovasc Interv* 70(5):760–764, 2007.
100. Bapat V, Attia R, Redwood S, et al: Use of transcatheter heart valves for a valve-in-valve implantation in patients with degenerated aortic bioprosthesis: technical considerations and results. *J Thorac Cardiovasc Surg* 144(6):1372–1379, discussion 1379–1380, 2012.
101. Dvir D, Webb J, Brecker S, et al: Transcatheter aortic valve replacement for degenerative bioprosthetic surgical valves results from the global valve-in-valve registry. *Circulation* 126(19):2335–2344, 2012.
102. Sarkar K, Ussia GP, Tamburino C: Transcatheter aortic valve implantation for severe aortic regurgitation in a stentless bioprosthetic valve with the CoreValve revalving system-technical tips and role of the Accutrak system. *Catheter Cardiovasc Interv* 78(3):485–490, 2011.
103. Seiffert M, Conradi L, Baldus S, et al: Transcatheter mitral valve-in-valve implantation in patients with degenerated bioprostheses. *JACC Cardiovasc Interv* 5(3):341–349, 2012.
104. Webb JG, Wood DA, Ye J, et al: Transcatheter valve-in-valve implantation for failed bioprosthetic heart valves. *Circulation* 121(16):1848–1857, 2010.
105. Cerillo AG, Chiaramonti F, Murzi M, et al: Transcatheter valve in valve implantation for failed mitral and tricuspid bioprosthesis. *Catheter Cardiovasc Interv* 78(7):987–995, 2011.
106. Seiffert M, Franzen O, Conradi L, et al: Series of transcatheter valve-in-valve implantations in high-risk patients with degenerated bioprostheses in aortic and mitral position. *Catheter Cardiovasc Interv* 76(4):608–615, 2010.
107. Descoutures F, Himbert D, Maisano F, et al: Transcatheter valve-in-ring implantation after failure of surgical mitral repair. *Eur J Cardiothorac Surg* 44(1):e8–e15, 2013.
108. Lange R, Bleiziffer S, Mazzitelli D, et al: Improvements in transcatheter aortic valve implantation outcomes in lower surgical risk patients: a glimpse into the future. *J Am Coll Cardiol* 59(3):280–287, 2012.
109. Wenaweser P, Stortecky S, Schwander S, et al: Clinical outcomes of patients with estimated low or intermediate surgical risk undergoing transcatheter aortic valve implantation. *Eur Heart J* 34(25):1894–1905, 2013.
110. D'Errigo P, Barbanti M, Ranucci M, et al: Transcatheter aortic valve implantation versus surgical aortic valve replacement for severe aortic stenosis: results from an intermediate risk propensity-matched population of the Italian OBSERVANT study. *Int J Cardiol* 167(5):1945–1952, 2013.
111. Latib A, Maisano F, Bertoldi L, et al: Transcatheter vs surgical aortic valve replacement in intermediate-surgical-risk patients with aortic stenosis: a propensity score-matched case-control study. *Am Heart J* 164(6):910–917, 2012.
112. Piazza N, Kalesan B, van Mieghem N, et al: A 3-center comparison of 1-year mortality outcomes between transcatheter aortic valve implantation and surgical aortic valve replacement on the basis of propensity score matching among intermediate-risk surgical patients. *JACC Cardiovasc Interv* 6(5):443–451, 2013.
113. Daneault B, Kirtane AJ, Kodali SK, et al: Stroke associated with surgical and transcatheter treatment of aortic stenosis: a comprehensive review. *J Am Coll Cardiol* 58(21):2143–2150, 2011.
114. Zegdi R, Lecuyer L, Achouh P, et al: Increased radial force improves stent deployment in tricuspid but not in bicuspid stenotic native aortic valves. *Ann Thorac Surg* 89(3):768–772, 2010.
115. Svensson LG: Aortic valve stenosis and regurgitation: an overview of management. *J Cardiovasc Surg (Torino)* 49(2):297–303, 2008.
116. Chiam PT, Chao VT, Tan SY, et al: Percutaneous transcatheter heart valve implantation in a bicuspid aortic valve. *JACC Cardiovasc Interv* 3(5):559–561, 2010.
117. Hayashida K, Bouvier E, Lefevre T, et al: Transcatheter aortic valve implantation for patients with severe bicuspid aortic valve stenosis. *Circ Cardiovasc Interv* 6(3):284–291, 2013.
118. Himbert D, Pontnau F, Messika-Zeitoun D, et al: Feasibility and outcomes of transcatheter aortic valve implantation in high-risk patients with stenotic bicuspid aortic valves. *Am J Cardiol* 110(6):877–883, 2012.
119. Kochman J, Huczek Z, Koltowski L, et al: Transcatheter implantation of an aortic valve prosthesis in a female patient with severe bicuspid aortic stenosis. *Eur Heart J* 33(1):112, 2012.
120. Wijesinghe N, Ye J, Rodes-Cabau J, et al: Transcatheter aortic valve implantation in patients with bicuspid aortic valve stenosis. *JACC Cardiovasc Interv* 3(11):1122–1125, 2010.
121. Yousef A, Simard T, Pourdjabbar A, et al: Performance of transcatheter aortic valve implantation in patients with bicuspid aortic valve: systematic review. *Int J Cardiol* 176(2):562–564, 2014.
122. Mylotte D: Transcatheter aortic valve replacement in bicuspid aortic valve disease. In American College of Cardiology (ACC)/i2 Scientific Session, Washington, DC, 2014.
123. Testa L, Latib A, Rossi ML, et al: CoreValve implantation for severe aortic regurgitation: a multicentre registry. *EuroIntervention* 10(6):739–745, 2014.
124. Seiffert M, Diemert P, Koschyk D, et al: Transapical implantation of a second-generation transcatheter heart valve in patients with noncalcified aortic regurgitation. *JACC Cardiovasc Interv* 6(6):590–597, 2013.
125. Genereux P, Head SJ, Van Mieghem NM, et al: Clinical outcomes after transcatheter aortic valve replacement using valve academic research consortium definitions: a weighted meta-analysis of 3,519 patients from 16 studies. *J Am Coll Cardiol* 59(25):2317–2326, 2012.
126. Eggebrecht H, Schmermund A, Voigtlander T, et al: Risk of stroke after transcatheter aortic valve implantation (TAVI): a meta-analysis of 10,037 published patients. *EuroIntervention* 8(1):129–138, 2012.
127. Hahn RT, Pibarot P, Webb J, et al: Outcomes with post-dilation following transcatheter aortic valve replacement: the PARTNER I trial (placement of aortic transcatheter valve). *JACC Cardiovasc Interv* 7(7):781–789, 2014.
128. Nombela-Franco L, Rodes-Cabau J, DeLarochelliere R, et al: Predictive factors, efficacy, and safety of balloon post-dilation after transcatheter aortic valve implantation with a balloon-expandable valve. *JACC Cardiovasc Interv* 5(5):499–512, 2012.
129. Athappan G, Gajulapalli RD, Sengodan P, et al: Influence of transcatheter aortic valve replacement strategy and valve design on stroke after transcatheter aortic valve replacement: a meta-analysis and systematic review of literature. *J Am Coll Cardiol* 63(20):2101–2110, 2014.
130. Amat-Santos IJ, Rodes-Cabau J, Urena M, et al: Incidence, predictive factors, and prognostic value of new-onset atrial fibrillation following transcatheter aortic valve implantation. *J Am Coll Cardiol* 59(2):178–188, 2012.
131. Kahlert P, Knipp SC, Schlamann M, et al: Silent and apparent cerebral ischemia after percutaneous transfemoral aortic valve implantation: a diffusion-weighted magnetic resonance imaging study. *Circulation* 121(7):870–878, 2010.
132. Van Mieghem NM, Schipper ME, Ladich E, et al: Histopathology of embolic debris captured during transcatheter aortic valve replacement. *Circulation* 127(22):2194–2201, 2013.
133. Athappan G, Patvardhan E, Tuzcu EM, et al: Incidence, predictors, and outcomes of aortic regurgitation after transcatheter aortic valve replacement: meta-analysis and systematic review of literature. *J Am Coll Cardiol* 61(15):1585–1595, 2013.
134. Genereux P, Head SJ, Hahn R, et al: Paravalvular leak after transcatheter aortic valve replacement: the new Achilles' heel? A comprehensive review of the literature. *J Am Coll Cardiol* 61(11):1125–1136, 2013.
135. Hahn RT, Pibarot P, Stewart WJ, et al: Comparison of transcatheter and surgical aortic valve replacement in severe aortic stenosis: a longitudinal study of echocardiography parameters in cohort A of the PARTNER trial (placement of aortic transcatheter valves). *J Am Coll Cardiol* 61(25):2514–2521, 2013.
136. Kodali S, Pibarot P, Douglas PS, et al: Paravalvular regurgitation after transcatheter aortic valve replacement with the Edwards SAPIEN Valve in the PARTNER trial: characterizing patients and impact on outcomes. *Eur Heart J* 2014. pii: ehu384 [Epub ahead of print].
137. Lerakis S, Hayek SS, Douglas PS: Paravalvular aortic leak after transcatheter aortic valve replacement: current knowledge. *Circulation* 127(3):397–407, 2013.
138. Tamburino C, Capodanno D, Ramondo A, et al: Incidence and predictors of early and late mortality after transcatheter aortic valve implantation in 663 patients with severe aortic stenosis. *Circulation* 123(3):299–308, 2011.
139. Nombela-Franco L, Ruel M, Radhakrishnan S, et al: Comparison of hemodynamic performance of self-expandable CoreValve versus balloon-expandable Edwards SAPIEN aortic valves inserted by catheter for aortic stenosis. *Am J Cardiol* 111(7):1026–1033, 2013.
140. Watanabe Y, Hayashida K, Yamamoto M, et al: Transfemoral aortic valve implantation in patients with an annulus dimension suitable for either the Edwards valve or the CoreValve. *Am J Cardiol* 112(5):707–713, 2013.
141. Gripari P, Ewe SH, Fusini L, et al: Intraoperative 2D and 3D transoesophageal echocardiographic predictors of aortic regurgitation after transcatheter aortic valve implantation. *Heart* 98(16):1229–1236, 2012.
142. John D, Buellesfeld L, Yuecel S, et al: Correlation of device landing zone calcification and acute procedural success in patients undergoing transcatheter aortic valve implantations with the self-expanding CoreValve prosthesis. *JACC Cardiovasc Interv* 3(2):233–243, 2010.
143. Marwan M, Achenbach S, Ensminger SM, et al: CT predictors of post-procedural aortic regurgitation in patients referred for transcatheter aortic valve implantation: an analysis of 105 patients. *Int J Cardiovasc Imaging* 29(5):1191–1198, 2013.
144. Detaint D, Lepage L, Himbert D, et al: Determinants of significant paravalvular regurgitation after transcatheter aortic valve: implantation impact of device and annulus discongruence. *JACC Cardiovasc Interv* 2(9):821–827, 2009.
145. Schultz C, Rossi A, van Mieghem N, et al: Aortic annulus dimensions and leaflet calcification from contrast MSCT predict the need for balloon post-dilatation after TAVI with the Medtronic CoreValve prosthesis. *EuroIntervention* 7(5):564–572, 2011.
146. Daneault B, Koss E, Hahn RT, et al: Efficacy and safety of postdilatation to reduce paravalvular regurgitation during balloon-expandable transcatheter aortic valve replacement. *Circ Cardiovasc Interv* 6(1):85–91, 2013.
147. Makkar RR, Jilaihawi H, Chakravarty T, et al: Determinants and outcomes of acute transcatheter valve-in-valve therapy or embolization: a study of multiple valve implants in the U.S. PARTNER trial (Placement of AoRTic TraNscathetER Valve Trial Edwards SAPIEN Transcatheter Heart Valve). *J Am Coll Cardiol* 62(5):418–430, 2013.
148. Aktug O, Dohmen G, Brehmer K, et al: Incidence and predictors of left bundle branch block after transcatheter aortic valve implantation. *Int J Cardiol* 160(1):26–30, 2012.
149. Piazza N, Onuma Y, Jesserun E, et al: Early and persistent intraventricular conduction abnormalities and requirements for pacemaking after percutaneous replacement of the aortic valve. *JACC Cardiovasc Interv* 1(3):310–316, 2008.
150. Erkapic D, De Rosa S, Kelava A, et al: Risk for permanent pacemaker after transcatheter aortic valve implantation: a comprehensive analysis of the literature. *J Cardiovasc Electrophysiol* 23(4):391–397, 2012.
151. Khatri PJ, Webb JG, Rodes-Cabau J, et al: Adverse effects associated with transcatheter aortic valve implantation: a meta-analysis of contemporary studies. *Ann Intern Med* 158(1):35–46, 2013.
152. Urena M, Webb JG, Tamburino C, et al: Permanent pacemaker implantation after transcatheter aortic valve implantation: impact on late clinical outcomes and left ventricular function. *Circulation* 129(11):1233–1243, 2014.

153. Genereux P, Kodali S, Leon MB, et al: Clinical outcomes using a new crossover balloon occlusion technique for percutaneous closure after transfemoral aortic valve implantation. *JACC Cardiovasc Interv* 4(8):861–867, 2011.
154. Hayashida K, Lefevre T, Chevalier B, et al: True percutaneous approach for transfemoral aortic valve implantation using the Prostar XL device: impact of learning curve on vascular complications. *JACC Cardiovasc Interv* 5(2):207–214, 2012.
155. Stortecky S, Wenaweser P, Diehm N, et al: Percutaneous management of vascular complications in patients undergoing transcatheter aortic valve implantation. *JACC Cardiovasc Interv* 5(5):515–524, 2012.
156. Cota L, Stabile E, Agrusta M, et al: Bioprostheses "thrombosis" after transcatheter aortic valve replacement. *J Am Coll Cardiol* 61(7):789–791, 2013.
157. Latib A, Messika-Zeitoun D, Maisano F, et al: Reversible Edwards SAPIEN XT dysfunction due to prosthesis thrombosis presenting as early structural deterioration. *J Am Coll Cardiol* 61(7):787–789, 2013.
158. Sorajja P, Booker JD, Rihal CS: Alcohol septal ablation after transaortic valve implantation: the dynamic nature of left outflow tract obstruction. *Catheter Cardiovasc Interv* 81(2):387–391, 2013.
159. Ribeiro HB, Webb JG, Makkar RR, et al: Predictive factors, management, and clinical outcomes of coronary obstruction following transcatheter aortic valve implantation: insights from a large multicenter registry. *J Am Coll Cardiol* 62(17):1552–1562, 2013.
160. Barbanti M, Yang TH, Rodes Cabau J, et al: Anatomical and procedural features associated with aortic root rupture during balloon-expandable transcatheter aortic valve replacement. *Circulation* 128(3):244–253, 2013.
161. Ribeiro HB, Urena M, Kuck KH, et al: Edwards CENTERA valve. *EuroIntervention* 8(Suppl Q):Q79–Q82, 2012.
162. Urena M, Doyle D, Rodes-Cabau J, et al: Initial experience of transcatheter aortic valve replacement with the St. Jude Medical Portico valve inserted through the transapical approach. *J Thorac Cardiovasc Surg* 146(4):e24–e27, 2013.
163. Kempfert J, Treede H, Rastan AJ, et al: Transapical aortic valve implantation using a new self-expandable bioprosthesis (ACURATE TA): 6-month outcomes. *Eur J Cardiothorac Surg* 43(1):52–56, discussion 57, 2013.
164. Mollmann H, Diemert P, Grube E, et al: Symetis ACURATE TF aortic bioprosthesis. *EuroIntervention* 9(Suppl):S107–S110, 2013.
165. Holzhey D, Linke A, Treede H, et al: Intermediate follow-up results from the multicenter engager European pivotal trial. *Ann Thorac Surg* 96(6):2095–2100, 2013.
166. Schofer J, Colombo A, Klugmann S, et al: Prospective multicenter evaluation of the direct flow medical transcatheter aortic valve. *J Am Coll Cardiol* 63(8):763–768, 2014.
167. Ensminger S: First results of the JUPITER Registy on long-term performance and safety of the transapical JenaValve. In EuroPCR, Paris, France, 2013.
168. Meredith IT: REPRISE II: A prospective registry study of transcatheter aortic valve replacement with a repositionable transcatheter heart valve in patients with severe aortic stenosis. In PCR London Valves, London, U.K., 2013.

30 Transcatheter Mitral Valve Intervention

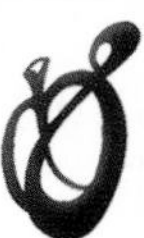

Saif Anwaruddin and Howard C. Herrmann

Section I: Mitral Stenosis

INTRODUCTION

Normal Mitral Valve Anatomy

To appreciate the complexity of the mitral valve is to understand its intricate anatomical and physiologic properties. The mitral valve can be divided into several components, each one important in maintaining proper valve functionality. The mitral valve consists of two leaflets, a posterior leaflet with three distinct scallops and a corresponding, but much larger, anterior leaflet. The two mitral valve leaflets are continuous with each other and maintain a connection at the commissures. The anterior leaflet is continuous with the ascending aorta and the membranous ventricular septum. The leaflets anchor to the myocardium by way of two papillary muscles, the anterolateral and posteromedial. The anterolateral papillary muscle is usually the larger of the two structures. The attachment between the papillary muscle and the valve leaflets occurs by way of chordae tendinae.

With systolic contraction of the left ventricular (LV) cavity, the resultant traction of the papillary muscles leads to valve closure by transmission of the force through the chordae. The chordae tendinae insert on the underside of the leaflet tissue. Blood in the ventricular chamber passes through interchordal spaces on its route from the left atrium.

The two mitral valve leaflets attach to the base of the left atrium to a thin ovoid-shaped membrane—the mitral valve annulus. The annulus itself is a nonplanar saddle-shaped structure, which functions to influence valve competency.[1] In close proximity to the anterior portion of the mitral valve annulus are two fibrous trigones, which are separated by the fibrous intertrigonal region. The posterior portion of the annulus is not surrounded by any fibrous tissue, however, and serves to separate the ventricular tissue from the atria.

The coronary sinus generally lies close to the posterior side of the mitral valve annulus. This anatomic relationship allows for the use of percutaneous annuloplasty techniques. There is variability in the relationship between the annulus and the coronary sinus and is likely influenced by the size of the left atrium and other factors. For the purpose of percutaneous interventions on the mitral valve apparatus, it is important to consider the relationship between the coronary sinus and the course of the left circumflex coronary artery. Cardiac computed tomography has been used to demonstrate that the left circumflex artery crosses between the mitral annulus and the coronary sinus in the vast majority of patients with significant variability in the location of crossover.[2]

Disease of the mitral valve can be primarily valvular, or secondary to other processes, notably those affecting the myocardium. The standard of care for treatment of mitral valve disease has been primarily surgical. Several percutaneous approaches to treating mitral valve disease have emerged and continue to evolve as possible alternatives to surgical treatment, particularly in those patients not considered appropriate surgical candidates. As such, an appreciation for the complexity of mitral valve anatomy is necessary to understand how, and why, percutaneous approaches work in treatment of mitral valve disease.

MITRAL VALVE DISEASE STATES: MITRAL STENOSIS

Etiologies of Mitral Stenosis

The primary disturbance in mitral stenosis is an obstruction to the inflow of blood from the left atrium into the left ventricle during diastole. Worldwide, the primary etiology of mitral stenosis is rheumatic heart disease. Rheumatic changes can affect the mitral valve itself and the subvalvular apparatus as well. Less common etiologies for mitral stenosis include congenital abnormalities such as cor triatriatum and parachute mitral valve, and noncongenital etiologies such as left atrial (LA) myxoma, endocarditis, carcinoid, mucopolysaccharidosis, rheumatoid arthritis, and systemic lupus erythematosus, among others.

Lutembacher syndrome denotes the presence of a secondary atrial septal defect and rheumatic mitral stenosis. In the elderly population, severe mitral annular calcifications can lead to varying degrees of mitral stenosis and mitral regurgitation. For the remainder of the discussion on mitral stenosis and its treatment by percutaneous balloon mitral valvuloplasty, we will focus only rheumatic mitral stenosis.

Pathology of Rheumatic Mitral Stenosis

As mentioned, the most common etiology for mitral stenosis, worldwide, is rheumatic heart disease. In patients with rheumatic mitral stenosis, as many as half of patients are not aware of a prior history of rheumatic fever. Following an episode of acute rheumatic fever, it may take several years prior to the development of mitral stenosis and many more years until the development of symptoms. Progression of disease and development of clinical symptoms correlate with episodes of rheumatic fever.[3] Ongoing inflammatory insults affecting the valve may result in eventual clinical manifestations.

The basis for the development of mitral stenosis following streptococcal infection is believed to be molecular mimicry. The similarity between streptococcal bacterial M protein and human cardiac proteins (myosin and others) is likely the reason for molecular mimicry between the two organisms. Humoral and cellular responses are important in the pathogenesis, and the CD4+ T cell response is the main culprit of the molecular mimicry response affecting cardiac tissue.[4]

In rheumatic mitral stenosis, there is diffuse fibrous thickening of the mitral valve leaflets with calcific deposits. In addition to fibrous thickening, there is fusion of the leaflet commissures along with shortening and fusion of the subvalvular chordae tendinae. The amount of calcification of the valve leaflets itself is variable. This process is not, however, limited to the valves as it affects the three layers of the heart as well with increased amounts of fibrous tissue.

Pathophysiology of Rheumatic Mitral Stenosis

In addition to the characteristic findings of mitral stenosis upon the valve, these structures can also be affected by concomitant calcification. In combination, these changes result in significant restriction in the opening of the mitral leaflet. As such, there is severe reduction in size of the mitral valve orifice leading to a funnel-shaped orifice often described as "fish mouth" in appearance. Also, there can be associated mitral regurgitation due to leaflet malcoaptation arising from fibrosis and shortening of the subvalvular apparatus, including the chordae.

The end result of these changes upon the mitral valve complex is a restriction of blood flow across the mitral valve orifice. The normal mitral valve has an orifice area of between 4 cm^2 to 6 cm^2. Mitral stenosis is a slowly progressive disease that worsens over the course of many years. With a reduction in mitral valve orifice area, a higher transvalvular pressure gradient may develop, leading to increased LA pressure. There is then transmission of elevated LA pressure into the pulmonary vasculature, eventually leading to the development of pulmonary venous pressures. Long standing mitral stenosis and increased LA pressures can lead to severe and irreversible pulmonary hypertension both from elevated LA pressures, pulmonary vascular constriction, and obliterative changes to the vasculature.

With chronically elevated pulmonary arterial pressures in long-standing and untreated mitral stenosis, patients can develop right ventricular dilation and dysfunction over time. With development of severe tricuspid valve regurgitation as a consequence, signs and symptoms of right heart failure can develop. Most patients will start to develop symptoms when the mitral valve area (MVA) is between 1.0 cm^2 and 1.5 cm^2 in area. It is important to understand that the process can affect other valves and the myocardium, leading to ventricular dysfunction, which can contribute to symptoms.

Clinical Presentation of Mitral Stenosis

Clinical Manifestations

Patients will often present with symptoms related to mitral stenosis several years to decades after their initial bout of rheumatic fever. In developing countries this may occur sooner due to repeat bouts of rheumatic fever. With development of symptoms, long-term survival is severely compromised.

According to the World Health Organization, reliable statistics on the incidence and prevalence of rheumatic fever are not easily available. However, the annual incidence in developing countries has been reported to vary between 1 per 100,000 school-age children to over 150 per 100,000 school-age children. The prevalence of rheumatic heart disease varies from between 0.5 per 1000 school-age children in developed countries to over 70 per 1000 school-age children in other developing countries. It is reported that rates vary even within developing countries, and hospital admissions for rheumatic heart disease vary between 12% and 65%.[5]

The diagnosis of rheumatic fever is made based on the Jones Criteria, first published by Dr. T. Duckett Jones in 1944, and since revised. The presence of two major, or one major and two minor, criteria must be met. The major criteria include carditis, polyarthritis, erythema marginatum, chorea, and subcutaneous nodules. The minor criteria include fever, arthralgias, elevated sedimentation rate, elevated C reactive protein, and a prolonged PR interval. These findings are used in the context of a documented Group A β-hemolytic streptococcal throat infection.

Although the progression in the rate of mitral valve stenosis is variable, it is estimated to be about a 0.1 cm^2 reduction in valve area per year.[6] The onset of clinical manifestations is also variable. The primary symptom in mitral valve stenosis is exertional dyspnea secondary to elevated LA pressures and elevated pulmonary venous and arterial pressures. This is often accompanied by orthopnea, coughing, and wheezing. Even when mitral stenosis is less advanced, co-existent conditions such as anemia, pregnancy, infection, atrial fibrillation, exertion, or fever can precipitate symptoms by decreasing diastolic filling time and increasing blood flow across the stenotic mitral orifice.

With progression of disease, patients can experience pulmonary edema, atrial fibrillation, pulmonary hemorrhage from rupture of dilated bronchial veins, and chest pain. Other less common symptoms include systemic embolization, clinical signs and symptoms of right heart failure, and hoarseness due to compression of the left recurrent

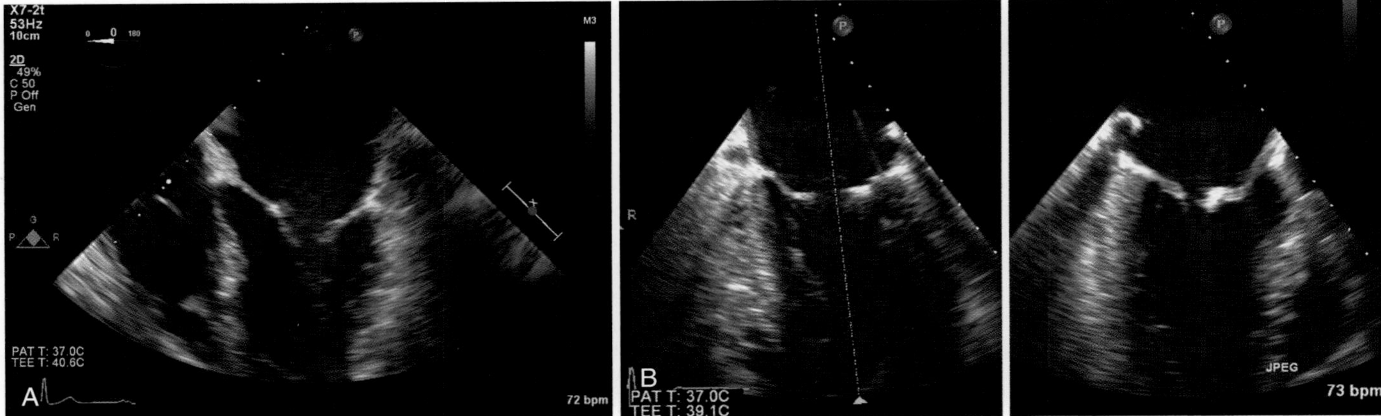

FIGURE 30-1 **A,** Transesophageal echocardiogram (TEE) demonstrating rheumatic mitral stenosis. Note the leaflet thickening and restricted opening of the valve leaflets. **B,** TEE of mitral valve opening and closing in a patient with rheumatic mitral stenosis.

laryngeal nerve by dilated pulmonary artery, enlarged lymph nodes, or an enlarged left atrium (Ortner's syndrome).

Clinical Assessment

History and Physical Examination

Oftentimes, obtaining a history in a patient with rheumatic mitral stenosis will not reliably reveal a prior history of rheumatic fever. Furthermore, given the slow progression of the disease, many patients will report being asymptomatic and deny frank exertional dyspnea. It is important to note that given the slow progression, patients will reduce their level of activity to remain without symptoms.

The patient with severe mitral stenosis will demonstrate purple and pink patches on the cheeks termed "mitral facies."[7] It is important to remember that in severe mitral stenosis, LA function may be normal and LA filling pressures may be low or normal. As such, palpation of the left ventricle will likely reveal a normal apical impulse. With palpation, a left parasternal right ventricular heave can sometimes be appreciated in the setting of pulmonary hypertension. Jugular venous pressure can be elevated in the setting of right ventricular dysfunction.

Auscultation of the patient with severe mitral stenosis will reveal several characteristics about the mitral valve itself. The characteristic findings on auscultation are that of a loud S1, an opening snap (OS), and a mid-diastolic murmur, described as a rumble. The opening snap follows A2 and can be best heard at the left lower sternal border. The pliability of anterior mitral leaflet is the source of the sound for the OS. The opening snap usually follows the A2 sound by 0.04 seconds to 0.12 seconds. During exhalation, it is possible to differentiate the physiologic splitting of the second heart sound from the OS, as the two sounds are that of the S2 followed by the OS. The duration of time between the A2 and the OS is also a marker of severity of disease. Specifically, increased pressure gradient or elevated LA pressure leads to faster opening of the mitral valve in diastole. As such, the time duration between A2 and OS will be markedly shorter in the setting of higher LA pressure and severity of mitral stenosis. Maneuvers that decrease venous blood return will serve to increase the A2 to OS interval.

The diastolic murmur of mitral stenosis is best appreciated with the patient in the left lateral decubitus position and is often described as a low pitch rumble at the apex. The duration of the murmur is a marker for severity of disease as it is driven by the gradient across the left atrium and ventricle. Maneuvers such as exhalation can accentuate the MS murmur and Valsalva can serve to decrease the intensity of the diastolic murmur due to a reduction in flow across the mitral valve.

Clinical Assessment with Diagnostic Tools

The diagnostic workup of the patient with mitral stenosis relies heavily on the echocardiographic findings. The electrocardiogram (ECG) and chest x-ray are at times helpful, but the diagnosis squarely rests on the results of noninvasive imaging. The ECG will often reveal findings consistent with LA enlargement and the chest x-ray can demonstrate LA enlargement as well as enlargement of the pulmonary vasculature and pulmonary edema, on occasion.

Echocardiography

Transthoracic (TTE) or transesophageal (TEE) echocardiography can be used to diagnose and to determine severity of mitral stenosis (**Figure 30-1AB**). TTE can be helpful in the assessment of the morphology, mobility, and function of the mitral valve itself. The characteristic thickening and doming, or "hockey stick" appearance, of the anterior mitral leaflet can be appreciated in the parasternal long axis on TTE. There is a reduction in leaflet mobility noted and TTE can also be used to quantify the degree of mitral regurgitation, if any. In addition, TTE can be useful in the assessment of the subvalvular apparatus, the degree of calcification of the valve leaflets, commissures and the subvalvular apparatus, pulmonary arterial pressures, and concomitant valvular disease.

Determining the morphology of the mitral valve and the subvalvular apparatus is important in preprocedural planning for balloon mitral valvuloplasty. The suitability of a valve for balloon mitral valvuloplasty can be determined using the Wilkins criteria, which scores four features of the valve including leaflet mobility, leaflet thickening, leaflet calcification, subvalvular calcification, and thickening. Each feature is assigned a score from 1 to 4 and higher valve scores (maximum of 16) predict unfavorable outcomes with mitral valvuloplasty.[8]

Assessment of mitral valve gradients is best performed with TTE in the apical-4 chamber view with the Doppler beam parallel to the mitral jet so as to obtain the most accurate gradients. Assessment of MVA with TTE can be

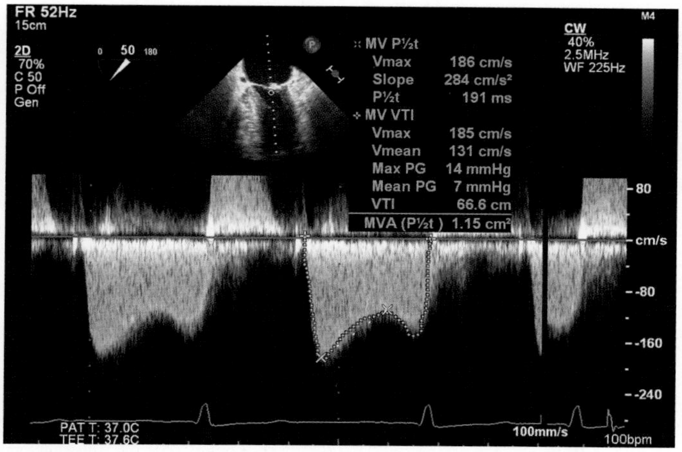

FIGURE 30-2 Calculating mitral valve area in a patient with rheumatic mitral stenosis using the pressure half-time formula.

performed with planimetry, continuity equation, or with pressure half-time (PHT) measurements. Planimetry of the mitral valve orifice is performed using the parasternal short axis view and it is important to start imaging at the apex and move upwards so as to identify the smallest mitral valve orifice for measurement. This method can at times lead to overestimation of the MVA if the imaging plane is proximal to the true orifice or due to irregularities in the orifice itself.

The PHT is a flow-dependent method that estimates MVA based on the time needed for the peak gradient across the valve to fall by half (**Figure 30-2**). The slope derived from this decrease is related to the degree of stenosis. With more severe stenosis, there is a larger gradient and a smaller mitral orifice, which will result in a longer time for pressure decline and a longer PHT. With PHT, one can calculate MVA as follows:

$$\mathbf{MVA = 220/PHT}$$

In situations where there is an alteration in the LA or LV pressures, the PHT measurement can be unreliable. In the setting of LV dysfunction with increased LVEDP, the PHT will be shortened, thus overestimating the MVA. In patients with severe aortic regurgitation, the rise in LV end-diastolic pressure (EDP) can also lead to shortening of the PHT and an overestimation of the MVA.

TEE can be used to further assess the morphology of the mitral valve and the subvalvular apparatus. Prior to catheter-based intervention, TEE can be used to assess for LA, or LA appendage thrombus, in patients with atrial fibrillation. TEE can also be used to help guide catheter-based interventions including safely crossing the atrial septum into the left atrium and to assess mitral valve morphology post-balloon valvuloplasty.

Exercise stress echocardiography can also be utilized in the assessment of mitral valve stenosis severity. It can be used to evaluate exercise tolerance in mitral stenosis patients who are otherwise asymptomatic or to assess severity of otherwise mild mitral stenosis at rest in patients with clear symptoms. Exercise testing can also be performed with a pulmonary artery catheter. Significant increases in PA systolic pressures or mean mitral valve gradients can help identify patients who would benefit from mitral valuloplasty.[9]

Cardiac Catheterization and Angiography

While echocardiography remains the mainstay of diagnosis, cardiac catheterization is not only a confirmatory diagnostic modality, as it serves to resolve discrepancies between clinical and noninvasive imaging findings, assess for coronary atherosclerosis as an etiology for symptoms, or prior to mitral valve surgery. It also serves to help determine the role of mitral stenosis in patients with concomitant lung disease.

Assessment of mitral valve gradients can be accomplished using an LV pigtail catheter and a PA catheter with pulmonary capillary wedge pressure (PCWP) measurements as a surrogate for LA pressure. The PCWP tends to overestimate the gradients across the mitral valve. The use of the PCWP may be unreliable in patients with pulmonary veno-occlusive disease. Direct measurement of the LA pressure can also be accomplished by crossing the atrial septum under fluoroscopic or echocardiographic guidance. Accurate gradients can be calculated using direct LA and LV measurements (**Figure 30-3AB**).

MVA can be calculated using the Gorlin formula. Cardiac output can be calculated using right heart catheterization with the thermodilution, or Fick measurements. In patients with low output or concomitant regurgitant valvular lesions, Fick measurements of cardiac output may be more accurate. The Gorlin formula is as follows:

$$\mathbf{MVA\ (cm^2) = [SV/DFP] / [K * (sq\ rt\ mean\ MV\ gradient)]}$$

Where SV equals stroke volume, DFP equals diastolic filling period (sec), and K is a constant, which is 37.7 for the MV. The Hakki formula can also be used to calculate MVA as follows:

$$\mathbf{MVA\ (cm^2) = CO/(sq\ rt\ mean\ MV\ gradient)}$$

In patients with mitral stenosis and atrial fibrillation, the mean mitral valve gradient should be averaged over 10 beats. Measurements of gradients and calculations of valve area are highly dependent on flow and heart rate. Elevated gradients will be noted in conditions that cause tachycardia or decrease the diastolic filling period.

MANAGEMENT OF MITRAL STENOSIS

Medical Therapy for Mitral Stenosis

Antibiotic therapy is the mainstay of therapy in patients with rheumatic fever and prophylaxis in certain populations to reduce the risk of recurrence. In patients with rheumatic heart disease, medical therapy is aimed at improving symptoms and reducing conditions that lead to tachycardia. Diuretics and careful restriction of sodium intake can be used for treatment of pulmonary edema and pulmonary venous congestion in symptomatic patients. Treatment of anemia, dehydration, concomitant thyroid disease, fever, infection, or other conditions can help to alleviate symptoms in patients with mitral stenosis.

The use of β-blockers and calcium channel blockers can be used to lower heart rate and increase diastolic filling time. In the setting of atrial fibrillation, which occurs not uncommonly in patients with mitral stenosis, the goals of treatment should be rate control with β-blockers, calcium channel blockers, digoxin, or consideration of electrical cardioversion after exclusion of LA thrombus by TEE. In situations where atrial fibrillation with rapid ventricular rates is

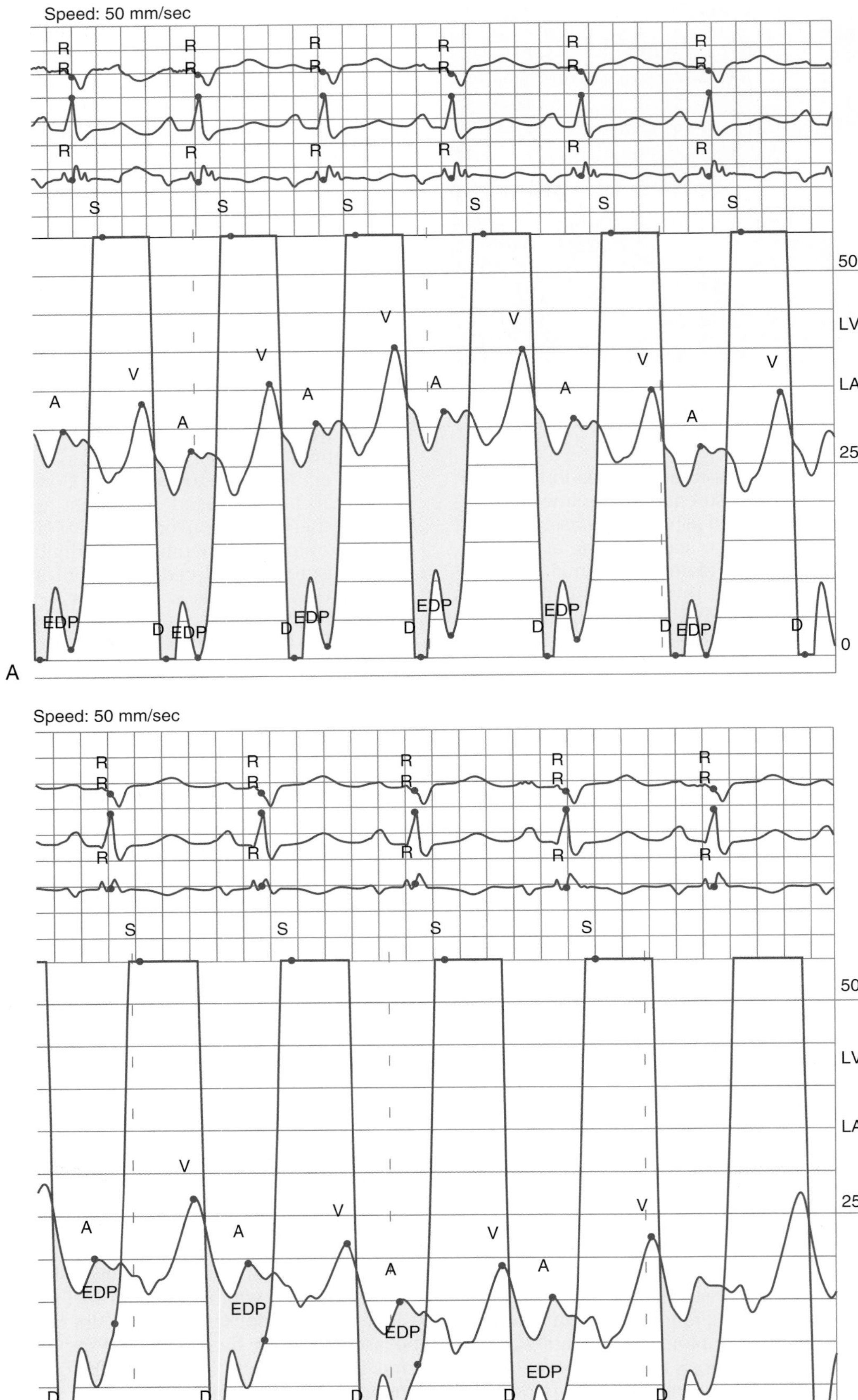

FIGURE 30-3 **A,** Direct left atrial (LA) and left ventricular (LV) pressure tracings demonstrating a gradient of 23 mm Hg from rheumatic mitral stenosis. **B,** Direct left atrial and left ventricular pressure tracings following a single inflation of a balloon in a percutaneous balloon mitral valvuloplasty on the same patient in **A.** The mean gradient is between 11 to 12 mm Hg. *EDP*, End-diastolic pressure.

not well tolerated hemodynamically, emergent cardioversion may be necessary in absence of an assessment for LA thrombus. Anticoagulation should be initiated in any patient with mitral stenosis and atrial fibrillation assuming no other contraindications. Given the risk of systemic embolization, anticoagulation has been suggested in mitral stenosis patients even without evidence of atrial fibrillation. Per the American College of Cardiology/American Heart Association (ACC/AHA) Guidelines, anticoagulation is a Class I indication in those patients with atrial fibrillation, prior embolic event, and with evidence for LA thrombus. Anticoagulation is a Class IIb recommendation in patients with severe MS and dilated left atrium, or with evidence of spontaneous echo contrast.[10] Post mitral valve intervention, atrial fibrillation can persist and will need to be managed appropriately.

Catheter-Based Treatment of Mitral Stenosis

Indications for Catheter-Based Treatment

Percutaneous mitral balloon valvuloplasty (PMBV) as a treatment for rheumatic mitral stenosis was first described separately both by Inoue and Lock in the mid-1980s. Prior to this, surgery was the only treatment modality. PMBV is indicated in symptomatic mitral stenosis patients who have at least moderate to severe mitral stenosis, favorable valve morphology for PMBV with the absence of LA thrombus, or moderate to severe mitral regurgitation. In patients with moderate to severe mitral stenosis without symptoms and favorable mitral valve morphology, PMBV can be used in treating patients with pulmonary hypertension (PASP at rest of at least 50 mm Hg or >60 mm Hg with exercise) assuming absence of LA thrombus, or moderate to severe mitral regurgitation. In patients with rheumatic mitral stenosis with calcified nonpliable valves and who are at high-risk or unsuitable for open surgery, PMBV is also a reasonable alternative in symptomatic patients with moderate to severe MS.

Per the ACC/AHA Updated Valve Guidelines, PMBV can be considered in an asymptomatic patient with moderate to severe mitral stenosis and new onset atrial fibrillation after excluding LA thrombus, or moderate to severe mitral regurgitation (IIb). In patients with symptoms and mild MS (MVA >1.5 cm^2), PMBV can be considered if there is evidence of significant mitral stenosis on exercise (IIb).[10]

The proposed mechanism of benefit for patients from PMBV is separation of the fused commissures, which acts to relieve the physical obstruction by reducing the gradient and increasing the MVA.

Patient Selection

Central to successful outcomes with any percutaneous or surgical procedure is optimal patient selection. In the case of mitral stenosis, optimal mitral valve and subvalvular morphology is very important in helping to ensure optimal outcomes with the PMBV procedure. The previously mentioned Wilkins echo score is a widely used assessment tool to determine suitability of the mitral valve for PMBV. Leaflet mobility, leaflet calcification, leaflet thickening, and subvalvular thickening and calcification are individually graded on a scale of 1 to 4. Typically unfavorable outcomes are predicted with scores >8.[8]

It should be noted that careful noninvasive assessment of the subvalvular apparatus is also an important procedural consideration. Evidence of subvalvular apparatus deformity on echo or absence of a c-wave on a LA pressure waveform can suggest severe deformity. Severe subvalvular deformity can potentially alter post-PMBV results.[11]

Absolute contraindications to PMBV include the presence of LA thrombus or moderate to severe mitral regurgitation. In the presence of LA thrombus, anticoagulation should be prescribed for 3 months and PMBV should be considered after resolution of thrombus.

Procedure

The transvenous antegrade transseptal route is most commonly used to gain access to the left atrium to perform PMBV. There are two main percutaneous techniques that have been described and widely used. The Inoue technique was first utilized in 1982 and described in 1984.[12] The Inoue technique utilizes a special balloon with a staged inflation technique. The double balloon technique is less commonly used, however, and utilizes two peripheral arterial balloons across the mitral valve with guidewires positioned in the left ventricle.

Transseptal Catheterization

Fundamental to successfully performing PMBV is the ability to gain access to the left atrium safely via the transseptal route. The transseptal procedure was developed and later modified in the late 1950s and 1960s. A careful understanding of septal anatomy is necessary to be able to carry out the procedure (**Figure 30-4AB**). While fluoroscopy is the mainstay for guiding the procedure, adjunct imaging with TEE and intracardiac echocardiography (ICE) has added value to the procedure both in terms of delineating anatomy and for safety.

With the patient in supine position, the atrial septum spans from the 1 o'clock to 7 o'clock position. The fossa ovalis lies posterior to the aortic root (often best appreciated in the right anterior oblique [RAO] view), and is bordered superiorly by a ridge (limbus). The lie and position of the interatrial septum and the fossa can become distorted in various disease states. In mitral stenosis, the plane of the septum can become more horizontal and the septum can become flat.

The transseptal procedure is performed using a Mullins sheath and dilator, which are advanced over a previously placed 0.032-inch J-wire. The wire should be placed into the superior vena cava (SVC), and used to insert and deliver the Mullins sheath/dilator into the SVC. The Brockenbrough needle is a curved needle that can be delivered through the Mullins sheath to allow for transseptal puncture. Additionally, a shield on the proximal end of the needle with an arrow indicates the direction of the curvature of the needle tip. It is imperative to confirm alignment between the arrow tip and the direction of the needle tip.

When the Mullins Sheath is positioned in the SVC, the 0.032-inch wire is removed and the Brockenbrough needle is carefully advanced into the dilator until the tip of the needle lies in the dilator. There should be approximately 2 cm of distance (approximately two finger widths) between the proximal portion of the dilator and the shield of the Brockenbrough needle. At this point, the stylet should be removed and the proximal end of the needle should be flushed and attached to a pressure transducer. Many operators obtain 4 Fr or 5 Fr femoral arterial access to place a pigtail catheter in the right coronary sinus to help delineate the position of the aorta.

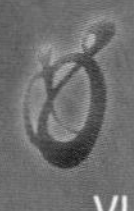

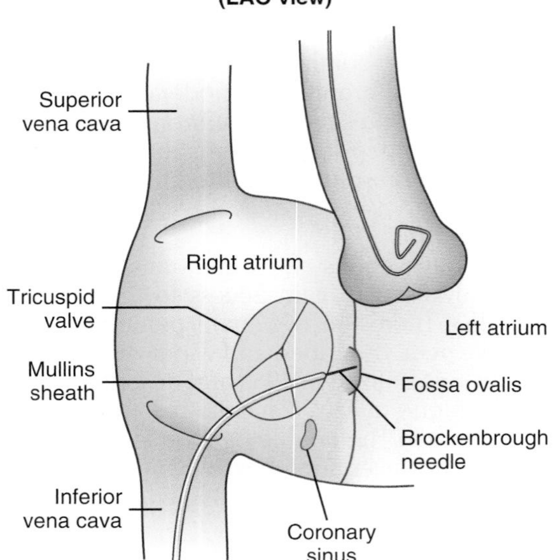

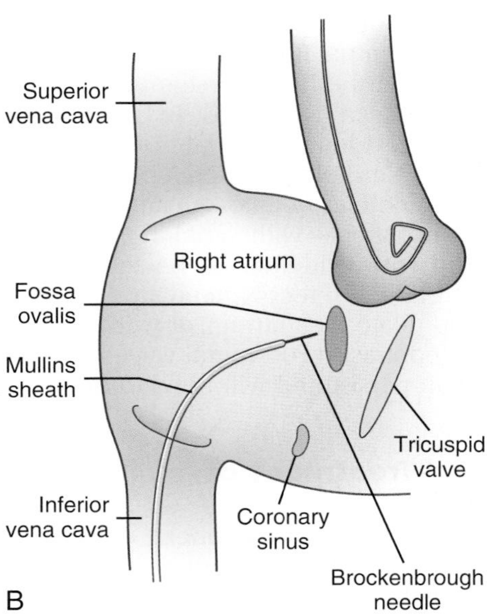

FIGURE 30-4 **Illustrations of the anatomy of the transseptal puncture. A,** Left anterior oblique (LAO) and right anterior oblique (RAO) **(B)** projections. *(Modified from Early M: Heart, 95:85–92, 2009.)*

Prior to puncture, it is important to verify needle position and maintain that the sheath and dilator are manipulated as one unit. Then, typically in the PA position, the entire unit is rotated clockwise until the arrow on the Brockenbrough needle is at the 4 o'clock position. The next step is to withdraw the unit into the fossa. On withdrawal, there are three sequential transitions that can be felt with this motion: first is the SVC/RA junction, next is the ascending aorta, and finally is the limbus of the fossa ovalis. Using a combination of fluoroscopic and echocardiographic imaging to obtain the best views, the operator should confirm accurate positioning of the Mullins sheath/dilator/Brockenbrough needle apparatus.

Once position is confirmed, the entire apparatus should be advanced into the fossa until there is dampening of the right atrial waveform. Some operators inject a small amount of contrast to demonstrate tenting of the septum by the needle. At this point, the apparatus should be advanced, often in the left anterior oblique (LAO) projection in which the needle should be pointing to the right of the screen, until entry into the left atrium is confirmed with pressure waveform and imaging guidance (Video 30-1). Use of contrast can help confirm position in the left atrium and exclude possibility of aortic or pericardial entry. Once entry is confirmed, the entire device is advanced approximately 1 cm using hemodynamic and imaging guidance until the tip of the Mullins dilator is in the left atrium. At this point, the needle is removed and the 0.032-inch J-wire is reinserted and placed in the left atrium. The sheath and dilator are advanced over the wire and then the wire and dilator are removed (Video 30-2). The sheath is flushed carefully and systemic anticoagulation with heparin is initiated.

Prior to the use of intracardiac or transesophageal echocardiography to guide the transseptal procedure, it was performed using fluoroscopy only. While single plane fluoroscopy can be used, the procedure is ideally performed using biplane fluoroscopy so as to identify the ideal position both in the PA and lateral views. Despite the advantages of biplane over single-plane fluoroscopy, there are several limitations to using only fluoroscopic guidance to perform the procedure. As such, the use of echocardiographic imaging as an adjunct has several distinct advantages over using fluoroscopy alone. Using echocardiographic guidance, confirming proper needle position prior to puncture can enhance procedural safety. Being able to determine the exact site of puncture can also be helpful in more complex procedures, such as percutaneous mitral valve repair, where the position of septal entry is important to the procedure itself. For percutaneous mitral valve repair using the mitraclip system, the desired location to enter the septum is high and posterior in the fossa ovalis to allow for device manipulation and delivery (Videos 30-3 and 30-4).

While transthoracic echocardiography (TTE) has been shown to be of utility in transseptal puncture, the use of TEE provides improved visualization of the interatrial septum and surrounding structures. Furthermore, it allows for precise entry across the septum so as to facilitate more complex procedures. TEE requires an additional operator and requires heavy sedation, or general anesthesia, to perform the procedure and should be considered as part of procedural planning (**Figure 30-5ABC**).

ICE can also be utilized to perform imaging of the fossa ovalis and to help guide the transseptal puncture. ICE provides excellent visualization of the septum in addition to being able to guide precise entry using direct visualization. In addition to superior imaging and unlike TEE, there is no need for general anesthesia, or heavy sedation, or an additional operator (**Figure 30-6AB**). The ICE catheter requires 8 Fr or 9 Fr contralateral venous access for delivery.

Transseptal puncture can be performed safely and effectively using meticulous technique and adjunctive imaging as a guide. With the use of echocardiographic imaging, hemodynamics, and fluoroscopy, transseptal puncture and catheterization can guide diagnostic procedures and complex therapeutic procedures while minimizing the risk of procedural complications. The decision as to which

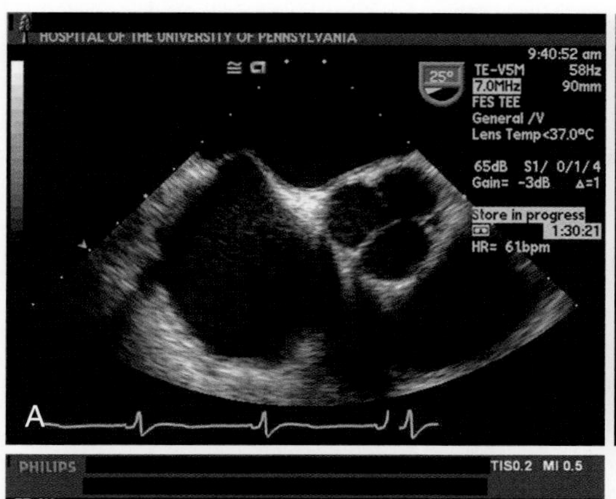

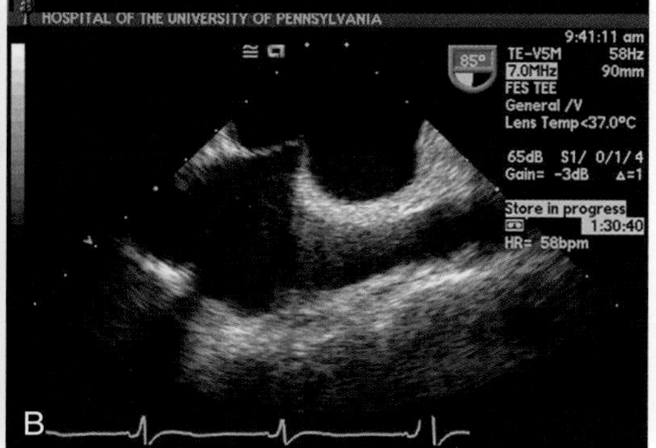

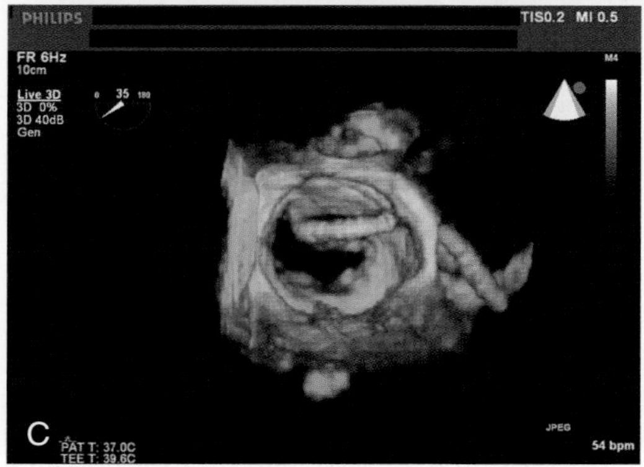

FIGURE 30-5 **Transesophageal echocardiogram (TEE) images of transseptal puncture. A,** TEE view of tenting of the Brockenbrough needle through the interatrial septum and its proximity to the aortic valve. **B,** TEE of Brockenbrough needle tenting the interatrial septum in caval view, and **(C)** 3D TEE view of the Mullins sheath in the left atrium following transseptal puncture.

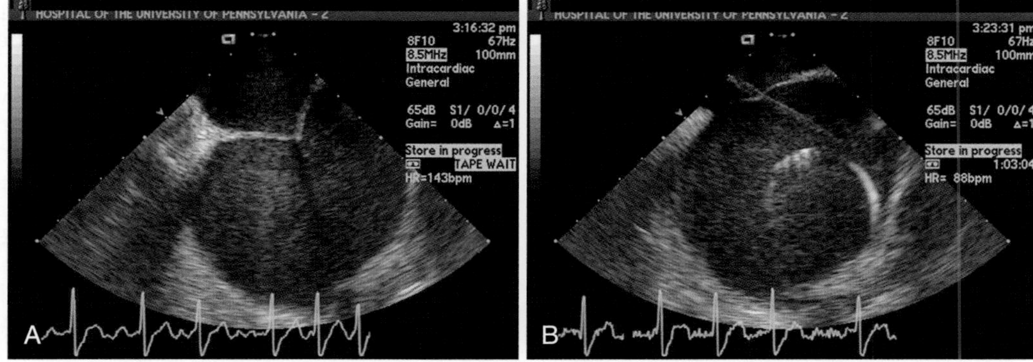

FIGURE 30-6 Intracardiac echo images of transseptal puncture. **A,** ICE image of the Brockenbrough needle tenting the interatrial septum, and **(B)** ICE image of the Mullins sheath and guidewire across the interatrial septum into the left atrium.

adjunct imaging modality to use will be heavily influenced by user preference and, ultimately, the planned procedure following transseptal puncture (see section on Procedural Imaging).

Inoue Technique

This Inoue balloon is a self-positioning latex balloon wrapped with a nylon mesh. There are several sizes to the Inoue balloon and because of its compliance the balloon size can vary up to 4 mm in diameter. Balloon size selection is based on patient's height. The catheter valve is elongated upon insertion through the femoral vein.

Following transseptal catheterization and dilation of the interatrial septum, the patient should receive therapeutic anticoagulation with IV heparin, and a wire is placed into the left atrium to facilitate placement of the balloon. Once the balloon is advanced into the left atrium, it is steerable to enable crossing of the stenotic mitral valve. When inflated the balloon has a sequential inflation of the distal part of the balloon followed by the entire balloon. The balloon has a characteristic hourglass or dumbbell shape that allows for positioning and stabilization. The balloon is compliant, allowing for incremental increase in balloon dilatation size without the need to exchange for a larger size.

Once the Inoue balloon has crossed the interatrial septum, the guidewire can be exchanged for a torque-able stylet, which is inserted into the balloon catheter. With the image intensifier in the 20- to 30-degree RAO position, the stylet can be used to align the balloon with the mitral valve orifice, usually with a counterclocking (anterior deflection) motion. At this point, the balloon catheter can be advanced across the mitral valve orifice while inflating the distal portion of the balloon. With inflation of the distal portion of the balloon (across the mitral orifice), the balloon is gently withdrawn back until it straddles the mitral orifice (using fluoroscopic and TEE guidance). At this point the balloon

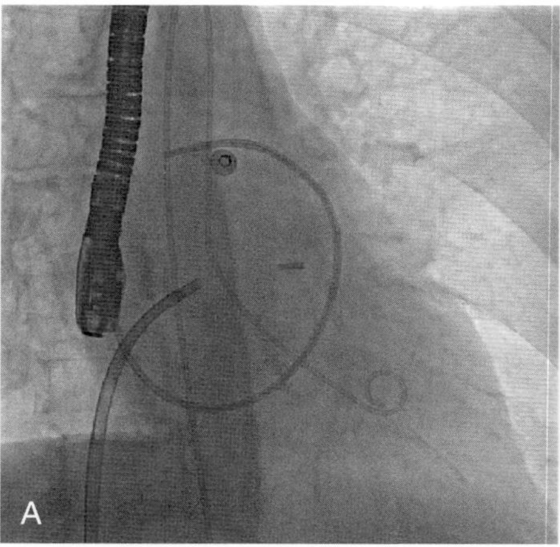

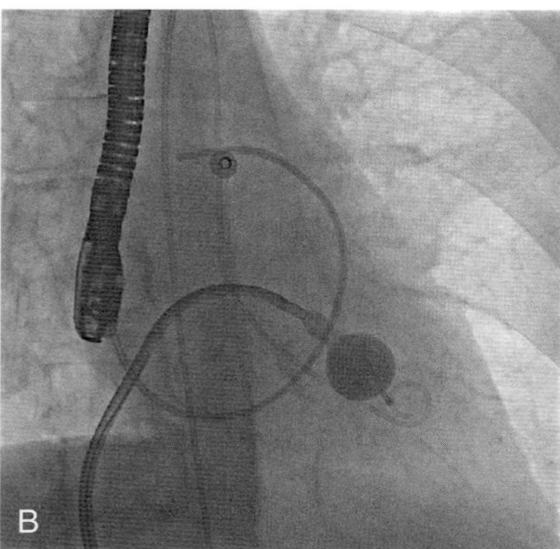

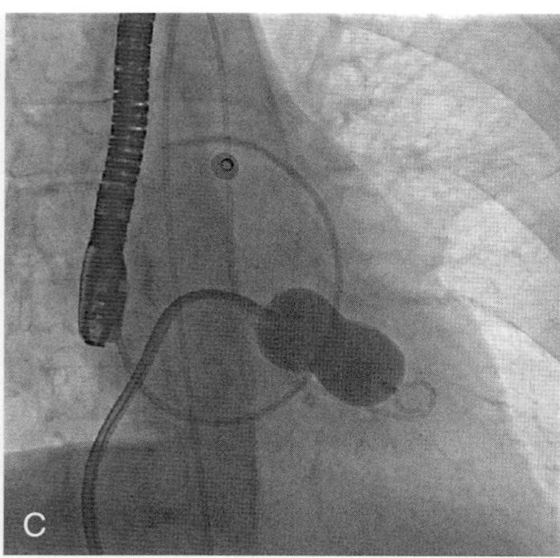

FIGURE 30-7 **A,** Fluoroscopic image demonstrating an Inoue balloon positioned across the atrial septum positioned in the left atrium. Also, note a pigtail catheter in the left ventricle, a Swan-Ganz catheter in right pulmonary artery, and a TEE probe for procedural imaging. **B,** Fluoroscopic image of inflation of the distal end of the Inoue balloon, and the balloon straddling the mitral valve orifice prior to complete inflation. **C,** Fluorosopic image of complete inflation of the Inoue balloon across a stenotic mitral valve during a balloon mitral valvuloplasty procedure.

is fully inflated for 4 seconds to 5 seconds and rapidly deflated. Following deflation, the balloon is withdrawn to the left atrium (**Figure 30-7ABC**).

After balloon inflation, the stylet can be removed and the balloon catheter can be attached to a pressure transducer (with care so as not to introduce air) to monitor LA pressure. TEE can be used to assess valve gradients, morphology, and degree of mitral regurgitation. Direct measurements of gradients with the catheters in both the LA and LV can provide information about residual gradients. A reduction in mean MV gradient by 50% or an increase in MVA >1.5 cm^2 is considered a successful result. An increase in mitral regurgitation by more than 1 Grade after balloon inflation should signal ending the procedure despite residual gradients. As such, it is important to carefully evaluate for severe commiussural calcium preprocedurally. Calcium does not split with balloon inflation but increases the potential for tearing the leaflet creating mitral regurgitation.

Double Balloon Technique

The double balloon technique is less widely used and has been mostly replaced by the Inoue technique, in part due to the lack of risk of LV perforation with the Inoue balloon. Following transseptal catheterization, and therapeutic anticoagulation, a balloon-tipped end-hole catheter is used to traverse the mitral valve via the transseptal puncture site. This catheter is navigated to the apex of the left ventricle and once positioned, a 260-cm guidewire is placed in the LV apex. The wire can also be tracked and placed into the descending aorta, although is certainly more time consuming. A second guidewire is placed using a similar technique, or by using a dual lumen catheter. An 18- or 20-mm dilation balloon is tracked and positioned on each wire and then advanced across the mitral valve orifice and inflated simultaneously to dilate the valve.[13,14]

Results

With PMBV, the initial success rate (MVA of >1.5 cm^2 and a decrease in LA pressure <18 mm Hg, without complications) in selected patients exceeds 80%. Over the long term, survival and event-free survival post-PMBV is influenced by valve morphology reflected by a Wilkins echo score >8. In 879 patients having undergone the PMBV with a mean follow-up of 4.2 ± 3.7 years, in patients with a Wilkins echo score <8, there was a greater immediate increase in MVA post-PMBV ($p < 0.0001$), and improved long-term survival (82% vs. 57%; $p < 0.0001$) in these patients. These patients with higher echo scores also have higher events in the long term including need for repeat PMBV, need for mitral valve surgery, and death. In a multivariate analysis, age, post-PMBV MR grade of ≥3+, prior surgical commissurotomy, NYHA Class IV symptoms, and elevated post-PMBV pulmonary arterial systolic pressures were all independently associated with worse outcome at follow-up.[15]

Prior to PMBV, surgical commissurotomy was the surgical treatment for patients with symptomatic mitral stenosis. With the advent of cardiopulmonary bypass, commissurotomy was performed as an open operation. Two studies examined the longer-term comparison between open commissurotomy versus PMBV. Cotrufo et al. examined 193 patients (111 PMBV with Inoue technique) who underwent either PMBV or open commissurotomy with a mean follow-up of 37 ± 22.9 months and a mean age of 46.5 ± 13.8 years. The mean echo score in the PMBV group was 7.63 ± 1.9, and 8.18 ± 1.93 in the surgical group. At follow-up both groups had similar risk and incidence of complications; however, those undergoing surgery had larger MVAs and better functional recovery.[16] A study by Ben Farhat et al.[17] compared PMBV, open commissurotomy, and closed commissurotomy. In this analysis, the mean patient age was lower, and the mean echo score was lower than the Cotrufo study. At 7-year follow-up, open commissurotomy (30 patients) and PMBV (30 patients) had comparable results in a more favorable patient population for PMBV.

The most common complication from PMBV is severe mitral regurgitation and can occur in 2% to 10% of procedures. The rates of severe mitral regurgitation after PMBV are not significantly different between the Inoue and double balloon techniques.[18] Overall procedural mortality is approximately 1%. Other less common procedural complications include pericardial tamponade, embolic events, vascular complications, arrhythmias, bleeding, stroke, myocardial infarction, residual atrial septal defect, and LA perforation. Due to the technically challenging nature of the procedure, operator experience should be taken into account when considering procedural success and complication rates.

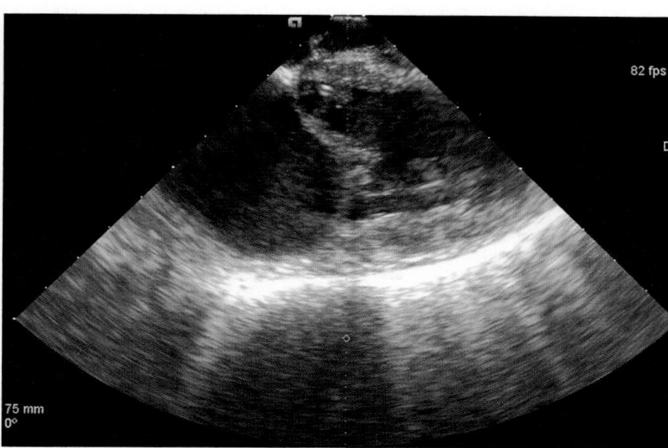

FIGURE 30-8 Intracardiac echo (ICE) view of the left atrium, left ventricle, and a rheumatic mitral valve prior to percutaneous mitral balloon valvuloplasty (PMBV) for mitral stenosis. Note that the ICE catheter is positioned in the right ventricle to obtain this view.

Procedural Imaging

The use of procedural imaging beyond fluoroscopy can assist the interventional operator to safely and effectively perform the PMBV procedure. Imaging is also helpful in the assessment of postprocedural results and complications such as acute severe mitral regurgitation. TEE is commonly used to guide the interventional procedure. Optimal TEE views can help facilitate balloon positioning during PMBV. Furthermore, TEE can be used to confirm residual gradients and assess post-inflation mitral regurgitation. This information may be of value in deciding for or against additional balloon inflation. Three-dimensional TEE (3D TEE) can provide a "surgeon's view" of the mitral valve and the fused commissures. The use of 3D TEE has been shown to be superior to TTE in reducing fluoroscopy time and time from first transseptal puncture to first balloon inflation time.[19] A scoring system has also been developed to assess suitability of the mitral valve for PMBV as well.[20]

An alternative to TEE is intracardiac echocardiography (ICE). An ICE catheter can be placed in the contralateral femoral vein through a sheath and placed in the RA, or RV, to help guide transseptal puncture and PMBV (**Figure 30-8**). Furthermore, ICE has been placed in the aorta via arterial access and has been shown to be safe and in most cases more helpful for the procedure than ICE positioned in the venous system.[21] Ideally, the decision regarding which imaging modality for the procedure should be based on operator experience and comfort, and patient-related factors. Optimal imaging guidance is of utmost importance for procedural success.

SPECIAL CONSIDERATIONS—PREGNANCY

There are several potential patient-related issues that add complexity to the treatment of severe rheumatic mitral stenosis. Given the young age of onset of rheumatic heart disease in many populations, patients can present with symptoms during pregnancy. Pregnancy can exacerbate symptoms in patients with mild or moderate mitral stenosis due to the increase in plasma volume and relative anemia. The resultant hemodynamic effects are decreased diastolic filling periods and increased mean transmitral pressure gradients. Mainstays of medical therapy for symptomatic patients include diuretic therapy and heart rate control. Caution must be used to select medications that are considered safe during pregnancy. Pregnancy patients with severe mitral stenosis should be referred to an experienced center for consideration of PMBV prior to delivery. The hemodynamic changes and fluid shifts that occur during delivery can lead to acute pulmonary edema and appropriate careful monitoring of patients at the time of delivery is necessary.

Section II: Mitral Regurgitation

PATHOPHYSIOLOGY

Unlike mitral stenosis, which is primarily caused by rheumatic fever, mitral regurgitation (MR) is a more diverse disease that results from dysfunction of any of the portions of the complex mitral valve apparatus, including the leaflets, chords, annulus, and left ventricle. It is often further classified as primary (organic or degenerative) disease, which primarily affects the leaflets (e.g., fibromuscular dysplasia, mitral valve prolapse, rheumatic disease) and secondary (ischemic or functional) diseases, which spare the leaflets (e.g., diseases of the atrium and ventricle, including ischemic dysfunction and dilated cardiomyopathy). Patients with severe MR have decreased survival, whether symptomatic or not, and surgery is often recommended.[22-24] In asymptomatic patients with preserved LV, a "watchful waiting" approach until the development of symptoms, LV dysfunction, pulmonary hypertension, or atrial fibrillation can be considered.[25] Current guidelines recommend surgery for symptomatic patients and asymptomatic patients with abnormal LV function, and surgery may also be considered for asymptomatic patients with normal LV function when there is a high likelihood of successful repair.[26]

Rationale for Transcatheter Therapy

Surgery improves survival in observational studies,[27] but is associated with mortality rates of 1% to 5% and additional morbidity rates of 10% to 20%, including stroke, reoperation, renal failure, and prolonged ventilation.[28] The risks of surgery are particularly high in patients who are elderly or have LV dysfunction. In one study of more than 30,000 patients undergoing mitral valve replacement, the mortality increased from 4.1% in those younger than 50 years to 17.0% in octogenarians.[29] The risks of surgery, particularly in consideration of morbidity and patient preference, have stimulated attempts to develop less invasive solutions.[30]

When considering percutaneous or transcatheter approaches for mitral repair, it is useful to classify them according to the major structural abnormality that they address.[31] Unlike the extensive toolbox available to the mitral surgeon, transcatheter approaches are much more limited and often only able to address a single major element of the dysfunctional valve that contributes to MR. **Table 30-1** lists some of the devices, their manufacturers, current state of development, and any available published reports.

Leaflet Repair with the MitraClip Device

MitraClip (Abbott Vascular, Redwood City, California) was the first transcatheter mitral valve repair technology to receive CE Mark approval and has now also received limited FDA approval for patients with primary (degenerative) MR and prohibitive surgical risk (**Figure 30-9**). This system

TABLE 30-1 Devices for Transcatheter Mitral Valve Therapy

Leaflet/chordal	MitraClip	Abbott Vascular, Abbott Park, Ill.	CE Mark Phase III (U.S.)
	NeoChord DS1000 System	Neochord, Inc., Eden Prairie, Minn.	Phase 1 (outside U.S.)
	Mitra-Spacer	Cardiosolutions, Inc., West Bridgewater, Mass.	Phase 1 (outside U.S.)
	MitraFlex	TransCardiac Therapeutics, LLC, Atlanta, Ga.	Preclinical
Indirect annuloplasty	CARILLON XE2 Mitral Contour System	Cardiac Dimensions, Inc., Kirkland, Wis.	CE Mark
	Kardium MR	Kardium, Inc., Richmond, British Columbia, Canada	Preclinical
	Cerclage annuloplasty	National Heart, Lung, and Blood Institute, Bethesda, Md.	Preclinical
Direct or left ventricular annuloplasty	Mitralign Percutaneous	Mitralign, Inc., Tewksbury, Mass.	Phase 1 (outside U.S.)
	Annuloplasty System GDS Accucinch System	Guided Delivery Systems, Santa Clara, Calif.	Phase 1 (outside U.S.)
	Boa RF Catheter	QuantumCor, Inc., Laguna Niguel, Calif.	Preclinical
	Cardioband	Valtech Cardio, Or-Yehuda, Israel	Preclinical
	Millipede system	Millipede LLC, Ann Arbor, Mich.	Preclinical
Hybrid surgical	Adjustable annuloplasty ring	Mitral Solutions, Fort Lauderdale, Fla.	Phase 1
	Dynaplasty ring	MiCardia Corporation, Irvine, Calif.	Phase 1
LV remodeling	The Basal Annuloplasty of the Cardia Externally (BACE)	Mardil Medical, Minneapolis, Minn.	Phase 1
	Tendyne Repair	Tendyne Holdings, Inc., Baltimore, Md.	Preclinical
Replacement	Endovalve	Micro Interventional Devices, Inc., Langhorne, Pa.	Preclinical
	CardiAQ	CardiAQ Valve Technologies, Inc., Irvine, Calif.	Preclinical
	Lutter	Universitatsklinikum, Kiel, Germany	Preclinical
	Tiara	Neovasc, Inc., Richmond, British Columbia, Canada	Preclinical
	Ventor Embracer	Medtronic, Inc., Minneapolis, Minn.	Preclinical
	PCS Mitral Valve	Percutaneous Cardiovascular Solutions, Pty, Ltd, Newcastle, New South Wales, Australia	Preclinical

From Chapter 22: Transcatheter mitral valve repair and replacement. In Otto and Bonow: Valvular heart disease, a companion to Braunwald's heart disease, ed 4, Table 22-1, page 343.

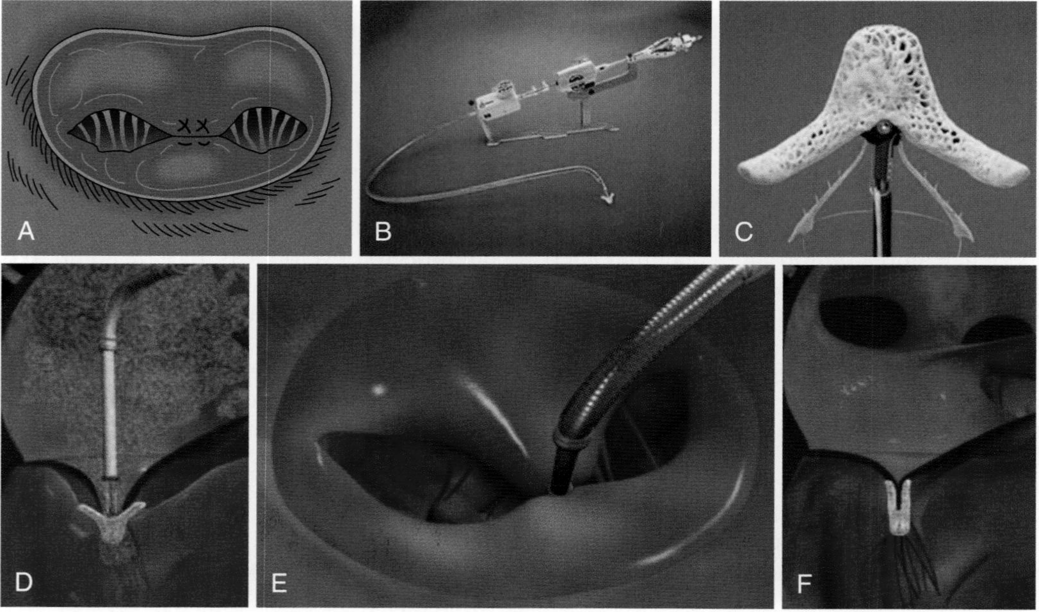

FIGURE 30-9 The MitraClip leaflet coaptation system. This device (Abbott Vascular, Inc.) creates a bridge between the P2 and A2 segments of the mitral valve similar to the Alfieri stitch operation **(A)** utilizing a clip delivery system **(B)** and the MitraClip **(C). D** and **E,** Side view and left atrial view of the clip delivery system as it is advanced through the mitral valve in the open position prior to grasping of the leaflets. **F,** The final result is illustrated after the clip has been released and the delivery system removed. *(From Chapter 22: Transcatheter mitral valve repair and replacement. In Otto and Bonow: Valvular heart disease, a companion to Braunwald's heart disease, ed 4. Figure 22-2, page 342.)*

replicates the Alfieri stich operation, in which the middle scallops of the posterior and anterior leaflets (P2 and A2, respectively) are sutured together to create a double-orifice mitral valve. This operation, though usually performed with adjunctive ring annuloplasty, has proved effective and durable in a wide variety of pathologies as well as in selected patients without annuloplasty.[32,33]

Trials with this device have confirmed its feasibility (Endovascular Valve Edge-to-Edge Repair Study [EVEREST] I), and its safety and efficacy were compared with those of surgical repair in a randomized trial (EVEREST II), providing a wealth of data on this technology.[34,35] The procedure is performed with standard catheterization techniques utilizing a transseptal approach from the right femoral vein.[36] The clip delivery system is introduced through a 24 Fr sheath into the left atrium, where it can be guided by TEE using a series of turning knobs under through the mitral valve into the left ventricle. A properly aligned and oriented clip can be placed on the P2 and A2 segments of leaflets, grasping them from the ventricular side to create leaflet opposition. Once leaflet insertion is confirmed by echocardiography, the clip can be released. If a suboptimal grasp occurs, the leaflet can be released, allowing repositioning prior to a second grasp attempt. Additionally, a second or more clips can be placed as needed for optimal MR reduction.[36]

In the 2:1 randomized EVEREST II trial, 184 patients were designated to receive MitraClip therapy, and 95 to undergo surgical repair or replacement. These patients were almost a decade older (mean age 67 years) than in usual surgical series and had more co-morbidities. Major adverse events at 30 days were significantly less frequent with MitraClip therapy (9.6% vs. 57% with surgery; $p < 0.0001$), although much of the difference could be attributed to the greater need for blood transfusions with surgery.[37] The freedom from the combined outcome of death, mitral valve surgery, and MR severity greater than 2 + at 12 months was higher with surgery (73%) than with MitraClip therapy (55%; $p = 0.0007$). Importantly, in patients with acute MitraClip therapy success, the result appears durable with a very low rate of later mitral valve surgery.

Subsequent analyses of this rich database have demonstrated persistent reductions in MR grade, improvement in New York Heart Association (NYHA) functional class, and reduction in LV dimensions with MitraClip therapy.[37] Other studies have demonstrated a lack of mitral stenosis, no effect of initial rhythm on results, and benefit in higher-risk subjects.[38-40]

Most recently, Lim and colleagues reported on 127 high-risk patients with degenerative MR with 1-year follow-up.[41] The patients were elderly (mean age 82 years) and at high surgical risk (STS score 13.2). The 30-day mortality was lower than predicted (6.3%), and the 83% of surviving patients had MR <2 + at 1 year with reduced LV volumes and improved quality of life. Importantly, there was a 73% reduction in hospitalization for heart failure in the year post-Mitraclip as compared with the year prior to Mitraclip implantation.

Although the EVEREST II trial failed to demonstrate efficacy equivalent to that of surgery for a diverse group of patients with varied risk and etiology, the EVEREST High-Risk Registry and Prohibitive-risk subset combined with the experience outside the United States point to a more appropriate role in high-risk patients with secondary functional and ischemic MR. A new randomized trial (Clinical Outcomes Assessment of the MitraClip Percutaneous Therapy for High Surgical Risk Patients [COAPT]) is under way to compare the device with medical therapy in these patients. Finally, there are several other devices designed to provide leaflet repair, including NeoChord, Mitra-Spacer, and MitraFlex in either preclinical or phase 1 evaluation.

Indirect Annuloplasty

The venous anatomy of the heart is of particular interest for treating MR because of the ease of access (from the right internal jugular vein) and the location of the great cardiac vein in proximity to the posterior mitral annulus. Some of the first attempts to treat MR without surgery did so by mimicking surgical ring annuloplasty through placement of devices in the coronary sinus, so-called indirect or percutaneous coronary sinus annuloplasty. The goal of this approach is to remodel the posterior annulus cinching the great cardiac vein, or pushing in on the posterior annulus from the vein, in order to improve leaflet co-aptation.

The CARILLON XE2 Mitral Contour System (Cardiac Dimensions, Inc. Kirkland, Washington) has CE Mark and uses novel anchors placed permanently in the coronary sinus that are pulled toward each other with a cinching device to reduce the mitral annular dimension by traction (**Figure 30-10**). Early evaluation in the Amadeus study demonstrated feasibility, with implantation in 30 of 48 patients and modest improvement in quantitative measures of MR with a small risk of coronary compromise (15%) and death (1 patient).[42] More recently, a redesigned device was tested in the Transcatheter Implantation of Carillon Mitral Annuloplasty Device (TITAN) trial.[43] Among 65 enrolled subjects with secondary MR (62% ischemic), the device was implanted successfully in 36 patients with a mean age of 62 years, mean ejection fraction 29%, with predominantly New York Heart Association functional Class III symptoms, and with 2 + (30%), 3 + (55%), or 4 + (15%) Grade MR. Quantitative measures of MR were better at 6 months and 12 months than in 17 patients who were enrolled in the trial and did not receive implants.

In general, indirect annuloplasty devices may be able to provide modest MR reduction in selected patients, but likely less than is achievable with surgery. Whether this level of efficacy will result in sufficient symptomatic improvement and LV remodeling to justify the procedure requires further study. The limited efficacy is related to the location of the coronary sinus relative to the annulus (up to 10 mm more cranial), great individual anatomic variability, and the limited benefit of partial annular remodeling.[44,45] Possibly, some "super-responders" may be able to be identified on the basis of anatomic considerations before the procedure.

The risks of this approach must also be considered. In addition to the risk for damage to the cardiac venous system, devices in this location can compress the left circumflex or diagonal coronary arteries, which traverse between the coronary sinus and the mitral annulus in most patients.[46]

In this regard, one novel indirect approach to reduce the septal-lateral dimension that deserves further consideration is the Cerclage annuloplasty technique (see **Figure 30-10**). This approach attempts to create a more complete circumferential annuloplasty by placing a suture from the coronary sinus through a septal perforator vein into the right atrium or ventricle, where it is snared and tensioned with the proximal end from the right atrium to create a closed

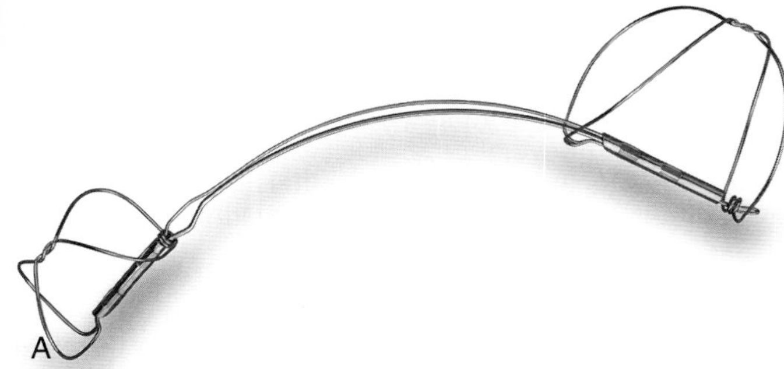

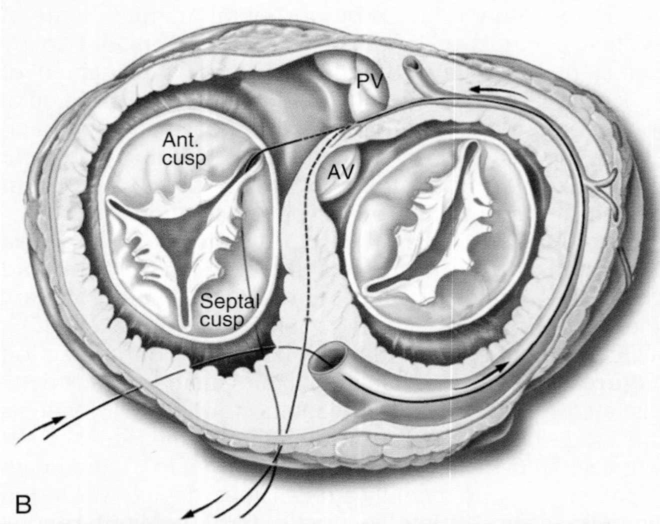

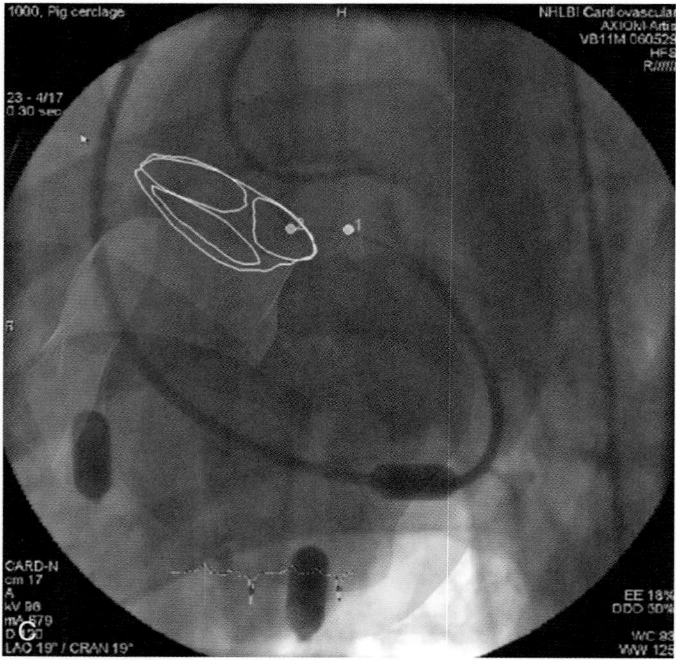

FIGURE 30-10 **Several indirect annuloplasty devices. A,** CARILLON XE2 Mitral Contour System (Cardiac Dimension, Inc., Kirkland, Washington) coronary sinus cinching device. Cerclage technique, shown in a schematic **(B)**, and an angiogram with superimposed magnetic resonance images **(C)**. *(B and C, from Kim JH, Kocaturk O, Ozturk C, et al: Mitral Cerclage annuloplasty, a novel transcatheter treatment for secondary mitral valve regurgitation: initial results in swine. J Am Coll Cardiol 54:638–651, 2009.) Also, from Chapter 22: Transcatheter mitral valve repair and replacement. In Otto and Bonow: Valvular heart disease, a companion to Braunwald's heart disease, ed 4. Figure 22-7B, F, G, page 346.)*

purse-string.[47] The procedure is guided by cardiac magnetic resonance and also uses a novel rigid protection device to avoid coronary compression.

Direct Annuloplasty and Left Ventricular Remodeling Techniques

Other devices have been developed to more directly remodel the mitral annulus, in part due to the limitations of indirect coronary sinus annuloplasty described above (**Figure 30-11**). The Mitralign Percutaneous Annuloplasty System (Mitralign, Inc., Tewksbury, Massachusetts) was originally based on the surgical techniques of Paneth's posterior suture plicaton.[48] In this procedure, a transaortic catheter is advanced to the left ventricle and used to deliver pledgeted anchors through the posterior annulus that can be pulled together to shorten (plicate) the annulus up to 17 mm (with two implants). In 16 patients treated in a phase 1 trial, septal-lateral dimension could be reduced up to 8 mm.[44] A CE Mark trial is planned. The Accucinch (Guided Delivery Systems, Santa Clara, California) device utilizes a similar catheter approach to place up to 12 anchors along the ventricular surface of the posterior mitral annulus. A cable running through the anchors is tensioned to create posterior placation. In a later development, the anchors have been placed in the ventricular myocardium just below the valve plane (percutaneous ventriculoplasty). This device has been characterized as more of a ventricular remodeling approach rather than one that is truly annular (see **Figure 30-11**).

In addition to these devices that have entered clinical investigation, a preclinical device that deserves mention is the QuantumCor device (QuantumCor Inc., Lake Forest, California). This technology uses low-radiofrequency energy delivered via a transseptal catheter (Boa RF Catheter) to shrink the collagen within the mitral annulus. In animals, a 20% to 25% reduction in anterior-posterior dimension was achieved with a durability to 6 months. A first-in-human validation study during open-heart surgery is planned.

Finally, the Cardioband (Valtech Cardio, Or-Yehuda, Israel) is an adjustable, catheter-delivered, sutureless device that is inserted transseptally or transatrially and anchored on the atrial side of the annulus with the potential for subsequent adjustment (see **Figure 30-11**). A successful first-in-human experience of 11 patients at three European centers with this device was recently reported.[49]

The basis for devices to treat MR by affecting the shape of the left ventricle arises from the pathophysiology of secondary ischemic or functional MR. Changes in the inferior and lateral left ventricle due to infarction can lead to tethering or tenting of the posterior leaflet, allowing anterior leaflet override as the mechanism of MR.[50,51] Similarly, failure of leaflet co-aptation due to global LV enlargement causing annular distension is the major mechanism for MR in dilated cardiomyopathy.[52] Although ring annuloplasty can often ameliorate MR caused by LV distortion, procedures that specifically address the underlying LV pathology may also be beneficial. The Basal Annuloplasty of the Cardia Externally (BACE) device (Mardil, Inc., Morrisville, North Carolina) is a surgically implanted external tension band placed around the heart externally at the time of CABG revascularization to treat ischemic MR. In a preliminary report of 11 patients treated in India, MR grade was reduced acutely from Grade 3.3 to 0.6.[53] Preclinical work with a transcatheter approach to approximate the papillary muscles is also in

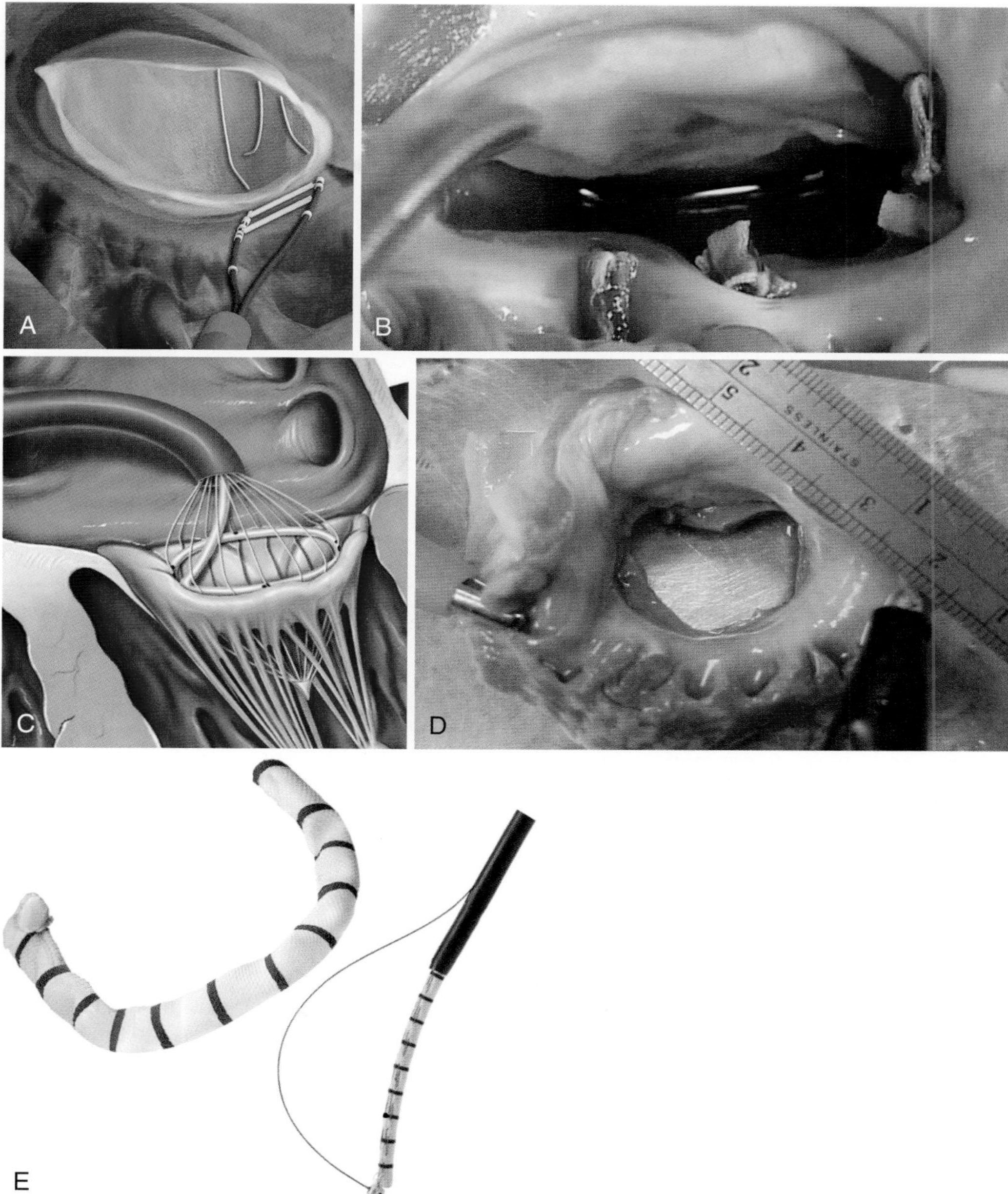

FIGURE 30-11 Devices that directly remodel a portion of either the posterior annulus or the left ventricular wall near the annulus. A, The Bident (Mitralign Inc., Tewksbury, Mass.) direct annuloplasty system and the result in an animal annulus **(B)**; **C,** the Boa radiofrequency collagen remodeling catheter is illustrated based on the QuantrumCor device; **D,** the results of heat remodeling of an animal's annulua in vitro. **E,** Cardioband (Valtech Cardio, Or-Yehuda, Israel). *(**A** to **E**, From Chapter 22: Transcatheter mitral valve repair and replacement. In Otto and Bonow: Valvular heart disease, a companion to Braunwald's heart disease, ed 4. Figure 22-8, page 347–348.)*

development (Tendyne Repair, Tendyne Holdings, Inc., Baltimore, Maryland).

Transcatheter Mitral Valve Replacement

The rationale for transcatheter mitral valve replacement has as its basis several lessons learned from surgical valve replacement.[54] Surgical valve replacement is the most effective method to reliably reduce MR. This is particularly apparent in comparisons with transcatheter repairs, which do not appear to reduce MR to the same extent as surgical repairs. Despite its proven efficacy, the risks of surgery may include significant morbidity and mortality related to the incision and the need for cardiopulmonary bypass.[28,29]

One of the most touted advantages of surgical repair over replacement is the improved survival related to better LV remodeling.[27] However, this and other observational comparisons may be confounded by differences in patient baseline characteristics and co-morbid conditions. In a recent randomized trial, 251 patients with severe ischemic MR underwent either surgical repair or chordal-sparing replacement.[55] At 12 months there was no difference in the primary endpoint of LA end-systolic volume index and more frequent recurrent MR in the repair group (32.6% with moderate or severe MR vs. 2.3% with replacement). This finding provides further rationale to consider transcatheter mitral valve replacement in this patient population as an alternative to open surgical repair.

Transcatheter mitral valve prostheses will likely first be used in elderly and other patients at high surgical risk for whom the benefits of repair are unproven and the risks of

TABLE 30-2 Transcatheter Mitral Valve-in-Valve Implantation

FIRST AUTHOR (YEAR)	N	ACCESS ROUTE (N)	PROCEDURE SUCCESS (N/TOTAL)	POSTPROCEDURE MR GRADE	RESIDUAL MEAN GRADIENT (MM HG)	30-DAY MORTALITY (%)	COMMENT
Seiffert (2010)[56]	1	TA	1/1	0-1+	2	100	
Webb (2010)[57]	7	Transseptal (1), transaortic (1), transapical (5)	6/7	0-1+	8	29	
Cerillo (2011)[58]	3	Transapical	2/3	1+	5	33	
Cheung (2011)[59]	11	Transaortic (1), transapical (10)	9/10	0-1+	7	10	Includes some patients[57]
Van Garsse (2011)[60]	1	Transapical	1/1	0	3	0	
De Weger (2011)[62]	1	Transapical	1/1	1+	4	0	Status after ring annuloplasty
Himbert (2011)[63]	1	Transseptal	1/1	1+	8	0	Status after ring annuloplasty
Gaia (2012)[61]	1	Transatrial	1/1	0	5	0	
Vahanian (2012)[64]	8	Transseptal					Status after ring annuloplasty (n = 6)

From Chapter 22: Transcatheter mitral valve repair and replacement. In Otto and Bonow: Valvular heart disease, a companion to Braunwald's heart disease, ed 4.

surgery are high. In this regard, early experience utilizing transcatheter aortic valve implantation (TAVI) devices in previously implanted, and now degenerating surgical bioprostheses and rings, has confirmed the feasibility of this approach (**Table 30-2**). Balloon expandable prostheses have been implanted in degenerating bioprostheses[56-61] and previous surgical annuloplasty rings[62-64] predominantly via a transapical approach. However, the feasibility of transseptal delivery[57,63,64] and transatrial[57,59] delivery has also been demonstrated. Complications, including valve embolization, bleeding, and death, have been reported, but the early results have been generally favorable with excellent reduction in MR grade and low residual transmitral gradients.

Despite these early demonstrations of the feasibility of transcatheter mitral valve-in-valve implantation, it is likely that de novo placement of such devices in native valves will be more challenging. The devices will need to be larger than most aortic devices, and fixation to the diseased mitral apparatus will be hampered by the greater valve complexity, the lack of calcium, the potential need for orientation, and the noncircular annular shape. Paravalvular leaks, already demonstrated to reduce survival after TAVI, will likely be even less well tolerated in the mitral valve, with the higher driving pressures and more common development of hemolysis. Finally, all such devices will need to preserve the subvalvular apparatus and not create LV outflow tract obstruction. Most current designs utilize a stent-based bioprosthesis that is self-expanding and inserted transseptally (CardiAQ Valve Technologies, Inc., Winchester, Massachusetts) or transapically (Tiara; Neovasc, Inc., Richmond, British Columbia, Canada, and The Engager Aortic Valve Bioprosthesis; Medtronic, Inc., Minneapolis, Minnesota).

One device that does not rely on radial force for fixation in the annulus (Lutter) may be advantageous to reduce the risk for outflow tract obstruction. Initial experience with this transapical, off-pump, porcine self-expanding stent prosthesis in pigs has been reported and highlights the challenges of this approach. Seven of the eight animals died because of paravalvular leaks, suboptimal positioning, or failure of fixation.[65] A subsequent bovine pericardial design with a ventricular tethering fixation system reduced embolization, but malpositioning and failure of ventricular fixation resulted in death in six of eight animals.[66]

CardiAQ Valve Technologies, Inc., is developing a transseptally inserted stent device with a foreshortening frame and anchor barbs. The device sits in the left atrium to a significant degree above the annulus, a characteristic that has hampered the experimental evaluation. Nonetheless, investigators reported on its use in 82 pigs with acute and subchronic MR, with delivery system failure in 36% and unsuccessful implant positions in 21% of the remaining completed procedures.[67] A first-in-human report demonstrated feasibility, but the patient did not survive and the device is undergoing re-design.

Finally, several self-expanding bovine pericardial prostheses for transapical delivery are also under development: Tiara (Neovasc, Inc.) and Ventor Engager (Medtronic, Inc.). Both these devices will benefit from the growing experience with transapical TAVI[68] and paravalvular leak closure.[69] Furthermore, several companies are developing transapical closure devices to simplify insertion of both aortic and mitral prostheses via catheters.

Both transseptal and transapical insertion of mitral valve replacement prostheses may be an attractive future option for patients for whom surgery poses a high risk. The potential advantages of this approach include the avoidance of both the surgical incision and the effects of cardiopulmonary bypass. Such devices could be fully sparing of the subvalvular apparatus and provide MR reduction that is equivalent to that achieved with surgical valve replacement.

CONCLUSIONS

The complexity of the mitral valve apparatus and the myriad causes of MR have caused the field of transcatheter mitral valve repair and replacement to develop more slowly than treatments for other valve diseases. The release of devices to treat MR in Europe and aortic stenosis throughout the world has re-energized the development of new transcatheter valve therapies. Fueled by the ever-growing prevalence of heart failure in the aging U.S. population[70]—most of these older patients with heart failure have significant MR—and aided by the ingenuity of physicians and engineers, transcatheter mitral valve therapies will probably also become an available option for such patients.

References

1. Gorman JH, 3rd, Jackson BM, Enomoto Y, et al: The effect of regional ischemia on mitral valve annular saddle shape. *Ann Thorac Surg* 77(2):544–548, 2004.
2. Choure AJ, Garcia MJ, Hesse B, et al: In vivo analysis of the anatomical relationship of coronary sinus to mitral annulus and left circumflex coronary artery using cardiac multidetector computed tomography: implications for percutaneous coronary sinus mitral annuloplasty. *J Am Coll Cardiol* 48(10):1938–1945, 2006.
3. Chandrashekar Y, Westaby S, Narula J: Mitral stenosis. *Lancet* 374:1271–1283, 2009.
4. Guilherme L, Fae KC, Oshiro SE, et al: Rheumatic Fever: how S. pyogenes-primed peripheral T cells trigger heart valve lesions. *Ann N Y Acad Sci* 1051:132–140, 2005.
5. WHO: *Rheumatic fever and rheumatic heart disease,* WHO Technical Report Series no 923, Geneva, 2001, www.who.int/cardiovascular_diseases/resources/en/cvd_trs923.pdf.
6. Gordon SP, Douglas PS, Come PC, et al: Two-dimensional and Doppler echocardiographic determinants of the natural history of mitral valve narrowing in patients with rheumatic mitral stenosis: implications for follow-up. *J Am Coll Cardiol* 19:968–973, 1992.
7. Zipes DP, Libby P, Bonow RO, et al: *Braunwald's Heart Disease: a Textbook of Cardiovascular Medicine*, ed 7, Philadelphia, 2005, Elsevier Saunders, pp 1553–1564.
8. Wilkins GT, Weyman AE, Abascal VM, et al: Percutaneous balloon dilatation of the mitral valve: an analysis of echocardiographic variables related to outcome and the mechanism of dilatation. *Br Heart J* 60:299–308, 1988.
9. Aviles RJ, Nishimura RA, Pellikka PA, et al: Utility of stress Doppler echocardiography in patients undergoing percutaneous mitral balloon valvotomy. *J Am Soc Echocardiogr* 14:676–681, 2001.
10. Bonow RO, Carabello BA, Chatterjee K, et al: 2008 focused update incorporated into the ACC/AHA 2006 Guidelines for the management of patients with valvular heart disease: a report of the American College of Cardiology/American Heart Association Task Force on Practice Guidelines (Writing Committee to revise the 1998 guidelines for the management of patients with valvular heart disease). Endorsed by the Society of Cardiovascular Anesthesiologists, Society for Cardiovascular Angiography and Interventions, and Society of Thoracic Surgeons. *J Am Coll Cardiol* 52:e1–e142, 2008.
11. Palacios IF, Block PC, Wilkins GT, et al: Follow-up of patients undergoing percutaneous mitral balloon valvotomy. Analysis of factors determining restenosis. *Circulation* 79:573–579, 1989.
12. Inoue K, Owaki T, Nakamura T, et al: Clinical application of transvenous mitral commissurotomy by a new balloon catheter. *J Thorac Cardiovasc Surg* 87:394–402, 1984.
13. Al Zaibag M, Al Kasab S, Ribiero RA, et al: Percutaneous double-balloon mitral valvotomy for rheumatic mitral valve stenosis. *Lancet* 1:757–761, 1986.
14. Palacios IF, Block PC, Brandi S, et al: Percutaneous balloon valvotomy for patients with severe mitral stenosis. *Circulation* 75:778–784, 1987.
15. Palacios IF, Sanchez PL, Harrell LC, et al: Which patients benefit from percutaneous mitral valvuloplasty? Prevalvuloplasty and postvalvuloplasty variables that predict long-term outcome. *Circulation* 105:1465–1471, 2002.
16. Cotrufo M, Renzulli A, Ismeno G, et al: Percutaneous mitral commissurotomy versus open mitral commissurotomy: a comparative study. *Eur J Cardiothorac Surg* 15:646–651, 1999.
17. Ben Farhat M, Ayari M, Maatouk F, et al: Percutaneous balloon versus surgical closed and open mitral commissurotomy: seven-year follow-up results of a randomized trial. *Circulation* 97:245–250, 1998.
18. Ruiz CE, Zhang HP, Macaya C, et al: Comparison of Inoue single-balloon versus double-balloon technique for percutaneous mitral valvotomy. *Am Heart J* 123:942–947, 1992.
19. Eng MH, Salcedo EE, Kim M, et al: Implementation of real-time three-dimensional transesophageal echocardiography for mitral balloon valvuloplasty. *Catheter Cardiovasc Interv* 82:994–998, 2013.
20. Anwar AM, Attia WM, Nosir YF, et al: Validation of a new score for the assessment of mitral stenosis using real-time three-dimensional echocardiography. *J Am Soc Echocardiogr* 23:13–22, 2010.
21. Akkaya E, Vuruskan E, Zorlu A, et al: Aortic intracardiac echocardiography-guided septal puncture during mitral valvuloplasty. *Eur J Cardiovasc Imaging* 15:70–76, 2014.
22. Bursi F, Enriquez-Sarano M, Nkomo VT, et al: Heart failure and death after myocardial infarction in the community: the emerging role of mitral regurgitation. *Circulation* 111:295–301, 2005.
23. Trichon BH, Felker GM, Shaw LK, et al: Relation of frequency and severity of mitral regurgitation to survival among patients with left ventricular systolic dysfunction and heart failure. *Am J Cardiol* 91:538–543, 2003.
24. Enriquez-Sarano M, Avierinos JF, Messika-Zeitoun D, et al: Quantitative determinants of the outcome of asymptomatic mitral regurgitation. *N Engl J Med* 352:875–883, 2005.
25. Rosenhek R, Rader F, Klaar U, et al: Outcome of watchful waiting in asymptomatic severe mitral regurgitation. *Circulation* 113:2238–2244, 2006.
26. Bonow RO, Carabello BA, Chatterjee K, et al: 2008 focused update incorporated into the ACC/AHA 2006 guidelines for the management of patients with valvular heart disease: a report of the American College of Cardiology/American Heart Association Task Force on Practice Guidelines (Writing Committee to revise the 1998 guidelines for the management of patients with valvular heart disease). Endorsed by the Society of Cardiovascular Anesthesiologists, Society for Cardiovascular Angiography and Interventions, and Society of Thoracic Surgeons. *J Am Coll Cardiol* 52:e1–e142, 2008.
27. Enriquez-Sarano M, Schaff HV, Orszulak TA, et al: Valve repair improves the outcome of surgery for mitral regurgitation: a multivariate analysis. *Circulation* 91:1022–1028, 1995.
28. Gammie JS, O'Brien SM, Griffith BP, et al: Influence of hospital procedural volume on care process and mortality for patients undergoing elective surgery for mitral regurgitation. *Circulation* 115:881–887, 2007.
29. Mehta RH, Eagle KA, Coombs LP, et al: Influence of age on outcomes in patients undergoing mitral valve replacement. *Ann Thorac Surg* 74:1459–1467, 2002.
30. Masson JB, Webb JG: Percutaneous treatment of mitral regurgitation. *Circ Cardiovasc Interv* 2:140–146, 2009.
31. Chaim PTL, Ruiz CE: Percutaneous mitral valve repair: a classification of the technology. *J Am Coll Cardiol Interv* 4:1–13, 2011.
32. Alfieri O, Maisano F, DeBonis M, et al: The double-orifice technique in mitral valve repair: a simple solution for complex problems. *J Thorac Cardiovasc Surg* 122:674–681, 2001.
33. Maisono F, Caldarola A, Blasio A, et al: Midterm results of edge-to-edge mitral valve repair without annuloplasty. *J Thoracic Cardiovasc Surg* 126:1987–1997, 2003.
34. Feldman T, Wasserman HS, Herrmann HC, et al: Percutaneous mitral valve repair using the edge-to-edge technique: six-month results of the EVEREST Phase 1 Clinical Trial. *J Am Coll Cardiol* 46:2134–2140, 2005.
35. Herrmann HC, Feldman T: Percutaneous mitral valve edge-to-edge repair with the Evalve MitraClip System: rationale and phase 1 results. *EuroIntervention* 1(Suppl A):A36–A39, 2006.
36. Silvestry FE, Rodriguez LL, Herrmann HC, et al: Echocardiographic guidance and assessment of percutaneous repair for mitral regurgitation with the Evalve MitraClip: lessons learned from EVEREST 1. *J Am Soc Echocardiogr* 20:1131–1140, 2007.
37. Feldman T, Foster E, Glower D, et al: Percutaneous repair or surgery for mitral regurgitation. *N Engl J Med* 364:1395–1406, 2011.
38. Herrmann HC, Kar S, Siegel R, et al: Effect of percutaneous mitral repair with the MitraClip device on mitral valve area and gradient. *EuroIntervention* 4:437–442, 2009.
39. Herrmann HC, Gertz ZM, Silvestry FE, et al: Effects of atrial fibrillation on treatment of mitral regurgitation in the EVEREST II Randomized Trial. *J Am Coll Cardiol* 59:A17–A20, 2012.
40. Whitlow PL, Feldman T, Pedersen WR, et al: Acute and 12-month results with catheter-based mitral valve leaflet repair. *J Am Coll Cardiol* 59:130–139, 2012.
41. Lim DS, Reynolds MR, Feldman T, et al: Improved functional status and quality of life in prohibitive surgical risk patients with degenerative mitral regurgitation after transcatheter mitral valve repair. *J Am Coll Cardiol* 64:182–192, 2014.
42. Schofer J, Siminiak T, Haude M, et al: Percutaneous mitral annuloplasty for functional mitral regurgitation: results of the Carillon Mitral Annuloplasty Device European Union Study. *Circulation* 120:326–333, 2009.
43. Goldberg S: Presentation at TransCatheter Therapeutics 23rd Annual Scientific Symposium, November 7-11, 2011, San Francisco.
44. Choure AJ, Barcia MJ, Hesse B, et al: In vivo analysis of the anatomical relationship of coronary sinus to mitral annulus and left circumflex coronary artery using cardiac multidetector computed tomography. *J Am Coll Cardiol* 48:1938–1945, 2006.
45. Maselli D, Guarracino F, Chiaramonti F, et al: Percutaneous mitral annuloplasty: an anatomic study of human coronary sinus and its relation with mitral valve annulus and coronary arteries. *Circulation* 114:377–380, 2006.
46. Spongo S, Bertrand OF, Philippon F, et al: Reversible circumflex coronary artery occlusion during percutaneous transvenous mitral annuloplasty with the Viacor system. *J Am Coll Cardiol* 59:288, 2012.
47. Kim JH, Kocaturk O, Ozturk C, et al: Mitral Cerclage annuloplasty, a novel transcatheter treatment for secondary mitral valve regurgitation: initial results in swine. *J Am Coll Cardiol* 54:638–651, 2009.
48. Tibayan FA, Rodriguez F, Liang D, et al: Paneth suture annuloplasty abolishes acute ischemic mitral regurgitation but preserves annular and leaflet dynamics. *Circulation* 108(Suppl II):II-128–II-133, 2003.
49. Maisano F: TCT 2013 presentation.
50. Chaput M, Handschumacher MD, Tournoux F, et al: Mitral leaflet adaptation to ventricular remodeling: occurrence and adequacy in patients with functional mitral regurgitation. *Circulation* 118:845–852, 2008.
51. Silbinger JJ: Mechanistic Insights into Ischemic Mitral regurgitation: echocardiographic and surgical implications. *J Am Soc Echocardiogr* 24:707–719, 2011.
52. Komeda M, Glasson JR, Bolger AF, et al: Geometric determinants of ischemic mitral regurgitation. *Circulation* 96(Suppl):II-128–II-133, 1997.
53. Raman J: Presentation at TransCatheter Therapeutics 23rd Annual Scientific Symposium, November 7-11, 2011, San Francisco.
54. Herrmann HC: Transcatheter mitral valve implantation. *Cardiac Interventions Today* August/September:82–85, 2009.
55. Acker MA, et al: *NEJM* 370:23–32, 2014.
56. Seiffert M, Franzen O, Conradi L, et al: Series of transcatheter valve-in-valve implantations in high-risk patients with degenerated bioprostheses in aortic and mitral position. *Cath Cardiovasc Interv* 76:608–615, 2010.
57. Webb JG, Wood DA, Ye J, et al: Transcatheter valve-in-valve implantation for failed bioprosthetic heart valves. *Circulation* 121:1848–1857, 2010.
58. Cerillo AG, Chiaramonti F, Murzi M, et al: Transcatheter valve in valve implantation for failed mitral and tricuspid bioprostheses. *Cath Cardiovasc Interv* 78:987–995, 2011.
59. Cheung AW, Gurvitch R, Ye J, et al: Transcatheter transapical mitral valve-in-valve implantations for a failed bioprosthesis: a case series. *J Thorac Cardiovasc Surg* 141:711–715, 2011.
60. Van Garsse LAFM, Gelsomino S, Van Ommen V, et al: Emergency transthoracic transapical mitral valve-in-valve implantation. *J Interv Cardiol* 24:474–476, 2011.
61. Gaia DF, Palma JH, de Souza JAM, et al: Transapical mitral valve-in-valve implant: an alternative for high risk and multiple reoperative rheumatic patients. *Int J Cardiol* 154:e6–e7, 2012.
62. de Weger A, Ewe SH, Delagado V, et al: First in man implantation of a transcatheter aortic valve in a mitral annuloplasty ring: novel treatment modality for failed mitral valve repair. *Eur J Cardiothorac Surg* 39:1054–1056, 2011.
63. Himbert D, Brochet E, Radu C, et al: Trans-septal implantation of a transcatheter heart valve in a mitral annuloplasty ring to treat mitral repair failure. *Circ Cardiovasc Interv* 4:396–398, 2011.
64. Himbert D, Descoutures F, Brochet E, et al: Transvenous mitral valve replacement after failure of surgical ring annuloplasty. *J Am Coll Cardiol* 60:1205–1206, 2012.
65. Lozonschi L, Quaden R, Edwards NM, et al: Transapical mitral valved stent implantation. *Ann Thorac Surg* 86:745–748, 2008.
66. Lozonschi L, Bombien R, Osaki S, et al: Transapical mitral valved stent implantation: a survival series in swine. *J Thorac Cardiovasc Surg* 140:4220–4226, 2010.
67. Mack M: Presentation at TransCatheter Therapeutics 23rd Annual Scientific Symposium, November 7-11, 2011, San Francisco.
68. Dewey TM, Thourani V, Bavaria JE, et al: Transapical aortic-valve replacement for critical aortic stenosis: results from the nonrandomized continued-access cohort of the PARTNER trial. Presented to Society of Thoracic Surgeons 48th Annual Meeting, January 30, 2012, Fort Lauderdale, Florida.
69. Sorajja P, Cabalks AK, Hagler DJ, et al: Percutaneous repair of paravalvular prosthetic regurgitation: acute and 30-day outcomes in 115 patients. *Circ Cardiovasc Interv* 4:314–321, 2011.
70. Roger VL, Go AS, Lloyd-Jones DM, et al: Heart disease and stroke statistics-2011 update. A report from the American Heart Association. *Circulation* 123:e18–e209, 2011.

31 Hypertrophic Cardiomyopathy

Shikhar Agarwal and E. Murat Tuzcu

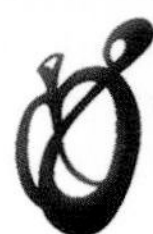

INTRODUCTION AND EPIDEMIOLOGY

Hypertrophic cardiomyopathy (HCM) is a complex cardiac disorder that has been the subject of intense scrutiny and scientific investigation for the past half century. HCM is a unique cardiac condition that has the potential to manifest during any phase of life, from infancy to the ninth decade. Despite the wide range of symptoms and ages of affected individuals, sudden and unexpected death in young people is perhaps the most devastating aspect of this disease. Despite a wealth of scientific data in this field, controversy continues with regard to diagnostic criteria, clinical course, and optimal management strategies for patients with HCM.

Since its first description in 1958,[1] HCM has been referred to by a wide variety of names reflecting lapses in understanding of this complex disease and its clinical heterogeneity. The terms like *idiopathic hypertrophic subaortic stenosis* (IHSS) or *hypertrophic obstructive cardiomyopathy* (HOCM) are misleading, since they encompass only a subset of patients who have left ventricular outflow tract (LVOT) obstruction. In fact, roughly three fourths of the patients have no LVOT gradient at rest, and one third of patients do not demonstrate any LVOT gradient at rest, or with provocative maneuvers.[2] With an improved understanding of the clinical heterogeneity of the disease, HCM is a more appropriate descriptive term that encompasses the overall disease spectrum.

HCM is a global disease and is the most common genetic cardiovascular disease encountered. The current prevalence of HCM in the adult population has been estimated to be 0.2% (1:500 adults),[3] with similar estimates for other parts of the world. Approximately 600,000 adults are currently believed to be suffering from HCM. However, HCM patients constitute no more than 1% of outpatients in a routine cardiology practice, implying that a large majority of these patients remain undiagnosed.[4] Due to the relatively infrequent prevalence of patients with HCM, most outpatient cardiologists care for only a few HCM patients and may not be aware of the contemporary management of this complex disease. This has led to an impetus for establishment of clinical programs of excellence, called "HCM Centers," which would be staffed with cardiologists and cardiac surgeons familiar with the contemporary diagnostic and treatment options for HCM. These should include comprehensive history and physical examination followed by transthoracic echocardiography (TTE), cardiac magnetic resonance (CMR) imaging, both surgical septal myectomy (SM) and alcohol septal ablation (ASA), along with management of arrhythmias, and implantation of implantable cardiac defibrillators (ICD), genetic testing, and counseling.

HALLMARKS AND DIFFERENTIAL DIAGNOSIS

HCM has been defined as a disease state characterized by unexplained LV hypertrophy without chamber dilation in the absence of another cardiac or systemic disease that is capable of producing hypertrophy to the observed degree, with the caveat that patients who are genotypically positive may be phenotypically negative without manifest LV hypertrophy. HCM is usually recognized by a maximal septal hypertrophy ≥15 mm on echocardiography, particularly in the presence of other compelling information like family history of HCM. The LV septal thickness of 13 to 14 mm is considered borderline. Most of the current literature in the field of HCM has quantified LV septal thickness using echocardiography, although the use of CMR has been increasing over the last few years,[5] and new data are likely to emerge in forthcoming years. In children, increased LV septal thickness is defined as thickness ≥2 standard deviations above the mean for age, sex, and body size. Despite these widely utilized cutoff points, it must be understood that any degree of LV wall thickness is compatible with the genetic substrate of HCM. An emerging subgroup within the broad clinical spectrum may be composed of family members with disease causing sarcomere mutations but without evidence of the disease phenotype.[6-9] These individuals are

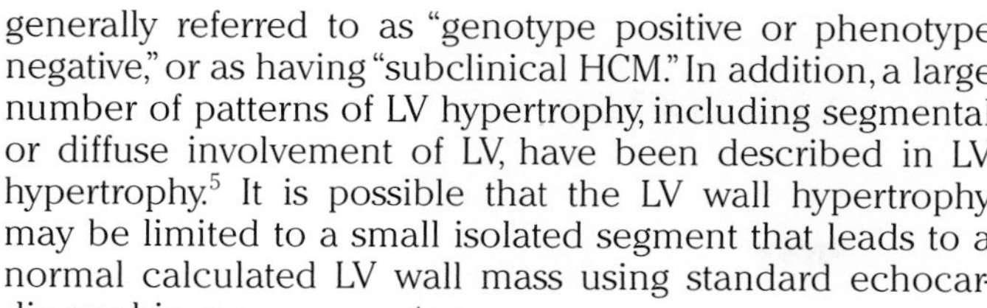

generally referred to as "genotype positive or phenotype negative," or as having "subclinical HCM." In addition, a large number of patterns of LV hypertrophy, including segmental or diffuse involvement of LV, have been described in LV hypertrophy.[5] It is possible that the LV wall hypertrophy may be limited to a small isolated segment that leads to a normal calculated LV wall mass using standard echocardiographic measurements.

The most common differential diagnoses of HCM include hypertensive heart disease and the physiologic remodeling of the heart seen among athletes (athlete's heart).[10-14] Mild morphologic expressions of HCM, or borderline HCM, pose the maximum degree of confusion with these diseases. In older individuals, HCM may even co-exist with hypertensive heart disease, which may pose further diagnostic challenges. The likelihood of HCM increases when the presentation is associated with a diagnostic sarcomere mutation, or inferred by marked LV thickness >25 mm and/or LVOT obstruction with systolic anterior motion (SAM) of the anterior mitral leaflet. The important distinction between pathologic LV hypertrophy seen in HCM and physiologic LV hypertrophy seen among athletes is the fact that the latter is usually associated with chamber enlargement (usually both LV and RV), and generally regresses when the high-level exercise routine is stopped. Besides ventricular dimensions, a detailed review of the family history, sarcomeric mutations, diastolic function, and pattern of LV hypertrophy may aid in the distinction of two states.

Several metabolic and infiltrative diseases may mimic HCM among babies, older children, and young adults—for example, mitochondrial diseases,[15,16] Fabry disease,[17] storage disease caused by mutations in genes encoding the γ-2 regulatory subunit of the adenosine monophosphate (AMP) activated protein kinase (PRKAG2), or the X-linked lysosome associated membrane protein gene (LAMP2; Danon disease).[18-21] Other mimics of HCM may be encountered in the context of multisystem disorder such as Noonan syndrome (craniofacial and congenital heart malformations) as well as LV hypertrophy from mutations in genes of the RAt Sarcoma (RAS) pathway[5,22] or distinct cardiomyopathies such as Pompe's disease (glycogen storage disorder II, due to deficiency of α-1, 4-glucosidase).[23-27]

NATURAL COURSE OF DISEASE AND CLINICAL PRESENTATION

The understanding of the natural history of HCM has been hampered by a significant selection bias in published literature. Earlier published studies from the tertiary and quaternary centers reported a high annual mortality rate of 3% to 6%.[3] Recent data from regional- and community-based centers suggest an annual mortality rate of ~1%.[28,29] Selected subpopulations who have high-risk features, or those who are symptomatic, may have a higher annual mortality rate averaging ~5%.[3] When mortality rates are reviewed, it is important to take into consideration the population that constitutes the denominator.

The clinical course of HCM is unpredictable in most scenarios. In addition, there are currently no therapies that prevent progression of this disease. Despite this, most affected individuals attain normal life expectancy without any disability or even a need for invasive therapeutic interventions. On the other hand, HCM disease progression may result in serious complications with a potential for premature death. Among those who do become symptomatic, there are three discrete clinical presentations of this disease.

- Sudden cardiac death (SCD) due to unpredictable and often refractory ventricular tachyarrhythmias. This is often encountered in young asymptomatic individuals <35 years of age (including competitive athletes).
- Heart failure with or without angina: This results in a progressively worsening exertional dyspnea. The earlier stages of HCM are characterized by diastolic heart failure without loss of systolic function. If left untreated, it may progress to the end-stage with LV remodeling and systolic dysfunction secondary to extensive myocardial scarring.
- Supraventricular tachycardia including atrial fibrillation (AF), which may be paroxysmal or permanent and leads to an increased risk of systemic thromboembolism including stroke. AF with rapid ventricular response may result in abrupt decompensation of an otherwise asymptomatic patient.

In the current era, the natural history of HCM can be altered by a number of therapeutic interventions: ICD implantation for prevention of SCD, medical therapy for managing heart failure symptoms, SM or ASA for progressive LVOT obstruction leading to sequelae, anti-arrhythmic or ablation therapies for management of AF, and lastly heart transplantation for end-stage HCM with refractory symptoms and systolic dysfunction.

PATHOPHYSIOLOGY

The pathophysiology of HCM is complex and involves interplay of multiple factors. It is important to understand and quantify the contribution of each of the following mechanisms to an individual patient's phenotype as the management strategies are largely dependent on these pathophysiologic mechanisms.

Left Ventricular Outflow Tract Obstruction

In patients with HCM, LVOT obstruction at rest has been demonstrated to be a strong, independent predictor of progression to severe symptoms of heart failure and of death.[30] In HCM, the peak instantaneous gradient rather than the mean gradient holds greater prognostic significance and influences treatment decisions. Based on the extent of obstruction, the entire HCM cohort can be divided into three groups. The first group includes those who have obstruction (defined as LVOT gradient ≥30 mm Hg) at resting conditions. The second group includes those who have labile physiologically provoked gradients (defined as LVOT gradient <30 mm Hg at rest and ≥30 mm Hg with physiologic provocation).[2] The final group includes those who have nonobstructive HCM, with LVOT gradient <30 mm Hg at rest and on provocation. Marked gradients ≥50 mm Hg at rest or with provocative maneuvers represent the conventional threshold for invasive management if symptoms are not controlled with medications alone.

LVOT obstruction in HCM is classically dynamic, varying with loading conditions and the loading conditions of the ventricle.[28] Increased myocardial contractility, decreased ventricular volume, or decreased afterload increases the degree of LVOT obstruction. Patients with low LVOT gradients at rest may generate marked LVOT obstruction with exercise, Valsalva maneuver, or with pharmacologic provocation with amyl nitrite[31,32] (**Figure 31-1**). There may be a large variation in the degree of LVOT obstruction based on

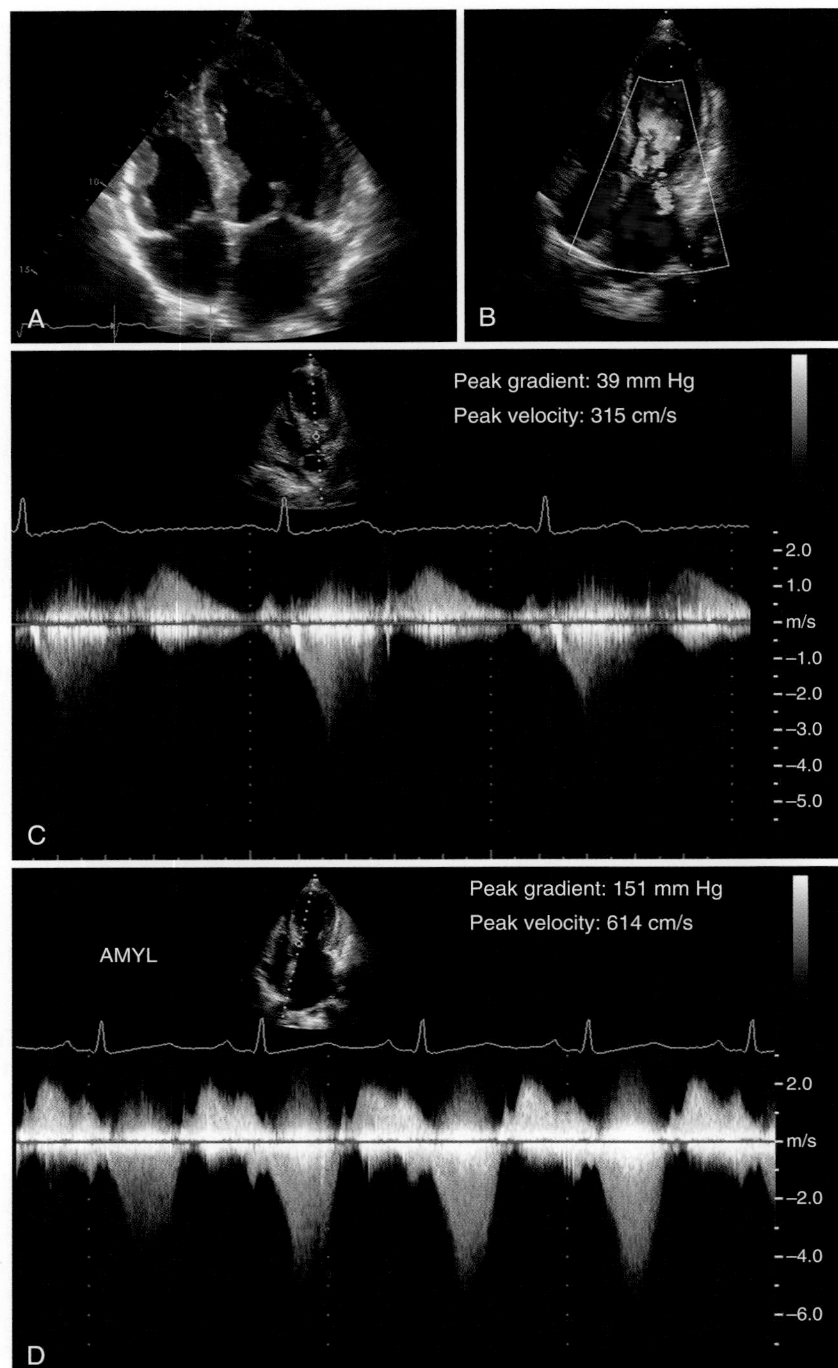

FIGURE 31-1 This figure demonstrates the measurement of left ventricular outflow tract (LVOT) gradient using continuous wave Doppler. **A,** demonstrates apical 4-chamber view of the heart showing significant upper septal hypertrophy. **B,** demonstrates color Doppler imaging showing flow acceleration across the LVOT and posteriorly directed jet of mitral regurgitation. **C,** demonstrates the measurement of resting peak gradient across the LVOT of 39 mm Hg. Upon administration of amyl nitrite, the peak gradient across the LVOT was measured to be 151 mm Hg, as seen in **D.**

day-to-day activities, even minute to minute, based on heart rate and blood pressure, or even with food or alcohol intake; exacerbation of symptoms during the postprandial period is not uncommon.[33]

LVOT obstruction leads to an increase in LV systolic pressure. This, in turn, leads to prolongation of ventricular relaxation, elevation of LV end-diastolic pressure, worsening mitral regurgitation (MR), myocardial ischemia, and a decrease in cardiac output. Although it was initially believed that LVOT obstruction primarily results from the systolic contraction of the hypertrophied basal ventricular septum encroaching on the LVOT, recent studies have demonstrated a greater involvement of the mitral valve leaflets in causing LVOT obstruction. LVOT obstruction generally occurs by virtue of systolic anterior motion (SAM) of anterior mitral leaflet and resultant mitral septal contact (**Figure 31-2**). Ventricular systole in HCM causes an abnormal drag force on anterior mitral leaflet that "sucks in" this leaflet into the LVOT, causing obstruction. Occasionally, presence of hypertrophied papillary muscle abutting the septum, or anomalous papillary muscle insertion

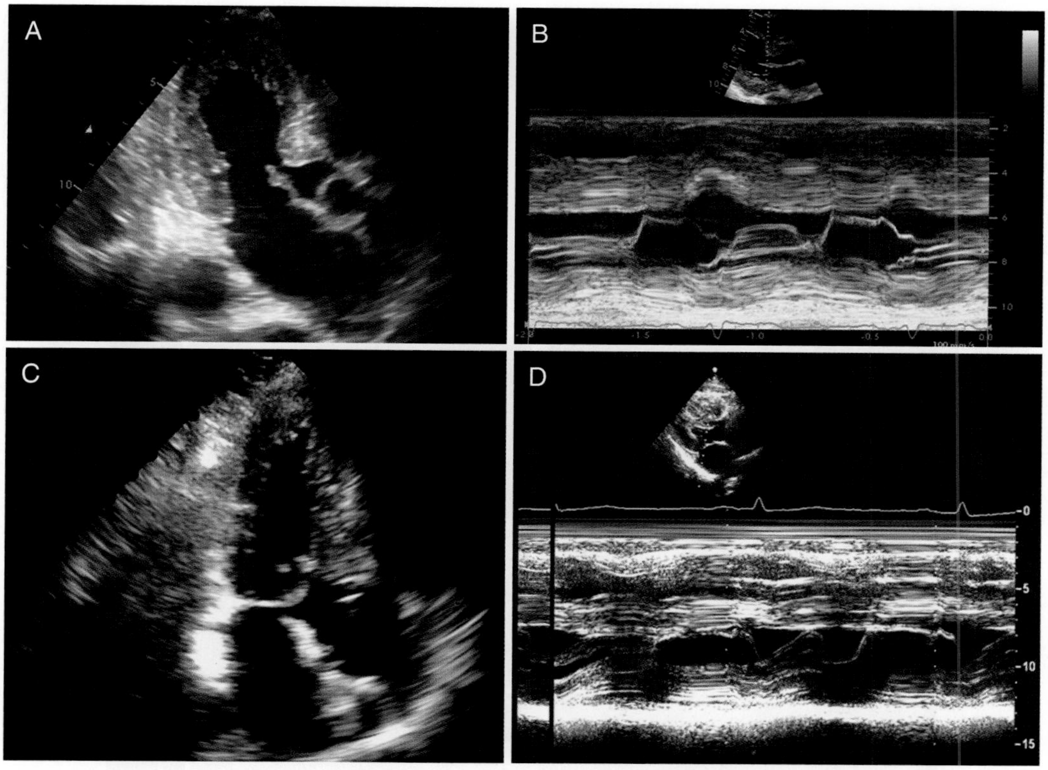

FIGURE 31-2 This figure demonstrates the systolic anterior motion (SAM) of the anterior mitral leaflet causing significant obstruction across the left ventricular outflow tract (LVOT). **A** and **B,** The apical long-axis view and the M-mode through the mitral valve leaflets in a patient with mild SAM. There is anterior motion of the mitral leaflet that can be clearly appreciated in **B. C,** The apical long-axis view and the M-mode through the mitral valve leaflets in a patient with severe SAM. There is an anterior motion of the mitral leaflet during systole with overt mitral-septal contact, which can be clearly seen in **D.**

into the anterior mitral leaflet, may cause significant midcavitary obstruction.[34,35]

The presence and degree of LVOT obstruction is assessed using two-dimensional echocardiography and continuous wave Doppler assessment (**Figure 31-1**). The peak instantaneous gradient derived from the late-peaking systolic velocity is what reflects the subaortic obstruction. If the resting outflow gradient is <50 mm Hg, provocative measures are employed to ascertain if higher gradients can be obtained. This can be demonstrated using exercise (stress echocardiography) or Valsalva maneuver, or by inhalation of amyl nitrite. In equivocal cases, where there is a considerable discordance between clinical presentation and echocardiography data, cardiac catheterization with isoproterenol infusion may further aid in eliciting a provocable gradient.[36]

Diastolic Dysfunction

Diastolic dysfunction is a major pathophysiologic mechanism in HCM that results in impairment of ventricular relaxation and chamber stiffness. The former results from systolic contraction against an obstructed LVOT, nonuniformity of ventricular contraction and relaxation, and a delayed inactivation caused by abnormal intracellular calcium reuptake. A marked increase in the LV wall thickness results in both impaired ventricular relaxation as well as increased chamber stiffness. Diffuse myocardial ischemia also potentiates the amount of diastolic dysfunction encountered in HCM. With exercise, there is a decrease in diastolic filling time and an increase in the amount of myocardial ischemia, which results in worsening of the diastolic dysfunction and may cause an increase in the pulmonary capillary wedge pressure resulting in dyspnea.

Myocardial Ischemia

Chest pain, both typical and atypical, is reported by roughly 80% of HCM patients.[37] In many cases, heart catheterization reveals normal coronary arteries. Despite this observation, several studies with functional assessment of ischemia using single photon emission computed tomography (SPECT), positron emission tomography (PET), and CMR technologies have demonstrated significant reversible and irreversible myocardial perfusion defects in HCM patients.[37-41] Autopsy data have reported that up to 15% of HCM patients may have findings of myocardial infarction, which may or may not be the reason for mortality. This discordance suggests that microvascular dysfunction may play an important role in the development of myocardial ischemia in these patients. The etiology of microvascular dysfunction is probably multifactorial. It may be partly due to arteriolar medial hypertrophy, resulting in reduced luminal diameter and an impaired coronary vasodilatory response. In addition, there is a demand supply mismatch that is created because of an abnormally thickened ventricle along with adverse loading conditions due to LVOT obstruction.

Autonomic Dysfunction

About a quarter of patients with HCM undergoing exercise stress testing demonstrate an abnormal blood pressure response to exercise characterized by a failure of systolic blood pressure to increase by at least 20 mm Hg at peak exercise, or a fall in systolic blood pressure.[42,43] This subset of patients has been shown to have poorer prognosis compared with others.[43,44] In addition to the potentiation of the dynamic LVOT gradient, it is speculated that autonomic dysregulation with resultant systemic vasodilation plays an

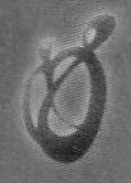

important role in this phenomenon. It is believed that autonomic dysregulation is present in these patients and the fall in blood pressure, and associated bradycardia, may be an abnormal reflex response secondary to LVOT obstruction.

Mitral Regurgitation

Mitral regurgitation (MR) is common in patients with HCM and may play a primary role in mediating the symptoms of dyspnea (**Figure 31-3**). The detailed mechanistic studies and the resolution of MR with SM suggest that MR is a secondary phenomenon in most patients with HCM.[31,32,45] MR is usually caused by distortion of mitral valve apparatus from SAM-induced drag forces. In this case, the jet of MR is generally directed posterolaterally (**Figure 31-3**). An anterior, or anteromedially, directed jet should suggest an intrinsic abnormality of the mitral valve apparatus. If the mechanism of MR is directly related to LVOT obstruction-induced SAM, changes in ventricular load and contractility would affect the degree of MR. It is very important to identify patients with intrinsic abnormality of mitral valve (prolapse

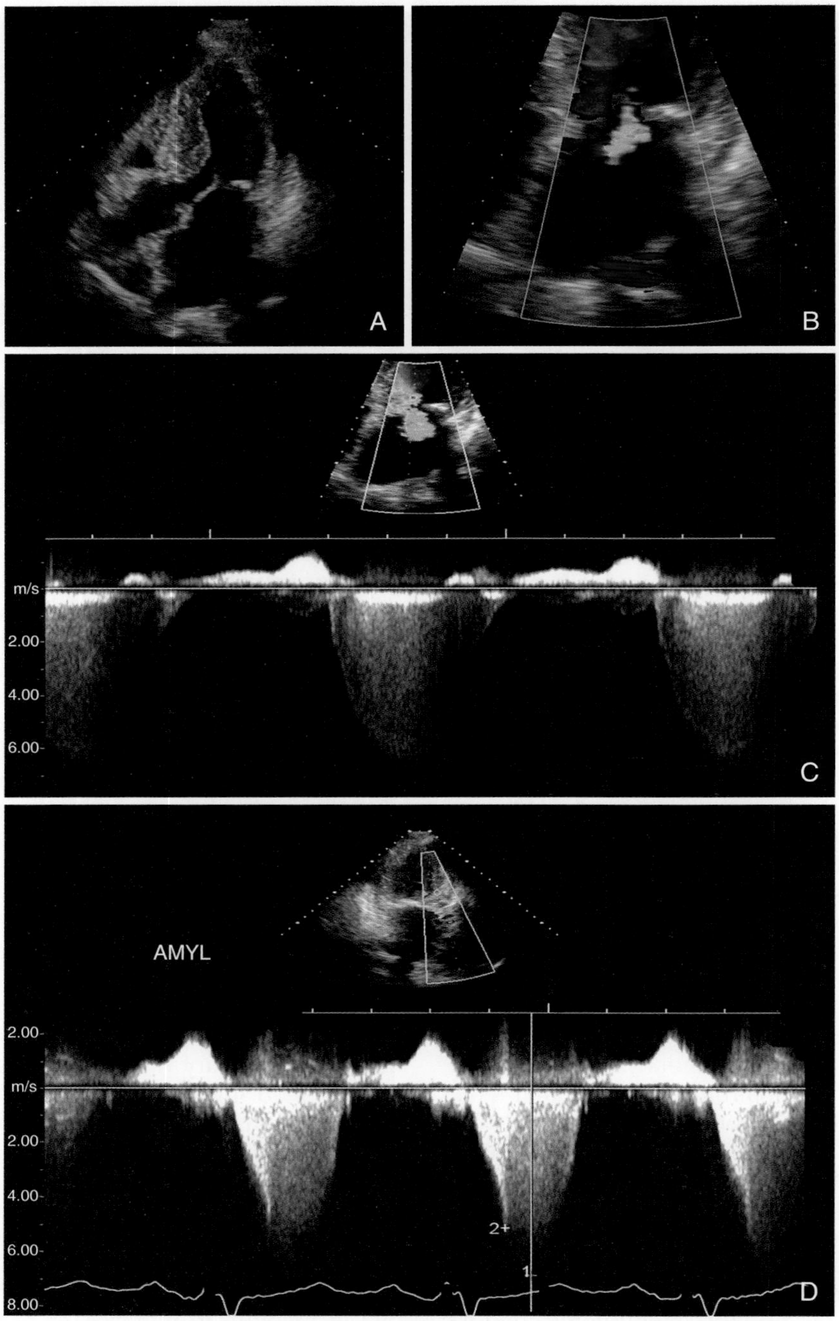

FIGURE 31-3 This figure demonstrates the importance of precise assessment of the left ventricular outflow tract gradient (LVOT) in the presence of severe mitral regurgitation (MR). It is important not to misinterpret the Doppler spectral display of MR for LVOT velocities given their close spatial orientations. **A,** Apical view of the heart demonstrating significant upper septal hypertrophy. **B,** Color Doppler imaging showing flow acceleration across the LVOT and posteriorly directed jet of MR. **C,** Continuous wave Doppler across the mitral valve to trace the Doppler spectral display of the MR jet. **D,** The Doppler spectral display of the LVOT velocities. Notice that it is contaminated by the MR Doppler display, as the two envelopes appear very similar to each other. The velocity labeled "1" (614 cm/s) represents the peak MR jet velocity and would erroneously overestimate the LVOT gradient. The actual LVOT velocity in this case is represented by velocity labeled "2" (420 cm/s), which is the peak of the early dense spectral display that overlies the MR spectral display.

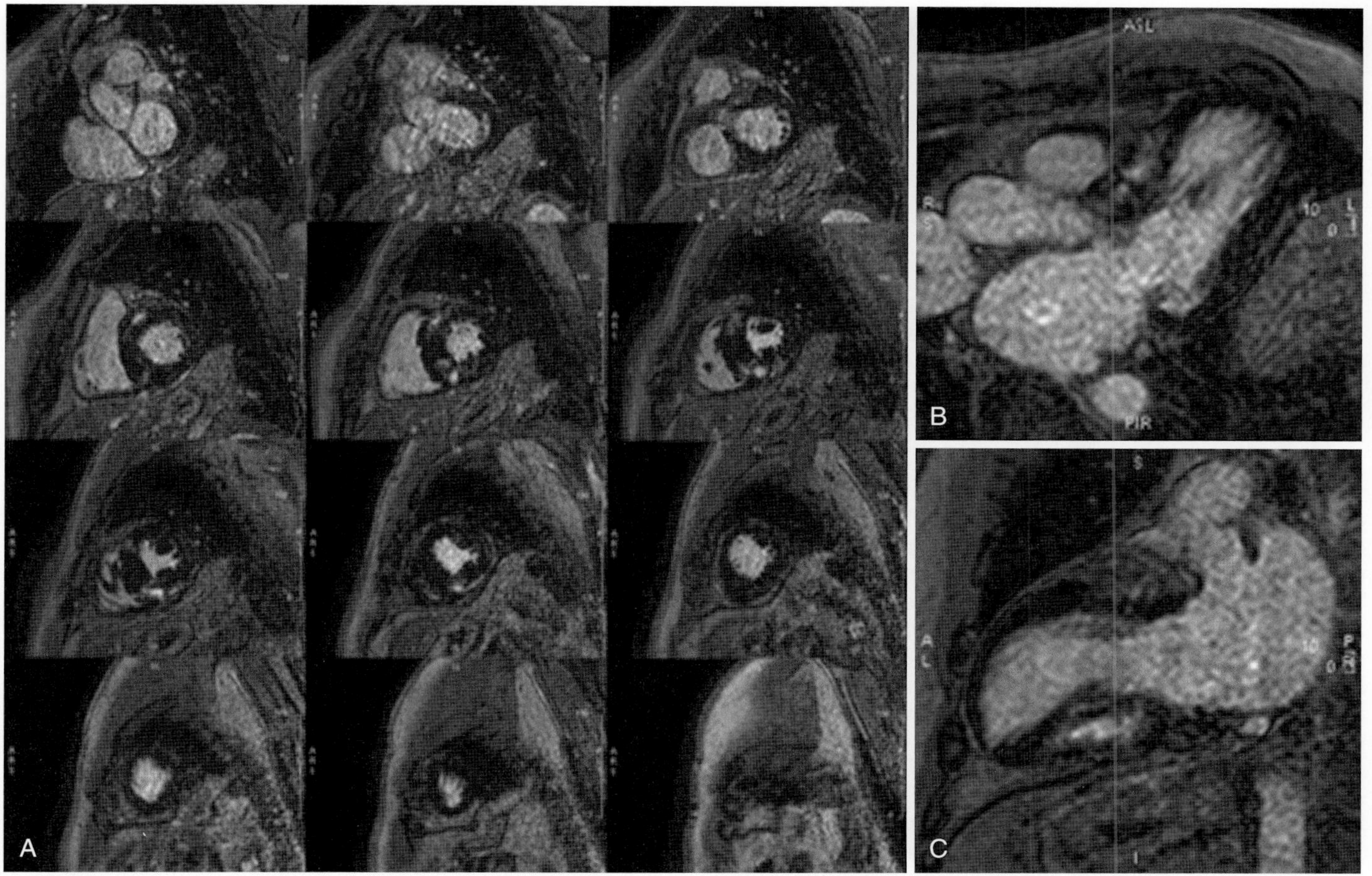

FIGURE 31-4 Cardiac magnetic resonance imaging with late gadolinium enhancement (LGE) indicative of extensive myocardial fibrosis. The left-sided panels **(A)** demonstrate consecutive short-axis images of the heart; the upper right panel **(B)** demonstrates a four-chamber representation; and the lower right panel **(C)** demonstrates a two-chamber representation. Collective interpretation of these images demonstrates a significant amount of scar involving the upper septum and inferior walls of the heart.

or flail leaflets) because this finding has a major implication on the choice of treatment strategy.

Myocardial Fibrosis

Histopathologic examination of myocardium affected by HCM typically demonstrates myocardial fiber disarray with markedly thickened cardiomyocytes, arranged in whirls and branches and an increased amount of fibrosis, especially in advanced cases. It may be speculated that this cellular disarray reduces the contractile force of the affected myocardium, which in turn stimulates the myocardial hypertrophy process. Assessment of fibrosis may be performed using biomarkers as well as cardiac imaging modalities like echocardiography and CMR. In HCM, extracellular matrix turnover also seems to be a determinant of cardiac remodeling. Accordingly, the ratio of PICP (C-terminal propeptide of type I procollagen, a marker for collagen synthesis) to C-terminal telopeptide of type I collagen (collagen degradation product) was increased in subjects with HCM, suggesting that collagen synthesis exceeds degradation in these patients.[46] The presence of fibrosis is suggested by late gadolinium enhancement (LGE) of affected myocardium observed on CMR (**Figure 31-4**). LGE imaging detects accumulation of contrast in areas of fibrosis due to slower contrast kinetics and greater volume of distribution in the extracellular matrix. However, it should be noted that not all areas of LGE represent scar, especially in HCM.[47] Areas of LGE identified in 40% to 80% of HCM patients may be helpful in the diagnosis of HCM versus other causes of LV wall thickening. Besides CMR, newer echocardiographic modalities like tissue Doppler imaging and speckle tracking can also help determine the extent of fibrosis in HCM. Low septal tissue velocity (<5 cm/s, normal >8 cm/s) corresponds to increased early diastolic stiffness of the fibrotic septum (**Figure 31-5**). Speckle tracking often shows markedly reduced septal strain as opposed to the normal systolic function of the less fibrotic lateral wall.

GENETICS AND ROLE OF GENETIC TESTING

Genetic studies have demonstrated that HCM is caused by dominant mutations in any one of the 11 or more genes encoding thick and thin contractile myofilament protein components of the sarcomere, or the adjacent Z-disc.[48] Of patients who have been genotyped, about 70% have mutations in two genes: β-myosin heavy chain (MYH7) and myosin binding protein C (MYBPC3). Troponin T (TNNNT2), troponin I (TNNI3), and several other genes account for 5% or less of all cases. Despite few of these mutations accounting for a large majority of cases, more than 1400 mutations (largely missense) have been identified that may be responsible for causing HCM. Some of these include α-myosin heavy chain (MYH6), titin (TTN), muscle LIM protein (CSRP3), telethonin (TCAP), vinculin (VCL), and junctophilin 2 (JPH2).

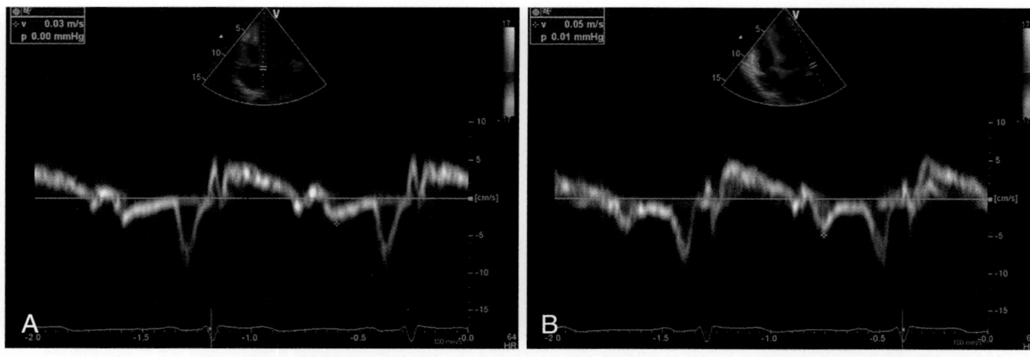

FIGURE 31-5 This figure shows tissue Doppler imaging in a patient with HCM. **A,** Markedly low early diastolic tissue velocities at the level of medial mitral valve annulus (3 cm/s). **B,** Markedly low early diastolic tissue velocities at the level of lateral mitral valve annulus (5 cm/s).

Genetic mutations that cause HCM are transmitted in an autosomal dominant fashion, implying that each offspring of an affected individual has a 50% chance of inheriting this disease. Sporadic cases may arise due to de novo mutations. The phenotypic heterogeneity that exists between individual cases suggests that the mutations of the sarcomeres are probably not the only determinant of the HCM phenotype. It is possible that modifier genes or environmental factors affect the final phenotype. Age-related penetrance can occasionally result in delayed appearance of LV hypertrophy during adulthood. Nevertheless, LV wall thicknesses evident in mid-life and at older ages are generally modest. Extreme LV hypertrophy is rare at advanced ages.

Rapid, automated DNA sequencing provides opportunities for comprehensive genetic testing and identification of mutations causing HCM. However, pathogenic mutations can be identified in fewer than half of clinically affected probands. In addition, DNA-based testing frequently identifies novel DNA sequence variants for which pathogenicity is unresolved. Such ambiguous variants have virtually no clinical use for family screening and promote confusion in interpretation of genetic testing results.

The American College of Cardiology (ACC) and American Heart Association (AHA) recommend genetic testing for evaluation of familial inheritance for all patients with diagnosed HCM (Class I).[49] Patients who undergo genetic testing should also undergo counseling by a cardiovascular genetics expert to review the implications of the results of their investigation (Class I).[49] Genetic and/or clinical screening of all first-degree family members of patients with HCM is recommended to identify those with undiagnosed disease (Class I).[49] Because familial HCM is a dominant disorder, the risk that an affected patient will transmit disease to each offspring is 50%. Because HCM mutations are highly penetrant, a mutation conveys substantial (>95%) risk for developing phenotypic expression of HCM. According to the current guidelines, the usefulness of genetic testing in the assessment of risk of SCD in HCM patients is considered uncertain (Class IIb).[49] Genetic testing is not indicated in relatives when the index patient does not have a definitive pathogenic mutation (Class III).[49]

DIAGNOSIS

Echocardiography

Two-dimensional echocardiography is the most common method for establishing the clinical diagnosis of HCM via identification of a thickened nondilated LV in the absence of other co-morbidities known to cause LV hypertrophy. According to the latest ACC/AHA guidelines, TTE is recommended in the initial evaluation of all patients with suspected HCM (Class I).[49] In addition, a TTE is recommended as a component of the screening algorithm for family members of patients with HCM (Class I).[49] For family members between 12 and 21 years, screening should be performed every 12 to 18 months. For relatives older than 21 years, imaging should be performed either at the onset of symptoms or possibly at 5-year intervals. More frequent intervals may be appropriate among families, where a malignant clinical course or history of late-onset HCM exists. For children <12 years of age, screening is optional unless the child is a competitive athlete in an intensive training program, or is symptomatic, or there is a malignant family history of premature death from HCM, or other adverse complications are present.

Although classically thought to involve the upper septum, HCM can result in any pattern of LV thickening.[50] While maximal wall thickness >15 mm is the traditional echocardiographic threshold utilized for defining HCM, the degree of LV hypertrophy often demonstrates considerable variability. It is important to note that the paucity of characteristic LV hypertrophy >15 mm on TTE does not exclude the presence of a gene mutation for HCM. Serial echocardiographic examinations are often necessary for monitoring the progression of LV hypertrophy and LVOT obstruction. In addition, there are considerable differences in the pattern of LV involvement between young and elderly patients. Elderly patients are often found to have an elliptical ventricular cavity with hypertrophy limited to the basal septum. In contrast, young patients often have a crescent-shaped LV cavity associated with diffuse hypertrophy of the interventricular septum.[51]

Resting LVOT obstruction is observed in approximately one third of patients with HCM. Subaortic obstruction is usually dynamic in nature and is secondary to SAM of the anterior mitral leaflet leading to mitral-septal contact during mid-systole. Obstruction is not present in resting conditions in another third of all patients but can be provoked by pharmacological maneuvers (like amyl nitrite), or by physiological maneuvers (like Valsalva, exercise). Significant MR frequently accompanies SAM owing to distortion of the valvular apparatus and malcoaptation of the anterior and posterior mitral leaflets during systole. Up to 30% of the patients with HCM may have intrinsic mitral valve abnormalities such as leaflet prolapse, chordal rupture, or leaflet calcification/fibrosis. Less commonly, a mid-cavity gradient may be present because of anomalous insertion of the anterolateral papillary muscle directly onto the anterior mitral leaflet or an exaggerated proliferation of the mid-ventricular papillary musculature coming into apposition with the ventricular septum. It is important not to misinterpret the Doppler spectral display of MR for LVOT velocities given their close spatial orientations (**Figure 31-3**). In the setting of SAM, the MR jet is generally posterolaterally directed into the left atrium, and it is often difficult to distinguish from the LVOT flow. It is useful to sweep anterior to posterior with continuous wave Doppler to distinguish these two flows.

Given the degree of LV hypertrophy seen in HCM, it is not uncommon to observe diastolic dysfunction on echocardiography. This may be manifested by reduced maximal flow velocity in early diastole (E wave), an increase in isovolumic relaxation time, and increased atrial contribution to the ventricular filling (A wave). Further, tissue Doppler imaging may demonstrate reduced velocities at the upper septal location suggestive of stiff fibrotic septum (**Figure 31-5**). These changes are often present in patients without significant LVOT obstruction, suggesting that diastolic dysfunction may be an earlier clinical manifestation in the spectrum of the disease process.

Electrocardiography

Although increased voltages consistent with LV hypertrophy and early repolarization abnormalities are commonly encountered in HCM, electrocardiographic (ECG) findings in HCM are quite heterogeneous. Although >90% of patients have abnormal ECGs, no pattern is highly specific for the condition. Besides increased voltages and repolarization abnormalities, there may be left axis deviation, left atrial enlargement, T wave inversion, or nonspecific ST segment abnormalities. The degree of LV hypertrophy in HCM does not appear to correlate with the magnitude of hypertrophy when assessed using TTE. In a subset of Japanese patients with hypertrophy limited to the ventricular apex, giant T wave inversions are frequently noted in the anterior leads; these are often termed Yamaguchi's disease.[52] Pathological Q waves may be seen in the inferolateral leads in about 50% of patients with HCM. Moreover, approximately a third of patients have delayed His-Purkinje conduction noted on electrophysiological studies, possibly owing to the strain on the anterior fascicle, which overlies the hypertrophied ventricle.

According to the current ACC/AHA guidelines, 24-hour ambulatory ECG monitoring is recommended in the initial evaluation of patients with HCM to detect ventricular tachycardia (VT), and identify patients who may be candidates for ICD therapy (Class I).[49] In addition, 24-hour ambulatory ECG monitoring or event recording is recommended in patients with HCM who develop palpitations or lightheadedness (Class I).[49] Furthermore, a 12-lead ECG is recommended as a screening tool for first-degree relatives of patients with HCM (Class I).[49] It is considered reasonable to perform serial ambulatory ECG monitoring on an annual or 2-year basis in patients who do not have ICDs, who are stable, and do not manifest arrhythmias on baseline 12-lead ECG and Holter monitoring (Class IIa).[49]

Stress Testing

Treadmill exercise testing is considered reasonable to determine functional capacity and response to therapy in patients with HCM (Class IIa).[49] In patients with HCM who do not have a resting LVOT gradient >50 mm Hg, exercise echocardiography is reasonable for detection and quantification of exercise-induced dynamic LVOT obstruction (Class IIa).[49] Exercise testing is useful in assessment of patients with HCM, as abnormal blood pressure response to exercise (defined as failure to increase systolic blood pressure by at least 20 mm Hg, or a drop in systolic blood pressure at peak exercise) has been shown to be associated with the risk of SCD.[43,44,49,53,54] Stress-testing modalities may include bicycle, treadmill testing using the Bruce protocol, or metabolic cardiopulmonary testing, with measurement of gradient either during or immediately after exercise.

Cardiac Magnetic Resonance Imaging

Cardiac magnetic resonance (CMR) imaging offers multiple advantages to better detect areas of LV hypertrophy that are not well visualized or missed by TTE. These include superior resolution with precise morphological characterization, enhanced tissue contrast capability, and production of three-dimensional images. The ACC/AHA currently recommend CMR for patients with suspected HCM, when echocardiography is inconclusive or equivocal for establishing diagnosis (Class I).[49] In addition, CMR imaging is indicated in patients with known HCM when additional information that may have an impact on management of decision making regarding invasive management such as magnitude and distribution of hypertrophy, or anatomy of the mitral valve apparatus, or papillary muscles are not adequately defined with echocardiography (Class I).[49] CMR imaging is considered reasonable in patients with suspected Yamaguchi's disease to define apical hypertrophy (Class IIa).[49]

The last few years have witnessed a growing use of contrast-enhanced CMR with LGE to identify areas of myocardial fibrosis in patients with HCM (**Figure 31-4**). A substantial proportion of patients with HCM have been shown to have LGE suggestive of areas with fibrosis that may occupy a significant volume of the LV myocardium.[35,55] Patients with presence of LGE on CMR imaging tend to have more markers of risk of SCD, such as nonsustained VT on ambulatory monitoring, as compared with those without LGE.[56,57] It is currently hypothesized that areas of LGE represent a substrate for generation of malignant ventricular tachyarrhythmias, which might be responsible for SCD. Several studies have already demonstrated that presence of LGE (rather than extent) may be associated with adverse cardiovascular events among patients with HCM.[58,59] The current evidence supports a potential role of contrast-enhanced CMR with LGE as an arbitrator in clinical decision making for primary prevention ICDs, where SCD risk stratification remains inconclusive.

Invasive Hemodynamic Assessment

Given the vast amount of diagnostic and prognostic information that can be derived with noninvasive modalities discussed above, cardiac catheterization is generally not required for the diagnosis of HCM. Invasive evaluation is generally employed in four scenarios, as follows:

- If noninvasive imaging is insufficient to qualify, or quantify, the degree of LVOT obstruction
- To rule out concomitant coronary artery disease among those that present with typical anginal chest discomfort, especially in presence of traditional cardiovascular risk

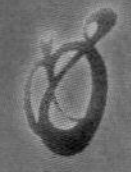

factors for atherosclerotic heart disease (intermediate-high likelihood of coronary artery disease) (Class I)[49]

- To evaluate the presence of coronary artery disease prior to planned surgical myectomy
- To evaluate the anatomy of the septal perforators prior to ASA

Coronary arteries are generally free of obstruction in patients with HCM. Due to significant hypertrophy of the septum, compression of the left anterior descending (LAD) artery may be seen during systole, resulting in a classically described "sawfish" appearance.[60] Myocardial bridging (or tunneling) may be present in up to 40% of patients with HCM.[61] Myocardial bridging may be responsible for causing angina in the absence of significant epicardial coronary artery stenosis. Although it has been suggested that intermittent ischemia as a result of myocardial bridging could be a potential mechanism for sudden death in HCM patients,[62] there has been no convincing evidence to support this hypothesis in adults or children.[63,64] Left ventriculography may demonstrate systolic cavity obliteration, MR, and occasionally hypertrophied septum prolapsing into the LVOT. Direct measurement and localization of the gradient may be performed by placing an end-hole catheter at the LV apex and then slowly withdrawing it while continuously monitoring the pressure waveform. Use of a wire placed via guide catheter helps maintain control during the pullback, and a more accurate determination of the level of obstruction. As opposed to aortic stenosis (AS), the gradient is seen to reduce before crossing the aortic valve. Measurement of gradient across the LVOT may also be performed by placement of a pigtail catheter in the aortic root and another pigtail catheter into the LV via the transseptal route, through the mitral valve, to allow for a simultaneous aortic and LV pressure waveform assessment, which is generally more accurate than the former technique.

Since the gradient across the LVOT is generally labile, various physiologic and pharmacologic maneuvers may need to be utilized to accentuate the LVOT obstruction. One of the classical signs described is the Brockenbrough-Braunwald-Morrow sign, or the postextrasystolic potentiation.[65] This refers to the augmentation of the LV pressure with a concomitant decrease in the aortic systolic and pulse pressures as a result of increased LVOT obstruction in the cardiac cycle that follows a premature ventricular contraction (PVC) (**Figure 31-6**). Postextrasystolic increase in the gradient between LV and aorta is seen in AS too, but unlike

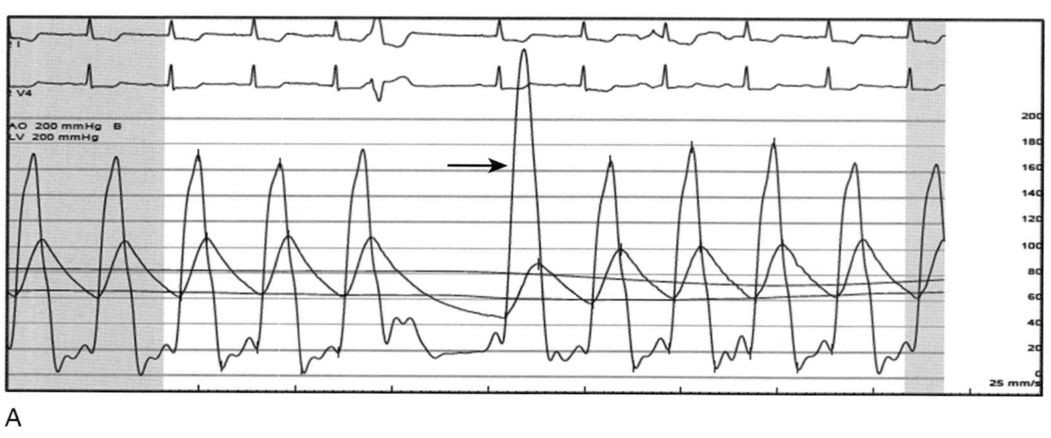

A

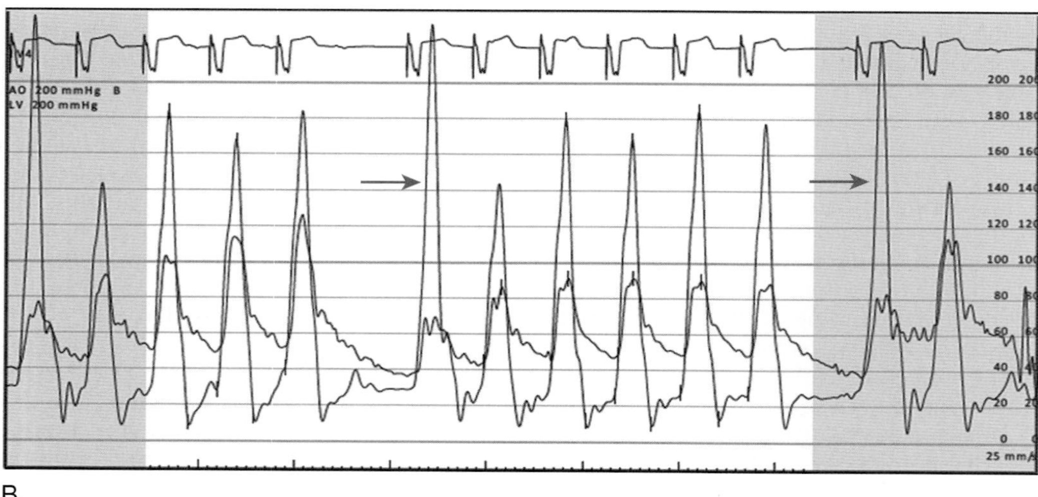

B

FIGURE 31-6 This figure shows the Brockenbrough-Braunwald-Morrow sign. The hemodynamic tracings shown in the two panels were obtained with simultaneous measurement of LV pressure waveform and aortic pressure waveform with two catheters. **A,** The classic sign with marked augmentation of the LV pressure with a concomitant decrease in the aortic systolic and pulse pressures as a result of increased left ventricular outflow tract (LVOT) obstruction in the cardiac cycle that follows a premature ventricular contraction (PVC) *(black arrow)*. **B,** A modified version of this sign in a patient with a dual chamber pacemaker, who was pacing in an "A-sense, V-pace" manner. It can be clearly appreciated that there are differing RR intervals secondary to irregular atrial activity. The *red arrows* demonstrate the beats following unusually long RR interval. The hemodynamic tracings mimic the classic sign, with an augmentation of the LV pressure with a decrease in the aortic systolic, and pulse pressure, during beats with long RR interval.

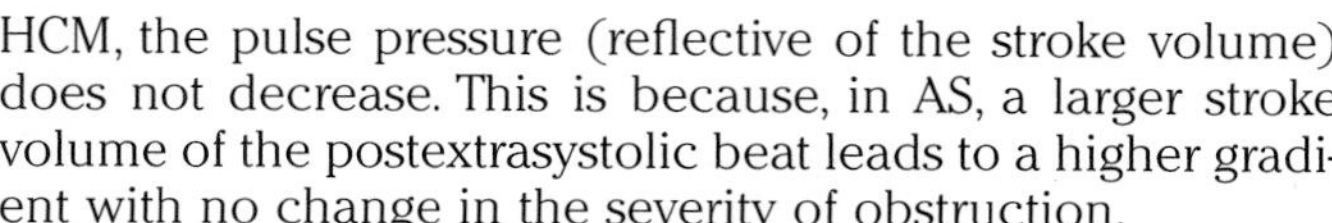

HCM, the pulse pressure (reflective of the stroke volume) does not decrease. This is because, in AS, a larger stroke volume of the postextrasystolic beat leads to a higher gradient with no change in the severity of obstruction.

MANAGEMENT OF HCM

Management of patients with HCM requires a thorough understanding of the complex pathophysiology and often needs to be individualized to the patient. The management decisions are based on presence and extent of obstructive physiology, symptoms and their persistence, LV systolic function, surgical candidacy, co-morbidities, and patient preferences.

Asymptomatic Patients

A large proportion of patients with HCM are asymptomatic and a majority of those generally achieve a normal life expectancy. Risk stratification for SCD must be performed meticulously in all patients with HCM, irrespective of symptomatology. Education is key, and it is essential to counsel all patients and their families about the disease process, screening of all first-degree relatives, and avoidance of strenuous activity in competitive athletes.[66] According to the current ACC/AHA guidelines, it is recommended that co-morbidities that contribute to atherosclerotic disease like hypertension, diabetes, hyperlipidemia, and obesity be aggressively treated in compliance with existing relevant guidelines (Class I).[49] This is because concomitant CAD has a significant adverse impact on survival in patients with HCM.[67] A low-intensity aerobic exercise regimen is reasonable to achieve optimal cardiovascular fitness.[49,68]

It is important to avoid dehydration and environmental circumstances that promote vasodilation among all asymptomatic patients with resting or provocable LVOT gradient. Hence, high-dose diuretics and vasodilators should be avoided in patients with HCM, as these may promote a smaller LV cavity and exacerbate the degree of obstruction. Although the usefulness of β-blockade and calcium channel blockade to alter the natural course of disease is not well established in asymptomatic patients, these agents may be utilized to treat relevant co-morbidities like hypertension (Class IIb).[49] Some preliminary data in animal models have demonstrated the efficacy of angiotensin-converting enzyme inhibitors or statins or calcium channel blockers[69] in halting progression of LV hypertrophy. However, similar data are not available in humans. Therefore, these agents should not be utilized for the intent of altering HCM-related clinical outcomes, but only for the control of symptoms or for control of relevant co-morbidities.

Septal reduction therapies are currently not recommended for asymptomatic patients with HCM with normal exercise capacity regardless of the extent of LVOT obstruction (Class III).[49,53,54] The indication of septal reduction therapy is to improve symptoms refractory to medical therapy resulting in significant impairment of quality of life. Therefore, they should not be performed in an asymptomatic patient solely based on the extent of resting or provocable LVOT gradient.

Symptomatic Patients

Medical Management

Medical therapy should be utilized as the initial therapeutic approach for treatment of symptomatic patients with HCM. Due to a relatively small number of cases, pharmacotherapy for HCM is largely based on expert opinion, clinical experience, and retrospective observational analyses. Patients with LVOT obstruction constitute the largest proportion of symptomatic obstruction. Besides these patients with manifest obstruction, a significant number of nonobstructing patients may also suffer consequences of diastolic dysfunction such as heart failure, angina, and atrial fibrillation,[66] which may require pharmacologic treatment. Due a greater utilization of genetic markers and echocardiography in diagnosis of HCM, it has become increasingly clear that a vast majority of patients with HCM remain asymptomatic for an extended period of time. Most available data suggest that this population does not warrant empiric therapy until and unless symptoms develop.

Beta-Blockers

According to the current ACC/AHA guidelines, β-blockers should be utilized as primary pharmacologic therapy for treatment for symptoms in adult patients with obstructive or nonobstructive HCM, and with caution in patients with sinus bradycardia, or severe conduction disease (Class I).[49] If low doses of β-blockers prove to be ineffective in controlling symptoms, it is often useful to titrate the dose to a resting heart rate <60 to 65 beats/minute (up to generally accepted and recommended maximum doses of individual agents) (Class I).[49] β-blockers are effective due to their negative inotropic effects and their ability to attenuate adrenergic-induced tachycardia. These effects significantly reduce myocardial oxygen demand, thereby reducing myocardial ischemia. The reduction in resting heart rate prolongs the diastolic filling period, which allows for more efficient inactivation of myocardial contractile proteins and improving diastolic filling mechanics.[69-71] Due to their negative chronotropic properties, these agents are especially helpful in patients with supraventricular tachycardia. The first agent initially utilized for treatment, propranolol, has largely been replaced by the newer generation, longer-acting, cardioselective agents such as metoprolol.

Calcium Channel Blockers

Nondihydropyridine calcium channel blocker verapamil has been traditionally utilized in patients with HCM. According to the current guidelines, verapamil therapy (beginning in low doses and titrating up to 480 mg/d) is recommended for treatment of symptoms in patients with obstructive or nonobstructive HCM who do not respond to β-blockers, or who have adverse effects or contraindications to the use of β-blockers (Class I).[49] In symptomatic patients, it is a common clinical practice to begin therapy using β-blockers rather than verapamil. Should the patient be intolerant of the side effects, or if symptoms persist despite adequate titration of the β-blocker therapy, consideration may be given to changing (or adding) therapy to verapamil. However, at the current time, there is no evidence to suggest that combination therapy with verapamil and β-blockers is more effective than either a β-blocker or verapamil alone. In case a decision for combination therapy is made, caution should be exercised because of the potential for high-grade atrioventricular (AV) conduction block.

Verapamil functions as a negative inotrope and a negative chronotope by blocking the intracellular migration of calcium ions. This results in a symptomatic improvement in patients, owing to increased diastolic filling time and enhanced diastolic ventricular relaxation without adversely affecting systolic function as well as ensuring reduced myocardial oxygen consumption.[72,73] In addition, verapamil has been shown to increase absolute myocardial blood flow during pharmacologic stress testing, while also reducing ischemic burden and improving exercise tolerance in HCM patients.[74,75] Although verapamil has classically been utilized in both obstructive as well as nonobstructive disease, caution should be exercised in those with a large resting LVOT gradient owing to reports of severe hemodynamic compromise resulting in cardiogenic shock and pulmonary edema.[49] The current guidelines recommend against the use of verapamil in patients with obstructive HCM in the setting of systemic hypotension or severe dyspnea (Class III).[49]

Although some preliminary data in animals have suggested the utility of diltiazem in preventing LV hypertrophy, there are scarce data in humans to suggest its usefulness in HCM.[69] However, in patients who do not tolerate beta-blockers or verapamil, diltiazem may be considered (Class IIb).[49] Nifedipine or other dihydropyridine calcium channel blockers are potentially harmful for treatment of symptoms in patients with HCM who have resting or provocable LVOT gradient (Class III).[49] This is because their vasodilatory effects may exacerbate the outflow obstruction, possibly leading to worsening of current symptoms.

Disopyramide

Disopyramide has been in the armamentarium for HCM for over three decades. It is a Class IA anti-arrhythmic agent that also functions as a negative inotropic effect and leads to a relative increase in the systemic vascular resistance. The current ACC/AHA guidelines consider it reasonable to combine disopyramide with β-blockers or verapamil in treatment of symptomatic obstructive HCM, in patients who do not respond to β-blockers or verapamil alone (Class IIa).[49] While it does not appear to have any effect on the diastolic dysfunction, disopyramide has been shown to effectively reduce the outflow obstruction due to SAM with improved symptomatic control in patients who are refractory to other forms of therapy.[76-78] The initiation of disopyramide therapy should be performed in hospital with cardiac monitoring for arrhythmias due to its QT prolonging effects. Anti-cholinergic side effects like dry mouth, urinary retention, and constipation might occur, which may be managed with dose reduction. The use of disopyramide alone without β-blockers or verapamil is potentially harmful in HCM patients with AF because disopyramide may enhance AV conduction and increase the ventricular rate during episodes of AF (Class III).[49]

Amiodarone

While current data appear to be conflicting with the use of amiodarone in HCM, it has been suggested that amiodarone might reduce the risk of SCD and improve survival in selected high-risk patients with nonsustained VT on ambulatory cardiac monitoring.[79] Although some reports have demonstrated its efficacy in improvement of symptoms and functional capacity, amiodarone may have a pro-arrhythmic effect and may theoretically lead to an increased risk of SCD due to VT.[80,81] However, recent data indicate that chronic low-dose amiodarone therapy (200 mg/d) in high-risk patients with recurrent nonsustained VT is not associated with any increase in long-term mortality.[82] At this dose, amiodarone has been demonstrated to be effective therapy for treatment and prevention of VT in patients with HCM.[83] Care should be exercised in selecting chronic VT suppression therapy with amiodarone, especially considering its attendant adverse effect profile, until more definitive data become available.

Other Agents

Although high-dose diuretics are generally contraindicated for fear of dehydration, it is considered reasonable to add low-dose oral diuretics in patients with nonobstructive or obstructive HCM when the symptoms of dyspnea persist despite the use of β-blockers or verapamil, or their combination (Class IIa).[49] Diuretics often afford symptomatic relief in patients with pulmonary edema, but judicious use is certainly warranted. The usefulness of angiotensin-converting enzyme inhibitors or angiotensin receptor blockers in treatment of symptomatic HCM patients with preserved systolic function is not well established, and these drugs should be cautiously used (if at all) in patients with resting or provocable LVOT obstruction (Class IIa).[49] Intravenous phenylephrine is recommended for treatment of acute hypotension in patients with obstructive HCM who fail to respond to intravenous fluid administration (Class I).[49] Use of norepinephrine, dopamine, dobutamine, or other positive inotropic agents is potentially harmful for treatment of hypotension in patients with symptomatic HCM and is not recommended (Class III).[49]

Invasive Management

The current ACC/AHA guidelines recommend that septal reduction therapy should be performed in *eligible patients* with severe drug refractory symptoms and LVOT obstruction as defined by the following core criteria

- Clinical: Severe angina or dyspnea (NYHA class III/IV) or other symptoms like syncope or near syncope that interfere with activities of daily living or adversely affect quality of life despite adequate medical therapy
- Hemodynamic: Resting or provocable LVOT gradient more than 50 mm Hg associated with septal hypertrophy and SAM of the mitral valve
- Anatomic: Targeted septal thickness sufficient to perform the procedure safely and effectively in the judgment of the individual operator.

Septal reduction therapy should not be done for patients who are asymptomatic with normal exercise tolerance or whose symptoms are minimized on optimal medical therapy (Class III).[49] Septal reduction therapies include SM and ASA. Although these are methodologically very different approaches and interventions, they have been treated similarly in ACC/AHA guidelines as well as European guidelines[84] as they are both accepted methods for relief of symptoms in patients with LVOT obstruction. There are some nuances in tailoring individual therapies among the affected population, which have been discussed further in this chapter. SM has been used for the last 50 years, and relief of LVOT obstruction can be achieved with minimal perioperative morbidity and mortality in experienced centers.[85,86] Given the duration of experience, long-term results, and established safety in experienced hands, SM is considered as the treatment of choice in most patients who meet criteria for invasive management of HCM. Considerations that lead to the choice of SM include younger age, greater septal thickness, and concomitant cardiac disease that require surgical correction like intrinsic mitral valve disease or coronary artery disease. Specific abnormalities of mitral valve apparatus can contribute significantly to the generation of LVOT gradient, suggesting the potential value of additional surgical approaches (e.g., plication, papillary muscle relocation, valvuloplasty). Although ASA has been around only for the past two decades, the number of these procedures performed has surpassed the number of myectomies performed in the last five decades. ASA causes a regional infarction of the basal septum, thereby initially decreasing contractility and eventually causing thinning of the basal septum and consequent widening of the LVOT. Among patients who meet core criteria for septal reduction therapy, considerations that favor the use of ASA over SM include advanced age, significant noncardiac co-morbidities that increase surgical risk, and the patient's desire to avoid open heart surgery after a thorough discussion of both options.

It has been recommended that both these procedures should only be performed by experienced operators, in the context of a comprehensive HCM clinical program. The ACC/AHA define an experienced operator as someone with a cumulative case volume of at least 20 procedures or an individual operator who is working in a dedicated HCM program with a cumulative total of at least 50 procedures.[49] In addition, given the data available from experienced centers, operators should aim to achieve mortality rates <1% and major complication rates <3%, with documented improvement in hemodynamics and symptoms of their treated HCM patients. Therefore, septal reduction therapy should only be performed as part of a program dedicated to the longitudinal and multidisciplinary care of patients with HCM.[49]

Septal Myectomy

Transaortic SM is currently considered the gold standard for the majority of patients with obstructive HCM and severe symptoms refractory to medical therapy. Although published literature demonstrate a considerable improvement in the surgical results over the last few decades, the data are limited to a relatively few centers with extensive experience and particular interest in the treatment of HCM. There has been a significant evolution in the spectrum of surgical therapy from the original isolated septal myotomy performed by Cleland[87] in 1960, to the more modern, and widely utilized Morrow myectomy.[88] The Morrow myectomy is performed via the transaortic approach so that the proximal septum is visualized and 5 to 15 g of myocardial tissue is resected from the base of the aortic valve to a region distal to the mitral leaflets such that the area of the mitral-septal contact that results in SAM is removed, consequently enlarging the LVOT.[88,89] It is critically important to correctly identify the involved portion of the LV septum and resect enough myocardium to relieve the LVOT gradient. Therefore, most experienced centers utilize transesophageal echocardiography (TEE) to assist with the localization of the desired region for resection, and to monitor the effect of resection on the LVOT gradient intraoperatively.

Despite its more aggressive nature, an alteration of the classic Morrow procedure has been described, which involves an extended myectomy with a partial excision and mobilization of the papillary muscles. This procedure results in amelioration of the LVOT obstruction, reduced tethering of the subvalvular mitral structures, and a more individualized surgical resection depending on the extent and location of the patient's LV hypertrophy. In patients with concomitant disorders like AF or coronary artery disease, SM may be combined with adjunctive procedures like surgical treatment for atrial fibrillation (MAZE) or coronary artery bypass grafting. Abnormalities of mitral valve apparatus such as elongated and flexible leaflets often contribute to the degree of LVOT obstruction in a minority of patients. These patients often benefit from leaflet plication at the time of myectomy to more effectively reduce the degree of LVOT obstruction that results from SAM and to reduce the associated MR. Mitral valve replacement is generally reserved for patients with significant primary valvular abnormalities such as myxomatous degeneration leading to mitral valve prolapse or severe MR. The surgical specimen obtained during the operation should be submitted for histopathological examination, not only to confirm the diagnosis of HCM, but also for special stains to rule out other storage disorders that can mimic HCM.

Patient Selection. Since SM is considered to be a gold standard for the treatment of symptomatic obstructive HCM, clinicians should favor this procedure in all patients who are deemed surgical candidates. Subjective assessment of operative risk by clinicians often results in an overestimation of risk, resulting in the denial of SM for eligible patients.[90] Considerations that lead to the choice of SM include younger age, greater septal thickness, and concomitant cardiac disease that require surgical correction like intrinsic mitral valve disease or coronary artery disease. Specific abnormalities of mitral valve apparatus can contribute significantly to the generation of LVOT gradient, suggesting the potential value of additional surgical approaches (e.g., plication, papillary muscle relocation, valvuloplasty).

Early Results. Based on the results from several experienced centers, SM has been established as the most efficacious procedure for reversing the consequences of heart failure, relief of LVOT obstruction, as well as restoration of exercise capacity and good quality of life in HCM patients who were symptomatic on maximal tolerated pharmacologic therapy.[91-97] Successful SM leads to an improvement in treadmill time, maximum workload, peak oxygen consumption, myocardial oxygen demand, and coronary blood flow.[54,98,99] SM leads to basal septal thinning leading to an enlargement of the LVOT area. This leads to a redirection of forward flow and abolition of drag and Venturi effect on the mitral valve, leading to loss of SAM and mitral-septal contact.[100-102] MR is usually eliminated without need for additional mitral valve surgery.[2] With SM, the LA size (and the risk of subsequent AF) is reduced and LV end-diastolic pressure along with LV wall stress is normalized.[54,85,103-105] In experienced centers the operative risk is particularly low and is estimated to be <1%.[106]

Late Results. It is believed that LVOT obstruction after SM might extend the longevity of patients with HCM.[85] Although randomized controlled trials comparing SM with medical therapy do not exist, nonrandomized studies have demonstrated that SM resulted in excellent long-term survival similar to that in the general population. After SM, actuarial survival was 99%, 98%, and 95% at 1 year, 5 years, and 10 years postmyectomy, respectively. This survival rate did not differ from that expected in a matched general U.S. population and was superior to that achieved by patients with obstructed HCM who did not undergo SM.[85] Although the rate of SCD or inappropriate ICD discharge following SM is very low (<0.9%), SM does not eliminate the need for

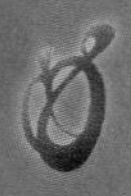

individual SCD risk assessment and consideration of placement of ICD in those with a significant risk burden.

Complications. In experienced hands, SM is a very safe procedure. The risk of operative mortality is <1%. Although left bundle branch block is relatively common after surgery, the risk of complete heart block is ~2% with SM. It is higher in patients with pre-existing right bundle branch block or those who have been subjected to alcohol septal ablation (ASA) in the past. In patients with prior ASA, the risk of complete heart block may be as high as 50% to 85%.[107] Iatrogenic ventricular septal defect is rare and occurs in <1% of cases. Finally, the risk of aortic valve or mitral valve injury is also low (<1%), particularly when an experienced operator performs the procedure.

Important Considerations. Abnormalities of the mitral valve apparatus may be identified preoperatively or intraoperatively using TEE. These include anomalous direct anterolateral papillary muscle insertion into anterior mitral leaflet or elongated mitral leaflets. These anomalies are generally correctable with modified mitral valve repair or extended myectomy without the need for valve replacement. With excellent early and late outcomes following extended SM for treatment of obstructive HCM, the requirement of mitral valve replacement has become rare.[89] Concomitant degenerative mitral valve disease can be treated with adjunctive mitral valve repair at the time of myectomy. Mitral valve repair techniques need to be modified in HCM according to the degree of contribution of an abnormal mitral valve to LVOT obstruction or MR.

Mitral valve replacement has been performed rarely when septal reduction therapy was judged unsafe or felt to be ineffective. When the basal septum is mildly hypertrophied (<16 mm), the risk of either iatrogenic ventricular septal defect from excessive muscular resection or residual postoperative LVOT obstruction from inadequate resection increases considerably. Mitral valve replacement may be an option in these rare patients.[108,109]

Alcohol Septal Ablation

First performed by Sigwart in 1995,[110] ASA was intended for symptomatic patients who do not wish to undergo invasive open heart surgery, are suboptimal surgical candidates due to co-morbidities, or are located in areas without sufficient surgical expertise. Through the selective infusion of absolute (100%) ethanol into either the first or second septal perforator arteries, the ASA technique attempts to mimic the effect of the traditional Morrow myectomy by inducing a controlled infarction in the basal portion of the hypertrophied septum, resulting in scarring, thinning, and akinesis, leading to a significant reduction in the LVOT gradient and SAM of the anterior mitral valve leaflet. Although there are no randomized control trials comparing ASA to SM or medical therapy, short-term observational studies have demonstrated a significant reduction in LVOT gradient, and improvement in symptoms and functional capacity, with a reported mortality similar to or lower than the SM.[98,111-115] The short-term success of this procedure combined with its minimally invasive character has led to a dramatic increase in the utilization of ASA for treatment of symptomatic obstructive HCM. It is estimated that ASA is performed 15 to 20 times more commonly than SM worldwide, relieving LVOT obstruction in symptomatic HCM patients.[66,116,117]

Patient Selection. ASA has the potential for a greater patient satisfaction because of its minimally invasive character, lack of surgical incision and general anesthesia, less overall discomfort, a much shorter recovery time, and a shorter hospital stay. It is well known that the perioperative risks and complications of cardiac surgery increase with age and therefore ASA might offer a selective advantage in older patients in whom surgical risk is high due to co-morbidities. ASA is not currently indicated in children.

There are several important considerations that physicians should discuss with their patients before a choice of ASA is made over SM. The likelihood of permanent pacemaker implantation postablation is 4 to 5 times higher as compared with SM. Clinical and hemodynamic benefit is achieved immediately after recovery from SM but may be delayed for up to 3 months after ASA; although a large majority of patients do achieve notable symptomatic benefit shortly after the procedure. In addition, patients with severe septal hypertrophy (>30 mm) derive limited or no benefit from ASA. In experienced hands, surgical myectomy is almost always predictable. However, the success of the ASA depends in part to distribution of the targeted septal perforator branch and the blood supply to the area of the septum that is aimed to be ablated. Before embarking on the choice of ASA, a thorough search should be made for concomitant abnormalities that are better addressed surgically. These include anomalous papillary muscle insertion into the mitral valve, anatomically abnormal mitral valve with long leaflet, co-existent coronary artery disease, primary valvular disease involving the mitral or aortic valve or subaortic membrane, or pannus, all of which would not be adequately addressed by ASA. In addition, abnormally elongated and flexible anterior mitral leaflet resulting in an anterior location of the co-aptation line and LVOT obstruction will not be correctable via ASA and would require SM with plication.[118] Furthermore, an appropriate septal anatomy amenable to intervention is imperative for a successful ASA procedure.

Procedural Technique (Video 31-1)**.** The procedure is generally performed under conscious sedation with special attention to pain control at the time of alcohol infusion into the septal perforator. The first step of the procedure is to perform a standard diagnostic coronary angiogram to clearly define the coronary anatomy and evaluate for concomitant atherosclerotic disease (**Figure 31-7**). For the clearest anatomical characterization of the septal anatomy coursing through the basal interventricular septum, the c-arm must be positioned in the right anterior oblique (RAO) cranial or the posteroanterior (PA) cranial projections. At times, the septal anatomy may vary such that one subdivision may run along the left side of the septum while another runs along the right side. Angiography in the left anterior oblique (LAO) cranial projection often helps determine the septal vessels' course along the septum (leftwards or rightwards). Selection of the left-sided subdivision is advised as there is a significantly less likelihood of complete heart block during ethanol infusion into the leftward branches as compared with the rightward branches. While in a majority of cases the septal perforators arise from the LAD, substantial anatomical variation has been described in which the vessels may be seen to arise from the left main trunk (LMT), ramus intermedius (RI), left circumflex (LCX), the diagonal branches, or even from the branch of the right coronary artery (RCA).[119] Once the image acquisition is completed, the operator should select the appropriate septal perforator branch to ablate.

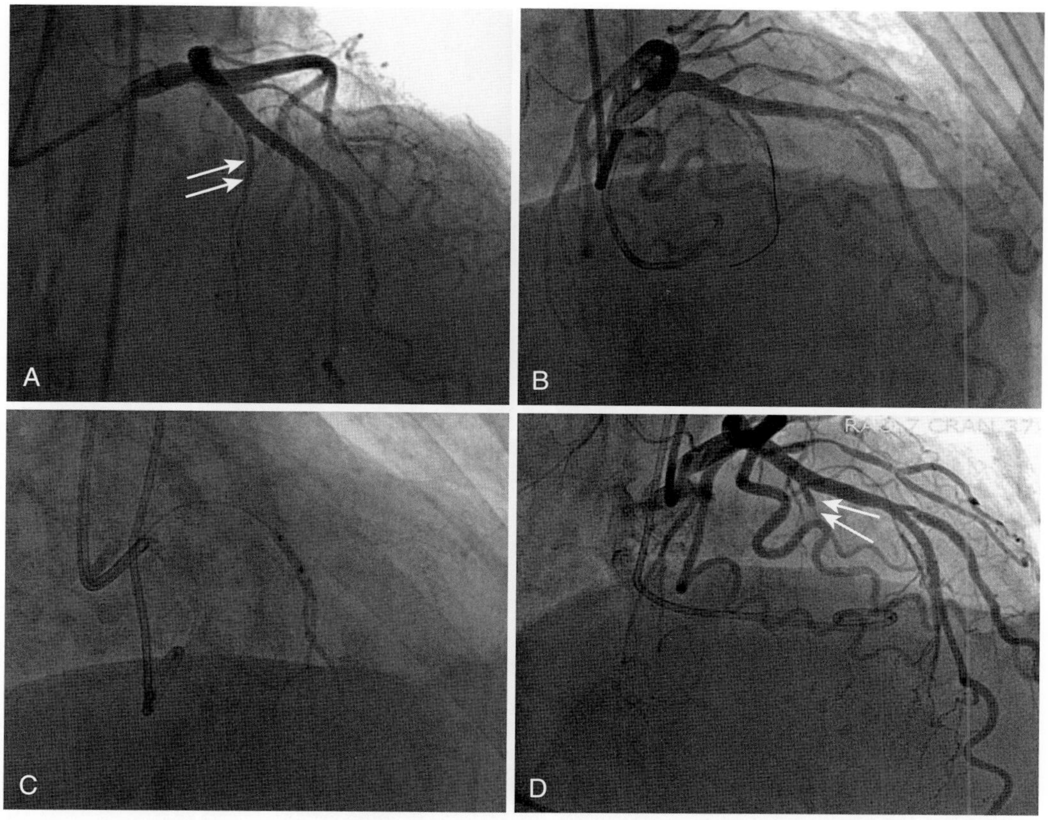

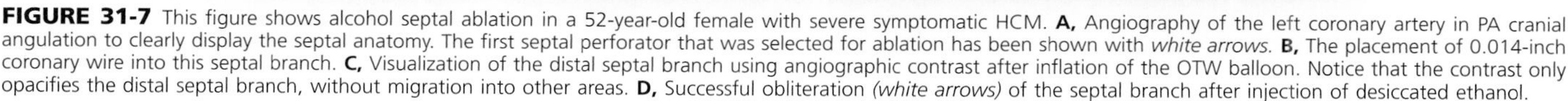

FIGURE 31-7 This figure shows alcohol septal ablation in a 52-year-old female with severe symptomatic HCM. **A,** Angiography of the left coronary artery in PA cranial angulation to clearly display the septal anatomy. The first septal perforator that was selected for ablation has been shown with *white arrows*. **B,** The placement of 0.014-inch coronary wire into this septal branch. **C,** Visualization of the distal septal branch using angiographic contrast after inflation of the OTW balloon. Notice that the contrast only opacifies the distal septal branch, without migration into other areas. **D,** Successful obliteration *(white arrows)* of the septal branch after injection of desiccated ethanol.

After completion of the diagnostic coronary angiography, a temporary transvenous pacemaker is placed as a prophylactic measure in case of development of complete heart block during or in the postprocedure period. Some operators prefer placing a screw-in active fixation lead via the right internal jugular vein. Since unfractionated heparin is generally utilized for anticoagulation, care should be taken to minimize the risk of bleeding during arterial sheath placement and pacemaker insertion. Following successful placement of the sheaths and pacemaker, heparin is administered intravenously to achieve activated clotting time of ≥300 to prevent thrombosis in the guiding catheters or wires.

Besides the characteristics mentioned above, there are several important considerations that must be included in the selection of the septal perforator for ablation. These include vessel size, vessel angulation, bifurcation of the septal perforator, and the myocardial territory served by the given vessel. Vessels with angulation >90 degrees are often technically challenging and may result in considerable difficulty in passing the balloon into the vessel, with frequent prolapse of the wire into the mid-LAD.[119] Specialized techniques using a catheter that allows control of the distal angle (Venture catheter, St. Jude Medical, Minnesota) may be useful in these rare cases. Assessment of myocardial territory supplied by the septal perforator is of paramount importance to avoid causing myocardial infarction in unintended territories. It has been demonstrated that there is substantial variation in the perforator anatomy in patients with HCM as compared with normal controls. In both angiographic and autopsy studies, it has been demonstrated that the first septal perforator may supply blood to regions other than the basal septum including the right ventricle.[119,120] At times, it may supply the basal septum incompletely and share this responsibility with the second septal perforator.[119,120] Accurate assessment of the myocardial territory supplied by a septal perforator is accomplished by the selective injection of dye under cine-acquisition and concomitant use of echocardiography utilizing injectable contrast material (**Figure 31-7**).

Following the angiographic assessment of the septal anatomy, a guiding catheter (usually a 6 Fr or 7 Fr XB catheter) is used to engage the LMT. Subsequently, a 0.014-inch guidewire with a soft tip is passed into the selected sepal perforator. A short over-the-wire (OTW) angioplasty balloon, usually 1.5 to 2 mm in diameter, is passed over the guidewire into the selected septal branch. Sometimes, there is difficulty in passing the balloon into the selected septal perforator, which may be overcome by using a stiffer guidewire. Following the placement of the angioplasty balloon, it is inflated to completely occlude the septal branch. It must be ensured that the balloon is placed deep enough and fully expanded so that injected alcohol does not reflux into the LAD. Conversely, if the balloon is seated very deeply into the septal branch, the injected ethanol might spare the basal septum, resulting in an unsuccessful procedure.

At this point, it is essential to verify the myocardial territory being supplied by the selected septal perforator, given a significant variation in the septal anatomy in HCM patients.

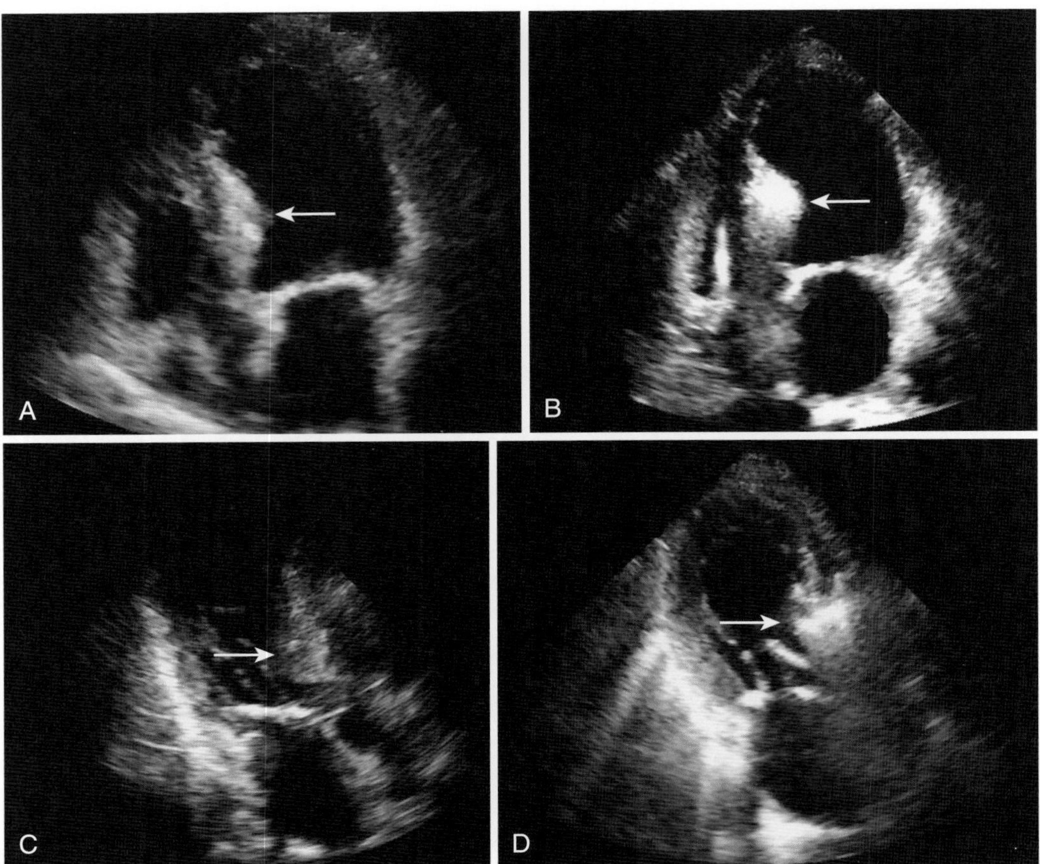

FIGURE 31-8 This figure shows echocardiographic characterization of the myocardial territory supplied by the targeted septal branch for alcohol ablation. **A** and **C,** The apical four-chamber and long-axis views prior to the echo contrast injection, showing the presence of severe septal hypertrophy. **B** and **D,** Respective images after injection of the echo contrast agent, delineating the myocardial territory supplied by the targeted septal branch. The *white arrows* point to the region of the upper septal hypertrophy.

Both angiographic as well as echocardiographic confirmation must be obtained prior to proceeding with alcohol injection. In order to obtain angiographic confirmation, the operator should inject 1 to 2 cc of contrast through the OTW balloon (**Figure 31-7**). Contrast should be injected slowly to mimic the anticipated alcohol injection. Three things must be observed. First, the operator should ensure that the selected perforator indeed supplies the basal septum that is responsible for LVOT obstruction. Second, the contrast does not reflux back into the mid-LAD. Third, the contrast does not reach the RCA circulation through septal collaterals, thereby leading to an inferior myocardial infarction. Following angiographic confirmation, further assessment of the septal distribution is obtained via contrast echocardiography. After carefully visualizing the septum in apical four-chamber and parasternal long-axis views, 1 to 2 cc of Albumex is injected into the septal perforator through the OTW balloon (**Figure 31-8**). Albumex is a first-generation echo contrast agent that is no longer available in several countries and has been replaced by second- and third-generation agents. These new agents have proven to be suboptimal due to their rapid passage through the capillary beds, which produces a large amount of echocardiographic shadowing from opacified ventricles. In our catheterization laboratory, the contrast vials are typically opened 10 to 15 minutes prior to the time of expected use to decrease their potency. Subsequently, the contrast agent is further diluted with sterile saline in a 1:5 to 1:10 mixture at the time of injection. Pulse wave Doppler with a low mechanical index is the method of choice to avoid destruction of the microbubbles with the higher frequency continuous wave ultrasound. The operator should expect appearance of the echo contrast in the basal septum responsible for greatest extent of septal-mitral contact. Appearance of contrast in the distal septum, right ventricle, or other areas of myocardium is a contraindication to ethanol infusion (**Figure 31-8**). As a final method of confirmation, a >30% reduction in the LVOT gradient on balloon inflation in the selected septal perforator is reassuring.

Before proceeding with ethanol injection, the operator should fluoroscopically verify that the balloon has not migrated and that the transvenous pacemaker continues to have a suitable pacing threshold. After this, the operator may proceed with the ethanol injection. Most experienced centers use between 1 to 2 mL of desiccated absolute ethanol. The volume may be adjusted based on the appearance of the septal anatomy and the degree of contrast washout. It has been demonstrated that a smaller amount of ethanol injection (1 to 2 mL) results in comparable mid-term clinical and hemodynamic outcomes, with reduced complication rates, especially permanent pacemaker requirement.[121] In cases where there is rapid contrast washout due to collateralization of the septal branch, the rate and volume of ethanol infusion should be reduced to prevent the alcohol from escaping to undesirable areas of the myocardium via the collaterals. The alcohol is generally

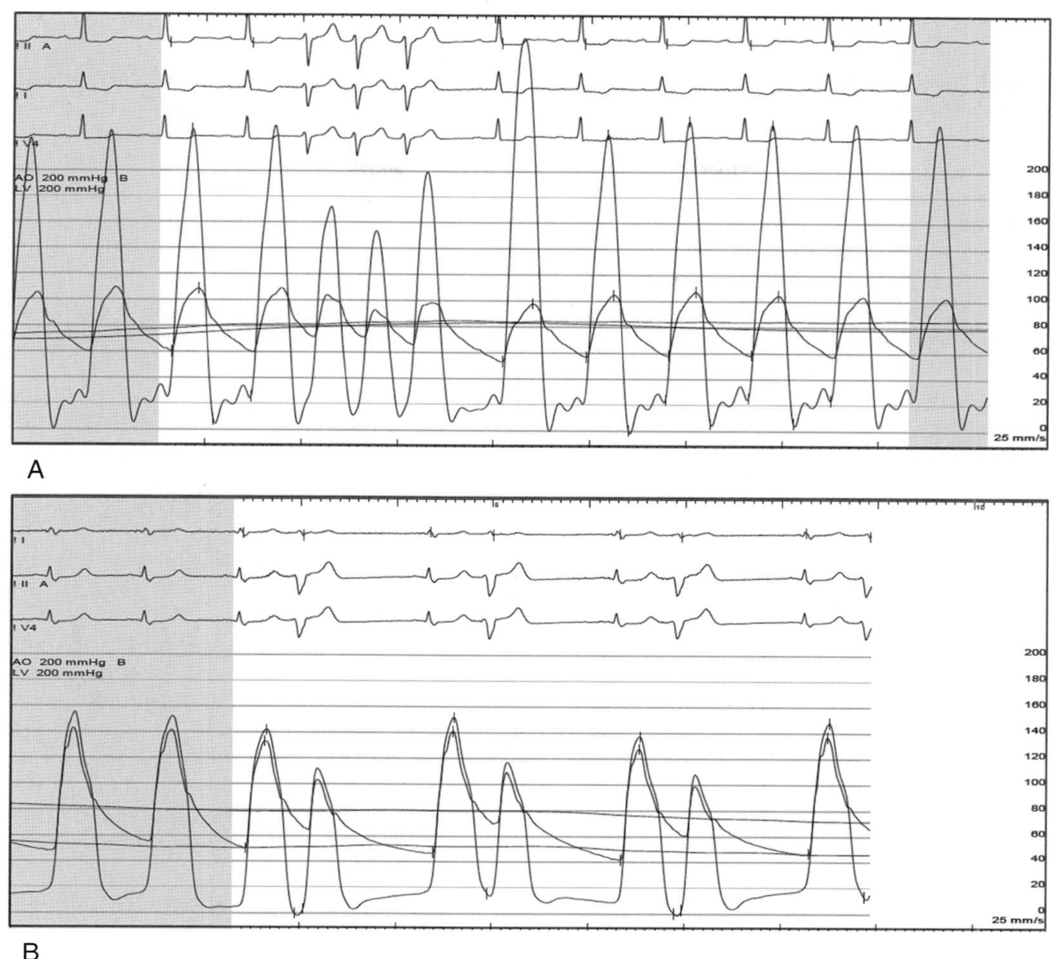

FIGURE 31-9 This figure shows hemodynamic tracings obtained from before **(A)** and after **(B)** successful alcohol septal ablation performed in a 52-year-old female with severe symptomatic HCM. The hemodynamic tracings shown in the two panels were obtained with simultaneous measurement of LV pressure waveform, and aortic pressure waveform with two catheters. The top panel shows a significant left ventricular outflow tract (LVOT) gradient with postextrasystolic potentiation after PVCs (Brockenbrough-Braunwald-Morrow sign). After a successful alcohol septal ablation procedure, there was a complete elimination of the LVOT gradient as well as the Brockenbrough-Braunwald-Morrow sign **(B)**.

injected over a 1- to 5-minute period with the balloon remaining inflated. Following the initial infusion, a reduction in the LVOT gradient to <30 mm Hg in the setting of a resting gradient >50 mm Hg, or a >50% reduction of a provocable gradient is considered indicative of a successful procedure (**Figure 31-9**). Before disengaging the balloon from the septal vessel, the guidewire is replaced into the septal branch to facilitate a smooth and quick removal of the balloon from the coronary circulation. As a final step, angiography of the left coronary artery is performed to document the occlusion of the septal branch and to verify the integrity of the rest of the coronary circulation.

Postprocedurally, all patients should be monitored in an intensive care unit setting for at least 48 hours. The transvenous pacing wire may be discontinued after 48 hours if there are no bradyarrhythmias or heart block that necessitates a longer observation or permanent pacemaker implantation. The amount of creatine kinase-MB (CK-MB) elevation postablation ranges between 800 IU/L to 1200 IU/L, although this is variable depending on the amount of alcohol injected, vessel size, and method of enzyme measurement. In most centers, the patient is transferred to a regular nursing floor for an additional 2 to 3 days to observe for postprocedural complications prior to discharge.

Results. Reduction in LVOT gradient after ASA demonstrates a triphasic response, and it may take up to 3 months to completely manifest its effect on LVOT gradient.[122] An acute reduction in LVOT gradient immediately after successful ASA is generally followed by an increase in the gradient to the baseline level within 3 days, followed by a decrease back to the immediate postablation level within 3 months. The acute decrease in the LVOT gradient reflects a loss of septal contractility caused by ischemia, necrosis, and stunning of the septal myocardium. The early recovery of gradient after ASA reflects the recovery of the septal myocardium from stunning along with myocardial edema that accompanies necrosis. Over the course of the next 3 months, there is thinning of the infarcted septum and LVOT remodeling, leading to sustained and more permanent reduction in gradients. Left atrial pressure is reduced, which may promote a decreased incidence of AF and amelioration of pulmonary hypertension.[123] The beneficial results of ASA have been reported to almost 5 years after the procedure with improved functional and anginal classes, exercise capacity, and quality of life.[111,113,114,124-126] However, the hemodynamic and symptomatic success is dependent on the ability to cannulate and ablate a septal perforator artery that supplies the area of the mitral-septal contact.

Complications. The complication rate following ASA is relatively low and comparable to SM. In contrast to the left bundle branch block commonly seen after SM, a right bundle branch block is observed in ~80% of cases after ASA.[112,119] The incidence of complete heart block ranges between 12% and 15% at most experienced centers.[112,113,119] The presence of a pre-existing left bundle branch block or a rapid bolus injection of ethanol during ablation has been correlated with high-degree AV block needing a permanent pacemaker implantation. Reflux or extravasation of contrast into mid-LAD is a rare but catastrophic complication of the procedure that leads to a mid to distal anterior wall myocardial infarction. Coronary dissection due to guiding catheters, pericardial tamponade from RV perforation from the transvenous pacemaker, and ventricular septal rupture from an injection of a generous quantity of alcohol are other rare complications. Ventricular arrhythmias can be seen during the procedure in the postprocedure period. Unlike SM, ASA results in a large myocardial scar that has been speculated to serve as a nidus for malignant ventricular tachyarrhythmias. However, this hypothesis is yet to garner substantial evidentiary support.

Comparison of Alcohol Septal Ablation and Septal Myectomy

Although there are no randomized controlled trials comparing SM and ASA and are highly unlikely to be in the future, meta-analyses of the existing observational studies have noted similar hemodynamic and functional improvement over 3 to 5 years with both techniques.[127] All studies published until now have compared their experience where the treatment allocation was not randomized. Despite age differences between the two groups with ASA patients on average ~10 years older in clinical practice, similar short-term and medium-term mortality rates have been reported with the two techniques.[127] The incidence of right bundle branch block as well as complete heart block requiring permanent pacemaker implantation after ASA has been reported to be significantly higher as compared with corresponding rates after SM.[127] Metaanalysis of observational studies comparing ASA and SM has demonstrated a similar NYHA functional class in both treatment categories. Although this metaanalysis demonstrated a significantly reduced LVOT gradient after SM as compared with ASA immediately after the procedure, it should be emphasized that complete benefit of ASA on LVOT gradient reduction is often realized several months after the procedure due to scar retraction and LVOT remodeling.[122] It is currently recommended that extensive discussions should be conducted with patients to explain the risks and benefits of the two procedures before embarking on the choice of therapy.

Role of Dual Chamber Pacing

Dual chamber pacing, as a less invasive alternative to the SM, was met with initial enthusiasm in the 1990s, when several observational studies demonstrated a significant reduction in the LVOT gradient, improvement in functional status, and quality of life.[128-130] While the exact mechanism is unclear, it has been proposed that activation of the RV apex results in dyssynchronous contraction of the interventricular septum, resulting in reduction in the LVOT gradient in the short-term and a positive ventricular remodeling in the long-term.[131] However, there have been three randomized cross-over trials in which patients received 2 to 3 months of continuous dual chamber (DDD) pacing but also underwent a backup AAI mode (no-pacing) as a control arm.[132-134] The overall reduction in the LVOT gradient was modest (25% to 40%), with a significant variation among individual patients. Although objective measurements of functional capacity were improved with DDD pacing, they were not significantly different from the control arm without pacing. This suggested that a placebo effect as well as a training effect probably contributed to the initial symptomatic improvement in patients undergoing DDD pacing. Overall, the proportion of patients with sustained symptomatic improvement is extremely variable (30% to 80%).[99,135-137] The overall success in terms of relief of symptoms as well as LVOT gradient reduction with DDD pacing is inferior as compared with SM. The mean LVOT gradient reduction after DDD pacing is ~10 mm Hg compared with 40 to 50 mm Hg reduction after SM.[128,132,133,136]

Based on these findings, the ACC/AHA recommends that in patients with HCM who have a dual chamber device implanted for non-HCM indications, it is reasonable to consider a trial of dual chamber AV pacing (from the RV apex) for the relief of symptoms attributable to LVOT obstruction (Class IIa).[49] In addition, permanent pacing might be considered in medically refractory symptomatic patients with obstructive HCM who are suboptimal candidates for septal reduction therapy (Class IIb).[49] However, permanent pacemaker implantation for the purpose of reducing LVOT gradient should not be performed in patients with HCM who are asymptomatic or whose symptoms are medically controlled (Class III).[49] In addition, a permanent pacemaker should not be implanted as a first-line therapy to relieve symptoms in medically refractory symptomatic patients with HCM and LVOT obstruction who are candidates for septal reduction therapy (Class III).[49] Furthermore, dual chamber pacing has not been shown to be beneficial for patients with nonobstructive HCM.[138]

Several considerations are important to realize the hemodynamic benefits of dual chamber pacing therapy. It is necessary to optimize the AV delay because an extremely short interval results in hemodynamic deterioration and an extremely long interval without complete pre-excitation of the ventricle leads to an inadequate response. The position of the RV lead is important, requiring distal apical capture for optimal hemodynamic results. In addition, programming of the rate adaptive packing is necessary so that full pre-excitation of the ventricle is obtained during exercise.

Management of Atrial Fibrillation

AF is an important co-morbidity in patients with HCM. Diagnosis of AF is often made using electrocardiogram (ECG) or ambulatory Holter monitoring. Anticoagulation with vitamin K antagonists (warfarin to achieve an international normalized ratio 2.0 to 3.0) is indicated in patients with paroxysmal, persistent or permanent AF, and HCM (Class I).[49] Anticoagulation with direct thrombin inhibitors like dabigatran may represent another therapeutic option to reduce the thromboembolic risk, but data for HCM patients are not currently available. High doses of β-blockers or nondihydropyridine calcium channel blockers may be required for achieving optimal ventricular rates in HCM patients who present with rapid ventricular rates (Class I).[49] The current guidelines consider disopyramide or amiodarone as reasonable anti-arrhythmic choices for rhythm control in patients with HCM (Class IIa).[49] Sotalol, dronaderone, and dofetilide might be considered as alternative anti-arrhythmic agents in patients with HCM, especially in those with ICD (Class IIb).[49] Radiofrequency ablation may be beneficial in patients who have refractory symptoms or who are unable to take anti-arrhythmic drugs (Class IIa).[49] MAZE procedure with excision or exclusion of left atrial appendage is reasonable in patients with HCM with a history of AF, either during SM or as an isolated procedure in selected individuals (Class IIa).[49]

Management of Systolic Dysfunction

Systolic dysfunction in HCM is uncommon and should prompt an investigation for known causes of LV dysfunction like coronary artery disease, unrelated valvular heart disease, or metabolic disorders. Systolic dysfunction in HCM patients might be a consequence of long-standing untreated disease, representing an end-stage in the natural course of HCM. Most randomized controlled trials evaluating the efficacy of therapies for heart failure exclude patients with HCM. Despite lack of data for this subset of patients, there is no compelling evidence to believe that highly effective, guideline-based therapies for systolic dysfunction need to be denied to HCM patients with systolic dysfunction.

The current ACC/AHA guidelines recommend that patients with nonobstructive HCM who develop LV dysfunction with ejection fraction <50% should be treated according to evidence-based medical therapy for adults with other forms of systolic heart failure, including β-blockers, angiotensin-converting enzyme inhibitors, angiotensin receptor blockers, and other efficacious drugs (Class I).[49] ICD implantation may be reasonable in patients with advanced heart failure (NYHA Class III/IV) and nonobstructive HCM, on maximal medical therapy with ejection fraction <50%, who do not otherwise have an indication for ICD (Class IIb).[49] For patients with HCM who develop LV dysfunction, it may be reasonable to reassess the use of negative inotropic agents previously indicated and consider discontinuing these therapies (Class IIb).[49]

Role of Heart Transplantation

According to the current guidelines, heart transplantation should be considered in patients with advanced heart failure and nonobstructive HCM and ejection fraction <50% who are not amenable to other interventions (Class I).[49] Most patients referred for heart transplant evaluation have extensive LV remodeling including cavity enlargement and wall thinning because of diffuse myocardial scarring. Although reduced ejection fraction is not a qualifying criterion, this treatment strategy is rarely recommended and performed in the presence of preserved ejection fraction. Symptomatic children with HCM with restrictive physiology who are not responsive to or appropriate candidates for other therapeutic interventions should also be considered for heart transplantation (Class I).[49] Heart transplantation should not be considered or performed in mildly symptomatic patients of any age with HCM (Class III).[49]

PREVENTION OF SUDDEN CARDIAC DEATH

All patients with HCM should undergo comprehensive risk stratification for sudden cardiac death (SCD) at initial evaluation. The established risk factors for SCD are[49]:

- Prior personal history of ventricular fibrillation, SCD, or sustained VT, including appropriate ICD therapy for ventricular tachyarrhythmias (Class I)
- Family history of SCD (Class I)
- Unexplained syncope (Class I)
- Documented nonsustained VT defined as 3 or more beats at >120 bpm on ambulatory ECG monitoring (Class I)
- Maximal LV wall thickness ≥30 mm (Class I)
- Abnormal blood pressure response during exercise (Class IIa)

Other potential SCD risk modifiers include[49]:

- Severity of LVOT obstruction (Class IIb)
- LGE on CMR imaging (Class IIb)
- Presence of LV apical aneurysm (Class IIb)
- "Malignant" genetic mutations including double and compound mutations (Class IIb)

Besides a personal history of cardiac arrest, other risk factors for SCD possess low positive predictive value (~10% to 20% each) and modestly high negative predictive value (~85% to 95%). Presence of multiple risk factors in an individual may suggest a greater risk of SCD; however, a majority of patients with ≥1 risk factor will not experience a SCD event in their lifetime. In the international HCM-ICD registry,[139] the number of risk factors failed to correlate with the rate of subsequent appropriate ICD discharges among presumably high-risk patients selected for ICD implantation. This suggests that presence of a single risk factor may be sufficient or insufficient to warrant ICD placement in some patients, but these decisions need to be individualized with regard to age, the strength of risk factor, and the risk-benefit of lifelong ICD therapy.[139,140] Invasive electrophysiologic testing as routine SCD risk stratification for patients with HCM is not currently indicated and should not be performed (Class III).[49]

Participation in Competitive Sports

In terms of participation in competitive or recreational sports, it is reasonable for patients with HCM to participate in low-intensity competitive sports (e.g., golf, bowling) (Class IIa).[49] However, patients with HCM should not participate in intense competitive sports regardless of age, sex, race, extent of LVOT obstruction, prior septal reduction therapy, or ICD implantation status. The ACC as well as the European Society of Cardiology (ESC) guidelines indicate that the risk of SCD is increased during the intense competitive sports and suggest that avoidance of these activities in affected individuals might significantly mitigate their risk.[49,84] This principle is the basis for disqualification of athletes with HCM from sanctioned high school and college sports. It should, however, be noted that these recommendations for competitive athletes are independent of those for noncompetitive, informal, recreational sporting activities.

General recommendations for informal recreational exercise should be tailored based on the patient's desires and abilities. There are some general guidelines that prevail, in order to aid the physician for providing recommendations to these patients.

- Aerobic exercise as opposed to isometric exercise is preferable.
- Patients should generally avoid recreational sports in which participation is intense and simulates competitive organized athletics.
- Burst exertion, in which an abrupt increase in heart rate is triggered (like sprinting), is less advisable than swimming laps or cycling.
- Patients should avoid physical exertion in extreme environmental conditions of heat, cold, or high humidity, with attention paid to maintaining adequate hydration status.

Role of ICD Implantation

The decision to implant an ICD in patients should include application of individual clinical judgment through discussion of strength of evidence, benefits, and risks to allow the informed and active participation of the patient in decision making. ICD implantation is recommended in patients with prior documented cardiac arrest, ventricular fibrillation, or hemodynamically significant VT (Class I).[49] It may be reasonable to consider an ICD in patients with HCM under the following circumstances[49]:

- Sudden death presumably caused by HCM in one or more first-degree relatives (Class IIa)
- Maximal LV wall thickness ≥30 mm (Class IIa)
- One or more recent, unexplained syncopal episodes (Class IIa)
- Nonsustained VT (particularly <30 years of age), in presence other SCD risk factors (Class IIa)
- Abnormal blood pressure response to exercise, in presence of other SCD risk factors (Class IIa)

It may be reasonable to consider ICD implantation in high-risk children with HCM, based on unexplained syncope, massive LV hypertrophy, or family history of SCD, after taking into account the relatively high-complication rate of long-term ICD implantation (Class IIa).[49] The usefulness of ICD is uncertain in certain scenarios, especially when there is only one risk factor present. The usefulness of ICD implantation is considered uncertain in patients with HCM with isolated bursts of nonsustained VT in the absence of other SCD risk factors (Class IIb).[49] Likewise, the usefulness of ICD implantation is uncertain in patients with an abnormal blood pressure response with exercise in the absence of other risk factors (Class IIb).[49] ICD implantation is not recommended as a routine strategy in patients without an indication of increased risk for SCD (Class III).[49] In addition, ICD implantation in patients with HCM in the absence of clinical manifestations of HCM is potentially harmful and should not be performed (Class III).[49] Furthermore, ICD placement as a strategy to permit patients with HCM to participate in intense competitive athletics is not recommended (Class III).[49]

In patients who meet indications for ICD placement, single-chamber devices are reasonable in younger patients without a need for atrial or ventricular pacing (Class IIa).[49] Dual chamber ICD implantation should be considered in patients with sinus bradycardia or paroxysmal AF (Class IIa).[49] In patients with HCM, who meet indications for ICD implantation, dual chamber ICD may be reasonable in patients with LVOT gradient >50 mm Hg and significant heart failure symptoms who may benefit from RV pacing (most commonly, but not limited to >65 years of age) (Class IIa).[49] In addition, ICD implantation should be considered in all patients with NYHA Class III/IV symptoms on maximal medical therapy and ejection fraction ≤50% who do not have any other indication for an ICD (Class IIb).[49]

CONCLUSIONS

HCM is a complex genetic disease with multiple heterogeneous phenotypes and clinical manifestations. Because of the considerable heterogeneity of the disease and lack of randomized controlled trials in this arena, there is variability encountered in the management of patients with HCM across the world. The management of any patient with HCM should ideally focus on the following aspects:

- Control of heart failure symptoms
- Assessment of risk of sudden death and appropriate risk management
- Treatment of AF
- Management of LVOT obstruction using invasive techniques, when indicated
- Screening of family members

Although the current guidelines provide an important framework that helps in evaluation and treatment of patients with HCM, the unique characteristics and preferences of each patient should play a vital role in the decision-making and management strategies.

Despite significant improvement in the understanding of disease pathophysiology in the last few decades, there are considerable gaps that need to be addressed to improve care in this patient population. Long-term data on ASA will define its precise role in relation to myectomy in management of medically refractory patients with HCM. Improvements in the risk stratification for SCD will more accurately identify patients with HCM at risk for SCD. Development of subcutaneous and leadless ICD systems will likely reduce complications and lower the threshold for device implantation in young patients. The role of genetic testing will also become clearer when genotyping becomes cheaper and more accessible. Further research is needed for a more thorough understanding of the genetic basis of this disease in order to develop greater and more widespread clinical utility of genotyping in HCM.

References

1. Teare D: Asymmetrical hypertrophy of the heart in young adults. *Br Heart J* 20(1):1–8, 1958.
2. Maron MS, Olivotto I, Zenovich AG, et al: Hypertrophic cardiomyopathy is predominantly a disease of left ventricular outflow tract obstruction. *Circulation* 114(21):2232–2239, 2006.
3. Maron BJ: Hypertrophic cardiomyopathy: a systematic review. *JAMA* 287(10):1308–1320, 2002.
4. Maron BJ, Peterson EE, Maron MS, et al: Prevalence of hypertrophic cardiomyopathy in an outpatient population referred for echocardiographic study. *Am J Cardiol* 73(8):577–580, 1994.
5. Maron MS, Maron BJ, Harrigan C, et al: Hypertrophic cardiomyopathy phenotype revisited after 50 years with cardiovascular magnetic resonance. *J Am Coll Cardiol* 54(3):220–228, 2009.
6. Christiaans I, Lekanne dit Deprez RH, van Langen IM, et al: Ventricular fibrillation in MYH7-related hypertrophic cardiomyopathy before onset of ventricular hypertrophy. *Heart Rhythm* 6:1366–1369, 2009.
7. Ho CY, Sweitzer NK, McDonough B, et al: Assessment of diastolic function with Doppler tissue imaging to predict genotype in preclinical hypertrophic cardiomyopathy. *Circulation* 105:2992–2997, 2002.
8. Ho CY, Lopez B, Coelho-Filho OR, et al: Myocardial fibrosis as an early manifestation of hypertrophic cardiomyopathy. *N Engl J Med* 363:552–563, 2010.
9. Nagueh SF, McFalls J, Meyer D, et al: Tissue Doppler imaging predicts the development of hypertrophic cardiomyopathy in subjects with subclinical disease. *Circulation* 108:395–398, 2003.
10. Maron BJ, Pelliccia A, Spirito P: Cardiac disease in young trained athletes: insights into methods for distinguishing athlete's heart from structural heart disease, with particular emphasis on hypertrophic cardiomyopathy. *Circulation* 91:1596–1601, 1995.
11. Maron BJ, Pelliccia A: The heart of trained athletes: cardiac remodeling and the risks of sports, including sudden death. *Circulation* 114:1633–1644, 2006.
12. Maron BJ: Distinguishing hypertrophic cardiomyopathy from athlete's heart physiological remodelling: clinical significance, diagnostic strategies and implications for preparticipation screening. *Br J Sports Med* 43:649–656, 2009.
13. Pelliccia A, Kinoshita N, Pisicchio C, et al: Long-term clinical consequences of intense, uninterrupted endurance training in Olympic athletes. *J Am Coll Cardiol* 55:1619–1625, 2010.
14. Pelliccia A, Di Paolo FM, De Blasiis E, et al: Prevalence and clinical significance of aortic root dilation in highly trained competitive athletes. *Circulation* 122:698–706, 2010.
15. Cox GF, Sleeper LA, Lowe AM, et al: Factors associated with establishing a causal diagnosis for children with cardiomyopathy. *Pediatrics* 118:1519–1531, 2006.
16. Scaglia F, Towbin JA, Craigen WJ, et al: Clinical spectrum, morbidity, and mortality in 113 pediatric patients with mitochondrial disease. *Pediatrics* 114:925–931, 2004.
17. Monserrat L, Gimeno-Blanes JR, Marin F, et al: Prevalence of Fabry disease in a cohort of 508 unrelated patients with hypertrophic cardiomyopathy. *J Am Coll Cardiol* 50:2399–2403, 2007.
18. Alcalai R, Seidman JG, Seidman CE: Genetic basis of hypertrophic cardiomyopathy: from bench to the clinics. *J Cardiovasc Electrophysiol* 19:104–110, 2008.
19. Arad M, Maron BJ, Gorham JM, et al: Glycogen storage diseases presenting as hypertrophic cardiomyopathy. *N Engl J Med* 352:362–372, 2005.
20. Maron BJ, Roberts WC, Arad M, et al: Clinical outcome and phenotypic expression in LAMP2 cardiomyopathy. *JAMA* 301:1253–1259, 2009.
21. Yang Z, McMahon CJ, Smith LR, et al: Danon disease as an underrecognized cause of hypertrophic cardiomyopathy in children. *Circulation* 112:1612–1617, 2005.
22. Maron BJ, Semsarian C: Emergence of gene mutation carriers and the expanding disease spectrum of hypertrophic cardiomyopathy. *Eur Heart J* 31:1551–1553, 2010.
23. Colan SD, Lipshultz SE, Lowe AM, et al: Epidemiology and cause-specific outcome of hypertrophic cardiomyopathy in children: findings from the Pediatric Cardiomyopathy Registry. *Circulation* 115:773–781, 2007.

24. Gelb BD, Tartaglia M: Noonan syndrome and related disorders: dysregulated RAS-mitogen activated protein kinase signal transduction. *Hum Mol Genet* R220–R226, 2006.
25. Montalvo AL, Bembi B, Donnarumma M, et al: Mutation profile of the GAA gene in Italian patients with late onset glycogen storage disease type II. *Hum Mutat* 27:999–1006, 2006.
26. Pandit B, Sarkozy A, Pennacchio LA, et al: Gain-of-function RAF1 mutations cause Noonan and LEOPARD syndromes with hypertrophic cardiomyopathy. *Nat Genet* 39:1007–1012, 2007.
27. van den Hout HM, Hop W, van Diggelen OP, et al: The natural course of infantile Pompe's disease: 20 original cases compared with 133 cases from the literature. *Pediatrics* 112:332–340, 2003.
28. Braunwald E, Lambert CT, Rockoff SD, et al: Idiopathic hypertrophic subaortic stenosis, I: a description of the disease based upon an analysis of 64 patients. *Circulation* 30:119, 1964.
29. Maron BJ: Hypertrophic cardiomyopathy: an important global disease. *Am J Med* 116:63–65, 2004.
30. Maron MS, Olivotto I, Betocchi S, et al: Effect of left ventricular outflow tract obstruction on clinical outcome in hypertrophic cardiomyopathy. *N Engl J Med* 348(4):295–303, 2003.
31. Wigle ED, Sasson Z, Henderson MA, et al: Hypertrophic cardiomyopathy: the importance of the site and the extent of hypertrophy: a review. *Prog Cardiovasc Dis* 28:1–83, 1985.
32. Wigle ED, Rakowski H, Kimball BP, et al: Hypertrophic cardiomyopathy: clinical spectrum and treatment. *Circulation* 92:1680–1692, 1995.
33. Geske JB, Sorajja P, Ommen SR, et al: Left ventricular outflow tract gradient variability in hypertrophic cardiomyopathy. *Clin Cardiol* 32:397–402, 2009.
34. Falicov RE, Resnekov L, Bharati S, et al: Mid-ventricular obstruction: a variant of obstructive cardiomyopathy. *Am J Cardiol* 37:432–437, 1976.
35. Maron BJ, Nishimura RA, Danielson GK: Pitfalls in clinical recognition and a novel operative approach for hypertrophic cardiomyopathy with severe outflow obstruction due to anomalous papillary muscle. *Circulation* 98:2505–2508, 1998.
36. Elesber A, Nishimura RA, Rihal CS, et al: Utility of isoproterenol to provoke outflow tract gradients in patients with hypertrophic cardiomyopathy. *Am J Cardiol* 101:516–520, 2008.
37. Maron BJ, Epstein SE, Roberts WC: Hypertrophic cardiomyopathy and transmural myocardial infarction without significant atherosclerosis of the extramural coronary arteries. *Am J Cardiol* 43(6):1086–1102, 1979.
38. Dilsizian V, Bonow RO, Epstein SE, et al: Myocardial ischemia detected by thallium scintigraphy is frequently related to cardiac arrest and syncope in young patients with hypertrophic cardiomyopathy. *J Am Coll Cardiol* 22(3):796–804, 1993.
39. Choudhury L, Mahrholdt H, Wagner A, et al: Myocardial scarring in asymptomatic or mildly symptomatic patients with hypertrophic cardiomyopathy. *J Am Coll Cardiol* 40(12):2156–2164, 2002.
40. Basso C, Thiene G, Corrado D, et al: Hypertrophic cardiomyopathy and sudden death in the young: pathologic evidence of myocardial ischemia. *Hum Pathol* 31(8):988–998, 2000.
41. Schwartzkopff B, Mundhenke M, Strauer BE: Alterations of the architecture of subendocardial arterioles in patients with hypertrophic cardiomyopathy and impaired coronary vasodilator reserve: a possible cause for myocardial ischemia. *J Am Coll Cardiol* 31(5):1089–1096, 1998.
42. Frenneaux MP, Counihan PJ, Caforio AL, et al: Abnormal blood pressure response during exercise in hypertrophic cardiomyopathy. *Circulation* 82:1995–2002, 1990.
43. Sadoul N, Prasad K, Elliott PM, et al: Prospective prognostic assessment of blood pressure response during exercise in patients with hypertrophic cardiomyopathy. *Circulation* 96:2987–2991, 1997.
44. Olivotto I, Maron BJ, Montereggi A, et al: Prognostic value of systemic blood pressure response during exercise in a community-based patient population with hypertrophic cardiomyopathy. *J Am Coll Cardiol* 33:2044–2051, 1999.
45. Wigle ED, Adelman AG, Auger P, et al: Mitral regurgitation in muscular subaortic stenosis. *Am J Cardiol* 24:698–706, 1969.
46. Fassbach M, Schwartzkopff B: Elevated serum markers for collagen synthesis in patients with hypertrophic cardiomyopathy and diastolic dysfunction. *Z Kardiol* 94(5):328–335, 2005.
47. Kuribayashi T, Roberts WC: Myocardial disarray at junction of ventricular septum and left and right ventricular free walls in hypertrophic cardiomyopathy. *Am J Cardiol* 70(15):1333–1340, 1992.
48. Richard P, Charron P, Carrier L, et al, EUROGENE Heart Failure Project: Hypertrophic cardiomyopathy: distribution of disease genes, spectrum of mutations, and implications for a molecular diagnosis strategy. *Circulation* 107(17):2227–2232, 2003.
49. Gersh BJ, Maron BJ, Bonow RO, et al, American College of Cardiology Foundation/American Heart Association Task Force on Practice Guidelines: 2011 ACCF/AHA Guideline for the Diagnosis and Treatment of Hypertrophic Cardiomyopathy: a report of the American College of Cardiology Foundation/American Heart Association Task Force on Practice Guidelines. Developed in collaboration with the American Association for Thoracic Surgery, American Society of Echocardiography, American Society of Nuclear Cardiology, Heart Failure Society of America, Heart Rhythm Society, Society for Cardiovascular Angiography and Interventions, and Society of Thoracic Surgeons. *J Am Coll Cardiol* 58(25):e212–e260, 2011.
50. Klues HG, Schiffers A, Maron BJ: Phenotypic spectrum and patterns of left ventricular hypertrophy in hypertrophic cardiomyopathy: morphologic observations and significance as assessed by two-dimensional echocardiography in 600 patients. *J Am Coll Cardiol* 26(7):1699–1708, 1995.
51. Lever HM, Karam RF, Currie PJ, et al: Hypertrophic cardiomyopathy in the elderly. Distinctions from the young based on cardiac shape. *Circulation* 79(3):580–589, 1989.
52. Yamaguchi H, Ishimura T, Nishiyama S, et al: Hypertrophic nonobstructive cardiomyopathy with giant negative T waves (apical hypertrophy): ventriculographic and echocardiographic features in 30 patients. *Am J Cardiol* 44(3):401–412, 1979.
53. Maron BJ: Hypertrophic cardiomyopathy: a systematic review. *JAMA* 287:1308–1320, 2002.
54. Maron BJ, McKenna WJ, Danielson GK, et al: American College of Cardiology/European Society of Cardiology clinical expert consensus document on hypertrophic cardiomyopathy. *J Am Coll Cardiol* 42:1687–1713, 2003.
55. Maron MS, Appelbaum E, Harrigan CJ, et al: Clinical profile and significance of delayed enhancement in hypertrophic cardiomyopathy. *Circ Heart Fail.* 1:184–191, 2008.
56. Adabag AS, Maron BJ, Appelbaum E, et al: Occurrence and frequency of arrhythmias in hypertrophic cardiomyopathy in relation to delayed enhancement on cardiovascular magnetic resonance. *J Am Coll Cardiol* 51:1369–1374, 2008.
57. Rubinshtein R, Glockner JF, Ommen SR, et al: Characteristics and clinical significance of late gadolinium enhancement by contrast-enhanced magnetic resonance imaging in patients with hypertrophic cardiomyopathy. *Circ Heart Fail.* 3:51–58, 2010.
58. O'Hanlon R, Grasso A, Roughton M, et al: Prognostic significance of myocardial fibrosis in hypertrophic cardiomyopathy. *J Am Coll Cardiol* 56:867–874, 2010.
59. Bruder O, Wagner A, Jensen CJ, et al: Myocardial scar visualized by cardiovascular magnetic resonance imaging predicts major adverse events in patients with hypertrophic cardiomyopathy. *J Am Coll Cardiol* 56:875–887, 2010.
60. Brugada P, Bär FW, de Zwaan C, et al: "Sawfish" systolic narrowing of the left anterior descending coronary artery: an angiographic sign of hypertrophic cardiomyopathy. *Circulation* 66(4):800–803, 1982.
61. Basso C, Thiene G, Mackey-Bojack S, et al: Myocardial bridging, a frequent component of the hypertrophic cardiomyopathy phenotype, lacks systematic association with sudden cardiac death. *Eur Heart J* 30:1627–1634, 2009.
62. Yetman AT, McCrindle BW, MacDonald C, et al: Myocardial bridging in children with hypertrophic cardiomyopathy: a risk factor for sudden death. *N Engl J Med* 339:1201–1209, 1998.
63. Sorajja P, Ommen SR, Nishimura RA, et al: Myocardial bridging in adult patients with hypertrophic cardiomyopathy. *J Am Coll Cardiol* 42:889–894, 2003.
64. Mohiddin SA, Begley D, Shih J, et al: Myocardial bridging does not predict sudden death in children with hypertrophic cardiomyopathy but is associated with more severe cardiac disease. *J Am Coll Cardiol* 36:2270–2278, 2000.
65. Brockenbrough EC, Braunwald E, Morrow AG: A hemodynamic technic for the detection of hypertrophic subaortic stenosis. *Circulation* 23:189–194, 1961.
66. Spirito P, Seidman CE, McKenna WJ, et al: The management of hypertrophic cardiomyopathy. *N Engl J Med* 336:775–785, 1997.
67. Sorajja P, Ommen SR, Nishimura RA, et al: Adverse prognosis of patients with hypertrophic cardiomyopathy who have epicardial coronary artery disease. *Circulation* 108:2342–2348, 2003.
68. Maron BJ, Chaitman BR, Ackerman MJ, et al: Recommendations for physical activity and recreational sports participation for young patients with genetic cardiovascular diseases. *Circulation* 109:2807–2816, 2004.
69. Semsarian C, Ahmad I, Giewat M, et al: The L-type calcium channel inhibitor diltiazem prevents cardiomyopathy in a mouse model. *J Clin Invest* 109:1013–1020, 2002.
70. Alvares RF, Goodwin JF: Non-invasive assessment of diastolic function in hypertrophic cardiomyopathy on and off beta adrenergic blocking drugs. *Br Heart J* 48:204–212, 1982.
71. Bourmayan C, Razavi A, Fournier C, et al: Effect of propranolol on left ventricular relaxation in hypertrophic cardiomyopathy: an echographic study. *Am Heart J* 109:1311–1316, 1985.
72. Bonow RO, Dilsizian V, Rosing DR, et al: Verapamil-induced improvement in left ventricular diastolic filling and increased exercise tolerance in patients with hypertrophic cardiomyopathy: short- and long-term effects. *Circulation* 72(4):853–864, 1985.
73. Bonow RO, Rosing DR, Bacharach SL, et al: Effects of verapamil on left ventricular systolic function and diastolic filling in patients with hypertrophic cardiomyopathy. *Circulation* 64(4):787–796, 1981.
74. Gistri R, Cecchi F, Choudhury L, et al: Effect of verapamil on absolute myocardial blood flow in hypertrophic cardiomyopathy. *Am J Cardiol* 74(4):363–368, 1994.
75. Udelson JE, Bonow RO, O'Gara PT, et al: Verapamil prevents silent myocardial perfusion abnormalities during exercise in asymptomatic patients with hypertrophic cardiomyopathy. *Circulation* 79(5):1052–1060, 1989.
76. Pollick C: Muscular subaortic stenosis: hemodynamic and clinical improvement after disopyramide. *N Engl J Med* 307(16):997–999, 1982.
77. Matsubara H, Nakatani S, Nagata S, et al: Salutary effect of disopyramide on left ventricular diastolic function in hypertrophic obstructive cardiomyopathy. *J Am Coll Cardiol* 26(3):768–775, 1995.
78. Sherrid M, Delia E, Dwyer E: Oral disopyramide therapy for obstructive hypertrophic cardiomyopathy. *Am J Cardiol* 62(16):1085–1088, 1988.
79. McKenna WJ, Oakley CM, Krikler DM, et al: Improved survival with amiodarone in patients with hypertrophic cardiomyopathy and ventricular tachycardia. *Br Heart J* 53(4):412–416, 1985.
80. Fananapazir L, Leon MB, Bonow RO, et al: Sudden death during empiric amiodarone therapy in symptomatic hypertrophic cardiomyopathy. *Am J Cardiol* 67(2):169–174, 1991.
81. Prasad K, Frenneaux MP: Hypertrophic cardiomyopathy: is there a role for amiodarone? *Heart* 79(4):317–318, 1998.
82. Cecchi F, Olivotto I, Montereggi A, et al: Prognostic value of non-sustained ventricular tachycardia and the potential role of amiodarone treatment in hypertrophic cardiomyopathy: assessment in an unselected non-referral based patient population. *Heart* 79(4):331–336, 1998.
83. Almendral JM, Ormaetxe J, Martínez-Alday JD, et al: Treatment of ventricular arrhythmias in patients with hypertrophic cardiomyopathy. *Eur Heart J* 14(Suppl J):71–72, 1993.
84. Maron BJ, McKenna WJ, Danielson GK, et al, American College of Cardiology Foundation Task Force on Clinical Expert Consensus Documents; European Society of Cardiology Committee for Practice Guidelines: American College of Cardiology/European Society of Cardiology Clinical Expert Consensus Document on Hypertrophic Cardiomyopathy. A report of the American College of Cardiology Foundation Task Force on Clinical Expert Consensus Documents and the European Society of Cardiology Committee for Practice Guidelines. *Eur Heart J* 24(21):1965–1991, 2003.
85. Ommen SR, Maron BJ, Olivotto I, et al: Long-term effects of surgical septal myectomy on survival in patients with obstructive hypertrophic cardiomyopathy. *J Am Coll Cardiol* 46:470–476, 2005.
86. Smedira NG, Lytle BW, Lever HM, et al: Current effectiveness and risks of isolated septal myectomy for hypertrophic obstructive cardiomyopathy. *Ann Thorac Surg* 85(1):127–133, 2008.
87. Goodwin JF, Hollman A, Cleland WP, et al: Obstructive cardiomyopathy simulating aortic stenosis. *Br Heart J* 22:403–414, 1960.
88. Morrow AG: Hypertrophic subaortic stenosis. Operative methods utilized to relieve left ventricular outflow obstruction. *J Thorac Cardiovasc Surg* 76(4):423–430, 1978.
89. Maron BJ, Dearani JA, Ommen SR, et al: The case for surgery in obstructive hypertrophic cardiomyopathy. *J Am Coll Cardiol* 44(10):2044–2053, 2004.
90. Bach DS, Siao D, Girard SE, et al: Evaluation of patients with severe symptomatic aortic stenosis who do not undergo aortic valve replacement: the potential role of subjectively overestimated operative risk. *Circ Cardiovasc Qual Outcomes.* 2:533–539, 2009.
91. Theodoro DA, Danielson GK, Feldt RH, et al: Hypertrophic obstructive cardiomyopathy in pediatric patients: results of surgical treatment. *J Thorac Cardiovasc Surg* 112:1589–1597, 1996.
92. McCully RB, Nishimura RA, Tajik AJ, et al: Extent of clinical improvement after surgical treatment of hypertrophic obstructive cardiomyopathy. *Circulation* 94:467–471, 1996.
93. Cohn LH, Trehan H, Collins JJ: Long-term follow-up of patients undergoing myotomy/myectomy for obstructive hypertrophic cardiomyopathy. *Am J Cardiol* 70:657–660, 1992.
94. McIntosh CL, Maron BJ: Current operative treatment of obstructive hypertrophic cardiomyopathy. *Circulation* 78:487–495, 1988.
95. Mohr R, Schaff HV, Puga FJ, et al: Results of operation for hypertrophic obstructive cardiomyopathy in children and adults less than 40 years of age. *Circulation* 80:I191–I196, 1989.
96. Robbins RC, Stinson EB: Long-term results of left ventricular myotomy and myectomy for obstructive hypertrophic cardiomyopathy. *J Thorac Cardiovasc Surg* 111:586–594, 1996.
97. Schulte HD, Borisov K, Gams E, et al: Management of symptomatic hypertrophic obstructive cardiomyopathy: long-term results after surgical therapy. *Thorac Cardiovasc Surg* 47:213–218, 1999.
98. Firoozi S, Elliott PM, Sharma S, et al: Septal myotomy-myectomy and transcoronary septal alcohol ablation in hypertrophic obstructive cardiomyopathy: a comparison of clinical, haemodynamic and exercise outcomes. *Eur Heart J* 23:1617–1624, 2002.
99. Ommen SR, Nishimura RA, Squires RW, et al: Comparison of dualchamber pacing versus septal myectomy for the treatment of patients with hypertrophic obstructive cardiomyopathy: a comparison of objective hemodynamic and exercise end points. *J Am Coll Cardiol* 34:191–196, 1999.
100. Schoendube FA, Klues HG, Reith S, et al: Long-term clinical and echocardiographic follow-up after surgical correction of hypertrophic obstructive cardiomyopathy with extended myectomy and reconstruction of the subvalvular mitral apparatus. *Circulation* 92(Suppl 9):II122–II127, 1995.
101. Maron BJ, Harding AM, Spirito P, et al: Systolic anterior motion of the posterior mitral leaflet: a previously unrecognized cause of dynamic subaortic obstruction in patients with hypertrophic cardiomyopathy. *Circulation* 68:282–293, 1983.
102. Spirito P, Maron BJ, Rosing DR: Morphologic determinants of hemodynamic state after ventricular septal myotomy-myectomy in patients with obstructive hypertrophic cardiomyopathy: Mmode and two-dimensional echocardiographic assessment. *Circulation* 70:984–995, 1984.

103. Yu EH, Omran AS, Wigle ED, et al: Mitral regurgitation in hypertrophic obstructive cardiomyopathy: relationship to obstruction and relief with myectomy. *J Am Coll Cardiol* 36:2219–2225, 2000.
104. Sherrid MV, Chaudhry FA, Swistel DG: Obstructive hypertrophic cardiomyopathy: echocardiography, pathophysiology, and the continuing evolution of surgery for obstruction. *Ann Thorac Surg* 75:620–632, 2003.
105. Nishimura RA, Holmes DR: Clinical practice. *N Engl J Med* 350:1320–1327, 2004.
106. Maron BJ: Controversies in cardiovascular medicine. *Circulation* 116:196–206, 2007.
107. Redberg RF, Benjamin EJ, Bittner V, et al: ACCF/AHA 2009 performance measures for primary prevention of cardiovascular disease in adults. *J Am Coll Cardiol* 54:1364–1405, 2009.
108. Krajcer Z, Leachman RD, Cooley DA, et al: Mitral valve replacement and septal myomectomy in hypertrophic cardiomyopathy: ten-year follow-up in 80 patients. *Circulation* 78:135–143, 1988.
109. McIntosh CL, Greenberg GJ, Maron BJ, et al: Clinical and hemodynamic results after mitral valve replacement in patients with obstructive hypertrophic cardiomyopathy. *Ann Thorac Surg* 47:236–246, 1989.
110. Sigwart U: Non-surgical myocardial reduction for hypertrophic obstructive cardiomyopathy. *Lancet* 346:211–214, 1995.
111. Faber L, Meissner A, Ziemssen P, et al: Percutaneous transluminal septal myocardial ablation for hypertrophic obstructive cardiomyopathy: long term follow up of the first series of 25 patients. *Heart* 83(3):326–331, 2000.
112. Gietzen FH, Leuner CJ, Raute-Kreinsen U, et al: Acute and long-term results after transcoronary ablation of septal hypertrophy (TASH). Catheter interventional treatment for hypertrophic obstructive cardiomyopathy. *Eur Heart J* 20(18):1342–1354, 1999.
113. Lakkis NM, Nagueh SF, Dunn JK, et al: Nonsurgical septal reduction therapy for hypertrophic obstructive cardiomyopathy: one-year follow-up. *J Am Coll Cardiol* 36(3):852–855, 2000.
114. Knight C, Kurbaan AS, Seggewiss H, et al: Nonsurgical septal reduction for hypertrophic obstructive cardiomyopathy: outcome in the first series of patients. *Circulation* 95(8):2075–2081, 1997.
115. Ruzyłło W, Chojnowska L, Demkow M, et al: Left ventricular outflow tract gradient decrease with non-surgical myocardial reduction improves exercise capacity in patients with hypertrophic obstructive cardiomyopathy. *Eur Heart J* 21(9):770–777, 2000.
116. Chimenti C, Pieroni M, Morgante E, et al: Prevalence of Fabry disease in female patients with late-onset hypertrophic cardiomyopathy. *Circulation* 110:1047–1053, 2004.
117. Andersen PS, Havndrup O, Hougs L, et al: Diagnostic yield, interpretation, and clinical utility of mutation screening of sarcomere encoding genes in Danish hypertrophic cardiomyopathy patients and relatives. *Hum Mutat* 30:363–370, 2009.
118. Klues HG, Maron BJ, Dollar AL, et al: Diversity of structural mitral valve alterations in hypertrophic cardiomyopathy. *Circulation* 85(5):1651–1660, 1992.
119. Holmes DR, Jr, Valeti US, Nishimura RA: Alcohol septal ablation for hypertrophic cardiomyopathy: indications and technique. *Catheter Cardiovasc Interv* 66(3):375–389, 2005.
120. Singh M, Edwards WD, Holmes DR, Jr, et al: Anatomy of the first septal perforating artery: a study with implications for ablation therapy for hypertrophic cardiomyopathy. *Mayo Clin Proc* 76(8):799–802, 2001.
121. Veselka J, Duchonová R, Procházková S, et al: Effects of varying ethanol dosing in percutaneous septal ablation for obstructive hypertrophic cardiomyopathy on early hemodynamic changes. *Am J Cardiol* 95(5):675–678, 2005.
122. Yoerger DM, Picard MH, Palacios IF, et al: Time course of pressure gradient response after first alcohol septal ablation for obstructive hypertrophic cardiomyopathy. *Am J Cardiol* 97(10):1511–1514, 2006.
123. Sorajja P, Nishimura RA, Ommen SR, et al: Effect of septal ablation on myocardial relaxation and left atrial pressure in hypertrophic cardiomyopathy an invasive hemodynamic study. *J Am Coll Cardiol Intv.* 1:552–560, 2008.
124. Fernandes VL, Nielsen C, Nagueh SF, et al: Follow-up of alcohol septal ablation for symptomatic hypertrophic obstructive cardiomyopathy: the Baylor and Medical University of South Carolina experience 1996 to 2007. *J Am Coll Cardiol Intv.* 1:561–570, 2008.
125. Kim JJ, Lee CW, Park SW, et al: Improvement in exercise capacity and exercise blood pressure response after transcoronary alcohol ablation therapy of septal hypertrophy in hypertrophic cardiomyopathy. *Am J Cardiol* 83:1220–1223, 1999.
126. Serber ER, Sears SF, Nielsen CD, et al: Depression, anxiety, and quality of life in patients with obstructive hypertrophic cardiomyopathy three months after alcohol septal ablation. *Am J Cardiol* 100:1592–1597, 2007.
127. Agarwal S, Tuzcu EM, Desai MY, et al: Updated meta-analysis of septal alcohol ablation versus myectomy for hypertrophic cardiomyopathy. *J Am Coll Cardiol* 55(8):823–834, 2010.
128. Fananapazir L, Epstein ND, Curiel RV, et al: Long-term results of dual-chamber (DDD) pacing in obstructive hypertrophic cardiomyopathy: evidence for progressive symptomatic and hemodynamic improvement and reduction of left ventricular hypertrophy. *Circulation* 90:2731–2742, 1994.
129. Jeanrenaud X, Goy JJ, Kappenberger L: Effects of dual-chamber pacing in hypertrophic obstructive cardiomyopathy. *Lancet* 339:1318–1323, 1992.
130. McDonald K, McWilliams E, O'Keeffe B, et al: Functional assessment of patients treated with permanent dual chamber pacing as a primary treatment for hypertrophic cardiomyopathy. *Eur Heart J* 9:893–898, 1988.
131. Posma JL, Blanksma PK, Van Der Wall EE, et al: Effects of permanent dual chamber pacing on myocardial perfusion in symptomatic hypertrophic cardiomyopathy. *Heart* 76(4):358–362, 1996.
132. Nishimura RA, Trusty JM, Hayes DL, et al: Dual-chamber pacing for hypertrophic cardiomyopathy: a randomized, double-blind, crossover trial. *J Am Coll Cardiol* 29(2):435–441, 1997.
133. Maron BJ, Nishimura RA, McKenna WJ, et al: Assessment of permanent dual-chamber pacing as a treatment for drug-refractory symptomatic patients with obstructive hypertrophic cardiomyopathy: a randomized, double-blind, crossover study (M-PATHY). *Circulation* 99:2927–2933, 1999.
134. Kappenberger L, Linde C, Daubert C, et al: Pacing in hypertrophic obstructive cardiomyopathy: a randomized crossover study. *Eur Heart J* 18:1249–1256, 1997.
135. Erwin JP, Nishimura RA, Lloyd MA, et al: Dual chamber pacing for patients with hypertrophic obstructive cardiomyopathy: a clinical perspective in 2000. *Mayo Clin Proc* 75:173–180, 2000.
136. Slade AK, Sadoul N, Shapiro L, et al: DDD pacing in hypertrophic cardiomyopathy: a multicentre clinical experience. *Heart* 75:44–49, 1996.
137. Gadler F, Linde C, Daubert C, et al: Significant improvement of quality of life following atrioventricular synchronous pacing in patients with hypertrophic obstructive cardiomyopathy: data from 1 year of follow-up. *Eur Heart J* 20:1044–1050, 1999.
138. Ralph-Edwards A, Woo A, McCrindle BW, et al: Hypertrophic obstructive cardiomyopathy: comparison of outcomes after myectomy or alcohol ablation adjusted by propensity score. *J Thorac Cardiovasc Surg* 129:351–358, 2005.
139. Maron BJ, Spirito P, Shen WK, et al: Implantable cardioverter-defibrillators and prevention of sudden cardiac death in hypertrophic cardiomyopathy. *JAMA* 298:405–412, 2007.
140. Lin G, Nishimura RA, Gersh BJ, et al: Device complications and inappropriate implantable cardioverter defibrillator shocks in patients with hypertrophic cardiomyopathy. *Heart* 95:709–714, 2009.

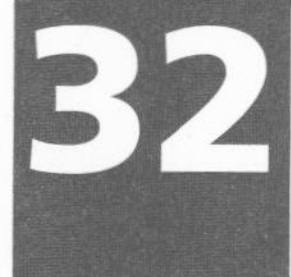

Patent Foramen Ovale, Atrial Septal Defect, Left Atrial Appendage, and Ventricular Septal Defect Closure

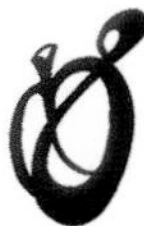

Sachin S. Goel, Lourdes R. Prieto, and Samir R. Kapadia

PATENT FORAMEN OVALE

Introduction

A potential causal relationship between patent foramen ovale (PFO) and stroke was first described by Cohnheim in 1877.[1] In the last two decades several studies have investigated the role of PFO in cryptogenic ischemic stroke, migraine headaches, platypnea-orthodeoxia, and decompression sickness.[2-4] Percutaneous PFO closure has emerged as a treatment option in the last decade, with significant controversy around its indications. Results of randomized trials of transcatheter PFO closure have only been recently reported.

Developmental Anatomy of the Atrial Septum (Figure 32-1)

During fetal life, there is a single atrial cavity. A septum primum (SP) develops from the cranial wall of the single atrium and grows toward the endocardial cushions, thereby dividing the single atrium into left- and right-sided chambers. The area between the SP and the endocardial cushions is known as ostium primum (OP). Fenestrations then develop in the middle of the septum primum and coalesce to form ostium secundum (OS). The OS allows right-to-left shunting of oxygenated blood. To the right of septum primum, another septum known as septum secundum (SS) then develops, and covers the OS and in most instances covers the OP as well. A flaplike valve known as PFO is formed between the two septae, which now allows oxygenated placental blood to cross over from right-to-left atrium during the remainder of intrauterine life. Spontaneous fusion of SP with SS occurs in about 75% of the individuals by 2 years of age, leading to closure of PFO. In the remaining individuals there is an oblique crescent-shaped defect resembling a tunnel, which is called PFO.[5] The prevalence of probe-patent PFO is about 27% in necropsy studies with decreasing prevalence for each decade of life.

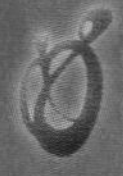

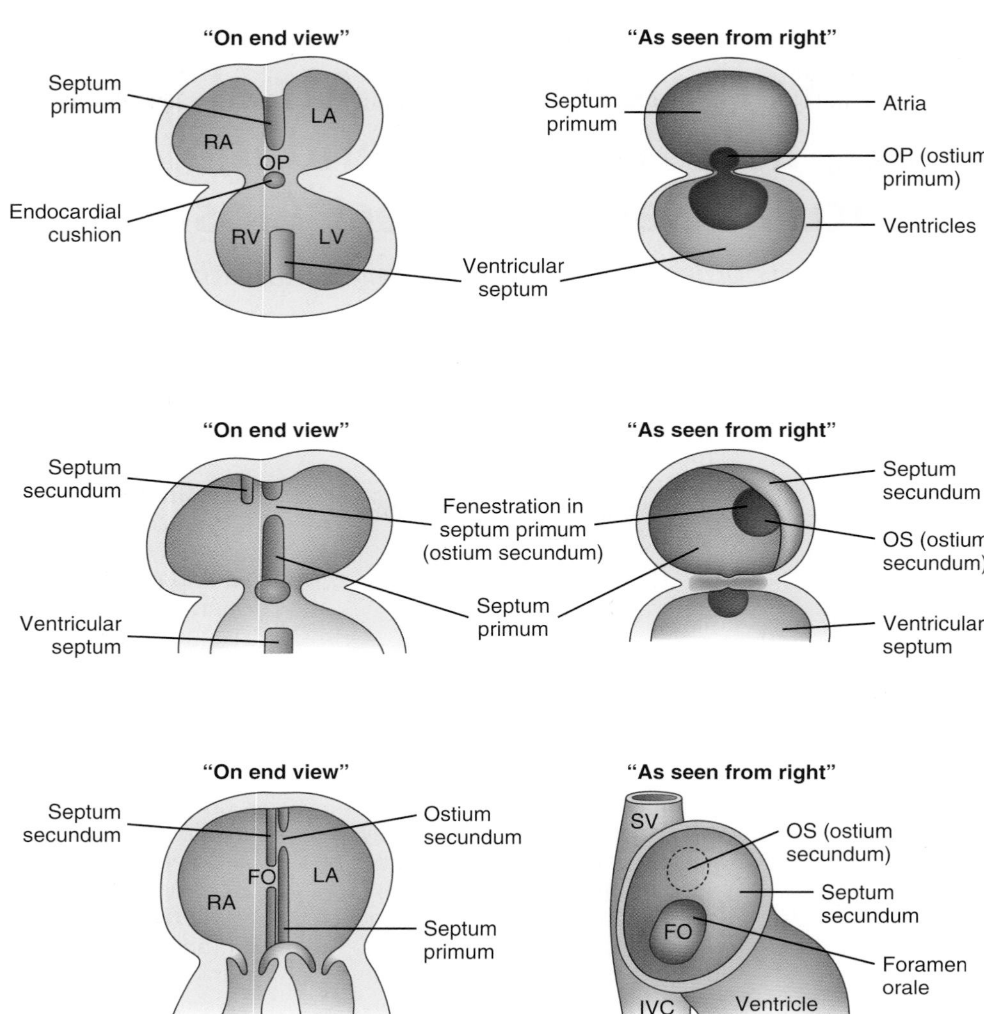

FIGURE 32-1 Development of the interatrial septum. *FO,* Foramen orale; *IVC,* inferior vena cava; *LA,* left atrium; *LV,* left ventricle; *RA,* right atrium; *RV,* right ventricle; *SV,* superior vena cava.

Clinical Presentation

Paradoxical embolism of a thrombus originating in pelvic or lower extremity veins has been implicated as a mechanism to explain association between PFO and ischemic stroke. The incidence of pelvic deep vein thrombosis (DVT) has been found to be significantly higher in patients with cryptogenic stroke and PFO compared with patients with stroke of determined origin.[6] Some PFOs have a long overlap between the SP and SS referred to as the tunnel. There are several reports of thrombus visualized "in transit" through PFO on transthoracic (TTE) as well as transesophageal echocardiography (TEE).[7,8] This has also led to speculation that stagnated blood in the tunnel may lead to thrombus formation, which may subsequently embolize in the systemic circulation—an explanation often referred to as the "lurking clot theory."[9] Studies have shown an association between the presence of atrial septal aneurysm (ASA) and risk of stroke.[4,10,11]

Platypnea-orthodeoxia is a rare clinical syndrome characterized by dyspnea and oxygen desaturation in the upright position that is relieved by lying down or recumbence. In the absence of elevated right-sided pressures, or lung disease, this can occur due to an anatomical abnormality that predisposes to right-to-left shunt from a PFO, such as a prominent eustachian valve that directs blood from the inferior vena cava (IVC) toward the interatrial septum, an aortic aneurysm, or an enlarged or elongated and horizontal aortic root that distorts the interatrial septum thereby predisposing to right-to-left shunting during upright position. TTE or TEE in the sitting position may be required to demonstrate flow across the septum by color or contrast if negative in supine position. Cardiac magnetic resonance imaging (MRI) or computed tomography (CT) may help demonstrate aortic abnormalities. Transcatheter PFO closure has been shown to be associated with marked improvement in symptoms.[12]

Decompression sickness occurs when a diver ascends from a dive and nitrogen bubbles entering venous circulation, which usually get diffused in the lungs, enter the systemic circulation via a right-to-left shunting source such as PFO, and embolize to the brain leading to ischemic lesions. A recent prospective study of 104 scuba divers with history of major decompression sickness showed that transcatheter PFO closure appears to prevent symptomatic and asymptomatic (ischemic brain lesions on MRI) decompression sickness.[13]

Migraine is a common disorder affecting about 10% of the adult population and is more common in women. In the last two decades, studies have shown an association between PFO and migraine, especially migraine with aura.[14] Several retrospective observational studies have reported an improvement in migraine after PFO closure.[15,16] In contrast, the only completed prospective randomized double blind trial (Migraine Intervention with STARFLEX Technology—MIST trial) in patients undergoing PFO closure primarily for migraine control failed to show any significant difference of PFO closure on the primary endpoint of migraine cessation, or secondary endpoints of improvement in migraine compared with a sham procedure.[17] However, the MIST trial was found to have several limitations including unrealistic endpoint of migraine cessation, inadequacy of TTE in screening for PFO as indicated by absence of PFO during closure, and shorter duration of follow-up. This implies that there may be some patients who benefit from device closure who remain to be identified. Recently, a significant reduction in frequency and severity of migraine was demonstrated with PFO closure in patients with large PFO (based on TCD) and subclinical brain MRI lesions.[18] These brain lesions may indicate silent thromboembolism and these patients may be high risk for future embolic events. Similarly, Rigatelli and colleagues recently showed that PFO closure resulted in significant reduction in migraine in patients with high-risk PFO characteristics such as curtain shunt pattern on TCD and TEE (implying larger degrees of shunting), right-to-left shunting during normal respiration, ASA, and presence of eustachian valve.[19] Not all patients with migraine have a PFO and not all patients with PFO suffer from migraine. The onus is on future trials to identify patients who would benefit most from PFO closure based on high-risk PFO morphology, which is best assessed with TEE, and possibly also those with subclinical lesions on brain imaging.

Diagnosis

PFO can be detected using various echocardiographic techniques, including TTE, TEE, and transcranial Doppler (TCD). More recently, three-dimensional echocardiography (3DE), CT, and MRI have been used, although none as the primary diagnostic tool in routine practice. Agitated saline is commonly used for diagnosing right-to-left shunts. Although the definition of positive contrast study on TTE or TEE remains controversial, it is generally accepted that a right-to-left shunt is diagnosed if at least 3 micro-bubbles appear in the left atrium, either spontaneously or after provocative maneuvers such as cough or Valsalva, within 3 cycles of complete opacification of the right atrium (**Figure 32-2**).[4] A provocative maneuver increases right atrial filling, thus increasing the RA pressure and opening the foramen ovale. Valsalva maneuver can be calibrated (40 mm Hg strain measured by spirometry and sustained for 10 seconds).[20] A good Valsalva maneuver is sometimes more difficult to obtain during TEE, especially if the patient is heavily sedated, as compared with TTE or TCD. Some studies have shown that sensitivity of detection of PFO was increased when a femoral vein was used for contrast injection instead of the antecubital vein.[21,22] This is likely due to different inflow pattern into the RA after injection through the femoral vein. Contrast through the inferior vena cava is directed toward the interatrial septum, often potentiated by a eustachian valve (**Figure 32-2**), whereas contrast through the superior vena cava is directed toward the tricuspid valve. Different morphological characteristics of PFO such as size, degree of shunting, and tunnel length should be taken into account when evaluating a patient with PFO and cryptogenic stroke (**Figure 32-2**).[23] TCD of the middle cerebral artery after injection of contrast can similarly be used to diagnose right-to-left shunting.

TEE has been shown to correlate very well with autopsy findings, with a sensitivity and specificity approaching 100% in the diagnosis of PFO.[24] Due to its high sensitivity and greater image resolution of the interatrial septal area allowing detailed characterization of PFO morphology, TEE is the current gold standard to diagnose and characterize PFO (**Figure 32-2**). The drawbacks of TEE are its semi-invasiveness and occasional inability to obtain a good Valsalva maneuver in sedated patients.

The 3DE using reconstruction techniques as well as real-time analysis have been used to evaluate a wide range of pathologies including patent foramen ovale. In a recent comparison, diagnostic accuracy of real-time 3D TTE was significantly higher than that of contrast TTE: sensitivity 83% versus 44% ($p < 0.001$) and close to that of contrast TEE.[25]

Small studies using contrast-enhanced MRI and cardiac CT (**Figure 32-2**) showed good concordance with TEE in the diagnosis of PFO. However, larger studies have shown both modalities to be inferior compared with TEE in detecting PFO.[26,27]

Management

Currently the best therapeutic modality for primary or secondary prevention of stroke in patients with PFO is debatable. There are data to suggest that PFO is more common in patients with cryptogenic stroke compared with those with a known cause of ischemic stroke.[2] However, a PFO is fairly common in the "control" population without stroke (prevalence of about 25%), and there are many unknown causes of "cryptogenic stroke." The available options include antiplatelet therapy, anticoagulant therapy with warfarin, transcatheter closure, and surgical closure. It is very likely that not all PFOs are "culprits" responsible for PTE, especially due to the high prevalence of PFO in the general population. Supporting this, a recent meta-analysis showed that one third of detected PFOs in patients with cryptogenic stroke are likely to be incidental and not benefit from closure, suggesting the importance of patient selection in therapeutic decision making.[28]

Medical Therapy

At present, there is no consensus regarding antiplatelet versus anticoagulant therapy in patients with cryptogenic stroke and PFO, as reflected by the heterogeneity in the medical arms of the published randomized PFO closure trials. Data from the Warfarin-Aspirin Recurrent Stroke Study (WARSS) show that there was no difference between treatment with warfarin or aspirin in the prevention of recurrent ischemic stroke or death in a large cohort of patients with cryptogenic stroke.[29] The Patent Foramen Ovale in Cryptogenic Stroke Study (PICSS), which is a substudy of WARSS with patients undergoing TEE examination, showed that there was a nonsignificant trend toward lower 2-year risk of stroke or death among warfarin-treated cryptogenic stroke patients with PFO compared with those receiving antiplatelet treatment (9.5% vs. 17.9%; hazard ratio [HR] 0.52; confidence interval [CI], 0.16-1.67).[30] In the PFO-ASA study, consisting of over 580 patients with ischemic stroke of unknown origin, recurrent stroke occurred more commonly despite aspirin therapy in patients with PFO and ASA compared with those with PFO, or ASA alone (HR for

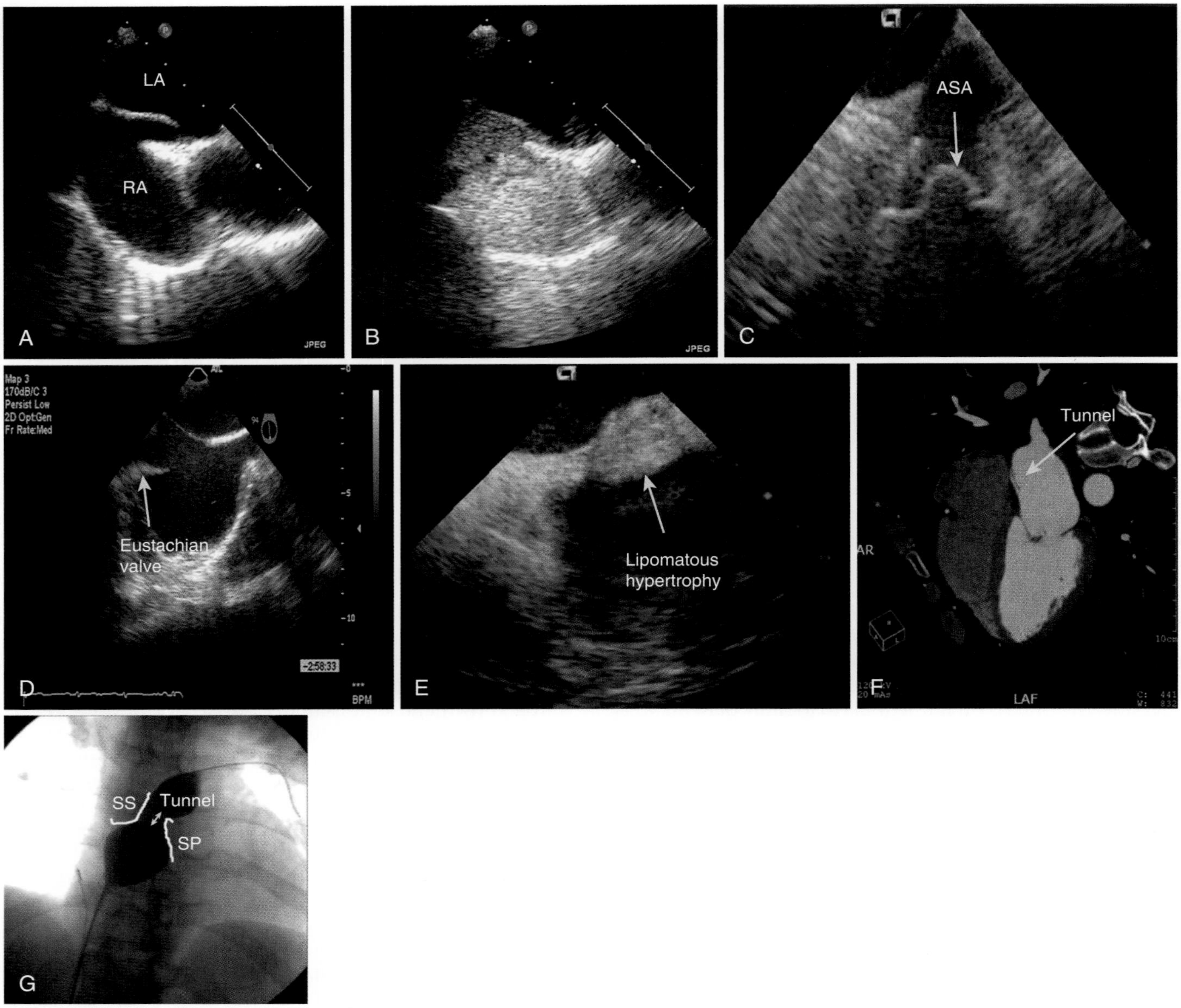

FIGURE 32-2 Diagnosis of PFO and associated morphological features. A, Patent foramen ovale (PFO) as visualized on transesophageal echocardiography. **B,** Positive bubble study on TEE through PFO. **C,** Atrial septal aneurysm. **D,** Eustachian valve. **E,** Lipomatous hypertrophy of the interatrial septum. **F,** PFO tunnel as visualized on cardiac computed tomography. **G,** PFO tunnel with balloon occlusion during transcatheter closure on fluoroscopy.

combination of PFO and ASA, 4.17; 95% CI, 1.47-11.84), suggesting that preventive strategies in addition to aspirin may be needed for such patients with high-risk PFO anatomy.[4] A recent meta-analysis of retrospective studies also suggests benefit of anticoagulation over antiplatelet therapy for prevention of recurrent neurologic events in patients with PFO and cryptogenic stroke.[31]

Transcatheter Patent Foramen Ovale Closure

Retrospective studies and meta-analyses have shown potential benefit of PFO closure in patients with cryptogenic stroke.[31] However, the completed prospective randomized trials failed to show such benefit as detailed below. This suggests that the real-world selection of high-risk patients where PFO-related PTE is the cause of stroke may potentially be a beneficial approach. Of course, results from retrospective studies, meta-analyses and randomized trials, and their limitations must be discussed with patients. Pending further studies, informed individualized therapeutic decisions should be made depending on patient preferences and perceived risk of PFO and recurrent stroke.

Randomized Trials of Patent Foramen Ovale Closure for Cryptogenic Stroke

In the first randomized report of transcatheter PFO closure, the CLOSURE 1 (Evaluation of the STARFlex septal closure system in patients with stroke and/or transient ischemic attack due to presumed paradoxical embolism through a PFO) trial, 909 patients with cryptogenic stroke or TIA were randomized to medical therapy or transcatheter PFO closure using the STARFlex device. With a success rate of 89% for closure, there was no difference in the outcomes of recurrent stroke (2.9% vs. 3.1%; p = 0.79) or TIA (3.1% vs. 4.1%; p = 0.44) with closure compared with medical therapy.[32] There were many limitations of the CLOSURE 1 trial. The majority of recurrent events in this study (20 of 23 patients in closure group and 22 of 29 patients in medical therapy group) were not related to PTE, and alternative explanations for recurrent neurologic events were observed, including atrial fibrillation, subcortical lacunar infarcts, aortic arch atheroma, complex migraine, vasculitis, etc. This increases the likelihood that the initial neurologic event may not have been related to PFO and PTE. Thus, patients in the CLOSURE 1 trial may not have been the ideal population to study PFO closure. Only a third of patients in this trial had high-risk features such as ASA, and only about a half had significant shunting. Closure of insignificant or incidental PFOs may have diluted the beneficial effects of PFO closure. Patients with hypercoagulable testing or DVT were excluded from this study, thus excluding patients in whom the mechanism of stroke was perhaps most likely to be related to PTE. Moreover, even though the CLOSURE trial is being viewed as a "negative" trial, it shows that PFO closure is an effective alternative to medical therapy in reducing stroke.

In RESPECT (Randomized evaluation of recurrent stroke comparing PFO closure to established current standard of care treatment) trial, 980 patients with cryptogenic stroke were randomized to medical therapy or transcatheter PFO closure.[33] In the intention-to-treat cohort, recurrent stroke occurred in 9 patients in the closure group and 16 in the medical therapy group (HR with closure 0.49; 95% CI, 0.22-1.11; p = 0.08). In contrast, there was statistically significant reduction in the risk of recurrent stroke with PFO closure when analyses were performed in prespecified per-protocol cohort (HR 0.37; 95% CI, 0.14-0.96, p = 0.03), and as-treated cohort (HR 0.27; 95% CI, 0.10-0.75, p = 0.007). In addition, closure was found to provide greater benefit in patients with severe right-to-left shunt and in those with an atrial septal aneurysm. Strengths of the RESPECT trial over CLOSURE 1 trial include longer follow-up, more stringent inclusion criteria with exclusion of patients with TIA and lacunar infarcts, and use of Amplatzer PFO occlude device, which provides more effective closure rates with much less device-related complications such as thrombosis and atrial fibrillation. Limitations of the RESPECT trial include high drop-out rate (17% in medical therapy group and 9% in closure group) and nonadherence to protocol in some patients with important implications on outcomes (3 out of 9 patients with recurrent ischemic stroke in the closure group of the intention-to-treat population did not have a device at the time of recurrent stroke).

In the PC (Comparing Percutaneous closure of PFO using the Amplatzer PFO Occluder with medical treatment in patients with cryptogenic embolism) trial, 414 patients were randomized to transcatheter PFO closure or medical therapy.[34] Recurrent stroke occurred less frequently in the closure group compared with the medical therapy group; however, this was not statistically significant (0.5% vs. 2.4%; HR, 0.20; 95% CI, 0.02-1.72; p = 0.14). Closure also did not reduce recurrent TIAs compared with medical therapy alone (2.5% vs. 3.3%; HR, 0.71; 95% CI, 0.23-2.24; p = 0.56). Limitations of the PC trial include inclusion of TIA in the primary endpoint and difficulty recruiting patients with a long recruitment period.

Despite lack of benefit in reduction of recurrent neurologic events with PFO closure compared with medical therapy in randomized trials, there are signals pointing toward benefit with closure, particularly in a select group of patients at high risk, such as those with ASA and large shunting. Whenever possible, patients with cryptogenic neurologic events and PFO must be enrolled in ongoing randomized trials such as Patent Foramen Ovale Closure or Anticoagulation versus Antiplatelet Therapy to Prevent Stroke Recurrence (CLOSE, ClinicalTrials.gov number, NCT00562289), Device Closure versus Medical Therapy for Cryptogenic Stroke Patients with High-Risk Patent Foramen Ovale (DEFENSE-PFO, NCT01550588), and Gore Helex Septal Occluder/Gore Septal Occluder for Patent Foramen Ovale (PFO) Closure in Stroke Patients (REDUCE, NCT00738894).

Indications for Transcatheter Patent Foramen Ovale Closure

In the United States, transcatheter PFO closure is not Food and Drug Administration (FDA) approved. As discussed, this procedure is still controversial, given discordance in retrospective and randomized trial data. Off-label PFO closure has been performed in patients with cryptogenic stroke, other paradoxical embolic events presumed to be related to PFO, platypnea-orthodeoxia syndrome, decompression sickness, and migraine headaches. The author found no difference in the risk of stroke in patients with PFO and an implantable intracardiac device such as pacemaker or defibrillator compared with those without an intracardiac device.[35] Another study found an increased risk of stroke/TIA in patients with implantable devices with PFO compared with those without PFO.[36] The authors study was different from this study in that the patient population consisted of PFO patients only with the goal of studying whether device implantation had any impact on the outcome of stroke in patients with PFO.[35] Additionally, the latter study included patients with prior stroke/TIA while the authors did not, as prior stroke itself is an important predictor of future stroke. The authors have also found no difference in stroke risk between patients with atrial fibrillation with and without PFO.[37] As such, PFO closure cannot be recommended in patients with pacemakers, implantable defibrillators, or atrial fibrillation.

Devices

Transcatheter PFO closure has been performed off-label with devices that are used for transcatheter atrial septal defect (ASD) closure (**Figure 32-3**). These include the Helex septal occlude (WL Gore, Flagstaff, Arizona), Amplatzer atrial septal occluder (ASO) (St. Jude Medical), Amplatzer multifenestrated, or cribriform ASO. In addition, Amplatzer PFO occluder, CardioSEAL, STARFlex, and Premere PFO closure system have also been used. Currently only the Amplatzer and Helex systems are used in the United States.

Amplatzer Devices

The Amplatzer PFO occluder, used in the RESPECT and PC trials, is a self-expanding, double-disk device made of 0.005-inch nitinol wire and polyester patches sewn within each disk to occlude blood flow (**Figure 32-3**). The waist is thin and mobile and the right atrial disk is larger than the left atrial disk as opposed to the Amplatzer ASO device. There are 3 device sizes available, based on the right atrial disk diameter—18, 25, and 35 mm. Device sizing depends on distance from the PFO to the SVC or aorta. The 25-mm device is used in the vast majority of cases. The Amplatzer cribriform ASO device, used for closure of fenestrated secundum ASDs, also has been used for PFO closure. It consists of a thin waist and equal-sized left and right atrial disks and is

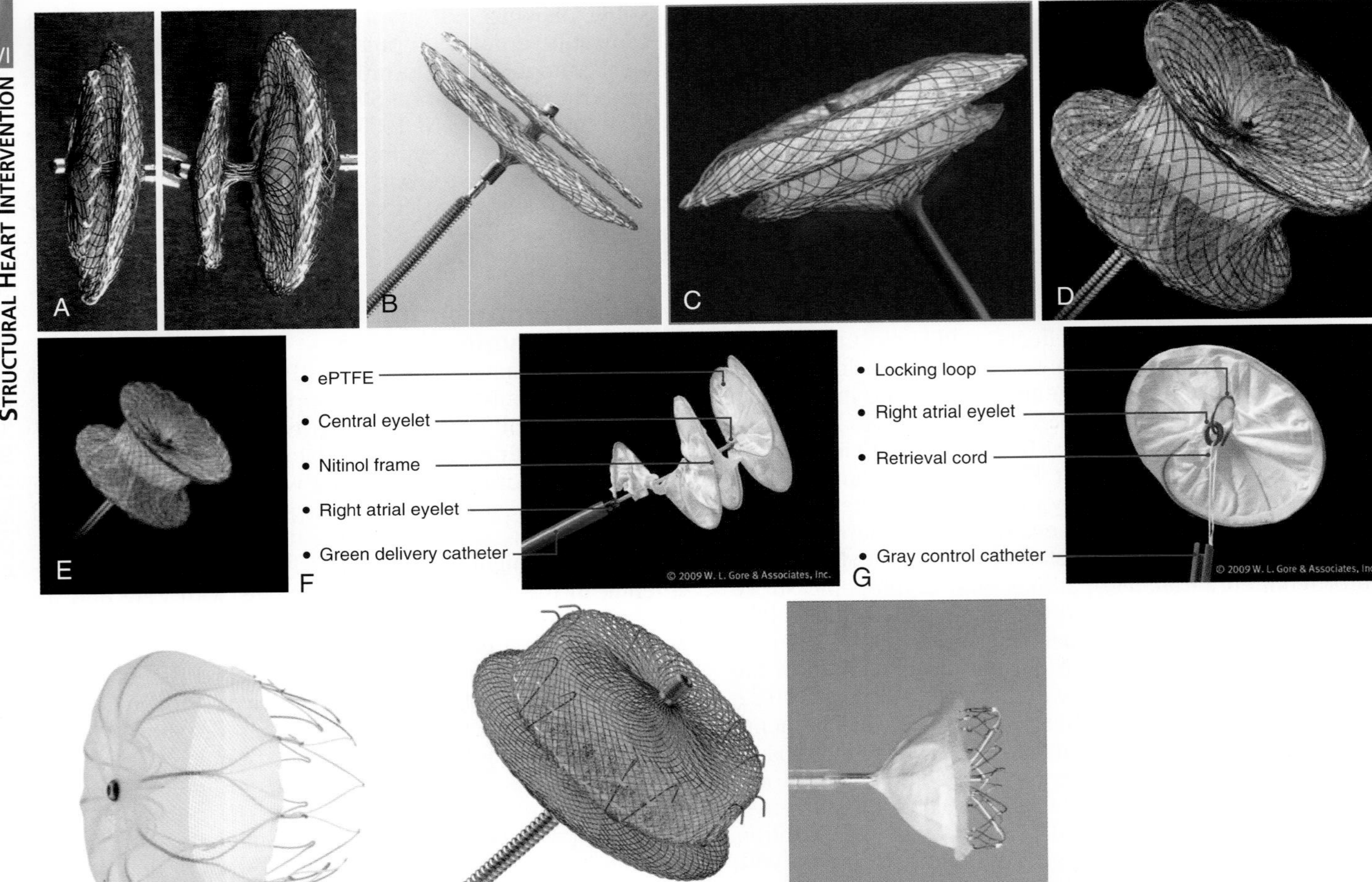

FIGURE 32-3 Devices for transcatheter closure of patent foramen ovale (PFO), atrial septal defect, left atrial appendage (LAA), and ventricular septal defect (VSD) closure discussed in this chapter. A, Amplatzer PFO occluder. **B,** Amplatzer multifenestrated "cribriform" occluder. **C,** Amplatzer septal occluder. **D,** Amplatzer muscular VSD occluder. **E,** Amplatzer post-myocardial infarction VSD occluder. **F, G,** Helex septal occluder. **H,** Watchman LAA occluder. **I,** Amplatzer cardiac plug. **J,** Coherex WaveCrest device.

available in 4 sizes—18, 25, 30, and 35 mm. The Amplatzer ASO device is discussed in the ASD closure section.

Helex Device

The Helex device is a nonself-centering double disk device composed of single nitinol wire covered with polytetrafluoroethylene (PTFE) with a left atrial eyelet, center eyelet, and right atrial eyelet (**Figure 32-3**). This device is FDA approved for closure of secundum ASDs >18 mm in diameter. The device is available in 5-mm increments, from 15 to 35 mm. The gray catheter attaches to the right atrial eyelet and is used to retract or extrude the device. The mandrel attaches to the left atrial eyelet and contains the locking loop; pulling the mandrel releases the device and locks it in place.

Procedural Details

Transcatheter PFO closure is performed in the cardiac catheterization laboratory under conscious sedation (we use midazolam and fentanyl) with fluoroscopic and ultrasound guidance (TEE, or now usually intracardiac echocardiography [ICE]) (**Figures 32-4 and 32-5**) (Videos 32-1 and 32-2). Aspirin 325 mg is usually administered before the procedure and Clopidogrel 600 mg loading dose at the end of the procedure. Femoral venous access is obtained in bilateral groins with an 8 Fr or 9 Fr sheath each (or both sheaths in the same vein), one of which is for ICE. We prefer a long 30-cm sheath for the ICE catheter to easily traverse the iliac vein into the inferior vena cava, particularly if inserted into the left vein. The ICE catheter is advanced into the right atrium and the interatrial septum adequately interrogated, and bubble study is performed through the contralateral femoral venous sheath. A Goodale-Lubin (GL) catheter is advanced with a 0.035-inch J-tipped guidewire into the SVC. The guidewire is removed and the GL catheter connected to the manifold. Right atrial angiography can then be performed if needed. The GL catheter is then directed toward the interatrial septum and the PFO crossed with or without the 0.035-inch J-tipped guidewire using ICE and fluoroscopic guidance. Once across the PFO, intravenous heparin is administered in order to achieve ACT >250 seconds. The catheter and guidewire are placed in the left superior pulmonary vein, taking care to ensure that the wire tip is not in the left atrial appendage to avoid perforation. The 0.035-inch J-tipped guidewire is exchanged for a 0.035-inch J-tipped Amplatz extra-stiff wire, again taking care to ensure that the tip is not in the appendage. PFO diameter is then measured with a sizing balloon, taking care to inflate

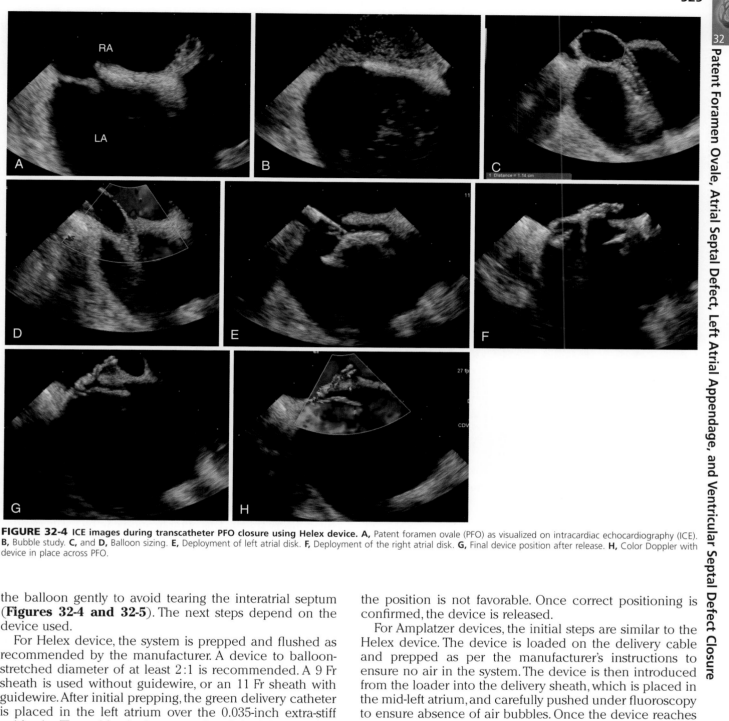

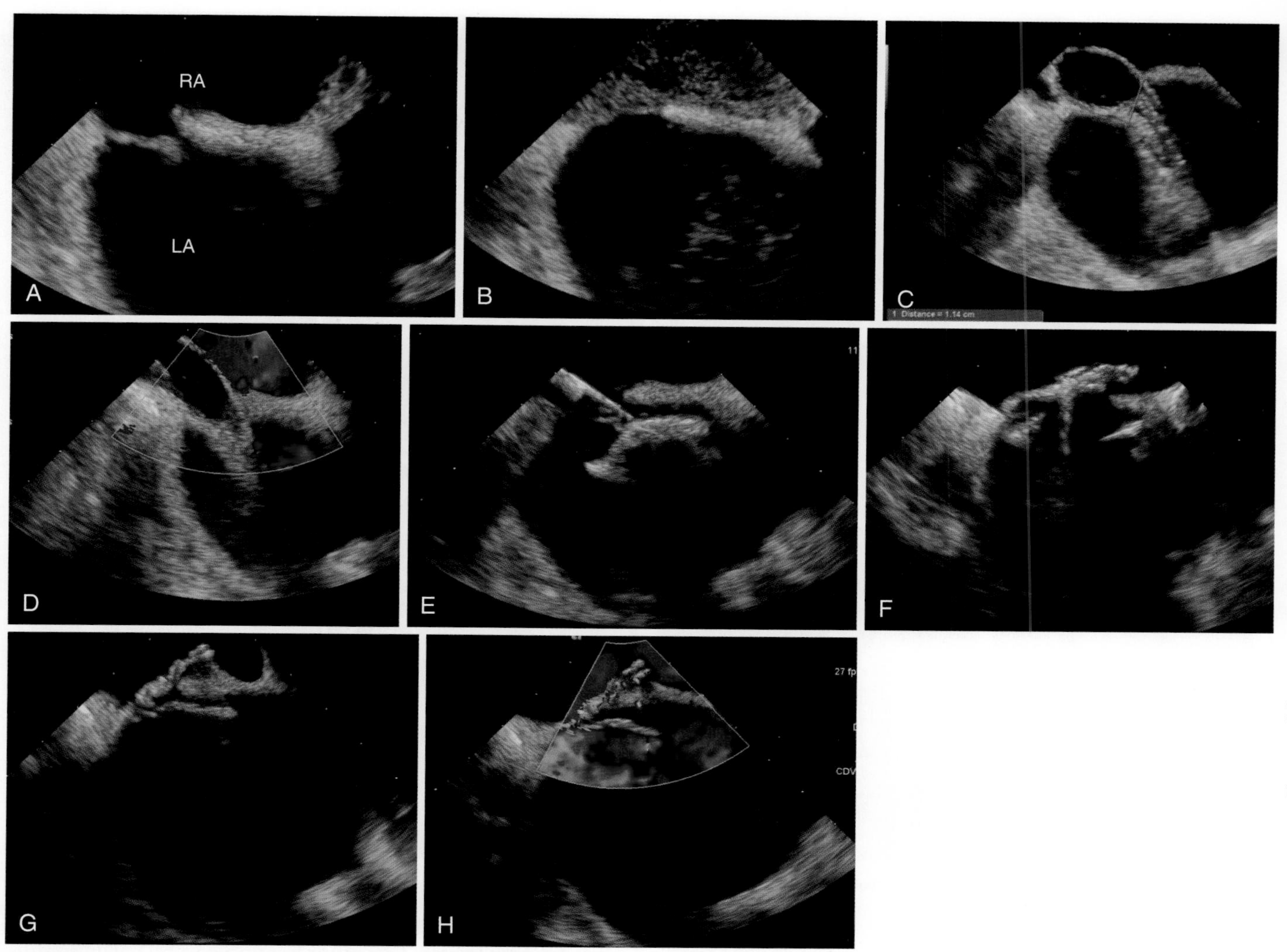

FIGURE 32-4 **ICE images during transcatheter PFO closure using Helex device. A,** Patent foramen ovale (PFO) as visualized on intracardiac echocardiography (ICE). **B,** Bubble study. **C,** and **D,** Balloon sizing. **E,** Deployment of left atrial disk. **F,** Deployment of the right atrial disk. **G,** Final device position after release. **H,** Color Doppler with device in place across PFO.

the balloon gently to avoid tearing the interatrial septum (**Figures 32-4 and 32-5**). The next steps depend on the device used.

For Helex device, the system is prepped and flushed as recommended by the manufacturer. A device to balloon-stretched diameter of at least 2:1 is recommended. A 9 Fr sheath is used without guidewire, or an 11 Fr sheath with guidewire. After initial prepping, the green delivery catheter is placed in the left atrium over the 0.035-inch extra-stiff guidewire. The guidewire is removed and the left atrial disk is deployed using the "push-pinch-pull" technique under fluoroscopic and ICE guidance to ensure positioning in the left atrium away from the roof and appendage. The entire system is then pulled against the left side of the interatrial septum. The right atrial disk is then deployed. Placement and positioning is confirmed with ICE, and left anterior oblique (LAO) projection on fluoroscopy, with the right and left atrial disks straddling the septum (**Figures 32-4 and 32-5**). Once acceptable placement is confirmed, the mandrel is pulled, which moves the locking loop off the left atrial eyelet to around the right atrial eyelet. The device can be retrieved and redeployed at any point prior to lock release. It can also be retrieved from the body after lock release if the position is not favorable. Once correct positioning is confirmed, the device is released.

For Amplatzer devices, the initial steps are similar to the Helex device. The device is loaded on the delivery cable and prepped as per the manufacturer's instructions to ensure no air in the system. The device is then introduced from the loader into the delivery sheath, which is placed in the mid-left atrium, and carefully pushed under fluoroscopy to ensure absence of air bubbles. Once the device reaches the tip of the delivery sheath, the sheath is withdrawn gently, exposing the left atrial disk, under fluoroscopic and ICE guidance. After making sure there is adequate opening of the left atrial disk in the left atrium, the system is pulled against the left atrial side of the interatrial septum such that the left atrial disk abuts the septum. The sheath is then withdrawn, exposing the right atrial disk on the right atrial side under fluoroscopic and ICE guidance. Once the device position is confirmed with fluoroscopy and ICE, and felt to be stable and fully expanded without obstruction or impingement of nearby structures, the device is released. Bubble study or right atrial angiogram may be performed at the end of the procedure. Femoral venous sheaths are removed and hemostasis achieved by manual compression.

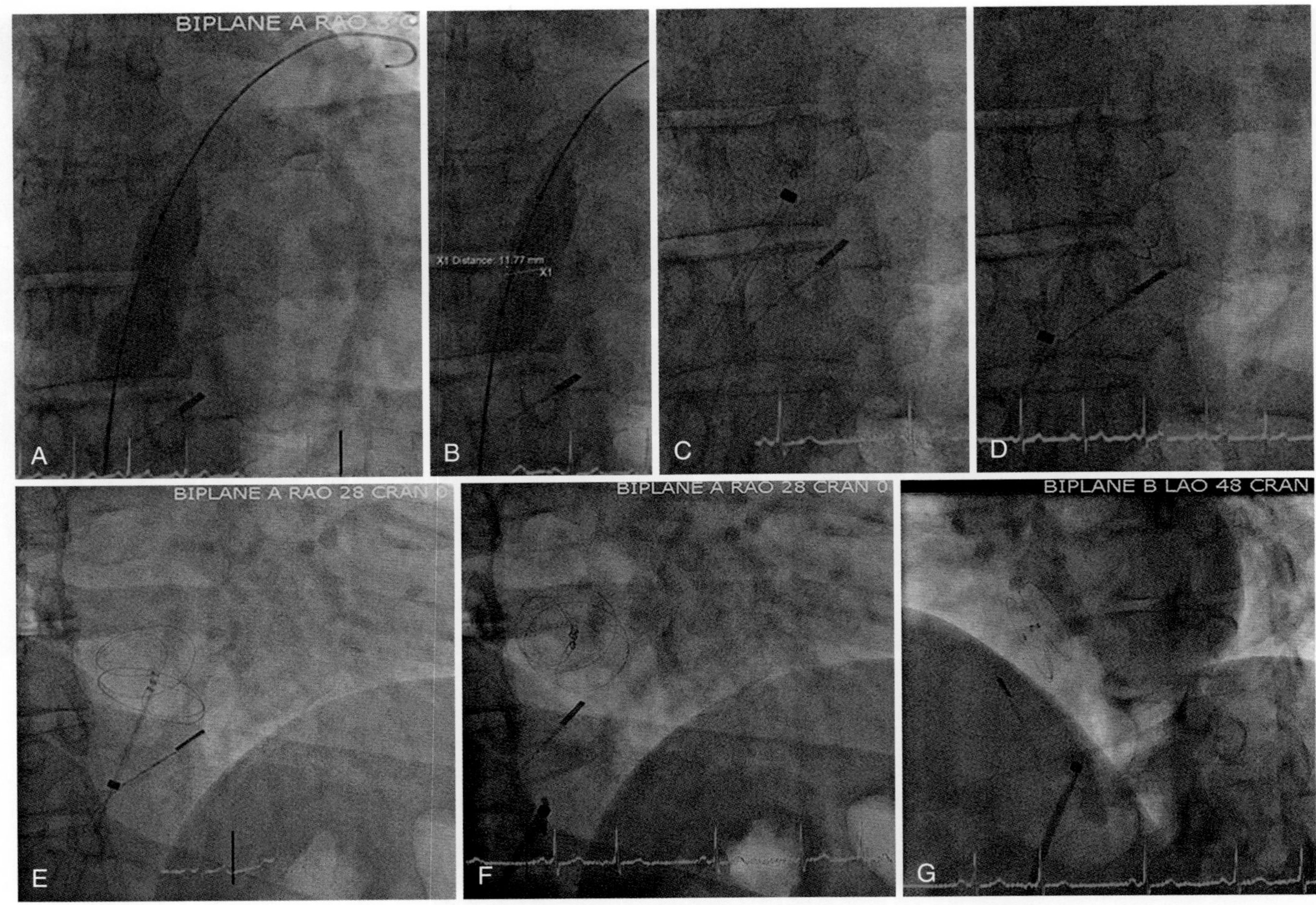

FIGURE 32-5 **Fluoroscopic images during transcatheter patent foramen ovale (PFO) closure using Helex device. A** and **B,** Balloon sizing. **C-E,** Device deployment. **F** and **G,** Final device position after release.

Postprocedure Care

It is our practice to administer two doses of antibiotics 12 hours apart. Patients are monitored with telemetry overnight, and chest x-ray and TTE with bubble study are performed the following morning to confirm accurate positioning. Aspirin 81 mg daily and Clopidogrel 75 mg daily for 6 months are prescribed. TTE with bubble study is repeated at 6 months. Endocarditis prophylaxis is advised for 6 months.

Complications

Transcatheter PFO closure is a safe procedure; however, complications can occur in 1% to 4% of patients with most complications being mild.[31,33,34] The most frequent reported complication after PFO closure is the occurrence of atrial arrhythmias including atrial fibrillation and atrial flutter. In retrospective studies, new atrial fibrillation (AF) was observed in 3.9% of patients,[31] while the rate of AF was very low in the RESPECT trial (0.2%). Device thrombosis occurs in 0.6% patients[31] and device embolization can occur in 0.07% of patients.[38] Device fracture was observed in older generation devices, but extremely rare in the current devices. Serious bleeding from vascular complications occurred in ≤0.5% in the RESPECT and PC trials. Pericardial effusion or tamponade has been reported in 0.3% of patients.[31,33] Air embolism is a potentially disastrous complication that can occur due to inadequate flushing of the device systems or while introducing the device systems into the delivery sheath. This complication can be easily avoided by careful flushing and paying meticulous attention to fluoroscopy while advancing the device through the delivery sheath.

ASD CLOSURE

Introduction

ASD is the most common congenital heart defect presenting in adults after bicuspid aortic valve and accounts for 6% to 10% of all defects at birth. It affects twice as many females as males. Left-to-right shunting at the atrial level with right-sided volume overload and eventually pulmonary vascular disease and pulmonary hypertension are responsible for the clinical presentation. Since FDA approval of a device for transcatheter ASD closure in December 2001, there has been a shift from surgical closure to transcatheter closure with excellent results and good prognosis in treated patients.

Anatomy

The development of the interatrial septum has been discussed in the section on PFO (**Figure 32-1**). There are 4 types of ASDs depending on location. The most common is secundum ASD (75% of all ASDs), which is a defect in the region of the fossa ovalis. The primum ASD (15% to 20%) is located in the inferior portion of the atrial septum near the crux of the heart and occurs due to deficiency of endocardial cushion tissue. It is often associated with a cleft in the anterior mitral valve leaflet or ventricular septal defect (common atrioventricular canal defects). The sinus venosus type of ASD (5% to 10%) is located in the superior or inferior part of the septum, near the entrance of the superior or inferior vena cava into the right atrium or SVC. The superior sinus venosus ASD is often associated with anomalous pulmonary venous drainage into the right atrium. Coronary sinus septal defect (<1%) is located in the wall separating the ostium of the coronary sinus from the left atrium. Only the secundum ASDs can be repaired by transcatheter closure; the other types require surgical closure. ASDs are associated with Down syndrome (particularly ostium primum ASD), Holt-Oram syndrome, and DiGeorge syndrome. In addition to the above, other associated lesions with ASD can include mitral valve prolapse and valvular pulmonic stenosis.

Pathophysiology

ASD leads to shunting at the atrial level. The magnitude and direction of shunting depends on defect size and the relative compliance of the ventricles. Usually the shunt is from left-to-right atrium due to higher compliance of the right ventricle. With increasing age, the left ventricular compliance decreases and left atrial pressure rises, and the magnitude of left-to-right shunt increases. This leads to volume overload and enlargement of the right atrium, right ventricle, and pulmonary artery. Over time, high pulmonary blood flow occurring for several years leads to pulmonary vascular bed remodeling, increase in pulmonary vascular resistance, and pulmonary hypertension. Left untreated, pulmonary vascular changes become irreversible, leading to severe pulmonary hypertension, right-sided pressure overload, and reversal of shunting leading to right-to-left shunting.

Clinical Presentation

During childhood, patients with ASD are usually asymptomatic and may have a pulmonary outflow murmur or fixed splitting of the second heart sound detected incidentally during routine examination. Some children may present with recurrent respiratory infections or even heart failure. Typically, most young adults have a prolonged asymptomatic course. With increasing age, symptoms of reduced exercise tolerance, progressive exertional dyspnea, and heart failure occur with progressive left-to-right shunting as a result of decreased left ventricular compliance and increased left atrial pressure. Arrhythmias including supraventricular arrhythmias, atrial fibrillation, or atrial flutter may be the presenting sign. Paradoxical embolism resulting in stroke or ischemia of other organ systems may also occur. Untreated ASDs can lead to pulmonary vascular disease and pulmonary hypertension in the absence of other causes, but typically not until adulthood.

Diagnosis

Physical exam findings that lead to evaluation for ASD include right ventricular heave, wide and fixed split of the second heart sound (due to delayed pulmonary valve closure), ejection systolic murmur best heard at the left sternal border (reflecting increased blood flow through the pulmonary valve), and loud pulmonic component of second heart sound in patients with pulmonary hypertension. Ostium primum ASDs may have associated mitral and tricuspid regurgitation murmurs. Electrocardiographic findings include right atrial enlargement (P-pulmonale), right axis deviation, right ventricular hypertrophy (tall R wave in V1), and incomplete right bundle branch block (rSR' or rsR' in leads V1-V3) in secundum ASD. In primum ASD, left axis deviation may be seen. First-degree atrioventricular block can be seen in any kind of ASD. Chest x-ray findings include right atrial and right ventricular enlargement, dilated pulmonary artery, and increased pulmonary plethora.

Echocardiography is the diagnostic modality of choice for ASD (**Figure 32-6**). In children TTE provides most of the information; however, in adults TEE is important for complete evaluation. The defect is usually seen on TTE from subcostal view of the interatrial septum or apical four-chamber view. Septal dropout is an important limitation of TTE, which can lead to false-positive diagnosis of ASD. Saline contrast echocardiography leads to accurate diagnosis in most cases. In addition to making a diagnosis, TTE demonstrates presence of right atrial and right ventricular enlargement and enables assessment of pulmonary artery pressure using the tricuspid regurgitation jet velocity. The magnitude of left-to-right shunt using noninvasive calculation of pulmonary to systemic blood flow ratio (Qp/Qs) can also be assessed, but is rarely used due to inaccuracies. Additionally, TTE allows evaluation for other associated congenital anomalies such as pulmonary valve disease, mitral valve prolapse, and pulmonary venous drainage. Prior to transcatheter ASD closure, complete assessment using TEE or ICE (usually performed just prior to closure) is critical (**Figure 32-6**). This allows assessment of various rims/margins for suitability for device closure, drainage of all four pulmonary veins, exclusion of sinus venosus-type ASDs, which can be missed by TTE, and detailed evaluation of mitral valve disease if present. Recently three-dimensional echocardiography has also been used for evaluating ASDs (**Figure 32-6**). MRI is another noninvasive imaging modality that can be used if echocardiography does not provide all required information. MRI enables direct visualization of the defect, pulmonary venous drainage, calculation of shunt size, and quantification of RV volume and function. Contrast-enhanced cardiac CT can also provide similar anatomic information.

Cardiac Catheterization

In the current era, cardiac catheterization is not required to establish a diagnosis in the presence of adequate noninvasive imaging. Right heart catheterization with measurement of oxygen saturations (shunt run) and measurement of pulmonary artery pressure and coronary angiography in patients >40 years of age are usually performed at the time of planned transcatheter closure. The author usually performs pulmonary angiogram to confirm absence of anomalous pulmonary venous drainage at the time of closure. Invasive hemodynamic assessment to determine shunt size may be needed when the hemodynamic significance is not clear by echocardiography and also when there is need to determine PVR and pulmonary vascular reactivity in the presence of pulmonary hypertension.

Management and Indications for Atrial Septal Defect Closure

Small ASDs with diameter <5 mm and no evidence of RV volume overload may not require closure as these do not usually impact the natural history. Unrepaired ASDs with significant shunting can result in right-sided volume overload, with progressive heart failure, arrhythmias, hemodynamically significant tricuspid regurgitation, pulmonary

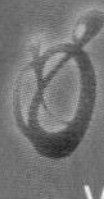

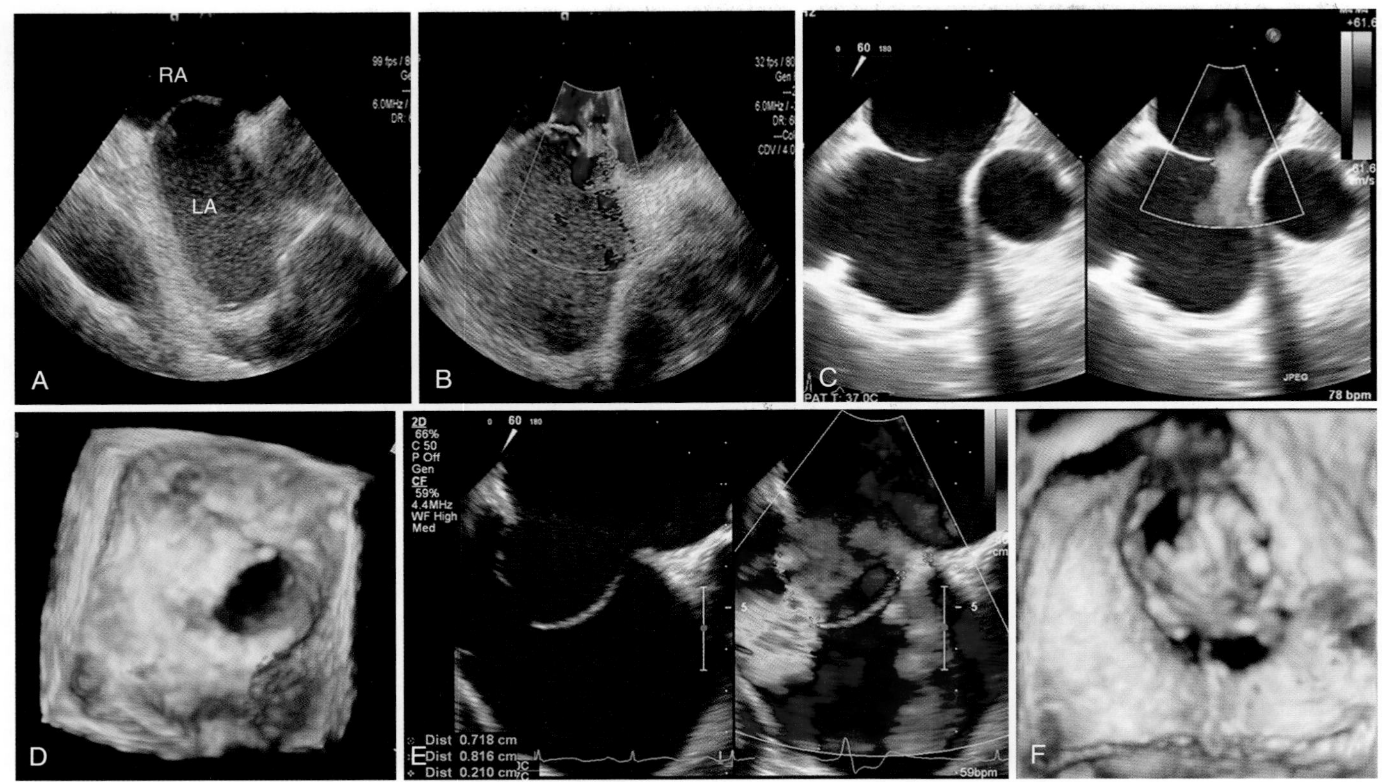

FIGURE 32-6 Diagnosis of atrial septal defect (ASD) by echocardiography. A, Secundum ASD as visualized by intracardiac echocardiography (ICE). **B,** Secundum ASD by ICE with color Doppler. **C,** Secundum ASD on transesophageal echocardiography (TEE) with deficient anterior rim. **D,** Secundum ASD as visualized by 3D echocardiography. **E,** Aneurysmal septum with cribriform ASD. **F,** Cribriform ASD on 3D echocardiography.

hypertension, and reduced survival. Current ACC/AHA guidelines recommend (Class I) ASD closure in the presence of right-sided volume overload, that is, right ventricular or right atrial dilatation in a symptomatic or asymptomatic patient.[39] Closure in presence of symptoms or right-sided heart enlargement prevents further deterioration and helps normalize the right-sided dilatation. Natural history studies of ASD closure show reduced survival after closure in patients older than 24 years of age or with pulmonary hypertension (systolic PAP ≥ 40 mm Hg).[40] Additionally, closure in patients over 40 years of age, while improving symptoms and mortality compared with a medically managed group, did not reduce the risk of atrial arrhythmias.[41] Therefore ASD closure should be performed in a timely fashion in appropriate patients to prevent long-term complications. An ASD other than secundum ASD should be repaired surgically. Closure of ASD may be considered in some patients regardless of evidence of right-sided enlargement, for example, in professional divers and patients undergoing pacemaker implantation due to risk of paradoxical embolism. Similarly, ASD closure may be considered prior to pregnancy. In patients with PAH, pulmonary vasodilator testing to assess for reversibility and test occlusion of ASD should be performed. Inhaled nitric oxide is used commonly as a pulmonary vasodilator. A positive vasoreactivity response is defined as a reduction of mean PAP of >10 mm Hg with resultant mean PAP of 40 mm Hg or less, without fall in cardiac output. Closure in such patients may be performed if there is net left-to-right shunting, PA pressure <2/3 systemic levels, PVR <2/3 SVR, or when responsive to either pulmonary vasodilator testing or test occlusion. A favorable response is indicated by a fall in mean pulmonary artery pressure with test occlusion with no decrease in cardiac output and no rise in right atrial pressure. In presence of unfavorable response, pulmonary vasodilator therapy should be initiated and hemodynamics reassessed a few months later. ASD closure is also indicated in presence of paradoxical embolism and documented platypnea-orthodeoxia. An absolute contraindication (Class III) for closure is irreversible PAH and no evidence of left-to-right shunt.

Devices for Atrial Septal Defect Closure

Percutaneous transcatheter closure has largely replaced surgical repair for a vast majority of secundum ASDs with appropriate morphology in the absence of any other associated defects due to good outcomes and low rates of complications. The two devices approved for transcatheter ASD closure are the Amplatzer ASO (AGA Medical Corporation, Golden Valley, Minnesota) device and the Helex septal occlude (discussed in the PFO section). The Amplatzer ASO is a self-expandable, double-disk device made of nitinol wire mesh that is tightly woven into 2 disks with a 3- to 4-mm connecting waist between the 2 disks (**Figure 32-3**). The super-elastic properties of nitinol allow the device to be stretched and delivered via sheath size of 6 Fr to 8 Fr. The device size is determined by the waist diameter and ranges from 4 to 40 mm (4 to 20 mm at 1-mm increments, 22 to 40 mm at 2-mm increments; the 40-mm device is not available in the United States). The disk diameters increase with increasing size and the left atrial disk is 6 to 8 mm larger than the right atrial disk depending on device size, as shunting is from left-to-right. The Amplatzer delivery system supplied separately from the device consists of a loader, hemostasis valve with extension tube and stopcock, delivery sheath of varying size and length (depending on device size to be used), a dilator, and a delivery cable. All delivery sheaths have a 45-degree tip (45-degree TorqVue Delivery Sheath). There are sheaths with 180-degree turn available but they are typically not used for ASD closure. A 60-degree angulated Hausdorf Sheath (Cook Medical, Bloomington, Indiana) can be used for ASD with poor posterior inferior rim.

Procedural Details

ASD closure is usually performed in the cardiac catheterization laboratory with conscious sedation and ICE and fluoroscopic guidance (**Figures 32-7 and 32-8**) (Videos 32-3 and 32-4). For complex septal anatomy, such as multiple ASDs, TEE may be preferred. Advantages of ICE over TEE

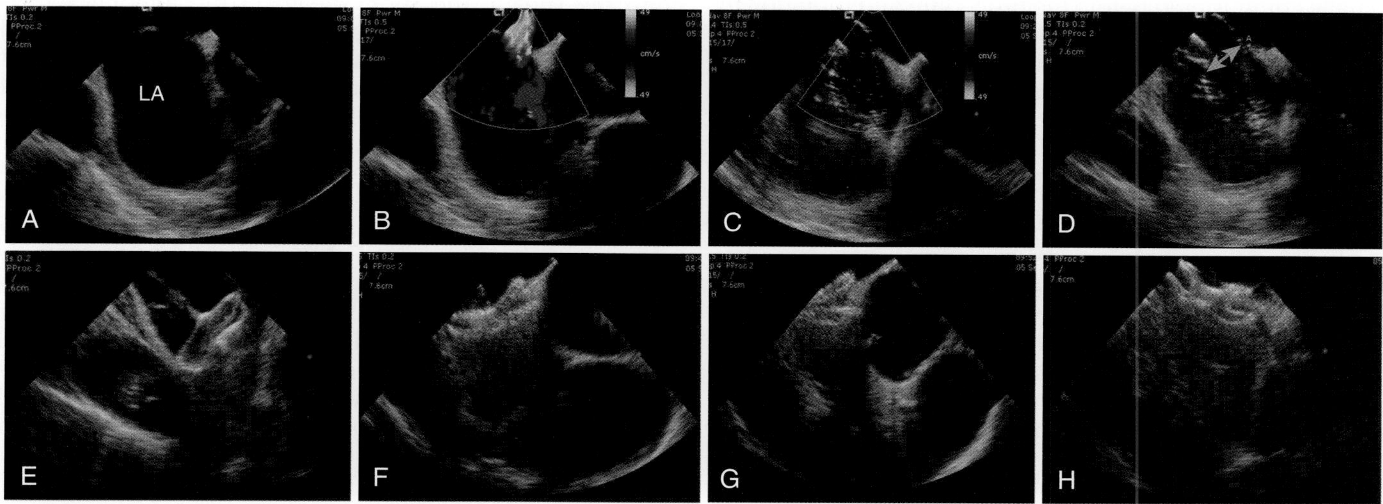

FIGURE 32-7 Intracardiac echocardiography (ICE) images during transcatheter secundum atrial septal defect (ASD) closure using Amplatzer ASO device. A and **B,** Secundum ASD with 2D and color Doppler by ICE. **C** and **D,** Balloon stop flow diameter, color Doppler, and 2D. **E,** Deployment of left atrial disk. **F,** Deployment of right atrial disk. **G,** Device splaying around aorta. **H,** Final device position.

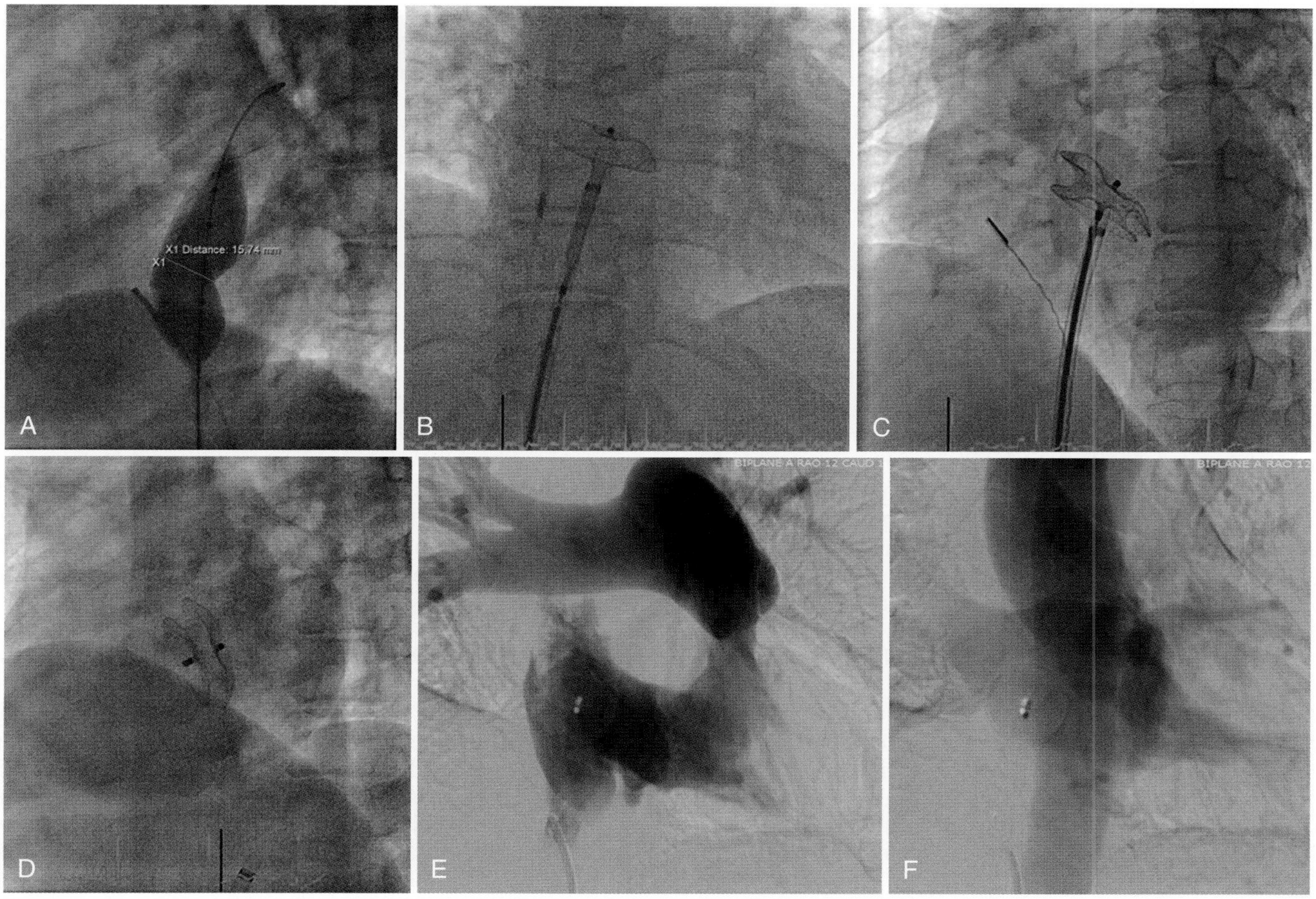

FIGURE 32-8 Fluoroscopic images during transcatheter secundum atrial septal defect (ASD) closure using Amplatzer ASO device. A, Balloon sizing. **B,** Deployment of left atrial disk. **C,** Deployment of right atrial disk. **D,** Final device position. **E** and **F,** Right atrial angiogram with levo phase imaging showing well-seated device.

include no need for general anesthesia or additional cardiologists to perform the procedure, better views of the posteroinferior part of the interatrial septum, and shorter procedure times. Most operators use the AcuNav ICE catheter (Siemens Medical Solutions distributed by Biosense Webster, Diamond Bar, California). The initial steps are similar to that described for PFO closure. Aspirin 325 mg is usually administered before the procedure and Clopidogrel 600 mg loading dose at the end of the procedure. Femoral venous access is obtained in bilateral groins with an 8 Fr or 9 Fr sheath each (or 2 sheaths in the same vein), one of which is for ICE. We prefer a 9 Fr 35-cm sheath for the ICE catheter to easily traverse the iliac vein into the inferior vena cava, particularly for left femoral vein insertion. Heparin is administered to maintain ACT >250 seconds and a dose of intravenous antibiotic is administered prior to device deployment.

A complete right heart catheterization is first performed to measure shunt fraction, pulmonary artery pressures, and pulmonary capillary wedge pressure. In patients older than 40 years, a coronary angiogram is also performed. We also perform pulmonary angiogram with levo phase imaging to assess drainage of all four pulmonary veins into the left atrium. Some operators perform right upper pulmonary vein angiogram in 35-degree LAO cranial projection, which provides an angiographic roadmap of the interatrial septum to facilitate closure.

The ICE catheter is advanced into the right atrium and the interatrial septum adequately interrogated for assessment of various rims, measuring defect size and confirming pulmonary venous drainage. A rim is considered to be deficient if its length is <5 mm, and absent if it is ≤1 mm. The rims should not be deficient (except anterior rim, as many patients lack the anterior rim and it is not a contraindication). The directions include a "warning" that a deficient aortic rim may incur increased risk of erosion, but data are insufficient as discussed later. After completion of hemodynamic assessment, angiography, and ICE assessment, a Goodale-Loubin (GL) catheter is advanced with a 0.035-inch J-tipped guidewire into the SVC. The GL catheter is moved in a caudal direction and then directed toward the interatrial septum and the ASD crossed with or without the 0.035-inch J-tipped guidewire using ICE and fluoroscopic guidance. The catheter and guidewire are placed in the left superior pulmonary vein, taking care to ensure that the wire tip is not in the left atrial appendage to avoid perforation. The 0.035-inch J-tipped guidewire is exchanged for a 0.035-inch 1-cm Amplatz super-stiff wire, again taking care to ensure that the tip is not in the appendage. Balloon sizing is the next step and is usually performed with an AGA sizing balloon or NuMed sizing balloon. Under fluoroscopic and ICE guidance, the balloon catheter is placed in the defect over the extra-stiff guidewire and the balloon is gently inflated until no flow is visualized by color Doppler on ICE imaging (**Figures 32-7 and 32-8**). It is very important to stop inflating when flow ceases (stop-flow diameter) to avoid oversizing the defect. This diameter is measured on ICE as well as fluoroscopy. For ASO, device size should be equal to but no larger than 1 to 2 mm above the stop-flow diameter. Helex septal occluder size should be at least twice the stop-flow diameter. For defects >18 mm, ASO is preferable over Helex device.

The next steps depend on the device used. For the ASO device, delivery sheath size ranges from 6 Fr to 12 Fr depending on device size chosen. The balloon-sizing catheter is removed, leaving the 0.035-inch wire in place. The delivery cable is passed through the loader and the device is screwed to the tip of the delivery cable. The device and loader are immersed in sterile saline solution and the device is pulled into the loader while flushing through the side arm. The delivery sheath is prepped and the dilator is inserted into the sheath. The short sheath in the femoral vein is removed and the delivery sheath/dilator is then advanced over the 0.035-inch wire, which has been placed in the left upper pulmonary vein. The dilator is removed once it reaches the right atrium and the sheath is de-aired. The sheath is then advanced over the wire into the left atrium, taking care to avoid suction of air in the system. The guidewire is removed and the sheath is flushed carefully. The loading device is then attached to the delivery sheath. Under fluoroscopic guidance, the device is advanced, carefully watching for any sign of air in the system. Once the device is at the tip of the delivery sheath in the left atrium, under fluoroscopic and echocardiography guidance the left atrial disk is deployed by retracting the sheath over the delivery cable. The device is gently pulled against the interatrial septum and with tension on the delivery cable; the sheath is retracted further to deploy the right atrial disk. After deployment, the position is checked by ICE and, if needed, a gentle "to and fro" motion (Minnesota wiggle) can be performed with the delivery cable to assure stable positioning. ICE assessment should include Doppler flow, which may still demonstrate flow through the waist (but should not be present around the disk), and evaluation for obstruction of adjacent structures including atrioventricular valves. If the positioning is unsatisfactory or there is impingement of adjacent structures, the device is retracted back into the delivery sheath and redeployed or replaced with a new device as appropriate. Device positioning can also be confirmed by angiography in LAO cranial projection, which allows separation of the left and right atrial disks. In cases where the device impinges or indents on the aortic root, there may be higher risk of erosion. Once satisfactory positioning is confirmed, the device is released by attaching the plastic vise to the delivery cable and rotating it counterclockwise. Deployment of the Helex septal occlude device is discussed in the section on PFO closure.

Postprocedure Care

After device deployment, sheaths are removed and hemostasis is achieved. We administer two doses of antibiotics 12 hours apart. Patients are monitored with telemetry overnight, and chest x-ray and TTE with bubble study are performed the following morning to confirm accurate positioning. The RV size and device are re-assessed at 6 months with TTE. Endocarditis prophylaxis is advised for 6 months.

Large Atrial Septal Defect with Deficient Rims

ASDs larger than 25 mm are most often associated with rim deficiency. The Helex device cannot be used to close large ASDs; hence most data exist for such defects with the ASO device. In cases of large ASDs with deficient superior, anterosuperior, or posteroinferior rims, the left atrial disk can prolapse through the defect during regular deployment. Several techniques have been described for these situations to increase chances of success. In pulmonary vein approach for large ASD with deficient anterior or posterior rim, the delivery sheath is placed in the left upper or right upper pulmonary vein and the left atrial disk is partially deployed in the pulmonary vein.[42] The sheath is then withdrawn and the remainder of the device is rapidly deployed, keeping the delivery cable fixed and stable. This technique allows the disks to be parallel to the septum. Similarly, in the left atrial roof approach, the delivery sheath is placed near the orifice of the right upper pulmonary vein (not inside the vein), and the left atrial disk deployed in the roof of the left atrium (disk is perpendicular to the spine). The right disk is then deployed by withdrawing the sheath. This allows the posterior edge of the left atrial disk to stay in the left atrium as the remainder of the device is deployed. Other approaches for closing large ASDs with deficient rims include sheath modifications or using special sheaths. The Hausdorf sheath (Cook Medical, Bloomington, Indiana) is a double curve sheath with an angled tip that keeps the disk parallel to the septum and away from the aortic rim. A modification of the Mullins sheath has been described for large ASDs with deficient anterior or posteroinferior rims, where the distal curved portion of the sheath is cut off, resulting in a straight side-hole (SSH) delivery sheath.[43] The sharp end of the cut sheath is then trimmed to reduce the risk of perforation. The SSH technique allows the device to exit the tip of the delivery sheath at an angle parallel to the septum. Other techniques for large ASDs with deficient posterior rims include using a right Judkins catheter technique or a steerable curved guiding catheter such as the Agilis catheter (St Jude Medical Inc., Minneapolis, Minnesota). The balloon-assisted technique consists of using a balloon as a buttress to prevent prolapse of the left atrial disk through the ASD during deployment.[44]

Multiple or Fenestrated Defects

Multiple defects are present in 10% of cases. These can often be treated with a single device. A second device is usually required if the distance between the primary and secondary defect is 7 mm or more. Other methods for closure with a single device include using a nonself-centering device such as Helex device or the Amplatzer cribriform device.

Complications

The vast majority of complications with transcatheter ASD closure are minor. The multicenter pivotal studies for both the ASO (St. Jude Medical Inc., St. Paul, Minnesota) and the HSO (W. L. Gore and Associates, Flagstaff, Arizona) showed differences in the efficacy between surgical and device closure of secundum ASD; however, there were differences in safety outcomes. The ASO pivotal study, which enrolled 442 patients in the device group and 152 patients in the surgical group, had a major adverse cardiac event (MACE) rate of 1.6% in the device group compared with 5.2% in the surgical group.[45] Similarly, in the Helex pivotal study, enrolling 119 patients in the device group and 128 patients in the surgical group, the MACE rate was lower in the device group compared with surgical group (5.9% vs. 10.9%).[46] Cardiac erosions are the most feared and life-threatening complications of ASD closure using ASO device.[47] There have not been any cases of erosions with the Helex device. The erosion rate has been reported to be 0.1% to 0.3% (1 to 3 per 1000 implants) with the ASO device.[47,48] Erosion most commonly occurs in the roof of the atria or the aorta. Large device size and lack of anterior or superior rims have been proposed as risk factors associated with erosion.[47,48] Lack of wiggle room in case of a large device with deficient rim can lead to constant impact on the atrial or aortic tissue from the edge of the device. A high-risk ASD is a large defect in the superior portion of the septum in close proximity to the aorta with absent or negligible aortic rim. Based on their findings, the AGA expert panel made recommendations regarding erosions, which include avoiding overstretching while balloon sizing, using stop-flow technique for sizing, gentle to and fro motion while assessing stability, and closer follow-up of those with large ASO (greater than 1.5 times native ASD size) and those with deformation of the ASO device at the aortic root with significant splaying of the device edges by the aorta. These are based on an expert opinion, and not verified conclusively in a prospective manner. There are still differences in opinion regarding risk of erosion. A survey of members of the Congenital Cardiovascular International Study Consortium (CCISC) showed that 71.7% felt that a device in which the disks approximated each other and touched/protruded into the aorta without splaying were at the highest risk of erosion.[49] The Circulatory System Devices Panel of the FDA met on May 24, 2012, to discuss current knowledge about the safety and effectiveness of the Amplatzer ASO device and Gore Helex ASD occlude as transcatheter ASD occluder devices used for the closure of secundum ASD. Since CE mark approval in 1998, there have been 97 cases of confirmed or presumed erosion worldwide in patients with on-label use of the ASO device. Within the 97 erosions, 8 deaths have occurred. Almost 90% of erosions occur within 1 year of being implanted, although one case of erosion was reported 8.5 years after the implant. All reported deaths occurred within 16 months following implant, and no deaths occurred in patients <16 years of age. The panel made some recommendations regarding more frequent follow-up in the first year after closure since events frequently occurred within 12 months, collection of ongoing device data for identification of risk factors for erosion, and thorough discussion of risks and benefits with patients.

Device malposition/embolization can potentially occur with any ASD closure. Various causes include large, eccentric defect, inadequate rims, improper sizing, and operator-related technical issues. Embolization is the most frequent complication reported at a rate of 0.5% to 3%.[50] An analysis of the device embolizations reported to the FDA's MAUDE database (Manufacturer and User Facility Device Experience) showed that in 77% of cases the device was retrieved using transcatheter approach and in 17% of cases surgical retrieval was needed.[51] There were two deaths related to device embolization. Most embolizations occur at the time of deployment or within 24 hours of the procedure. The operator must be familiar with transcatheter retrieval techniques using a gooseneck snare or bioptome. The most common site of embolization is left atrium, followed by right atrium, pulmonary artery, right ventricle, left ventricle, and aorta.[50] If the device is stuck in the ventricle and entangled within the atrioventricular valve apparatus, the patient should be referred for surgical removal. Device embolization appears to be more frequent with the Helex device compared with ASO device.

Other complications include wire frame fracture in the case of Helex device, thrombus formation on the device, new onset atrial arrhythmias, and impingement of adjacent structures including the atrioventricular valves.

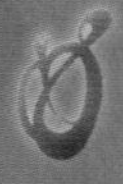

Clinical Trial Data

Results are excellent with both Amplatzer and Helex devices. Closure rates with the Amplatzer ASO device are >95% at 1-year follow-up, and >91% with Helex device.[46,52,53] Safety outcomes and complications have been discussed previously. Overall, the risk of complications is lower with the transcatheter closure approach compared with surgical approach.[45,54]

LEFT ATRIAL APPENDAGE CLOSURE

Introduction

Atrial fibrillation (AF) is the most common cardiac arrhythmia affecting 7 million patients in the United States.[55] The lifetime risk of developing AF is one in four in men and women over 40 years of age. Stroke, the most feared and serious complications of AF, is the third leading cause of death in the United States and the leading cause of disability. Patients with AF have a fivefold increased risk of stroke compared with the general population. The risk of stroke increases with age, 1.5% at 50 to 59 years, and nearly >20% at 80 to 89 years have AF.[56] Strokes related to AF have been associated with higher morbidity and mortality compared with non-AF-related strokes.

Medical Therapy for Stroke Prevention in Atrial Fibrillation

A number of risk models have been developed to stratify the risk of stroke in patients with AF. For example, the most widely used CHADS2 score consists of one point each for age >75 years, history of congestive heart failure, hypertension, and diabetes, and two points for prior embolic event.[57] The score ranges from 0 to 6, and the risk of stroke increases in an incremental fashion with increasing score (0.5% per year with score 0 to almost 7% per year with score 6, without warfarin).[58] The only medical option until recently for stroke prevention in patients with AF has been anticoagulation with warfarin, which reduces the risk of stroke by 60% compared with placebo, and by 30% to 40% when compared with aspirin alone.[59] Of note, the risk of both intracranial and extracranial hemorrhage was higher with warfarin compared with aspirin. Warfarin has also been shown to be superior in stroke prevention when compared with dual antiplatelet therapy with aspirin and Clopidogrel.[60] Despite its efficacy, warfarin has several drawbacks. It has a narrow therapeutic range, and requires frequent blood tests for monitoring. There is a significant risk of major bleeding of over 10% per year associated with warfarin use.[61] Additionally, the efficacy of anticoagulation is variable due to interactions with foods and other medications, and despite frequent monitoring and dosage adjustments, less than 50% of patients treated with warfarin have international normalized ratios (INRs) in the therapeutic range of 2.0 to 3.0. In addition, 40% of patients with AF have contraindications to warfarin.[62]

Newer anticoagulants have emerged in the last few years. The oral direct thrombin inhibitor, dabigatran was evaluated in the randomized evaluation of long-term anticoagulation therapy (RELY trial).[63] In this study, 18,113 patients with AF and increased risk of stroke (mean CHADS2 score of 2) were randomized to treatment with warfarin or dabigatran (110 or 150 mg twice daily) in a noninferiority design with primary endpoint of stroke or systemic embolism. The 110-mg dose of dabigatran proved noninferior to warfarin with respect to the primary endpoint with less major bleeding, whereas the 150-mg dose was associated with lower rate of the primary endpoint with similar major bleeding. A recent analysis from the RELY trial suggested that in patients ≥75 years, intracranial bleeding risk is lower, but extracranial bleeding risk is similar or higher with both doses of dabigatran compared with warfarin.[64] Similarly, other newer agents such as Apixaban and Rivaroxaban have been studied for stroke prevention in AF; however, these agents also carry the risk of bleeding as well as higher cost.[65,66]

Left Atrial Appendage Anatomy

The left atrial appendage (LAA) is an important cardiac structure located anterolaterally in the atrioventricular groove between the left ventricle and the left upper pulmonary vein. It originates from primordial atrial tissue and consists of trabeculated pectinate muscles, mostly in the mid and distal segments. There is wide variability in the shape, number of lobes, and volume of the LAA. An autopsy study of 500 hearts showed that 54% of LAA had two lobes, whereas 23% had three lobes unrelated to age or gender.[67] There is usually an elliptical ostial segment that is free of trabeculations. In sinus rhythm, the LAA has contractile function with an emptying velocity that can be distinctly recorded by TEE. In AF, there is stasis of blood in the LAA as a result of decreased contractility in conjunction with left atrial enlargement, leading to formation of thrombus. The LAA is the source of thrombus in the vast majority of patients (>90%) with nonvalvular AF and thromboembolic events as demonstrated by echocardiography.[68] Due to the several issues outlined above with anticoagulant therapy, surgical and recently percutaneous exclusion of the LAA has been developed.

Surgical Left Atrial Appendage Exclusion

Surgical LAA exclusion has been performed concomitantly in patients with AF undergoing heart surgery, such as aortic or mitral valve surgery along with maze procedure. There are several surgical techniques for LAA consisting of either excision or exclusion of the LAA. Excision is performed by removal of the LAA, either by scissors or a stapling device.[69] Exclusion of the LAA is performed by closing the orifice of the LAA surgically with a suture or by stapling. A high rate of late LAA patency after surgical techniques has been reported.[70] In one study, using TEE after surgery, the rate of successful LAA closure was found to be only 40% with greater rate of successful closure with excision (73%) than suture exclusion (23%).[71] Additionally, concerns remain for increased postoperative bleeding after surgical LAA exclusion or excision.

Percutaneous Left Atrial Appendage Closure

Many devices have emerged for percutaneous LAA closure. The devices and the data available are summarized here.

Imaging for Left Atrial Appendage Closure

Percutaneous LAA closure is performed under fluoroscopic and TEE guidance. While these modalities provide "real-time" imaging, they are limited by the two dimensional (2D) nature of data obtained. Multidetector CT (MDCT) acquires a 3D dataset, which allows reconstruction and provides more precise procedural planning as compared with 2D planning for structural interventions such as transcatheter aortic valve replacement (TAVR). A recent study outlined the use of MDCT for preprocedural planning for LAA closure.[72] In this study poor correlation was found between TEE measurements and those provided by MDCT. A strategy for assessing the LAA anatomy for percutaneous LAA closure was outlined and various measurements defined such as: distance from the fossa ovalis to the LAA ostium in three planes, distance from the LAA to the surrounding structures, assessment of sphericity of the LAA ostium, angulation of the appendage with reference to the ostial plane, and methods to predict optimal fluoroscopic views during percutaneous LAA closure procedure. It is possible that better assessment of 3D anatomy by MDCT will help in optimal sizing of the LAA closure device and reduce the chances of complications by minimizing manipulation of wires and devices in the left atrium.

PLAATO Device

The Percutaneous Left Atrial Appendage Transcatheter Occlusion (PLAATO) device (Appriva Medical, Plymouth, Massachusetts) was the first to be developed.[73] This device was a self-expanding nitinol cage with a polytetrafluoroethylene membrane and hooks to anchor in the LAA. Ostermayer et al. reported the results of LAA closure using the PLAATO device in 111 patients with AF and contraindication for anticoagulation.[74] Device implantation was successful in 97.3% of patients and 3 patients developed pericardial effusion requiring pericardiocentesis. At 6 months, successful LAA occlusion was observed in 98% of patients by TEE. The annual stroke rate was 2.2% (compared with CHADS2 predicted stroke rate of 6.3%), which led to a 65% relative risk reduction in stroke. At 5 years, stroke rate was 3.8% (compared with CHADS2 predicted rate of 6.6% per year).[75] This device is no longer available. Newer devices have been developed for percutaneous LAA closure as discussed later.

Watchman Device

The Watchman device (Boston Scientific, Natick, Massachusetts) is a self-expanding nitinol frame with fixation barbs and polyester membrane covering the frame on the left atrial side. The device is available in 5 sizes with diameters ranging from 21 to 33 mm. The Watchman device is the most studied percutaneous LAA closure device with over 2000 implants worldwide. This device has been evaluated in the PROTECT-AF trial, CAP registry, and the PREVAIL trial.

Procedure

The procedure is performed under TEE and fluoroscopic guidance (**Figure 32-9**). After transseptal puncture is performed in standard fashion (posterior and not high), a pigtail catheter is advanced into the LAA to perform an LAA angiogram. Using angiography, TEE (and preprocedural CT as described above), the appropriate size of the device to be used is determined. The LAA ostium is often ellipsoid[72] and the device is generally sized 10% to 20% larger than the LAA ostium. The device is advanced via the delivery system

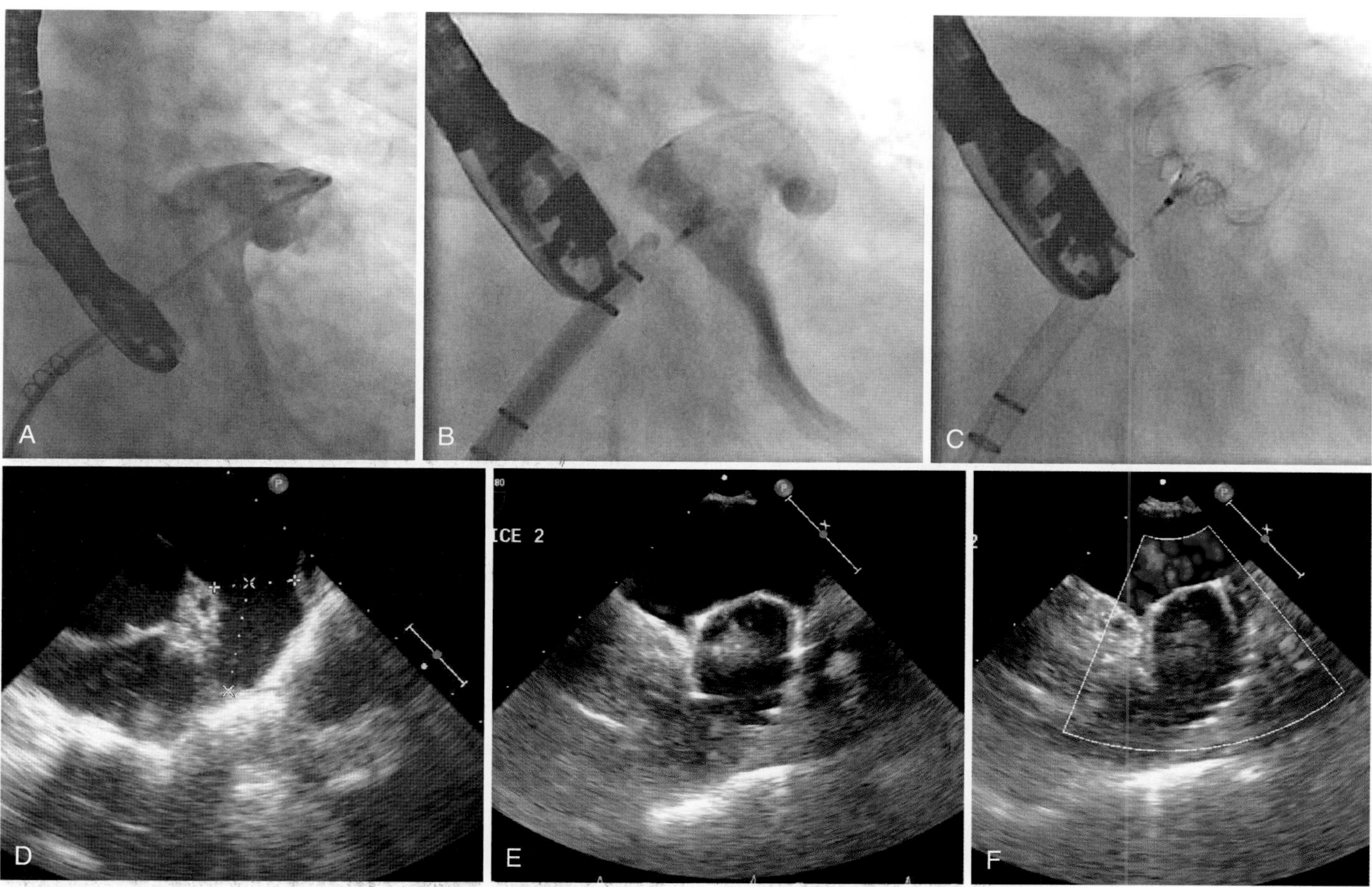

FIGURE 32-9 Fluoroscopic and transesophageal echocardiography (TEE) images during transcatheter left atrial appendage (LAA) closure using Watchman device. A, LAA angiogram with pigtail. **B,** LAA angiogram with Watchman device in position in LAA. **C,** Device deployment. **D,** LAA measurements using TEE for device sizing. **E** and **F,** 2D and color Doppler TEE image showing Watchman device in LAA.

through a 12 Fr transseptal sheath (outer diameter 14 Fr). The device is positioned and stability verified by fluoroscopy and TEE prior to release.

Data for Watchman Device

The PROTECT AF (WATCHMAN left atrial appendage system for embolic protection in patients with atrial fibrillation) study was the first prospective randomized controlled trial that examined the safety and efficacy of percutaneous LAA closure compared with anticoagulant therapy with warfarin (noninferiority study) in patients with nonvalvular AF.[76] Patients aged 18 years or older with paroxysmal, persistent, or permanent AF and CHADS2 score ≥1 were included. Patients with contraindications to warfarin, LAA thrombus, PFO with ASA and R-L shunt, mobile aortic atheroma, and symptomatic carotid artery disease were excluded. 707 patients were randomized in a 2:1 ratio to percutaneous LAA closure and subsequent discontinuation of warfarin 45 days later (intervention group, n = 463) followed by dual antiplatelet therapy for 6 months, then aspirin monotherapy or to warfarin therapy with target INR between 2.0 and 3.0 (control group, n = 244). At 1065 patient-years of follow-up (mean follow-up per patient was 18 months), the primary efficacy event rate (composite of stroke, cardiovascular death, and systemic embolism) was 3.0 per 100 patient-years (95% CI, 1.9 to 4.5) in the intervention group and 4.9 per 100 patient-years (95% CI, 2.8 to 7.1) in the control group (Rate ratio [RR], 0.62; 95% CI, 0.35 to 1.25) with a probability of noninferiority of the intervention >99.9%. The primary composite safety endpoint (bleeding or procedure-related complications such as serious pericardial effusion, device embolization, procedure-related stroke) occurred more frequently in the intervention group compared with the control group (7.4 per 100 patient-years; 95% CI, 5.5 to 9.7, vs. 4.4 per 100 patient-years, 95% CI, 2.5 to 6.7; RR 1.69, 1.01 to 3.19). The most frequent complication in the intervention group was serious pericardial effusion (defined as the need for percutaneous or surgical drainage), which occurred in 22 (4.8%) of patients, of which 15 patients were treated with pericardiocentesis and 7 underwent surgical intervention. Device embolization occurred in 3 patients (0.6%), and procedure-related stroke occurred in 5 patients (1.1%). There was a learning curve as reflected in the decline in rate of serious pericardial effusion with increasing operator experience at each site. Since patients who were not candidates for warfarin therapy were excluded, PROTECT AF did not address the role of percutaneous LAA closure in patients with contraindications to warfarin therapy.

The continued access protocol (CAP) registry, which evaluated 460 patients undergoing LAA closure with the Watchman device after PROTECT AF study was completed, demonstrated significant decline in procedure-related complications with greater operator experience.[77] The registry showed a significantly lower rate of serious pericardial effusion (2.2%, a 58% RR reduction from PROTECT AF), procedure-related stroke (0%), and overall procedure/device-related safety adverse events (3.7%). The Watchman device is also being evaluated in the PREVAIL (Evaluation of the Watchman LAA closure device in patients with atrial fibrillation versus long term warfarin therapy) randomized trial.

The ASAP (Aspirin Plavix Feasibility Study with Watchman Left Atrial Appendage Closure Technology) study was the first study to assess the safety and efficacy of LAA closure in patients with nonvalvular AF who were ineligible for warfarin therapy.[78] In this multicenter, prospective, nonrandomized study, 150 patients with AF and CHADS2 score >1 who were ineligible for warfarin due to history of bleeding or high-risk for bleeding underwent LAA closure with the Watchman device. Over mean follow-up of 14.4 ± 8.6 months, the rate of all-cause stroke or systemic embolism was 2.3% per year, ischemic stroke 1.7% per year, and hemorrhagic stroke 0.6% per year. Based on the mean CHADS2 score of 2.8, the annual ischemic stroke rate was expected to be 7.3% with aspirin alone. The observed rate of 1.7% represents 77% risk reduction. Pericardial effusion with tamponade requiring percutaneous drainage occurred in 1.3% of patients and device embolization occurred in 1.3% of patients. The ASAP study showed that LAA closure with the Watchman device can be safely performed without warfarin transition, and can be used in patients with AF at high risk for bleeding and unable to tolerate oral anticoagulation.

Amplatzer Cardiac Plug

The Amplatzer cardiac plug (ACP) (St. Jude Medical, Minneapolis, Minnesota) is a self-expandable device made from braided nitinol wires, consisting of a distal lobe and proximal disk connected by an articulating waist. There are 8 sizes, ranging from 16 to 30 mm, corresponding to the lobe diameter. The lobe has a fixed length of 6.5 mm and the disk diameter ranges from 20 to 36 mm. The lobe has up to 6 stabilizing hooks that help anchor the device in the LAA. It can be delivered via a 9 Fr, 10 Fr, or 13 Fr sheath depending on device size. The main potential advantages of the ACP device over the Watchman device are the ability to reposition, its shape with fixed lobe length of 6.5 mm, and a broad disk allowing implantation in a wide range of LAA anatomy including shallow LAAs and those with a broad diameter.[79]

Data for Amplatzer Cardiac Plug Device

The initial European experience of LAA closure with ACP device in 143 patients showed a procedural success rate of 96% and major complication rate of 7% including 3 patients with ischemic stroke, 2 patients with device embolization, and 5 patients with clinically significant pericardial effusions.[80] In a single-center 10-year experience consisting of ACP implantation in 120 patients with nonvalvular AF, the combined rate of death, stroke, and systemic embolization was 7% during follow-up and the periprocedural rate of complications including pericardial effusion, device embolization, procedure-related stroke, and major bleeding was 6.7%.[81] Similarly, in the Belgian registry evaluating 90 patients undergoing LAA closure with ACP device in seven centers, technical success was achieved in 95% of patients with periprocedural complication rate of 4.4% including three tamponades (resulting in death in one case).[82] In that study, the 30-day and 1-year survivals were 99% and 94%, respectively, with no deaths related to ACP device during follow-up, and the observed stroke rate was 2.14% per year in contrast to expected stroke rate of 5.08% per year according to the CHA2DS2-VASc score.[82] A single operator registry of 100 patients with contraindications to anticoagulant therapy undergoing LAA occlusion with ACP showed procedural success rate of 100% with only one case of pericardial tamponade and one periprocedural pulmonary edema.[83] A recent multicenter study from Canada reported outcomes in 52 patients with nonvalvular AF with contraindications to anticoagulation therapy who underwent LAA closure with the ACP device.[84] The mean age was 74 years, and the median CHADS2 score was 3 in this population. Procedural success was achieved in 98% of patients. At a mean follow-up of 20 months, the rates of death, stroke, systemic embolism, pericardial effusion, and major bleeding were 5.8%, 1.9%, 0%, 1.9%, and 1.9%, respectively.

LARIAT Device

The LARIAT (Sentre HEART, Redwood City, California) is a percutaneous epicardial suture device for LAA exclusion. It consists of 0.025-inch and 0.035-inch, magnet-tipped guidewires (FindrWire), a 15-mm compliant occlusion balloon catheter (EndoCATH), and a 12 Fr suture delivery device (Lariat). A preprocedural CTA is very useful in assessing the size, shape, and orientation of the LAA and also in guidance of the pericardial access. Since the width of the Lariat is 40 mm, LAA width >40 mm is a contraindication for this technique. Other contraindications include very superiorly oriented LAA or LAAs with apex directed behind the pulmonary trunk. The first step is percutaneous pericardial access, which is obtained via midline approach with a 17 G (gauge) epidural needle. This is often performed with a pigtail in the right ventricular apex, to keep the needle on the anterior surface of the heart. Once epicardial access is confirmed with small contrast injection, a 0.035-inch guidewire is advanced into the pericardial space. After dilating, a 14 Fr soft-tipped epicardial sheath is placed. The next step is transseptal access with preferentially an inferior and posterior puncture under fluoroscopic and TEE guidance. An 8.5 Fr SL1 catheter (St. Jude Medical, St. Paul, Minnesota) is then advanced into the ostium of the LAA. The 0.025-inch endocardial guidewire is then advanced through the balloon catheter to the apex of the LAA. An LAA angiogram is then performed through the lumen of the balloon catheter. The 0.035-inch epicardial wire is then placed through the 14 Fr epicardial sheath to achieve end-to-end magnetic union with the endocardial guidewire. This union is visualized fluoroscopically in the anteroposterior and lateral projections, and the Lariat device is then advanced over the epicardial wire followed by the LAA. The balloon is then inflated in the LAA and is used to position the snare at the LAA ostium. After confirming position, the snare is closed. LAA angiogram is performed to confirm closure. The endocardial wire and balloon are then removed and final tightening of the suture is performed. The Lariat device is removed and the suture is cut near the LAA ostium using a Lariat suture cutter. A pericardial drain is left in place overnight.

In a single-center prospective series consisting of 89 patients with nonvalvular AF and contraindications to warfarin therapy undergoing LAA ligation using Lariat device, 85 patients (96%) had successful procedure with 81 patients having complete closure (defined as <1 mm jet by color flow Doppler) immediately.[85] Complete closure of the LAA was observed in 98% of patients undergoing 1-year follow-up. There were three access-related complications—two during pericardial access and one related to transseptal catheterization. Severe pericarditis occurred in two patients post-procedure. Other smaller series have demonstrated similar feasibility and low incidence of complications.[86,87] Further studies are needed to determine the safety and efficacy of LAA exclusion with Lariat device.

Next Generation Left Atrial Appendage Closure Devices

Watchman Generation 5

The Watchman generation 5 device has a closed distal end, which is potentially less traumatic, thereby reducing the risk of cardiac tamponade. It can be recaptured and redeployed. It will be available in more sizes, thereby allowing wider range of LAAs to be treated.

Amulet

The Amulet device (St. Jude Medical, Minneapolis, Minnesota), a self-expanding device consisting of a nitinol mesh with two polyester patches sewn on to a distal lobe and a proximal disk connected by a short waist, received CE mark approval in Europe in 2013. It has several differences compared with the ACP. It has a larger disk diameter, longer lobe and waist length, more sizes available (up to 34 mm), and a stiffer stabilizing wire system. The Amulet device also has a recessed end-screw to reduce risk of thrombus formation, has more stabilizing wires, and is preloaded in the delivery system. These modifications were made to improve implantation and sealing with the device.

Coherex

The Coherex WaveCrest Left Atrial Appendage Occluder (Coherex Medical, Salt Lake City, Utah) consists of a nitinol frame supporting a polyurethane foam and ePTFE membrane. There are independent and retractable anchors to stabilize the device and a distal injection port to assess device stability during implantation. The device is positioned first and the anchors are rolled out subsequently. There are three sizes (22, 27, and 32 mm) to accommodate LAA sizes between 18 and 30 mm.

VENTRICULAR SEPTAL DEFECT

Introduction

Ventricular septal defect (VSD) is the most common congenital heart defect presenting at birth with a prevalence of almost 4 per 1000 live births.[88] The frequency varies with age at detection, since many small defects present at birth may close spontaneously with time. VSD is often a part of complex congenital anomalies such as Tetralogy of Fallot, transposition of great vessels, aortic co-arctation, etc. These are usually diagnosed and treated during childhood. We will focus on isolated VSD in this chapter.

Anatomy

VSDs are classified based on their location in the interventricular septum (**Figure 32-10**).[39] VSDs in the outflow portion of the right ventricle are Type 1 VSDs and are also referred to as subpulmonary, infundibular, supracristal, or doubly committed juxta-arterial VSDs. These account for about 6% of defects and rarely close spontaneously. Defects in the membranous septum, adjacent to the septal leaflet of the tricuspid valve, are referred to as Type 2, or perimembranous VSDs. These account for almost 80% of all VSDs and can be associated with adherence of the septal leaflet of the tricuspid valve to the defect, leading to formation of a pouch or "aneurysm" of the septum. Type 3, or inlet VSDs, occur in the inlet septum separating the mitral and tricuspid valves and area called atrioventricular septal defects. Type 4, or muscular VSDs (5% to 20% of VSDs), can be located anywhere in the muscular septum and are surrounded by

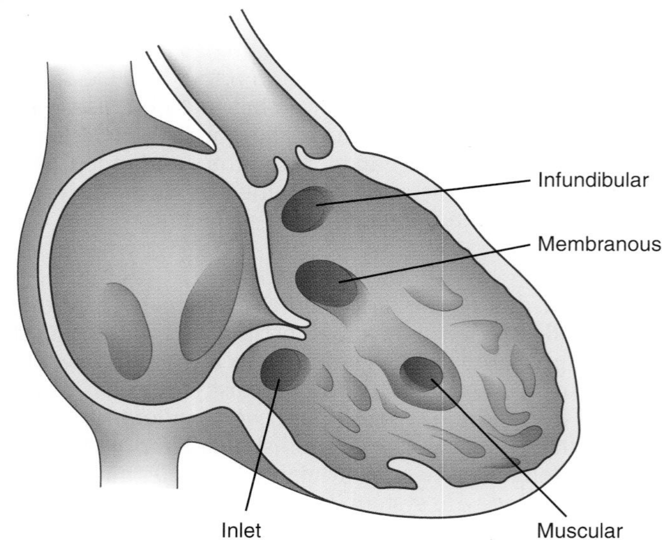

FIGURE 32-10 Location of various types of ventricular septal defects (VSDs) viewed from the right ventricular aspect.

muscular rims. These can be multiple and spontaneous closure is common. Acquired muscular VSDs are most often related to an acute myocardial infarction (MI) or trauma. Anterior infarctions are more likely to cause apical VSDs and inferior or lateral infarctions are more likely to cause basal defects at the junction of the septum and the posterior wall.

Pathophysiology

VSD leads to shunting at the ventricular level. Factors affecting the hemodynamic impact of VSD include size of the defect, pressure in the right and left ventricles, and the relative resistances of the pulmonary and systemic vascular beds. Small defects that are less than 25% the size of the aortic annulus have small net left-to-right shunt and are sometimes referred to as restrictive defects. With larger or nonrestrictive defects, the shunt volume is determined primarily by the size of the defect and pulmonary vascular resistance. At birth there may be minimal left-to-right shunting due to high pulmonary vascular resistance. As the pulmonary vascular resistance falls, left-to-right shunting increases and the defect becomes clinically apparent. In the absence of pulmonary hypertension or right ventricular outflow obstruction, the direction of shunting is left-to-right with consequent left atrial and left ventricular volume overload. In the presence of pulmonary hypertension or right ventricular outflow obstruction, shunting may be right-to-left, depending on the pressure difference. Eisenmenger's physiology results from chronic left-to-right shunting with structural changes in the pulmonary vasculature resulting in irreversible pulmonary hypertension and reversal of shunt and consequent systemic desaturation and cyanosis. Secondary abnormalities related to VSD include prolapse of the right cusp of the aortic valve with resultant aortic regurgitation in case of infundibular VSD, and tricuspid aneurysm formation secondary to adherent tricuspid valve leaflet into a perimembranous VSD. In cases of post-MI VSD, large left-to-right shunting occurs acutely, often leading to hemodynamic instability and circulatory collapse, depending on the size of the defect, presence of right ventricular infarction, and stunning of the right ventricle from volume overload.

Clinical Presentation

Adults with VSD usually have a prior diagnosis and/or evaluation. VSD may present in several possible ways: patients with a small left-to-right shunt due to a restrictive VSD may remain asymptomatic and present with a systolic murmur, patients with moderate-sized VSD may remain asymptomatic or develop symptoms of heart failure in childhood, and patients with large VSDs typically develop symptoms of heart failure during infancy. Other presentations include infective endocarditis, new diastolic murmur secondary to aortic regurgitation in cases of aortic valve prolapse with infundibular VSDs and Eisenmenger syndrome with cyanosis, clubbing, and marked exercise intolerance in late childhood or adulthood.

Diagnosis

Clinical examination is characterized by a systolic murmur at the left lower sternal border. The intensity and duration of murmur depends on the size of the VSD and right ventricular pressure. Smaller defects are loudest. With low right ventricular pressure, the murmur is usually holosystolic. Pulmonary hypertension and high right ventricular pressure is usually associated with a right ventricular heave, accentuated pulmonary component of second heart sound, and diminished, or no murmur. The ECG can be normal in patients with small VSDs. In patients with large VSD, there may be evidence of left-sided volume overload in the form of left ventricular hypertrophy (LVH), or biventricular hypertrophy in those with associated pulmonary hypertension.

Echocardiography is the main imaging modality for diagnosis of VSD. TTE is very useful in delineating the location, size, and number of defects, and in assessing the hemodynamic impact of the defect by estimating the right ventricular systolic pressure, left and right ventricular size and function, and associated abnormalities such as aortic regurgitation, tricuspid regurgitation and RV, or LV outflow obstruction. TEE may be necessary in patients with poor TTE windows. Three-dimensional echocardiography can be useful for quantifying shunts and for assessing defects that are difficult to visualize by 2D echocardiography. MRI can be used to evaluate VSDs with associated complex congenital lesions and to calculate shunt fraction.

Cardiac catheterization is recommended in patients with VSD and pulmonary hypertension to accurately measure pulmonary vascular resistance, pulmonary reactivity, and degree of shunting.[39] Angiography can show the location of the defect but is usually not required as echocardiography delineates this well.

Management and Indications for Ventricular Septal Defect Closure

The treatment of patients with VSD depends on the size and type of defect, pulmonary artery pressure and resistance, and associated acquired complications including double-chambered right ventricle and aortic regurgitation. A small VSD in the absence of symptoms or evidence of left ventricular volume overload does not require any intervention. Careful follow-up and monitoring is required in patients with VSD without signs of left ventricular volume overload. Medical management is recommended in patients with large defects and irreversible pulmonary hypertension or Eisenmenger syndrome. Such patients should be cared for in specialized centers with expertise in managing a wide range of medical conditions that could arise in these cases.

Vasodilator therapy can be an important adjunct and can provide functional improvement. In the current era, most adults presenting with unrepaired VSD likely have a small defect without left ventricular volume overload or have residual shunt after previous operation. According to the ACC/AHA guidelines, the indications for VSD closure include the following:

Class I: pulmonary to systemic blood flow ratio (Qp/Qs) of 2 or more and clinical evidence of LV volume overload, history of infective endocarditis.

Class IIa: closure of VSD is reasonable when net left-to-right shunting is present at a QP/Qs greater than 1.5 with pulmonary artery pressure less than two thirds of systemic pressure and PVR less than two thirds of systemic vascular resistance, or Qp/Qs greater than 1.5 in presence of LV systolic or diastolic failure.

Class III: VSD closure is not recommended in patients with severe irreversible pulmonary hypertension.

Primary surgical repair of VSD includes patch closure with a synthetic material (e.g., Dacron, polytetrafluoroethylene) and concomitant repair of associated defects if present, such as resection of right ventricular outflow obstruction in case of double-chambered right ventricle, aortic valve repair, or replacement in cases of aortic regurgitation. Intraoperative TEE is indicated to evaluate for additional defects and to assess adequacy of repair. Observational data suggest that surgical closure decreases the risk of endocarditis by at least 50%, reduces pulmonary artery pressure, and improves long-term survival.[89-91] Early mortality is low in the absence of elevated PVR and late survival is excellent in the presence of normal ventricular function. In a series of 516 patients who underwent surgical VSD repair, the 25-year survival was 83%.[92] However, long-term survival is significantly lower when repair is performed at older age, or in the presence of pulmonary hypertension.[90,91] Despite good prognosis after surgical repair of uncomplicated VSDs, long-term sequelae can occur and include arrhythmias, residual VSD, endocarditis, tricuspid and aortic regurgitation, ventricular dysfunction, and pulmonary hypertension.

Over the last decade, transcatheter techniques for VSD closure have been developed. Indications for transcatheter VSD closure include muscular VSD, particularly when it is remote from the tricuspid valve and aorta and associated with evidence of left ventricular volume overload.[39] Other indications include residual defects after prior surgical repair, traumatic or iatrogenic defects after surgical aortic valve replacement, patients at high surgical risk, multiple previous cardiac surgical interventions, and poorly accessible muscular VSDs.[39] Transcatheter VSD closure is not approved by the FDA in the United States for perimembranous VSD.

Devices for Transcatheter Ventricular Septal Defect Closure

There are mainly 3 devices in use currently for transcatheter VSD closure—the Amplatzer Muscular VSD Occluder, the Amplatzer Membranous VSD Occluder, and the Amplatzer Post Infarction Muscular VSD Occluder (St. Jude Medical) (**Figure 32-3**). The latter two are not approved for use in the United States. The Amplatzer Muscular VSD Occluder is a self-expandable, symmetrical double-disk device made from a Nitinol wire mesh, with a connecting 7-mm long waist with a diameter corresponding to the size of the VSD. The available waist diameters (and hence device sizes) range from 4 to 18 mm, in 2-mm increments. The delivery sheaths range from 6 Fr to 9 Fr in diameter, depending on device diameter. The Amplatzer Membranous VSD Occluder consists of two disks with a 1.5-mm-long waist. The left-sided disk is asymmetrical, with the aortic end being 0.5 mm larger than the waist and the ventricular end 5.5 mm larger than the waist. The ventricular side of the left-sided disk has a platinum marker to guide proper device deployment. The screw on the right-sided disk has a flat part that should align with the flat part on the capsule of the delivery cable to ensure proper positioning such that the platinum marker on the left-sided disk faces the ventricular apex. The device is available in sizes ranging from 4 to 18 mm in diameter (waist diameter) in 1-mm increments and can be delivered through 7 Fr to 9 Fr sheaths depending on size. The Amplatzer Post Infarction VSD Occluder has two symmetrical disks with a 10-mm long connecting waist, and is available in sizes ranging from 16 to 24 mm, in 2-mm increments. It can be delivered via a 9 Fr or 10 Fr sheath, depending on device size.

Contraindications for Closure (Muscular Ventricular Septal Defect)

The Amplatzer Muscular VSD Occluder is contraindicated for use in patients with defects less than 4 mm distance from the aortic, pulmonary, mitral or tricuspid valve, irreversible pulmonary hypertension, perimembranous or postinfarction VSD, active endocarditis, and in patients with contraindications to antiplatelet agents.

Procedural Details (Muscular Ventricular Septal Defect)

VSD closure is usually performed in the cardiac catheterization laboratory with general anesthesia or conscious sedation and TEE guidance (Video 32-5). The initial steps are similar to that described for ASD closure. Femoral or jugular venous and femoral arterial access is obtained. Generally, VSDs in the upper portion of the septum can be approached from the femoral vein, whereas lower/apical defects may be more amenable to closure by jugular venous approach. Heparin is administered to maintain ACT >250 seconds and a dose of intravenous antibiotic is administered prior to device deployment. Right and left heart catheterization is performed for shunt calculation and assessment of PVR. Biplane left ventriculography is performed (typically in LAO cranial projection and either straight lateral or orthogonal projection depending on VSD anatomy) to assess the location, size, and number of defects (**Figure 32-11**). TEE provides additional imaging and guides device placement. The Amplatzer Muscular VSD Occluder chosen should be up to 2 mm larger than the VSD size as assessed by TEE or angiography at end diastole. The VSD is crossed with a guidewire, usually an angled glide wire, using arterial or venous approach (superior or inferior vena cava), depending on the location of the VSD. Once the defect is crossed, the wire is advanced into the pulmonary artery, where it is snared and exteriorized via jugular venous or femoral venous approach, thus creating an arteriovenous loop. Over this exteriorized wire, the delivery sheath and dilator are advanced across the defect from the right-to-left ventricle. The delivery cable is passed through the loader and the Amplatzer Muscular VSD Occluder is attached to the tip of the delivery cable by rotating the device clockwise and rotating one eighth of a turn counterclockwise at the end.

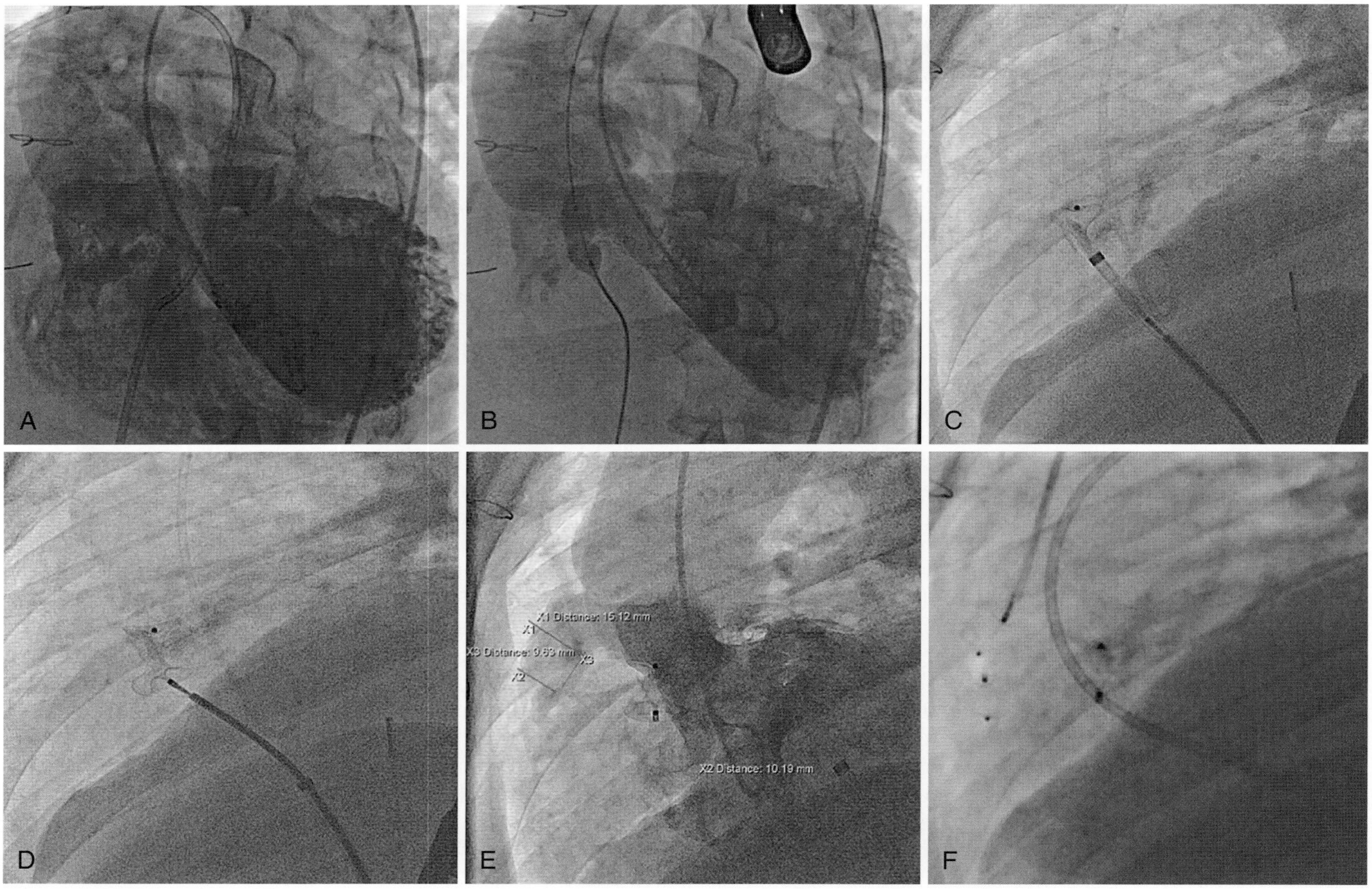

FIGURE 32-11 **Fluoroscopic images during transcatheter ventricular septal defects (VSDs) closure. A,** Left ventriculogram demonstrating VSD patch leak and subaortic VSD. **B,** Sizing balloon. **C** and **D,** Deployment of Amplatzer muscular VSD occluder. **E,** Left ventriculogram demonstrating second VSD in subaortic position. **F,** Second VSD closed with two Amplatzer vascular plugs.

The device and loader are immersed in sterile saline solution, and the device is then retracted into the loader. The dilator and guidewire are then gently removed allowing for back-bleeding to purge air from the system. The loader is then connected to the delivery sheath and advanced to the tip of the delivery sheath. Using TEE and fluoroscopy as a guide, the delivery sheath is slowly retracted to deploy the distal disk. The entire system (delivery sheath and cable) is then pulled into the defect and then the sheath is retracted to deploy the waist. After positioning is confirmed on echocardiography (and/or angiography), the sheath is then retracted further to deploy the proximal disk. Once appropriate positioning is confirmed, the device is released by rotating the delivery cable counterclockwise until it separates from the device. Echocardiography and angiography are again used to assess the device, residual shunting and additional lesions if present, and valve function.

Complications

Complications can occur during transcatheter VSD closure. The most common complications include rhythm or conduction disturbances. Complete heart block requiring permanent pacemaker implantation has been reported in 5.7% of patients undergoing percutaneous closure of perimembranous VSD closure.[93] Other rarer complications include device embolization/migration, pericardial effusion secondary to guidewire perforation, hemolysis, and valvular regurgitation due to impingement by the device. Snaring techniques can be useful for percutaneous retrieval in case of embolized device. Surgical retrieval should, however, be considered in such cases when there is risk of damaging the atrioventricular valve during percutaneous retrieval.

Clinical Trial Data

Successful VSD closure via the transcatheter route has been reported in 95% to 100% of selected patients.[94,95] In the multicenter European registry, consisting of 430 patients undergoing transcatheter VSD closure, procedural success was achieved in 95% of cases.[96] In 109 patients undergoing transcatheter perimembranous VSD closure, procedural success was 96%.[93] However, the relatively high incidence of complete high block has precluded FDA approval in the United States.

POST-MYOCARDIAL INFARCTION VENTRICULAR SEPTAL DEFECT

The incidence of post-MI VSD has decreased from 1% to 3% to about 0.2% after the advent of emergent reperfusion strategies including thrombolysis and primary percutaneous coronary intervention (PCI).[97] However, mortality among patients with post-MI VSD remains high (40% to 80%).[97,98] In the contemporary series such as GUSTO-1 (Global Utilization of Streptokinase and TPA for Occluded Coronary

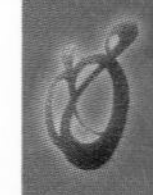

Arteries) trial, and APEX-AMI (Assessment of Pexelizumab in Acute Myocardial Infarction) trials, the median time to identification of VSD after MI was less than 24 hours.[97,99] The risk factors for post-MI VSD include advanced age, female gender, prior stroke, heart failure, and chronic kidney disease.[98,100] VSD develops after a transmural infarction of the ventricular septum with equal frequency in anterior and inferior/lateral infarctions. Anterior infarctions usually cause apical defects and inferior/lateral infarctions cause basal defects at the junction of the septum and the posterior wall. Clinical presentation can vary from stability to frank hemodynamic collapse depending on the size of the defect, presence of right ventricular infarction, ongoing RV ischemia, and stunning of the right ventricle from volume overload. Clinically, a harsh systolic murmur or a palpable thrill may be present, but this may be difficult to detect in the presence of cardiogenic shock or low output state. The diagnosis is most often made by 2D echocardiography or by the presence of step up in oxygen saturation at the ventricular level during right heart catheterization. Left ventriculography in LAO projection should be considered in a patient who continues to be in shock despite emergent revascularization in the catheterization laboratory to evaluate for shunting across the septum.

Management

Management should include prompt revascularization, afterload reduction with sodium nitroprusside and intra-aortic balloon pump insertion, and consultation for urgent surgical repair. Definitive surgery is the treatment of choice; however, it is a challenging operation with high early mortality. Surgical repair involves transinfarct ventriculotomy followed by debridement of infarcted tissue and using appropriately sized patch to avoid tension on the repair. Repair of posterior VSD is more challenging as it requires elevation of the heart for adequate exposure and the posterior descending artery and the posteromedial papillary muscle are in close proximity. In both anterior and posterior VSD, the ventriculotomy is closed primarily or with a patch.

A recent review from the STS (Society of Thoracic Surgeons) database showed an operative mortality of 43% among 2876 patients who underwent surgical repair for post-MI VSD.[101] Importantly, mortality varied depending on the timing of surgery. Patients who underwent surgery within 7 days of presentation had a mortality rate of 54.1% compared with 18.4% mortality if repair was delayed until after 7 days. This is likely due to survival bias. In the early phase, infarcted myocardium is friable and likely to hold sutures poorly, increasing the risk of tearing despite repair. Early surgery is most likely performed in the sickest patients and better outcome with delayed surgery may represent evolution of the infarct and increased stability of the tissue leading to more effective repair. Only 886 of 2876 patients (30.8%) in the STS database had surgery more than 7 days after presentation, suggesting that a minority of patients survive until elective repair. In addition, the number of patients deemed ineligible for surgery is unknown. The GUSTO-1 trial demonstrated 47% mortality at 30 days among 34 patients who underwent prompt surgical repair (median time 3.5 days) compared with 94% mortality in 35 patients who were managed without surgery.[97] Data on the use of extracorporeal membrane oxygenation (ECMO), LVAD (left ventricular assist device), or Tandem Heart as bridge to surgery or heart transplant are limited to case reports.[102-104] In the absence of large-scale data, the risks of emergent surgery must be balanced against the risk of postponing surgery in a case-by-case fashion using a multidisciplinary team approach.

Transcatheter Post-Myocardial Infarction Ventricular Septal Defect Closure

Transcatheter techniques for closure of post-MI VSD have recently evolved.[105-110] These have largely been used in patients at very high risk from surgical repair, either as definitive therapy or as a bridge to surgical repair after stabilization.

There are no specific devices for post-MI VSD closure available in the United States. Devices used for ASD and muscular VSD closure have been used for post-MI VSD closure. The Amplatzer post-MI VSD occluder is not approved in the United States (although it is available under HDE use). Several considerations are taken into account when deciding the type and size of device to be implanted. Typically, a defect <15 mm in size is considered optimal for transcatheter closure, due to device sizes available and the size of the septum. Inferior/posterior defects are very challenging for transcatheter closure, due to lack of adequate rim and proximity to the septal leaflet of the tricuspid valve. Additionally, serpiginous defects can also be technically very difficult to close. For the largest Amplatzer ASO device (38 mm), the left-sided disk diameter is 54 mm, whereas for the largest post-MI VSD occluder (24 mm), the left-sided disk diameter is 32 mm. The left-sided disk diameter for the largest (18 mm) Amplatzer Muscular VSD occluder available in the United States is 26 mm, which can be too small to fully cover post-MI VSD. The waist length ranges from 4 mm for Amplatzer ASO device to 7 mm for Amplatzer Muscular VSD occluder, and 10 mm for Amplatzer post-MI VSD occluder. The Amplatzer Cribriform device has both disks of equal diameter, with fixed short waist length and diameter, and the device size is based on disk diameter (18, 25, 30, and 35 mm). It is important to keep in mind that the necrotic rims of the VSD are often friable and the guide catheter and/or wire can tear through the septum while delivering the device. Also, a device with wide waist, such as Muscular VSD occluder or ASO device, can exert pressure on the rims and tear the borders. Due to size, the muscular VSD device may not be sufficient to close the VSD completely. Post-MI VSDs are often complex and tend to have multiple exit points in addition to a thin septum. The Amplatzer Cribriform device can be very helpful if the defects are irregular and multiple where the device is placed from the largest or most central defect (**Figure 32-12**). Incomplete release of the right-sided disk with persistent shunting has been described with Amplatzer ASO device (Cobra phenomenon).[106] Therefore, using a transseptal approach to deploy the right-sided disk first by "pushing it out" may help to prevent this complication as well as prevent tricuspid regurgitation from immobilizing the septal leaflet of tricuspid valve. As healing progresses, the VSD can sometimes enlarge in size, leading to device malapposition or embolization mainly to the right ventricle. Imaging with echocardiography (TTE, TEE, and sometimes ICE) is critical in assessing anatomic features to determine feasibility of transcatheter closure and the type and size of device to be used.

A retrograde approach from the aortic valve or a transseptal approach to cross from MV is preferable depending on the location of the defect. A soft 0.035-inch wire such as

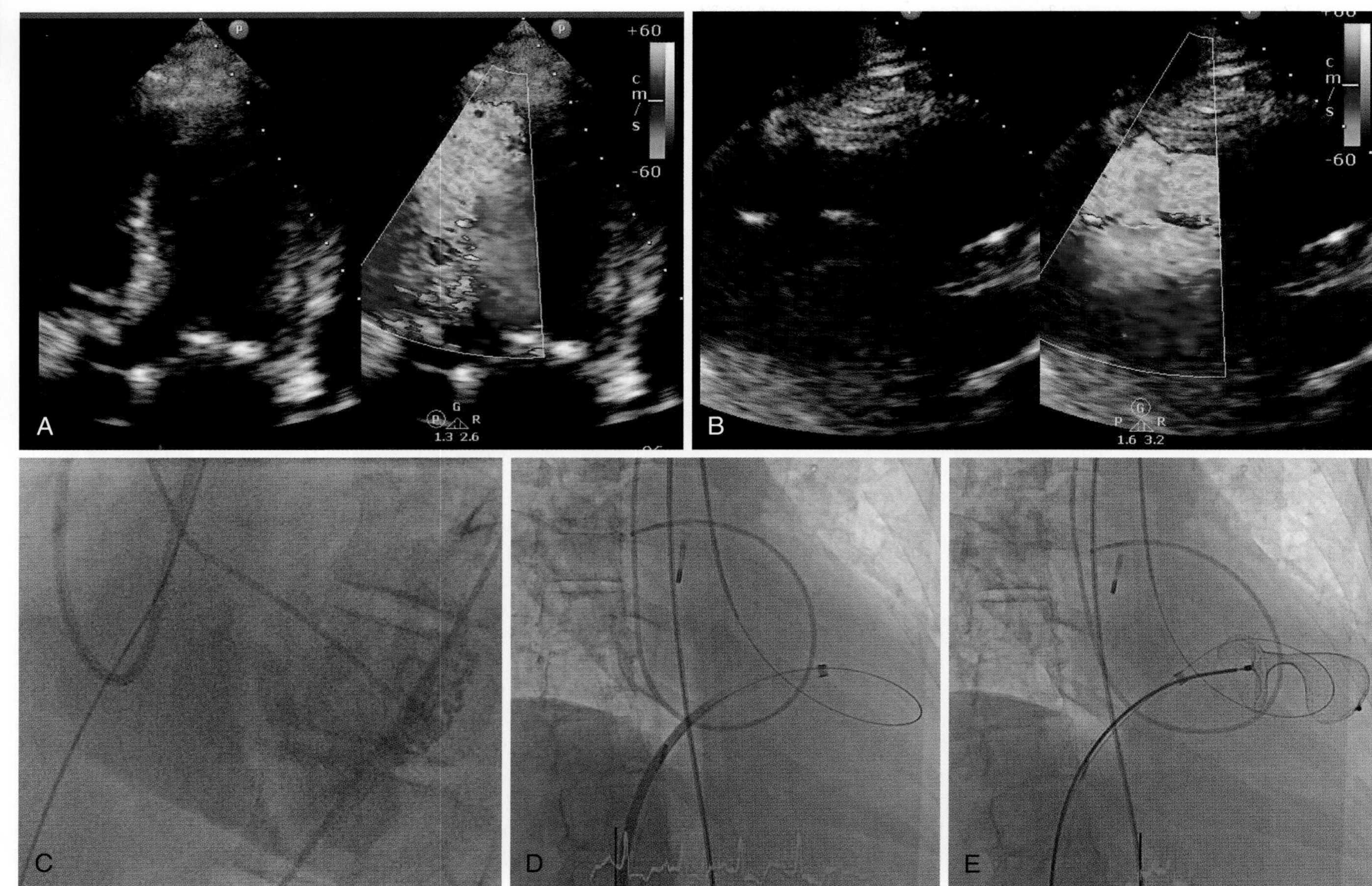

FIGURE 32-12 Transesophageal echocardiography (TEE) demonstrating apical post-myocardial infarction (MI) ventricular septal defect (VSD), and fluoroscopic images during transcatheter post-MI VSD closure using Amplatzer cribriform device. A and **B,** Four-chamber and parasternal short axis TTE demonstrating apical post-MI VSD. **C,** Left ventriculogram in LAO projection showing VSD. **D,** Creation of arteriovenous loop through the VSD. **E,** Device deployment across the VSD.

a Wholey wire is passed across the defect from LV to the RV. The wire is then snared in the pulmonary artery via jugular or femoral venous approach and externalized. We prefer the femoral venous approach. The delivery sheath can be advanced from the venous side and across the VSD into the LV from the right side, or from the LA across the VSD into the RV. The device deployment therefore can be performed from right ventricle or left ventricle. Both have advantages and disadvantages. The deployment from transseptal approach can cause hemodynamic instability from MR, whereas the "cobra phenomenon," or TR, can be potentially less likely from this approach. An alternative approach involves a hybrid procedure wherein the device can be placed under fluoroscopic guidance after an introducer is directly placed in the RA or RV after a standard thoracotomy or under direct visualization. The potential advantages of hybrid approach include direct approach, potential sparing of TV, and securing the device with additional sutures or patches. Patients are typically on cardiopulmonary bypass with arrested heart and the device is deployed with fluoroscopic guidance. This approach obviates the need for left ventriculotomy and repair compared with conventional surgery.

Case series of transcatheter closure of post-MI VSD have reported 30-day mortality ranging from 23% to 65%.[105,106,111] Transcatheter closure techniques can also be useful in cases of residual leak after primary surgical repair.

There are several challenges in managing patients with post-MI VSD. It is important to discuss in a multidisciplinary fashion (based on hemodynamic status and co-morbidities) whether or not patients are candidates for surgical repair and, if so, the timing of surgery. In stable patients with post-MI VSD, delayed elective surgery may be considered. If patients are not candidates for immediate surgery, transcatheter closure and/or supportive measures such as ECMO and percutaneous ventricular assist device should be considered. Transcatheter closure may offer an opportunity to stabilize patients who are not candidates for immediate surgical repair, although the data are currently limited. Further developments in device and delivery techniques in conjunction with multicenter studies may be needed to find optimal management strategies for patients with post-MI VSD.

CONCLUSIONS

PFO, ASD, LAA, and VSD closure are evolving rapidly as the field of structural heart intervention matures. Continued improvement in these types of devices, increased technical proficiency, and better adjunctive imaging are making these procedures safer. Ongoing studies will help refine which specific types of patients benefit most from these technologies. PFO, ASD, LAA, and VSD closure have become an important part of interventional cardiology.

References

1. Schrader R: Indication and techniques of transcatheter closure of patent foramen ovale. *J Interv Cardiol* 16:543–551, 2003.
2. Handke M, Harloff A, Olschewski M, et al: Patent foramen ovale and cryptogenic stroke in older patients. *N Engl J Med* 357:2262–2268, 2007.
3. Lechat P, Mas JL, Lascault G, et al: Prevalence of patent foramen ovale in patients with stroke. *N Engl J Med* 318:1148–1152, 1988.
4. Mas JL, Arquizan C, Lamy C, et al: Recurrent cerebrovascular events associated with patent foramen ovale, atrial septal aneurysm, or both. *N Engl J Med* 345:1740–1746, 2001.
5. Hara H, Virmani R, Ladich E, et al: Patent foramen ovale: current pathology, pathophysiology, and clinical status. *J Am Coll Cardiol* 46:1768–1776, 2005.
6. Cramer SC, Rordorf G, Maki JH, et al: Increased pelvic vein thrombi in cryptogenic stroke: results of the Paradoxical Emboli from Large Veins in Ischemic Stroke (PELVIS) study. *Stroke* 35:46–50, 2004.
7. Meacham RR, 3rd, Headley AS, Bronze MS, et al: Impending paradoxical embolism. *Arch Intern Med* 158:438–448, 1998.
8. Srivastava TN, Payment MF: Images in clinical medicine. Paradoxical embolism—thrombus in transit through a patent foramen ovale. *N Engl J Med* 337:681, 1997.
9. Meier B, Lock JE: Contemporary management of patent foramen ovale. *Circulation* 107:5–9, 2003.
10. Cabanes L, Mas JL, Cohen A, et al: Atrial septal aneurysm and patent foramen ovale as risk factors for cryptogenic stroke in patients less than 55 years of age. A study using transesophageal echocardiography. *Stroke* 24:1865–1873, 1993.
11. Lamy C, Giannesini C, Zuber M, et al: Clinical and imaging findings in cryptogenic stroke patients with and without patent foramen ovale: the PFO-ASA Study. Atrial Septal Aneurysm. *Stroke* 33:706–711, 2002.
12. Guerin P, Lambert V, Godart F, et al: Transcatheter closure of patent foramen ovale in patients with platypnea-orthodeoxia: results of a multicentric French registry. *Cardiovasc Intervent Radiol* 28:164–168, 2005.
13. Billinger M, Zbinden R, Mordasini R, et al: Patent foramen ovale closure in recreational divers: effect on decompression illness and ischaemic brain lesions during long-term follow-up. *Heart* 97:1932–1937, 2011.
14. Schwedt TJ, Demaerschalk BM, Dodick DW: Patent foramen ovale and migraine: a quantitative systematic review. *Cephalalgia* 28:531–540, 2008.
15. Wilmshurst PT, Nightingale S, Walsh KP, et al: Effect on migraine of closure of cardiac right-to-left shunts to prevent recurrence of decompression illness or stroke or for haemodynamic reasons. *Lancet* 356:1648–1651, 2000.
16. Reisman M, Christofferson RD, Jesurum J, et al: Migraine headache relief after transcatheter closure of patent foramen ovale. *J Am Coll Cardiol* 45:493–495, 2005.
17. Dowson A, Mullen MJ, Peatfield R, et al: Migraine Intervention With STARFlex Technology (MIST) trial: a prospective, multicenter, double-blind, sham-controlled trial to evaluate the effectiveness of patent foramen ovale closure with STARFlex septal repair implant to resolve refractory migraine headache. *Circulation* 117:1397–1404, 2008.
18. Vigna C, Marchese N, Inchingolo V, et al: Improvement of migraine after patent foramen ovale percutaneous closure in patients with subclinical brain lesions: a case-control study. *JACC Cardiovasc Interv* 2:107–113, 2009.
19. Rigatelli G, Dell'Avvocata F, Ronco F, et al: Primary transcatheter patent foramen ovale closure is effective in improving migraine in patients with high-risk anatomic and functional characteristics for paradoxical embolism. *JACC Cardiovasc Interv* 3:282–287, 2010.
20. Desai AJ, Fuller CJ, Jesurum JT, et al: Patent foramen ovale and cerebrovascular diseases. *Nat Clin Pract Cardiovasc Med* 3:446–455, 2006.
21. Gin KG, Huckell VF, Pollick C: Femoral vein delivery of contrast medium enhances transthoracic echocardiographic detection of patent foramen ovale. *J Am Coll Cardiol* 22:1994–2000, 1993.
22. Hamann GF, Schatzer-Klotz D, Frohlig G, et al: Femoral injection of echo contrast medium may increase the sensitivity of testing for a patent foramen ovale. *Neurology* 50:1423–1428, 1998.
23. Goel SS, Tuzcu EM, Shishehbor MH, et al: Morphology of the patent foramen ovale in asymptomatic versus symptomatic (stroke or transient ischemic attack) patients. *Am J Cardiol* 103:124–129, 2009.
24. Schneider B, Zienkiewicz T, Jansen V, et al: Diagnosis of patent foramen ovale by transesophageal echocardiography and correlation with autopsy findings. *Am J Cardiol* 77:1202–1209, 1996.
25. Monte I, Grasso S, Licciardi S, et al: Head-to-head comparison of real-time three-dimensional transthoracic echocardiography with transthoracic and transesophageal two-dimensional contrast echocardiography for the detection of patent foramen ovale. *Eur J Echocardiogr* 11:245–249, 2010.
26. Nusser T, Hoher M, Merkle N, et al: Cardiac magnetic resonance imaging and transesophageal echocardiography in patients with transcatheter closure of patent foramen ovale. *J Am Coll Cardiol* 48:322–329, 2006.
27. Hur J, Kim YJ, Lee HJ, et al: Cardiac computed tomographic angiography for detection of cardiac sources of embolism in stroke patients. *Stroke* 40:2073–2078, 2009.
28. Alsheikh-Ali AA, Thaler DE, Kent DM: Patent foramen ovale in cryptogenic stroke: incidental or pathogenic? *Stroke* 40:2349–2355, 2009.
29. Mohr JP, Thompson JL, Lazar RM, et al: A comparison of warfarin and aspirin for the prevention of recurrent ischemic stroke. *N Engl J Med* 345:1444–1451, 2001.
30. Homma S, Sacco RL, Di Tullio MR, et al: Effect of medical treatment in stroke patients with patent foramen ovale: patent foramen ovale in Cryptogenic Stroke Study. *Circulation* 105:2625–2631, 2002.
31. Agarwal S, Bajaj NS, Kumbhani DJ, et al: Meta-analysis of transcatheter closure versus medical therapy for patent foramen ovale in prevention of recurrent neurological events after presumed paradoxical embolism. *JACC Cardiovasc Interv* 5:777–789, 2012.
32. Furlan AJ, Reisman M, Massaro J, et al: Closure or medical therapy for cryptogenic stroke with patent foramen ovale. *N Engl J Med* 366:991–999, 2012.
33. Carroll JD, Saver JL, Thaler DE, et al: Closure of patent foramen ovale versus medical therapy after cryptogenic stroke. *N Engl J Med* 368:1092–1100, 2013.
34. Meier B, Kalesan B, Mattle HP, et al: Percutaneous closure of patent foramen ovale in cryptogenic embolism. *N Engl J Med* 368:1083–1091, 2013.
35. Poddar KL, Nagarajan V, Krishnaswamy A, et al: Risk of cerebrovascular events in patients with patent foramen ovale and intracardiac devices. *JACC Cardiovasc Interv* 7:1221–1226, 2014. Accepted for publication.
36. DeSimone CV, Friedman PA, Noheria A, et al: Stroke or transient ischemic attack in patients with transvenous pacemaker or defibrillator and echocardiographically detected patent foramen ovale. *Circulation* 128:1433–1441, 2013.
37. Nagarajan V, Goel SS, Kapadia SR: Is patent foramen ovale (PFO) and independent risk factor for stroke in patients with atrial fibrillation? *Circulation* 126:A18026, 2012.
38. Goel SS, Aksoy O, Tuzcu EM, et al: Embolization of patent foramen ovale closure devices: incidence, role of imaging in identification, potential causes, and management. *Tex Heart Inst J* 40:439–444, 2013.
39. Warnes CA, Williams RG, Bashore TM, et al: ACC/AHA 2008 guidelines for the management of adults with congenital heart disease: a report of the American College of Cardiology/American Heart Association Task Force on Practice Guidelines (Writing Committee to Develop Guidelines on the Management of Adults With Congenital Heart Disease). Developed in Collaboration With the American Society of Echocardiography, Heart Rhythm Society, International Society for Adult Congenital Heart Disease, Society for Cardiovascular Angiography and Interventions, and Society of Thoracic Surgeons. *J Am Coll Cardiol* 52:e143–e263, 2008.
40. Murphy JG, Gersh BJ, McGoon MD, et al: Long-term outcome after surgical repair of isolated atrial septal defect. Follow-up at 27 to 32 years. *N Engl J Med* 323:1645–1650, 1990.
41. Gatzoulis MA, Freeman MA, Siu SC, et al: Atrial arrhythmia after surgical closure of atrial septal defects in adults. *N Engl J Med* 340:839–846, 1999.
42. Amin Z: Transcatheter closure of secundum atrial septal defects. *Catheter Cardiovasc Interv* 68:778–787, 2006.
43. Kutty S, Asnes JD, Srinath G, et al: Use of a straight, side-hole delivery sheath for improved delivery of Amplatzer ASD occluder. *Catheter Cardiovasc Interv* 69:15–20, 2007.
44. Dalvi BV, Pinto RJ, Gupta A: New technique for device closure of large atrial septal defects. *Catheter Cardiovasc Interv* 64:102–107, 2005.
45. Du ZD, Hijazi ZM, Kleinman CS, et al: Comparison between transcatheter and surgical closure of secundum atrial septal defect in children and adults: results of a multicenter nonrandomized trial. *J Am Coll Cardiol* 39:1836–1844, 2002.
46. Jones TK, Latson LA, Zahn E, et al: Results of the U.S. multicenter pivotal study of the HELEX septal occluder for percutaneous closure of secundum atrial septal defects. *J Am Coll Cardiol* 49:2215–2221, 2007.
47. Amin Z, Hijazi ZM, Bass JL, et al: Erosion of Amplatzer septal occluder device after closure of secundum atrial septal defects: review of registry of complications and recommendations to minimize future risk. *Catheter Cardiovasc Interv* 63:496–502, 2004.
48. Crawford GB, Brindis RG, Krucoff MW, et al: Percutaneous atrial septal occluder devices and cardiac erosion: a review of the literature. *Catheter Cardiovasc Interv* 80:157–167, 2012.
49. El-Said HG, Moore JW: Erosion by the Amplatzer septal occluder: experienced operator opinions at odds with manufacturer recommendations? *Catheter Cardiovasc Interv* 73:925–930, 2009.
50. Levi DS, Moore JW: Embolization and retrieval of the Amplatzer septal occluder. *Catheter Cardiovasc Interv* 61:543–547, 2004.
51. DiBardino DJ, McElhinney DB, Kaza AK, et al: Analysis of the US Food and Drug Administration Manufacturer and User Facility Device Experience database for adverse events involving Amplatzer septal occluder devices and comparison with the Society of Thoracic Surgery congenital cardiac surgery database. *J Thorac Cardiovasc Surg* 137:1334–1341, 2009.
52. Masura J, Gavora P, Podnar T: Long-term outcome of transcatheter secundum-type atrial septal defect closure using Amplatzer septal occluders. *J Am Coll Cardiol* 45:505–507, 2005.
53. Fischer G, Stieh J, Uebing A, et al: Experience with transcatheter closure of secundum atrial septal defects using the Amplatzer septal occluder: a single centre study in 236 consecutive patients. *Heart* 89:199–204, 2003.
54. Butera G, Carminati M, Chessa M, et al: Percutaneous versus surgical closure of secundum atrial septal defect: comparison of early results and complications. *Am Heart J* 151:228–234, 2006.
55. Roger VL, Go AS, Lloyd-Jones DM, et al: Heart disease and stroke statistics—2011 update: a report from the American Heart Association. *Circulation* 123:e18–e209, 2011.
56. Wolf PA, Abbott RD, Kannel WB: Atrial fibrillation as an independent risk factor for stroke: the Framingham Study. *Stroke* 22:983–988, 1991.
57. Gage BF, Waterman AD, Shannon W, et al: Validation of clinical classification schemes for predicting stroke: results from the National Registry of Atrial Fibrillation. *JAMA* 285:2864–2870, 2001.
58. Go AS, Hylek EM, Chang Y, et al: Anticoagulation therapy for stroke prevention in atrial fibrillation: how well do randomized trials translate into clinical practice? *JAMA* 290:2685–2692, 2003.
59. Hart RG, Benavente O, McBride R, et al: Antithrombotic therapy to prevent stroke in patients with atrial fibrillation: a meta-analysis. *Ann Intern Med* 131:492–501, 1999.
60. Connolly S, Pogue J, Hart R, et al: Clopidogrel plus aspirin versus oral anticoagulation for atrial fibrillation in the Atrial fibrillation Clopidogrel Trial with Irbesartan for prevention of Vascular Events (ACTIVE W): a randomised controlled trial. *Lancet* 367:1903–1912, 2006.
61. Wysowski DK, Nourjah P, Swartz L: Bleeding complications with warfarin use: a prevalent adverse effect resulting in regulatory action. *Arch Intern Med* 167:1414–1419, 2007.
62. Bungard TJ, Ghali WA, Teo KK, et al: Why do patients with atrial fibrillation not receive warfarin? *Arch Intern Med* 160:41–46, 2000.
63. Connolly SJ, Ezekowitz MD, Yusuf S, et al: Dabigatran versus warfarin in patients with atrial fibrillation. *N Engl J Med* 361:1139–1151, 2009.
64. Eikelboom JW, Wallentin L, Connolly SJ, et al: Risk of bleeding with 2 doses of dabigatran compared with warfarin in older and younger patients with atrial fibrillation: an analysis of the randomized evaluation of long-term anticoagulant therapy (RE-LY) trial. *Circulation* 123:2363–2372, 2011.
65. Granger CB, Alexander JH, McMurray JJ, et al: Apixaban versus warfarin in patients with atrial fibrillation. *N Engl J Med* 365:981–992, 2011.
66. Patel MR, Mahaffey KW, Garg J, et al: Rivaroxaban versus warfarin in nonvalvular atrial fibrillation. *N Engl J Med* 365:883–891, 2011.
67. Veinot JP, Harrity PJ, Gentile F, et al: Anatomy of the normal left atrial appendage: a quantitative study of age-related changes in 500 autopsy hearts: implications for echocardiographic examination. *Circulation* 96:3112–3115, 1997.
68. Blackshear JL, Odell JA: Appendage obliteration to reduce stroke in cardiac surgical patients with atrial fibrillation. *Ann Thorac Surg* 61:755–759, 1996.
69. Gillinov AM, Pettersson G, Cosgrove DM: Stapled excision of the left atrial appendage. *J Thorac Cardiovasc Surg* 129:679–680, 2005.
70. Healey JS, Crystal E, Lamy A, et al: Left Atrial Appendage Occlusion Study (LAAOS): results of a randomized controlled pilot study of left atrial appendage occlusion during coronary bypass surgery in patients at risk for stroke. *Am Heart J* 150:288–293, 2005.
71. Kanderian AS, Gillinov AM, Pettersson GB, et al: Success of surgical left atrial appendage closure: assessment by transesophageal echocardiography. *J Am Coll Cardiol* 52:924–929, 2008.
72. Krishnaswamy A, Patel NS, Ozkan A, et al: Planning left atrial appendage occlusion using cardiac multidetector computed tomography. *Int J Cardiol* 158:313–317, 2012.
73. Sievert H, Lesh MD, Trepels T, et al: Percutaneous left atrial appendage transcatheter occlusion to prevent stroke in high-risk patients with atrial fibrillation: early clinical experience. *Circulation* 105:1887–1889, 2002.
74. Ostermayer SH, Reisman M, Kramer PH, et al: Percutaneous left atrial appendage transcatheter occlusion (PLAATO system) to prevent stroke in high-risk patients with non-rheumatic atrial fibrillation: results from the international multi-center feasibility trials. *J Am Coll Cardiol* 46:9–14, 2005.
75. Block PC, Burstein S, Casale PN, et al: Percutaneous left atrial appendage occlusion for patients in atrial fibrillation suboptimal for warfarin therapy: 5-year results of the PLAATO (Percutaneous Left Atrial Appendage Transcatheter Occlusion) Study. *JACC Cardiovasc Interv* 2:594–600, 2009.
76. Holmes DR, Reddy VY, Turi ZG, et al: Percutaneous closure of the left atrial appendage versus warfarin therapy for prevention of stroke in patients with atrial fibrillation: a randomised non-inferiority trial. *Lancet* 374:534–542, 2009.
77. Reddy VY, Holmes D, Doshi SK, et al: Safety of percutaneous left atrial appendage closure: results from the Watchman Left Atrial Appendage System for Embolic Protection in Patients with AF (PROTECT AF) clinical trial and the Continued Access Registry. *Circulation* 123:417–424, 2011.
78. Reddy VY, Mobius-Winkler S, Miller MA, et al: Left atrial appendage closure with the Watchman device in patients with a contraindication for oral anticoagulation: the ASAP study (ASA Plavix Feasibility Study With Watchman Left Atrial Appendage Closure Technology). *J Am Coll Cardiol* 61:2551–2556, 2013.

79. Rodes-Cabau J, Champagne J, Bernier M: Transcatheter closure of the left atrial appendage: initial experience with the Amplatzer cardiac plug device. *Catheter Cardiovasc Interv* 76:186–192, 2010.
80. Park JW, Bethencourt A, Sievert H, et al: Left atrial appendage closure with Amplatzer cardiac plug in atrial fibrillation: initial European experience. *Catheter Cardiovasc Interv* 77:700–706, 2011.
81. Nietlispach F, Gloekler S, Krause R, et al: Amplatzer left atrial appendage occlusion: single center 10-year experience. *Catheter Cardiovasc Interv* 82:283–289, 2013.
82. Kefer J, Vermeersch P, Budts W, et al: Transcatheter left atrial appendage closure for stroke prevention in atrial fibrillation with Amplatzer cardiac plug: the Belgian Registry. *Acta Cardiol* 68:551–558, 2013.
83. Meerkin D, Butnaru A, Dratva D, et al: Early safety of the Amplatzer Cardiac Plug for left atrial appendage occlusion. *Int J Cardiol* 168:3920–3925, 2013.
84. Urena M, Rodes-Cabau J, Freixa X, et al: Percutaneous left atrial appendage closure with the AMPLATZER cardiac plug device in patients with nonvalvular atrial fibrillation and contraindications to anticoagulation therapy. *J Am Coll Cardiol* 62:96–102, 2013.
85. Bartus K, Han FT, Bednarek J, et al: Percutaneous left atrial appendage suture ligation using the LARIAT device in patients with atrial fibrillation: initial clinical experience. *J Am Coll Cardiol* 62:108–118, 2013.
86. Massumi A, Chelu MG, Nazeri A, et al: Initial experience with a novel percutaneous left atrial appendage exclusion device in patients with atrial fibrillation, increased stroke risk, and contraindications to anticoagulation. *Am J Cardiol* 111:869–873, 2013.
87. Stone D, Byrne T, Pershad A: Early results with the LARIAT device for left atrial appendage exclusion in patients with atrial fibrillation at high risk for stroke and anticoagulation. *Catheter Cardiovasc Interv* 2013.
88. Hoffman JI, Kaplan S: The incidence of congenital heart disease. *J Am Coll Cardiol* 39:1890–1900, 2002.
89. Gersony WM, Hayes CJ, Driscoll DJ, et al: Bacterial endocarditis in patients with aortic stenosis, pulmonary stenosis, or ventricular septal defect. *Circulation* 87:I121–I126, 1993.
90. Ellis JH, Moodie DS, Sterba R, et al: Ventricular septal defect in the adult: natural and unnatural history. *Am Heart J* 114:115–120, 1987.
91. Otterstad JE, Erikssen J, Froysaker T, et al: Long term results after operative treatment of isolated ventricular septal defect in adolescents and adults. *Acta Med Scand Suppl* 708:1–39, 1986.
92. Kidd L, Driscoll DJ, Gersony WM, et al: Second natural history study of congenital heart defects. Results of treatment of patients with ventricular septal defects. *Circulation* 87:I38–I51, 1993.
93. Butera G, Carminati M, Chessa M, et al: Transcatheter closure of perimembranous ventricular septal defects: early and long-term results. *J Am Coll Cardiol* 50:1189–1195, 2007.
94. Fu YC, Bass J, Amin Z, et al: Transcatheter closure of perimembranous ventricular septal defects using the new Amplatzer membranous VSD occluder: results of the U.S. phase I trial. *J Am Coll Cardiol* 47:319–325, 2006.
95. Arora R, Trehan V, Thakur AK, et al: Transcatheter closure of congenital muscular ventricular septal defect. *J Interv Cardiol* 17:109–115, 2004.
96. Carminati M, Butera G, Chessa M, et al: Transcatheter closure of congenital ventricular septal defects: results of the European Registry. *Eur Heart J* 28:2361–2368, 2007.
97. Crenshaw BS, Granger CB, Birnbaum Y, et al: Risk factors, angiographic patterns, and outcomes in patients with ventricular septal defect complicating acute myocardial infarction. GUSTO-I (Global Utilization of Streptokinase and TPA for Occluded Coronary Arteries) Trial Investigators. *Circulation* 101:27–32, 2000.
98. Moreyra AE, Huang MS, Wilson AC, et al: Trends in incidence and mortality rates of ventricular septal rupture during acute myocardial infarction. *Am J Cardiol* 106:1095–1100, 2010.
99. French JK, Hellkamp AS, Armstrong PW, et al: Mechanical complications after percutaneous coronary intervention in ST-elevation myocardial infarction (from APEX-AMI). *Am J Cardiol* 105:59–63, 2010.
100. Menon V, Webb JG, Hillis LD, et al: Outcome and profile of ventricular septal rupture with cardiogenic shock after myocardial infarction: a report from the SHOCK Trial Registry. SHould we emergently revascularize Occluded Coronaries in cardiogenic shocK? *J Am Coll Cardiol* 36:1110–1116, 2000.
101. Arnaoutakis GJ, Zhao Y, George TJ, et al: Surgical repair of ventricular septal defect after myocardial infarction: outcomes from the Society of Thoracic Surgeons National Database. *Ann Thorac Surg* 94:436–443, discussion 43–44, 2012.
102. Loyalka P, Cevik C, Nathan S, et al: Closure of post-myocardial infarction ventricular septal defect with use of intracardiac echocardiographic imaging and percutaneous left ventricular assistance. *Tex Heart Inst J* 39:454–456, 2012.
103. Tsai MT, Wu HY, Chan SH, et al: Extracorporeal membrane oxygenation as a bridge to definite surgery in recurrent postinfarction ventricular septal defect. *ASAIO J* 58:88–89, 2012.
104. Kar B, Gregoric ID, Basra SS, et al: The percutaneous ventricular assist device in severe refractory cardiogenic shock. *J Am Coll Cardiol* 57:688–696, 2011.
105. Assenza GE, McElhinney DB, Valente AM, et al: Transcatheter closure of post-myocardial infarction ventricular septal rupture. *Circ Cardiovasc Interv* 6:59–67, 2013.
106. Thiele H, Kaulfersch C, Daehnert I, et al: Immediate primary transcatheter closure of postinfarction ventricular septal defects. *Eur Heart J* 30:81–88, 2009.
107. Maltais S, Ibrahim R, Basmadjian AJ, et al: Postinfarction ventricular septal defects: towards a new treatment algorithm? *Ann Thorac Surg* 87:687–692, 2009.
108. Bialkowski J, Szkutnik M, Zembala M: Ventricular septal defect closure—importance of cardiac surgery and transcatheter intervention. *Kardiol Pol* 65:1022–1024, 2007.
109. Demkow M, Ruzyllo W, Kepka C, et al: Primary transcatheter closure of postinfarction ventricular septal defects with the Amplatzer septal occluder—immediate results and up-to 5 years follow-up. *EuroIntervention* 1:43–47, 2005.
110. Holzer R, Balzer D, Amin Z, et al: Transcatheter closure of postinfarction ventricular septal defects using the new Amplatzer muscular VSD occluder: Results of a U.S. Registry. *Catheter Cardiovasc Interv* 61:196–201, 2004.
111. Jones BM, Kapadia SR, Smedira NG, et al: Ventricular septal rupture complicating acute myocardial infarction: a contemporary review. *Eur Heart J* 35:2060–2068, 2014. Accepted for publication.

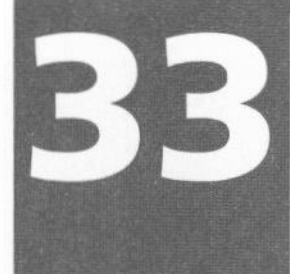

Interventions for Advanced Heart Failure

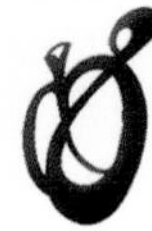

Navin K. Kapur and Marwan F. Jumean

INTRODUCTION

Heart disease remains the number one cause of mortality in the United States. Over the past 50 years, pharmacologic advancements for cardiovascular risk factors and device innovation for the management of coronary disease including acute myocardial infarction (AMI) have radically changed the landscape of heart disease. No longer is AMI considered a terminal event as in-hospital mortality rates have been reduced to less than 10% and more individuals are now surviving their incident and subsequent heart attacks. However, with each myocardial insult, nearly 25% of individuals develop chronic heart failure after an AMI leading to a growing number of patients with heart failure entering the catheterization laboratory (cath lab).[1,2]

An estimated 2.6% of the total American population and nearly 11% of the elderly population over age 80 suffer from heart failure, which is defined as "a syndrome caused by cardiac dysfunction, generally resulting from myocardial muscle dysfunction or loss and characterized by either LV (left ventricle) dilation or hypertrophy or both."[3] Of the 10.5 million emergency department visits for acute heart failure each year, nearly 50% occur in patients with preserved systolic function. By 2030, more than 8 million people in the United States (1 in every 33) will be diagnosed with heart failure. Direct and indirect costs for heart failure are projected to increase from $31 billion in 2012 to $70 billion in 2030.[4] The increasing population of individuals with heart failure has also increased the number of coronary and noncoronary procedures being performed in patients with high-risk features including advanced age, low ejection fraction, renal insufficiency, and decompensated hemodynamics. The approach to this high-risk interventional population now requires a better understanding of their heart failure status. There exists a growing demand for operators trained in invasive hemodynamics who can interface with a heart failure/mechanical support/cardiac transplant program and who have experience with emerging cutting-edge techniques for the management of advanced heart failure.

DEFINING ADVANCED HEART FAILURE

Symptoms of heart failure may occur secondary to disease of the myocardium, endocardium, pericardium, cardiac valves, systemic vasculature, and metabolic or neurohormonal stress. Several classification systems for heart failure exist. First, heart failure can be broadly categorized as being associated with reduced (HFrEF) or preserved (HFpEF) left ventricular ejection. HFrEF is defined as symptoms of heart failure in patients with a left ventricular ejection fraction (LVEF) ≤40%. HFpEF may be further categorized as diastolic heart failure (LVEF >50%), borderline HFpEF (LVEF 41% to 49%), or improved HFpEF (prior HFrEF). Second, the New York Heart Association (NYHA) functional classification categorizes patients based on symptom severity (**Table 33-1**). Third, the American College of Cardiology and the American Heart Association have defined progressive stages of heart failure with specific goals and strategies to facilitate management at each level of heart failure (**Table 33-1**). Fourth, the term "advanced heart failure" is often reserved for Stage D patients who exhibit symptoms refractory to guideline-based management strategies. The European Society of Cardiology has defined advanced heart failure using several criteria (**Table 33-2**). For Stage D patients being considered for surgical ventricular assist devices the Interagency for Mechanically Assisted Circulatory Support

Dr. Kapur has received preclinical research support from Heartware Inc. and Cardiac-Assist Inc. and has worked as a speaker and consultant for Maquet and Thoratec Inc.

TABLE 33-1 Heart Failure Definition, Stages, and New York Heart Association Classification

		HEART FAILURE DEFINITION	LVEF %	DESCRIPTION
Heart failure definition based on ejection fraction		**(HF*r*EF)HF*p*EF** **HF*p*EF, *borderline***	≤40 ≥50 41-49	Referred to as "systolic heart failure" Referred to as "diastolic heart failure"
		HF*p*EF, *improved*	>40	Outcomes appear similar to HF*p*EF patients Subset of HF*p*EF with previous HF*r*EF
ACC/AHA heart failure stages		**Stage A:** At risk for HF but without evidence of structural heart disease or HF symptoms **Stage B:** Structural heart disease but without signs or symptoms of HF **Stage C:** Structural heart disease with prior or current symptoms of HF **Stage D:** Refractory HF requiring specialized interventions		
New York Heart Association classification		**Class I:** No limitations to physical activity. No symptoms of HF with ordinary activity **Class II:** Slight limitation to physical activity. Symptoms of HF with ordinary activity **Class III:** Marked limitation to physical activity. Symptoms of HF with less than ordinary exertion **Class IV:** Inability to carry on any physical activity. Symptoms of HF at rest		
ESC definition of heart failure	**Diagnosis of HFrEF requires the following three conditions to be satisfied**	• Symptoms typical of HF • Signs typical of HF • Reduced LVEF		
	Diagnosis of HFpEF requires the following four conditions to be satisfied	• Symptoms typical of HF • Signs typical of HF • Normal or only mildly reduced LVEF, non-dilated LV • Relevant structural heart disease: LV hypertrophy, LA enlargement, and/or diastolic dysfunction		

HF, Heart failure; *HFrEF,* heart failure with reduced ejection fraction; *HFpEF,* heart failure with preserved ejection fraction; *LA,* left atrium; *LV,* left ventricular; *LVEF,* left ventricular ejection fraction.

TABLE 33-2 Definition of Advanced Heart Failure

Markers of advanced heart failure (ACC/AHA)	• ≥2 Hospitalizations or emergency department visits for HF in past 12 months • Persistent NYHA class IV symptoms • Progressive weight loss • Hypotension • Inability to tolerate ACE inhibitors or beta-blockers, increasing diuretic dose • Progressive decline in renal function • Progressive hyponatremia • Frequent ICD shocks

ESC definition of advanced heart failure	• Persistent NYHA class III-IV symptoms
	• ≥1 HF hospitalization in past 6 months
	• Episodes of fluid retention and/or systemic hypoperfusion at rest
	• Evidence of severe cardiac dysfunction
	  • LVEF <30%
	  • Pseudonormal or restrictive mitral inflow pattern
	  • Mean PCWP >16 mm Hg and/or CVP >12 mm Hg
	  • High BNP or NT-proBNP plasma levels
	• Impaired functional capacity
	  • Inability to exercise
	  • Peak VO_2 <12-14 mL/kg/min
	  • 6-Minute walk distance <300 m

ACE, Angiotensin converting enzyme; *BNP,* brain natriuretic peptide; *CVP,* central venous pressure; *HF,* heart failure; *ICD,* implantable cardioverter defibrillators; *LVEF,* left ventricular ejection fraction; *NT-proBNP,* N-terminal-pro-brain natriuretic peptide; *NYHA,* New York Heart Association; *PCWP,* pulmonary capillary wedge pressure.

TABLE 33-3 INTERMACS Profiles—Updated Version

INTERMACS PATIENT PROFILE	DEFINITION
Profile 1	Critical cardiogenic shock despite escalating support
Profile 2	Progressive decline despite inotropes
Profile 3	Clinically stable but inotrope dependent
Profile 4	Recurrent, not refractory, advanced heart failure
Profile 5	Exertion intolerant, comfortable at rest
Profile 6	Exertion limited, can perform mild activity
Profile 7	Advanced NYHA class III

NYHA, New York Heart Association.

(INTERMACS) has further defined distinct patient profiles for risk stratification (**Table 33-3**).[5-7]

HEMODYNAMICS OF HEART FAILURE

Nearly all approaches to treat heart failure reduce ventricular wall stress, which is defined by the law of Laplace as the product of ventricular pressure and volume (i.e., LV diameter) and is inversely related to wall thickness (**Figure 33-1**). Across all phases of heart failure progression, from an inciting event (i.e., myocardial infarction) to chronic dilated cardiomyopathy, increased left ventricular pressure and volume promotes LV wall stress. Increased wall stress, in turn, activates multiple signaling cascades that stimulate myocardial hypertrophy, fibrosis, and inflammation. Both pharmacologic and mechanical therapies for heart failure limit LV wall stress by reducing LV volume and pressure.

The hemodynamics of heart failure and the effect of therapeutic interventions can be represented in the pressure-volume (PV) domain using data derived from a conductance catheter. Each pressure-volume loop represents one cardiac cycle (**Figure 33-2**). Various pharmacologic interventions such as increasing preload with volume resuscitation, increasing afterload with vasopressors, or increasing inotropy will modulate ventricular PV relationships differently. In most cases, these interventions are adequate to stabilize hemodynamics, augment native stroke volume, and increase vital organ perfusion. However, the net effect of each of these therapies is increased LV wall stress (**Figure 33-3**), which increases myocardial oxygen demand, promotes myocardial ischemia, and can trigger ventricular arrhythmias.

In 1914, Ernest Starling extended findings from Otto Frank and defined the Frank-Starling mechanism, which describes the intrinsic ability of the heart to increase stroke volume in response to increases in LV pressure or volume. Numerous studies have confirmed these early observations and further shown that in heart failure the slope of the operating curve defined by LV pressure and volume is reduced and small changes in LV pressure or volume can lead to hypotension or pulmonary congestion (**Figure 33-4**). At each of these stages (acute heart failure, stable chronic heart failure, and decompensated heart failure/cardiogenic shock), the objectives of therapy are to improve stroke volume and reduce intracardiac volume and pressure overload, while maintaining an adequate mean arterial pressure to support end-organ tissue perfusion. For these reasons, careful timing and selection of pharmacologic therapy can impact patient outcomes. Invasive diagnostic evaluation and monitoring can guide therapy in advanced heart failure management (**Table 33-4**).

PERCUTANEOUS MECHANICAL CIRCULATORY SUPPORT

The use of surgically implanted left ventricular assist devices (LVADs) as an approach to "bridge" patients to recovery or cardiac transplantation or as "destination therapy" has

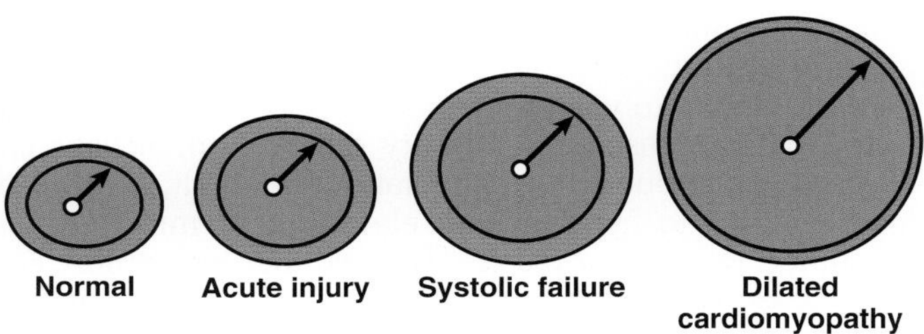

FIGURE 33-1 Hemodynamics of heart failure. Cardiac remodeling is a term that broadly refers to changes in myocardial structure and function in response to injury. Irrespective of the injurious mechanism (i.e., myocardial infarction, hypertensive heart disease, valvulopathy, myocarditis, or primary myocyte failure), a decline in ventricular function activates the sympathetic nervous system and the renin-angiotensin-aldosterone system, which increase left ventricular end-systolic (ESP) and end-diastolic pressure. Sustained neurohormonal activation promotes systolic failure and can lead to a dilated cardiomyopathy, where left ventricle end-diastolic volume (EDV) is increased. Ventricular afterload is defined as wall stress generated during systolic ejection. The law of Laplace quantifies ventricular wall stress, which can be represented as the product of ESP and EDV. *EDP,* End-diastolic pressure; *EDV,* end-diastolic volume; *ESP,* end-systolic pressure; *LV,* left ventricle.

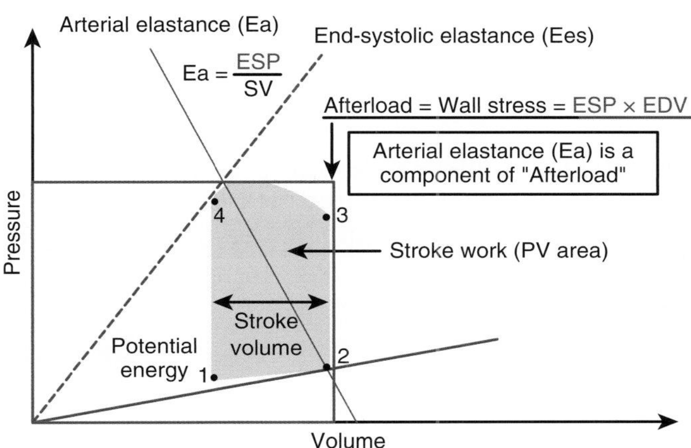

FIGURE 33-2 Cardiac hemodynamics in the pressure-volume domain. Each pressure-volume loop represents one cardiac cycle. Beginning at the end of isovolumic relaxation (Point 1), left ventricular (LV) volume increases during diastole (Phase 1 to 2). At end-diastole (Point 2), LV volume is maximal and isovolumic contraction (Phase 2 to 3) begins. At the peak of isovolumic contraction, LV pressure exceeds aortic pressure and blood begins to eject from the LV into the aorta (Point 3). During this systolic ejection phase, LV volume decreases until aortic pressure exceeds LV pressure and the aortic valve closes, which is known as the end-systolic pressure-volume point (ESPV) (Point 4). Stroke volume is represented by the width of the PV loop as the difference between end-systolic and end-diastolic volumes (Point 1—Point 2). Load-independent contractility, also known as elastance at end-systole (Ees), is defined as the maximal slope of the ESPV point under various loading conditions, known as the ESPV relationship (ESPVR). Effective arterial elastance (Ea) is defined as the ratio of end-systolic pressure and stroke volume. Under steady state conditions, optimal LV pump efficiency occurs when the ratio of Ea : Emax approaches 1 (Ref). Arterial elastance is a component of afterload, which is defined as the resistance to LV ejection throughout systole and can be represented as the product of end-systolic pressure (ESP) and end-diastolic volume (EDV). *EDV,* End-diastolic volume; *ESP,* end-systolic pressure; *LV,* left ventricle; *PV,* pressure-volume; *SV,* stroke volume.

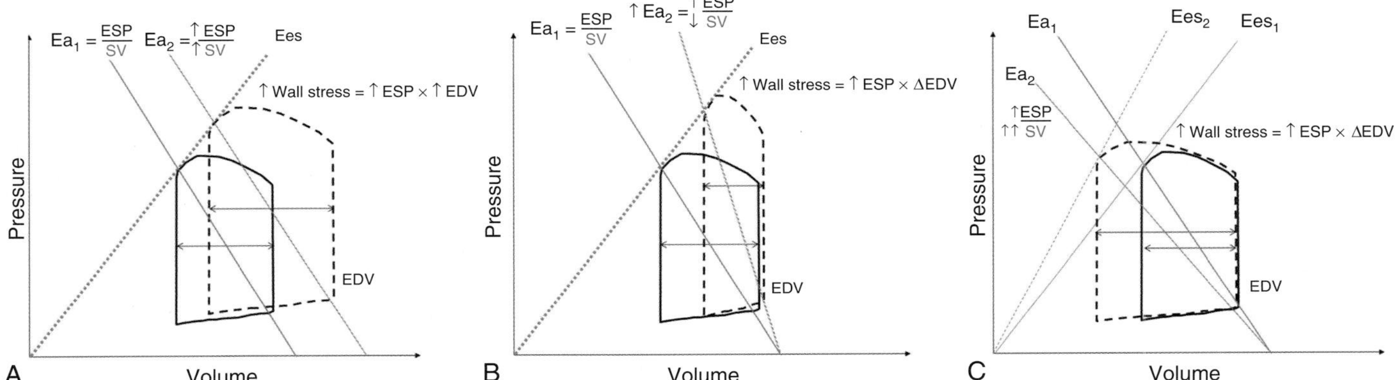

FIGURE 33-3 Impact of modulating preload, afterload, and inotropy on pressure-volume relationships in the left ventricle. A, Increasing preload augments left ventricular (LV) stroke volume (SV; *horizontal arrows*) and increases both end-systolic pressure (ESP) and end-diastolic volume (EDV) without changing elastance at end-systole (Ees) or arterial elastance (Ea). The net effect is increased LV wall stress (i.e. afterload) due to increased ESP and EDV. **B,** Vasopressors increase ESP and reduce SV without affecting EDV or Ees. Both Ea and LV wall stress are increased due to elevated ESP. **C,** Inotropes increase myocardial contractility (Ees), ESP, and SV without affecting EDV. Ea is decreased due to increased SV, but LV wall stress is increased due to increased ESP. Inotropes also increase heart rate and promote myocardial oxygen demand. Solid lines represent baseline conditions (1). Dashed lines represent modulated conditions (2).

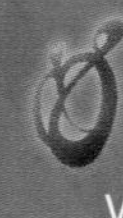

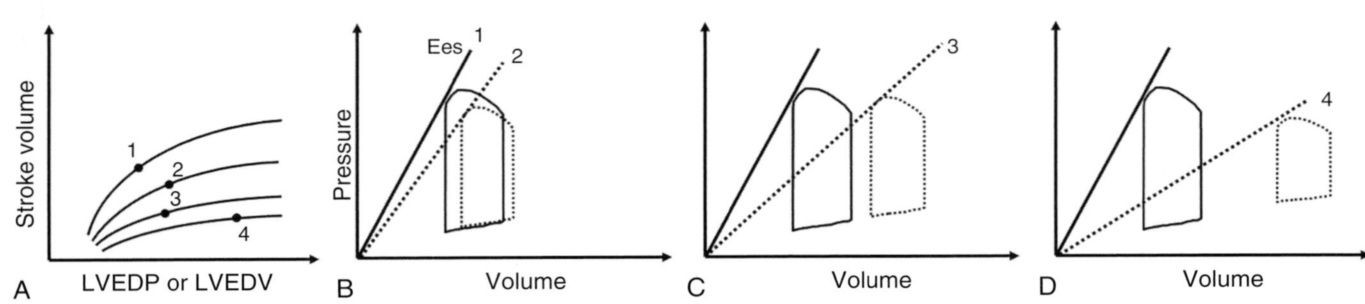

FIGURE 33-4 Hemodynamic conditions associated with stages of cardiac injury and treatment profiles. A, Frank-Starling curves represent the relationship (slope) between stroke volume (or cardiac output) and left ventricular end-diastolic pressure or end-diastolic volume (LVEDP or LVEDV). **B-D,** Pressure-volume (PV) loops represent the relationship between LV pressure and LV volume. A-D) Resting conditions are represented by Slope 1 and solid-lined PV loops. Increased LVEDP or LVEDV is associated with increased stroke volume. **B,** Acute cardiac injury reduces the Frank-Starling curve (Slope 2) and elastance at end-systole (Ees; *dashed line*) and increases end-diastolic volume and pressure. **C,** Chronic systolic heart failure is associated with a reduced Frank-Starling curve (Slope 3) and Ees. Patients with compensated systolic heart failure may demonstrate preserved stroke volume (width of the PV loop), increased LVEDV, and normal or mildly increased LVEDP. Increased LVEDP or LVEDV is associated with small increases in stroke volume. **D,** Decompensated systolic heart failure or cardiogenic shock is associated with reduced Ees and a flat Frank-Starling curve (Slope 4). In this condition, increased LVEDP or LVEDV is not associated with increased stroke volume.

TABLE 33-4 Guidelines for the Use of Pulmonary Artery Catheters in Advanced Heart Failure

RECOMMENDATIONS	COR
Monitoring with a pulmonary artery catheter should be performed in patients with respiratory distress or impaired systemic perfusion when clinical assessment is inadequate	I
Invasive hemodynamic monitoring can be useful for carefully selected patients with acute HF with persistent symptoms and/or when hemodynamics are uncertain	IIa
When ischemia may be contributing to HF, coronary arteriography is reasonable	IIa
Endomyocardial biopsy can be useful in patients with HF when a specific diagnosis is suspected that would influence therapy	IIa
Routine use of invasive hemodynamic monitoring is not recommended in normotensive patients with acute HF	III: No Benefit
Endomyocardial biopsy should not be performed in the evaluation of HF	III: Harm

Reproduced with permission from Yancy CW, Jessup M, Bozkurt B, et al: 2013 ACCF/AHA Guideline for the Management of Heart Failure: a report of the American College of Cardiology Foundation/American Heart Association Task Force on Practice Guidelines. J Am Coll Cardiol 62:e147–e239, 2013.
COR, Class of recommendation; *HF*, heart failure; *LOE*, level of evidence.

opened new opportunities for patients with advanced heart failure whose condition might otherwise have been rendered medically futile. Guidelines for the management of Stage D advanced heart failure recommend considering inotropic therapy, mechanical support, or cardiac transplantation (**Table 33-5**).[7] Nearly 2000 LVADs are implanted annually in the United States alone.[5] LVADs have evolved from large, bulky, pulsatile systems to smaller, compact, fully implantable continuous flow (CF) pumps that generate minimally pulsatile blood flow when functioning optimally. These CF-LVADs use rotodynamic pumps to transfer kinetic energy from a circulating impeller to the bloodstream, thereby generating forward flow. CF-LVADs can be divided into two categories: axial-flow and centrifugal-flow pumps. In both cases, blood is pulled into the impeller of the pump via an inlet cannula connected to the left ventricular apex and delivered to the systemic circulation via an outflow cannula connected to either the ascending or descending aorta (**Figure 33-5**; Video 33-1).

In parallel to the evolution of surgical LVADs, percutaneously delivered mechanical circulatory support (pMCS) systems have also grown from counterpulsation balloon systems to centrifugally driven circuits, or catheter-mounted axial-flow pumps. Both surgical LVADs and pMCS systems are subject to changes in preload and afterload. Inadequate LV preload due to volume depletion, poor right ventricular function, hypotension, pulmonary obstruction, or valvular disease will reduce flow generation. Similarly, increased afterload due to hypertension, elevated systemic vascular resistance, or valvular disease will reduce device flow. For these reasons, careful hemodynamic interrogation before, during, and after initiation of pMCS is essential for optimal device function.

The overall goals of pMCS systems are to: (1) increase vital organ perfusion, (2) augment coronary perfusion, and (3) reduce ventricular volume and filling pressures, thereby reducing wall stress, stroke work, and myocardial oxygen consumption. Clinical scenarios where these devices are commonly used include: cardiogenic shock, mechanical complications after AMI, high-risk coronary and noncoronary intervention, and for high-risk electrophysiologic ablations. Percutaneous circulatory support devices can be categorized by the type of pump used as either pulsatile or continuous blood flow devices. Each device impacts native ventricular function in a unique way and requires adequate preload for optimal use.

Intra-aortic Balloon Pump Counterpulsation

The intra-aortic balloon counterpulsation pump (IABP) is the most widely used MCS device with over 4 decades of clinical experience and registry data supporting its use.[8-12] The IABP is a catheter-mounted balloon that augments pulsatile blood flow by inflating during diastole, which displaces blood volume in the descending aorta and increases mean aortic pressure, thereby potentially augmenting coronary perfusion. Upon deflation, during systole, the IABP generates a pressure sink, which is filled by ejecting blood from the heart. Optimal IABP function should increase diastolic aortic pressure, reduce aortic and LV systolic pressure, increase systemic mean arterial pressure, reduce LV diastolic volume and pressure, and increase coronary perfusion pressure. The hemodynamic effect of an IABP can be directly measured using tracings obtained from the IABP

TABLE 33-5 Guidelines for the Management of Stage D, Advanced Heart Failure

RECOMMENDATIONS	COR	LOE	REFERENCES
Inotropic support			
Cardiac shock pending definitive therapy or resolution	I	C	N/A
BTT or MCS in stage D refractory to GDMT	IIa	B	647, 648
Short-term support for threatened end-organ dysfunction in hospitalized patients with stage D and severe HFrEF	IIb	B	592, 649, 650
Long-term support with continuous infusion palliative therapy in select stage D HF	IIb	B	651-653
Routine intravenous use, either continuous or intermittent, is potentially harmful in stage D HF	III: Harm	B	416, 654-659
Short-term intravenous use in hospitalized patients without evidence of shock or threatened end-organ performance is potentially harmful	III: Harm	B	592, 649, 650
MCS			
MCS is beneficial in carefully selected* patients with stage D HF in whom definitive management (e.g., cardiac transplantation) is anticipated or planned	IIa	B	660-667
Nondurable MCS is reasonable as a "bridge to recovery" or "bridge to decision" for carefully selected* patients with HF and acute profound disease	IIa	B	668-671
Durable MCS is reasonable to prolong survival for carefully selected* patients with stage D HFrEF	IIa	B	672-675
Cardiac transplantation			
Evaluation for cardiac transplantation is indicated for carefully selected patients with stage D HF despite GDMT, device, and surgical management.	I	C	680

Reproduced with permission from Yancy CW, Jessup M, Bozkurt B, et al: 2013 ACCF/AHA Guideline for the Management of Heart Failure: A Report of the American College of Cardiology Foundation/American Heart Association Task Force on Practice Guidelines. J Am Coll Cardiol 62:e147–e239, 2013.

BTT, bridge to transplantation; *GDMT,* guideline-directed medical therapy; *HF,* heart failure; *HFrEF,* heart failure with reduced ejection fraction; *MCS,* mechanical circulatory support.

*Although optimal patient selection for MCS remains an active area of investigation, general indications for referral for MCS therapy include patients with LVEF <25% and NYHA class III-I functional status despite GDMT, including, when indicated, CRT, with either high predicted 1- to 2-year mortality (eg, as suggested by markedly reduced peak oxygen consumption and clinical prognostic scores) or dependence on continuous parenteral inotropic support. Patient selection requires a multidisciplinary team of experienced advanced HF and transplantation cardiologists, cardiothoracic surgeons, nurses and ideally, social workers and palliative care clinicians.

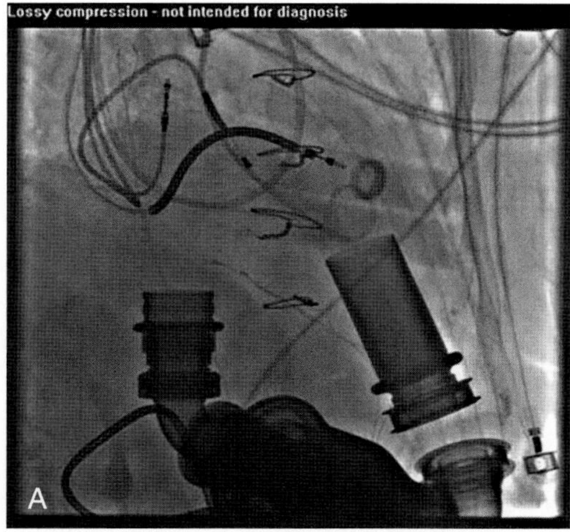

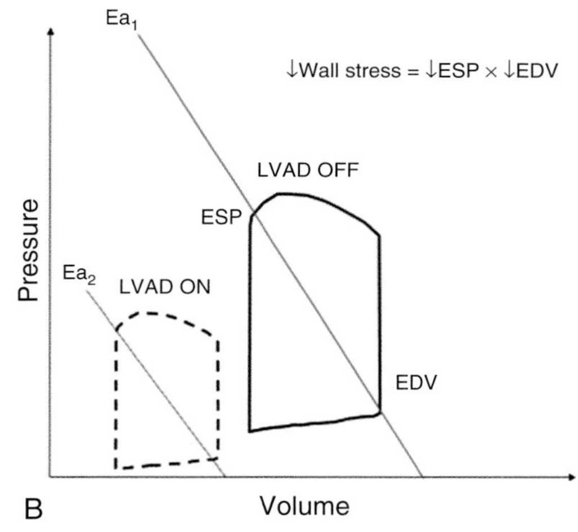

FIGURE 33-5 Hemodynamic profile of continuous flow left ventricular assist devices (CF-LVAD). A, Fluoroscopic image of a HeartMate-II CF-LVAD (Thoratec Corp., Pleasanton, Calif.). **B,** Activation of a continuous flow LVAD reduces left ventricular end-systolic pressure, end-diastolic pressure, and end-diastolic volume with no significant change in arterial elastance, but a significant reduction in wall stress. *Ea,* Arterial elastance; *EDV,* end-diastolic volume; *ESP,* end-systolic pressure; *LVAD,* left ventricular assist devices.

console to determine the magnitude of systolic unloading and diastolic augmentation (**Figure 33-6**).

The pioneering work of Kantrowitz, Weber, Janicki, Sarnoff, Schreuder, Kern, and many others have established that the hemodynamic impact of balloon counterpulsation is primarily determined by four factors: (1) the magnitude of diastolic pressure augmentation, (2) the magnitude of reduced systolic pressure, (3) the magnitude of volume displacement, and (4) the timing of balloon inflation and deflation.[11-18] IABP balloon capacity ranges from 34 cc to 50 cc. Larger capacity IABPs potentially offer better hemodynamic support than standard 40 cc IABPs.[19] In addition to balloon capacity, the hemodynamic effects of IABP are determined by frequency and timing of IABP inflation and deflation, its position in the descending aorta, shape and occlusivity, as well as biologic factors including heart rate, blood pressure, and aortic compliance.[20-23]

IABP advantages include its relative cost compared with other assist devices, ease of insertion, and widespread familiarity with its insertion technique. However, its use in the

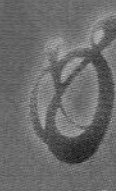

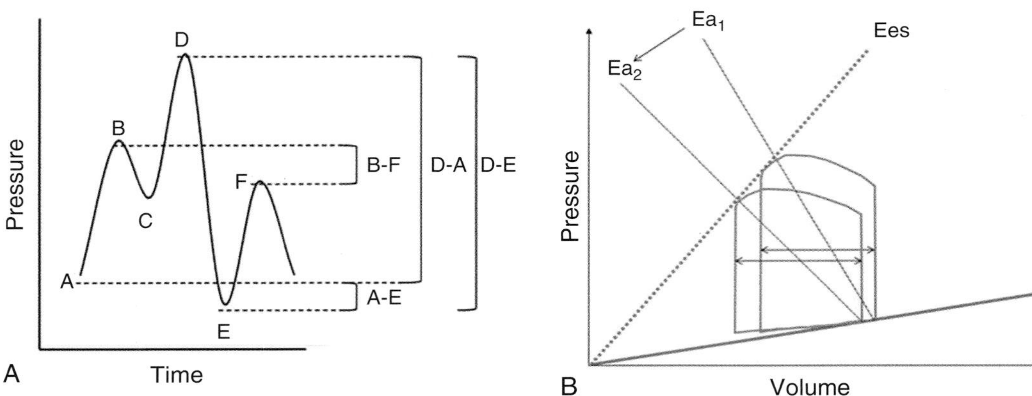

FIGURE 33-6 Hemodynamic profile of intra-aortic balloon counterpulsation pumps (IABPs). A, IABP tracings acquired at a balloon to heart beat synchronization ratio of 1 : 2 can identify nonaugmented diastolic (A) and systolic (B) pressures, dicrotic-notch pressure (C), augmented diastolic (D) pressure, reduced aortic end-diastolic pressure (E), and augmented or reduced systolic pressure (F). Systolic unloading can be calculated as the difference between nonaugmented and augmented systolic pressures (B-F). Diastolic augmentation is the difference between non-augmented and augmented diastolic pressures (D-A). Diastolic unloading can be calculated as the difference between nonaugmented diastolic pressure and reduced aortic end-diastolic pressure (A-E). The change in aortic pressure at balloon deflation (deflation pressure) is measured as the difference between augmented diastolic pressure and reduced aortic end-diastolic pressure (D-E). The slope of deflation pressure is measured as the deflation pressure divided by time. **B,** Optimal IABP function reduces left ventricular end-systolic pressure (ESP) and end-diastolic volume (EDV), while increasing stroke volume. Arterial elastance is reduced due to increased stroke volume and reduced ESP. Wall stress is reduced due to decreased ESP and EDV.

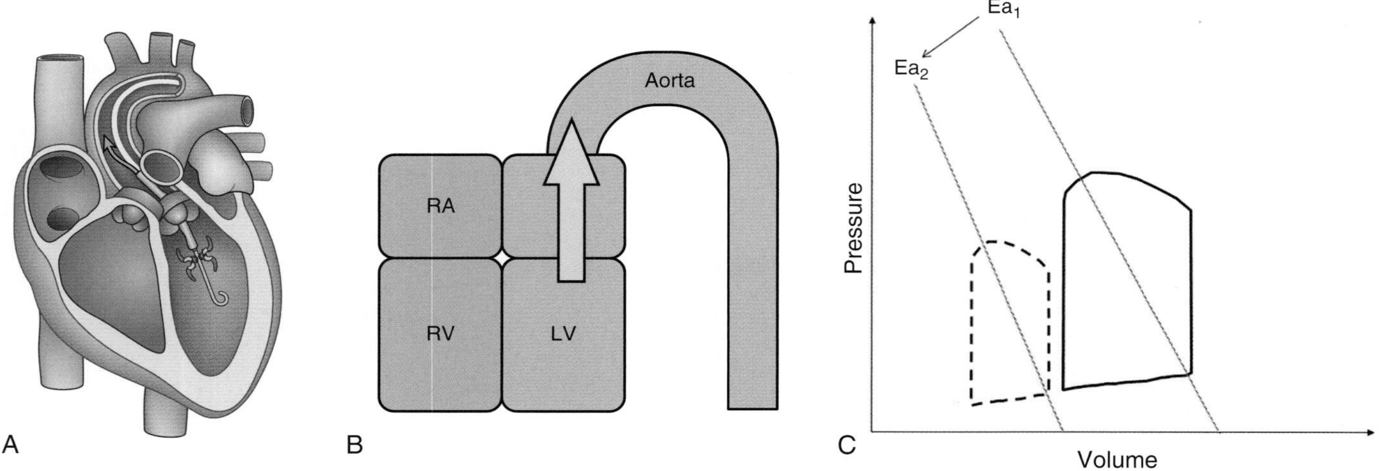

FIGURE 33-7 Hemodynamic profile of the Impella pump. A-B, The Impella pump is an intracorporeal axial-flow catheter deployed into the arterial circulation via either percutaneous or surgical access. The pump rests across the aortic valve and withdraws blood from the LV into the ascending aorta. **C,** Optimal Impella pump function reduces left ventricular ESP and EDV, while decreasing native left ventricular stroke volume by directly displacing blood from the LV. Ea is slightly increased due to reduced stroke volume; however, LV afterload or wall stress is reduced due to decreased ESP and EDV. *Ea,* Arterial elastance; *EDV,* end-diastolic volume; *ESP,* end-systolic pressure; *LV,* left ventricular; *RA,* right atrium; *RV,* right ventricular.

setting of cardiogenic shock is best when deployed early in the management of cardiogenic shock and decompensated heart failure. Major complications, including acute limb ischemia, severe bleeding, IABP failure or leak, or death directly related to IABP insertion, occurred at a frequency of 2.6% in 16,909 patient case records in the Benchmark Registry.[24] Clinician expertise, sheathless insertion, and smaller IABPs are associated with decreased incidence of vascular complications.[25,26]

Percutaneous Rotodynamic Pumps

Both the Impella (Abiomed Inc., Danvers, Massachusetts) and TandemHeart (CardiacAssist Inc., Pittsburgh, Pennsylvania) devices are rotodynamic pumps that generate continuous, minimally pulsatile blood flow when functioning optimally. The Impella devices are catheter-mounted axial-flow pumps that are placed into the left ventricle in retrograde fashion across the aortic valve. The pump transfers kinetic energy from a circulating impeller to the bloodstream, which results in continuous blood flow from the left ventricle to ascending aorta. The Impella 2.5 LP and CP devices can be deployed without the need for surgery, while the Impella 5.0 device requires surgical vascular access (**Figure 33-7**; Video 33-2; Video 33-3). At present, there is growing experience with the CP device in the United States. In contrast, the TandemHeart device is an extracorporeal centrifugal flow pump that reduces left ventricular preload by transferring oxygenated blood from the left atrium to the descending aorta via two cannulas: a transseptal inflow cannula in the left atrium and an arterial outflow cannula in the femoral artery. The net effect of these devices is to reduce native left ventricular volume and pressure, while increasing mean arterial pressure without greatly influencing ventricular afterload (**Figure 33-8**; Video 33-4; Video 33-5). An advantage of the Impella 2.5 and CP devices is ease of insertion via a single arterial access, while an

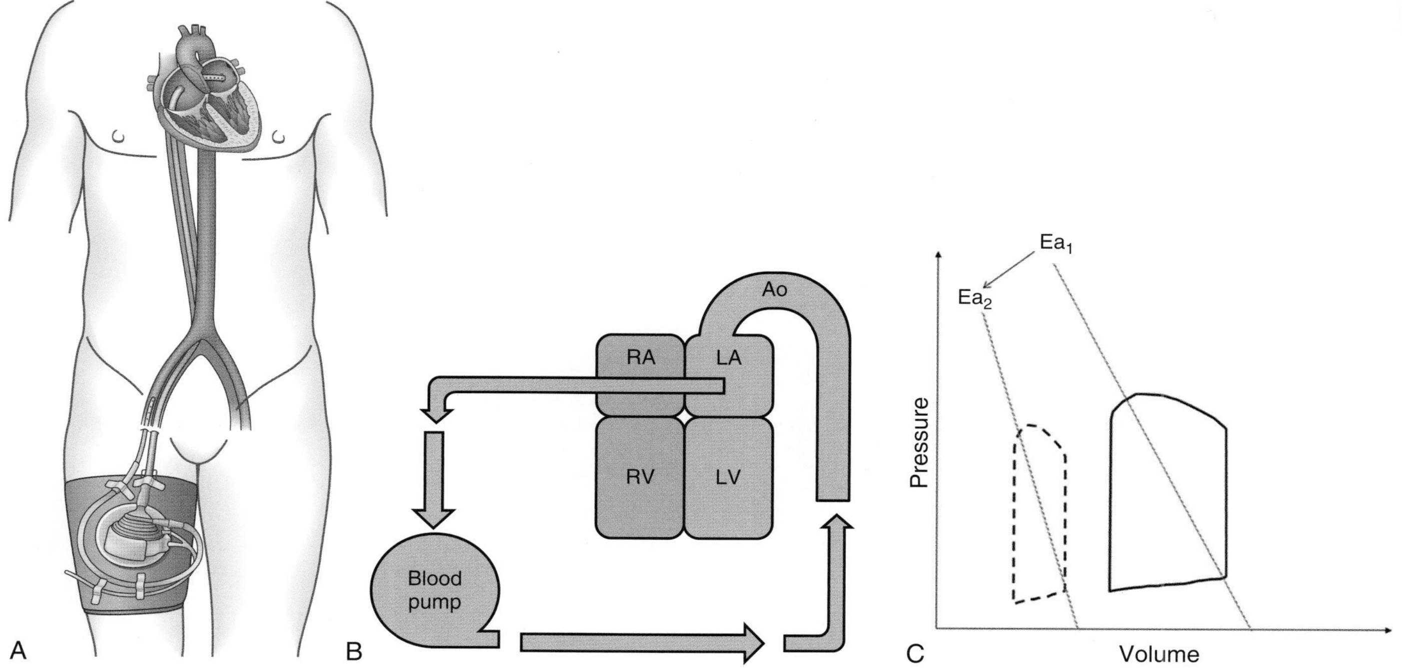

FIGURE 33-8 Hemodynamic profile of the TandemHeart pump. A and **B,** The TandemHeart pump is an extracorporeal, centrifugal-flow pump that delivers oxygenated blood from the LA via a transseptal inflow cannula into the systemic circulation via a femoral arterial outflow cannula. **C,** Optimal TandemHeart pump function reduces LV ESP and EDV, while decreasing native left ventricular stroke volume by reducing LV preload. Ea is slightly increased due to reduced stroke volume; however, LV afterload or wall stress is reduced due to decreased ESP and EDV. *Ea,* Arterial elastance; *EDV,* end-diastolic volume; *ESP,* end-systolic pressure; *LA,* left atrium; *LV,* left ventricular; *RA,* right atrium; *RV,* right ventricular.

TABLE 33-6 Advantages and Disadvantages of Percutaneous Mechanical Circulatory Support Devices

PERCUTANEOUS ASSIST DEVICE	ADVANTAGES	DISADVANTAGES
IABP	• Ease of insertion • Widespread familiarity with insertion technique • Relative cost compared with other devices • Bedside placement is feasible • Improves coronary perfusion • Anticoagulation is recommended but not required	• Moderate hemodynamic support in moderate to severe cardiogenic shock • Contraindicated in severe aortic insufficiency
Impella devices	• Provides up to 3.5 L/minute of flow (surgical 5.0 implant provides 5.0 L/minute) • Ease of insertion • Improves coronary perfusion	• Requires fluoroscopy for placement • Impella 5.0 requires surgical cutdown for placement • Requires systemic anticoagulation • Contraindicated in mechanical aortic valves or severe aortic stenosis • Contraindicated in patients with LV thrombus
TandemHeart	• Provides up to 5.0 L/minute of flow • Can be used to support left and/or right ventricles • Can be used in severe aortic insufficiency • No surgical cutdown necessary for placement • Improves coronary perfusion	• Requires fluoroscopy for placement • Transseptal puncture for LV support • Requires systemic anticoagulation
VA-ECMO	• Ease of insertion • Does not require fluoroscopy for placement • Offers complete cardiopulmonary support	• Requires systemic anticoagulation • Acute increase in LV afterload necessitating venting of the LV • Requires a perfusionist at bedside • Does not improve coronary perfusion

IABP, Intraaortic balloon pump; *LV,* left ventricular; *VA-ECMO,* venoarterial extracorporeal membrane oxygenation.

advantage of the TandemHeart device is the magnitude of support provided without the need for surgical vascular access (**Table 33-6**). No studies comparing these continuous flow devices head-to-head exist.

Other centrifugal pumps include the Centrimag (Thoratec Inc., Pleasanton, California), Rotaflow (Maquet Getinge Group, Wayne, New Jersey), and Biomedicus (Medtronic, Minneapolis, Minnesota) pumps, which are more commonly implanted surgically or used to provide flow for venoarterial extracorporeal membrane oxygenation (VA-ECMO). VA-ECMO is more commonly used to enhance systemic oxygenation during cardiorespiratory collapse or biventricular failure. The major effect of VA-ECMO is to displace blood volume from the venous to the arterial circulation. As a result, a reduction in both right and left ventricular volumes can be observed with a concomitant increase in mean arterial pressure and both LV systolic and diastolic pressures. This increase in LV afterload or wall stress occurs

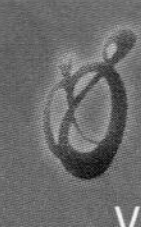

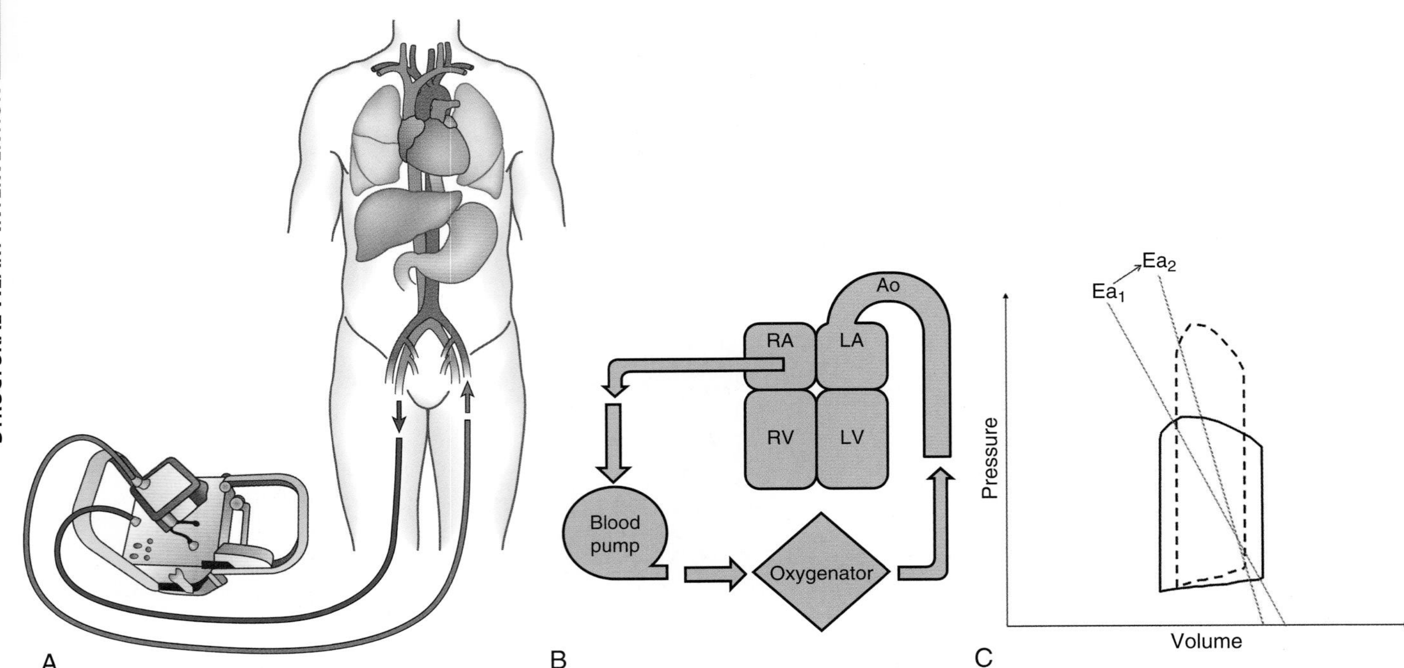

FIGURE 33-9 Hemodynamic profile of venoarterial extracorporeal membrane oxygenation. A and **B,** Venoarterial extracorporeal membrane oxygenation (VA-ECMO) is an extracorporeal, centrifugal-flow pump that delivers deoxygenated blood from the venous system via an inflow cannula through an oxygenator and into the systemic circulation via a femoral arterial outflow cannula. **C,** Optimal VA-ECMO pump function reduces LV stroke volume and increases ESP and EDP. Ea and LV afterload or wall stress are significantly increased due to increased ESP. *Ea,* Arterial elastance; *ESP,* end-systolic pressure; *LA,* left atrium; *LV,* left ventricular; *RA,* right atrium; *RV,* right ventricular.

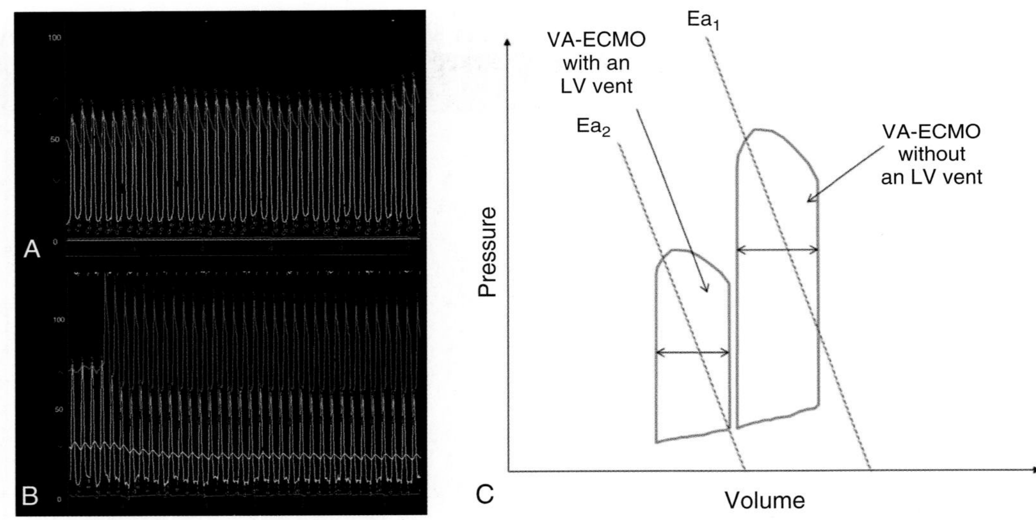

FIGURE 33-10 Hemodynamic profile of venoarterial extracorporeal membrane oxygenation with and without left ventricular venting. A, A double-lumen pigtail catheter during activation of venoarterial extracorporeal membrane oxygenation (VA-ECMO) shows increased LV systolic pressure and reduced aortic pulse pressure. **B,** Initiation of an IABP with VA-ECMO shows reduced LV systolic pressure (venting) and elevated aortic diastolic pressure. **C,** Venting of the LV with either an IABP, Impella device, or transseptal left atrial cannula during VA-ECMO support reduces LV end-systolic pressure and end-diastolic volume. *Ea,* Arterial elastance; *LV,* left ventricular.

in contrast to the Impella or TandemHeart devices since there is no direct venting of the left ventricle with VA-ECMO (**Figure 33-9**; Video 33-6). For this reason, operators have combined VA-ECMO with either an IABP, Impella device, or a transseptal left atrial cannula to negate the effect of increased left ventricular afterload during VA-ECMO support (**Figure 33-10**). Advantages of VA-ECMO include the relative ease of insertion, the ability to support systemic oxygenation or biventricular failure, and the ability to provide cardiopulmonary support during ventricular tachycardia or fibrillation (**Table 33-7**).

TABLE 33-7 Hemodynamic Effects of Percutaneous Mechanical Circulatory Support Devices

	ESP	EDV	WALL STRESS	STROKE WORK	MAP	EDP
IABP	↓	↓	↓	↓	↑	↓
Impella 5.0	↓↓	↓	↓↓	↓↓	↑↑	↓
TandemHeart	↓	↓↓	↓↓	↓↓	↑↑	↓↓
VA-ECMO	↑↑	←	↑	↑	↑↑	↓

IABP, Intraaortic balloon pump; *VA-ECMO,* venoarterial extracorporeal membrane oxygenation.

CIRCULATORY SUPPORT FOR CARDIOGENIC SHOCK AND ADVANCED HEART FAILURE

Cardiogenic shock (CS) is a major cause of global morbidity and mortality in patients diagnosed with an acute myocardial infarction (AMI). Shock from any cause is characterized by tissue hypoperfusion leading to end-organ damage. CS is defined as tissue hypoperfusion secondary to cardiac failure despite adequate circulatory volume and left ventricular filling pressure. Specifically, hemodynamic criteria for CS include: a systolic blood pressure <90 mm Hg for >30 minutes or a fall in mean arterial blood pressure greater than 30 mm Hg below baseline with a cardiac index (CI) of <1.8 L/min (m^2) without hemodynamic support or <2.2 L/min (m^2) with support and a pulmonary capillary wedge pressure (PCWP) >15 mm Hg.[27]

The incidence of CS after acute myocardial infarction has remained relatively stable over the past 30 years and ranges between 7% and 9%.[28,29] A recent evaluation of the National Registry of Myocardial Infarction (NRMI) reported that CS occurred in 8.6% of patients presenting with AMI, defined as ST-segment elevation or new left bundle branch block, between June 1995 and May 2004. In this study, only 29% of patients presented with CS upon presentation, while 71% developed CS after admission.[28] In the landmark SHould we emergently revascularize Occluded Coronary arteries for cardiogenic shocK (SHOCK) trial registry time from onset of AMI to CS was 7 hours.[30] In the Trandalopril Cardiac Evaluation (TRACE) registry, early development of CS within 48 hours of admission was associated with significantly lower 30-day mortality than patients with late-development of CS.[31]

Mortality associated with CS is high. In the SHOCK trial registry, in-hospital mortality was 60%. This finding was consistent with reported in-hospital mortality rates from the NRMI, which ranged from 60.3% in 1995 to 47.9% in 2004.[28,30] Importantly, CS can develop in both ST-elevation myocardial infarction (STEMI) and non-ST-elevation myocardial infarction (NSTEMI). The Global Use of Strategies to Open Occluded Coronary Arteries (GUSTO)-IIb trial reported CS in 4.2% of STEMI and 2.5% of NSTEMI subjects. The mean time to onset of CS after STEMI was 9.6 hours compared with 76.3 hours after NSTEMI. Despite variable times to onset, in-hospital mortality was not significantly different between the two groups.[32]

Several historic classification schemes for CS after an AMI exist including the Killip and Forrester classes. Killip classes were first defined in 1967 in an observational series of 250 patients presenting with an AMI and without cardiac arrest. Killip Class IV defines CS and was associated with a 67% 30-day mortality rate.[33] In 1977, Forrester and colleagues expanded the Killip definitions to include hemodynamic parameters such as PCWP and CI.[34] Given the advances in treatment for AMI and the increasing number of patients with heart failure, more commonly applied classification systems for the use of MCS include the New York Heart Association Class and Interagency Registry for Mechanically Assisted Circulatory Support (INTERMACS) Class.[5] No predictive tools or classification schemes to identify candidates for percutaneous MCS in advanced heart failure or cardiogenic shock exist.

Clinical trials examining the clinical utility of percutaneous circulatory support devices have failed to identify reduced in-hospital mortality in high risk PCI or cardiogenic shock. No large randomized studies examining the utility of any percutaneous MCS device in advanced heart failure exist. Registry data have historically supported the use of IABPs[9,35,36]; however, recent studies attempting to identify optimal candidates for IABP support in high-risk PCI, acute MI, or cardiogenic shock have shown no significant benefit associated with elective IABP insertion. The Counterpulsation Reduces Infarct Size Acute Myocardial Infarction (CRISP-AMI) trial showed that IABP implantation immediately prior to revascularization for an anterior STEMI does not reduce infarct size or improve short-term survival.[37] The IABP-SHOCK II study suggested that not all patients presenting with an ACS with marginal blood pressures and clinical evidence of hypoperfusion benefit from IABP activation.[38] In HR-PCI patients, the prospective, randomized clinical trial of hemodynamic support with Impella 2.5 versus intra-aortic balloon pump in patients undergoing high-risk percutaneous coronary intervention (PROTECT II) showed no difference in major adverse cardiovascular events between IABP and the Impella 2.5 axial-flow catheter.[39] The Balloon Pump Assisted Coronary Intervention Study (BCIS)-1 also showed no reduction in short-term mortality with IABP insertion prior to HR-PCI; however, follow-up data suggested a possible long-term benefit up to five years after PCI.[40,41]

For the Impella device, the recently published PROTECT II study was terminated early due to a determination of futility. No difference in major adverse cardiovascular events was observed between IABP and Impella 2.5 for patients undergoing high-risk PCI.[39] Subsequent analysis of the PROTECT II study has generated potentially important insight into the timing of device activation for high-risk PCI and the potential benefits of multi-vessel revascularization with concomitant MCS. Further studies are required to confirm these observations. Furthermore, a meta-analysis of smaller studies evaluating these devices for cardiogenic shock showed improved hemodynamic profiles associated with the Impella, and TandemHeart devices compared with IABP, however, showed no impact on short-term mortality.[42] The use of VA-ECMO in prolonged cardiac arrest with reversible disease and severe cardiogenic shock has shown promising results in several observational studies and small case series, with survival rates ranging from 20% to 40%.[43-47]

INTERVENTIONAL THERAPY FOR RIGHT HEART FAILURE

While most clinical and preclinical science has focused on left ventricular (LV) failure, the importance of right ventricular (RV) function has become more apparent over the past few decades. Causes of RV failure can be broadly categorized into three groups: (1) direct RV myocyte injury in the setting of myocardial infarction, myocarditis, or after cardiac surgery, (2) volume overload secondary to right-sided valvular insufficiency or after placement of a left ventricular assist device (LVAD), and (3) pressure overload due to pulmonary hypertension, pulmonic valve stenosis, or a pulmonary embolus. Irrespective of the mechanism, the presence of RV dysfunction is a primary determinant of functional capacity and prognosis.

Several studies have examined the clinical importance of RV failure in the setting of an AMI. RV dysfunction as defined by echocardiography can be identified in up to 50% of patients presenting with an acute inferior wall myocardial infarction (IWMI).[48-50] Of these patients, 15% to 25%

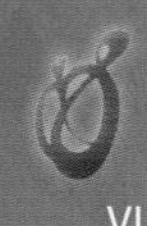

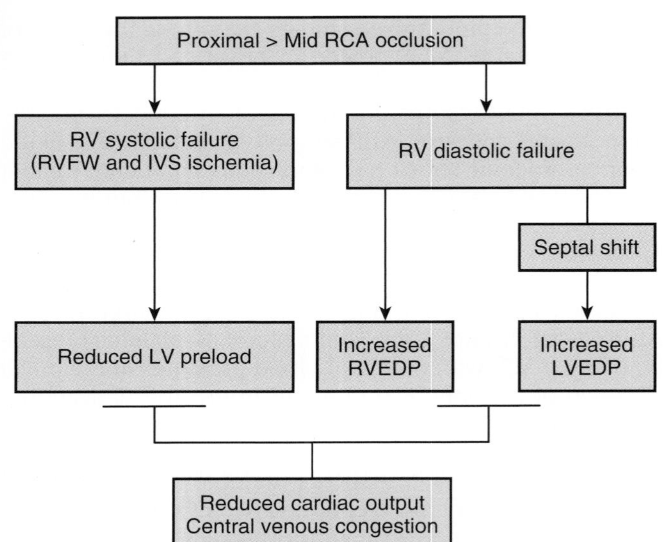

FIGURE 33-11 Pathophysiology of right ventricular myocardial infarction. *LV,* Left ventricular; *LVEDP,* left ventricular end-diastolic pressure; *RCA,* right coronary artery; *RV,* right ventricular; *RVEDP,* right ventricular end-diastolic pressure; *RVFW,* right ventricular free wall.

will exhibit hemodynamic instability suggestive of RV involvement, yet histologic infarction of the RV free wall occurs in only 3% to 5% of patients with an acute IWMI.[51] In a sub-study of the SHOCK trial, RV-dominant cardiogenic shock was associated with similar in-hospital mortality rates as LV-dominant cardiogenic shock (53.1% vs. 60.8%, p = 0.3) despite a younger age, lower rate of anterior MI, and higher likelihood of single-vessel disease among RV-dominant shock patients.[52] Furthermore, a meta-analysis of several studies showed significantly higher in-hospital mortality and higher incidence of shock, ventricular arrhythmias, and advanced atrio-ventricular block if AMI involved the RV.[53]

Acute RV failure can occur in the setting of ischemia, due to either a coronary occlusion or after open heart surgery, and can occur after direct myocyte injury secondary to myocarditis (**Figure 33-11**). In these settings, RV failure is characterized by both RV systolic and biventricular diastolic failure. More commonly after acute proximal right coronary artery (RCA) occlusion, both RV free-wall and interventricular septal ischemia reduce RV cardiac output and a subsequent reduction in LV preload.[54] RV ischemia also impairs RV diastolic function, which in combination with RV systolic failure causes RV pressure and volume overload with subsequent RV dilation.[55] After LVAD implantation, increased venous return to the RV can cause volume overload and lead to RV dilatation.[56] In the setting of primary or secondary pulmonary hypertension, increased RV afterload leads to RV hypertrophy and fibrosis, which ultimately contributes to adverse cardiac remodeling and progressive RV failure. Irrespective of the primary cause of RV failure, in the presence of an intact pericardium, RV dilation compresses the LV cavity, thereby equalizing biventricular diastolic filling pressures. The combination of RV systolic and biventricular diastolic dysfunction reduces systemic cardiac output, worsens renal and hepatic congestion, and impairs global coronary blood flow.

Contemporary management of RV failure includes reversal of the primary cause, volume resuscitation, inotropic support, and pulmonary vasodilation, which serve to maintain RV preload, enhance RV contractility, and reduce RV afterload, respectively.[57] In refractory RV failure, treatment options are limited to surgical RV assist devices (RVAD), VA-ECMO, atrial septostomy, and cardiac transplantation. Percutaneously delivered circulatory support for RV failure is an emerging field with several investigational options including the intra-aortic balloon pump (IABP), the TandemHeart centrifugal flow pump, and the axial-flow Impella RP catheter.[58] Appropriate patient-device selection, timing of device utilization, weaning parameters, and the hemodynamic impact of each device remains poorly understood and represents a new era in percutaneous therapies for the advanced heart failure patient.

Over the past three decades, mechanical support devices for right heart failure have passed through several generations of development. First-generation, surgically implanted RV pumps were pulsatile with valves located within the inflow and outflow segments.[59] Early attempts at dedicated RV support devices include pulmonary artery balloon counterpulsation (PABCP) to reduce RV afterload, which required surgical implantation and thus had limited clinical application.[60] By the early 1990s, continuous flow RVADs demonstrated better hemodynamic support and clinical outcomes compared with pulsatile devices for RVF.[61] Second- and third-generation surgical devices now include rotodynamic pumps that transfer rotational kinetic energy to the bloodstream and involve either multiple moving parts (impeller and bearings) or a single moving part (impeller), respectively.[59]

Percutaneously delivered assist devices that specifically address RV failure are relatively new. Historically, percutaneous mechanical support for RVF has been limited to the IABP. Nordhaug and colleagues performed one of the few preclinical studies examining the impact of IABP use in a model of acute RV failure caused by microembolization of the RCA. In this study, IABP activation caused a small, but statistically significant increase in systemic mean arterial pressure, total cardiac output, and biventricular stroke volume, while reducing both left and right ventricular afterload. Furthermore, a trend toward increased RCA flow was observed with IABP application. These data support the use of IABPs in the setting of acute RVMI; however, the hemodynamic impact is small and does not provide optimal RV unloading.[62]

In 2006, the first successful implantation of a percutaneously delivered RVAD in the setting of RV failure after AMI[63] using the TandemHeart centrifugal flow pump was reported (**Figure 33-12**). Since then, the TandemHeart right ventricular assist device (TH-RVAD) has been implanted for RV failure in the setting of AMI,[64] post-LVAD implantation,[65] severe pulmonary hypertension,[66] and cardiac rejection after orthotopic heart transplantation.[67] As a centrifugal pump that generates continuous flow with a minimal, low-amplitude pulsatile component, the TH-RVAD may more closely approximate native RV function and may have hemodynamic benefits over more common used surgically placed, pulsatile RVADs. Furthermore, percutaneous application of a mechanical circulatory support device provides the opportunity for early intervention in the cascade of refractory RV failure without the need for surgery.

Another mechanical option for acute RV failure is VA-ECMO, which enhances systemic oxygenation during cardio-respiratory collapse and reduces RV stroke work while

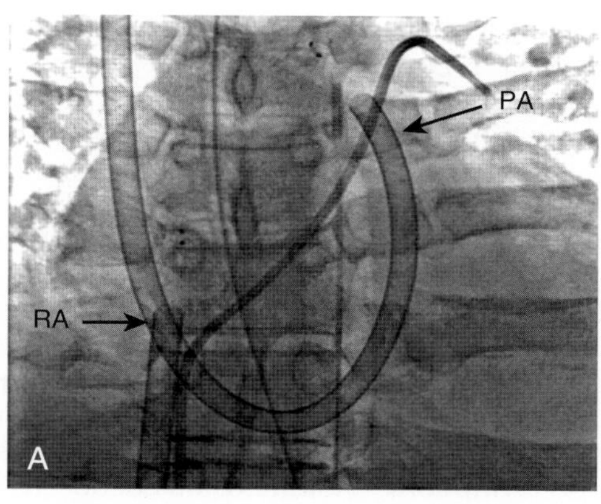

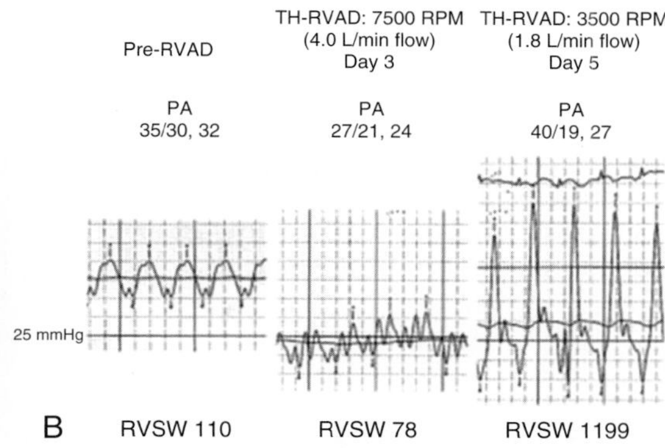

FIGURE 33-12 Hemodynamic profile of the TandemHeart pump as a right ventricular support device (TH-RVAD). A, The TandemHeart pump is an extracorporeal, centrifugal-flow pump that delivers blood from the right atrium (RA) into the pulmonary artery (PA), thereby bypassing the right ventricle (RV). **B,** PA tracings show a narrow pulse pressure and low RV stroke work (RVSW) before RVAD implantation. During TH-RVAD support, the PA pulse pressure narrows and both mean PA pressure and RVSW are reduced. After recovery of the RV, the TH-RVAD is weaned to a low flow setting, which reveals improved PA pulse pressure and RVSW.

maintaining adequate mean pulmonary pressures and LV preload. VA-ECMO is particularly beneficial in cases of biventricular failure or refractory ventricular arrhythmias.

More recently, the Impella RP (Abiomed Inc., Danvers, Massachusetts) axial-flow catheter has been developed and is currently undergoing evaluation as a support option for RV failure.[68] Whether axial- or centrifugal-flow pumps provide better support for RV failure remains unknown. The Recover Right Study is currently under way to examine the safety and feasibility of the Impella RP catheter. One potential advantage of centrifugal-flow pumps is the ability to splice an oxygenator into the circuit and thereby provide ECMO support while unloading the RV, while an advantage of the Impella RP may be the ability to deploy the device using a single venous access site.

At present, minimal data exploring the clinical utility of percutaneous RV support devices exist. Several studies have shown the potential benefits of centrifugal-flow pumps in RV failure using surgical and hybridized surgical-percutaneous deployment with the Centrimag (Thoratec Inc., Pleasanton, California)[69] and the Rotaflow (Maquet Getinge Group, Wayne, New Jersey)[70] pumps, respectively. We recently reported our single-center experience with fully percutaneous deployment of the TH-RVAD in 9 patients with medically refractory RV failure and identified that compared with preprocedural values, mean arterial pressure (57 ± 7 vs. 75 ± 19; $p < 0.05$), right atrial pressure (22 ± 3 vs. 15 ± 6; $p < 0.05$), cardiac index (1.5 ± 0.4 vs. 2.3 ± 0.5; $p < 0.05$), mixed venous oxygen saturation (40 ± 14 vs. 58 ± 4; $p < 0.05$), and right ventricular stroke work (3.4 ± 3.9 vs. 9.7 ± 6.8; $p < 0.05$) improved significantly within 24 hours of TH-RVSD implantation. In-hospital mortality among 9 patients was 44% (n = 4). Time from admission to TH-RVSD placement was lower in subjects who survived to hospital discharge (0.9 ± 0.8 vs. 4.8 ± 3.5 days; $p = 0.04$, survivors vs. nonsurvivors). In this report, no mechanical complications were observed during or after device implantation, suggesting that TH-RVSD is clinically feasible and may not be associated with excess risk.[71]

The TandemHeart in RIght VEntricular support (THRIVE) study was a retrospective, observational registry of 46 patients receiving a TH-RVAD for RV failure in eight tertiary care centers in the United States. The central finding of this report was that implantation of the TH-RVAD is clinically feasible via both surgical and percutaneous routes and is associated with acute hemodynamic improvement in RV failure across a broad variety of clinical presentations. This study also identified that evaluation of RV failure in real-world practice did not always involve quantitative measures of RV function and further does not always include comprehensive evaluation and management of concomitant left ventricular dysfunction. In-hospital mortality varied widely among different indications for mechanical RV support and was lowest among patients with RV failure in the setting of AMI or after LVAD implantation. Increased age, biventricular failure, and TIMI major bleeding were more commonly observed in patients not surviving to hospital discharge.[72]

Since the TH-RVSD provides centrifugal flow from the RA to main PA, penetration of cannulas into the heart is required to bypass a poorly functioning RV. Close monitoring for evidence of cannula migration is essential and can be prevented by marking cannula depths at the skin incision site, minimizing patient mobility, and stabilizing cannulas during patient transport. Echocardiographic and daily chest radiographs to confirm cannula position also reduce the likelihood of cannula migration. Antegrade migration into a secondary branch of the pulmonary arteries could present as hypoxic respiratory failure, hemothorax, hemoptysis, decreased cardiac output, and an acute decrease in TH-RVAD flows. Retrograde migration into the RV may result in decreased cardiac output due to tricuspid regurgitation, reduced TH-RVAD flows, or ventricular arrhythmia. While antegrade or retrograde cannula migration are possible, no institutions in the THRIVE study reported migration as a device-associated complication.[72] TIMI major bleeding was the most common complication associated with the TH-RVSD and is likely to be secondary to the need for continuous anticoagulation and sheathless deployment of the device cannulas. Bleeding is best controlled by close monitoring of anticoagulation and minimizing patient movement while on support. Mechanical complications associated with the TH-RVSD were rare and included isolated cases of injury to the main pulmonary artery (PA) during surgical deployment only and an isolated case of retroperitoneal bleed associated with peripheral venous cannulation. The development of deep venous thrombosis was reported in three cases despite required anticoagulation during device support and may be due to severe multiorgan dysfunction or partial obstruction of venous flow by cannulas in the inferior vena cava.

With the introduction of RV support options, the field of percutaneous mechanical circulatory support represents an important approach to the management of advanced heart failure and provides an opportunity to rapidly deliver univentricular or biventricular (**Figure 33-13**) mechanical support as either a bridge to definitive therapy or recovery as advances in coronary intervention, cardiac surgery, pulmonary hypertension, transplant medicine, and VAD technology provide more options for patients surviving cardiogenic shock.

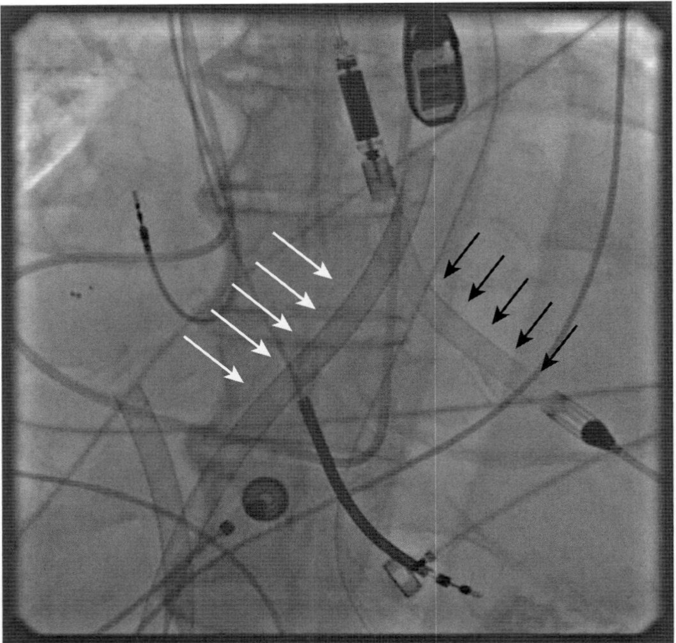

FIGURE 33-13 Percutaneous biventricular circulatory support. Fluoroscopic image showing an Impella 5.0 VAD implanted via the axillary artery across the aortic valve *(black arrows),* and a TandemHeart VAD implanted for simultaneous right ventricular support with an inflow cannula positioned in the inferior vena cava/right atrium junction and an outflow cannula in the main pulmonary artery *(white arrows).*

Emerging Percutaneous Circulatory Support Devices

Innovation in device therapy for advanced heart failure continues to push the envelope. Emerging devices for acute circulatory support include the Percutaneous Heart Pump (PHP; Thoratec Inc.), which is a catheter-mounted, self-expanding axial-flow pump that can conceptually generate up to 4.5 L/min of flow through a 13 Fr arterial access site (**Figure 33-14**). Minimally invasive device therapy is also expanding to target patients with Stage C, NYHA class III-IV, and INTERMACS profile 3 and 4 patients. Emerging device options for these chronically ill patients include the Procyrion (Texas), NuPulse (Arizona), Sunshine Heart (Minnesota), Symphony (Abiomed, Massachusetts), and CircuLite devices. The Procyrion device is an implantable, stent-based, axial-flow pump deployed in the descending aorta that is designed to reduce LV afterload. The NuPulse, Symphony, and Sunshine Heart systems are counterpulsation technologies that displace blood volume using implantable balloons, respectively. CircuLite is an implantable, hybrid, axial-centrifugal flow pump that transfers blood from the left atrium to ascending aorta.

PERCUTANEOUS CORONARY INTERVENTION (PCI) IN THE HEART FAILURE PATIENT

General guidelines for surgical and interventional management of coronary and structural heart disease in patients with advanced heart failure have been recently published (**Table 33-8**). Ischemic cardiomyopathy is the most common cause of HFrEF in developed countries. The introduction of myocardial viability assessment over the past two decades has advanced our ability to identify patients who would potentially benefit from coronary revascularization. Observational studies estimate the prevalence of myocardial viability in patients with reduced LVEF to be as high as 50% of patients, depending on the assessment modality chosen.[73,74] Several studies published prior to the STICH trial (Surgical Treatment for Ischemic Heart Failure) reported improved symptoms, functional class, and reduced mortality after

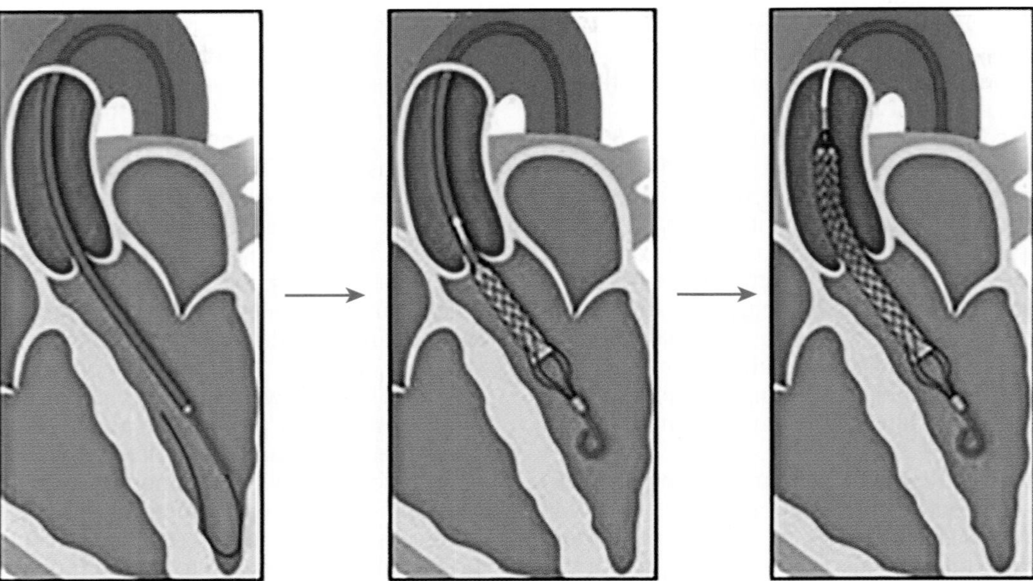

FIGURE 33-14 Emerging percutaneous circulatory support device. The percutaneous heart pump (PHP; Thoratec Inc), which is a catheter-mounted, self-expanding axial-flow pump. This device is investigational.

TABLE 33-8 Guidelines for the Management of Coronary Disease, Valvular Heart Disease, or Ventricular Dilatation in Advanced Heart Failure

RECOMMENDATIONS	COR	LOE	REFERENCES
CABG or percutaneous intervention is indicated for HF patients on GDMT with angina and suitable coronary anatomy, especially significant left main stenosis or left main equivalent	I	C	10, 12, 14, 848
CABG to improve survival is reasonable in patients with mild to moderate LV systolic dysfunction and significant multivessel CAD or proximal LAD stenosis when viable myocardium is present	IIa	B	848-850
CABG or medical therapy is reasonable to improve morbidity and mortality for patients with severe LV dysfunction (EF <35%), HF, and significant CAD	IIa	B	309, 851
Surgical aortic valve replacement is reasonable for patients with critical aortic stenosis and a predicted surgical mortality of no greater than 10%	IIa	B	852
Transcatheter aortic valve replacement is reasonable for patients with critical aortic stenosis who are deemed inoperable	IIa	B	853
CABG may be considered in patients with ischemic heart disease, severe LV systolic dysfunction, and operable coronary anatomy whether or not viable myocardium is present	IIb	B	307-309
Transcatheter mitral valve repair or mitral valve surgery for functional mitral insufficiency is of uncertain benefit	IIb	B	854-857
Surgical reverse remodeling or LV aneurysmectomy may be considered in HFrEF for specific indications, including intractable HF and ventricular arrhythmias	IIb	B	858

Reproduced with permission from Yancy CW, Jessup M, Bozkurt B, et al: 2013 ACCF/AHA Guideline for the Management of Heart Failure: a report of the American College of Cardiology Foundation/American Heart Association Task Force on Practice Guidelines. J Am Coll Cardiol 62:e147–e239, 2013.

CABG, Coronary artery bypass graft; *CAD,* coronary artery disease; *COR,* class of recommendation; *EF,* ejection fraction; *GDMT,* guideline-directed medical therapy; *HF,* heart failure; *HFrEF,* heart failure with reduced ejection fraction; *LAD,* left anterior descending; *LOE,* level of evidence; *LV,* left ventricular.

revascularization of viable myocardium.[75-78] A meta-analysis of nonrandomized studies including over 3000 patients with a mean LVEF of 32% (±8%) demonstrated a 79.6% reduction in annual mortality (16% vs. 3.2%, chi-square = 147; p <0.0001) in patients with myocardial viability demonstrated on noninvasive testing who undergo revascularization compared with medical therapy alone.[79] Furthermore, patients with viability showed a direct relationship between severity of LV dysfunction and magnitude of benefit with revascularization (p <0.001).[79] The STICH randomized controlled trial examined 1212 coronary artery disease (CAD) patients with an LVEF ≤35% treated with coronary artery bypass grafting (CABG) and optimal medical therapy (OMT) or OMT alone and reported no significant difference in death from any cause after 56 months of follow-up. However, CABG was superior to medical therapy for the secondary endpoints including death from any cause or recurrent hospitalizations.[80] In contrast to prior observational studies and meta-analyses, assessment of myocardial viability in the viability substudy of STICH did not identify patients with a differential survival benefit from CABG, as compared with OMT alone.[81] Several studies following STICH, though nonrandomized, demonstrate the usefulness of viability testing prior to revascularization and improved survival in patients with viability using newer imaging modalities such as FDG-PET and cardiac magnetic resonance imaging.[82-84]

Most patients in the studies mentioned above underwent CABG as the primary means of revascularization. Studies assessing the relative efficacy of PCI among patients with low LVEF are limited. The Bypass Angioplasty Revascularization Investigation (BARI) study reported that survival among patients with three-vessel disease and reduced LVEF (mean 41 ± 6%) was not significantly different between CABG and percutaneous balloon angioplasty (70% vs. 74%; p = 0.6). When diabetics were excluded from the analysis, survival was not significantly different between CABG and percutaneous balloon angioplasty, irrespective of LVEF.[85] Similarly, no difference in mortality was noted between CABG versus PCI in 94 patients with a mean LVEF of 25% from a post hoc analysis of 454 patients in the AWESOME randomized trial of CABG versus PCI who had medically refractory unstable or provocable ischemia after stabilization with medical therapy. Similar results were noted in patients with an LVEF <35% in the nonrandomized AWESOME registry.[86]

PCI in patients with depressed LV function is considered "high risk." Several studies have reported increased mortality, myocardial infarction, stent thrombosis, and target lesion revascularization following PCI in patients with reduced LVEF.[87-91] O'Keefe et al. reported that among 700 patients who underwent balloon angioplasty and followed longitudinally, LVEF of ≤40% was a predictor of both in-hospital mortality and survival at 5-year follow-up compared with subjects with preserved LV function (89% vs. 81%, respectively for survival; p = 0.05).[92] In addition, a stepwise increase in hospital mortality with declining pre-PCI LVEF was noted in a retrospective study of over 55,000 patients undergoing elective PCI. Compared with patients with preserved LVEF, odds ratio for in-hospital mortality was1.56 (95% confidence interval [CI], 1.06 to 2.30) for patients with an LVEF of 36% to 45%, 2.17 (95% CI, 1.42 to 3.31) in those with an LVEF of 26% to 35%, and 3.85 (95% CI, 2.46 to 6.01) for those with an LVEF ≤25 (**Figure 33-15**).[89]

Careful preprocedural planning can potentially mitigate risk associated with PCI and improve both the ability to complete the procedure and clinical outcomes. Identification of high-risk patients based on patient characteristics, coronary anatomy, and clinical presentation is crucial in estimating the likelihood of technical, procedural, and clinical success of PCI. Multiple multivariable risk models have been developed and validated over the years to estimate periprocedural risk of death and major adverse cardiac events (MACE), all of which include reduced LVEF as a risk factor.[93-98] Among 5463 procedures between 1996 and 1999 in the Mayo Clinic model, five clinical and three angiographic variables predicted the occurrence of major adverse cardiac events or death, including (in decreasing predictive

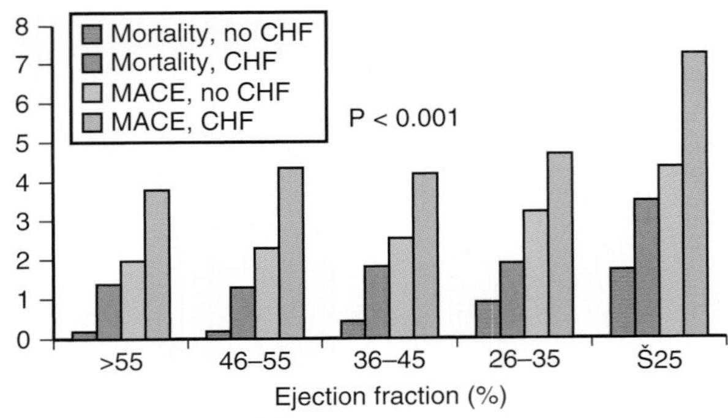

FIGURE 33-15 Hospital mortality or MACE among 55,709 patients undergoing elective PCI. Reduced left ventricular ejection fraction increases the risk of hospital mortality or MACE. *CHF,* Clinical heart failure; *MACE,* major adverse cardiac events. *(Reprinted with permission from Wallace TW, Berger JS, Wang A, et al: Impact of left ventricular dysfunction on hospital mortality among patients undergoing elective percutaneous coronary intervention. Am J Cardiol 103:355–360, 2009.)*

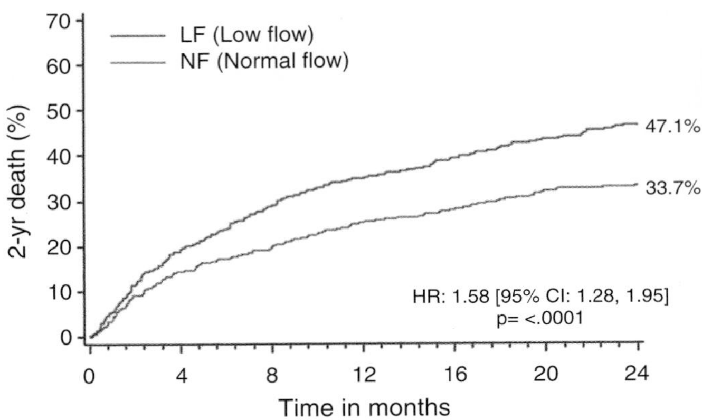

FIGURE 33-16 Kaplan-Meier all-cause mortality analysis at 2 years in patients with low flow versus normal flow. *CI,* Coincidence interval; *HR,* heart rate. *(Reused with permission from Herrmann HC, Pibarot P, Hueter I, et al: Predictors of mortality and outcomes of therapy in low-flow severe aortic stenosis: a Placement of Aortic Transcatheter Valves (PARTNER) trial analysis. Circulation 127:2316–2326, 2013.)*

power) cardiogenic shock, left main disease, renal insufficiency, urgent or emergent procedure, New York Heart Association functional class greater than or equal to three, thrombus, multi-vessel disease, and increasing age.[98] Similarly, the National Heart, Lung, and Blood Institute (NHLBI) Dynamic Registry of 4448 patients revealed seven predictive variables, with five of seven overlapping with Mayo Clinic predictors, including (in decreasing predictive power) cardiogenic shock, renal insufficiency, active heart failure, attempted total coronary occlusion, urgent or emergent procedure, number of attempted lesions, and increasing age.[96] Other models that closely approximate the accuracy of the Mayo Clinic model include the New York state model,[94] the Northern New England model,[95] and the Cleveland Clinic model.[93] A subsequent study from the Mayo Clinic that included 9035 PCIs performed on 7640 patients between 2000 and 2005 developed two risk-prediction models that successfully predicted the risk for MACE and in-hospital mortality. The model consisted of seven baseline clinical and noninvasive variables that included age, myocardial infarction (MI) within the past 24 hours, preprocedural shock, serum creatinine, LVEF, heart failure, and peripheral artery disease.[97]

Existing risk calculators fail to capture essential components of the evaluation and management of patients with advanced heart failure referred for high-risk PCI. First, many patients with advanced heart failure have established relationships with a heart failure/transplant physician and have discussed the options of cardiac transplantation, circulatory support, or palliation. A detailed discussion with the patient and family about the risks, benefits, and alternatives to PCI including the potential need for surgical or percutaneous circulatory support is required. Second, any hemodynamic instability should be addressed before PCI, including management of poor systemic perfusion, pulmonary edema, hypotension, and arrhythmias. Stabilizing patients before PCI may require intravenous diuretics, inotropes, vasopressors, vasodilators, or elective endotracheal intubation. Third, most risk calculators use LVEF as a measure of heart failure severity; however, many patients with mildly depressed LVEF (40% to 50%) may have severely deranged cardiac filling pressures depending on their loading conditions and therefore be at higher risk for impaired myocardial perfusion or pulmonary congestion during high-risk PCI. Future studies examining the role of invasive hemodynamics during high-risk PCI are required. Finally, postprocedural management of patients with advanced heart failure after PCI is equally as important as pre- and intraprocedural care. Intermittent periods of myocardial ischemia contribute to deranged hemodynamics that persist after successful coronary revascularization. For this reason, assessing hemodynamic status after PCI should be considered. If a pMCS device is used to support PCI, weaning the device to a lower support setting and monitoring hemodynamic conditions in the catheterization laboratory may identify whether a patient is stable for decannulation of the pMCS system.

VALVULAR INTERVENTIONS IN ADVANCED HEART FAILURE

Transcatheter Aortic Valve Replacement in Advanced Heart Failure

Transcatheter aortic valve replacement (TAVR) has emerged over the past several years as an alternative to conventional surgical valve replacement in patients with severe symptomatic aortic stenosis (AS) who are deemed nonsurgical candidates due to technical considerations or perceived high surgical risks.[99] Reduced LVEF is a marker of disease progression and portrays a worse outcome in patients with severe aortic stenosis.[100] Low-flow (defined as LV stroke volume index ≤35 mL/m^2), low-gradient (transvalvular pressure gradient ≤40 mm Hg) severe aortic stenosis occurs either in the setting of LV systolic dysfunction with reduced LVEF or due to reduced ventricular volumes and LV hypertrophy in preserved LVEF.[101] Careful evaluation of hemodynamic changes in response to cardiac output augmentation with pharmacologic interventions using dobutamine or nitroprusside can be used to distinguish true aortic stenosis from pseudostenosis. Of particular concern are patients with low flow but preserved LVEF, as those patients have worse survival than those with normal flow (**Figure 33-16**).[102,103]

Reduced LVEF as a predictor of worse outcomes in severe AS patients was demonstrated in some studies. In an Italian multicenter prospective study of 663 consecutive patients who underwent TAVR with the third-generation 18 Fr CoreValve device (Medtronic Inc., Minnesota), the cumulative mortality was 5.3% at 30 days and 15% at one year. In addition to major access site complications, diabetes mellitus, prior stroke, and moderate to severe paravalvular leak, reduced LVEF (<40%) was an independent predictor of mortality in this study, with an odds ratio (OR) of 3.51.[104]

Among 971 patients in the PARTNER trial, low flow was observed in 55% of patients; low flow and reduced LVEF of <50% was observed in 23%; and low flow low LVEF and low gradient was observed in 15%. The 2-year mortality was significantly higher in patients with low flow compared with those with normal flow (47% vs. 34%; HR of 1.5; 95% CI, 1.25 to 1.89; p = 0.006). Interestingly, low flow but not reduced LVEF or low gradient was an independent predictor of mortality in all patient cohorts.[105] Similarly, low flow but not low LVEF or low gradient was noted to be an independent predictor of 30-day and 2-year mortality following TAVR in 334 severe AS patients.[106]

Preprocedural planning and intraprocedural considerations should be made should hemodynamic decompensation occur. This includes assessment of hemodynamics with a right heart catheterization to avoid hypovolemia and to maintain adequate filling pressure, the use of inotropic support in those with reduced cardiac output or with pulmonary hypertension, and ensuring a mean arterial pressure of >75 mm Hg prior to initiation of rapid ventricular pacing. In patients with marginal hemodynamics and reduced LVEF, consideration should be made for direct valve deployment instead of predeployment balloon valvuloplasty to avoid multiple rapid pacing runs that can be detrimental. In addition, careful positioning of the guidewire during transapical TAVR is critical to avoid traction of the subvalvular apparatus of the mitral leading to acute mitral regurgitation. Lastly, a contingency plan should be in place in case of hemodynamic compromise, including percutaneous mechanical support and full cardiopulmonary bypass.

Percutaneous Approaches for Functional Mitral Regurgitation

In contrast to primary anatomic abnormalities causing regurgitation in degenerative mitral valve disease (DMR), functional mitral regurgitation (FMR) in patients with dilated cardiomyopathies results from altered left ventricular geometry and distortion of the normal spatial relationship of the mitral valve to its subvalvular apparatus, which includes progressive mitral annular dilation, apical, and lateral papillary muscle displacement, and tethering and tenting of the mitral valve leaflets.[107-109] Furthermore, FMR mediates further ventricular remodeling as it poses a hemodynamic load on the left ventricle, leading to progressive eccentric hypertrophy and dilation, potentially exacerbating the degree of FMR as well.[107,110,111]

Varying degrees of FMR are virtually seen in all patients with a dilated cardiomyopathy[112,113]; however, moderate to severe FMR is seen in 17% up to 50% of patients with reduced LVEF[114-116] and considered an independent predictor of 1-year mortality as demonstrated in a retrospective review of over 1200 patients with a hazard ratio of 1.85.[112] Furthermore, the presence of FMR is associated with reduced 5-year survival, reduced functional capacity, and increased heart failure exacerbations (**Figure 33-17**).[114,117-120]

Percutaneous mitral valve repair offers an attractive alternative to surgical repair in high-risk surgical candidates. Based on the Alfieri technique, which creates a double mitral orifice by means of stitching the central part of the mitral valve leaflets,[121] percutaneous mitral valve repair using the MitraClip (Abbott Vascular, Illinois) has been recently introduced in clinical practice in Europe and currently under investigational use in the United States for the management of both DMR and FMR.[122,123] The 4-mm-wide cobalt-chromium implant is delivered percutaneously and aligned over the origin of the regurgitant jet under fluoroscopic and transesophageal echocardiographic guidance.[124-126] In a subgroup analysis of 65 patients with FMR enrolled in the EVEREST II trial, there was no difference in the primary outcome at 12 months (freedom from death, mitral-valve surgery, and from grade 3+ or 4+ mitral regurgitation) in those randomized to percutaneous versus surgical repair of the mitral valve.[124] Despite suboptimal results when compared with surgical mitral valve repair, data thus far demonstrate improved overall functional capacity and degree of residual mitral regurgitation with percutaneous mitral valve repair in FMR. However, data regarding survival benefit with surgical or transcatheter repair of FMR, particularly in those patients with severe left ventricular systolic dysfunction, are still controversial. As a result, the 2013 American College of Cardiology (ACC)/American Heart Association (AHA) guidelines for surgical or percutaneous repair of FMR provide no formal recommendations; rather they indicate that such interventions on FMR should be considered on a case-by-case basis.[7]

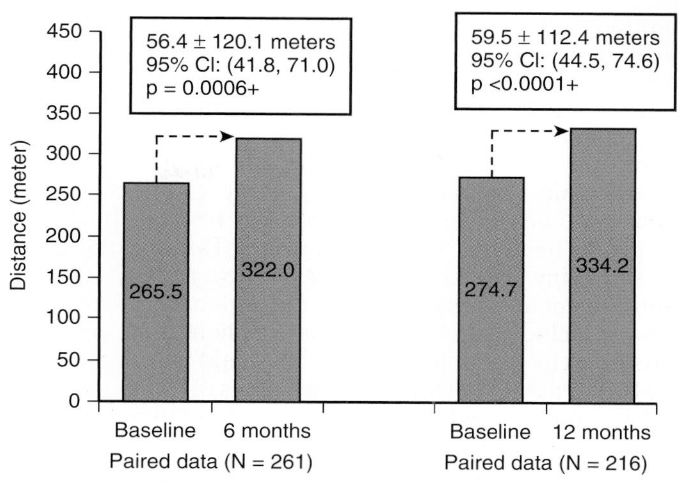

FIGURE 33-17 Changes in 6-min walk distance from baseline to 6 and 12 months in patients with functional mitral regurgitation and degenerative mitral valve disease. *(Reprinted with permission from Maisano et al., JACC 2013, license number 3372110267854.)*

EMERGING INTERVENTIONAL APPROACHES FOR HEART FAILURE

Percutaneous Ventricular Volume Reduction

As described above, all existing pharmacologic and device-based therapies are designed to reduce LV "load" by optimizing LV volume and pressure. The prognostic significance of LV volume was established in the 1980s by White and Wild who reported that a LV end-systolic volume index (LVESVI) >60 mL/m^2 is a predictor of survival after MI.[127] A more contemporary meta-analysis by Kramer and Udelson showed that remodeling indices such as end-systolic volume (ESV) and end-diastolic volume (EDV) also predict mortality after therapeutic intervention for chronic systolic heart failure.[128] Once the LVESVI exceeds 25 mL/m^2, optimal medical therapy for heart failure offers limited benefit.[129] Based on these observations, several studies examined the role of surgical ventricular restoration (SVR) therapy as an approach to reduce LV cavity size and improve outcomes in ischemic cardiomyopathy.[129] Despite extensive registry data supporting the potential benefit of SVR, the STICH (Surgical Treatment for Ischemic Heart Failure) trial failed to show any benefit of CABG + SVR over CABG alone.[115] Subsequent analysis of the STICH trial identified major limitations including: (1) enrollment of patients with relatively preserved LV ejection fraction (>35%) and no prior myocardial infarction, (2) inconsistent measures of LV volumes, and (3) few patients achieving a reduction in LVESVI >30% of preoperative values.[129]

The Parachute device (CardioKinetix Inc., California) is a percutaneously delivered LV partitioning system that is designed to reduce ESV and EDV in patients with chronic heart failure due to infarction in the territory of the left anterior descending artery. The device is comprised of three main parts: a self-expanding nitinol frame, an expandable polytetrafluoroethylene (ePTFE) membrane, and an apically positioned foot. Studies in a sheep model of chronic ischemic cardiomyopathy showed reduced LV volumes and improved mechanical LV efficiency, defined as the percentage of total mechanical energy converted to external work (**Figure 33-18**). Based on these findings, several early clinical studies have been completed. The PARACHUTE Cohort A (14 implants) and PARACHUTE US feasibility study (17 implants) showed improved hemodynamics and functional status at 12 months after implantation. Enrollment for the PARACHUTE Cohort B and postmarketing studies in the European Union (PARACHUTE III) are complete and the US pivotal trial (PARACHUTE IV) is currently under way.[130]

Interventions for Heart Failure With Preserved Ejection Fraction

Of the nearly 6 million individuals with heart failure in the United States, approximately one half have a preserved ejection fraction above 40%. Interventions for heart failure with preserved ejection fraction (HFpEF) are more common in elderly individuals (over age 70), women, and in patients with co-morbid illnesses, which include hypertension, diabetes mellitus, coronary disease, chronic renal insufficiency, and obesity.[7,131-133] Mortality due to HFpEF approximates values associated with HFrEF; however, no therapy to specifically target HFpEF exists. The lack of treatment options is likely due to the fact that mechanisms behind HFpEF remain poorly understood. Proposed cardiac mechanisms include: ischemia, excess cardiac fibrosis, dysregulated hypertrophy, cardiomyocyte stiffness, oxidative stress, and abnormal calcium handling.[132,133] In addition to primary cardiac causes, volume overload and vascular dysfunction contribute to HFpEF by promoting inefficient ventricular function.

Interventional approaches for HFpEF are emerging and may include the use of one-way valves positioned along the inter-atrial septum to off-load excess volume from the left atrium.[134] In addition, renal sympathetic denervation as an approach to limit systemic hypertension may limit the onset and progression of HFpEF.[135] Future studies are required to validate these emerging approaches.

Invasive Approaches for Patients Requiring Left Ventricular Assist Device Support

The rising use of machines to support heart function has led to increased awareness of device-associated complications. The cardiac cath lab offers a platform for invasive hemodynamic assessment to diagnose a variety of those complications in addition to an emerging number of therapeutic interventions (**Table 33-9**). An evolving field in interventional cardiology is the development of techniques to percutaneously manage some of these complications. Emerging approaches to patients with advanced heart failure being supported by LVADs include catheter-based thrombolysis for LVAD thrombosis, stenting of obstructed LVAD outflow grafts (**Figure 33-19**), coronary revascularization for active ischemia during LVAD support, percutaneous aortic valve therapy for aortic insufficiency, percutaneous

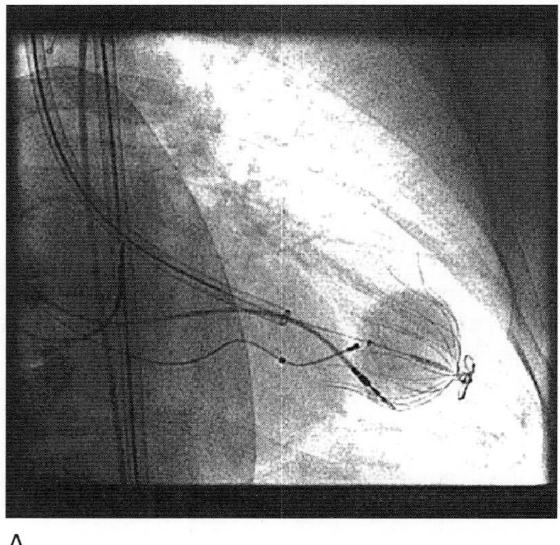

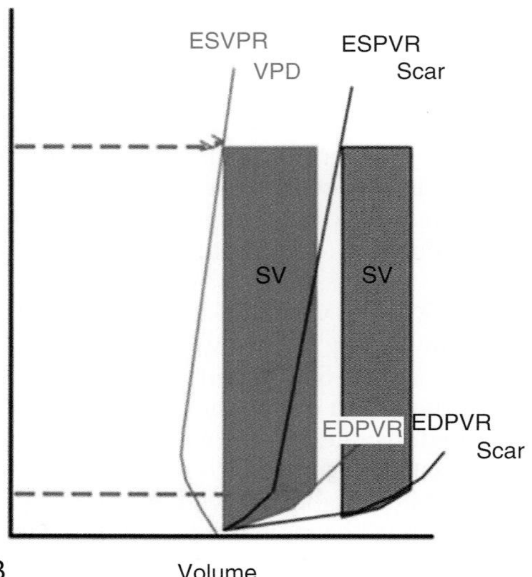

FIGURE 33-18 Percutaneous ventricular restoration. A, Fluoroscopic image of the investigational parachute device in the left ventricle. **B,** Delivery of this ventricular portioning device (VPD) is designed to reduce left ventricular volume, thereby improving the slope of end-diastolic pressure-volume relationship (EDPVR) and augmenting stroke volume (SV).

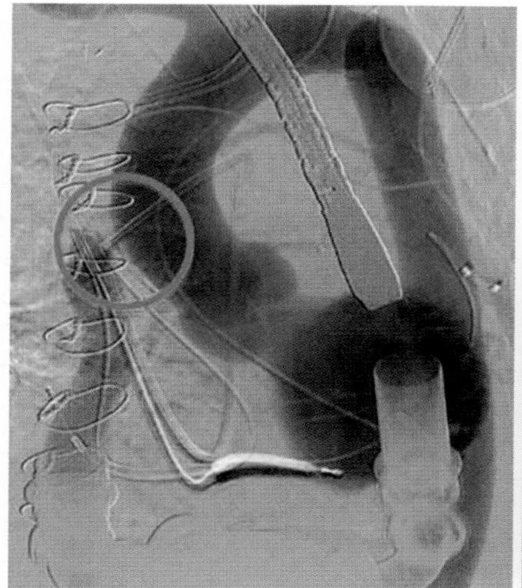

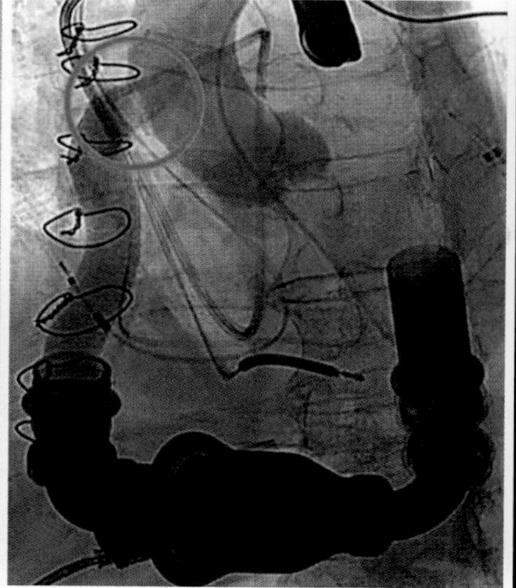

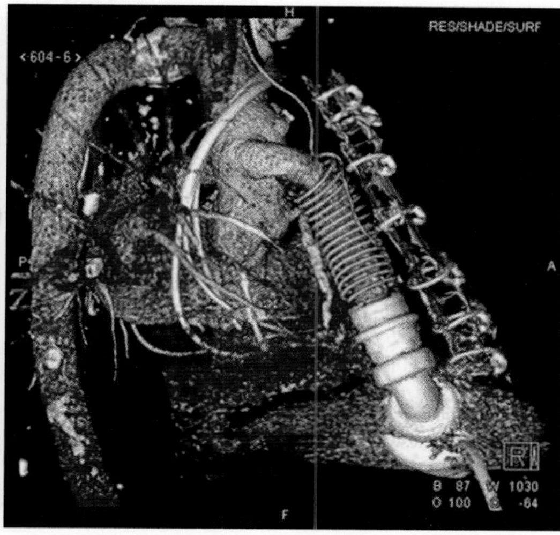

FIGURE 33-19 Left ventricular outflow tract (LVOT) graft stenosis in a patient supported by a HeartMate-II continuous flow left ventricular assist device (CF-LVAD). Pressure gradient across the anastomosis of the LVOT graft to the aorta was 50 mm Hg. After percutaneous stent deployment, the LVOT graft stenosis was relieved and the pressure gradient decreased to less than 5 mm Hg. A computerized tomographic reconstruction of the stent in the LVOT graft is shown.

TABLE 33-9 Emerging Indications and Contraindications for Cardiac Catheterization in LVAD Recipients

Diagnostic Indications
• Left heart failure • Right heart failure • Chest pain • LVAD alarms • Recurrent arrhythmias • Hypotension • Valvular heart disease (i.e., aortic insufficiency)
Therapeutic Interventions
• Percutaneous right ventricular support • Percutaneous coronary revascularization • Catheter-based intra-cavitary thrombolysis • Outflow graft stenting • Percutaneous aortic valve therapy • Ventricular tachycardia ablation • Atrial septal defect closure
Contraindications
• Aortic valve or root thrombosis • Coagulopathy • Inability to prevent catheter or wire entrapment in the conduits or pump rotor

LVAD, Left ventricular assist device.

closure for inter-atrial septal defects, and ablation of ventricular arrhythmias on LVAD support. Larger studies are needed to better define the role of invasive approaches in the treatment algorithm of patients requiring chronic LVAD support.

CONCLUSIONS

Heart failure was once considered a terminal diagnosis, and management focused on symptom management, palliation, and the rare opportunity for cardiac transplantation. Armed with an improved understanding of the hemodynamic mechanisms governing heart failure and better invasive diagnostic and therapeutic options, the light at the end of the tunnel has become brighter for patients with advanced heart failure. The role of the interventional cardiologist as an integral participant of the team approach to managing advanced heart failure will grow by: (1) providing the ability to perform a comprehensive invasive hemodynamic and angiographic evaluation of complex pathophysiologic states, (2) understanding and communicating the clinical implications of diagnostic results, and (3) implementing advanced treatment strategies as part of a team approach for all stages and types of the heart failure spectrum. Given the growing number of patients with heart failure and increasing therapeutic options available to them, the next generation of invasive operators will be asked to think more like heart failure specialists when managing this complex patient population.

References

1. Roger VL, Go AS, Lloyd-Jones DM, et al: Executive summary: heart disease and stroke statistics–2012 update: a report from the American Heart Association. *Circulation* 125(1):188–197, 2012.
2. Loehr LR, Rosamond WD, Chang PP, et al: Heart failure incidence and survival (from the Atherosclerosis Risk in Communities study). *Am J Cardiol* 101(7):1016–1022, 2008.
3. Roger VL, Go AS, Lloyd-Jones DM, et al: Heart disease and stroke statistics–2012 update: a report from the American Heart Association. *Circulation* 125(1):e2–e220, 2012.
4. Heidenreich PA, Albert NM, Allen LA, et al: Forecasting the impact of heart failure in the United States: a policy statement from the American Heart Association. *Circ Heart Fail* 6(3):606–619, 2013.
5. INTERMACS Interagency Registry for Mechanically Assisted Circulatory Support quarterly statistical report. Implant dates: June 23 M, 2011. Available from: http://www.uab.edu/ctsresearch/intermacs/DocumentLibrary/INTERMACS Federal Partners Quarterly Report 03 2011 web site.pdf.
6. McMurray JJ, Adamopoulos S, Anker SD, et al: ESC guidelines for the diagnosis and treatment of acute and chronic heart failure 2012: the Task Force for the Diagnosis and Treatment of Acute and Chronic Heart Failure 2012 of the European Society of Cardiology. Developed in collaboration with the Heart Failure Association (HFA) of the ESC. *Eur J Heart Fail* 14(8):803–869, 2012.
7. Yancy CW, Jessup M, Bozkurt B, et al: 2013 ACCF/AHA Guideline for the Management of Heart Failure: a report of the American College of Cardiology Foundation/American Heart Association Task Force on Practice Guidelines. *J Am Coll Cardiol* 62(16):e147–e239, 2013.
8. Cohen M, Urban P, Christenson JT, et al: Intra-aortic balloon counterpulsation in US and non-US centres: results of the Benchmark Registry. *Eur Heart J* 24(19):1763–1770, 2003.
9. Stone GW, Ohman EM, Miller MF, et al: Contemporary utilization and outcomes of intra-aortic balloon counterpulsation in acute myocardial infarction: the benchmark registry. *J Am Coll Cardiol* 41(11):1940–1945, 2003.
10. Williams DO, Korr KS, Gewirtz H, et al: The effect of intraaortic balloon counterpulsation on regional myocardial blood flow and oxygen consumption in the presence of coronary artery stenosis in patients with unstable angina. *Circulation* 66(3):593–597, 1982.
11. Kern MJ, Aguirre F, Bach R, et al: Augmentation of coronary blood flow by intra-aortic balloon pumping in patients after coronary angioplasty. *Circulation* 87(2):500–511, 1993.
12. Kern MJ, Aguirre FV, Tatineni S, et al: Enhanced coronary blood flow velocity during intraaortic balloon counterpulsation in critically ill patients. *J Am Coll Cardiol* 21(2):359–368, 1993.

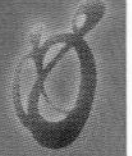

13. Braunwald E, Sarnoff SJ, Case RB, et al: Hemodynamic determinants of coronary flow: effect of changes in aortic pressure and cardiac output on the relationship between myocardial oxygen consumption and coronary flow. *Am J Physiol* 192(1):157–163, 1958.
14. Sarnoff SJ, Braunwald E, Welch GH, Jr, et al: Hemodynamic determinants of oxygen consumption of the heart with special reference to the tension-time index. *Am J Physiol* 192(1):148–156, 1958.
15. Sarnoff SJ, Case RB, Welch GH, Jr, et al: Performance characteristics and oxygen debt in a nonfailing, metabolically supported, isolated heart preparation. *Am J Physiol* 192(1):141–147, 1958.
16. Welch GH, Jr, Braunwald E, Case RB, et al: The effect of mephentermine sulfate on myocardial oxygen consumption, myocardial efficiency and peripheral vascular resistance. *Am J Med* 24(6):871–881, 1958.
17. Schreuder JJ, Castiglioni A, Donelli A, et al: Automatic intraaortic balloon pump timing using an intrabeat dicrotic notch prediction algorithm. *Ann Thorac Surg* 79(3):1017–1022, discussion 22, 2005.
18. Schreuder JJ, Maisano F, Donelli A, et al: Beat-to-beat effects of intraaortic balloon pump timing on left ventricular performance in patients with low ejection fraction. *Ann Thorac Surg* 79(3):872–880, 2005.
19. Majithia A, Jumean M, Shih H, et al: The hemodynamic effects of the MEGA intra-aortic balloon counterpulsation pump. *J Heart Lung Transplant* 32(4S):S226, 2013.
20. Charitos CE, Nanas JN, Kontoyiannis DA, et al: The efficacy of the high volume counterpulsation technique at very low levels of aortic pressure. *J Cardiovasc Surg (Torino)* 39(5):625–632, 1998.
21. Weber KT, Janicki JS, Walker AA: Intra-aortic balloon pumping: an analysis of several variables affecting balloon performance. *Trans Am Soc Artif Intern Organs* 18(0):486–492, 1972.
22. Papaioannou TG, Mathioulakis DS, Nanas JN, et al: Arterial compliance is a main variable determining the effectiveness of intra-aortic balloon counterpulsation: quantitative data from an in vitro study. *Med Eng Phys* 24(4):279–284, 2002.
23. Stamatelopoulos SF, Nanas JN, Saridakis NS, et al: Treating severe cardiogenic shock by large counterpulsation volumes. *Ann Thorac Surg* 62(4):1110–1117, 1996.
24. Ferguson JJ, 3rd, Cohen M, Freedman RJ, Jr, et al: The current practice of intra-aortic balloon counterpulsation: results from the Benchmark Registry. *J Am Coll Cardiol* 38(5):1456–1462, 2001.
25. Eltchaninoff H, Dimas AP, Whitlow PL: Complications associated with percutaneous placement and use of intraaortic balloon counterpulsation. *Am J Cardiol* 71(4):328–332, 1993.
26. Erdogan HB, Goksedef D, Erentug V, et al: In which patients should sheathless IABP be used? An analysis of vascular complications in 1211 cases. *J Card Surg* 21(4):342–346, 2006.
27. Reynolds HR, Hochman JS: Cardiogenic shock: current concepts and improving outcomes. *Circulation* 117(5):686–697, 2008.
28. Babaev A, Frederick PD, Pasta DJ, et al: Trends in management and outcomes of patients with acute myocardial infarction complicated by cardiogenic shock. *JAMA* 294(4):448–454, 2005.
29. Jeger RV, Radovanovic D, Hunziker PR, et al: Ten-year trends in the incidence and treatment of cardiogenic shock. *Ann Intern Med* 149(9):618–626, 2008.
30. Hochman JS, Buller CE, Sleeper LA, et al: Cardiogenic shock complicating acute myocardial infarction–etiologies, management and outcome: a report from the SHOCK Trial Registry. SHould we emergently revascularize Occluded Coronaries for cardiogenic shocK? *J Am Coll Cardiol* 36(3 Suppl A):1063–1070, 2000.
31. Lindholm MG, Boesgaard S, Torp-Pedersen C, et al: Diabetes mellitus and cardiogenic shock in acute myocardial infarction. *Eur J Heart Fail* 7(5):834–839, 2005.
32. Holmes DR, Jr, Berger PB, Hochman JS, et al: Cardiogenic shock in patients with acute ischemic syndromes with and without ST-segment elevation. *Circulation* 100(20):2067–2073, 1999.
33. Killip T, 3rd, Kimball JT: Treatment of myocardial infarction in a coronary care unit. A two year experience with 250 patients. *Am J Cardiol* 20(4):457–464, 1967.
34. Forrester JS, Diamond G, Chatterjee K, et al: Medical therapy of acute myocardial infarction by application of hemodynamic subsets (second of two parts). *N Engl J Med* 295(25):1404–1413, 1976.
35. Abdel-Wahab M, Saad M, Kynast J, et al: Comparison of hospital mortality with intra-aortic balloon counterpulsation insertion before versus after primary percutaneous coronary intervention for cardiogenic shock complicating acute myocardial infarction. *Am J Cardiol* 105(7):967–971, 2010.
36. Curtis JP, Rathore SS, Wang Y, et al: Use and effectiveness of intra-aortic balloon pumps among patients undergoing high risk percutaneous coronary intervention: insights from the National Cardiovascular Data Registry. *Circ Cardiovasc Qual Outcomes* 5(1):21–30, 2012.
37. Patel MR, Smalling RW, Thiele H, et al: Intra-aortic balloon counterpulsation and infarct size in patients with acute anterior myocardial infarction without shock: the CRISP AMI randomized trial. *JAMA* 306(12):1329–1337, 2011.
38. Thiele H, Schuler G, Neumann FJ, et al: Intraaortic balloon counterpulsation in acute myocardial infarction complicated by cardiogenic shock: design and rationale of the Intraaortic Balloon Pump in Cardiogenic Shock II (IABP-SHOCK II) trial. *Am Heart J* 163(6):938–945, 2012.
39. O'Neill WW, Kleiman NS, Moses J, et al: A prospective, randomized clinical trial of hemodynamic support with Impella 2.5 versus intra-aortic balloon pump in patients undergoing high-risk percutaneous coronary intervention: the PROTECT II study. *Circulation* 126(14):1717–1727, 2012.
40. Perera D, Stables R, Clayton T, et al: Long-term mortality data from the balloon pump-assisted coronary intervention study (BCIS-1): a randomized, controlled trial of elective balloon counterpulsation during high-risk percutaneous coronary intervention. *Circulation* 127(2):207–212, 2013.
41. Perera D, Stables R, Thomas M, et al: Elective intra-aortic balloon counterpulsation during high-risk percutaneous coronary intervention: a randomized controlled trial. *JAMA* 304(8):867–874, 2010.
42. Cheng JM, den Uil CA, Hoeks SE, et al: Percutaneous left ventricular assist devices vs. intra-aortic balloon pump counterpulsation for treatment of cardiogenic shock: a meta-analysis of controlled trials. *Eur Heart J* 30(17):2102–2108, 2009.
43. Shin TG, Choi JH, Jo IJ, et al: Extracorporeal cardiopulmonary resuscitation in patients with inhospital cardiac arrest: a comparison with conventional cardiopulmonary resuscitation. *Crit Care Med* 39(1):1–7, 2011.
44. Chen YS, Lin JW, Yu HY, et al: Cardiopulmonary resuscitation with assisted extracorporeal life-support versus conventional cardiopulmonary resuscitation in adults with in-hospital cardiac arrest: an observational study and propensity analysis. *Lancet* 372(9638):554–561, 2008.
45. Combes A, Leprince P, Luyt CE, et al: Outcomes and long-term quality-of-life of patients supported by extracorporeal membrane oxygenation for refractory cardiogenic shock. *Crit Care Med* 36(5):1404–1411, 2008.
46. Massetti M, Tasle M, Le Page O, et al: Back from irreversibility: extracorporeal life support for prolonged cardiac arrest. *Ann Thorac Surg* 79(1):178–183, discussion 83–84, 2005.
47. Younger JG, Schreiner RJ, Swaniker F, et al: Extracorporeal resuscitation of cardiac arrest. *Acad Emerg Med* 6(7):700–707, 1999.
48. Alam M, Wardell J, Andersson E, et al: Right ventricular function in patients with first inferior myocardial infarction: assessment by tricuspid annular motion and tricuspid annular velocity. *Am Heart J* 139(4):710–715, 2000.
49. Engstrom AE, Vis MM, Bouma BJ, et al: Right ventricular dysfunction is an independent predictor for mortality in ST-elevation myocardial infarction patients presenting with cardiogenic shock on admission. *Eur J Heart Fail* 12(3):276–282, 2010.
50. Masci PG, Francone M, Desmet W, et al: Right ventricular ischemic injury in patients with acute ST-segment elevation myocardial infarction: characterization with cardiovascular magnetic resonance. *Circulation* 122(14):1405–1412, 2010.
51. O'Rourke RA, Dell'Italia LJ: Diagnosis and management of right ventricular myocardial infarction. *Curr Probl Cardiol* 29(1):6–47, 2004.
52. Jacobs AK, Leopold JA, Bates E, et al: Cardiogenic shock caused by right ventricular infarction: a report from the SHOCK registry. *J Am Coll Cardiol* 41(8):1273–1279, 2003.
53. Mehta SR, Eikelboom JW, Natarajan MK, et al: Impact of right ventricular involvement on mortality and morbidity in patients with inferior myocardial infarction. *J Am Coll Cardiol* 37(1):37–43, 2001.
54. Greyson CR: Pathophysiology of right ventricular failure. *Crit Care Med* 36(1 Suppl):S57–S65, 2008.
55. Goldstein JA: Acute right ventricular infarction: insights for the interventional era. *Curr Probl Cardiol* 37(12):533–557, 2012.
56. John R, Lee S, Eckman P, et al: Right ventricular failure–a continuing problem in patients with left ventricular assist device support. *J Cardiovasc Transl Res* 3(6):604–611, 2010.
57. Piazza G, Goldhaber SZ: The acutely decompensated right ventricle: pathways for diagnosis and management. *Chest* 128(3):1836–1852, 2005.
58. Haddad F, Doyle R, Murphy DJ, et al: Right ventricular function in cardiovascular disease, part II: pathophysiology, clinical importance, and management of right ventricular failure. *Circulation* 117(13):1717–1731, 2008.
59. Patel SM, Allaire PE, Wood HG, et al: Methods of failure and reliability assessment for mechanical heart pumps. *Artif Organs* 29(1):15–25, 2005.
60. Flege JB, Jr, Wright CB, Reisinger TJ: Successful balloon counterpulsation for right ventricular failure. *Ann Thorac Surg* 37(2):167–168, 1984.
61. Taylor AJ, Edwards FH, Macon MG, et al: A comparative evaluation of pulmonary artery balloon counterpulsation and a centrifugal flow pump in an experimental model of right ventricular infarction. *J Extra Corpor Technol* 22(2):85–90, 1990.
62. Nordhaug D, Steensrud T, Muller S, et al: Intraaortic balloon pumping improves hemodynamics and right ventricular efficiency in acute ischemic right ventricular failure. *Ann Thorac Surg* 78(4):1426–1432, 2004.
63. Atiemo AD, Conte JV, Heldman AW: Resuscitation and recovery from acute right ventricular failure using a percutaneous right ventricular assist device. *Catheter Cardiovasc Interv* 68(1):78–82, 2006.
64. Prutkin JM, Strote JA, Stout KK: Percutaneous right ventricular assist device as support for cardiogenic shock due to right ventricular infarction. *J Invasive Cardiol* 20(7):E215–E216, 2008.
65. Takagaki M, Wurzer C, Wade R, et al: Successful conversion of TandemHeart left ventricular assist device to right ventricular assist device after implantation of a HeartMate XVE. *Ann Thorac Surg* 86(5):1677–1679, 2008.
66. Rajdev S, Benza R, Misra V: Use of Tandem Heart as a temporary hemodynamic support option for severe pulmonary artery hypertension complicated by cardiogenic shock. *J Invasive Cardiol* 19(8):E226–E229, 2007.
67. Bajona P, Salizzoni S, Brann SH, et al: Prolonged use of right ventricular assist device for refractory graft failure following orthotopic heart transplantation. *J Thorac Cardiovasc Surg* 139(3):e53–e54, 2010.
68. Cheung A, Freed D, Hunziker P, et al: TCT-371 First clinical evaluation of a novel percutaneous right ventricular assist device: the Impella RP. *J Am Coll Cardiol* 60(17S): 2012. doi: 10.1016/j.jacc.2012.08.399.
69. Hsu PL, Parker J, Egger C, et al: Mechanical circulatory support for right heart failure: current technology and future outlook. *Artif Organs* 36(4):332–347, 2012.
70. Loor G, Khani-Hanjani A, Gonzalez-Stawinski GV: Use of RotaFlow (MAQUET) for temporary right ventricular support during implantation of HeartMate II left ventricular assist device. *ASAIO J* 58(3):275–277, 2012.
71. Kapur NK, Paruchuri V, Korabathina R, et al: Effects of a percutaneous mechanical circulatory support device for medically refractory right ventricular failure. *J Heart Lung Transplant* 30(12):1360–1367, 2011.
72. Kapur NK, Paruchuri V, Jagannathan A, et al: Mechanical circulatory support for right ventricular failure. *JACC Heart Fail* 1(2):127–134, 2013.
73. Ragosta M, Beller GA, Watson DD, et al: Quantitative planar rest-redistribution 201Tl imaging in detection of myocardial viability and prediction of improvement in left ventricular function after coronary bypass surgery in patients with severely depressed left ventricular function. *Circulation* 87(5):1630–1641, 1993.
74. Auerbach MA, Schoder H, Hoh C, et al: Prevalence of myocardial viability as detected by positron emission tomography in patients with ischemic cardiomyopathy. *Circulation* 99(22):2921–2926, 1999.
75. Di Carli MF, Asgarzadie F, Schelbert HR, et al: Quantitative relation between myocardial viability and improvement in heart failure symptoms after revascularization in patients with ischemic cardiomyopathy. *Circulation* 92(12):3436–3444, 1995.
76. Marwick TH, Zuchowski C, Lauer MS, et al: Functional status and quality of life in patients with heart failure undergoing coronary bypass surgery after assessment of myocardial viability. *J Am Coll Cardiol* 33(3):750–758, 1999.
77. Pagley PR, Beller GA, Watson DD, et al: Improved outcome after coronary bypass surgery in patients with ischemic cardiomyopathy and residual myocardial viability. *Circulation* 96(3):793–800, 1997.
78. Meluzin J, Cerny J, Frelich M, et al: Prognostic value of the amount of dysfunctional but viable myocardium in revascularized patients with coronary artery disease and left ventricular dysfunction. Investigators of this Multicenter Study. *J Am Coll Cardiol* 32(4):912–920, 1998.
79. Allman KC, Shaw LJ, Hachamovitch R, et al: Myocardial viability testing and impact of revascularization on prognosis in patients with coronary artery disease and left ventricular dysfunction: a meta-analysis. *J Am Coll Cardiol* 39(7):1151–1158, 2002.
80. Velazquez EJ, Lee KL, Deja MA, et al: Coronary-artery bypass surgery in patients with left ventricular dysfunction. *N Engl J Med* 364(17):1607–1616, 2011.
81. Bonow RO, Maurer G, Lee KL, et al: Myocardial viability and survival in ischemic left ventricular dysfunction. *N Engl J Med* 364(17):1617–1625, 2011.
82. Kwon DH, Hachamovitch R, Popovic ZB, et al: Survival in patients with severe ischemic cardiomyopathy undergoing revascularization versus medical therapy: association with end-systolic volume and viability. *Circulation* 126(11 Suppl 1):S3–S8, 2012.
83. Gerber BL, Rousseau MF, Ahn SA, et al: Prognostic value of myocardial viability by delayed-enhanced magnetic resonance in patients with coronary artery disease and low ejection fraction: impact of revascularization therapy. *J Am Coll Cardiol* 59(9):825–835, 2012.
84. Ling LF, Marwick TH, Flores DR, et al: Identification of therapeutic benefit from revascularization in patients with left ventricular systolic dysfunction: inducible ischemia versus hibernating myocardium. *Circ Cardiovasc Imaging* 6(3):363–372, 2013.
85. Chaitman BR, Rosen AD, Williams DO, et al: Myocardial infarction and cardiac mortality in the Bypass Angioplasty Revascularization Investigation (BARI) randomized trial. *Circulation* 96(7):2162–2170, 1997.
86. Sedlis SP, Ramanathan KB, Morrison DA, et al: Outcome of percutaneous coronary intervention versus coronary bypass grafting for patients with low left ventricular ejection fractions, unstable angina pectoris, and risk factors for adverse outcomes with bypass (the AWESOME Randomized Trial and Registry). *Am J Cardiol* 94(1):118–120, 2004.

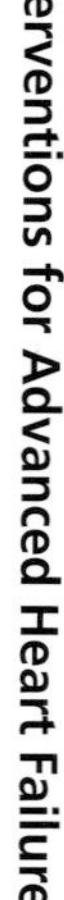

87. Sardi GL, Gaglia MA, Jr, Maluenda G, et al: Outcome of percutaneous coronary intervention utilizing drug-eluting stents in patients with reduced left ventricular ejection fraction. *Am J Cardiol* 109(3):344–351, 2012.
88. Goto M, Kohsaka S, Aoki N, et al: Risk stratification after successful coronary revascularization. *Cardiovasc Revasc Med* 9(3):132–139, 2008.
89. Wallace TW, Berger JS, Wang A, et al: Impact of left ventricular dysfunction on hospital mortality among patients undergoing elective percutaneous coronary intervention. *Am J Cardiol* 103(3):355–360, 2009.
90. Keelan PC, Johnston JM, Koru-Sengul T, et al: Comparison of in-hospital and one-year outcomes in patients with left ventricular ejection fractions <or = 40%, 41% to 49%, and >or = 50% having percutaneous coronary revascularization. *Am J Cardiol* 91(10):1168–1172, 2003.
91. Lindsay J, Jr, Grasa G, Pinnow EE, et al: Procedural results of coronary angioplasty but not late mortality have improved in patients with depressed left ventricular function. *Clin Cardiol* 22(8):533–536, 1999.
92. O'Keefe JH, Jr, Rutherford BD, McConahay DR, et al: Multivessel coronary angioplasty from 1980 to 1989: procedural results and long-term outcome. *J Am Coll Cardiol* 16(5):1097–1102, 1990.
93. Ellis SG, Weintraub W, Holmes D, et al: Relation of operator volume and experience to procedural outcome of percutaneous coronary revascularization at hospitals with high interventional volumes. *Circulation* 95(11):2479–2484, 1997.
94. Hannan EL, Racz M, Ryan TJ, et al: Coronary angioplasty volume-outcome relationships for hospitals and cardiologists. *JAMA* 277(11):892–898, 1997.
95. O'Connor GT, Malenka DJ, Quinton H, et al: Multivariate prediction of in-hospital mortality after percutaneous coronary interventions in 1994–1996. Northern New England Cardiovascular Disease Study Group. *J Am Coll Cardiol* 34(3):681–691, 1999.
96. Holmes DR, Selzer F, Johnston JM, et al: Modeling and risk prediction in the current era of interventional cardiology: a report from the National Heart, Lung, and Blood Institute Dynamic Registry. *Circulation* 107(14):1871–1876, 2003.
97. Singh M, Rihal CS, Lennon RJ, et al: Bedside estimation of risk from percutaneous coronary intervention: the new Mayo Clinic risk scores. *Mayo Clin Proc* 82(6):701–708, 2007.
98. Singh M, Lennon RJ, Holmes DR, Jr, et al: Correlates of procedural complications and a simple integer risk score for percutaneous coronary intervention. *J Am Coll Cardiol* 40(3):387–393, 2002.
99. Zajarias A, Cribier AG: Outcomes and safety of percutaneous aortic valve replacement. *J Am Coll Cardiol* 53(20):1829–1836, 2009.
100. Lund O, Flo C, Jensen FT, et al: Left ventricular systolic and diastolic function in aortic stenosis. Prognostic value after valve replacement and underlying mechanisms. *Eur Heart J* 18(12):1977–1987, 1997.
101. Bonow RO, Carabello BA, Chatterjee K, et al: 2008 Focused update incorporated into the ACC/AHA 2006 guidelines for the management of patients with valvular heart disease: a report of the American College of Cardiology/American Heart Association Task Force on Practice Guidelines (Writing Committee to Revise the 1998 Guidelines for the Management of Patients With Valvular Heart Disease): endorsed by the Society of Cardiovascular Anesthesiologists, Society for Cardiovascular Angiography and Interventions, and Society of Thoracic Surgeons. *Circulation* 118(15):e523–e661, 2008.
102. Clavel MA, Dumesnil JG, Capoulade R, et al: Outcome of patients with aortic stenosis, small valve area, and low-flow, low-gradient despite preserved left ventricular ejection fraction. *J Am Coll Cardiol* 60(14):1259–1267, 2012.
103. Hachicha Z, Dumesnil JG, Bogaty P, et al: Paradoxical low-flow, low-gradient severe aortic stenosis despite preserved ejection fraction is associated with higher afterload and reduced survival. *Circulation* 115(22):2856–2864, 2007.
104. Tamburino C, Capodanno D, Ramondo A, et al: Incidence and predictors of early and late mortality after transcatheter aortic valve implantation in 663 patients with severe aortic stenosis. *Circulation* 123(3):299–308, 2011.
105. Herrmann HC, Pibarot P, Hueter I, et al: Predictors of mortality and outcomes of therapy in low-flow severe aortic stenosis: a Placement of Aortic Transcatheter Valves (PARTNER) trial analysis. *Circulation* 127(23):2316–2326, 2013.
106. Le Ven F, Freeman M, Webb J, et al: Impact of low flow on the outcome of high-risk patients undergoing transcatheter aortic valve replacement. *J Am Coll Cardiol* 62(9):782–788, 2013.
107. Lancellotti P, Marwick T, Pierard LA: How to manage ischaemic mitral regurgitation. *Heart* 94(11):1497–1502, 2008.
108. Trichon BH, O'Connor CM: Secondary mitral and tricuspid regurgitation accompanying left ventricular systolic dysfunction: is it important, and how is it treated? *Am Heart J* 144(3):373–376, 2002.
109. Yiu SF, Enriquez-Sarano M, Tribouilloy C, et al: Determinants of the degree of functional mitral regurgitation in patients with systolic left ventricular dysfunction: a quantitative clinical study. *Circulation* 102(12):1400–1406, 2000.
110. Spoor MT, Geltz A, Bolling SF: Flexible versus nonflexible mitral valve rings for congestive heart failure: differential durability of repair. *Circulation* 114(1 Suppl):I67–I71, 2006.
111. Romano MA, Bolling SF: Update on mitral repair in dilated cardiomyopathy. *J Card Surg* 19(5):396–400, 2004.
112. Koelling TM, Aaronson KD, Cody RJ, et al: Prognostic significance of mitral regurgitation and tricuspid regurgitation in patients with left ventricular systolic dysfunction. *Am Heart J* 144(3):524–529, 2002.
113. Strauss RH, Stevenson LW, Dadourian BA, et al: Predictability of mitral regurgitation detected by Doppler echocardiography in patients referred for cardiac transplantation. *Am J Cardiol* 59(8):892–894, 1987.
114. Agricola E, Stella S, Figini F, et al: Non-ischemic dilated cardiopathy: prognostic value of functional mitral regurgitation. *Int J Cardiol* 146(3):426–428, 2011.
115. Jones RH, Velazquez EJ, Michler RE, et al: Coronary bypass surgery with or without surgical ventricular reconstruction. *N Engl J Med* 360(17):1705–1717, 2009.
116. Bouma W, van der Horst IC, Wijdh-den Hamer IJ, et al: Chronic ischaemic mitral regurgitation. Current treatment results and new mechanism-based surgical approaches. *Eur J Cardiothorac Surg* 37(1):170–185, 2010.
117. Lamas GA, Mitchell GF, Flaker GC, et al: Clinical significance of mitral regurgitation after acute myocardial infarction. Survival and Ventricular Enlargement Investigators. *Circulation* 96(3):827–833, 1997.
118. Bursi F, Enriquez-Sarano M, Nkomo VT, et al: Heart failure and death after myocardial infarction in the community: the emerging role of mitral regurgitation. *Circulation* 111(3):295–301, 2005.
119. Grigioni F, Detaint D, Avierinos JF, et al: Contribution of ischemic mitral regurgitation to congestive heart failure after myocardial infarction. *J Am Coll Cardiol* 45(2):260–267, 2005.
120. Grigioni F, Enriquez-Sarano M, Zehr KJ, et al: Ischemic mitral regurgitation: long-term outcome and prognostic implications with quantitative Doppler assessment. *Circulation* 103(13):1759–1764, 2001.
121. Alfieri O, Maisano F, De Bonis M, et al: The double-orifice technique in mitral valve repair: a simple solution for complex problems. *J Thorac Cardiovasc Surg* 122(4):674–681, 2001.
122. Fann JI, St Goar FG, Komtebedde J, et al: Beating heart catheter-based edge-to-edge mitral valve procedure in a porcine model: efficacy and healing response. *Circulation* 110(8):988–993, 2004.
123. St Goar FG, Fann JI, Komtebedde J, et al: Endovascular edge-to-edge mitral valve repair: short-term results in a porcine model. *Circulation* 108(16):1990–1993, 2003.
124. Feldman T, Foster E, Glower DD, et al: Percutaneous repair or surgery for mitral regurgitation. *N Engl J Med* 364(15):1395–1406, 2011.
125. Feldman T, Kar S, Rinaldi M, et al: Percutaneous mitral repair with the MitraClip system: safety and midterm durability in the initial EVEREST (Endovascular Valve Edge-to-Edge REpair Study) cohort. *J Am Coll Cardiol* 54(8):686–694, 2009.
126. Silvestry FE, Rodriguez LL, Herrmann HC, et al: Echocardiographic guidance and assessment of percutaneous repair for mitral regurgitation with the Evalve MitraClip: lessons learned from EVEREST I. *J Am Soc Echocardiogr* 20(10):1131–1140, 2007.
127. White HD, Norris RM, Brown MA, et al: Left ventricular end-systolic volume as the major determinant of survival after recovery from myocardial infarction. *Circulation* 76(1):44–51, 1987.
128. Kramer DG, Trikalinos TA, Kent DM, et al: Quantitative evaluation of drug or device effects on ventricular remodeling as predictors of therapeutic effects on mortality in patients with heart failure and reduced ejection fraction: a meta-analytic approach. *J Am Coll Cardiol* 56(5):392–406, 2010.
129. Buckberg G, Athanasuleas C, Conte J: Surgical ventricular restoration for the treatment of heart failure. *Nat Rev Cardiol* 9(12):703–716, 2012.
130. Costa MA, Pencina M, Nikolic S, et al: The PARACHUTE IV trial design and rationale: percutaneous ventricular restoration using the parachute device in patients with ischemic heart failure and dilated left ventricles. *Am Heart J* 165(4):531–536, 2013.
131. Bench T, Burkhoff D, O'Connell JB, et al: Heart failure with normal ejection fraction: consideration of mechanisms other than diastolic dysfunction. *Curr Heart Fail Rep* 6(1):57–64, 2009.
132. Borlaug BA, Paulus WJ: Heart failure with preserved ejection fraction: pathophysiology, diagnosis, and treatment. *Eur Heart J* 32(6):670–679, 2011.
133. Grossman W, Paulus WJ: Myocardial stress and hypertrophy: a complex interface between biophysics and cardiac remodeling. *J Clin Invest* 123(9):3701–3703, 2013.
134. Søndergaard L, Reddy V, Kaye D, et al: Transcatheter treatment of heart failure with preserved or mildly reduced ejection fraction using a novel interatrial implant to lower left atrial pressure. *Eur J Heart Fail* 16(7):796–801, 2014.
135. Bernard S, Maurer MS: Heart failure with a Normal Ejection Fraction: treatments for a complex syndrome? *Curr Treat Options Cardiovasc Med* 14(4):305–318, 2012.

34 Endomyocardial Biopsy

James B. Young and Deepak L. Bhatt

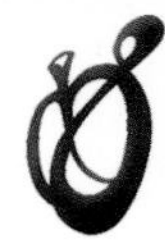

INTRODUCTION

Endomyocardial biopsy has long been used in patients with cardiovascular disease to diagnose disease, guide treatments, and assist with prognostication. To better understand the role of this invasive diagnostic procedure, reviewing the history of the procedure, approach to patients, safety, and its utility are important. Assessment of the risk/benefit ratio of the procedure is dependent on understanding the nuances of our experience with its application. Clinicians, investigators, and professional societies have all addressed this issue, and guideline recommendations to help with expert clinical practice have been developed. Nonetheless, one will sometimes encounter a pejorative comment that endomyocardial biopsy is "a procedure looking for an indication." That is not the case.

DEVELOPMENT OF THE PROCEDURE—A HISTORIC PERSPECTIVE

Linking pathologic information obtained during post mortem examination of the heart or tissue specimens removed at the time of cardiac surgery has given insight into myocardial pathology.[1] Linking these findings to clinical scenarios is a foundation of medical practice. Histologic, histobiochemical, immune histochemical, and nuclear protein analysis of cardiac tissue can more precisely characterize disease in many patients premortem, particularly when a clinical diagnosis is challenging to make. However, examination of biopsy specimens could only be performed after cardiac tissue was obtained at the time of thoracic or beating heart surgery. In the 1950s, a limited thoracotomy approach was sometimes used to obtain samples of myocardium. The first percutaneous, nonsurgical, transthoracic, needle biopsy approaches to heart biopsy were reported in the late 1950s.[2-4] These adventures were associated with an incidence of major complications including cardiac tamponade, coronary artery laceration, and pneumothorax in almost 10% of procedures. Direct percutaneous needle biopsy of the heart was limited by these problems as well as the difficulty of obtaining adequate tissue samples using relatively small needle puncturing and cutting devices as were used for percutaneous biopsy of the liver and kidney. The beating heart with a high pressure blood-filled system proved a difficult target. Multiple passes into the myocardium to obtain adequate tissue increased risk. Sutton's report of a percutaneous transthoracic biopsy approach noted that insufficient tissue for examination was the outcome in almost a quarter of the patients.[5] Often, no endomyocardial tissue could be obtained during these procedures. It was the development of a bioptome that could be utilized with a transvenous, or transarterial, approach to the right or left ventricle via the left basilica, and either femoral vein or from the left axillary, or either femoral artery and then into the heart that first allowed more reliable examination of adequate endomyocardial tissue. This facilitated diagnoses that were made after autopsy or direct surgical recovery of specimens.[6] Sakakibara and Konno used a flexible bioptome with retractable and then grasping terminus cutting cusps to pinch off pieces of myocardium during an endovascular approach to the left ventricle. Subsequently, Caves, utilizing a modified Konno biopsy forceps (subsequently coming to be known as the Stanford Caves-Shulz bioptome, which evolved to the Scholten apparatus), to obtain tissue after passing the instrument through the right internal jugular vein with only local anesthesia used, and rapid tissue.[6] This promoted procedure safety and success.[7-10] The motivation for development of this device was diagnosing cardiac transplant allograft rejection so that immunosuppression could be modified in order to optimize transplant heart function and prevent or treat potentially catastrophic rejection. This tool was reusable and

Dr. Deepak L. Bhatt discloses the following relationships: **Advisory Board**: Cardax, Elsevier Practice Update Cardiology, Medscape Cardiology, Regado Biosciences; **Board of Directors**: Boston VA Research Institute, Society of Cardiovascular Patient Care; **Chair**: American Heart Association Get With The Guidelines Steering Committee; **Data Monitoring Committees**: Duke Clinical Research Institute, Harvard Clinical Research Institute, Mayo Clinic, Population Health Research Institute; **Honoraria**: American College of Cardiology (Senior Associate Editor, Clinical Trials and News, ACC.org), Belvoir Publications (Editor in Chief, Harvard Heart Letter), Duke Clinical Research Institute (clinical trial steering committees), Harvard Clinical Research Institute (clinical trial steering committee), HMP Communications (Editor in Chief, Journal of Invasive Cardiology), Journal of the American College of Cardiology (Associate Editor; Section Editor, Pharmacology), Population Health Research Institute (clinical trial steering committee), Slack Publications (Chief Medical Editor, Cardiology Today's Intervention), WebMD (CME steering committees); **Other**: Clinical Cardiology (Deputy Editor); **Research Funding**: Amarin, AstraZeneca, Bristol-Myers Squibb, Eisai, Ethicon, Forest Laboratories, Ischemix, Medtronic, Pfizer, Roche, Sanofi Aventis, The Medicines Company; **Unfunded Research**: FlowCo, PLx Pharma, Takeda.

underwent subsequent modification that improved tissue biopsy while becoming the standard management system for heart transplant patients that subsequently morphed into multiple disposable and reusable instruments used today.[11] The Stanford Caves-Shulz system had the advantage over the Konno bioptome in that it did not require a cutdown to facilitate entry into the saphenous or basilic vein (or the femoral or brachial artery if left ventricular tissue was the target).[7,8] With fluoroscopic or echocardiographic (subsequently) imaging, the bioptome could be safely advanced to the endocardial surface with the jaws closed, the catheter slightly withdrawn and the jaws opened, followed by the catheter being re-advanced onto the endocardial surface (usually signaled by premature ventricular contractions, ectopy couplets, or short runs of nonsustained ventricular tachycardia). After closure of the clasps and then gentle tugging back the closed-jaw bioptome, withdrawal of tissue was usually successful and a few cubic millimeters in size. Crush artifact was not often a problem and, unless significant fibrotic endocardium was at the biopsy site, adequate samples of heart tissue were obtained. The Stanford Caves-Shulz bioptome could be utilized for many procedures (often more than 50) without reconstructive maintenance or sharpening. Subsequently, the King bioptome became utilized as well and was a modification of biopsy forceps used for bronchoscopic transbronchial biopsy.[12] This flexible shaft bioptome could be introduced through a catheter into the right or left ventricle and, utilizing the same technique with the jaw-opening mechanism, allowed retrieval of several samples from slightly varying locations in the ventricle during several reinsertions and passes at the myocardium. Subsequent modification of biopsy catheters allowed disposal of single-use bioptomes and improved flexibility, which allowed greater percutaneous positioning and mobility of the catheter.[11]

TECHNIQUE OF THE PROCEDURE

Today, the right internal jugular vein is most commonly accessed with a puncture and sheath-based catheter system for right ventricular endomyocardial biopsy.[13-16] Some experts routinely approach the patient by accessing the femoral vein using longer bioptomes and sheath systems.[11] This approach has the disadvantage of requiring the patient to remain supine for some time after the procedure to ensure that the puncture site does not bleed. Usually when doing the procedure from the neck or subclavian site, the patient can sit up and walk immediately post biopsy. Also, this approach, because the catheter system is quite long, makes manipulation and proper placement of the bioptome in the ventricle more challenging. Utilizing sonographic imaging of the internal jugular vein has remarkably decreased the challenges of doing endomyocardial biopsy.[17] The number of attempts required for successful venipuncture, complications, and duration of the procedure have been improved with the ability to image the great veins of the neck and mediastinum by facilitating determination of vessel size, patency, and phasic respiratory variation of the target size and location.[17-20] Of course, ultrasound guidance for femoral vein puncture can also be utilized and might be particularly helpful in patients who have unusual femoral triangle anatomy or scarring in this region from prior catheterization procedures. For central venous puncture some operators place the patient in a reverse Trendelenburg position during the internal jugular vein approach to facilitate venous engorgement, or simply place a wedging device under the patient's legs. This should be removed after successful venous access has been achieved, particularly if right heart hemodynamic measurements are to be assessed. Having the patient do a Valsalva maneuver during the puncture in order to engorge and, thus, expand the internal jugular vein to a more sizeable dimension may facilitate safe and successful vascular access. During the procedure, the patient is monitored from an electrocardiographic, systemic blood pressure, and pulse oximetric perspective. If the internal jugular venous system is atretic or occluded for one reason or another, the subclavian vein is an option. With a natural "C" curvature formed with the bioptome, utilization of the left subclavian vein seems preferable to the right, although both approaches are relatively straightforward and feasible. If left ventricular tissue, for one reason or another, is desirable, the approach usually employs a sheath placed into a femoral artery.[11] Constant positive pressure is maintained during this approach to avoid blood stasis and clot formation within the sheath with its risk of subsequent embolization, particularly when the system end-hole is in the left ventricle or aortic arch. The sheath system can be pushed across the aortic valve and positioned near the endocardium with the bioptome then passed repeatedly through it to obtain samples, again with care taken to avoid air or thrombus embolization.

Guidance of the biopsy catheter into the heart is generally done under fluoroscopic surveillance in a cardiac catheterization laboratory or radiologic procedure room but two-dimensional echocardiography has also been employed.[18,19] Portable echocardiographic and fluoroscopic units can facilitate the biopsy procedures being done at the bedside, usually in an intensive care unit for critically ill, hospitalized patients. Arguably, fluoroscopy generally provides more information than echocardiography (some bioptomes commercially available are not very echogenic). With the patient in the PA (posterior-anterior) fluoroscopic view the course of the bioptome through the great thoracic vessels as it crosses the tricuspid, or aortic, valve and then enters the right or left ventricular cavity can be monitored (**Figure 34-1**, Video 34-1A). During fluoroscopy the image can be rotated into the LAO (left anterior oblique) position to assist with confirmation that bioptome jaws are facing the interventricular septum rather than the free left ventricular wall (**Figure 34-2**, Video 34-1B). The main challenge of echocardiographic-guided endomyocardial biopsy is imaging the bioptome, and particularly the jaws of the device. This can be a function of the device echogenicity and the ease of obtaining echocardiographic images in any particular patient. When successful images are obtained, however, endomyocardial biopsy can be made safer and provide better target images. An apical four-transthoracic echocardiographic view can allow a panoramic image of the right ventricle and help with target identification for the bioptome jaws. It is particularly important to avoid the free right ventricular wall, if at all possible, to decrease the likelihood of ventricular perforation. This is particularly important in the nonheart transplant patient (Video 34-1C). Also helpful is the fact that echocardiographic images can identify the papillary muscles and give insight into where chordae tendinae might lay such that biopsy of these structures (particularly the tip of the papillary muscle) is avoided, specifically in the cardiac allograft where multiple biopsies

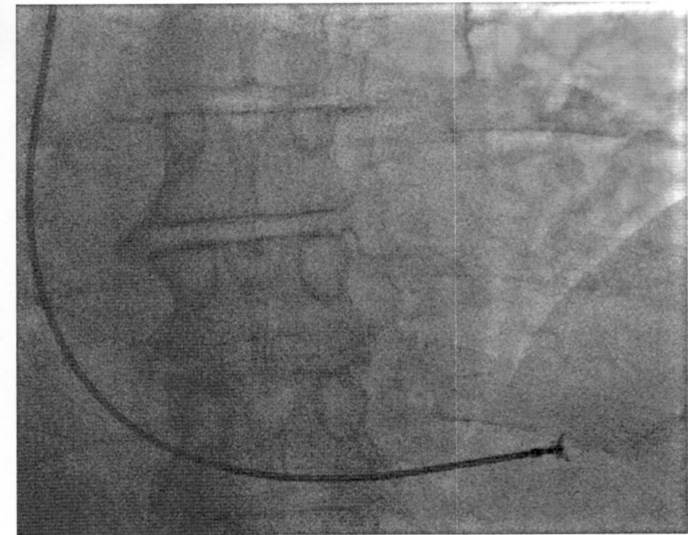

FIGURE 34-1 The posterior-anterior projection is used to position the bioptome in the right ventricle.

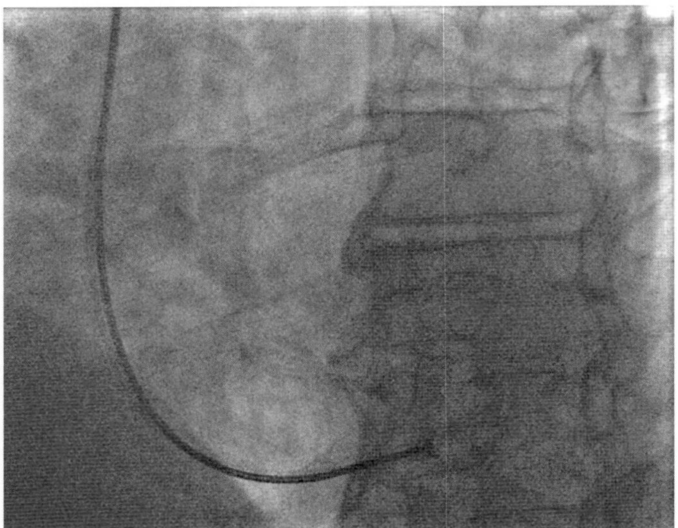

FIGURE 34-2 The left anterior oblique projection is used to confirm the bioptome is facing the right ventricular septum.

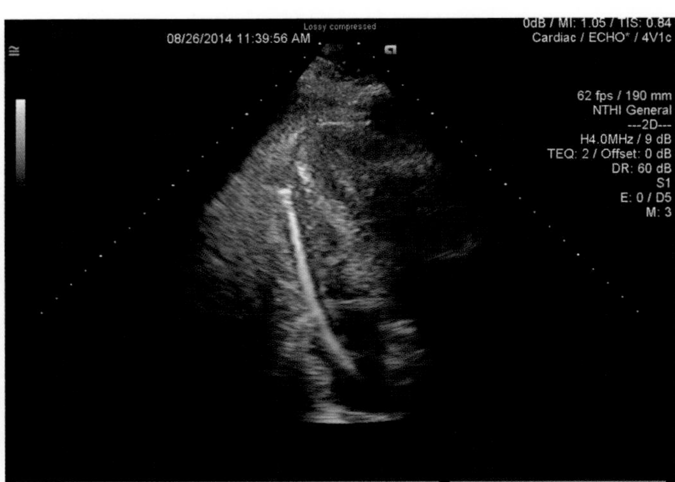

FIGURE 34-3 Echocardiography shows that the bioptome is pointing toward the right ventricular free wall and needs to be repositioned toward the right ventricular septum.

over time are required. Another approach to lessening the risk of biopsy-induced tricuspid insufficiency is to utilize a longer sheath system, one which can be placed as a guiding sheath across the triscupid valve. This would likely prevent damage to the valve itself from the rigid and relatively unforgiving bioptome as it is pushed through the tricuspid valve. Perhaps this is more important when repeated biopsies are done on a cardiac allograft, but some would argue that it is more important when doing a biopsy in a native heart. Unfortunately, sometimes when the sheath is left across the tricuspid valve during the biopsy procedure it limits mobility of the bioptome when it is trying to be placed against the right ventricular target. With either fluoroscopic or echocardiographic guidance, after confirmation that the bioptome jaws are opposing the interventricular septum, the device is advanced into the septum, premature ventricular are induced (usually), with the jaws then quickly and firmly closed and specimen removed with a gentle tug (Video 34-1D).

Employing both fluoroscopic and echocardiographic monitoring when a specific location in the ventricle is the target can be helpful (**Figure 34-3**, Video 34-2). Prior to the biopsy procedure, computed tomographic (CT) or cardiac magnetic resonance (CMR) imaging of the heart might be helpful with making a pathologic diagnosis and give the operator insight into precise cardiac anatomy, particularly the angle of the intraventricular septum in relationship to the superior or inferior vena cava, and specific location of target areas for biopsy.[14-16,20-24] It has been noted that knowledge of anatomic relationships characterized by multimodal imaging may lessen the risk of inadvertent free right ventricular wall biopsy during a fluoroscopic-directed procedure, which could decrease the likelihood of right ventricular perforation and subsequent problematic pericardial effusion and cardiac tamponade. It should be noted that using MRI to help target focal disease location that might allow bioptome navigation into areas of interest is challenging. Three-dimensional echocardiography has also been utilized to assist with the procedure and obviate the need for fluoroscopy but limited data are available comparing this approach to the others.

SAFETY OF ENDOMYOCARDIAL BIOPSY

Today, the vast majority of endomyocardial biopsies are done to monitor cardiac allograft rejection after heart transplant.[14,15,23-25] This relates to the importance of knowing allograft rejection status, relative safety of the procedure, and reasonable diagnostic accuracy. As with any invasive procedure, the likelihood of an adverse experience or event seems dependent on the experience of the operator and team doing the procedure.[14,15,25] This is further influenced by the clinical status or stability of the patient, bioptome utilized, vascular access approach chosen, presence or absence of left bundle branch block, location in the ventricle biopsied, and underlying disease. **Table 34-1** summarizes potential difficulties occurring during endomyocardial biopsy. Risks that develop acutely include problems associated with vascular access such as inadvertent puncture of central or peripheral arteries, biopsy site hematoma formation, creation of peripheral arterial-venous fistula, or

TABLE 34-1 Risks of Endomyocardial Biopsy

Potential Difficulties

- Vascular access
  - Inadvertent arterial puncture while obtaining venous access
  - Horner's syndrome (hoarseness with unilateral ptosis, injected conjunctiva, anisocoria, and anhidrosis of the face) due to caudal migration of local anesthetic when inadvertently injected into the carotid—internal jugular vascular sheath with sympathetic-parasympathetic nerve action disrupted
  - Vasovagal reaction
  - Air embolism during internal jugular approach
  - Puncture site bleeding and neck hematoma
  - Pneumothorax
- Biopsy procedure
  - Innominate vein perforation
  - Tricuspid valve injury
    - Tricuspid valve leaflet injury/perforation
    - Severing tricuspid valve chordae tendinae
    - Flail tricuspid valve leaflets
    - Tricuspid valve insufficiency
  - Arrhythmias/conduction disturbances
    - Premature atrial and ventricular contractions
    - Atrial flutter/fibrillation
    - Nonsustained/sustained ventricular tachycardia
    - Ventricular fibrillation
    - Bundle branch blocks
    - Heart block
    - Ventricular free wall perforation (with/without pain)
    - Pericardial effusion
    - Cardiac tamponade
    - Cardiac arrest
- Death
- Inability to obtain tissue/inadequate sample

arterial-venous fistulae within the heart itself related to coronary artery injury.[14,15,18,23-26] One usually transient and generally minor difficulty is nerve paralysis related to anesthesia infiltration of tissue overlying the vascular access site with dissection down the arterial-venous tissue sheath running into the mediastinum where recurrent laryngeal nerve paralysis can develop. Ventricular or supraventricular arrhythmias can be seen, including paroxysmal supraventricular tachycardia and atrial fibrillation (usually transient) as well as isolated ventricular arrhythmias, sustained ventricular tachycardia, and ventricular fibrillation with frank cardiac arrest (which is rare). Vasovagal reactions can occur in the nonheart transplant population where the hearts remain innervated, though rarely has been noted in patients with orthotopic cardiac allografts if re-innervation of the graft is present. Sudden heart block can develop and may be more frequent in patients with left bundle branch block, or trifascicular right bundle branch block. Pneumothorax and hemothorax are substantial risks but lessened by utilizing sonographic imaging of the neck and mediastinal great vessels to help guide venous access and catheter journey. Pulmonary embolization can occur, including air embolization. The operator must be ever mindful of this potential difficulty and take efforts to not allow air into the venous system, particular during deep inspiration by the patient. Long term, perhaps one of the more devastating difficulties can be disruption of tricuspid valve integrity, particularly after repeated right ventricular endomyocardial biopsies during follow-up of heart transplant patients. Indeed, tricuspid valve leaflets can be punctured or torn by the sheath, bioptome, chordae tendinae biopsy, or tissue removal from the tip of a papillary muscle. This can produce substantial tricuspid insufficiency. Utilizing a long sheath that can be placed into the right ventricle across the tricuspid valve may decrease the risk of tricuspid valve trauma; however, biopsy of tricuspid valve chordae tendineae may still occur even when a sheath is utilized. The operator must be ever alert to the possibility of bleeding into the pericardium, particularly when it is vigorous enough to cause cardiac tamponade after right ventricular free wall puncture. Fortunately, most right ventricular perforations seal off without sequelae after the culprit catheter is pulled back into the ventricle because of myocardial elasticity. However, the thin free wall of the right ventricle or areas of substantive scar tissue can produce challenges in some patients when perforation occurs. One must be vigilant postprocedure and remember that delayed complications can be seen and include access site bleeding (particularly when an artery is inadvertently punctured during the procedure, or the patient is anticoagulated or on antiplatelet agents), late cardiac tamponade, access site venous thrombosis, and, as mentioned, tricuspid insufficiency severe enough to cause hemodynamic alterations. The precise frequency of long-term adverse events, such as tricuspid regurgitation, is not well characterized.

Data are available to give insight into the complications noted during right ventricular endomyocardial biopsy.[14-16,20,24-26] Overall, when large registry-based data are reviewed, the complication rate for access site acquisition is in the 2% to 3% range and with actual biopsy procedure 3% to 4% (**Table 34-1**). The most common complication during access site approach is unplanned arterial puncture during infusion of local anesthesia or inadvertent insertion of access catheters, or bioptomes, into an artery (around 2%), vasovagal reaction (less than 1%), and prolonged venous oozing after bioptome and sheath removal (well under 1%). The most common adverse events associated with obtaining tissue is arrhythmia excluding isolated premature contractions (around 2% when conduction abnormalities are included), undiagnosed perforation manifesting as chest pain (less than 1% though more frequently patients report sharp pain or pleuritic pain when specimens are removed), and definite perforation manifest by pericardial fluid and rarely cardiac tamponade (also well under 1%). Despite these low numbers it should be noted that deaths can occur after perforation of the ventricle with cardiac tamponade or development of malignant, hemodynamically unstable arrhythmias. Patients having a higher risk of ventricular perforation include those with increased right ventricular systolic pressure, blood clotting abnormalities, on anticoagulants or antiplatelet agents, or having right ventricular enlargement, which can be associated with right ventricular wall thinning. Whenever the operator is concerned about myocardial perforation because of a pain syndrome, hypotension, or tachycardia, before central venous access is removed and the patient leaves the diagnostic laboratory, echocardiography should be performed to confirm, or refute, presence of pericardial fluid and document any imaging evidence of hemodynamic compromise. The capability to surgically address substantive pericardial effusions, particularly those with hemodynamic compromise, from a surgical or pericardiocentesis approach should be present and immediately available at any center performing endomyocardial biopsy.

Many risks can be diminished by utilizing ultrasound imaging for access site and catheter guidance, as noted, but also by avoiding the immediate supraclavicular approach with a higher internal jugular puncture technique. Rarely is heart block a permanent problem, but in patients with left bundle branch block, when the bioptome or guiding catheter is placed into the right ventricle and pressed against the intraventricular septum, it can develop. Most of the time simply pulling back on the sheath, or bioptome, is enough to allow normal conduction to reappear and only on rare occasions will a patient require temporary pacing. Horner syndrome with vocal paresis and sometimes diaphragmatic excursion limitation can be noted with large volume lidocaine infusion into the jugular venous and carotid sheath but does not generally result in permanent damage and resolves quickly. Trauma from the puncture needle itself can also cause this difficulty and, perhaps, more permanent impairment. Again, one of the troubling problems in heart transplant patients is development of tricuspid insufficiency, or worsening of this problem after exposure to multiple serial biopsies.[25]

PROCESSING ENDOMYOCARDIAL TISSUE SPECIMENS

By convention, 5 to 10 passes into the ventricle are made to obtain, generally, 5 specimens. Usually, the pieces are 1 to 2 mm in size.[16] The 2011 consensus statement on endomyocardial biopsy from the Association for European Cardiovascular Pathology and the Society for Cardiovascular Pathology suggested "three, preferably four" fragments 1 to 2 mm in size should be obtained and then immediately fixed in a 10% buffered formalin solution and kept at room temperature to prevent contraction band formation.[16] In addition, one or two additional specimens should be "snap" frozen in liquid nitrogen for molecular testing, or other esoteric but more specific staining procedures based on the patients' clinical presentation. Finally, the consensus statement points out that one fragment should be fixed in a 2.5% glutaraldehyde or Karnovsky solution so that it can be used for cellular ultrastructural analysis if desired.

Pathologic examination would include light microscopy routinely performed on formalin fixed and paraffin imbedded samples with hematoxylin-eosin, and a variety of other staining techniques for more specific evaluations. This might include Masson or Mallory trichrome stain, Movat pentichrome stain, and Weigert-Van Gieson stain for collagen and elastin fibers. PAS (periodic-acid Schiff) stain with and without diastase is helpful for evaluating glycogen storage diseases, which might better be performed on frozen sections. Because amyloidosis is a frequent indication for endomyocardial biopsy, attention to Congo-red sulfate, alcian-blue, or S/T thioflavin staining is important. PERLS iron stain is also useful when evaluating possible infiltrative cardiomyopathies. Histochemical, histomorphologic, and immunohistochemical stains supplement the more routine evaluation and are, in particular, helpful when inflammatory myocarditis or cellular infiltration is anticipated.[27] Monitoring cardiac allograft patients is helped by knowledge of certain immunohistochemical reactions. These stains would include CD45, 20, 3, 4, 8, 68, and HLA-DR and -ABC. Transthyreitin, κ and λ chains, apolipoprotein, and amyloid A stains are helpful for amyloid typing. Certain antibodies can characterize neoplasia and some genetic cardiomyopathies can be demonstrated with dystrophin, lamin A/C, desmin, plakoglobin, and N-cadherin in some patients. Immunohistochemical stains including those used to type amyloid infiltration may be performed on frozen tissue. In certain circumstances frozen tissue appears preferable for immunohistochemistry analysis of dystrophin and HLA-ABC.

Because of the importance of myocarditis in causing acute and chronic cardiomyopathy syndromes, great attention has been played to the molecular detection of viral genomic "footprints" in the myocardium, which might suggest a specific viral attack on the heart with subsequent contractility impairment.[27-31] Many studies have demonstrated evidence that a wide variety of viruses including enteroviruses, adenoviruses, cytomegalovirus, herpes simplex virus, and Epstein-Barr virus have infected the myocardium. Most frequently, adenovirus and enterovirus genomes are noted. There is a significant limitation in interpretation of viral genome data, however, because the sensitivity is not well characterized for these investigations. A positive polymerase chain reaction (PCR) test, for example, appears diagnostic but a negative examination would not necessarily exclude a viral disease pathology. Furthermore, very small viral loads have been reported in some patients and the clinical significance of this can be unclear. Linking viral footprint evidence of residence may not explain the etiology of a cardiomyopathy syndrome completely. The 2007 scientific statement from the American Heart Association (AHA), the American College of Cardiology (ACC), and the European Society of Cardiology pointed out that, because of these uncertainties, centers not experienced in techniques of viral load analysis should avoid exploration of myocardial tissue in this fashion.[14] Furthermore, the lack of consensus regarding treatment of patients with viral myocarditis, both acutely and chronically, emphasizes, arguably, the limited value today of this approach.[28-31]

While performing the procedure and obtaining samples the operator must be mindful of the fact that transmission electron microscopic examination on glutaraldehyde, or Karnovsky, solution-fixed specimens is important for some difficulties such as Adriamycin-induced cardiomyopathy. Special attention needs to be paid to proper preservation of the tissue for this type of analysis.

INDICATIONS FOR ENDOMYOCARDIAL BIOPSY

The 2011 consensus statement on endomyocardial biopsy focused on three broad categories of patients likely to benefit from the procedure.[16] In the first category, the importance of diagnosing a specific etiology of heart failure is the leading question. After other diagnostic procedures are employed and various diseases excluded, endomyocardial biopsy may provide a very specific clinical diagnosis (**Table 34-2**). The second category includes the necessity of making a decision regarding the importance of obtaining a definitive diagnosis, which would then dictate specific therapies (such as, arguably, for acute myocarditis) rather than nonspecific therapies (beta adrenergic drugs or angiotensin receptor blockers), or clinical management (the safety of administering an anthracycline compound in an individual with recurrent malignancy treated previously with such an agent for example). The third general category is linked to the first two because of the importance of linking clinical diagnosis with therapeutic plans. This category focused on managing new onset (less than 6 months) of unexplained heart failure, significant cardiac arrhythmias that might be related to myocarditis or sarcoidosis, chronic heart failure caused by hypertrophic or restrictive diseases, investigation

TABLE 34-2 Diagnostic Potential for Endomyocardial Biopsy: 2011 Consensus Statement

Definite diagnosis can be made:
• **Cardiac sarcoidosis:** noncaseous granulomas
• **Cardiac amyloidosis:** myocardial amyloid infiltration
• **Iron overload:** intracellular iron deposition
• **Desmin cardiomyopathy:** abnormal granulomatous aggregates of desmin-type intermediate filaments in the cytoplasm of cardiomyocytes and at the Z band level
• **Dystrophin cardiomyopathy (Duchenne dystrophy):** absence of dystrophin in myocyte sarcolemma
• **Loeffler endocarditis (acute phase)/endomyocardial fibrosis:** degranulated eosinophilic endomyocardial infiltrates and endomyocardial thrombosis with evidence of endocardial fibrous thickening and subendocardial myocyte abnormalities
• **Cardiac tumors:** cellular evidence of tumor pathology
• **Cardiac allografts:** acute cellular rejection, antibody-mediated rejection, post-transplant lymphoproliferative disease, unusual infections (toxoplasma gondii, cytomegalovirus inclusion bodies)
Probable diagnosis can be made:
• **"Toxic" myocardial disease (anthracycline)/hypersensitivity disease:** eosinophilic myocarditis, and myocyte degeneration with intra-mitochondrial inclusion bodies
• **Anderson-Fabry disease:** hypertrophic vaculated cells with dislocation of contractile elements to the periphery of myocytes
• **Mitochondrial cardiomyopathies:** morphologically altered mitochondria noted on electron microscopy
• **Glycogen storage diseases (Pompe, Cori, Andersen, Danon disease):** diffuse intracellular glycogen deposits
• **Arrhythmogenic right ventricular cardiomyopathy:** fibrous or fibro-fatty replacement and myocardial atrophy from biopsy of the right ventricular outflow tract
Possible diagnosis:
• **Hypertrophic cardiomyopathy:** myocyte hypertrophy, perhaps myocyte disarray, interstitial, or substitutive fibrosis
• **Idiopathic dilated cardiomyopathy:** myocyte hypertrophy, nuclear alterations, perinuclear halo with/without fibrosis
• **Idiopathic restrictive cardiomyopathy:** normal myocardium, and/or fibrosis, and/or disarray
• **Laminopathies (lamin A/C):** interstitial/replacement fibrosis, myocyte hypertrophy and vacuolization, enlarged and irregular-shaped nuclei

of cardiac masses, and assessment of cardiac transplant allograft rejection. **Table 34-2** summarizes the diagnostic potential for endomyocardial biopsy as outlined in the 2011 consensus statement,[16] pointing out when definite, probably, and possible diagnoses can be achieved.

A different approach was taken by the 2007 endomyocardial biopsy scientific statement from the AHA/ACC/and European Society of Cardiology (ESC).[15] It was much more specific with respect to the procedure's role in fourteen clinical scenarios that were crafted to characterize the most common patient presentations clinicians might face while considering endomyocardial biopsy in any particular circumstance. The consensus statement included the "level of recommendation" and "level of evidence" supporting the class of recommendation. This statement utilized the usual AHA/ACC approach to this with a Class I recommendation, meaning there is evidence or general agreement that a procedure is beneficial, useful, and effective, while a Class II indication is based on conflicting evidence or a divergence of opinion about the usefulness of a procedure, and further subdivided into Class II-A where the weight of evidence is in favor of usefulness and Class II-B where support for a procedure's usefulness is less well established. A Class III recommendation suggests there is evidence or general agreement that a procedure is not useful and may even be harmful. Level A evidence provides the highest and least controversial data and is generally obtained from multiple randomized clinical trials. Level B evidence generally comes from limited numbers of randomized trials, nonrandomized studies, and registries whereas the lowest level of evidence (LOE), Level C, has been pejoratively termed "expert opinion."

One can juxtapose the 2007 scientific statement with the 2011 one, based on the clinical scenarios presented, to see where consensus is consistent among professional organizations.[15,16] The most solid evidence and highest class of recommendation for utilizing endomyocardial biopsy from the 2007 scientific statement is new onset of heart failure of less than 2 weeks' duration associated with a normal-sized or dilated left ventricle and hemodynamic compromise, which received a Class I recommendation with an LOE assigned B. This recommendation Class and LOE also was assigned to patients with new onset heart failure of 2 weeks' to 3 months' duration associated with a dilated left ventricle and new ventricular arrhythmias, second- or third-degree heart block, or failure to respond to usual care within 1 to 2 weeks. Of course, when making a decision about proceeding to endomyocardial biopsy, the clinician should weigh the risks and benefits of the procedure in light of information guiding the practitioner to a definitive diagnosis, which can then influence treatment plans. Subsequent scenarios getting a II-A recommendation but rating only "expert opinion" (Class C LOE) includes patients with heart failure of greater than 3 months' duration associated with a dilated left ventricle and new ventricular arrhythmia, second- or third-degree heart block, or failure to respond to usual care within 1 to 2 weeks. Heart failure associated with a dilated cardiomyopathy of any duration that is seen in an individual with suspected allergic reaction and/or eosinophilia, heart failure associated with suspected anthrocycline cardiomyopathy, heart failure with unexplained restrictive cardiomyopathy, suspected cardiac tumors, and unexplained cardiomyopathy in children fall into this recommendation class and LOE as well. A Class II-B recommendation, where there is evidence, or general agreement, that endomyocardial biopsy is not useful and, in some cases, may be harmful, includes individuals with the new onset of heart failure of 2 weeks to 3 months' duration associated with a dilated left ventricle, without new ventricular arrhythmias or second- or third-degree heart block, who respond to usual care within 1 to 2 weeks, or heart failure of greater than 3 months' duration associated with a dilated ventricle without new ventricular arrhythmias or second- or third-degree heart block that responds to care within 1 to 2 weeks. Additionally, heart failure associated with unexplained hypertrophic cardiomyopathy, suspected arrhythmogenic right ventricular dysplasia, and patients with unexplained ventricular arrhythmias also fall into the II-B category. A Class III recommendation, indicating there was general agreement that the procedure was not useful, was put forth for those patients with unexplained atrial fibrillation. One of the obvious problems with making "clinical scenario-based recommendations" of this sort is the imprecise time course determinations that are included in the recommendation. The concept of driving decision making by a presentation of less than or more than "3 months" or "2 weeks to 3 months" seems arbitrary, however.

Giving a different perspective on the utility of endomyocardial biopsy in diagnosing cardiac disease, the 2011 consensus statement lists several specific disease processes with a "definite" diagnostic potential (**Table 34-2**). The majority of diagnostic challenges occur in patients where a "definitive diagnosis" can be made but requires tissue that has pathognomonic findings of a disease that may be distributed unevenly in the myocardium and therefore prone to sampling error when biopsy specimens are obtained.

On the other hand, cardiac allograft rejection is more diffuse and, therefore, endomyocardial biopsy, particularly when done serially over time, becomes attractive. Data obtained from these tissue specimens allow staging of rejection severity in addition to making a diagnosis. Other pathology that can be noted on heart biopsies from cardiac allografts include post-transplant lymphoproliferative disease and some opportunistic infections that can trouble an immunocompromised patient. In addition to routine tissue staining, CD4 immunohistochemical and immunofluorescence stains for antibody-mediated rejection, as opposed to lymphocytic or cell-mediated rejection, should be done. Sometimes, however, severe myocardial dysfunction is noted with pathologically unremarkable endomyocardial biopsy findings and this creates a perplexing situation.[25] At the present time serial endomyocardial biopsy in the heart transplant recipient remains the best and most valued method of following these patients for allograft rejection.

Cardiac amyloidosis can definitively be diagnosed when amyloid infiltration plus histomorphological findings of extracellular space expansion and collagen fiber deposition is noted. Cytoplasmic vacuolization and reduced myofibrils are also seen. Congo-red, modified sulfated alcian-blue, or thioflavin-T stains are recommended while immunomicroscopy, protein sequencing, or mass spectrometry to establish the type of amyloid is required.[16] Recently, great strides have been taken with the application of CMR imaging to the diagnosis and prognosis of amyloid heart disease and this procedure might replace routine endomyocardial biopsy in patients with heart failure due to restrictive myocardial disease.[23,32-36] Though echocardiography can give insight into the possible presence of cardiac amyloidosis, it is not sensitive or specific enough to solely rely on. Unfortunately, CMR cannot be done in everyone suspected of having cardiac amyloidosis because of the frequent use of pacemakers and defibrillators in this population. Furthermore, as Kwong and Jerosch-Herold point out, much more work must be done to characterize the precise parameters to make the diagnosis, determine amyloid subtype, and allow prognostication.[36]

A definitive diagnosis of cardiac sarcoidosis can be made when noncaseous granulomatous myocarditis is noted. The problem with making this diagnosis is the spotty or patchy infiltration of the heart that is characteristic of cardiac sarcoidosis. Biopsies not sampling regions infiltrated by granuloma will not allow the diagnosis to be made.[20] Some have suggested that computerized tomographic or CMR imaging in conjunction with echocardiography can define areas of wall motion abnormality that should attract interest of the operator who, theoretically, can guide the bioptome into these zones.[21,22] The reality of this occurring on a regular basis is, however, limited.

When tissue is removed in the zone of a cardiac tumor, a definite diagnosis can be made. Sometimes immunohistochemical stains can be useful for tumor typing. As with sarcoidosis, it is difficult to direct the bioptome precisely to the location of a suspected tumor. Operators should be cautioned about biopsying sessile masses in the heart as these might be thrombus formation and there is risk of embolization. Masses having the appearance of a myxoma are generally very difficult to biopsy with currently available bioptomes.

A definitive diagnosis of desmin cardiomyopathy can be made based on ultrastructural findings, which includes an abnormal granulofilamentous aggregation of desmin-type intermediate filaments in the cytoplasm of the cardiomyocytes and the Z-Band. Electron microscopy is necessary as is immunoelectron microscopy to confirm that these aggregates are formed by desmin.

The absence of dystrophin in myocyte sarcolemma will make a definitive diagnosis of Duchenne muscular dystrophy while the extensive irregularities and discontinuities of dystrophin in the myocyte sarcolemma provide support for a diagnosis of Becker muscular dystrophy. Immunohistochemical staining and immunofluorescent studies are required. Of course, the clinical diagnoses of these syndromes are paramount.

Cardiac iron overload can be definitively determined by noting intracellular iron deposition with iron staining procedures. It is recommended that iron staining routinely be done for all endomyocardial biopsy specimens from patients with unexplained dilated cardiomyopathy undergoing this procedure.

Loeffler endocarditis can be definitively diagnosed in the acute phase when endomyocardial eosinophilic infiltration and endocardial fibrosis are noted. A possible diagnosis in the chronic phase is supported by the finding of endocardial fibrous thickening and subendocardial myocyte abnormalities. Timing of the biopsy is linked to the diagnostic probability, with biopsy utility decreasing over the course of time in this situation.

Inflammatory cardiomyopathy can be definitively diagnosed when lymphocytic, granulocytic, polymorphous, eosinophilic, necrotizing eosinophilic, giant cell, and granulomatous formation is observed with or without associated myocyte necrosis or damage.[27] The diagnostic criteria and classification for myocarditis are summarized in **Table 34-3**. The so-called "Dallas Criteria" was developed in 1986 for the Myocarditis Treatment Trial and not linked to more sophisticated immunohistochemical studies or "viral footprint" tracking. There is substantial inter-observer and intra-observer variability in making the diagnosis when using the Dallas criteria. Furthermore, patients treated in the Myocarditis Treatment Trial based on endomyocardial biopsy data and this diagnostic scheme fared no better than those not getting immunosuppressive drugs.[37] Timing of the endomyocardial biopsy in the course of the disease may have impacted diagnostic sensitivity and specificity. Still, the Dallas Criteria remains in use for the diagnosis of inflammatory cardiomyopathy.

Those conditions where endomyocardial biopsy can make a "probable" diagnosis include Anderson-Fabry disease, which is likely present if hypertrophic vacuolated cells with dislocation of contractile elements to the periphery of myocytes are noted. Electron microscopic study should be done to assess electron dense concentric lamellar bodies to assist with the diagnosis.

Arrhythmogenic right ventricular cardiomyopathy is probably present when fibrous or fibro-fatty replacement and myocardial atrophy are noted in the right ventricular outflow tract. Unfortunately, endomyocardial biopsies from

TABLE 34-3 "Dallas" Criteria and Classification for the Pathologic Diagnosis of Myocarditis

Definition: Inflammatory infiltrate of the myocardium with necrosis and/or degeneration of adjacent myocytes not typical of the ischemic damage associated with coronary artery disease

Dallas criteria and classification:

- First biopsy
  - Myocarditis with/without fibrosis
  - Borderline myocarditis
  - No myocarditis
- Subsequent biopsy
  - Ongoing (persistent) myocarditis with or without fibrosis
  - Resolving (healing) myocarditis with or without fibrosis
  - Resolved (healed) myocarditis with or without fibrosis
- Descriptions
  - Inflammatory infiltrate
    - Distribution—focal, confluent, diffuse
    - Extent—mild, moderate, severe
    - Type—lymphocytic, eosinophilic, granulomatous, giant cell, neutrophilic, mixed
  - Fibrosis
    - Distribution—endocardial, interstitial
    - Extent—mild, moderate, severe
    - Type—perivascular, replacement

Problems:

- Substantial interobserver/intraobserver variability during specimen review
- Sampling error possible because of patchy infiltrates
- Variance with other viral and immune activation markers
- Patient outcomes not improved with therapies studied in the myocarditis treatment trial
- Criteria unlikely sensitive enough to adequately identify patients with viral-mediated disease
- Criteria (developed in 1986 for the myocarditis treatment trial) not linked to more sophisticated immunohistochemical studies or "viral footprint" tracking developed subsequently

the interventricular septum may not be informative as the pathologic findings tend to be in the outflow tract, which is generally a thin-walled and, therefore, dangerous zone to biopsy.

A probable diagnosis of drug-induced "toxic" myocardial disease can be seen with hypersensitivity myocarditis or findings of excessive anthracycline exposure manifest by characteristic electron microscopic study. Indeed, electron microscopy is essential for making the diagnosis of anthracycline cardiomyopathy.

A probable diagnosis can be made of glycogen storage diseases including Pompe disease (type II glycogenoses), Cori disease (type III glycogenoses), Anderson disease (type V glycogenoses), and Dannon disease when diffuse intracellular glycogen storage abnormalities are noted. Electron microscopy and histochemical stains are useful to assess the type of intracellular deposits observed.

In mitochondrial cardiomyopathies morphologically altered mitochondria noted on electron microscopic evaluation often with enlarged myocytes and extensive cytoplasmic vacuolization suggest the diagnosis of a mitochondrial cardiomyopathy.

For "laminopathies" interstitial fibrotic replacement noted on an endomyocardial biopsy specimen accompanied by myocyte hypertrophy and vacuolization with enlarged and irregular-shaped nuclei are helpful.

"Possible" diagnoses can be made in hypertrophic cardiomyopathy where myocyte hypertrophy, interstitial fibrosis, so-called myocyte disarray, and small vessel disease can be noted. Idiopathic restrictive cardiomyopathy can be

TABLE 34-4 Restrictive Cardiomyopathy Where Endomyocardial Biopsy Might Provide Clinical Insight

Myocardial disease

- **Infiltrative cardiomyopathies**: amyloidosis,* fatty infiltration,* Gaucher's disease,* Hurler's disease, sarcoidosis*
- **Noninfiltrative cardiomyopathies**: diabetic, familial hypertrophic, idiopathic, pseudoxanthoma elasticum, scleroderma
- **Other**: hemochromatosis,* Fabrey's disease, glycogen storage disease*

Endomyocardial disease

- **Syndromes**: endomyocardial fibrosis,* hypereosinophilic syndrome,* carcinoid heart disease, metastatic tumors,* radiation, toxic effects of anthracycline*
- **Drugs causing fibrous endocarditis**: busulfan, ergotamine, mercurial agents, methysergide, serotonin

Leone O, Veinot JP, Angelini A, et al: 2011 Consensus statement on endomyocardial biopsy from the Association for European Cardiovascular Pathology and the Society for Cardiovascular Pathology. Cadiovasc Pathol 21:245–275, 2012.

*Biopsy can provide definite diagnosis based on 2011 Consensus Statement on Endomyocardial Biopsy from the Association for European Cardiovascular Pathology and the Society for Cardiovascular Pathology.

suggested when hemodynamic findings of restriction are present but the myocyte is normal in the presence of interstitial fibrosis. Making a precise diagnosis in the setting of restrictive myocardial disease can be difficult and **Table 34-4** summarizes situations where endomyocardial biopsy can provide clinical insight. Idiopathic dilated cardiomyopathy is associated with myocyte hypertrophy, nuclear alterations, perinuclear halo, and often, but not always, significant fibrosis. The findings in hypertrophic cardiomyopathy, idiopathic restrictive cardiomyopathy, and idiopathic dilated cardiomyopathy are nonspecific and routine endomyocardial biopsy is not routinely performed in these patients.

UTILITY OF ENDOMYOCARDIAL BIOPSY IN CARDIAC TRANSPLANT ALLOGRAFTS

The International Society for Heart and Lung Transplantation adapted in 1990 a scheme for diagnosing and staging acute cell-mediated rejection after heart transplant. The most recent revision of the grading scheme was in 2004.[25] These staging criteria have become internationally adopted by the heart transplant community and assist with day-to-day patient management as well as investigations into immunosuppression strategies. For acute cellular rejection, when no cellular infiltration is noted, Grade 0 is assigned. Grade 1R is characterized as "mild" acute cellular rejection and is diagnosed by interstitial and/or perivascular inflammatory infiltrates with up to one focus of myocyte damage. Grade 2R or "moderate" rejection is when two or more foci of inflammatory infiltrates associated with myocyte damage are seen, with Grade 3R being "severe" acute cellular rejection and reflecting diffuse inflammatory infiltrates with multifocal myocyte damage and/or edema, hemorrhage, and vasculitis. Antibody-mediated rejection is currently classed as Grade 0 when immunohistochemical stains are negative, or Grade 1 when stains are positive and histologic features of myocardial capillary injury (endothelial swelling and intravascular macrophages), interstitial edema and hemorrhage, neutrophils in and around the capillaries, intravascular thrombi, and myocyte necrosis are noted. Immunofluorescence or immunoperoxidase staining for antibody-mediated rejection should include immunoglobulin stains

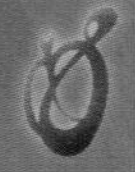

(IGG, IGM, and/or IGA), and compliment (C3D, C4D, and/or C1Q) deposition on cells and capillaries or macrophages (CD68) in capillaries, and compliment (C4D) deposition on capillary endothelium by immunohistochemistry.

"Nonrejection" post-transplant myocardial injury can also be noted on endomyocardial biopsy. Indeed, so-called "chronic" allograft rejection, basically small vessel atherosclerotic disease that undoubtedly reflects long-term perturbation of the immunologic situation, can cause ischemic injury. Early perioperative ischemic injury can also be noted on the first postoperative biopsy caused by cold preservation storage required during donor organ retrieval. A mixed inflammatory infiltrate of neutrophils, lymphocytes, macrophages, and eosinophils may present a challenge in distinguishing this particular process from acute cellular rejection. Late ischemic injury can be suggested by observation of small vessel arteriolar occlusion observation and substantial scarring in territories believed to be ischemic. One unusual finding has been called the "Quilty" effect, named after the first heart transplant patient at Stanford University with this finding.[25] The effect is an intense focus of endocardial infiltrate that has a nodular quality extending some into the underlying myocardium with or without significant myocyte damage. This endocardial infiltrate often is associated with prominent vascularity and an intense lymphocytic beehive appearance. The relationship of the Quilty effect to substantial pathologic difficulties, if any, after heart transplant is not clear.

EXPERT PRACTICE SUMMARY

Endomyocardial biopsy can be a valuable diagnostic procedure. Endomyocardial biopsy can cause egregious complications and even death. Its utility focuses on the evaluation of myocardial tissue, particularly for monitoring patients after cardiac transplantation. In the proper setting, it is helpful while trying to make a diagnosis of inflammatory heart disease, cardiac drug toxicity, unexplained or cryptogenic cardiomyopathies, certain arrhythmias, secondary myocardial involvement in systemic diseases, and for the diagnosis of cardiac masses or myocardial tumor infiltration. Many disease states can be definitively diagnosed, particularly cardiac allograft rejection, myocarditis, and some infiltrative as well as "myocardial storage" diseases. Because of the focal nature of some diseases such as sarcoidosis, it is less helpful when biopsy findings pathognomonic of the disease are absent. To best manage patients with amyloidosis, hemochromatosis, Anderson-Fabrey disease, and myocarditis, endomyocardial biopsy information is essential. Though multimodal cardiac imaging is gaining greater respect with regard to diagnosing several difficulties, having tissue for pathologic evaluation still seems preferable. **Table 34-5** summarizes data from a creative clinical study that examines the clinical study that examines the clinical utility of endomyocardial biopsy by relating the number of biopsies that were pathologically diagnostic and altered management strategies in 851 nonheart transplant patients who were categorized according the 14 clinical scenarios outlined in the ACC/AHA Scientific Statement regarding the role of endomyocardial biopsy.[20] The study confirmed the fact that the procedure was generally safe and, overall, provided a specific diagnosis and influenced alteration in medical management plans about 26% of the time. Diagnostic success rates ranged from 0% (in unexplained atrial fibrillation patients) to 50% (in suspected anthracycline toxicity patients) while the range for biopsy result-driven alteration of medical management was 11% (new onset of dilated cardiomyopathy without arrhythmia) to 38% (again in suspected anthracyclinie toxicity patients).

TABLE 34-5 Diagnostic Yield and "Clinical Utility" of Endomyocardial Biopsies in 851 Nonheart Transplant Patient Scenarios

CLINICAL SCENARIO	% BIOPSY DIAGNOSTIC	% BIOPSY-ALTERED MANAGEMENT
Suspected anthracycline toxicity (24)	50	38
Acute HF w/ HYD compromise (109)	39	28
DCM with "allergic reaction" suspected (9)	33	33
"Restrictive" CM (286)	29	26
Unexplained HCM (28)	25	29
Unexplained ventricular arrhyth (8)	25	13
Suspected ARVD (62)	24	39
Suspected cardiac tumor (4)	25	25
New DCM, arrhyth, poor response (29)	21	28
Chronic DCM, arrhyth, poor response (26)	19	12
Unexplained pediatric CM (29)	17	26
Stable chronic DCM, no arrhyth (134)	16	13
New onset DCM, no arrthyth (100)	14	11
Unexplained atrial fibrillation (3)	0	
OVERALL (851 total cases)	26	26

Modified from Bennett MK, Gilotra NA, Harrignton C, et al: Evaluation of endomyocardial biopsy in 851 patients with unexplained heart failure from 2000-2009. Circ Heart Failure 6:676–684, 2013.
arrhyth, Arrhythmia; *CM,* cardiomyopathy; *D,* dilated; *HF,* heart failure; *HYD,* hemodynamic compromise.

CONCLUSIONS

Though endomyocardial biopsy procedures have evolved dramatically over time and, relatively speaking, are safe, major complications and rarely death occur during, or shortly after, the procedure. Long-term adverse sequelae of repeated biopsies, particularly in patients after heart transplantation, are noted and operators must be sensitive to that fact, particularly the clinical scenario of deteriorating right ventricular function in a setting of substantive tricuspid valve insufficiency. Endomyocardial biopsy is not a procedure "looking for an indication," but wisdom must guide its application and performance in carefully selected patients and be done by experienced operators having adequate infrastructure for procedure performance and, equally important, tissue evaluation.

References

1. McManus BM: *Atlas of Cardiovascular Pathology for the Clinician*, ed 2, New York, 2008, Springer.
2. Melvin KR, Mason JW: Endomyocardial biopsy: it's history, techniques and current indications. *Can Med Assoc J* 126:1381–1386, 1982.
3. Brock R, Milstein BB, Ross DN: Percutaneous left ventricular puncture in the assessment of aortic stenosis. *Arch Surg* 76:825–829, 1958.

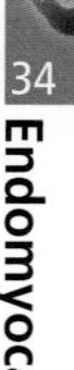

4. Weinberg M, Fell EH, Lynfield J: Diagnostic biopsy of the pericardium and myocardium. *AMA Arch Surg* 76:825–829, 1958.
5. Sutton DC, Sutton GC, Kent G: Needle biopsy of the human ventricular myocardium. *Q Bull Northwest Univ Med Sch* 30:212, 1969.
6. Sakakibara S, Konno S: Endomyocardial biopsy. *Jpn Heart J* 3:537–543, 1962.
7. Konno S, Sekiguchi M, Sakakibara S: Catheter biopsy of the heart. *Radiol Clin North Am* 3:491–510, 1971.
8. Caves PK, Stinson EB, Billingham M, et al: Percutaneous transvenous endomyocardial biopsy in human heart recipients. *Ann Thorac Surg* 16:325–336, 1973.
9. Mackay EH, Littler WA, Sleight P: Critical assessment of diagnostic value of endomyocardial biopsy. *Br Heart J* 40:69–78, 1978.
10. Shirey EK, Proudfit WL, Hawk WA: Primary myocardial disease: correlation with clinical findings, angiographic and biopsy diagnosis. *Am Heart J* 99:198–207, 1980.
11. Scholten Surgical Instruments, Inc. <http://bioptome.com> accessed 2/13/2014.
12. Richardson PJ: King's endomyocardial bioptome. *Lancet* 303:660–661, 1974.
13. Fowler NO: Classification and differential diagnosis of the myocardiopathies. *Prog Cardiovasc Dis* 7:1–16, 1964.
14. Yancy CW, Jessup M, Bozkurt B, et al: 213 ACCF/AHA Guideline for the management of heart failure: a report of the American College of Cardiology Foundation/American Heart Association Task Force on Practice Guidelines. *Circulation* 128:e240–e327, 2013.
15. Cooper LT, Baughman KL, Feldman AM, et al: The role of endomyocardial biopsy in the management of cardiovascular disease: a scientific statement from the American Heart Association, the American College of Cardiology, and the European Society of Cardiology. *Circulation* 116:2216–2233, 2007.
16. Leone O, Veinot JP, Angelini A, et al: 2011 Consensus statement on endomyocardial biopsy from the Association for European Cardiovascular Pathology and the Society for Cardiovascular Pathology. *Cadiovasc Pathol* 21:245–275, 2012.
17. Keenan SP: Use of ultrasound to place central lines. *J Crit Care* 17:126–137, 2002.
18. Miller LW, Labovitz AJ, McBride LA, et al: Echocardiography guided endomyocardial biopsy: a 5-year experience. *Circulation* 78(Pt 2):III99–III104, 1988.
19. Jang SY, Cho Y, Song JH, et al: Complication rate of transfemoral endomyocardial biopsy with fluoroscopic and two-dimensional echocardiographic guidance: a 10 year experience of 228 consecutive procedures. *J Korean Med Sci* 28:1323–1328, 2013.
20. Bennett MK, Gilotra NA, Harrignton C, et al: Evaluation of endomyocardial biopsy in 851 patients with unexplained heart failure from 2000-2009. *Circ Heart Fail* 6:676–684, 2013.
21. Patel MR, Cawley PJ, Heitner JF, et al: Detection of myocardial damage in patients with sarcoidosis. *Circulation* 120:1969–1977, 2009.
22. Blankstein R, Osborne M, Naya M, et al: Cardiac positron emission tomography enhances prognostic assessments of patients with suspected cardiac sarcoidosis. *J Am Coll Cardiol* 63:329–336, 2014.
23. Aljaroudi WA, Desai MY, Tang WH, et al: Role of imaging in the diagnosis and management of patients with cardiac amyloidosis: state of the art review and focus on emerging nuclear techniques. *J Nucl Cardiol* 21:271–283, 2014.
24. Aaron M, Maleszewski JJ, Rihal CS: Current status of endomyocardial biopsy. *Mayo Clin Proc* 86:1095–1102, 2011.
25. Writing Committee for the International Society of Heart and Lung Transplantation: Guidelines for the care of heart transplant recipients. *J Heart Lung Transplant* 29:914–956, 2010.
26. Chimenti C, Frustaci A: Contribution and risks of left ventricular endomyocardial biopsy in patients with cardiomyopathies. *Circulation* 128:1531–1541, 2013.
27. Basso C, Calabrese F, Angelini A, et al: Classification and histological, immunohistochemical, and molecular diagnosis of inflammatory myocardial disease. *Heart Fail Rev* 18:673–681, 2013.
28. Kindermann I, Barth C, Mahford F, et al: Update on myocarditis. *J Am Coll Cardiol* 59:779–792, 2012.
29. Mason JW: Basic research on myocarditis. *J Am Coll Cardiol* 19:1746–1747, 2013.
30. Hazebrock MR, Everaerts K, Heymans S: Diagnostic approach of myocarditis: strike the golden mean. *Neth Heart J* 22:80–84, 2014. published on line 08 January 2014.
31. Baughman KL: Diagnosis of myocarditis: death of the dallas criteria. *Circulation* 113:593–595, 2006.
32. Dungu JN, Valencia O, Pinney JH, et al: CMR-based differentiation of AL and ATTR cardiac amyloidosis. *JACC Cardiovasc Imaging* 7:133–142, 2014.
33. White JA, Kim HW, Shah D, et al: CMR imaging with rapid visual T1 assessment predicts mortality in patients suspected of cardiac amyloidosis. *JACC Cardiovasc Imaging* 7:143–156, 2014.
34. Fontana M, Banypersad MB, Treible TA, et al: Native T1 mapping in transthyretin amyloidosis. *JACC Cardiovasc Imaging* 7:157–165, 2014.
35. Kwong RY, Jerosch-Herold M: CMR and amyloid cardiomyopathy. Are we getting closer to the biology? *JACC Cardiovasc Imaging* 7:166–168, 2014.
36. Hahn EA, Artz VL, Moon TE, et al: The myocarditis treatment trial: design methods and patient enrollment. *Eur Heart J* 16(Suppl O):162–167, 1995.
37. Mason JW, O'Connell JB, Herskowitz A, et al: A clinical trial of immunosuppressive therapy for myocarditis. *N Engl J Med* 333:269–275, 1995.

Pericardiocentesis and Pericardial Intervention

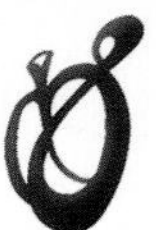

Ronan Margey and Igor F. Palacios

INTRODUCTION

Pericardial disease reflects a wide range of clinical presentations and pathologies, from acute pericarditis to cardiac tamponade. Unlike coronary artery disease, heart failure, or valvular heart disease, however, there are few randomized clinical trial data to guide physicians and interventionalists in its management. There are currently no American College of Cardiology guidelines on management of pericardial disease, with only European Society of Cardiology guidelines available to aid in the diagnosis and management of these conditions.[1]

The clinical presentations of pericardial effusions are variable, with some patients being completely asymptomatic while others develop cardiac tamponade and hemodynamic collapse.[2-4] Pericardiocentesis is a catheter-based technique utilizing a needle to aspirate the pericardial fluid, usually under electrocardiographic (EKG), fluoroscopic, and/or echocardiographic guidance. Percutaneous balloon pericardiotomy is a relatively novel catheter-based technique that offers patients a less invasive technique than conventional surgical pericardial window to relieve recurrent pericardial effusions or malignant effusions. Improvements in the technique to access the pericardial space, and the concomitant use of pericardioscopy, have led to the development of a number of novel interventional techniques over the past two decades to perform a number of procedures: from percutaneous biopsy of the percardium, to epicardial electrophysiological ablation procedures, and most recently, percutaneous ligation of the left atrial appendage as a method of stroke prevention in individuals with permanent atrial fibrillation in whom anticoagulation is contraindicated.

These pericardial techniques, their indications and supporting clinical evidence, and procedural complications will be discussed in detail in this chapter.

THE NORMAL PERICARDIUM

The pericardium is a relatively avascular fibroelastic sac that surrounds the heart and is composed of two layers: a visceral and a parietal layer separated by a potential space containing 15 mL to 35 mL of straw-colored serous fluid.[3] The visceral pericardium is composed of a single layer of mesothelial cells adherent to the myocardial surface. The parietal pericardium is a fibrous structure composed primarily of collagen and a lesser amount of elastin.

As a result of its fibrous inelastic qualities, the normal pericardium has a relatively steep pressure-volume curve. It is distensible when the intrapericardial volume is small but becomes gradually inextensible when the volume increases. In the presence of a pericardial effusion, the intrapericardial pressure depends on the relationship between the absolute volume of the effusion, the speed of accumulation of the

TABLE 35-1 Causes of Pericardial Effusion

INFECTIOUS	NEOPLASTIC	INFLAMMATORY	METABOLIC AND MISCELLANEOUS
Viral: coxsackievirus, echovirus, cytomegalovirus, Epstein-Barr, herpes, varicella, hepatitis	Primary mesothelioma, fibrosarcoma	Acute rheumatic fever	Idiopathic
Bacterial: tuberculosis, staphylococcus, streptococcus, gram-negative bacteria, gonococcus, rickettsia	Metastatic lung cancer, melanoma, breast cancer, lymphoma, leukemia	Rheumatoid arthritis	Myxedema
Fungal: histoplasma, coccidioides, candida, aspergillus, blastomyces, actinomyces		Systemic lupus erythematosus	Uremia
Parasitic infection: entamoeba, echinococcosis toxoplasmosis, trypanosomiasis		Systemic sclerosis	Adverse drug reactions
		Still's disease	Radiation
		Dressler's syndrome	Traumatic
		Other vasculitides	Aortic dissection
		Mixed connective tissue disease	Postcardiac surgery
			Chylopericardium
			Myocardial infarction

fluid, and the intrinsic pericardial elasticity. Therefore, the clinical presentation of pericardial effusion depends not only on the volume of the effusion, but also on the rapidity of fluid accumulation.[5,6]

PERICARDIAL EFFUSION AND TAMPONADE

Pericardial effusion may result from a variety of clinical conditions (see **Table 35-1**). Transudative fluids result from obstruction of fluid drainage through lymphatic channels. Exudative fluids occur secondary to inflammatory, infectious, malignant, or autoimmune processes. The frequency of specific etiologies varies greatly based on geography. In developed countries, both malignancy and infection are the most common causes of pericardial effusion. A pericardial effusion is associated with a known systemic disease in approximately 60% of cases.[7-9]

Pericardial effusions may be asymptomatic or manifest a wide range of clinical symptoms. Patients can report pericarditis-related chest pain, which is typically relieved by sitting up and worsened by lying supine and deep breathing. They may report palpitations most frequently due to atrial arrhythmias. They may manifest generalized symptoms such as dyspnea and cough, presyncope or syncope, dysphagia, abdominal fullness, anxiety, cyanosis, and fever. Large pericardial effusions in the absence of inflammatory signs and symptoms are often neoplastic.[10]

Cardiac tamponade is a life-threatening condition that results from the accumulation of intrapericardial fluid that impairs ventricular diastolic filling.[6] Ultimately, cardiac chambers are compressed and fail to fill when their pressures are exceeded by the intrapericardial pressure. Because of their lower pressures, the right heart chambers are more prone to compression. The intrapericardial pressure depends on the volume of the effusion, the speed of accumulation, and the pericardial elasticity.[11] Rapidly accumulating effusions result in cardiac tamponade at relatively small volumes because the pericardium does not have adequate time to stretch. When effusions accumulate slowly, pericardial compliance gradually increases, allowing the pericardium to accommodate large volumes (as much as 2 to 3 L). Malignancy is the most common cause of pericardial effusion with tamponade (~50%).

In all cases of cardiac tamponade, the initial treatment consists of removing pericardial fluid by prompt pericardiocentesis and drainage.[8] Reaccumulation is common, especially in malignant effusions, and is traditionally an indication for surgical pericardial window. Autopsy and surgical studies have demonstrated myocardial or pericardial metastatic deposits in approximately 50% of patients presenting with malignant effusion-related cardiac tamponade. Although the short-term survival of patients with tamponade depends on its early diagnosis and prompt treatment, long-term survival is dictated by the prognosis of the underlying primary illness, regardless of the surgical technique or interventional procedure performed.[7,12]

CLINICAL DIAGNOSIS OF PERICARDIAL TAMPONADE

Clinical findings suggestive of pericardial tamponade include:

- Beck's triad of tamponade: hypotension, distant heart sounds, jugular venous distention.
- Pulsus paradoxus: A decrease in systolic blood pressure of more than 10 mm Hg with inspiration due to a reduction in cardiac output during inspiration. With inspiration, negative intrathoracic pressures increase venous return and filling of the right-sided chambers. The interventricular septum consequently bows to the left, reducing left ventricular filling and output. This is quantified during the physical examination using a manual sphygmomanometer cuff during normal respirations by listening for Korotkoff sounds. As the cuff pressure is slowly reduced, Korotkoff sounds will initially be intermittent and become continuous with further reduction in the cuff pressure. The difference in the pressure measurement at which Korotkoff sounds are first audible and become continuous define the pulsus.
- Elevated jugular venous pressure with loss of the Y descent of the jugular venous pulse.

A pericardial friction rub is associated with acute pericarditis and can occur with effusions. This high-pitched, scratching sound is best auscultated at the left lower sternal border with the patient leaning forward. A rub typically consists of three components, namely, ventricular systole, ventricular diastole, and atrial systole. Frequently, only one or two of the components are audible. Additionally, the patient may demonstrate tachycardia and tachypnea and have signs of venous congestion with ascites, hepatosplenomegaly, and lower extremity edema.[8]

On the EKG, pericarditis with an effusion may produce typical EKG changes:

- Widespread ST-segment elevation (>25% of the height of the T-wave)
- PR depression (elevation is often seen in lead aVR)
- Low voltage can be indicative of a large pericardial effusion
- Electrical alternans may result as the heart swings within a large pericardial effusion.

INDICATIONS FOR PERICARDIOCENTESIS

Pericardiocentesis is the technique of catheter-based aspiration and drainage of pericardial fluid. It may serve both as a diagnostic and potentially therapeutic procedure in patients with pericarditis with pericardial effusion, chronic pericardial effusion, effusive-constrictive pericardial effusion, and pericardial effusion with cardiac tamponade.

Many asymptomatic large pericardial effusions do not require pericardiocentesis by themselves if they do not produce hemodynamic compromise, unless there is a need to perform fluid analysis to aid diagnosis. The yield of pericardial fluid analysis in determining the cause of pericardial effusion is low. Prospective long-term follow-up of patients with large idiopathic chronic pericardial effusions has demonstrated that these effusions can be well tolerated for long periods in the majority of cases, although the risk of developing tamponade is unpredictable. Although pericardiocentesis may be effective at draining the fluid collection, it frequently reaccumulates. Therefore, in this situation, it is recommended that the patients be considered for early definitive pericardiotomy or pericardial window creation.[10,13,14]

In patients with pretamponade or overt cardiac tamponade, emergency drainage of pericardial fluid is a life-saving therapy, avoiding hemodynamic collapse and cardiac arrest with pulseless electrical activity. In situations of impending circulatory collapse or overt tamponade, pericardiocentesis can be performed blindly using anatomic landmarks, but in more stable circumstances, it is advisable to ultilize EKG, echocardiographic, and fluoroscopic guidance.[3,15]

When performing pericardiocentesis, several objectives should be achieved:

1. Relief of tamponade, if present
2. Obtaining fluid for appropriate diagnostic analysis
3. Assessment of pericardial and right heart hemodynamics before and after fluid drainage to assess for effusive-constrictive pericarditis.

Elective pericardiocentesis is contraindicated in patients receiving systemic anticoagulation, in patients with platelet or bleeding disorders, in patients with a platelet count of less than 50,000/μL, and in suspected hemorrhagic pericardial effusion from acute aortic dissection. Additionally, pericardiocentesis should be performed with caution in persons with organized or loculated pericardial effusions or significant pericardial adhesions from prior surgery. Consideration in these cases should be given to surgical pericardiotomy or pericardioscopic assisted pericardial access.

PERICARDIOCENTESIS TECHNIQUE

Pericardiocentesis is most often performed within the catheterization laboratory under fluoroscopic and electrocardiographic guidance. However, the procedure can also be safely performed at the bedside under echocardiographic guidance and some operators prefer using both fluoroscopy and echocardiography.[15]

The most common approach is subxiphoid, although apical and parasternal approaches are also feasible. The subxiphoid is the safest approach when echocardiographic guidance is not available.

The skin in the subxiphoid area is shaved and sterilized with a topical antiseptic solution. The patient is then draped with an aperture drape sheet. The patient is placed on continuous cardiac and blood pressure monitoring. Prophylactic broad spectrum antimicrobial antibiotics should be administered, using a single intravenous dose of a second or third generation cephalosporin antibiotic or vancomycin if the patient has a penicillin allergy or is colonized with methicillin-resistant *Staphylococcus aureus*.

An electrocardiography (ECG) electrode is attached to a large-bore needle at least 5 cm in length using an alligator clip. Most operators use either a Tuohy spinal needle or Pajunk needle for pericardial access. Pericardiocentesis utilizes the Seldinger technique of catheter insertion.

After administration of local anesthetic, the needle is slowly advanced toward the pericardial space. For the subxiphoid approach, the needle is inserted in the angle between the xiphoid process and the left costal margin and advanced at a 45° angle toward the left shoulder. For the apical approach, echocardiography is often used to identify the spot at which the pericardium is closest to the skin. Alternatively, the needle is inserted 1 cm outside the point of maximal impulse within the intercostal space and directed toward the right shoulder. For the parasternal approach, the needle is inserted immediately adjacent to the sternum, usually in the fifth intercostal space, with care being taken to avoid the vessels coursing along the inferior border of each rib.

Regardless of approach, the needle is slowly advanced with periodic attempts to gently aspirate fluid. While advancing the needle, special attention is given to the attached ECG electrode lead. Elevation of the ST or PR segment is seen when the needle is in direct contact with the myocardium. Atrial or ventricular ectopic beats can also be seen. If this occurs, slow withdrawal of the needle until ECG changes resolve should position the needle tip within the pericardial space.

A discrete pop is often felt upon entering the pericardial space. Once the pericardial space is entered, contrast or agitated saline injection can confirm needle position using either fluoroscopy or echocardiography, respectively (**Figure 35-1** and Video 35-1). This is especially recommended if hemorrhagic fluid is obtained. Alternatively, the aspirate can be injected into a cup. Pericardial fluid, even when hemorrhagic, will not clot, whereas intracardiac blood will.

A stiff guidewire is introduced into the pericardial space through the needle. A dilator is used to dilate the soft tissue

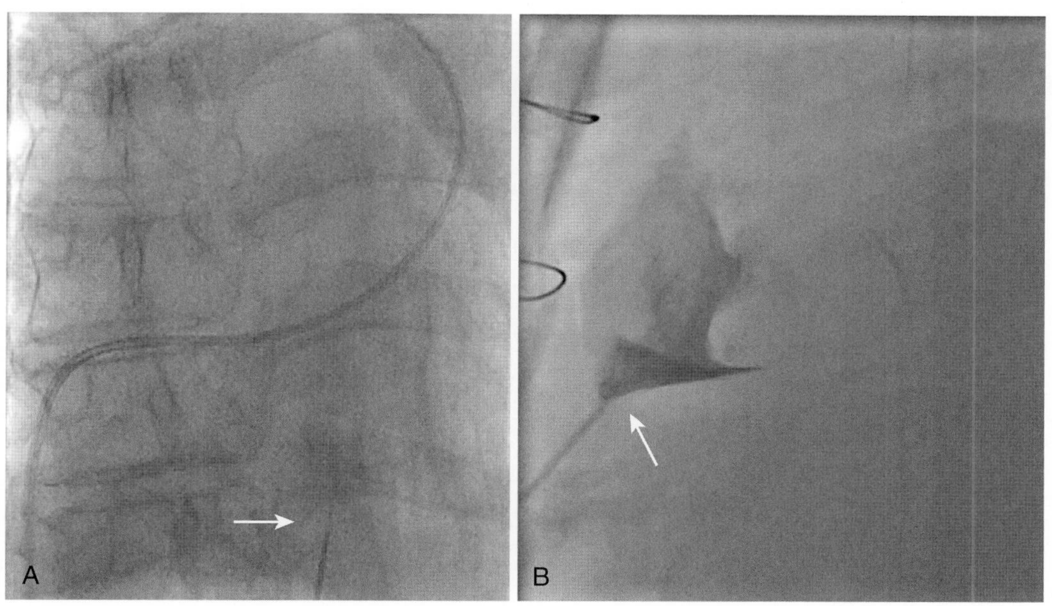

FIGURE 35-1 **Subxiphoid needle access for pericardiocentesis. A** and **B,** Anteroposterior and lateral projections of needle access to the pericardial space. Contrast injection through the access needle can be used to confirm successful pericardial space access on fluoroscopy *(arrows)*. Alternatively, agitated saline can be injected and visualized on echocardiography.

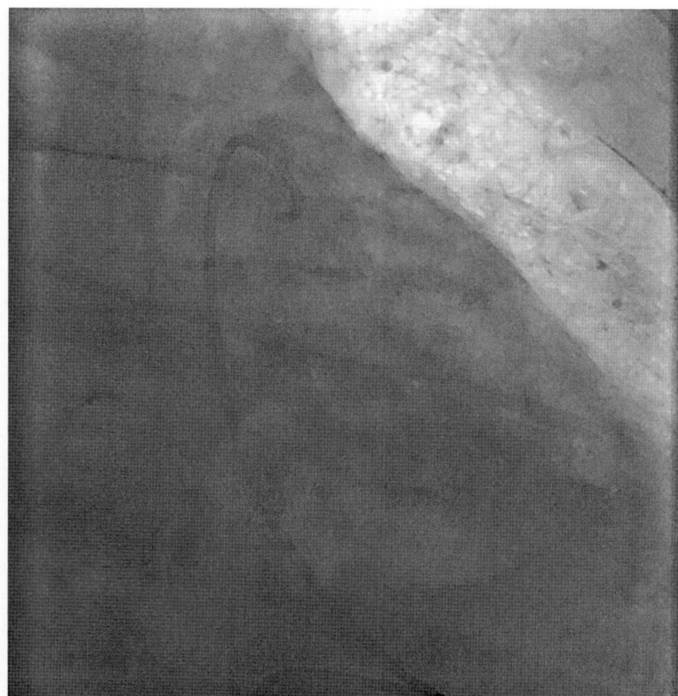

FIGURE 35-2 **Successful placement of a pigtail pericardial drainage catheter.**

tract and a pigtail pericardial drainage catheter is then inserted over the stiff guidewire (**Figure 35-2**). In the catheterization laboratory, the intrapericardial pressures should then be documented by transducing the pericardial catheter. Additionally, radiographic contrast material can be injected through the catheter to confirm position and freedom within the pericardial space.

The pericardial fluid is then drained. **Table 35-2** outlines the basic biochemical, microbiologic, and pathologic analyses pericardial fluid should be tested for. Once complete, pericardial pressures are often reassessed to document the degree of improvement. The pericardial catheter is often left in place to allow for continuous drainage or as a route to allow percutaneous pericardial window creation and/or instillation of sclerosing or chemotherapeutic agents. In this situation, the catheter is sutured in place and a sterile dressing applied.

Echocardiographic-guided pericardiocentesis is a safe and effective alternative to conventional EKG and fluoroscopic guidance. In a case series of 1127 therapeutic echo-guided pericardiocentesis procedures performed in 977 patients at the Mayo Clinic from 1979 to 1998, the procedural success rate was 97%, with an overall complication rate of 4.7%. Echocardiography guidance is particularly useful in organized loculated effusions and often utilizes a left anterior chest wall approach rather than the conventional subxiphoid approach.[3]

POSTPERICARDIOCENTESIS CATHETER MANAGEMENT

Pericardiocentesis may not completely remove the effusion in most cases, and therefore it is not unusual for the drainage catheter to be kept in place for 24 hours to 72 hours following the procedure.

Attempts to drain the pericardium should continue until <50 cc of fluid is drained within a 24-hour period. However, the catheter should be removed as soon as possible in order to minimize the risk of infection within the pericardial space.

The patient is usually maintained on continuous cardiac monitoring and the volume and rate of catheter drainage are recorded. The pericardial catheter can be drained by gravity continuously or alternatively drained manually using sterile technique every 4 to 8 hours. Heparinized saline (2 to 3 cc) should be instilled into the catheter after each drainage attempt. Follow-up echocardiography can be

TABLE 35-2 Pericardial Fluid Analysis: Typical Biochemical, Microbiologic and Pathologic Testing of Pericardial Fluid

BIOCHEMISTRY	EXUDATIVE EFFUSION IS CHARACTERIZED BY	MICROBIOLOGY	PATHOLOGY	SPECIALIZED TEST
Total protein	Total protein fluid : serum >0.5	Gram stain	Fluid cytology	Viral PCR
Glucose	LDH: fluid : serum >0.6 and/or LDH >300 U/dL	Aerobic and anaerobic cultures	Fluid immunohistochemistry	TB PCR
Specific gravity	LDH fluid level >two thirds the upper limit of normal serum level	Acid fast bacilli staining		Adenosine deaminase
LDH	Glucose: fluid : serum <1	Tuberculous cultures		Tumor markers
Fluid hematocrit	Specific gravity >1.015	Viral cultures		
Cell count	Total protein >3.0 mg/dL			

LDH, Lactic acid dehydrogenase; *PCR,* polymerase chain reaction.

useful to determine resolution of the collection. Intravenous antibiotics are given while the drain remains in place for prophylaxis against pericardial infection. It is our institutional practice to administer cefotaxime 1 gram every 8 hours or vancomycin 500 to 1000 mg every 12 hours if the patient has a penicillin allergy or methicillin-resistant *Staphylococcus aureus* colonization.

Patients who continue to drain more than 75 to 100 mL daily 3 days after catheter placement or who reaccumulate with recurrence of tamponade should be considered for additional therapeutic strategies including intrapericardial sclerosing or chemotherapy agents, radiotherapy, percutaneous balloon pericardial window (as outlined below), and surgical pericardial window.

COMPLICATIONS OF PERICARDIOCENTESIS

While pericardiocentesis can be performed safely, there is the potential to traumatize surrounding structures, perforate cardiac chambers, and lacerate coronary arteries or veins.

Most often, cardiac perforation involves the right ventricle when using the subxiphoid approach for pericardiocentesis. Bleeding from a right ventricular puncture is often not severe due to the chamber's relatively low pressures. However, the thin right ventricular wall is vulnerable to laceration, which frequently leads to substantial bleeding. This is especially possible in patients with pulmonary arterial hypertension and right ventricular dysfunction.

Ectopic atrial or ventricular beats may occur when the pericardiocentesis needle is in direct contact or perforates the myocardium. Sustained arrhythmias are also possible, although less common.

Coronary arterial injury or spasm can occur also. The right coronary artery is most frequently perforated or lacerated during the subxiphoid approach. The left anterior descending artery and its branches can similarly be injured during apical pericardiocentesis. The internal mammary artery and inferior phrenic arteries are prone to injury during the parasternal and subxiphoid approaches, respectively.

Acute pulmonary edema can occur rarely when the pericardial effusion is decompressed too rapidly. Pneumothorax from puncture of the left pleura and lingula has also been described. Pneumopericardium can occur from introduction of air at the time of catheter placement. Additionally, it may be possible to cause a systemic air embolism if air is introduced into a cardiac chamber inadvertently. Injury to intercostal, internal mammary, or phrenic arteries may result in hemothorax. Needle perforation of the inferior vena cava, liver, stomach, and colon have all been described.

MALIGNANT, RECURRENT, OR PERSISTENTLY DRAINING PERICARDIAL EFFUSIONS

The management of chronic or recurrent pericardial effusions represents a challenge for both interventional cardiologists and cardiac surgeons due to the general moribund state of patients with this condition. In the industrialized world, chronic or recurrent pericardial effusions are most likely malignant (25% to 50% of cases depending on case series) or infectious (27%).[7,10,16]

Cancers that commonly cause malignant pericardial effusions in decreasing frequency include lung carcinoma, breast carcinoma, lymphoma or leukemia, pancreatic carcinoma, ovarian carcinoma, carcinoma of unknown primary, and melanoma. Primary pericardial tumors such as fibrosarcomas or mesotheliomas are rare.

Autopsy series of patients with a preexisting diagnosis of malignancy demonstrate pericardial metastatic involvement in up to 15% to 30%. However, only about 20% of patients with malignant pericardial disease present with effusion, and in up to two thirds, the pericardial effusion can be due to other nonmalignant mechanisms.

Malignancy can result in pericardial effusion by a number of mechanisms: direct invasion, metastasis from distant primary cancers, lymphatic obstruction, chemotherapy- or radiation-induced toxicities (such as cyclophosphamide-induced myopericarditis or radiation-induced effusive-constrictive pericarditis) or opportunistic infection from chemotherapy-induced immunosuppression (such as tuberculous, fungal, or cytomegalovirus [CMV] pericarditis).

Following catheter drainage as described above, malignancy-related pericardial effusion will reaccumulate in 15% to 50% of cases. Additionally, malignant effusions will recur in approximately 5% of patients after surgical subxiphoid pericardial windowing. Neither treatment has been demonstrated to reduce mortality (determined by the underlying malignancy).[10,12,17]

Persistent pericardial drainage is defined as >100 mL/24 hour drainage 3 days following pericardial catheter placement. Guidelines recommend more aggressive therapy for patients with persistent drainage or reaccumulation, including chemotherapeutic or sclerosant agents, percutaneous balloon pericardiotomy, or surgical pericardiotomy. (level of evidence B; class of recommendation IIb.)[1]

Systemic chemotherapy or radiation therapy following catheter drainage has been shown to prevent reaccumulation in malignant effusions, reducing reaccumulation rates to approximately 30% to 40%.

Intrapericardial chemotherapeutic or sclerosant agents have also been used. A number of agents have been used including tetracyclines, bleomycin, cisplatinum, nitrogen mustard, fluorouracil, teniposide, and thiopeta with varying morbidities and success rates. One reported advantage of intrapericardial therapy is that it avoids spread of malignant cells into other body cavities as can occur with surgical or percutaneous approaches. Overall, however, reaccumulation rates in malignancy remain disappointing at 40%.[10]

Three surgical approaches to malignant effusion have been described: (1) subxiphoid pericardial window, (2) thoracotomy with creation of a pleuropericardial window, and (3) thoracotomy with pericardiectomy. Surgery has the additional advantage of allowing tissue to be obtained for diagnostic purposes. However, surgical window procedures while successful, have reported reaccumulation rates of up to 15% depending on the technique, and substantial morbidity (30%) and mortality (up to 13.8%). Patients with advanced malignancy are often poor candidates for general anesthesia and surgery. In addition, malnutrition and chemotherapy-related side effects increase the risk of infection and other perioperative complications.[14]

Finally, overall prognosis is poor in this group of patients, with mortality related to the underlying malignancy estimated at 80% in the reported case series, and increasing their length of hospital stay associated with a surgical procedure may compromise the quality of their remaining lifespan.

In 1991 Palacios et al. first proposed percutaneous balloon pericardiotomy under local anesthesia with conscious sedation as a less invasive alternative technique to surgical pericardial window procedures.[18]

TECHNIQUE OF SINGLE BALLOON PERCUTANEOUS BALLOON PERICARDIOTOMY

Patients undergoing percutaneous balloon pericardiotomy should undergo informed consent with discussion of pain and discomfort during the procedure, as well as potential complications including cardiac chamber, coronary artery or cardiac venous injury, pneumothorax, pleural effusion post procedure, arrhythmia, infection, bleeding, need for emergent cardiac surgery, and death.

The patient's preoperative complete blood count, renal profile (contrast administration and platelet dysfunction), and coagulation profile should be checked in advance of the procedure. The patient's most recent transthoracic echocardiogram should be reviewed in detail. Organized or loculated effusions are best managed with surgical pericardial window creation.

Patients typically receive antibiotic prophylaxis with a broad spectrum cephalosporin antibiotic or vancomycin in cases of pencillin allergy or methicillin-resistant *Staphylococcus aureus*.

Percutaneous balloon pericardiotomy (PBP) can be significantly painful during balloon inflation and can produce pericarditis-type chest pain following the procedure.

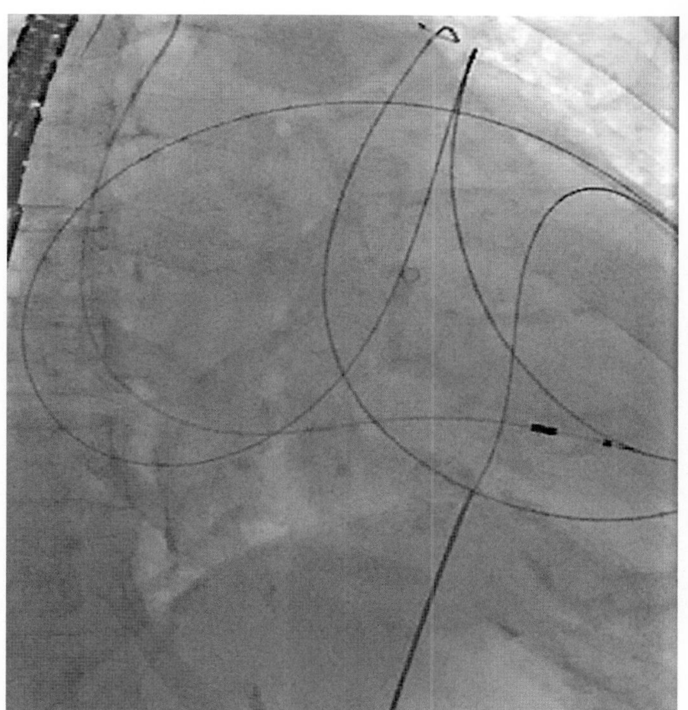

FIGURE 35-3 Successful needle access to the pericardium. This figure highlights the creation of a guidewire loop within the pericardium caused by the guidewire wrapping around the pericardial reflections. This confirms the guidewire is within the pericardial space. If the needle access was inadvertently into a cardiac chamber, there may be ectopy, injury current visible on the EKG, and the guidewire may pass beyond the cardiac border into the pulmonary artery.

Copious local anesthesia to the skin tract as well as generous conscious sedation is recommended.

PBP can be performed in patients with an existing pericardial drainage catheter and ongoing persistent drainage, and de novo for the first time in patients presenting for initial pericardiocentesis. In patients with a preexisting pericardial drainage pigtail catheter, the catheter can be removed over a stiff J-tipped 0.035-inch or 0.038-inch Amplatz guidewire, leaving the guidewire in the pericardial space. As with pericardiocentesis, the guidewire position should be confirmed by forming a loop within the pericardial space (**Figure 35-3**).

The skin tract into the parietal pericardium should be dilated usually up to 10 Fr over the guidewire to allow passage of the dilating balloon catheter. This may cause pain.

Typically a 12- to 20-mm-diameter balloon (Maxi Balloon, Cordis), 3 to 4 cm in length, is advanced over the guidewire to straddle the parietal pericardium. A number of variations on this standard technique have been described, including apical puncture, adjacent side-by-side pericardial balloon placement, double balloon pericardiotomy, Inoue balloon pericardiotomy, and use of a combination of a long and short dilating balloon.[19-24]

It is important to ensure the proximal end of the balloon is within the subcutaneous tissue and not extending through the skin, which can cause extreme discomfort. The optimal balloon position is confirmed by gentle inflation of the balloon to reveal a waist at the location of the parietal pericardium. The balloon is then manually inflated until the waist disappears. We advocate two to three inflations in order to ensure successful PBP (**Figure 35-4**).

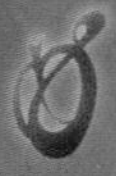

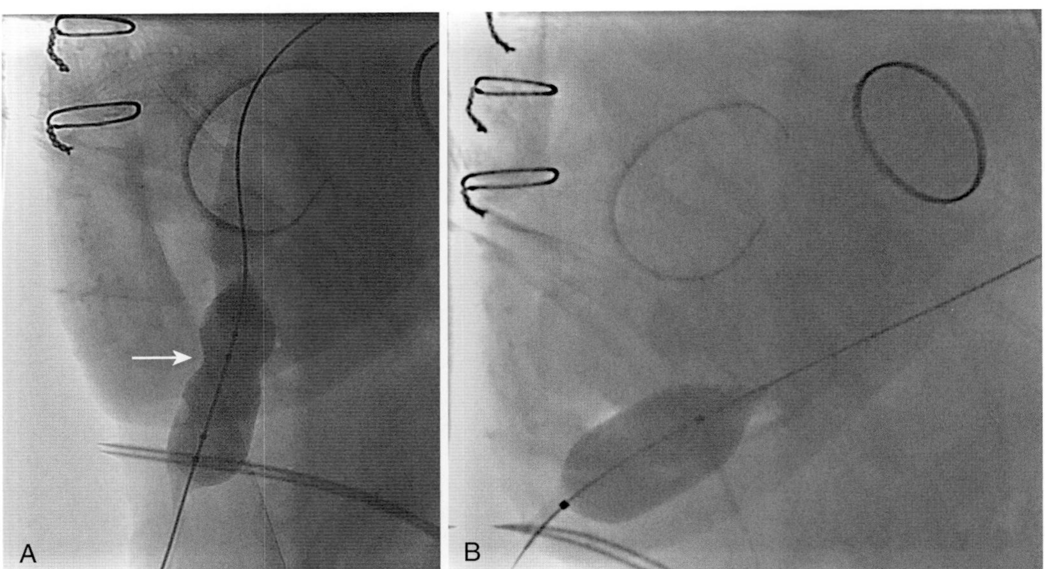

FIGURE 35-4 Percutaneous balloon pericardiotomy using a single balloon technique. A and **B,** Single balloon technique of percutaneous pericardial window creation using a 20 × 40-mm balloon in this case. Note the pericardial outline created by contrast injection into the pericardial space and the residual waist on the balloon *(white arrow)* at the site of the parietal pericardial layer.

Biplane fluoroscopy, if available, should be used to allow fluoroscopic confirmation of the correct positioning of the balloon. If there is difficulty in identifying the parietal pericardium, 5 to 15 mL of radiographic contrast can be injected to identify the pericardial borders. In a left lateral projection, the midpoint of the balloon should be positioned across the parietal pericardial layer.

If the parietal pericardium is adherent to the chest, with failure of proximal balloon inflation, then a countertraction technique can be used to pull the skin and tissue away from the pericardium as the balloon is advanced forward.

After balloon dilatation, the balloon catheter is removed over the stiff 0.035-inch guidewire and replaced with a new pigtail catheter, which is sutured in place.

In the setting of de novo pericardiotomy at the time of pericardiocentesis, the pericardium is entered in standard fashion and a drainage catheter placed to allow pericardial pressure measurement. After confirming the opening pericardial pressure, most of the pericardial fluid is aspirated, although some may be left behind to allow ease of position of the balloon dilatation catheter.

Following PBP, the pericardial catheter should be managed according to the protocol outlined in the pericardiocentesis section. Once there is no significant persistent drainage (<75 to 100 mL/24 hours), the catheter can be removed. Follow-up transthoracic echocardiography should be performed 48 hours after drainage catheter removal. Additionally, chest x-ray imaging should be performed to assess for possible pleural effusion development post PBP drainage.

The mechanism by which PBP works remains unclear. It is assumed that localized tearing of the parietal pericardium produces a communication between the pericardial space and the pleural space and/or the peritoneum. Prior pericardioscopy and radiographic contrast injection analysis have demonstrated a communication between the pericardium and the pleural space.[25] Additionally, Chow et al. showed an oval 18.6 × 16.4-mm window after 23-mm Inoue balloon inflation.[22,26] It is unlikely that a permanent communication persists. It is much more likely that drainage of the pericardial fluid allows the visceral and parietal pericardium to undergo inflammatory fusion.

TECHNIQUE OF DOUBLE BALLOON PERCUTANEOUS BALLOON PERICARDIOTOMY

The double balloon technique has emerged as the preferred strategy for balloon pericardiotomy over recent years. In theory, the double balloon technique creates a larger pericardial window and is better tolerated from a pain perspective than a single large balloon or Inoue balloon. Additionally, balloon rupture is less frequent, removing the risk of the ruptured balloon becoming lodged in the subcutaneous tissues and the possibility of retained balloon fragments.[27]

Again, similar to the single balloon technique, the patient should undergo preprocedural planning with review of the patient's complete blood count, renal profile, and coagulation profile, in addition to review of the patient's echocardiogram. Again, loculated effusions should be avoided.

The procedural complications of bleeding, infection, emergent cardiac surgery, pneumothorax, pneumopericardium, persistent left pleural effusion, hemothorax, cardiac vein and coronary artery injury, and cardiac chamber perforation are similar to both pericardiocentesis and the single balloon technique.

The patient should receive appropriate prophylactic antibiotic coverage as outlined earlier and appropriate periprocedural pain management.

A range of techniques are advocated to access the pericardium. Under EKG, echo, and/or fluoroscopic guidance, a 4 Fr micropuncture needle, Tuohy needle, or Pajunk needle can be used to access the pericardial space. Once the needle tip or tip of the micropuncture sheath is within the pericardial space, agitated saline can be infused and visualized on echocardiography or contrast can be injected to assure correct positioning in the pericardial space.

The skin tract is then serially dilated and ultimately a 7 Fr 13-cm sidearm sheath can be placed into the pericardium.

Following this, two 0.035-inch guidewires are introduced into the pericardial space and their position confirmed on fluoroscopy. The authors advocate using either soft-tipped stiff Amplatz Super or Extra stiff guidewires (Cook Medical, Bloomington, Indiana), or Supracore guidewires (Abbott Vascular, Santa Clara, California).

With both guidewires positioned in the pericardial space, the 7 Fr sheath is removed and replaced with two appropriately sized sheaths to accommodate the balloon diameters to be used. Next, an 8- to 12-mm by 20-mm balloon dilatation catheter is advanced over one of the guidewires while a second 8- to 12-mm by 40-mm balloon dilatation catheter is advanced over the second guidewire.

Under fluoroscopy, the position where the two guidewires begin to separate from each other represents the parietal pericardial layer. The balloons are then advanced sequentially to rest across the parietal pericardial layer.

Following positioning, the balloons are then inflated sequentially. Each balloon should be inflated slowly in order to reposition across the parietal pericardium and to ensure they are free of the subcutaneous space. Then the balloons should be maximally inflated. Both balloons should be inflated fully until the balloon waist disappears. Next, with the longer balloon anchored in position, the inflated shorter balloon should be advanced and retracted across the parietal pericardium several times in order to ensure there is an adequate pericardial window created.

The balloons should then be deflated, removed, and a standard drainage pigtail catheter placed over either guidewire. Depending on operator preference, contrast media may be injected into the pericardial space to document drainage via the newly created pericardial window into the pleural space. The second guidewire can be removed at this point.

The pericardial drainage catheter should be sutured in position until drainage is minimal. The patient should continue on prophylactic antibiotics and should undergo a postprocedure chest x-ray to ensure there is no procedural-induced pneumothorax.

OUTCOMES AFTER PERCUTANEOUS BALLOON PERICARDIOTOMY

Palacios et al. first described their initial experience with PBP in eight patients with malignant effusion/tamponade. Procedural success was 100%. There were no immediate or late complications attributed to the procedure. The mean time to development of a new or significantly increased left pleural effusion was 2.9 ± 0.4 days. The mean follow-up was 6 ± 2 months. No patients had recurrent pericardial effusion or tamponade. However, the prognosis of these patients was poor in keeping with their underlying primary diagnosis, with death occurring in five cases.[18]

A subsequent multicenter registry evaluated the therapeutic role of PBP in 130 patients in 16 centers from 1987 to 1996. Of these, 85% had a known diagnosis of malignancy (majority lung carcinoma), with 58% presenting with cardiac tamponade and had already undergone pericardiocentesis. PBP was defined as success if there was no recurrence of effusion on echocardiography and if there were no procedural complications. A total of 85% (111/130) were successful, with no effusion recurrences during a mean follow-up of 5 months ± 5.8 months. Chest tube placement was required in 15% of patients with preexisting effusions, compared with 9% in patients without a prior effusion. Of the 104 patients with malignancy, 86 died at a mean time of 3.8 ± 3.3 months after PBP. There were no predictors of survival or freedom from effusion reaccumulation.[28]

PBP should be avoided in loculated pericardial effusions as it is unlikely to provide complete drainage. Intrapericardial administration of urokinase or mechanical disruption of fibrinous debris using guidewires and pigtail catheters remains controversial.

Additionally, PBP should be avoided in patients with tenuous pulmonary function as it may result in a significant left pleural effusion further compromising their lung function.

PERCUTANEOUS PERICARDIAL BIOPSY

As outlined in the earlier sections, large pericardial effusion is a common clinical presentation of a number of disease states. The first step toward definitive diagnosis is pericardiocentesis.

Although helpful, pericardiocentesis provides a definitive diagnosis in only about 25% of cases. Tuberculosis is the most commonly missed diagnosis. In malignant pericardial effusions, fluid cytology is positive in 50% to 85% of cases, although cell typing remains limited, albeit improving with immunohistochemical staining. To increase diagnostic yield, pericardial biopsy is often required.

Traditionally, this has required open surgical biopsy under general anesthesia.[16] Percutaneous techniques for obtaining multiple pericardial tissue samples have been described over the past 20 years.

Percutaneous pericardial biopsy was first performed by Endrys et al. in 1988, who reported a series of 18 consecutive patients who needed pericardiocentesis for large pericardial effusion.[29] Using a subxiphoid approach, the authors advanced a 7 Fr Teflon sheath into the pericardial space and drained the pericardial effusion. This sheath was then exchanged for an 8 Fr Teflon sheath with a curved tip and multiple side holes. An endomyocardial bioptome was inserted through the sheath and air was allowed to enter the pericardium to delineate the visceral and parietal pericardium layers. An average of eight separate samples was obtained, with no complications. At the end of the procedure, the air was aspirated and a drainage catheter placed as usual. In 9 of the 18 cases a definitive diagnosis could be obtained from the biopsy specimens.

Mehan et al. noted that the floppy nature of the bioptome made it difficult to direct toward an appropriate target in the pericardial cavity. Therefore, they modified Endrys' technique to use the distal portion of 9 Fr Judkins coronary guiding catheter to target specific sites.[30]

Ziskind et al. subsequently used a similar fluoroscopic approach but used a special pericardial bioptome with a central needle and serrated jaws. They did not instill air into the pericardial cavity, but rather maintained visceral-parietal pericardial separation by not removing all the pericardial fluid at the start of the procedure. In their study of 15 patients, tissue adequate for a diagnosis was obtained in all patients. For patients with a history of malignancy, the addition of biopsy to cytology increased the diagnostic yield from 46%

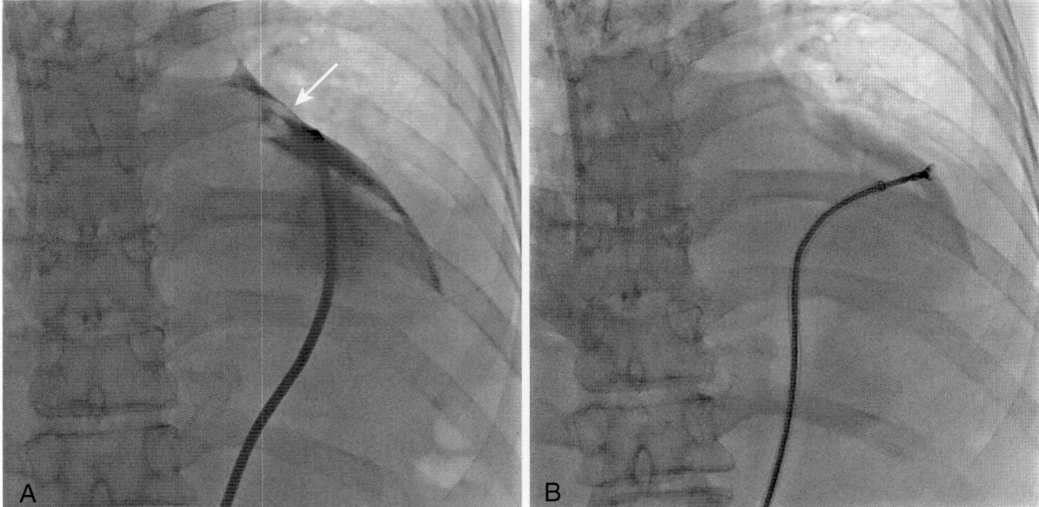

FIGURE 35-5 Percutaneous pericardial biopsy. Panel A depicts contrast injection through the 8 Fr sheath demonstrating the parietal pericardial layer. Panel B depicts the BiPal biopsy forceps placed through the sheath and directed toward the parietal pericardium, away from the cardiac surface.

to 62%.[31] Selig et al. further modified the technique using echocardiographic rather than fluoroscopic guidance for biopsy.[32]

Finally, Margey et al. recently described the outcome of pericardial biopsy in seven consecutive patients presenting with suspected malignant effusion. After drainage of the pericardial fluid under fluoroscopic and EKG guidance, they exchanged the pigtail drainage catheter for an 8 Fr 23-cm braided sheath and subsequently passed a 7 Fr BiPal biopsy forceps (Cordis, Johnson and Johnson, New Jersey) through the sheath and away from the cardiac shadow to the lateral parietal pericardial wall. They obtained a total of five biopsy specimens per procedure without any complications and demonstrated that pericardial biopsy adds incremental diagnostic yield to cytology alone. In this series, biopsy confirmed no malignant invasion in four patients with known malignancy and the presence of lymphocytic and organizing effusive pericarditis in one and two patients, respectively.[33]

Percutaneous pericardial biopsy is therefore a less invasive procedure than surgical pericardial biopsy and may be particularly useful in improving the yield of pericardial fluid analysis, especially in malignant and tuberculosis pericardial disease.

TECHNIQUE OF PERCUTANEOUS PERICARDIAL BIOPSY

Pericardial biopsy can either be performed in the setting of a previously drained pericardial effusion with a pigtail catheter still in place or at the same time as de novo pericardiocentesis.

Standard pericardiocentesis is performed as outlined above. Care is made to ensure that not all of the fluid is drained completely. This is best ascertained on echocardiography or by injection of 5 to 15 cc of radiographic contrast material into the pericardial space.

Adjunctive use of pericardioscopy, outlined below, may help improve the yield of pericardial biopsy by identifying areas of pericardial disease and deposits with direct visualization to target with biopsy.

The pigtail catheter is exchanged over a J-tipped 0.035-inch or 0.038-inch Amplatz Stiff guidewire for a 7 Fr or 8 Fr 23-cm braided sheath. The sheath is advanced into the retrocardiac pericardial space, aspirated, and flushed. Further local installation of radiographic contrast material can be performed to outline the visercal pericardial layer.

Subsequently, a 7 Fr BiPal Cordis bioptome is advanced through the sheath, the jaws opened, and angled by rotation away from the cardiac shadow toward the parietal pericardial layer. Ideally, this is confirmed in two fluoroscopic planes, usually an anteroposterior and lateral projection (**Figure 35-5** and Videos 35-2 and 35-3). Biplane cineangiography capability is useful for this reason. Once the operator is satisfied that the biopsy jaws are not directed toward the visceral pericardial layer, up to five biopsy specimens are obtained.

Following successful biopsy, the guidewire is readvanced through the sheath into the pericardial space and the sheath exchanged for a new drainage pigtail catheter. As outlined above, the pigtail is removed once the total drainage is <75 to 100 cc/24 hours.

While percutaneous pericardial biopsy is less invasive than surgery, it still carries the potential for serious adverse events, particularly when performed without pericardioscopic guidance. If separation of the visceral and parietal pericardial layers cannot be obtained, there is a risk of cardiac laceration or perforation and coronary arterial or venous injury. Additionally, ventricular ectopy, pain, and fever can also occur.

ROLE OF PERICARDIOSCOPY

Seferovic et al. reported their experience on the use of pericardioscopy in conjunction with pericardial biopsy to improve the diagnostic yield of isolated fluoroscopy-guided biopsy.[34] This paper included 49 patients with large pericardial effusion undergoing percutaneous biopsy. In 12 cases, standard fluoroscopy was used to guide biopsy, with 3 to 6 biopsy samples obtained per case. In 22 patients, 4 to 6 biopsies were obtained using pericardioscopy guidance with a 16 Fr flexible endoscope. Finally, in 15 patients, extensive pericardial sampling guided by pericardioscopy was performed, with 18 to 20 samples obtained. Sampling efficiency was significantly better with pericardioscopy versus fluoroscopy (84.9%, 84.2%, vs. 43.7%). Pericardial biopsy in the extensive sampling group had a much higher yield than fluoroscopy alone in establishing etiology (53.3% vs. 8.3%; $p < 0.05$). The addition of the 16 Fr endoscope access port did not result in any complications.

Therefore, direct visualization of the pericardium for pericardial infiltration or disease deposits may help target biopsy to areas of disease while minimizing the risk of iatrogenic injury.

PERCUTANEOUS EPICARDIAL ACCESS FOR ELECTROPHYSIOLOGY STUDIES AND ABLATION

Epicardial scar-related re-entry circuits have been recognized as an important cause of ventricular tachycardia.[35,36] Approximately 30% of all ventricular tachycardia circuits in nonischemic cardiomyopathies, including hypertrophic cardiomyopathy and dilated cardiomyopathy, and 10% to 15% of ventricular tachycardias in ischemic cardiomyopathy arise from an epicardial circuit. In addition, ventricular tachycardia in arrhythmogenic right ventricular cardiomyopathy and Chagas' cardiomyopathy is typically epicardial in origin.[37-39] Catheter-based intervention techniques in the pericardial space have gained traction since the original series published by Sosa et al. in 1996 as a modality to perform electrical mapping and ablation of ventricular tachycardia.[40]

Additionally, epicardial mapping and ablation also have a role in some atrioventricular re-entrant tachycardias; atrial fibrillation (in cases where there is failure to create a transmural lesion by endocardial approaches or if it is not possible to create full isolating encircling lesions around the pulmonary veins due to the pericardial reflections); atrial tachycardia, especially those arising from the left atrial appendage; and inappropriate sinus tachycardia.[36]

A recent multicenter US and separate European registry of epicardial access and ablation reported that epicardial access and ablation are performed in 12% to 17% of all ventricular tachycardia (VT) ablation procedures in tertiary referral centers.[41]

Traditionally, epicardial mapping and ablation have been recommended for cases with prior failed endocardial ablation of ventricular tachycardia or in conditions like Chagas' disease, where the circuit is typically epicardial. However, recently epicardial or a combined endoepicardial approach as a first-line therapy has been recommended in cases where there is an ECG morphology consistent with an epicardial origin, or internal electrocardiograms suggestive of an epicardial circuit, or in circumstances of intracardiac thrombus or a mechanical valve prosthesis that precludes endocardial access.[35,42,43] Recent multicenter registry data have demonstrated a growing confidence with epicardial ablation as a first-line therapy, with 35% of all epicardial mapping and ablation occurring as a first-line treatment, and 65% of cases occurring in patients with prior failed endocardial ablation. Long-term freedom from ventricular tachycardia can be achieved in 70% to 75% of epicardial ablation procedures.[41]

Epicardial access and ablation are usually contraindicated in patients with significant pericardial adhesions from prior cardiac surgery. However, if pericardioscopy or a hybrid surgical subxiphoid pericardial window is performed, then the pericardial adhesions can be divided, and successful epicardial ablation can be performed.[44,45]

TECHNIQUE OF PERICARDIAL ACCESS AND EPICARDIAL MAPPING AND ABLATION

A standard subxiphoid approach is most commonly used to access the pericardial space. Depending on the location of the electroanatomic substrate (inferior scar vs. anterior or lateral scar), either an anterior or inferior (along the diaphragmatic surface) approach with the needle to the pericardial space can be performed.

Typically, either a Tuohy spinal needle with a trochar or a Pajunk needle is used to minimize trauma. Under fluoroscopic and/or echocardiographic guidance, the needle is advanced toward the pericardium. Typically, the operator works from a shallow left anterior oblique (LAO) projection while checking the right anterior oblique (RAO) view intermittently. It is important to puncture over the mid right ventricle to avoid the base of the heart, where the coronary arteries and veins course, and the apex, which would limit catheter manipulation. Single or biplane projections can be used (**Figure 35-6**).

Once a "give" is felt as the needle enters the pericardial space, the needle trochar can be removed and the Luer-Lok syringe with contrast media can be attached. A small injection of contrast is used to demonstrate characteristic layering of fluid within the pericardial space. It is important not to use excessive contrast volumes as this will make the needle tip difficult to visualize during further attempts.

The right ventricle is inadvertently entered in up to 17% of cases. If recognized, it rarely results in bleeding especially if only the needle tip has entered the ventricular wall. However, if not recognized, then in approximately half of cases, there will be substantial pericardial bleeding and possible tamponade.

Once successful access to the pericardial space has been confirmed, the syringe can be removed and a standard 0.032-inch or 0.035-inch Amplatz guidewire can be advanced into the pericardial space. Demonstration of typical guidewire motion, the absence of premature ventricular ectopics, and tracking of the guidewire across both sides of the septum in the LAO projection help to confirm access to the pericardial space.

Laham et al. described a variant of this standard approach in a large animal model of epicardial access. A subxiphoid approach and fluoroscopy guidance, continuous positive pressure of 20 to 30 mm Hg, and saline infusion through the access needle were used to push the right ventricular wall away from the needle's path and create a potential space to puncture into. In their study of this technique in 49 pigs, no adverse events and no right ventricular injury occurred. However, this technique has not been widely adopted in clinical practice.[46]

Once the guidewire position is confirmed, a soft-tip 7 Fr or 8 Fr sheath is usually placed into the pericardial space. Soft-tip sheaths are recommended to avoid traumatic coronary artery or vein injury. Furthermore, some authors recommend that the access sheath should not be left empty in the pericardium to prevent trauma. Either the guidewire or a pigtail catheter can be placed through the sheath into the pericardial space. It is recommended to avoid preformed

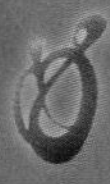

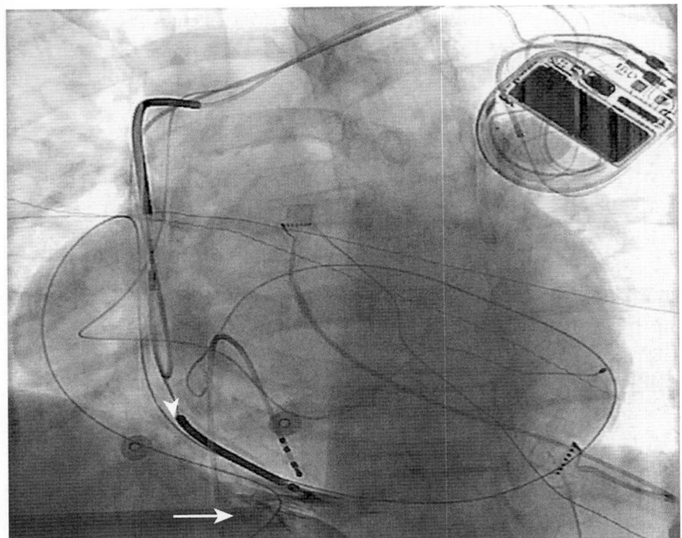

FIGURE 35-6 Pericardial access for epicardial ventricular tachycardia ablation. Note the contrast staining and layering to demarcate the location of the parietal pericardium *(white arrow)*. Also note the J-tipped guidewire coiled within the pericardial reflections *(white arrowhead)*. *(Image courtesy Dr. Edmond Cronin, Electrophysiologist, Hartford Hospital, Hartford, Conn.)*

angled or curved access sheaths, as these are much more likely to result in cardiac trauma or perforation. If directional support is required, then deflectable-tip catheter sheaths such as the Agilis EPI catheter (St. Jude Medical, Minneapolis, Minnesota) can be used.

Electroanatomic mapping can be performed using standard endocardial mapping systems or with a single mapping catheter introduced through the pericardial sheath. Irrigated tip radiofrequency ablation catheters are preferred as they deliver high-power output with less thermal injury. However, because of the continuous irrigation saline infused, the pericardial space should be intermittently drained through the sheath sidearm to prevent fluid accumulation and tamponade. Cryoablation catheters have also been used for epicardial ablation.[47]

Following completion of the ablation procedure, the sheath is usually left in place, with a pigtail catheter remaining in the pericardial space to minimize cardiac trauma. If there is minimal bleeding and no pericardial aspirate following the procedure, it can be removed. Otherwise, it can be left in place for 24 hours to drain any procedural bleeding.

Most operators instill intrapericardial steroid into the pericardial space to minimize sheath and ablation-induced inflammation and pericarditis.[48]

LIMITATIONS AND POTENTIAL COMPLICATIONS OF PERICARDIAL ACCESS AND EPICARDIAL ABLATION

There are some technical limitations of epicardial ablation. It may not be possible to access all of the posterior pericardial space due to pericardial reflections. Even with current endocardial and epicardial approaches and technologies, some ventricular tachycardias arising from the mid-myocardial level may not be possible to ablate. Epicardial fat may attenuate electrocardiogram signals and insulate the underlying muscle, making it impossible to effectively deliver ablation energy to the underlying myocardium.

Some degree of subxiphoid and retrosternal pain and discomfort is ubiquitous; however, 30% of patients will experience pericarditis following epicardial procedures. This may be associated with pericardial effusion or even hemorrhagic pericardial effusion. Intrapericardial injection of steroids has been demonstrated to reduce postprocedural pain and pericarditis.[48]

Major complications have been reported in approximately 5% of cases, with minor complications reported in 7% to 8% of cases. Complications can be related to the pericardial access or to the mapping and ablation procedures.[49]

Major complications include right ventricular perforation and major pericardial bleeding with tamponade. Dry right ventricular perforation from needle access is reported in up to 17% of cases. Right ventricular free wall rupture has also been reported secondary to sheath tip trauma. Other major complications include epicardial bleeding from coronary artery or coronary venous injury requiring emergent surgery, coronary vasospasm and myocardial ischemia, diaphragmatic arterial injury with hemoperitoneum, liver laceration and hepatic hematoma, liver perforation with hemoperitoneum, right ventricular pseudoaneursym, and rarely, right ventricular to peritoneal fistula. Any unexplained intraprocedural hypotension in the absence of pericardial effusion on echocardiography should be investigated further to assess for intrapericardial clot or intraabdominal hemorrhage.

Most operators advocate performing coronary angiography prior to delivery of ablation therapy to ensure there is no risk of coronary arterial injury with ablation. There is also the risk of phrenic nerve injury, and most operators will perform phrenic stimulation testing with high-output pacing via the ablation catheter to ensure no phrenic nerve stimulation prior to delivering energy.

Minor complications include postprocedural pain, drainable hemopericardium, dry right ventricular puncture with no bleeding, and rarely, left bundle branch block or transient complete heart block.

Increasingly, however, epicardial approaches for ablation in the hands of experienced operators has grown in volume and become safer overall.

PERCUTANEOUS PERICARDIAL ACCESS FOR TRANSCATHETER LEFT ATRIAL APPENDAGE LIGATION

Atrial fibrillation (AF) is the most common arrhythmia worldwide, with a current prevalence of over 3 million adults in the United States.[50] An estimated 12 to 16 million Americans will have a diagnosis of AF by 2050.[51] AF carries a significantly increased risk of morbidity and mortality, with embolic stroke being the most severe manifestation.[52,53] In patients with AF, there is a fivefold increased risk of stroke. The risk of stroke attributable to AF increases with age, from 1.5% in persons aged 50 to 59 years old, to 23.5% in persons aged 80 to 89 years old. The annual incidence of stroke in persons with untreated AF is 4.5%.

The left atrial appendage (LAA) is the prominent source of thrombi in AF, accounting for 90% of thrombi observed in persons undergoing cardioversion.[54]

Currently, oral anticoagulation is the most effective treatment option from stroke prevention (Class I, level of evidence A).[55] Unfortunately, only 50% to 60% of patients eligible for warfarin are maintained in the therapeutic window, and there are several drug and dietary interactions with warfarin, making long-term compliance difficult. Novel oral anticoagulant drugs, including dabigatran, apixaban, and rivaroxaban, have demonstrated noninferiority and/or superiority to warfarin in stroke prevention, without the need for regular blood monitoring. However, these agents still pose a risk of hemorrhagic complications, and no antidote or reversal agent is available for these medications.[56]

Those at highest risk of stroke, in whom anticoagulation is most recommended, can be identified using the Congestive Heart Failure, Hypertension, Age >75 years, Diabetes, Stroke,Vascular disease,Age 65 to 74 years, and sex category (CHADS2-Vasc) risk score.[57,58]

While anticoagulation is effective at stroke prevention, it does carry a risk of fatal and nonfatal bleeding complications. The risk of bleeding complications rises with age, and therefore, the patients who will benefit most from stroke prevention are also the patients most likely to experience bleeding complications.

Therefore, alternative methods of stroke prevention are required in patients with bleeding contraindications to anticoagulation or at high risk of bleeding events, such as patients with recurrent syncope and falls. Exclusion of the LAA has therefore emerged as a potential treatment alternative.[59-61]

Surgical exclusion of the LAA has been advocated for patients intolerant of anticoagulation, as part of a surgical MAZE atrial fibrillation ablation, or at the time of concomitant coronary artery bypass surgery or especially in patients undergoing mitral valve surgery. A number of different surgical techniques and devices are available, ranging from simple suture ligation, stapling devices, to minimally invasive thorascopically assisted or robotic assisted epicardial LAA occlusion using the AtriCureatriclip system (AtriCure, Cincinnati, Ohio). However, the rate of successful occlusion is variable, ranging from 60% to 80% success rates, with residual embolic stroke risk. Additionally, surgical ligation is associated with the risk of postoperative bleeding, perioperative stroke, and LAA laceration.

Several percutaneous approaches to LAA exclusion have therefore emerged. There are at least three endovenous transseptal closure devices developed for LAA exclusion at or completed clinical trial evaluation—the Watchman device (Boston Scientific, Natick, Massachusetts), Amplatz Cardiac Plug (St. Jude Medical, Minneapolis, Minnesota), and the PLAATO device (eV3 Medical, Plymouth, Minnesota), which is no longer in production. These devices are effective at occluding the LAA in patients with suitable LAA morphology and are as effective as and safer than long-term anticoagulation with warfarin. However, there are risks of device embolization, device erosion, infection, and thrombus formation on the endovenous side of these devices, which has slowed their widespread adoption.

In 2009, Bartus et al. published the description of a novel endocardial and epicardial approach to suture-mediated LAA exclusion in 26 dogs.[62] The device effectively closed the LAA in 100% of cases. This device, the LARIAT percutaneous suture ligation of the LAA (SentreHeart, Redwood, California), received Food and Drug Administration (FDA) approval for soft tissue closure and is currently marketed for LAA exclusion. It has been evaluated in a large single center observational study consisting of 119 patients assessing the efficacy of the LAA closure and procedural safety. Due to anatomic contraindications or intracardiac thrombus, only 85 patients received the LAA exclusion device. Of these, 96% of LAA ligations resulted in complete LAA closure, with the remaining cases having less than 2-mm leak on echocardiographic follow-up at 1 year.[63,64]

PREPROCEDURAL CONSIDERATIONS

As this procedure requires access to the anterior pericardial space, patients with pectus excavatum, pericardial adhesions and scarring from prior cardiac surgery, radiation, or inflammatory pericardial disease cannot undergo this procedure.

All patients undergo cardiac computed tomography (CT) angiography of the heart and LAA with three-dimensional reconstructions of the appendage. This is helpful to define the shape and size of the appendage. If the width of the appendage is greater than 40 mm, then the device will not be able to pass over the LAA body to ligate its neck or ostium. A larger device for LAA up to 50 mm may be available in the near future. Additionally, the CT helps to identify the orientation of the appendage—a superiorly oriented appendage with the LAA apex directed behind the pulmonary trunk is a contraindication to this technique. Last, bilobed or multilobed LAA in which the lobes are oriented in different planes exceeding 40 mm is also not eligible for this device.

Finally, the preprocedural CT scan helps the interventionalist determine the orientation of the LAA and therefore how lateral or anterior the guide sheath needs to be in order to have the most direct line approach to the distal end of the appendage to position the suture at the LAA ostium. Additionally, the CTA helps to identify the true deepest apex of the LAA in order to position the LAA endovascular guidewire as optimally as possible.

Preprocedural and intraprocedural transesophageal echocardiography is not only useful in assessing closure effectiveness but also, most importantly, in checking for intracardiac and LAA thrombus before embarking on closure. The presence of intracardiac thrombus is a contraindication to the procedure.

TECHNIQUE OF PERCUTANEOUS TRANSPERICARDIAL LEFT ATRIAL APPENDAGE EXCLUSION

In the majority of institutions, the procedure is performed in the cardiac catheterization laboratory under general anesthesia with transesophageal echocardiography guidance. Single-plane or biplane fluoroscopy can be used.

The patient should receive broad spectrum antibiotic prophylaxis with a second or third generation cephalosporin or with vancomycin in cases of penicillin allergy or methicillin-resistant *Staphylococcus aureus*. The patient should discontinue anticoagulation in advance of the procedure.

The LARIAT device consists of three components:

1. A 15-mm to 20-mm compliant occlusion balloon, EndoCath balloon
2. 0.025-inch and 0.035-inch magnet-tipped guidewires (FindrWIRE)
3. A 12 Fr to 14 Fr suture delivery device (LARIAT) with the snare

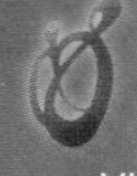

The procedure involves four basic steps:

1. Pericardial and transseptal access
2. Placement of the endocardial magnet-tipped guidewire in the apex of the LAA with balloon identification of the LAA ostium
3. Connection of the epicardial and endocardial magnet-tipped guidewires for stabilization of the LAA
4. Snare capture of the LAA with closure confirmation and release of the pretied suture

The technique of pericardial access is similar to that described earlier. Using either a Tuohy spinal needle or a Pajunk needle, from a standard subxiphoid approach, under fluoroscopic guidance, the needle is advanced toward the pericardium. It is essential the anterior pericardium is accessed. Right ventricular angiography can be performed to help identify the right ventricle border as a landmark. Small injections of contrast through the needle can be administered to see typical layering of contrast when the pericardium is entered. Anteroposterior and lateral fluoroscopic projections can be used to help aid visualization. After accessing the pericardial space, a standard 0.035-inch Amplatz guidewire is advanced into the space and confirmed on fluoroscopy. Over this guidewire, the skin tract is dilated and a 6 Fr sheath can be placed. A second guidewire can then be introduced and left as a precaution in case urgent pericardial drainage is required (**Figure 35-7** and Video 35-4). At this point, the 12 Fr to 14 Fr Softip delivery guiding catheter can be advanced over the guidewire into the pericardial space. Transeosphageal echocardiography should be used to confirm location and to assess for effusion or RV compression by the sheath.

Following this, transseptal puncture under transeosphageal echocardiography guidance is performed and access to the left atrium is established. The ideal location to cross the fossa for this procedure is slightly more posterior and superior than usual. Once access to the left atrium is established, the patient should be heparinized with an activate clotting time (ACT) goal of greater than 250 seconds. An SL-1 sheath can be used to direct anteriorly toward the LAA, and with a pigtail catheter, a left atriogram is performed. This is typically performed in an RAO projection to help identify the ostium and the body of the LAA (**Figure 35-8** and Videos 35-5 and 35-6).

Once left atrial access has been obtained, the 0.025-inch FindrWIRE (SentreHeart Inc., Redwood, California) with a small curve for steerability is backloaded into the EndoCath (SentreHeart Inc., Redwood, California) balloon catheter. They are both manipulated to the apex of the LAA under fluoroscopic guidance. The FindrWIRE should be advanced into the distalmost aspect of the LAA, and the proximal balloon marker should be placed just distal to the coronary sinus and circumflex coronary.

The 0.035-inch FindrWIRE magnet-tipped guidewire is then inserted into the pericardial sheath and advanced to the endocardial guidewire in the LAA apex in all form a pathway for the LARIAT snare delivery.

Once the wires have been connected, the LARIAT is placed over the epicardial guidewire (**Figure 35-9** and Video 35-7). The LARIAT is advanced toward the LAA, and the snare is opened and advanced over the LAA. The distal snare loop of the LARIAT should align with the proximal balloon marker. The balloon is inflated with a 50:50 mixture of contrast and saline. Transesophageal echocardiography is then used to identify the origin of the LAA. The LARIAT snare is then closed completely. A repeat atriogram and transesophageal echocardiogram are used to confirm closure and correct snare placement (**Figure 35-10** and Video 35-8).

The 0.025-inch FindrWIRE is then withdrawn into the tip of the balloon. The balloon is deflated and both the EndoCATH and the FindrWIRE are withdrawn as a single unit.

Once placement is satisfactory, the LARIAT suture is released and tightened until resistance is met. Two final tightenings are then performed with a suture-tension force gauge, the TenSURE device (SentreHeart, Redwood, California).

Both transesophageal echocardiography and left atriograms in an RAO and LAO projection can be performed to assess closure. Once the LAA is completely excluded, the red suture-release tab is cut and withdrawn over the LAA with snare completely open. Both the LARIAT delivery system and the 0.035-inch FindrWIRE are removed from the

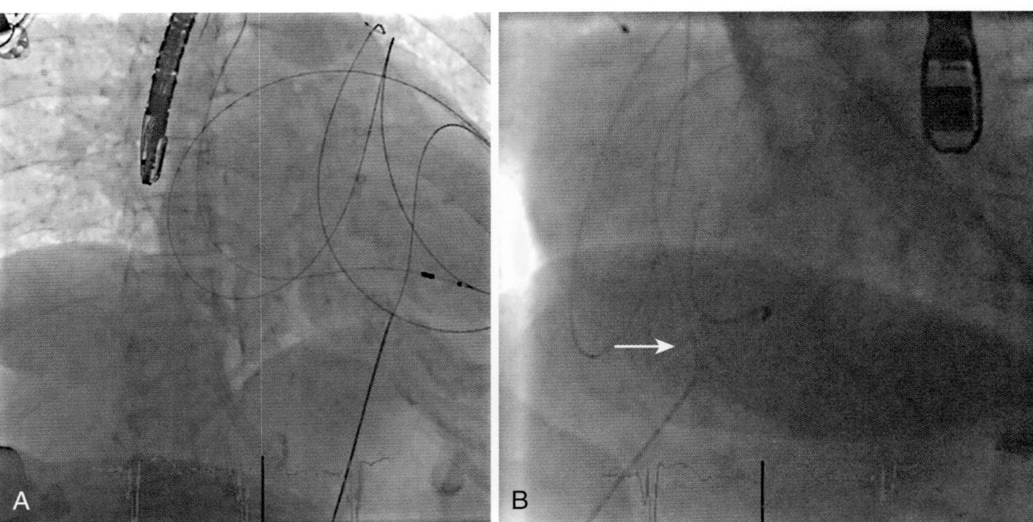

FIGURE 35-7 Percutaneous pericardial left atrial appendage occlusion—importance of location of needle access to the pericardium. A and **B**, The two panels depict successful needle access to the pericardium, with coiling of the guidewire within the pericardial space. Note the anterior location and trajectory of the access *(white arrow)*. This helps to direct the epicardial delivery sheath and, ultimately, the snare delivery system to the left atrial appendage.

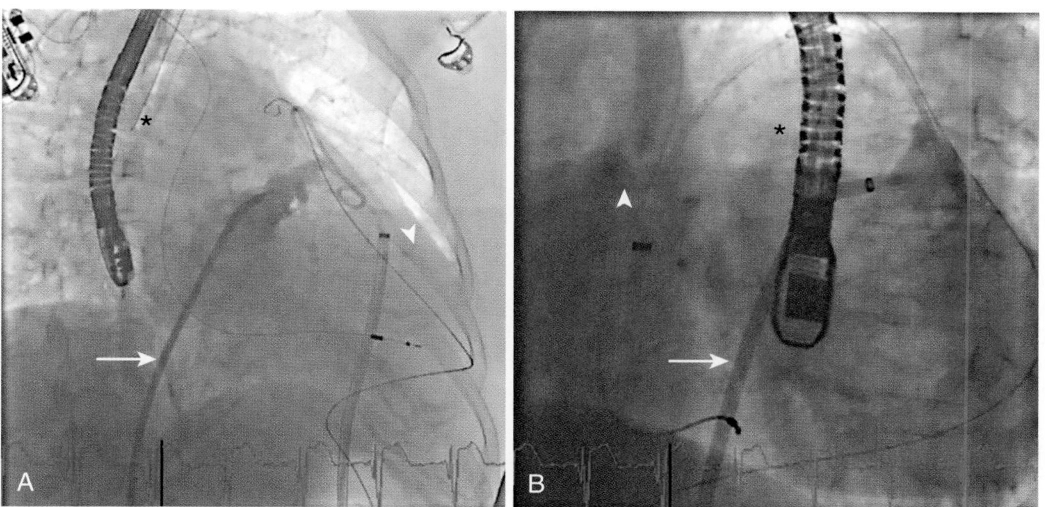

FIGURE 35-8 Percutaneous pericardial left atrial appendage occlusion—baseline left atriography. A demonstrates a right anterior oblique projection and **B** demonstrates a left anterior oblique projection. Note the transseptal SL-1 sheath *(white arrow)* placed at the ostium of the left atrial appendage. Note also the softip guiding sheath of the LARIAT delivery system in the pericardial space *(white arrowheads)*. Note that there is a pigtail catheter within this to minimize the risk of iatrogenic trauma to a coronary vessel. The procedure is usually performed under transesophageal guidance *(asterisk)*. Last, note that there is a second guidewire within the pericardium in case of emergency complications to facilitate prompt pericardial drainage.

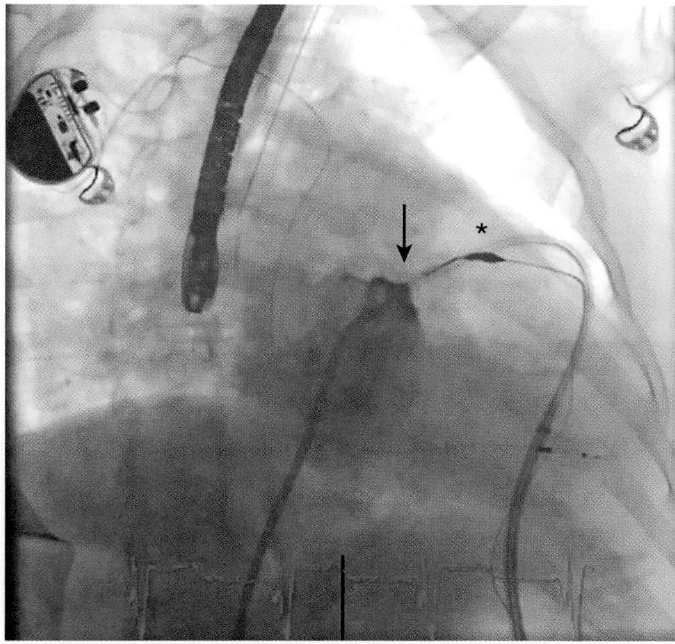

FIGURE 35-9 Percutaneous pericardial left atrial appendage occlusion—successful guidewire connection and advancement of the LARIAT snare device over the base of the left atrial appendage. After the 0.025-inch and the 0.035 magnetized FindrWIRE guidewires are connected at the apex of the LAA *(asterisk)*, the Soft-tip LARIAT delivery system and snare are advanced over the guidewires and slid over the inflated EndoCATH balloon to ensure capture of the true LAA ostium *(white arrow)*. Left atriography can be used to help identify the correct positioning of the delivery system. *LAA,* Left atrial appendage.

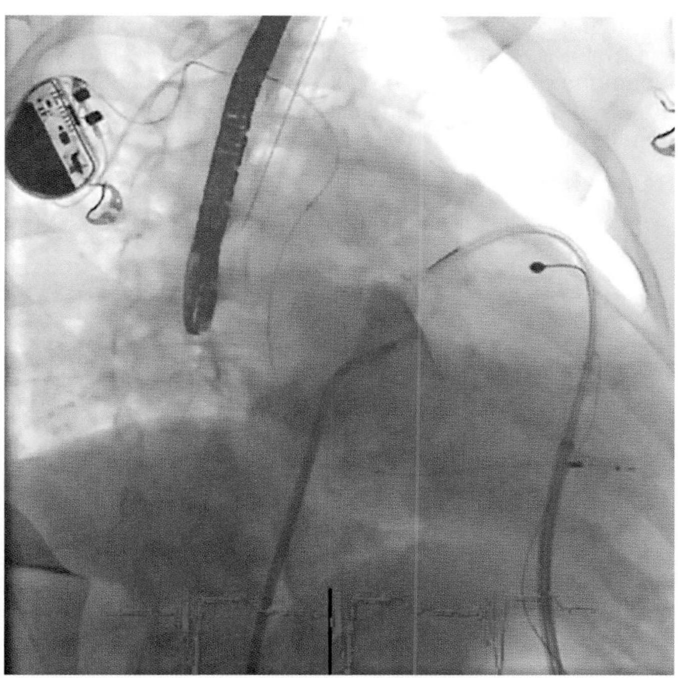

FIGURE 35-10 Percutaneous pericardial left atrial appendage occlusion—successful deployment of the LARIAT snare with completion left atriography. After confirmation of satisfactory positioning on fluoroscopy, atriography, and transesophageal echocardiography, the suture device is tightened and the snare delivery system is disconnected and withdrawn out of the pericardium.

guiding cannula, and the remnant suture tail is cut with a remote suture cutter.

Most centers advocate leaving a pericardial drainage catheter in place for at least 6 hours. If there is no drainage at that point, it can be removed safely. If there was inadvertent RV injury or evidence of hemorrhagic effusion, the catheter should remain in place. It is common for patients to develop pericarditis and pericarditis-related pericardial effusion. Intrapericardial steroids in addition to regular nonsteroidal anti-inflammatories can be used. Follow-up transesophageal echocardiography is recommended at 1 and 6 months as there are case reports of thrombus formation within small residual LAA leaks.

PROCEDURAL COMPLICATIONS

The most common procedural side effect is intense pericarditis, which is reported in up to 30% of patients undergoing

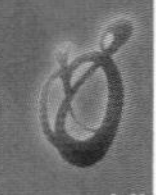

the procedure. This can result in pericarditis-related pericardial effusion. There are rare reports of effusive-constrictive pericarditis after the procedure.[63,64] As with any pericardial access technique, there is the potential to injure cardiac chambers, coronary arteries, and cardiac veins, resulting in hemorrhagic effusion, tamponade, and emergent cardiac surgery. With epicardial access there is the risk of diaphragmatic arterial, hepatic, or inferior vena cava puncture and bleeding. There is also the risk of lacerating the LAA, requiring emergent cardiac surgery. Last, there are isolated reports of persistent LAA leak after LARIAT closure requiring endocardial device occlusion and reports of thrombus formation on the surface of the ligated LAA, usually if there is a small residual pocket.[65-70]

CONCLUSIONS

In the course of the past two decades, transpericardial access and interventional techniques, both in structural heart disease and electrophysiology, have rapidly evolved and established themselves in the mainstream. In the future, use of the pericardial route to access the heart will continue to develop with local drug delivery, pacemaker lead delivery for cardiac resynchronization therapy, intrapericardial echocardiography, and further developments in epicardial electrophysiology and structural interventions.[71,72] The basic technique of accessing the pericardium, which all interventionalists should be familiar and comfortable with, will remain unchanged.

References

1. Maisch B, Seferovic PM, Ristic AD, et al: Guidelines on the diagnosis and management of pericardial diseases executive summary; the task force on the diagnosis and management of pericardial diseases of the European Society of Cardiology. *Eur Heart J* 25(7):587–610, 2004.
2. Hoit BD: Management of effusive and constrictive pericardial heart disease. *Circulation* 105(25):2939–2942, 2002.
3. Jneid H, Maree A, Palacios I: Pericardial tamponade: clinical presentation, diagnosis and catheter-based therapies. In Parillo J, Dellinger P, editors: *Critical Care Medicine*, ed 3, Philadelphia, 2008, Elsevier.
4. Little WC, Freeman GL: Pericardial disease. *Circulation* 113(12):1622–1632, 2006.
5. Reddy PS, Curtiss EI, O'Toole JD, et al: Cardiac tamponade: hemodynamic observations in man. *Circulation* 58(2):265–272, 1978.
6. Roy CL, Minor MA, Brookhart MA, et al: Does this patient with a pericardial effusion have cardiac tamponade? *JAMA* 297(16):1810–1818, 2007.
7. Flannery EP, Gregoratos G, Corder MP: Pericardial effusions in patients with malignant diseases. *Arch Intern Med* 135(7):976–977, 1975.
8. Jneid H, Maree A, Palacios I: Acute pericardial disease: pericardiocentesis and percutaneous pericardiotomy. In Mebazza A, Gheorghiade M, Zannad F, et al, editors: *Acute Heart Failure*, New York, 2008, Springer.
9. Sagrista-Sauleda J, Angel J, Permanyer-Miralda G, et al: Long-term follow-up of idiopathic chronic pericardial effusion. *N Engl J Med* 341(27):2054–2059, 1999.
10. Shepherd FA, Morgan C, Evans WK, et al: Medical management of malignant pericardial effusion by tetracycline sclerosis. *Am J Cardiol* 60(14):1161–1166, 1987.
11. Sagrista-Sauleda J, Angel J, Sambola A, et al: Low-pressure cardiac tamponade: clinical and hemodynamic profile. *Circulation* 114(9):945–952, 2006.
12. Laham RJ, Cohen DJ, Kuntz RE, et al: Pericardial effusion in patients with cancer: outcome with contemporary management strategies. *Heart* 75(1):67–71, 1996.
13. Soler-Soler J, Sagrista-Sauleda J, Permanyer-Miralda G: Management of pericardial effusion. *Heart* 86(2):235–240, 2001.
14. Fontenelle LJ, Cuello L, Dooley BN: Subxiphoid pericardial window. A simple and safe method for diagnosing and treating acute and chronic pericardial effusions. *J Thorac Cardiovasc Surg* 62(1):95–97, 1971.
15. Callahan JA, Seward JB: Pericardiocentesis guided by two-dimensional echocardiography. *Echocardiography* 14(5):497–504, 1997.
16. Selig MB: Percutaneous transcatheter pericardial interventions: aspiration, biopsy, and pericardioplasty. *Am Heart J* 125(1):269–271, 1993.
17. Marcy PY, Bondiau PY, Brunner P: Percutaneous treatment in patients presenting with malignant cardiac tamponade. *Eur Radiol* 15(9):2000–2009, 2005.
18. Palacios IF, Tuzcu EM, Ziskind AA, et al: Percutaneous balloon pericardial window for patients with malignant pericardial effusion and tamponade. *Cathet Cardiovasc Diagn* 22(4):244–249, 1991.
19. Bahl VK, Bhargava B, Chandra S: Percutaneous pericardiotomy using Inoue balloon catheter. *Cathet Cardiovasc Diagn* 36(1):98–99, 1995.
20. Bertrand O, Legrand V, Kulbertus H: Percutaneous balloon pericardiotomy: a case report and analysis of mechanism of action. *Cathet Cardiovasc Diagn* 38(2):180–182, 1996.
21. Chow WH, Chow TC, Cheung KL: Nonsurgical creation of a pericardial window using the Inoue balloon catheter. *Am Heart J* 124(4):1100–1102, 1992.
22. Chow WH, Chow TC, Yip AS, et al: Inoue balloon pericardiotomy for patients with recurrent pericardial effusion. *Angiology* 47(1):57–60, 1996.
23. Fakiolas CN, Beldekos DI, Foussas SG, et al: Percutaneous balloon pericardiotomy as a therapeutic alternative for cardiac tamponade and recurrent pericardial effusion. *Acta Cardiol* 50(1):65–70, 1995.
24. Thanopoulos BD, Georgakopoulos D, Tsaousis GS, et al: Percutaneous balloon pericardiotomy for the treatment of large, nonmalignant pericardial effusions in children: immediate and medium-term results. *Cathet Cardiovasc Diagn* 40(1):97–100, 1997.
25. Sugimoto JT, Little AG, Ferguson MK, et al: Pericardial window: mechanisms of efficacy. *Ann Thorac Surg* 50(3):442–445, 1990.
26. Chow LT, Chow WH: Mechanism of pericardial window creation by balloon pericardiotomy. *Am J Cardiol* 72(17):1321–1322, 1993.
27. Iaffaldano RA, Jones P, Lewis BE, et al: Percutaneous balloon pericardiotomy: a double-balloon technique. *Cathet Cardiovasc Diagn* 36(1):79–81, 1995.
28. Ziskind AA, Pearce AC, Lemmon CC, et al: Percutaneous balloon pericardiotomy for the treatment of cardiac tamponade and large pericardial effusions: description of technique and report of the first 50 cases. *J Am Coll Cardiol* 21(1):1–5, 1993.
29. Endrys J, Simo M, Shafie MZ, et al: New nonsurgical technique for multiple pericardial biopsies. *Cathet Cardiovasc Diagn* 15(2):92–94, 1988.
30. Mehan VK, Dalvi BV, Lokhandwala YY, et al: Use of guiding catheters to target pericardial and endomyocardial biopsy sites. *Am Heart J* 122(3 Pt 1):882–883, 1991.
31. Ziskind AA, Rodriguez S, Lemmon C, et al: Percutaneous pericardial biopsy as an adjunctive technique for the diagnosis of pericardial disease. *Am J Cardiol* 74(3):288–291, 1994.
32. Selig MB: Percutaneous pericardial biopsy under echocardiographic guidance. *Am Heart J* 122(3 Pt 1):879–882, 1991.
33. Margey R, Suh W, Witzke C, et al: Percutaneous pericardial biopsy—a novel interventional technique to aid diagnosis and management of pericardial disease. TCT 477 poster presentation, transcatheter therapeutics 2010. *J Am Coll Cardiol* 56(Suppl):B110, 2010. [TCT 477].
34. Seferovic PM, Ristic AD, Maksimovic R, et al: Diagnostic value of pericardial biopsy: improvement with extensive sampling enabled by pericardioscopy. *Circulation* 107(7):978–983, 2003.
35. Berruezo A, Mont L, Nava S, et al: Electrocardiographic recognition of the epicardial origin of ventricular tachycardias. *Circulation* 109(15):1842–1847, 2004.
36. d'Avila A, Koruth JS, Dukkipati S, et al: Epicardial access for the treatment of cardiac arrhythmias. *Europace* 14(Suppl 2):ii13–ii18, 2012.
37. Tung R, Michowitz Y, Yu R, et al: Epicardial ablation of ventricular tachycardia: an institutional experience of safety and efficacy. *Heart Rhythm* 10(4):490–498, 2013.
38. Sarkozy A, Tokuda M, Tedrow UB, et al: Epicardial ablation of ventricular tachycardia in ischemic heart disease. *Circ Arrhythm Electrophysiol* 6(6):1115–1122, 2013.
39. Pisani CF, Lara S, Scanavacca M: Epicardial ablation for cardiac arrhythmias: techniques, indications and results. *Curr Opin Cardiol* 29(1):59–67, 2014.
40. Sosa E, Scanavacca M, d'Avila A, et al: A new technique to perform epicardial mapping in the electrophysiology laboratory. *J Cardiovasc Electrophysiol* 7(6):531–536, 1996.
41. Della Bella P, Brugada J, Zeppenfeld K, et al: Epicardial ablation for ventricular tachycardia: a European multicenter study. *Circ Arrhythm Electrophysiol* 4(5):653–659, 2011.
42. Arenal A, Perez-David E, Avila P, et al: Noninvasive identification of epicardial ventricular tachycardia substrate by magnetic resonance-based signal intensity mapping. *Heart Rhythm* 11(8):1456–1464, 2014.
43. Fernandez-Armenta J, Berruezo A: How to recognize epicardial origin of ventricular tachycardias? *Curr Cardiol Rev* 10(3):246–256, 2014.
44. Tschabrunn CM, Haqqani HM, Cooper JM, et al: Percutaneous epicardial ventricular tachycardia ablation after noncoronary cardiac surgery or pericarditis. *Heart Rhythm* 10(2):165–169, 2013.
45. Soejima K, Couper G, Cooper JM, et al: Subxiphoid surgical approach for epicardial catheter-based mapping and ablation in patients with prior cardiac surgery or difficult pericardial access. *Circulation* 110(10):1197–1201, 2004.
46. Laham RJ, Simons M, Hung D: Subxyphoid access of the normal pericardium: a novel drug delivery technique. *Catheter Cardiovasc Interv* 47(1):109–111, 1999.
47. Nagashima K, Watanabe I, Okumura Y, et al: Epicardial ablation with irrigated electrodes—effect of bipolar vs. unipolar ablation on lesion formation. *Circ J* 76(2):322–327, 2012.
48. Dyrda K, Piers SR, van Huls van Taxis CF, et al: Influence of steroid therapy on the incidence of pericarditis and atrial fibrillation following percutaneous epicardial mapping and ablation for ventricular tachycardia. *Circ Arrhythm Electrophysiol* 7:992, 2014.
49. Koruth JS, Aryana A, Dukkipati SR, et al: Unusual complications of percutaneous epicardial access and epicardial mapping and ablation of cardiac arrhythmias. *Circ Arrhythm Electrophysiol* 4(6):882–888, 2011.
50. Wolf PA, Abbott RD, Kannel WB: Atrial fibrillation as an independent risk factor for stroke: the Framingham study. *Stroke* 22(8):983–988, 1991.
51. Miyasaka Y, Barnes ME, Gersh BJ, et al: Secular trends in incidence of atrial fibrillation in Olmsted County, Minnesota, 1980 to 2000, and implications on the projections for future prevalence. *Circulation* 114(2):119–125, 2006.
52. Benjamin EJ, Wolf PA, D'Agostino RB, et al: Impact of atrial fibrillation on the risk of death: the Framingham Heart Study. *Circulation* 98(10):946–952, 1998.
53. Risk factors for stroke and efficacy of antithrombotic therapy in atrial fibrillation. analysis of pooled data from five randomized controlled trials. *Arch Intern Med* 154(13):1449–1457, 1994.
54. Thambidorai SK, Murray RD, Parakh K, et al: Utility of transesophageal echocardiography in identification of thrombogenic milieu in patients with atrial fibrillation (an ACUTE ancillary study). *Am J Cardiol* 96(7):935–941, 2005.
55. Fuster V, Ryden LE, Cannom DS, et al: 2011 ACCF/AHA/HRS focused updates incorporated into the ACC/AHA/ESC 2006 guidelines for the management of patients with atrial fibrillation: a report of the American College of Cardiology Foundation/American Heart Association task force on practice guidelines. *Circulation* 123(10):e269–e367, 2011.
56. Eikelboom JW, Wallentin L, Connolly SJ, et al: Risk of bleeding with 2 doses of dabigatran compared with warfarin in older and younger patients with atrial fibrillation: an analysis of the randomized evaluation of long-term anticoagulant therapy (RE-LY) trial. *Circulation* 123(21):2363–2372, 2011.
57. Gage BF, Waterman AD, Shannon W, et al: Validation of clinical classification schemes for predicting stroke: results from the national registry of atrial fibrillation. *JAMA* 285(22):2864–2870, 2001.
58. Puwanant S, Varr BC, Shrestha K, et al: Role of the CHADS2 score in the evaluation of thromboembolic risk in patients with atrial fibrillation undergoing transesophageal echocardiography before pulmonary vein isolation. *J Am Coll Cardiol* 54(22):2032–2039, 2009.
59. Al-Saady NM, Obel OA, Camm AJ: Left atrial appendage: structure, function, and role in thromboembolism. *Heart* 82(5):547–554, 1999.
60. Veinot JP, Harrity PJ, Gentile F, et al: Anatomy of the normal left atrial appendage: a quantitative study of age-related changes in 500 autopsy hearts: implications for echocardiographic examination. *Circulation* 96(9):3112–3115, 1997.
61. Faletra FF, Nucifora G, Regoli F, et al: Anatomy of pulmonary veins by real-time 3D TEE: implications for catheter-based pulmonary vein ablation. *JACC Cardiovasc Imaging* 5(4):456–462, 2012.
62. Lee RJ, Bartus K, Yakubov SJ: Catheter-based left atrial appendage (LAA) ligation for the prevention of embolic events arising from the LAA: initial experience in a canine model. *Circ Cardiovasc Interv* 3(3):224–229, 2010.
63. Bartus K, Bednarek J, Myc J, et al: Feasibility of closed-chest ligation of the left atrial appendage in humans. *Heart Rhythm* 8(2):188–193, 2011.

64. Bartus K, Han FT, Bednarek J, et al: Percutaneous left atrial appendage suture ligation using the LARIAT device in patients with atrial fibrillation: initial clinical experience. *J Am Coll Cardiol* 62(2):108–118, 2013.
65. Baker MS, Paul Mounsey J, Gehi AK, et al: Left atrial thrombus after appendage ligation with LARIAT. *Heart Rhythm* 11(8):1489, 2014.
66. Briceno DF, Fernando RR, Laing ST: Left atrial appendage thrombus post LARIAT closure device. *Heart Rhythm* 11(9):1600–1601, 2014.
67. Keating VP, Kolibash CP, Khandheria BK, et al: Left atrial laceration with epicardial ligation device. *Ann Thorac Cardiovasc Surg* 2013.
68. Koneru JN, Badhwar N, Ellenbogen KA, et al: LAA ligation using the LARIAT suture delivery device: tips and tricks for a successful procedure. *Heart Rhythm* 11(5):911–921, 2014.
69. Koranne KP, Fernando RR, Laing ST: Left atrial thrombus after complete left atrial appendage exclusion with LARIAT device. *Catheter Cardiovasc Interv* 2014.
70. Mosley WJ, 2nd, Smith MR, Price MJ: Percutaneous management of late leak after LARIAT transcatheter ligation of the left atrial appendage in patients with atrial fibrillation at high risk for stroke. *Catheter Cardiovasc Interv* 83(4):664–669, 2014.
71. d'Avila A, Neuzil P, Thiagalingam A, et al: Experimental efficacy of pericardial instillation of anti-inflammatory agents during percutaneous epicardial catheter ablation to prevent postprocedure pericarditis. *J Cardiovasc Electrophysiol* 18(11):1178–1183, 2007.
72. Laham RJ, Hung D, Simons M: Therapeutic myocardial angiogenesis using percutaneous intrapericardial drug delivery. *Clin Cardiol* 22(1 Suppl 1):I6–I9, 1999.

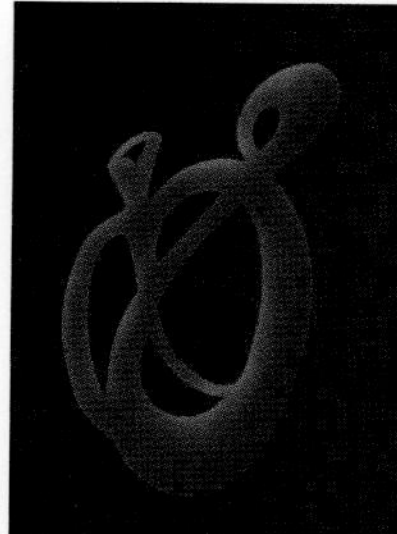

PART VII CONGENITAL HEART DISEASE

36 Congenital Heart Disease

John F. Rhodes, Jr.

INTRODUCTION

Congenital heart disease (CHD) has an incidence of approximately 0.8% or approximately 8 out of every 1000 live births.[1] These defects are derangements secondary to altered embryonic cardiovascular anatomy or the failure of a structure to progress beyond early stages of fetal development. Currently, nearly one million adults have CHD in the United States,[2] and although many adults with CHD live with only a mild or repaired derangement, some have more severe conditions that if left untreated can be life threatening. In addition, many of these patients require multiple surgical and/or catheter-based interventions during childhood and potentially also in adulthood.[3] Therefore, some of these important catheter-based interventions will be described in this chapter.

Catheterizations for patients with CHD are performed with either general anesthesia or moderate sedation with a combination of opiates and benzodiazepines. These procedures are performed using standard Seldinger technique in the femoral vein and femoral artery. Alternative venous access options include the internal jugular veins (high or low approach), subclavian veins, direct right atrial puncture, or a transhepatic vein approach. Arterial access may also be obtained from the arteries of the upper extremities (radial/axillary arteries) or the carotids. Anticoagulation is managed with heparin 100 units per kg body weight (maximum 5000-7000 units) for a goal activated clotting time (ACT) ≥200 to 250 seconds, depending on the procedure to be performed. Antibiotics are given to patients who receive an implanted device or who are deemed higher risk for bacterial endocarditis.

In general, baseline hemodynamic data are obtained in room air, precluding the need for a pulmonary vein PO_2. Subsequently, the ratio of pulmonary blood flow (Q_p) to systemic blood flow (Q_s) is calculated according to the following formula: $Q_p/Q_s = [(Ao_2 - MVo_2)/(PVo_2 - Pao_2)]$, where Ao_2 is the aortic oxygen saturation, MVo_2 is the mixed venous oxygen saturation, Pao_2 is the pulmonary arterial saturation, and PVo_2 is the pulmonary venous saturation. After hemodynamics, angiography is performed to further delineate the anatomy or lesion severity. For therapeutic procedures, a catheter is passed across the target area, such as stenosis, or abnormal shunt. A guidewire is then passed through the catheter to provide a track over which the delivery sheath and therapeutic devices are delivered. Balloon catheters are threaded directly, whereas stents and occlusion devices are protected or constrained within long delivery sheaths.

CATHETER-BASED INTERVENTIONS FOR CONGENITAL HEART DISEASE

Coarctation of the Aorta—Native or Restenosis for Intervention

Coarctation of the aorta occurs with a frequency of 8% of all congenital heart defects.[4,5] Although usually diagnosed in early childhood, many patients are diagnosed and treated as adults. The natural history suggests that isolated coarctation may represent one aspect of more diffuse arteriopathy. Diffuse arterial wall stiffness and renal hypoperfusion lead to a resetting of the renin-angiotensin system and a hyperrenin state that, unfortunately, may not abate even after relief of the obstructed aorta.[6] Also, although uncommon, cerebrovascular events from rupture of berry aneurysms may occur before or after relief of coarctation.[7,8] An associated bicuspid aortic valve is present in 50% to 85% of patients with aortic coarctation,[9] and a significant aortic gradient is particularly important to exclude when deciding on definitive therapy. Life expectancy beyond the sixth decade is unusual if the coarctation is not relieved, with a mean survival of approximately 35 years.[10] The coarctation site is typically at the isthmus just beyond the origin of the left subclavian artery across from the ampulla of the ligamentum arteriosus. Collateral circulation often is present to bypass the obstructed aortic segment and provide blood flow to the lower body. The most common origins for these collateral are from the subclavian arteries through the internal thoracic arteries and the thyrocervical and costocervical branches. These vessels communicate with the intercostal arteries, which then perfuse the descending aorta distal to the obstructed aortic segment. This can produce diminished but palpable lower extremity pulses and also mask a severely obstructed aorta.

Prior to the catheterization and during follow-up, transthoracic echocardiography (TEE) can be used to interrogate the descending aorta, with a resting peak systolic velocity ≥3.2 m/s or a diastolic velocity of ≥1.0 m/s suggestive of significant aortic obstruction. Echocardiography also allows interrogation of the aortic valve and assessment of the ascending aortic root. More recently, magnetic resonance imaging (MRI) has become the imaging modality of choice (**Figure 36-1**) both pre- and postcatheterization to assess the aorta and evaluate the coarctation segment anatomy. It also provides anatomical data regarding the aortic valve and ascending aorta. In the event of a contraindication to MRI (pacemaker or claustrophobia), or the lack of availability, computed tomography (CT) with contrast provides an acceptable alternative. In particular, multidimensional CT allows for 3D reconstruction similar to magnetic resonance angiographic methods.

Asymptomatic patients with a peak-to-peak gradient over 20 to 30 mm Hg across the coarctation site, by direct measurement in the catheterization laboratory, are considered for intervention. Also, symptomatic patients with a lesser gradient associated with a low cardiac output, or upper extremity hypertension and left ventricular (LV) hypertrophy, should be considered for intervention therapy. Other evolving indications for treatment include the presence of aortic aneurysms and symptomatic aneurysms of the circle of Willis. Young women who wish to bear children are also at risk, as there may be inadequate placental flow should they become pregnant.

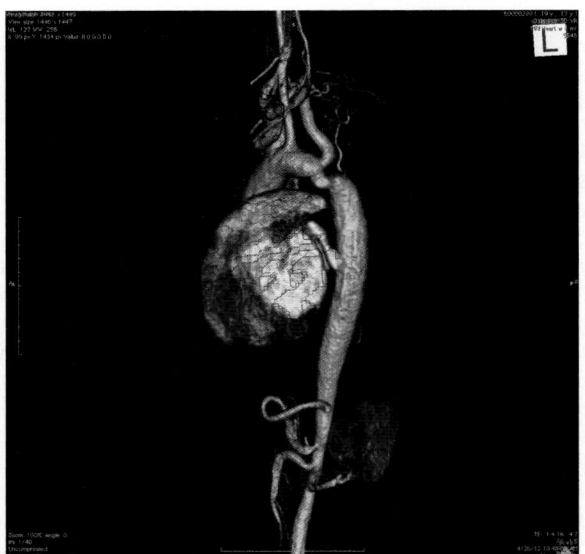

FIGURE 36-1 Three-dimensional reconstruction of a native coarctation of the aorta using cardiac magnetic resonance imaging.

Coarctation of the aorta after surgical repair of the aorta is referred to as "restenosis" as opposed to a native lesion. Often this occurs after an end-to-end surgical repair at the isthmus and can be due to aortic narrowing within the surgical site or potentially the transverse arch proximal to the surgical site. These later obstructive lesions are subcategorized as either proximal transverse arch (between the innominate artery and left carotid artery) or distal transverse arch (between the left carotid artery and left subclavian artery). Although few data exist regarding stent angioplasty within the transverse aortic arch, general experience has been that this is a safe and effective procedure.[11] An arterial monitoring catheter is placed in the right upper extremity and a 4 Fr sheath is used to advance a 4 Fr pigtail to the aorta from the right radial artery. This catheter is used to monitor pressures during stent angioplasty of the distal transverse arch and to cineangiograms to determine appropriate stent placement distal to the origin of the left carotid artery. Transcatheter stent angioplasty for postoperative re-coarctation of the aorta at the isthmus has been demonstrated to be safe and effective.[4,5,12] The technique usually involves a femoral arterial approach. The exchange length wire is placed in the ascending aorta or right subclavian artery. A high-pressure angioplasty balloon is used that is equal to or less than the diameter of the normal aortic segments around the stenosis (distal transverse arch or isthmus) and/or the diameter of the descending thoracic aorta near the diaphragm. The stent is mounted on an angioplasty balloon and delivered through a sheath at least 1 Fr to 2 Fr larger than is required by the angioplasty balloon. The stent length is dependent on the lesion length but is usually at least 35 mm to 40 mm in older patients. The stent can be fully dilated, but sometimes it is deemed safer to dilate the lesion over two procedures with 4 to 6 months between dilations.

Percutaneous angioplasty for coarctation has been performed since 1982, and the availability of stents has recently led to improved outcomes, to the extent that percutaneous intervention is now considered the procedure of choice in patients with re-coarctation following surgery.[4] More recently aortic stents of adequate size have been available, and these are particularly effective in preventing complications from recoil of the aorta following angioplasty (**Figure 36-2**). The size of the stent is never larger than the native aorta. Intravascular ultrasound has been useful in ensuring that there is adequate apposition of the stent against the aortic wall. A successful stent procedure is usually defined as a reduction in the peak gradient to near zero or less than 5 mm Hg.[13]

Postcoarctation aneurysm formation was particularly a concern early in the experience of using angioplasty for native coarctation; resulting in the recommendation that native coarctation is better treated with surgical intervention.[11] This concern has lessened more recently with the greater use of stenting, and many advocate a percutaneous approach in both native and postoperatively re-coarctation if the anatomy is suitable for stent placement. In general native coarctation should still be approached cautiously. For selected patients, stent placement may be considered as the primary intervention for native coarctation (**Figure 36-3**) but should be considered in light of the need for growth of the aorta and risk for aneurysm formation.[13]

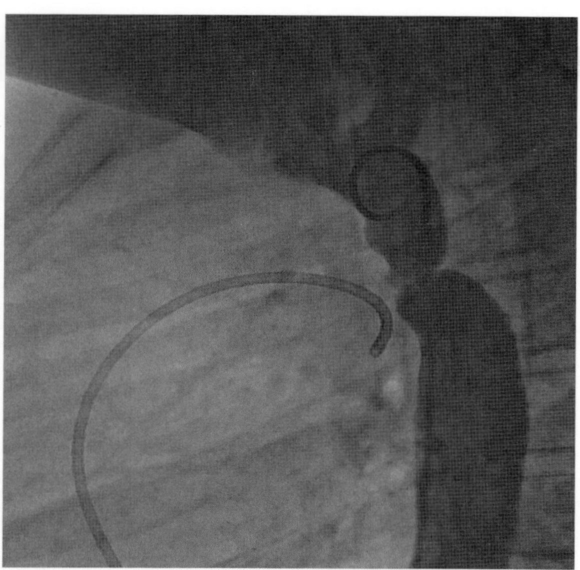

FIGURE 36-2 Lateral projection of aortic angiography demonstrating native coarctation of the aorta.

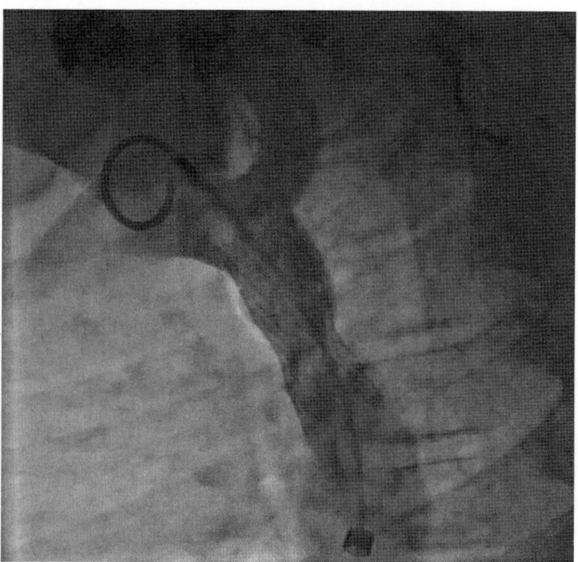

FIGURE 36-3 Lateral projection of aortic angiography demonstrating stent angioplasty for native coarctation of the aorta in the same patient as Figure 36-2.

Also, the long-term outcome into late adulthood after stent placement has yet to be determined, and investigation continues.[10]

Arteriovenous Fistulae or Malformations

Coronary Artery Fistulae

Coronary artery fistulae (CAF) are connections between the coronary arteries and a cardiac chamber or great vessel resulting in a "bypass" of the myocardial capillary bed. CAF occur in isolation (without other congenital heart defects), and the exact incidence is unknown. Most often they are discovered during routine coronary angiography, are clinically asymptomatic, and require no therapy.[14] More than half of cases of CAF originate from the proximal right coronary artery, with the proximal left anterior descending coronary artery being the next most frequently involved (one third of cases), followed by the proximal circumflex coronary artery.[15] Most of the CAF from either coronary artery terminate into the right side of the heart. The right ventricle (RV) is the most common site for drainage followed by the right atrium, coronary sinus, and pulmonary arteries (Video 36-1).

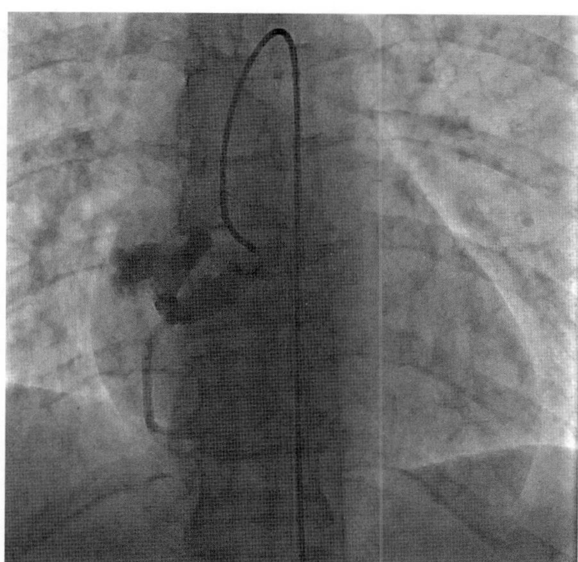

FIGURE 36-4 Selective coronary angiography in a patient with a large coronary artery fistula off of the right coronary artery to the right atrium.

Since most of the patients with CAF are asymptomatic, the diagnosis is usually suspected when a continuous murmur is detected during routine visit or during examination for other reasons. On rare occasions the steal from the coronary bed will be of significance and result in angina symptoms. This poor distal coronary perfusion can usually be demonstrated during exercise testing with imaging methods. It is uncommon for coronary fistulae to be large enough that a substantial left-to-right shunt is present, and often no oximetric step-up can be demonstrated at catheterization even in angiographically appearing large fistulae.[16] Reported symptoms due to a CAF include steal from the adjacent myocardium causing myocardial ischemia, thrombosis and embolism, cardiac failure, atrial fibrillation, rupture, endarteritis, and arrhythmias.[17-21] Other reported rare complications include thrombosis within the fistula leading to acute myocardial infarction, atrioventricular arrhythmias, and spontaneous rupture of the aneurysmal fistula causing hemopericardium.[22]

Access can be obtained in either the femoral or radial artery. A venous sheath is also placed in the event a rail technique or retrograde approach to deliver the occlusion device is deemed necessary. Selective coronary angiography is performed to confirm the diagnosis and delineate the anatomy of the CAF (**Figure 36-4**). Detailed angiographic views in multiple projections are essential to the safe and effective treatment of a CAF.

Transcatheter intervention is indicated when there is evidence for coronary steal and clinical symptoms (**Table 36-1**). CAF occlusion can be accomplished using various implantation techniques including various types of coils or vascular plugs (**Figure 36-5**), depending on a favorable vessel size and shape in order to position without embolization.[18] The main goal of treatment of CAF is complete

TABLE 36-1 Adult Congenital Interventions for Vascular Occlusion

	INDICATION	METHODS	ACUTE SUCCESS	COMMENTS
Coronary fistulae	Evidence of coronary steal	Coil occlusion	Technically high	Complications include unwanted branch occlusion or embolization
Pulmonary arteriovenous fistulae	Cyanosis Evidence of paradoxical emboli	Coil occlusion Occasionally Amplatzer or other occluder if fistula large	Technically high in selected lesions	Often multiple small fistulae present that are not amenable to coil occlusion Regrowth of collaterals high
Venovenous collaterals	Evidence of systemic hypoxemia or systemic embolic events	Coil occlusion if small or Amplatzer plug/PDA device if large collateral	Technically high in selected lesions	High long-term success rate Complications include residual leak, hemolysis, and embolization

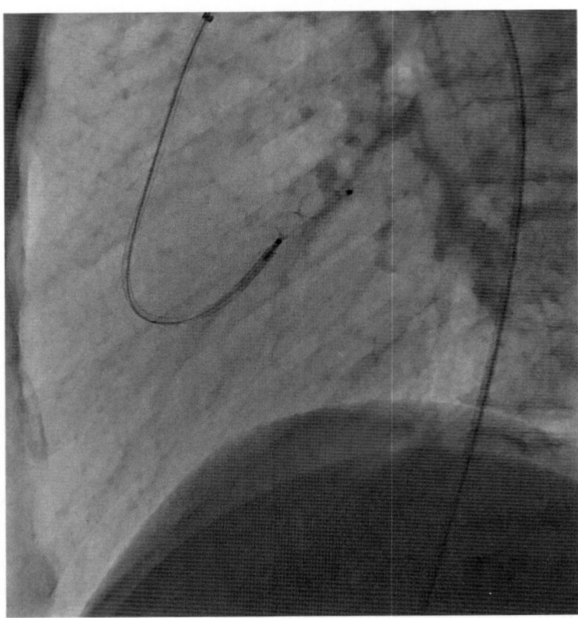

FIGURE 36-5 Deployment of an Amplatzer Vascular Plug II for closure of a coronary artery fistula.

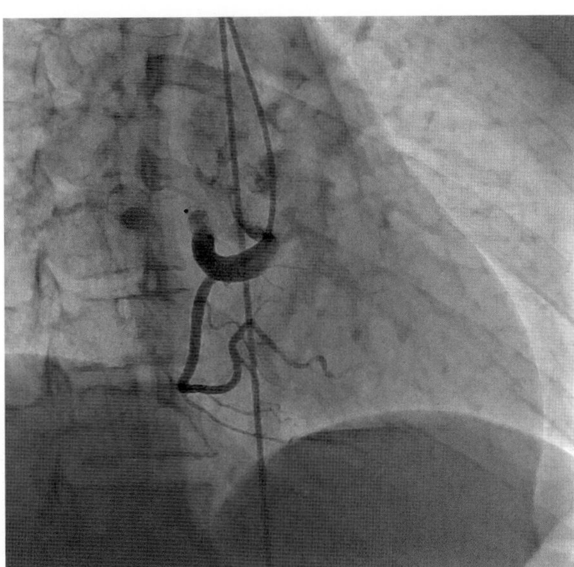

FIGURE 36-6 Selective coronary angiography demonstrating complete occlusion of a coronary artery fistula.

occlusion with no residual fistulae. Catheter closure should be as distal to the end point of the fistula as possible to avoid possible occlusion of coronary branches to normal myocardium.

The recommended technique is a coaxial system using a coronary guide catheter of proper size and shape (usually 6 Fr to 8 Fr) is advanced to the ostium of the involved coronary artery, with a second catheter within this guide catheter (4 Fr or 5 Fr hemodynamic catheter), to advance a wire distally within the CAF. A rail technique from the venous access is often necessary to secure the wire position. Then an end-hole wedge balloon catheter is passed over this wire (retrograde or antegrade), leaving the guide catheter at the ostium of the coronary artery. The balloon is positioned distal to the last viable myocardial branch and is inflated with contrast to temporarily occlude the vessel for 5 to 10 minutes to assess the risk of ischemia with fistula occlusion. With large CAF this may not be possible to accomplish. If no detectable ischemic changes are noted, then the choice of occlusion technique is based on the size and shape of the CAF. Coils or devices can be used to close the CAF. If coils are chosen, they are usually deployed retrograde (going from the guide catheter inside the delivery catheter positioned distal), and if devices are chosen, usually the wire is snared and exteriorized from either the femoral or jugular vein and the proper size sheath is advanced into the fistula. Then the device is advanced from the vein to the fistula. The guide catheter is used for selective injections to guide the deployment site and to look for other feeding vessels.

Complete occlusion of the fistula may be achieved in more than 95% of the patients (**Figure 36-6**). In the remaining patients, either further procedures may be required or managed conservatively if the residual fistulas are small. Procedurally related serious adverse events are uncommon but include embolization (within the coronary arteries), neurological events (systemic embolus), transient bundle branch block and myocardial infarction.[21] Coil or thrombus migration remains the most common serious adverse event, and thus recent recommendations are to consider the use of detachable coils and use antiplatelet agents or anticoagulation post occlusion to prevent thrombosis and closure of the larger main coronary arteries. Currently, catheter closure of the CAF is considered to be a safe and effective alternative to surgery.[3]

Pulmonary Arteriovenous Malformations

Pulmonary arteriovenous malformations (PAVM) are abnormal communications between pulmonary arteries and pulmonary veins.[23] PAVM can either be congenital or acquired but this particular etiology is often difficult to differentiate. PAVM is especially common in patients with inadequate pulmonary blood flow containing systemic hepatic venous

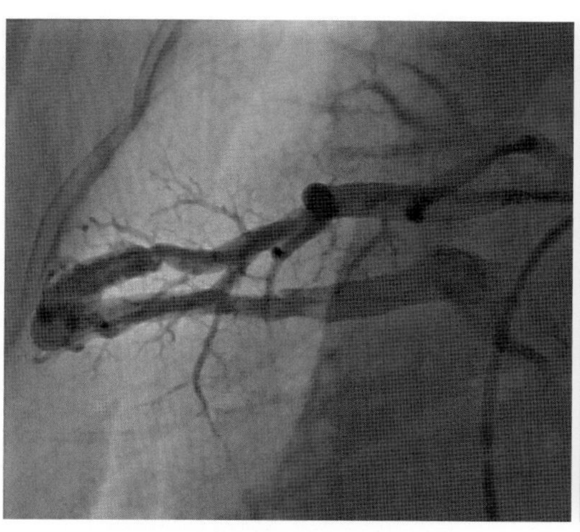
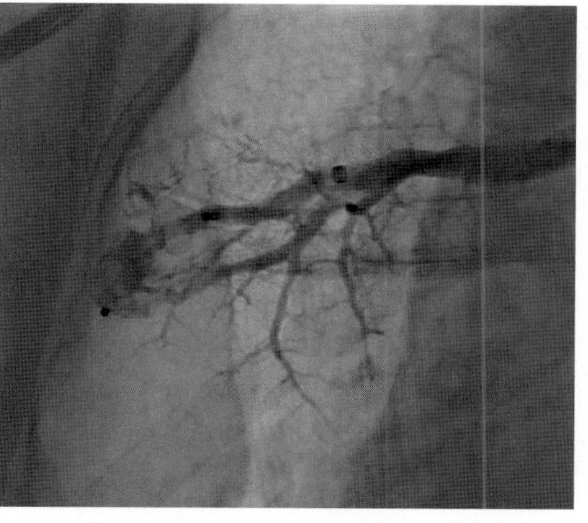

FIGURE 36-7 Side-by-side comparison of a right lung pulmonary arteriovenous malformation (AVM) and the same pulmonary AVM following placement of an Amplatzer Vascular Plug II with complete occlusion.

return. This occurs with various congenital heart defects but is common after a bidirectional Glenn (superior vena cava (SVA) anastomosed to the right pulmonary artery) for single ventricular physiology[24] (Video 36-2). PAVM are also particularly common in patients with hereditary hemorrhagic telangiectasia (Osler-Weber-Rendu syndrome)[24-26] and are found in nearly 5% of patients with migraine headache with aura.[27] Multiple small fistulae may also be seen in patients with hepato-pulmonary syndrome.[24] The clinical presentation varies between no symptoms and severe illness. The most common clinical presentation includes epistaxis, dyspnea, and hemoptysis. Systemic hypoxemia may occur from the right-to-left shunt, and the resultant shunt may lead to paradoxical embolus resulting in stroke or transient ischemic attack (TIA).

When the PAVM are large enough (>2.5 to 3.0 mm) and/or create either systemic hypoxemia or evidence for systemic embolization, then transcatheter occlusion[25,26,28-30] may be used (**Figure 36-7**). Transcatheter occlusion of PAVM is considered the mainstay of treatment[28-30] and the technique is similar to closure of the CAF. The most commonly used technique utilizes detachable coils or the vascular plug. Embolization of all entry vessels to the malformation is critical to prevent recanalization. The risk of migration through the malformation into systemic circulation has been decreased significantly with these more recent occlusion devices.

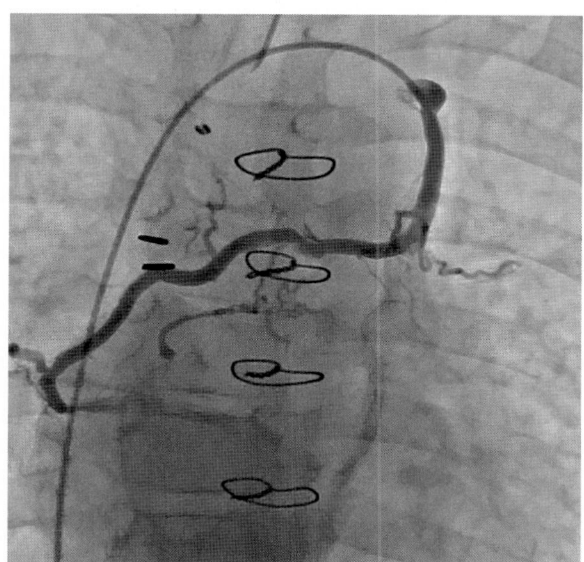

FIGURE 36-8 Anterior-posterior image of a venovenous collateral off of the distal left innominate vein in a patient with single ventricle physiology that bifurcates with one vessel draining into the right pulmonary veins and a persistent left superior vena cava (SVA) that is draining into the coronary sinus.

Anomalous Venovenous Connections Causing Systemic Hypoxemia

Anomalous venovenous connections may occur in patients with elevated systemic venous pressures, such as those who have had the Glenn or Fontan operation, or patients with stenoses or occlusions of the main systemic veins. Often these collaterals connect the left or right innominate vein or other systemic venous structures to the pulmonary veins or directly to the left atrium (**Figure 36-8**). Similar to patients who have a persistent fenestration, the patient with venovenous collaterals will manifest clinically as systemic hypoxemia, with or without exercise, or a route for systemic embolic events. The standard angiograms to assess the systemic venous circuit for these malformations is a 10- to 25-cc biplane cineangiogram in the inferior vena cava (IVC) distal to the hepatic veins, a biplane cineangiogram at the proximal anastomosis of the Fontan or Glenn pathway, a biplane cineangiogram in the left innominate vein for the patient with a right-sided Glenn shunt, and angiograms in both SVA in those patients with bilateral Glenn shunts (Video 36-3). If these angiograms do not demonstrate the explanation for the patients' systemic hypoxemia or embolic events we recommend agitated saline injections in the proximal right and left pulmonary arteries with simultaneous TEE, or chest wall echocardiography, to assess for tiny arteriovenous malformations in either lung. The lung with the least or no blood from the hepatic veins is most likely to have these later malformations. Transcatheter closure of the venovenous fistulae or larger arteriovenous malformations can be performed using Gianturco coils, vascular plugs, or vascular occlusion devices.[31] Final angiography or agitated saline injections can be utilized to assess for immediate closure and systemic oxygen saturations at rest, or during follow-up exercise testing, can be checked to confirm

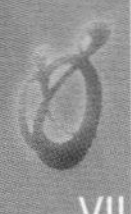

improvement and future risk for embolic events. Transcatheter coil occlusion of these anomalous channels has been used successfully to reduce the right-to-left shunt.

Valvular Heart Disease Secondary to Congenital Etiology

Pulmonary Valvuloplasty

Isolated valvar pulmonary stenosis (PS) represents 8% to 10% of all patients with CHD. The stenotic valve is usually dome-shaped with diffuse thickening and commissural fusion. Since transcatheter balloon pulmonary valvuloplasty for valvar PS was first reported[32,33] in the early 1980s it has become the first line of therapy, with a recommended balloon annulus ratio of 120%. Patients with mild to moderate valvar PS are often clinically asymptomatic. The diagnosis is usually made during physical examination with audible ejection systolic murmur in the position of the pulmonary valve. Patients with severe valvar PS may have dyspnea during exertion or also be asymptomatic irrespective of the severity of their obstruction. Treatment is indicated in those asymptomatic patients with a valvar PS gradient >40 to 60 mm Hg or in symptomatic patients with evidence of RV dysfunction irrespective of the gradient. Femoral venous access and right heart catheterization to assess the hemodynamics are performed. Femoral artery access is rarely needed. In neonatal critical PS, umbilical vein access may be used. RV angiography is performed in both anterior-posterior and lateral projections to identify the pulmonary valve and measure the annular size (between the hinge points) (**Figure 36-9**).

The reported success rate is >90% with major adverse events occurring in <1% of the procedures.[3] Hemodynamic measurements include the RV pressures in comparison to systemic arterial pressures and the peak-to-peak gradient across the pulmonary valve. Indications for balloon pulmonary valvuloplasty are at least moderate pulmonary valve stenosis. A useful guideline is the "rule of 50," defined as a peak RV systolic pressure of >50 mm Hg or >50% of the systemic pressure and a peak-to-peak gradient across the pulmonary valve of >50 mm Hg.

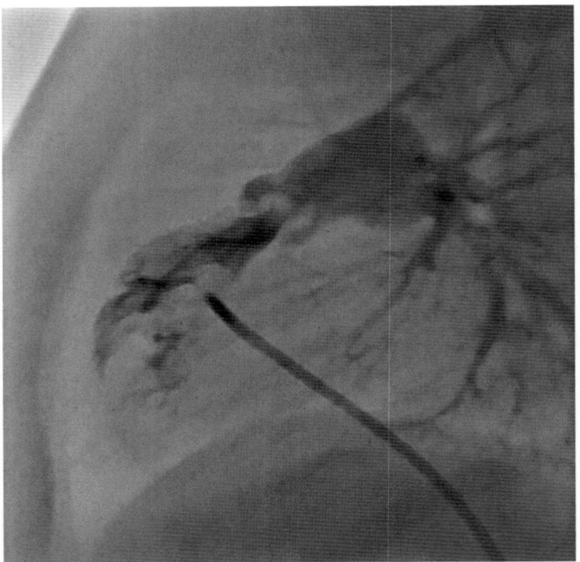

FIGURE 36-9 Lateral projection demonstrating doming and thickened pulmonary valve leaflets with limited mobility in an infant with severe pulmonary valve stenosis.

The balloon size is selected to be no more than 1.2 times the diameter of the valve annulus. A balloon end-hole catheter is advanced to the distal right or left pulmonary artery. A stiff-exchange length guidewire is then placed in the branch pulmonary artery. The desired balloon is introduced over the guidewire and is centered at the pulmonary valve. Adjustment of the balloon position may be performed by repeated small pressure inflations and waist verification. The balloon is then inflated rapidly until the waist disappears and is deflated immediately (Video 36-4). If suboptimal results are obtained, repositioning of the balloon and repeating the previous steps may be done. Larger balloon size may be used for the second inflation if optimal results are not achieved and no pulmonary regurgitation is observed.

Transcatheter Pulmonary Valve Placement

Similar to isolated valvar PS, RV outflow tract obstruction is also a common mechanism for pulmonary valve disease and manifests as pulmonary atresia, truncus arteriosus, or severe obstruction (tetralogy of Fallot) that has been treated with RV outflow tract surgical reconstruction using a conduit or bioprosthetic valve. Unfortunately, due to calcification or scar formation leading to valve dysfunction, conduits have limited durability, and progressive conduit dysfunction may lead to pulmonary outflow stenosis, and/or regurgitation.[34] Transcatheter pulmonary valve replacement has evolved into a viable alternative to surgical conduit[35] or bioprosthetic valve replacement.[36] This procedure has become the basis for a more advanced approach to congenital and structural interventional cardiology. Although many successes have been noted, so many challenges with this procedure including 18 Fr to 24 Fr delivery systems, the need for a "landing zone" for the valve as well as presenting optimal timing for intervening to prevent RV dysfunction, and atrial or ventricular arrhythmias continue to exist.

Cardiac magnetic resonance (CMR) imaging has been used to help determine timing of pulmonary valve intervention given this imaging modality's ability to quantify RV ejection fraction, ventricular volumes, and pulmonary regurgitation. Currently surgical intervention is indicated with indexed RV end-diastolic volumes (RVEDV) >150 mL/m^2 based on recently published data, as studies have suggested an indexed RVEDV that exceeds 150 mL/m^2 may lead to irreversible RV dilation.[37]

In 2000, Bonhoeffer et al. reported the concept of the transcatheter pulmonary valve replacement with a valve mounted on a balloon expandable stent in an ovine model.[38] Transcatheter pulmonary valve insertion was successful via the internal jugular approach in 7 out of 11 lambs. Although the overall success rate was only 36% due to some late failure of the valve, these attempts provided the platform for the first human transcatheter implantation in the pulmonary position.[39] Bonhoeffer's valve design was eventually acquired by Medtronic and renamed the Melody Valve (Medtronic Inc., Minneapolis, Minnesota). More recently, efforts have focused on assessing the safety and effectiveness of the transcatheter pulmonary valve as well as its longevity.

The Melody valve is made from a bovine jugular vein valve, which provides compliant and flexible leaflets. It is sewn into a platinum iridium stent and preserved in a proprietary sterilant of glutaraldehyde and alcohol.[38-40] The valve comes in one size, 18-mm diameter; length, 28 mm, that is crimped to 6 mm and can be re-expanded up to 22 to 24 mm. The company reports some success with the valve at deployed diameters as small as 12 mm.

The procedure is performed under general endotracheal anesthesia and access is usually obtained from the femoral vein. However, the procedure may also be performed via the internal jugular vein. After obtaining the access, the patient is given intravenous heparin, targeting an ACT of >200 to 250 seconds. Standard right heart catheterization is performed to assess the preprocedural saturations and pressures and the pressure gradient across the dysfunctional conduit. Angiography is then performed as follows: straight lateral and frontal with 20- to 30-degree cranial. Selective coronary angiography is performed simultaneously with a noncompliant angioplasty balloon (>8 to 10 atm) in the RV outflow tract (RVOT) conduit. Adequate angiographic distance (at least 10 mm) from the edge of the inflated balloon to the origin of the left coronary artery must exist to place the valve safely without compression of the coronary arteries. Angiographic assessment of the RVOT size, anatomy, as well as RV function is of paramount importance to ensure that valve delivery is feasible. Prestenting of the RVOT with a bare-metal stent prior to valve delivery has become standard (to reduce the incidence of stent fracture) when implanting the Melody valve. The bare-metal stent is usually deployed on a BiB (balloon-in-balloon) catheter (NuMED Inc., Hopkinton, New York) over a stiff guidewire, Meier wire (Boston Scientific Corporation, Natick, Massachusetts), or Lunderquist wire (Cook Medical, Bloomington, Indiana), which is placed preferably in the left pulmonary artery (**Figure 36-10**). Multiple angiograms are performed prior to balloon inflation to ensure proper position of the stent (Video 36-5).

The Medtronic Ensemble delivery system (Medtronic Inc., Minneapolis, Minnesota), comprises a delivery sheath, made of polytetrafluoroethylene (PTFE), which contains a BiB catheter onto which the valve is front-loaded and crimped by hand. Careful attention is paid to ensure that the valve is placed on the balloon in the correct position, to ensure the inflow and outflow of the valve is oriented appropriately. Once orientation of the balloon is confirmed, the valve is covered by the delivery sheath and advanced over the wire to its final position, before it is uncovered prior to deployment. Three sizes of the outer balloon are available: 18 mm, 20 mm, and 22 mm.

Clinical studies have reported that this procedure is safe and effective in eliminating pulmonary outflow stenosis or regurgitation and reducing the indexed RV volumes as well as improving patients' New York Heart Association (NYHA) functional class[36-41] (**Figure 36-11**). In addition, a multicenter prospective US clinical trial demonstrated freedom from Melody valve dysfunction or reintervention of 95.4% at 1-year follow-up with a high rate of procedural success (124/136), and improvement in NYHA functional class.[35]

Hemostasis is achieved after the procedure with either manual compression or Perclose sutures (Abbott Vascular, Abbott Park, Illinois) that should have been inserted prior to inserting the large sheath (pre-close) or simply by figure-of-eight suturing technique.[42,43]

Following the procedure, the patient is admitted to the intensive care unit for close observation overnight. Complete physical examination, ECG, chest x-ray, and echocardiography are performed prior to patient discharge. Aspirin 81 mg is advised for at least 3 to 6 months. Follow-up outpatient visits are recommended at 1, 6, and 12 months and yearly thereafter. Chest radiograph is obtained at 6 months to look for valve/stent position and any potential stent fracture. Echocardiography is routinely used to evaluate RV function, regurgitation, and/or stenosis with each visit. CT or CMR is also part of follow-up protocol when clinically indicated.

Procedural complications may necessitate conversion to surgery; these include valve migration, homograft rupture, guidewire injury to a distal branch pulmonary artery, damage to the tricuspid valve, and arrhythmia. Initial reports associated with these complications were documented to be as high as 12% in early studies[38,39]; however, recent studies have demonstrated a reduction in major complications to 5% to 6%.[40,41] A study published by Bonhoeffer's group in 2008 reported that, after their first 50 patients, procedural complications decreased from 6% to 2.9%.[40]

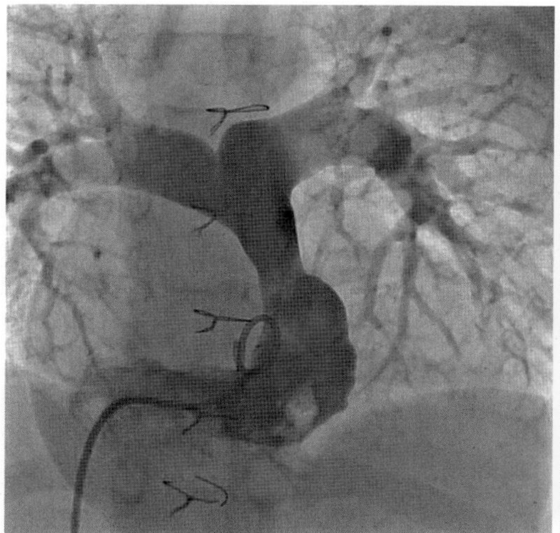
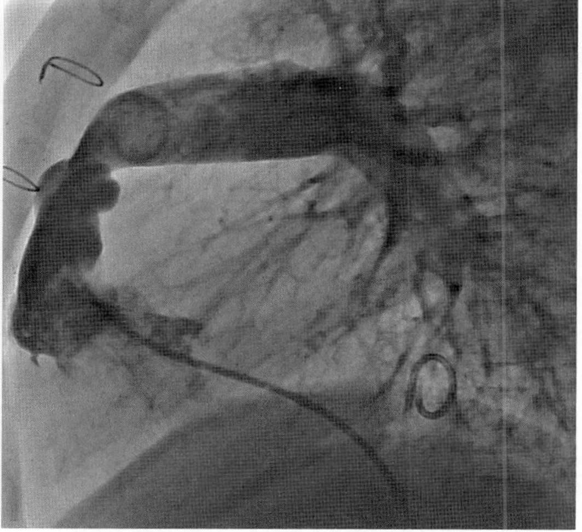

FIGURE 36-10 Anterior-posterior and lateral image of a stenotic RV to pulmonary artery conduit.

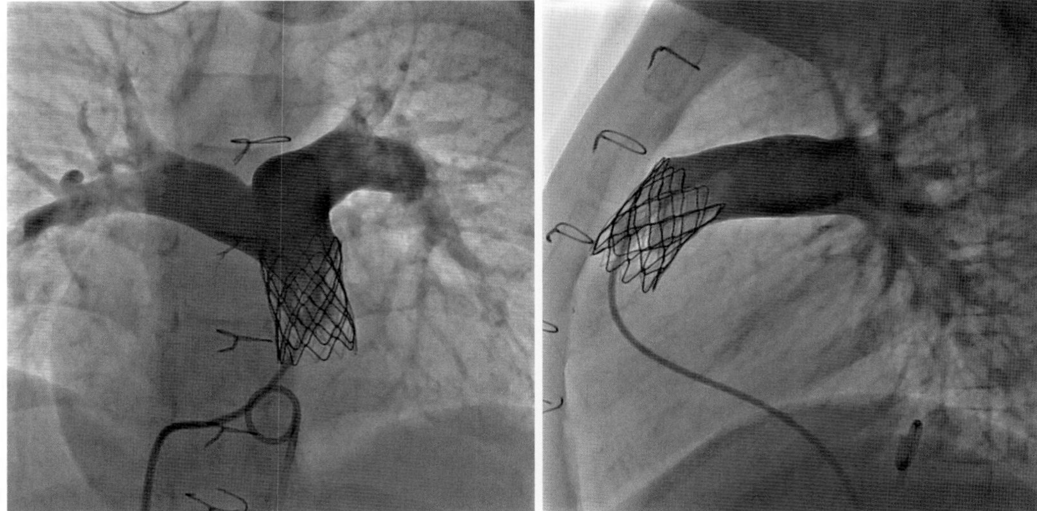

FIGURE 36-11 Anterior-posterior and lateral image of the final angiogram after Melody valve placement in the same patient.

A recent study demonstrated that 4.4% of the US cohort possessed unsuitable anatomy for valve implantation due to concerns regarding potential coronary artery compression.[44] This issue may be resolved by using CT/MRA, which may indicate the distance between the coronary artery and conduit; however, this should not be relied upon as stent implantation will distort the preexisting anatomy, and selective coronary angiography with a noncompliant balloon inflated in the RVOT should always be performed prior to attempted stent/valve implantation.

Conduit rupture has also been reported[41] as well as infective endocarditis.[45] Risk factors have yet to be fully elucidated. Increasingly covered stents are being used with aggressive prestenting of heavily calcified conduits. In the event of conduit rupture, self-expanding stents have been used to create a seal and prevent further risk of bleeding.[46]

In summary, many patients are now being treated with transcatheter valve implantation using the Melody valve. The multicenter study for Melody valve implantation demonstrated safety and efficacy for this procedure and the FDA approved the Melody valve in January 2010 for transcatheter valve replacement under the HDE (Humanitarian Device Exemption) pathway.[35] In addition, the 2010 American Heart Association statement on the Indications for Cardiac Catheterization and Intervention in Pediatric Cardiac Disease was expanded to include a Class IIa indication for transcatheter pulmonary valve replacement.[3]

Aortic Valve

Valvar aortic stenosis (AS) occurs in approximately 3% to 6% of patients with CHD.[47] The stenotic valve is usually secondary to minor to severe degrees of aortic valve maldevelopment with increased thickening and rigidity of the valve tissue and variable degrees of commissural fusion. Compensatory ventricular hypertrophy is proportional to the degree of obstruction. With severe hypertrophy and valvar obstruction, myocardial ischemia may result from the combination of limited cardiac output, reduced coronary perfusion, and increased myocardial oxygen consumption. Valvar AS can be classified into two groups, those with severe disease that presents at birth or within 1 to 2 years of age (10% to 15%) and those who are not diagnosed until after 2 years of age and will progress more slowly.[48] The mortality and need for intervention are significantly skewed toward the younger group. As with pulmonary stenosis, noninvasive imaging techniques have advanced to the point that nearly all anatomical and functional information about the valve may be obtained without catheterization, and catheterization is performed for valves that clearly merit intervention or when symptoms and imaging findings are incomplete or confounding.

Aortic valve stenosis is classified into the following categories: trivial, mild, moderate, severe, and critical. Critical aortic stenosis is not defined by a specific pressure gradient or valve orifice size but on the basis of physiological manifestations. If the stenosis is such that the patient is unable to produce and maintain an adequate cardiac output, the stenosis is critical. Patients in this group may have a low valve gradient, measured by echo, due to decreased cardiac function and low cardiac output. Although some controversy still exists as to the most beneficial treatment method for this population (surgical valvotomy vs. percutaneous balloon valvuloplasty) most centers have adopted balloon valvuloplasty as the initial treatment of choice. Patients in this category do not tolerate the stress of any procedure well, but catheterization has immediate results (reduction in gradient and resultant valve regurgitation) that are comparable to surgery and a shorter postprocedure intensive care unit course and overall hospital stay (Videos 36-6 to 36-8). Balloon valvuloplasty has been associated with an increased rate of reintervention over surgical valvotomy, secondary to recurrent stenosis or worsening regurgitation.[47-50] Given that residual aortic valve disease, especially regurgitation, may progress over time, recommendations for valvuloplasty technique are more conservative, with a smaller maximal balloon diameter (80% to 100% of the annulus) than that recommended for the pulmonary valve (100% to 120%). The valve may be approached retrograde from the aorta, using a soft-tipped J-wire to cross the narrowed valve orifice, with arterial access in the femoral (more common) or carotid artery. The valve may also be approached prograde, by crossing an existing atrial communication or by performing a transseptal puncture to access the left heart. Once in the LV, angiography is performed to measure the annulus of the valve and obtain landmarks for valvuloplasty. The diameter of the balloon should not exceed 80% to 90% of the valve annulus. The smaller balloon diameter, compared with a similar sized pulmonary valve annulus, is recommended to decrease the amount of valve tearing and resultant regurgitation. Many centers have adopted rapid RV pacing at the time of balloon inflation. This rapid pacing transiently reduces cardiac output and the shearing force transmitted to the balloon as it is inflated across the valve annulus. The goal is to reduce the motion on the fragile valve leaflets and prevent excessive damage and regurgitation. Repeat angiography and echocardiography following the inflation are essential to evaluate the success of the valvuloplasty and monitor for regurgitation or other complications. The differentiation among noncritical stenosis categories is made by noninvasive echocardiographic measurements of valve area and Doppler gradient. Normal valve area is 2 cm^2/m^2. Mild obstruction is consistent with valve areas less than 2 cm^2/m^2 but above 0.7 cm^2/m^2 and severe obstruction at valve areas less than 0.5 cm^2/m^2. Mean echocardiographic Doppler gradients are good predictors of the peak-to-peak pressure gradient measured at catheterization. Gradients less than 25 mm Hg are considered trivial, 25 to 50 mm Hg are mild, 50 to 75 mm Hg are moderate, and severe is >75 mm Hg. These measurements are made with the understanding that the cardiac function and cardiac output are normal. Catheterization is not recommended for trivial or mild stenosis. Moderate and severe stenoses are approached with primary balloon valvuloplasty.

Pulmonary Hypertension in Congenital Heart Disease

Overview

Changes in the pulmonary vasculature are common in patients with CHDs and can be related to increased blood flow secondary to left-to-right shunting, distortion of the pulmonary arteries due to shunts or others.[51] Right heart catheterization and pulmonary angiography are frequently performed to rule out pulmonary branch stenosis (proximal, distal, bilateral, or unilateral), assess pulmonary capillary wedge pressures, evaluate response of pulmonary pressures to vasodilator tests, and rule out pulmonary veno-occlusive disease. Catheterization will help in the decision-making process of selection for heart or heart and lung transplantation in selected patients (**Table 36-2**). If patients have a secundum atrial septal defect with elevated pulmonary vascular resistance or LV diastolic dysfunction, closure of this defect should be carefully evaluated before proceeding with device placement. Transient balloon occlusion of the defect can be performed to assess the changes in cardiac output and left atrial pressure. In patients with transposition of the great arteries after an atrial switch operation (Mustard or Senning) and pulmonary hypertension, pulmonary venous baffle obstruction or leak must be ruled out.

TABLE 36-2 Clinical Guidelines for Hemodynamic Evaluation

Pulmonary hypertension:
Mild: Mean PA >20 mm Hg
Moderate: Mean PA >30 mm Hg
Severe: Mean PA >45 mm Hg
PVR: Normal = 1-4 Wood units/m^2
High-risk levels of PVR: PVR >7.0 Wood units/m^2 is generally inoperable
Vaso-activity response to pulmonary vasodilators: >20% drop in PVR and mean PA pressure <45 mm Hg
Shunt magnitude: Intervene generally when Qp/Qs >1.5:1
Inoperable when there is shunt reversal and less than 1.5:1 left-to-right shunt

PA, Pulmonary artery; *PVR*, pulmonary vascular resistance.

Eisenmenger Syndrome/Secondary Pulmonary Hypertension

Unrepaired congenital heart defects can result in a long-standing state of increased pulmonary blood flow resulting from a left-to-right shunt. This insult over time can produce progressive structural changes in the pulmonary vasculature.[52] These changes will consist of medial thickening and hypertrophy, endothelial damage, and in situ thrombosis, resulting in an increase in pulmonary vascular resistance due to the decrease in the cross-sectional area of the pulmonary circulation and vasoconstriction. As the pulmonary pressures continue to increase, the degree of left-to-right shunt will diminish, and eventually there will be right-to-left shunting, resulting in systemic hypoxemia and cyanosis. Eisenmenger syndrome refers to reversal of a left-to-right shunt to a right-to-left shunt caused by the development of pulmonary vascular disease. Patients can present with syncope, cyanosis, palpitation, hyperviscosity symptoms, hemoptysis, stroke, or brain abscess.

The diagnosis is based on physical examination, which will disclose clubbing, cyanosis, a right parasternal heave, and loud P2 with a high-pitched decrescendo diastolic murmur of pulmonary valve regurgitation. The right ventricle can develop systolic and diastolic failure, thus resulting in signs of right-sided heart failure, with worsening tricuspid valve regurgitation.

Patients are advised to avoid dehydration, heavy exertion, or systemic vasodilators that can increase the right-to-left shunting. If a surgical procedure is planned, careful anesthetic management (cardiac anesthesia) should be available, and use of an air filter in all intravenous access to avoid paradoxical air embolism is mandatory.

Avoidance of hypotension is important; otherwise, the degree of right-to-left shunting will increase and progressive hypoxemia will develop, with the risk of death. If coronary angiography is needed, the most experienced operator should perform the procedure with minimal contrast to minimize the risk of kidney failure. Cyanotic patients are more susceptible to developing nephropathy with the use of contrast, NSAIDs, or other drugs such as aminoglycosides.[52]

FUTURE DIRECTIONS

Covered Stent Technology

Currently the COAST I and COAST II clinical trials have completed enrollment and are awaiting possible FDA approval for stent angioplasty (**Figure 36-12**) of native or recurrent coarctation.[5] These prospective data should complement the several large retrospective series for balloon angioplasty alone or balloon stent angioplasty that suggests that the success rate is between 65% and 100% and the serious adverse event rate is less than 3%.[12] Problems to monitor for include re-coarctation and aneurysm formation at the site of intervention and persistent blood pressure elevation. Older patients and those with an associated bicuspid aortic valve are at greatest risk for long-term complications.[7] Endocarditis prophylaxis is indicated.

Investigational Transcatheter Pulmonary Valve Technology

The SAPIEN (Edwards Lifesciences, Irvine, California) transcatheter heart valve is produced from three equal sized bovine pericardial leaflets that are hand sewn to a stainless steel balloon expandable stent (**Figure 36-13**). The valve is preserved in low-concentration solutions of buffered glutaraldehyde and is processed with the Edwards Thermafix (Edwards Lifesciences, Irvine, California) anticalcification pretreatment that is also utilized in the Carpentier-Edwards PERIMOUNT Magna (Edwards Lifesciences, Irvine, California) surgical valve. This process involves heat treatment of the tissue in glutaraldehyde and uses ethanol and polysorbate-80. The valve is available in 23 mm, with a stent height of 14.3 mm, and 26 mm, with a stent height of 16 mm.[53] The valve is mounted on a custom-made 3-cm-length volume expansion balloon. The Retroflex 3 delivery system (Edwards Lifesciences, Irvine, California) consists of a balloon catheter and a deflectable guiding catheter and requires a 22 Fr (for the 23 mm) and a 24 Fr (for the 26 mm) hydrophilic 35-cm-long sheath. A specialized Edwards crimper is used to symmetrically crimp the valve onto the balloon.

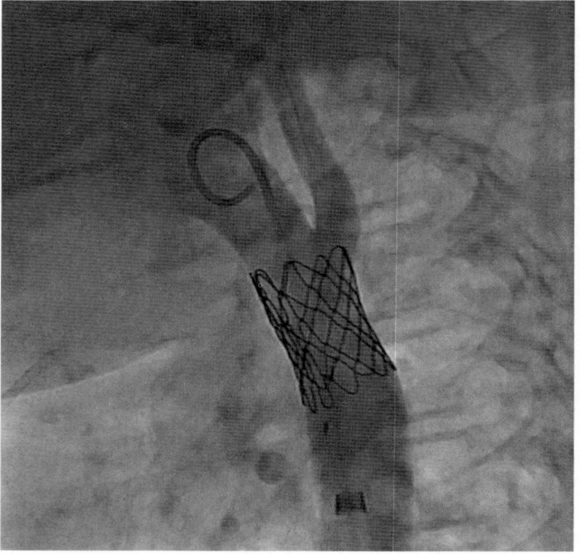

FIGURE 36-12 Lateral image of a COAST covered stent for primary stent angioplasty of the aorta in a patient with Turner's syndrome and bicuspid aortic valve.

The SAPIEN transcatheter heart valve was introduced as a transcatheter valve alternative to surgical aortic valve replacement in older adults with severe calcified aortic valve stenosis.[53] Also, an initial report outlined successful deployment in the pulmonary position in the United States in 2006,[54] and the ongoing prospective clinical trial (COMPASSION Trial) reported effective reduction in RV outflow tract gradients, improved clinical symptoms, and sustained pulmonary valve competence at 6-month follow-up. This clinical trial is continuing to enroll patients for pulmonary valve implantation using the Edwards transcatheter valve.

The PARTNER II trial is currently evaluating the next generation valve and the stent material has changed from stainless steel to a cobalt chromium alloy, which allows a smaller delivery profile and sheath size. Currently the valve is available in Europe and is also available in a diameter of 29 mm with a stent height of 19.1 mm. The delivery system, Novoflex catheter (Edwards Lifesciences, Irvine, California) is unique because it decreases the required sheath size secondary to its capability to load the valve onto the balloon inside the body. There are no available data for this valve in the pulmonic position.

Each valve has its own advantages; although the SAPIEN transcatheter heart valves are available in larger sizes and shorter heights that may be appropriate for larger conduits and challenging anatomy, it has a larger delivery system than the Melody valve that may render it more difficult to deliver. Interestingly, the SAPIEN transcatheter heart valve system does not use a covering sheath; therefore once it exits its delivery sheath (35 cm long) it may be difficult to retract inside the sheath. On the other hand, the Melody system is less bulky and has a retractable sheath that protects the

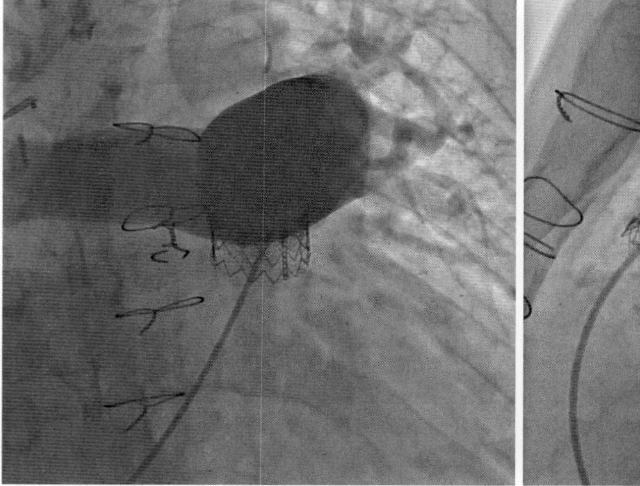

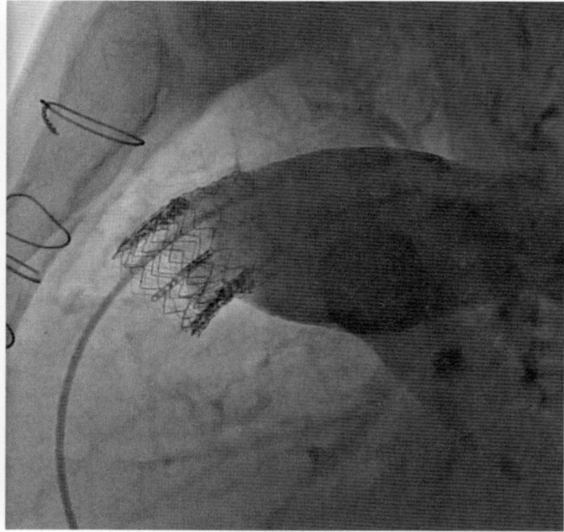

FIGURE 36-13 Anterior-posterior and lateral image of an Edwards SAPIEN valve implanted in the pulmonary position in a patient with repaired pulmonary atresia/VSD.

valve until it is deployed, but its limitation to 22 mm makes it less valuable for those with larger conduits.

Research is ongoing to broaden the use of this technology when treating patients with dilated RV outflow tracts, and early experience with a self-expanding valve model has been reported. Affordability is an important factor that must be considered especially in developing nations.

CONCLUSIONS

CHD in the adult population, more than any other type of congenital problem, is outgrowing the current medical facilities established to care for it. With better surgical options during childhood most of these patients are entering adulthood with needs for ongoing medical care. Catheter-based interventions are rarely curative, and that is why a lifetime of care will be required. Clinical systems designed for the transition of these patients out of the pediatric clinics, where many continue to receive their care, and into organized, regional ACHD centers of excellence will facilitate this process. As the catheter-based technology continues to advance regarding CHD, more and more patients will be coming to the catheterization laboratory for palliative interventions such as device deployment or stent valve angioplasty.

Cardiac catheterization for CHD has evolved from its early days as an exclusively diagnostic tool to a dynamic and continuously growing field of therapeutic interventional procedures for children and adults with cardiac abnormalities. The physicians and industry have a history of working together to push the field forward, finding novel solutions to difficult problems, while making the products to accomplish these goals smaller and safer. The interventional cardiologist and cardiothoracic surgeon have truly become an organized team in the treatment of once uniformly fatal conditions to offer longer and better quality of life to a diverse group of complex and rewarding patients.

This chapter summarized some of the interventional techniques used in the catheterization laboratories in CHD. Treatment of adults with CHD is a growing field and requires skilled personnel trained in both adult diseases and CHD to be able to understand the physiology, and the anatomy, of the cardiac lesion and hence to intervene.

The practice of interventional cardiology in adults or in children with CHD requires special training and a fully equipped catheterization laboratory to help minimize the risks of such procedures. Surgical backup is crucial in any institution practicing congenital cardiac intervention. Last, cardiac intervention is a rapidly growing and expanding field that now involves at its far end percutaneous valve placement and repair. The near future will bring further advances in this field.

ACKNOWLEDGMENT

The author would like to acknowledge Amanda Green, MSN, ARNP, from the Heart Program at Miami Children's Hospital for her help with this chapter.

References

1. Hoffman JI, Kaplan S, Liberthson RR: Prevalence of congenital heart disease. *Am Heart J* 147:425–439, 2004.
2. Warnes CA, Liberthson R, Danielson GK, et al: Task force 1: the changing profile of congenital heart disease in adult life. *J Am Coll Cardiol* 37:1170–1175, 2001.
3. Feltes TF, Bacha E, Beekman RH, et al: Indications for cardiac catheterization and intervention in pediatric cardiac disease: a scientific statement from the American Heart Association. *Circulation* 123(22):2607–2652, 2011. 10.1161/CIR.0b013e31821b1f10.
4. Forbes TJ, Garekar S, Amin Z, et al: The Congenital Cardiovascular Interventional Study Consortium (CCISC): procedural results and acute complications in stenting native and recurrent coarctation of the aorta in patients over 4 years of age: a multi-institutional study. *Catheter Cardiovasc Interv* 70(2):276–285, 2007.
5. Forbes TJ, Moore P, Pedra CA, et al: Intermediate follow-up following intravascular stenting for treatment of coarctation of the aorta. *Catheter Cardiovasc Interv* 70(4):569–577, 2007.
6. de Divitiis DM, Pilla C, Kattenhorn M, et al: Ambulatory blood pressure, left ventricular mass, and conduit artery function late after successful repair of coarctation of the aorta. *J Am Coll Cardiol* 41(12):2259–2265, 2003.
7. Oliver JM, Gallego P, Gonzalez A, et al: Risk factors for aortic complications in adults with coarctation of the aorta. *J Am Coll Cardiol* 44(8):1641–1647, 2004.
8. Connolly HM, Huston J, Brown RD, et al: Intracranial aneurysms in patients with coarctation of the aorta: a prospective magnetic resonance angiographic study of 100 patients. *Mayo Clin Proc* 78(12):1491–1499, 2003.
9. Fernandes SM, Khairy P, Sanders SP, et al: Bicuspid aortic valve morphology and interventions in the young. *J Am Coll Cardiol* 49(22):2211–2214, 2007.
10. Mathew P, Moodie DS, Blechman G, et al: Long-term follow-up of aortic coarctation in infants, children, and adults. *Cardiol Young* 3:20–26, 1993.
11. Cowley CG, Orsmond GS, Feola P, et al: Long-term, randomized comparison of balloon angioplasty and surgery for native coarctation of the aorta in childhood. *Circulation* 111(25):3453–3456, 2005.
12. Fawzy ME, Awad M, Hassan W, et al: Long-term outcome (up to 15 years) of balloon angioplasty of discrete native coarctation of the aorta in adolescents and adults. *J Am Coll Cardiol* 43(6):1062–1067, 2004.
13. Zabal C, Attie F, Rosas M, et al: The adult patient with native coarctation of the aorta: balloon angioplasty or primary stenting? *Heart* 89(1):77–83, 2003.
14. Harikrishnan S, Jacob SP, Tharakan J, et al: Congenital coronary anomalies of origin and distribution in adults: a coronary arteriographic study. *Indian Heart J* 54(3):271–275, 2002.
15. Wilde P, Watt I: Congenital coronary artery fistulae: six new cases with a collective review. *Clin Radiol* 31:301–311, 1980.
16. Lacombe P, Rocha P, Marchand X, et al: High flow coronary fistula closure by percutaneous coil packing. *Cathet Cardiovasc Diagn* 28(4):342–346, 1993.
17. Skimming JW, Walls JT: Congenital coronary artery fistula suggesting a "steal phenomenon" in a neonate. *Pediatr Cardiol* 14:174–175, 1993.
18. Qureshi SA: Coronary arterial fistulas. *Orphanet J Rare Dis* 1:51, 2006.
19. Ramo OJ, Totterman KJ, Harjula AL: Thrombosed coronary artery fistula as a cause of paroxysmal atrial fibrillation and ventricular arrhythmia. *Cardiovasc Surg* 2:720–722, 1994.
20. Alkhulaifi AM, Horner SM, Pugsley WB, et al: Coronary artery fistulas presenting with bacterial endocarditis. *Ann Thorac Surg* 60:202–204, 1995.
21. Kharouf R, Cao QL, Hijazi ZM: Transcatheter closure of coronary artery fistula complicated by myocardial infarction. *J Invasive Cardiol* 19:E146–E149, 2007.
22. Bauer HH, Allmendinger PD, Flaherty J, et al: Congenital coronary arteriovenous fistula: spontaneous rupture and cardiac tamponade. *Ann Thorac Surg* 62:1521–1523, 1996.
23. White RI, Jr, Lynch-Nyhan A, Terry P, et al: Pulmonary arteriovenous malformations: techniques and long-term outcome of embolotherapy. *Radiology* 169:663–669, 1988.
24. Vettukattil JJ: Pathogenesis of pulmonary arteriovenous malformations: role of hepatopulmonary interactions. *Heart* 88:561–563, 2002.
25. Rath PC, Tripathy MP, Panigrahi NK, et al: Successful coil embolization and follow-up result of a complex pulmonary arterio-venous fistula. *J Invasive Cardiol* 11(2):83–86, 1999.
26. Bialkowski J, Zabal C, Szkutnik M, et al: Percutaneous interventional closure of large pulmonary arteriovenous fistulas with the Amplatzer duct occluder. *Am J Cardiol* 96(1):127–129, 2005.
27. Dowson A, Mullen M, Peatfield R, et al: Migraine Intervention With STARFlex Technolody (MIST) trial. *Circulation* 117:1397–1404, 2008.
28. Dutton JA, Jackson JE, Hughes JM, et al: Pulmonary arteriovenous malformations: results of treatment with coil embolization in 53 patients. *AJR Am J Roentgenol* 165:1119–1125, 1995.
29. Lee DW, White RI, Jr, Egglin TK, et al: Embolotherapy of large pulmonary arteriovenous malformations: long-term results. *Ann Thorac Surg* 64:930–940, 1997.
30. Mager JJ, Overtoom TT, Blauw H, et al: Embolotherapy of pulmonary arteriovenous malformations: long-term results in 112 patients. *J Vasc Interv Radiol* 15:451–456, 2004.
31. Beekman RH, III, Shim D, Lloyd TR: Embolization therapy in pediatric cardiology. *J Interv Cardiol* 8(5):543–556, 1995.
32. Lababidi Z, Wu JR: Percutaneous balloon pulmonary valvuloplasty. *Am J Cardiol* 52:560–562, 1983.
33. Kan JS, White RI, Jr, Mitchell SE, et al: Percutaneous transluminal balloon valvuloplasty for pulmonary valve stenosis. *Circulation* 69:554–560, 1984.
34. Kaza AK, Lim HG, Dibardino DJ, et al: Long-term results of RV outflow tract reconstruction in neonatal cardiac surgery: options and outcomes. *J Thorac Cardiovasc Surg* 138(4):911–916, 2005.
35. McElhinney DB, Hellenbrand WE, Zahn EM, et al: Short-and medium-term outcomes after transcatheter pulmonary valve placement in the expanded multicenter US Melody valve trial. *Circulation* 122:507–516, 2010.
36. Gillespie MJ, Rome JJ, Levi DS, et al: Melody valve implant within failed bioprosthetic valves in the pulmonary position: a multicenter experience. *Circ Cardiovasc Interv* 5(6):862–870, 2012.
37. Buechel ER, Dave HH, Kellenberger CJ: Remodeling of the right ventricle after early pulmonary valve replacement in children with repaired tetralogy of Fallot: assessment by cardiovascular magnetic resonance. *Eur Heart J* 26:2721–2727, 2005.
38. Bonhoeffer P, Boudjemline Y, Saliba Z, et al: Percutaneous placement of pulmonary valve in a right-ventricle to pulmonary artery prosthetic conduit with valve dysfunction. *Lancet* 356:1403–1405, 2000.
39. Bonhoeffer P, Boudjemline Y, Quereshi S, et al: Percutaneous insertion of the pulmonary valve. *J Am Coll Cardiol* 39:1664–1669, 2002.
40. Lurz P, Coats L, Khambadkone S, et al: Percutaneous pulmonary valve implantation. Impact of evolving technology and learning curve on clinical outcome. *Circulation* 117:1964–1972, 2008.
41. Zahn EM, Hellenbrand WE, Lock JE, et al: Implantation of the Melody transcatheter pulmonary valve in patients with a dysfunctional RV outflow tract conduit. *J Am Coll Cardiol* 54:1722–1729, 2009.
42. Mahadevan VS, Jimeno S, Benson LN, et al: Pre-closure of femoral venous access sites used for large-sized sheath insertion with the Perclose device in adults undergoing cardiac intervention. *Heart* 94:571–572, 2008.
43. Cilingiroglu M, Salinger M, Zhao D, et al: Technique of temporary subcutaneous "figure-of-eight" sutures to achieve hemostasis after removal of large-caliber femoral venous sheaths. *Catheter Cardiovasc Interv* 78(1):155–160, 2001.
44. Morray BH, McElhinney DB, Cheatham JP, et al: Risk of coronary artery compression among patients referred for transcatheter pulmonary valve implantation: a multicenter experience. *Circ Cardiovasc Interv* 6(5):535–542, 2013.
45. McElhinney DB, Benson LN, Eicken A, et al: Infective endocarditis after transcatheter pulmonary valve replacement using the Melody valve: combines results of 3 prospective North American and European studies. *Circ Cardiovasc Interv* 6:292–300, 2013.
46. Sosnowski C, Kenny D, Hijazi Z: Bail out use of the Gore Excluder following pulmonary conduit rupture during transcatheter pulmonary valve replacement. *Catheter Cardiovasc Interv* 81(2):331–334, 2013.
47. Miyague NI, Cardoso SM, Meyer F, et al: Epidemiological study of congenital heart defects in children and adolescents. *Arq Bras Cardiol* 80:269–278, 2003.

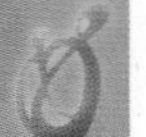

48. Vida VL, Bottio T, Milanesi O, et al: Critical aortic stenosis in early infancy: surgical treatment for residual lesions after balloon dilation. *Ann Thorac Surg* 79:47–52, 2005.
49. Moore P, Egito E, Mowrey H, et al: Midterm results of balloon dilation of congenital aortic stenosis: predictors of success. *J Am Coll Cardiol* 27:1257–1263, 1996.
50. Pedra CA, Sidhu R, McCrindle BW, et al: Outcomes after balloon dilation of congenital aortic stenosis in children and adolescents. *Cardiol Young* 14:315–321, 2004.
51. Deanfield J, Thaulow E, Warnes C, et al: Management of grown up congenital heart disease. Task Force on the Management of Grown Up Congenital Heart Disease, European Society of Cardiology; ESC Committee for Practice Guidelines. *Eur Heart J* 24(11):1035–1084, 2003.
52. Berman EB, Barst RJ: Eisenmenger syndrome: current management. *Prog Cardiovasc Dis* 45(2):129–138, 2002.
53. Garay F, Webb J, Hijazi ZM: Percutaneous replacement of pulmonary valve using the Edwards-Cribier percutaneous heart valve: first report in a human patient. *Catheter Cardiovasc Interv* 67:659–662, 2006.
54. Kenny D, Hijazi Z, Kar S: Percutaneous implantation of the Edwards Sapien Transcatheter Heart Valve for Conduit Failure in the Pulmonary Position: early phase I results from an international multicenter clinical trial. *J Am Coll Cardiol* 58(21):2248–2256, 2011.

Index

Page numbers followed by "*f*" indicate figures, and "*t*" indicate tables.

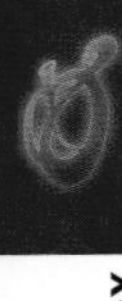

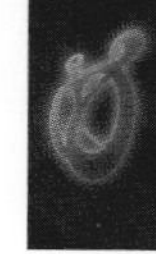

C

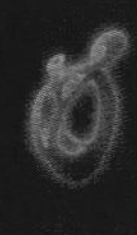

F

G

H

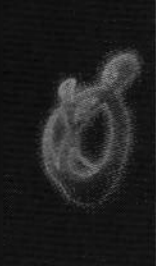

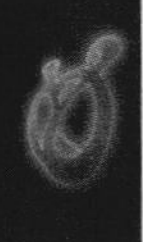

M

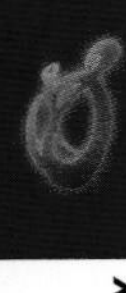

N

O

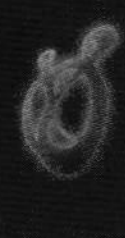

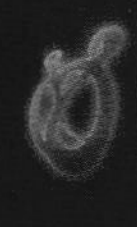

T

U

V